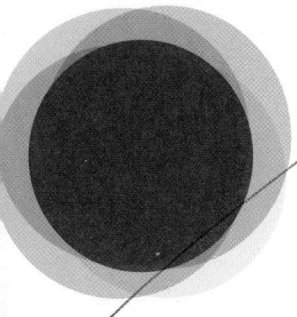

# An Invitation to Health:

## Build Your Future

**DIANNE HALES**

**15TH EDITION**

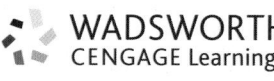
**WADSWORTH**
CENGAGE Learning

Australia • Brazil • Japan • Korea • Mexico • S               United States

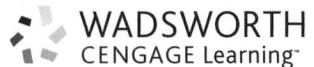
WADSWORTH
CENGAGE Learning

*An Invitation to Health: Build Your Future,*
**15th Edition, International Edition**
**Dianne Hales**

Publisher: Yolanda Cossio

Acquisitions Editor: Aileen Berg

Developmental Editor: Nedah Rose/Jake Warde

Assistant Editor: Kristina Chiapella

Editorial Assistant: Shannon Elderon

Media Editor: Katie Walton

Marketing Manager: Tom Ziolkowski

Marketing Assistant: Jing Hu

Marketing Communications Manager: Linda Yip

Content Project Manager: Carol Samet

Creative Director: Rob Hugel

Art Director: John Walker

Print Buyer: Karen Hunt

Rights Acquisitions Specialist: Tom McDonough

Production Service: Lachina Publishing Services

Text Designer: Yvo Riezebos Group

Photo Researcher: Alexa Orr, Bill Smith Group

Copy Editor: Lachina Publishing Services

Cover Image: Mark A. Johnson/Corbis

Compositor: Lachina Publishing Services

Library of Congress Control Number: 2011932623

International Student Edition:
ISBN-13: 978-1-111-99081-7
ISBN-10: 1-111-99081-6

Cengage Learning International Offices

**Asia**
www.cengageasia.com
tel: (65) 6410 1200

**Australia/New Zealand**
www.cengage.com.au
tel: (61) 3 9685 4111

**Brazil**
www.cengage.com.br
tel: (55) 11 3665 9900

**India**
www.cengage.co.in
tel: (91) 11 4364 1111

**Latin America**
www.cengage.com.mx
tel: (52) 55 1500 6000

**UK/Europe/Middle East/Africa**
www.cengage.co.uk
tel: (44) 0 1264 332 424

**Represented in Canada by**
**Nelson Education, Ltd.**
www.nelson.com
tel: (416) 752 9100 / (800) 668 0671

Cengage Learning is a leading provider of customized learning solutions with office locations around the globe, including Singapore, the United Kingdom, Australia, Mexico, Brazil, and Japan. Locate your local office at: **www.cengage.com/global**.

Cengage Learning products are represented in Canada by Nelson Education, Ltd.

For product information: **www.cengage.com/international**
Visit your local office: **www.cengage.com/global**
Visit our corporate website: **www.cengage.com**

Printed in Canada
1  2  3  4  5  6  7  15  14  13  12  11

# Brief Contents

# Contents

Contents

# Key Features

## MAKING CHANGE HAPPEN

## YOUR STRATEGIES FOR CHANGE

## YOUR STRATEGIES FOR PREVENTION

# Preface

## To the Student

How healthy are you? In nationwide surveys, most college students rate their health as good or excellent. Whether you're male or female, a traditional-age undergraduate or older, you're likely to say the same.

Ask yourself another question: How long do you think you will stay healthy? Through the next two decades? Until you turn fifty? Up to retirement age? Into your seventies or eighties? The answer, to a greater extent than you might imagine, depends on the choices you make and the behaviors you adopt now.

More than 40 percent of undergraduates are already overweight or obese. Twenty percent have at least one risk factor for cardiovascular disease. An estimated 70 to 85 percent do not exercise regularly. Most eat diets that are high in fats and sugar and low in fruits, vegetables, and grains. Nine in ten report feeling stressed. If you add the risks of smoking, binge drinking, and drug use, college itself can seem hazardous to a student's health.

Yet the years when you prepare for your professional life can also be the best time to build your future—one that's happy, healthy, and fulfilling. Every day you make choices that can affect both how long and how well you live. The knowledge you acquire in this course will help you make better choices, ones that will have a direct impact on how you look, feel, and function—now and for decades to come.

Perhaps you think you know all you need to know about how to take care of yourself. If so, take a minute and ask yourself some questions:

- How well do you understand yourself? Are you able to cope with emotional upsets and crises? Do you often feel stressed out?

- How strong are your social relationships?

- How nutritiously do you eat? Are you always going on—and off—diets?

- Do you exercise regularly?

- How solid and supportive are your relationships with others? Are you conscientious about birth control and safe-sex practices?

- Do you occasionally get drunk or high? Do you smoke?

- What do you know about your risk for infectious diseases, heart problems, cancer, or other serious illnesses?

- Are you a savvy health-care consumer? Do you know how to evaluate medical products and health professionals?

- How much do you know about complementary and alternative medicine?

- If you needed health care, do you know where you'd turn or how you'd pay?

- Have you taken steps to ensure your personal safety at home, on campus, and on the streets?

- Can you improve your odds for living a long and healthy life?

- What are you doing today to prevent physical, psychological, social, and environmental problems in the future?

Chances are there are some aspects of health you haven't considered before—and others you feel you don't have to worry about for years. Yet the choices you make and the actions you take now will have a dramatic impact on your future.

Your health is your personal responsibility. Over time, your priorities and needs will inevitably change, but the connections between various dimensions of your well-being will remain the same: The state of your mind will affect the state of your body, and vice versa. The values that guide you through today can keep you mentally, physically, and spiritually healthy throughout your lifetime. Your ability to cope with stress will influence your decisions about alcohol and drug use. Your commitment to honest, respectful relationships will affect the nature of your sexual involvements. Your eating and exercise habits will determine whether you develop a host of medical problems.

This edition of *An Invitation to Health: Build Your Future* is packed with information, advice, recommendations, and research, and provides the first step in taking full charge of your own well-being. Ultimately, the power to shape your destiny belongs to you—and it's a lot easier than you might think. You could simply add a walk or workout to your daily routine. You could snack on fruit instead of high-fat foods. You could cut back on alcohol. You could buckle your seat belt whenever you get in a car. These are small changes and relatively easy ones to make. They may not seem like a big deal now, yet they could make a crucial difference in determining how active and fulfilling the rest of your life will be.

Knowledge alone can't assure you a lifetime of well-being. The rest depends on you. The skills you acquire, the habits you form, the choices you make, the ways you live day by day will all shape your health and your future. You cannot simply read this book and study health the way you study French or chemistry. You must decide to make it part of your daily life.

This is our invitation to you.

—*Dianne Hales*

## To the Instructor

Most college students, regardless of their gender, ages, or ethnic backgrounds, think of themselves as healthy. Some even think they are invincible—too young, too strong, too energetic to worry about illness or injury. They may assume that they know all they need to know to stay that way.

You know better. And you know that the choices students make, the knowledge they gain, and the habits they form in college can make a difference for decades to come. This is why the theme of the new edition of *An Invitation to Health* is "Build Your Future." My message to students is that the future doesn't begin tomorrow, or next year, or on graduation day. It starts now.

The twenty chapters in the latest edition provide building blocks for a healthy, happy, fulfilling future. In addition to the most current scientific findings on the traditional aspects of health, I have included new topics that range from relationships in emerging adulthood to dangerous trends, such as distracted driving and cyberbullying. A ground-breaking chapter on Social Health explores the impact of digital communications and social networking on physical and psychological health.

To a greater extent than has ever been possible, this *Invitation* is truly interactive. A new "How Do You Compare?" feature provides current data on how undergraduates feel, sleep, eat, exercise, drink, and behave so students can get a better sense of real campus life. "Health in the Headlines" introduces students to Cengage's comprehensive "Global Health Watch" website with assignments that hone research skills. "Health in Action" gives students step-by-step guidance on how to apply what they're learning in their daily lives. Each chapter ends with a "Build Your Future" checklist that reinforces key behavioral changes that can enhance and safeguard health.

Because journaling can be a key element of the self-awareness that can lead to healthy change, several of the features include a direction to the students to use an online journal in which to record their responses to the activities in the feature. Many of your students may have an existing blog that they could use for these activities. If not, your school may provide students with access to a blogging platform that students can use; or, there are a number of free resources that can be used for journaling, such as WordPress, Blogger, TypePad, Tumblr, Posterous, LiveJournal, and many, many more. We encourage you and your students to explore them.

This textbook is an invitation to you as an instructor. I invite you to share your passion for education and to enter into a partnership with the editorial team at Wadsworth Cengage Learning. We welcome your feedback and suggestions. Please let us hear from you at **www.cengage.com/health**. I personally look forward to working with you toward our shared goal of preparing a new generation for a healthful future.

# What's New in *An Invitation to Health: Build Your Future*

Some things don't change: As always, this *Invitation* presents up-to-date, concise, research-based coverage of all the dimensions of health. As always, it defines health in the broadest sense of the word—not as an entity in itself, but as an integrated process for discovering, using, and protecting all possible resources within the individual, family, community, and environment.

What is new is the theme that threads through every chapter: preparing students for a healthy, happy, and fulfilling future. One of the most important building blocks is behavioral change, which has always been fundamental to *An Invitation to Health*. The one feature that has appeared in every edition—and that remains the most popular—is "Your Strategies for Change." In this edition every chapter concludes with "Making Change Happen," a preview of the four-step labs (such as Chapter 2's "Soul Food," Chapter 6's "Mind over Platter," and Chapter 19's "Going Green"), developed for our *Invitation to Personal Change* supplement.

The twenty chapters have been reorganized in response to reviewers' suggestions. We now discuss nutrition (including the new federal dietary guidelines) and weight management before fitness, and we've moved the chapter on Sexually Transmitted Infections to the section on Responsible Sexuality.

Completely new is a chapter on Social Health, which includes material on communicating, friendships, intimate relationships, marriage, and families. Also covered are issues related to social networking, including the Facebook phenomenon, self-disclosure and privacy in a digital age, relationships in emerging adulthood, hooking up, and online dating.

Throughout this edition, the focus is on students, with real-life examples, the latest statistics on undergraduate behaviors and attitudes, and coverage of new campus health risks, including hookah (waterpipe) smoking, the combination of binge drinking and disordered drinking, and the potent drugs known as "bath salts."

Every chapter includes several new interactive features:

- "How Do You Compare?," which showcases the latest research on student behavior, including their sleep habits (Chapter 2), stress levels (Chapter 4), weights (Chapter 7), and sexual experiences (Chapter 9).

- "Health in the Headlines," which directs students to Cengage's Global Health Watch website to research a key topic in each chapter, such as campus drinking (Chapter 13), alternative therapies (Chapter 17), or Alzheimer's disease (Chapter 20).

- "Health in Action," a practical learn-it, live-it lab that applies lessons from each chapter on such subjects as assessing a relationship (Chapter 5), kicking a tobacco habit (Chapter 14), or infection protection (Chapter 16).

- "Build Your Future," an end-of-the-chapter checklist that students can use to assess their current status and work toward a healthier future, whether by creating better relationships (Chapter 5), preventing serious illnesses (Chapter 15), or taking charge of their health (Chapter 17).

Other popular features that have been retained and updated include "Health on a Budget," "Consumer Alert," and a "Self-Survey" at the end of each chapter. Other end-of-chapter resources include "Review Questions," "Critical Thinking Questions," and "Key Terms." At the end of the book is a full Glossary, and on "CourseMate," you will find the *Hales Health Almanac*, which includes a directory of resources, emergency procedures, and a guide to common medical tests.

As in previous editions, icons indicate material related to students and campus life and to cultural or racial diversity.

Because health is an ever-evolving field, this edition includes many new topics, including insights into the teenage and twenty-something brain, autism spectrum disorders, caffeinated alcoholic beverages, the relationship between binge drinking and disordered eating, and insulin resistance and prediabetes. All of the chapters have been updated with the most current research, including many citations published in 2011 and incorporating the latest available statistics. The majority come from primary sources, including professional books; medical, health, and mental health journals; health education periodicals; scientific meetings, federal agencies and consensus panels; publications from research laboratories and universities; and personal interviews with specialists in a number of fields. In addition, "Internet Connections" presents reliable Internet addresses where students can turn for additional information.

As I tell students, *An Invitation to Health: Build Your Future* can serve as an owner's manual to their bodies and minds. By using this book and taking your course, they can acquire a special type of power—the power to make good decisions, to assume responsibility, and to create and follow a healthy lifestyle. This textbook is our invitation to them to live what they learn and make the most of their health and their future.

# An Overview of Changes

Following is a chapter-by-chapter listing of some of the key topics that have been added, expanded, or revised for this edition:

**Chapter 1:** Your Invitation to a Healthy Future
**New Sections:** Healthy People 2020 • The Perils of Young Adulthood

**Updated Sections:** Health and Wellness • The Dimensions of Health • A Report Card on the Health of Americans • Health Disparities • A Report Card on the Health of College Students • Student Health Norms

**Chapter 2:** Mind, Body, and Spirit
**New Sections:** Emotional and Mental Health • Develop Self-Compassion

**Updated Sections:** The Lessons of Positive Psychology • Happiness 101 • Become Optimistic • Sleepless on Campus

**Expanded Sections:** Enrich Your Spiritual Health • Cultivate Gratitude

**Chapter 3:** Caring for Your Mind
**New Sections:** The Teenage and Twenty-Something Brain • Students at Risk • The Toll on Students • Depression in Children and Teens • Minor Depression • Autism and Autism Spectrum Disorders • Getting Help for Psychological Problems

**Updated Sections:** Understanding Mental Health • Mind-Body Connection • Exercise Prescription • Mental Health on Campus • Depressive Disorders • Treating Depression • Attention Disorders • Suicide • Suicide on Campus

**Chapter 4:** Personal Stress Management
**New Sections:** The Cognitive Transactional Model • The Life Events Model • Psychological Responses to Stress • Managing Stress • Yoga

**Updated Sections:** Stress and the Heart • Stress and Immunity • Stress and Digestion • Stress on Campus • Gender Differences • Economic Stress • Meditation and Mindfulness • Posttraumatic Stress Disorder • Overcoming Procrastination

**Chapter 5:** Social Health
**New Sections:** The Social Dimension of Health • Learning to Listen • Being Agreeable and Assertive • Social Networking • The Facebook Phenomenon • Self-Disclosure and Privacy in a Digital Age • Shyness and Social Anxiety • Building a Health Community • Meeting People • Loving and Being Loved • Intimate Relationships • Partnering Across the Lifespan • Relationships in Emerging Adulthood • Unmarried Parents

**Updated Sections:** Communicating and Relating • Friendship • Dating on Campus • Hooking Up • Dysfunctional Relationships • Cohabitation • Long-Term Same-Sex Relationships • Marriage • The Benefits of Marriage • Issues Couples Confront

**Chapter 6:** Personal Nutrition
**New Sections:** Balancing Calories to Manage Weight • MyPlate • Foods and Food Components to Reduce • Foods and Nutrients to Increase • Building Healthy Eating Patterns

**Updated Sections:** Protein • Fiber • Vitamin D • Calcium • Dietary Supplements • Dietary Guidelines for Americans • Energy Drinks • Food Allergies

**Chapter 7:** Managing Your Weight
**New Sections:** Living in an "Obesogenic" Environment • Weight and the College Student

**Updated Sections:** Supersized Nation • How Did We Get So Fat? • Weight Loss Diets • Maintaining Weight Loss • Obesity Surgery • Who Develops Eating Disorders

**Chapter 8:** The Joy of Fitness
**Updated Section:** Physical Activity and Health

**Chapter 9:** Personal Sexuality
**New Section:** Teen Sexual Activity

**Updated Sections:** Circumcision • Premenstrual Syndrome • Making Sexual Decisions

**Chapter 10:** Reproductive Choices
**New Section:** Contraception on Campus

**Updated Section:** Hormonal Contraceptives

**Chapter 11:** Sexually Transmitted Infections
**New Section:** Biological Methods of Preventing HIV Infection

**Updated Sections:** STIs on Campus • HPV Incidence • HPV Vaccination • HIV and AIDS Incidence

**Chapter 12:** Addictions
**New Sections:** Drugged Driving • Synthetic Stimulants • Dissociative Drugs • Salvia

**Updated Section:** Gambling on Campus

**Chapter 13:** Alcohol
**New Sections:** Alcohol Expectancy • Defensive Drinking • Binge Drinking and Disordered Drinking • Caffeinated Alcoholic Beverages

**Updated Sections:** Drinking on Campus • Why Students Drink • How Schools Are Sobering Up • Moderate Alcohol Use • Cancer • Alcoholism Treatments

**Chapter 14:** Tobacco
**New Sections:** Water Pipes: Hookahs • Thirdhand Smoke

**Updated Sections:** Social Smoking • Health Effects on Students • Virtual Support • Medications • Health Effects of Secondhand Smoke

**Chapter 15:** Major Diseases
**Updated Sections:** Overweight/Obesity • Waist Circumference • Metabolic Syndrome • Insulin Resistance • Prediabetes • Risk Factors • Diabetes Mellitus • Hypertension • Lowering High Blood Pressure • Your Lipoprotein Profile • The Heart of a Woman • Aspirin and the Heart • Cancer

**Chapter 16:** Infectious Illnesses
**New Sections:** Seasonal Influenza • H1N1 Influenza • The Threat of a Pandemic

**Updated Sections:** Immunizations for Adults • Common Cold • Influenza • Hepatitis B • Hepatitis C • Herpes Gladiatorum (Mat Herpes, Wrester's Herpes, Mat Pox) • The "Superbug" Threat • Preventing MRSA • MRSA: Who Is at Risk?

**Chapter 17:** Traditional and Non-Traditional Health Care
**Updated Section:** Types of CAM

**Chapter 18:** Personal Safety
**New Sections:** Safety on the Road • Avoid Distracted Driving • Cyberbullying and Sexting

**Updated Sections:** Don't Text or Talk • Safe Cycling • Dating Violence • Nonvolitional Sex and Sexual Coercion

**Chapter 19:** A Healthier Environment
**New Section**: Hearing Loss

**Updated Sections**: Climate Change • Global Warming • The Health Risks • The Impact of Pollution • The Air You Breathe • Indoor Pollutants: The Inside Story • Environmental Tobacco Smoke • Secondhand Smoke • Thirdhand Smoke • Radon • Cell Phones • Your Hearing Health

**Chapter 20:** A Lifetime of Health
**Updated Sections**: How Long Can You Expect to Live? • Women at Midlife • Menopause • Hormone Therapy • Alzheimer's Disease

# Supplemental Resources

Throughout the text you will see references to "Labs for IPC." These labs are part of *An Invitation to Personal Change (IPC)*, coauthored by Dianne Hales and Kenneth W. Christian, Ph.D., a psychologist with more than 30 years of experience in personal change and maximum potential. Based on decades of psychological research and clinical practice, *IPC* serves as a curriculum for change, inviting students to take appropriate action in simple, compellingly straightforward ways.

The references throughout this book signal links to *Labs for An Invitation to Personal Change*, which present step-by-step blueprints for creating healthier habits, eliminating harmful behaviors, maximizing performance, and achieving greater physical, psychological, and spiritual well-being. The labs focus on key dimensions of personal health, including:

- Psychological and spiritual well-being ("The Grateful Thread," "Soul Food," "Your Psychological Self-Care Pyramid," "Defusing Test Stress," "Rx: Relax," "Taming a Toxic Temper," "Finity").

- Healthy habits ("Excise Exercise Excuses," "Thinking Thinner," "Mind over Platter," "Sleep Power").

- Behavioral choices ("Do It Now," "Don't Go There," "Your Alcohol Audit," "Butt Out," "The Seduction of Safer Sex," "To Have or Have Not").

- Communication skills ("Listen Up," "Help Yourself," "What's Your Intimacy Quotient?").

- Social dimensions of health ("Health Assurance," "Your Guardian Angel," "YourSpace"). We invite you to sample *An Invitation to Personal Change* by going to **servicedirect .cengage.com**.

## CourseMate™ with eBook

The CourseMate brings course concepts to life with interactive learning, study, and exam preparation tools that support the printed textbook. The CourseMate includes an interactive eBook, and interactive teaching and learning tools including quizzes, flashcards, videos, and more. It also contains the Engagement Tracker, a first-of-its-kind tool that monitors student engagement in the course.

## WebTutor with eBook on Blackboard and WebCT

WebTutor enables you to quickly and easily jumpstart your course with customizable, rich text-specific content within your learning management system. Using WebTutor allows you to assign online labs, provide access to a robust eBook, and deliver online text-specific quizzes and tests to your students. Give your students all their course materials through WebTutor from Cengage Learning.

## CengageNOW™ with eBook and InfoTrac®

Get instant access to CengageNOW™. This exciting online resource is a powerful learning companion that helps students gauge their unique study needs—and provides them with a personalized learning plan that enhances their problem-solving skills and conceptual understanding. A click of the mouse allows students to access online assessments, an interactive eBook, videos and other interactive learning tools whenever they choose, with no instructor setup necessary. CengageNOW also includes the Behavior Change Planner, which guides students through a behavior change process tailored specifically to their needs and personal motivation. An excellent tool to give as a project, this plan is easy to assign, track, and grade, even for large sections.

## Online Instructor's Manual with Test Bank

This comprehensive resource provides learning objectives, detailed chapter outlines integrated with critical thinking questions, discussion questions, and student activities. The Test Bank provides matching, multiple-choice, short answer, and critical thinking questions. Available for download on the password-protected instructor website and included on the PowerLecture DVD.

## PowerLecture DVD with ExamView® Computerized Testing

Designed to make lecture preparation easier, this DVD includes over 500 customizable PowerPoint® presentation slides with images from the text, new BBC video clips, and electronic versions of the Instructor's Manual and Test Bank. Also included is the ExamView® Computerized Test Bank, which allows you to create, deliver, and customize tests (both print and online) in minutes with this easy-to-use assessment and tutorial system.

## eCompanion

An eCompanion is now available to accompany the eBook for *Invitation to Health: Build Your Future*. Students can carry this light-weight manual to class and use it to help synthesize their understanding of key concepts from the text. Features include chapter objectives and summaries, key terms, an interactive "Concept Check" section, review questions, and space for note-taking. A comprehensive study tool, the eCompanion assists in exam preparation, allows students to follow along in class without the printed book or computer, and reinforces the concepts presented in the text.

## Global Health Watch

Updated with today's current headlines, Global Health Watch is your one-stop resource for classroom discussion and research projects. This resource center provides access to thousands of trusted Health sources, including academic journals, magazines, newspapers, videos, podcasts, and more. It is updated daily to offer the most current news about topics related to your Health course.

## Diet Analysis Plus

Take control. Reach your goals. Experience Diet Analysis +. Diet Analysis + allows students to track their diet and physical activity, and analyze the nutritional value of the food they eat so they can adjust their diets to reach personal health goals—all while gaining a better understanding of how nutrition relates to, and impacts, their lives. Diet Analysis Plus includes a 20,000+ food database; customizable reports; new assignable labs; custom food and recipe features; the latest Dietary Reference Intakes; and goals and actual percentages of essential nutrients, vitamins, and minerals. New features include enhanced search functionality with filter option, easy-to-use instructor page, and resources tab with helpful information.

## Careers in Health, Physical Education, and Sport, 2e

This unique booklet takes students through the complicated process of picking the type of career they want to pursue; explains how to prepare for the transition into the working world; and provides insight into different career paths, education requirements, and reasonable salary expectations. A designated chapter discusses some of the legal issues that surround the workplace, including discrimination and harassment. This supplement is complete with personal-development activities designed to encourage students to focus on and develop better insight into their future.

## Walk4Life® Pedometer

Provided through an alliance with Walk4Life, the Walk4Life Elite Model pedometer tracks steps, elapsed time, and distance. A calorie counter and a clock are included in this excellent class activity and tool to encourage students to track their steps and walk toward better fitness awareness.

## Instructor's Manual and Test Bank

These two essential ancillaries are bound together for your convenience. The Instructor's manual provides learning objectives, chapter summaries, lecture outlines, chapter-specific labs, discussion questions, classroom activities, and references/readings/resources. The Test Bank provides multiple choice, completion, matching, essay, and true/false questions. Test questions are ranked according to Bloom's Taxonomy.

## eCompanion

An eCompanion is now available to accompany the eBook for *An Invitation to Health*, 15th edition. Students can carry this light-weight manual to class and use it to help synthesize their understanding of key concepts from the text. Features include chapter objectives and summaries, key terms, an interactive "concept check" section, review questions, and space for note-taking. A comprehensive study tool, the eCompanion assists in exam preparation, allows students to follow along in class without the printed book or computer, and reinforces the concepts presented in the text.

## Student Course Guide for Journey to Health

This guide accompanies the "Journey to Health" telecourse produced by Dallas TeleLearning of the LeCroy Center for Educational Telecommunications. The *Journey to Health* course explores health in its broadest sense. Students are encouraged to use critical thinking and problem solving skills to develop their own healthy lifestyle using the most current information in the health and wellness field. The telecourse components consist of 26 half-hour video programs, the Hales *An Invitation to Health* text, the student telecourse guide, a faculty manual, and text-specific teaching and learning tools, including testing.

## Behavior Change Workbook

*The Behavior Change Workbook* includes a brief discussion of the current theories behind making positive lifestyle changes, along with exercises to help students effect those changes in their everyday lives.

## BBC Videos for Health and Wellness

These videos, available on the PowerLecture DVD, allow you to integrate the newsgathering and programming power of the BBC News networks into the classroom to show students the relevance of course topics to their everyday lives. The videos include news clips correlated directly with the text and can help you launch a lecture, spark a discussion, or demonstrate an application. Students can see firsthand how the principles they learn in the course apply to the stories they hear in the news.

# Acknowledgments

One of the joys of writing *An Invitation to Health: Build Your Future* is the opportunity to work with a team I consider the very best of the best in textbook publishing.

I thank Yolanda Cassio, our inspiring leader, for her unwavering support. Nedah Rose, our Senior Development Editor, has been endlessly supportive and enthusiastic and has made every step of the process of creating this edition go smoothly.

I thank Jake Warde for his skillful editing, and Shannon Elderon, our editorial assistant, who provided endless help—with endless patience and good humor. Thanks to Carol Samet, Senior Content Project Manager, for expertly shepherding this edition from conception to production, to Yvo Riezebos and his crew at RHDG | Riezebos Holzbaur for his vibrant new design, and Bonnie Briggle of Lachina Publishing Services for her supervision of the production process. Alexa Orr, our photo researcher, has provided us with dazzling, dynamic images that capture the diversity and energy of today's college students. I appreciate the skill and dedication of copy editor Carolyn Crabtree.

My thanks to Tom Ziolkowski, Senior Marketing Manager, for his enthusiastic support, to Linda Yip for her work on the promotional materials, to Kristina Chiapella, who guided the ancillaries, and to Julia Hales, my research assistant. Special thanks go to Susanne Wood, for her expert revising of the chapter learning objectives.

Finally, I would like to thank the reviewers whose input has been so valuable through these many editions. For this edition of *Invitation*, I thank the following for their comments and helpful assistance:

Jewel Carter-McCummings, *Montclair State University*
Matthew Flint, *Utah Valley University*
Margaret Kenrick, *Los Medanos College*
Claudia Mihovk, *Georgia Perimeter College*
Susan Milstein, *Montgomery College*
David Oster, *Jefferson College*
Joel Rogers, *West Hills Community College District*
Jennifer Vickery, *Winthrop College*

Thanks also to the reviewers who gave feedback about the supplements for this edition:

Ches Jones, *University of Arkansas*
Sherm Sowby, *Brigham Young University*
Maria Decker, *Marian Court College*
Debbie Hogan, *Tri County Community College*
Walter Justice, *Southwestern College*
Lisa Alastuey, *University of Houston*
Julia VanderMolen, *Davenport University*
Claudia Mihovk, *Georgia Perimeter College*
Olga Comissiong, *Kean University*
Veena Sallan, *Owensboro Community & Technical College*
Dena Pistor, *Rollins College*
Shanyn Olpin, *Weber State University*
Conswella Byrd, *California State University East Bay*
Margaret Hollinger, *Reading Area Community College*

For their help with earlier editions, I offer my gratitude to:

Ghulam Aasef, *Kaskaskia College*
Andrea Abercrombie, *Clemson University*
Daniel Adame, *Emory University*
Carol Allen, *Lone Community College*
Lana Arabas, *Truman State University*

Judy Baker, *East Carolina University*
Marcia Ball, *James Madison University*
Jeremy Barnes, *Southeast Missouri State University*
Rick Barnes, *East Carolina University*
Lois Beach, *SUNY-Plattsburg*
Liz Belyea, *Cosumnes River College*
Betsy Bergen, *Kansas State University*
Nancy Bessette, *Saddleback College*
Carol Biddington, *California University of Pennsylvania*
David Black, *Purdue University*
Jill M. Black, *Cleveland State University*
Cynthia Pike Blocksom, *Cincinnati Health Department*
Laura Bounds, *Northern Arizona University*
James Brik, *Willamette University*
Mitchell Brodsky, *York College*
Jodi Broodkins-Fisher, *University of Utah*
Elaine D. Bryan, *Georgia Perimeter College*
James G. Bryant, Jr., *Western Carolina University*
Marsha Campos, *Modesto Junior College*
Richard Capriccioso, *University of Phoenix*
James Lester Carter, *Montana State University*
Peggy L. Chin, *University of Connecticut*
Patti Cost, *Weber State University*
Maxine Davis, *Eastern Washington University*
Laura Demeri, *Clark College*
Lori Dewald, *Shippensburg University of Pennsylvania*
Julie Dietz, *Eastern Illinois University*
Robert Dollinger, *Florida International University College of Medicine*
Sarah Catherine Dunsmore, *Idaho State University*
Gary English, *Ithaca College*
Melinda K. Everman, *The Ohio State University*
Michael Felts, *East Carolina University*
Lynne Fitzgerald, *Morehead State University*
Kathie C. Garbe, *Kennesaw State College*
Gail Gates, *Oklahoma State University*
Dawn Graff-Haight, *Portland State University*
Carolyn Gray, *New Mexico State University*
Mary Gress, *Lorain County Community College*
Janet Grochowski, *University of St. Thomas*
Jack Gutierrez, *Central Community College*
Stephen Haynie, *College of William and Mary*
Amy Hedman, *Mankato State University*
Ron Heinrichs, *Central Missouri State University*
Michael Hoadley, *University of South Dakota*
Harold Horne, *University of Illinois at Springfield*
Linda L. Howard, *Idaho State University*
Mary Hunt, *Madonna University*
Kim Hyatt, *Weber State University*
Dee Jacobsen, *Southeastern Louisiana University*
John Janowiak, *Appalachian State University*
Peggy Jarnigan, *Rollins College*
Jim Johnson, *Northwest Missouri State University*
Chester S. Jones, *University of Arkansas*
Herb Jones, *Ball State University*
Jane Jones, *University of Wisconsin, Stevens Point*
Lorraine J. Jones, *Muncie, Indiana*
Becky Kennedy-Koch, *The Ohio State University*
Mark J. Kittleson, *Southern Illinois University*

Anthony F. Kiszewski, *Bentley University*
Darlene Kluka, *University of Central Oklahoma*
John Kowalczyk, *University of Minnesota, Duluth*
Debra A. Krummel, *West Virginia University*
Roland Lamarine, *California State University, Chico*
David Langford, *University of Maryland, Baltimore County*
Terri Langford, *University of Central Florida*
Beth Lanning, *Baylor University*
Norbert Lindskog, *Harold Washington College*
Loretta Liptak, *Youngstown State University*
David G. Lorenzi, *West Liberty State College*
S. Jack Loughton, *Weber State University*
Rick Madson, *Palm Beach Community College*
Ashok Malik, *College of San Mateo*
Michele P. Mannion, *Temple University*
Jerry Mayo, *Hendrix College*
Jessica Middlebrooks, *University of Georgia*
Kim H. Miller, *University of Kentucky*
Esther Moe, *Oregon Health Sciences University*
Kris Moline, *Lourdes College*
Rosemary Moulahan, *High Point University*
Richard Morris, *Rollins College*
Sophia Munro, *Palm Beach Community College*
John W. Munson, *University of Wisconsin–Stevens Point*
Anne O'Donnell, *Santa Rosa Junior College*
Terry Oehrtman, *Ohio University*
Randy M. Page, *University of Idaho*
Carolyn P. Parks, *University of North Carolina*
Anthony V. Parrillo, *East Carolina University*
Lorraine Peniston, *Hartford Community College*
Miguel Perez, *University of North Texas*
Pamela Pinahs-Schultz, *Carroll College*
Rosanne Poole, *Tallahassee Community College*
Janet Reis, *University of Illinois at Urbana-Champaign*
Pamela Rost, *Buffalo State College*
Sadie Sanders, *University of Florida*
Steven Sansone, *Chemeketa Community College*
Debra Secord, *Coastline College*
Behjat Sharif, *California State University–Los Angeles*
Andrew Shim, *Southwestern College*
Agneta Sibrava, *Arkansas State University*
Steve Singleton, *Wayne State University*
Larry Smith, *Scottsdale Community College*
Teresa Snow, *Georgia Institute of Technology*
Carl A. Stockton, *Radford University*
Linda Stonecipher, *Western Oregon State College*
Ronda Sturgill, *Marshall Univeristy*
Rosemarie Tarara, *High Point University*
Laurie Tucker, *American University*
Emogene Johnson Vaughn, *Norfolk State University*
Andrew M. Walker, *Georgia Perimeter College*
David M. White, *East Carolina University*
Sabina White, *University of California–Santa Barbara*
Robert Wilson, *University of Minnesota*
Roy Wohl, *Washburn University*
Martin L. Wood, *Ball State University*
Sharon Zackus, *City College of San Francisco*

# About the Author

Dianne Hales is one of the most widely published and honored freelance journalists in the country. She has written 14 trade books, including *La Bella Lingua*, *Think Thin*, *Just like a Woman*, and *Caring for the Mind*, as well as articles for many national publications such as *Family Circle*, *Fitness*, *Glamour*, *Good Housekeeping*, *Health*, *Mademoiselle*, *McCall's*, *New York Times*, *Psychology Today*, *Reader's Digest*, *Redbook*, *Science Digest*, *Self*, *Seventeen*, *Washington Post*, *Woman's Day*, and *World Book*. She has served as a contributing editor for *Parade*, *Ladies Home Journal*, *Working Mother*, and *American Health*.

Dianne Hales has received writing awards from the American Psychiatric Association, the American Psychological Association, an EMMA (Exceptional Media Merit Award) for health reporting from the National Women's Political Caucus and Radcliffe College, three "EDI" (Equality, Dignity, Independence) awards for print journalism from the National Easter Seal Society, the National Mature Media Award, Arthritis Foundation, California Psychiatric Society, CHADD (Children and Adults with Attention Deficit/Hyperactivity), Council for the Advancement of Scientific Education, and the New York City Public Library.

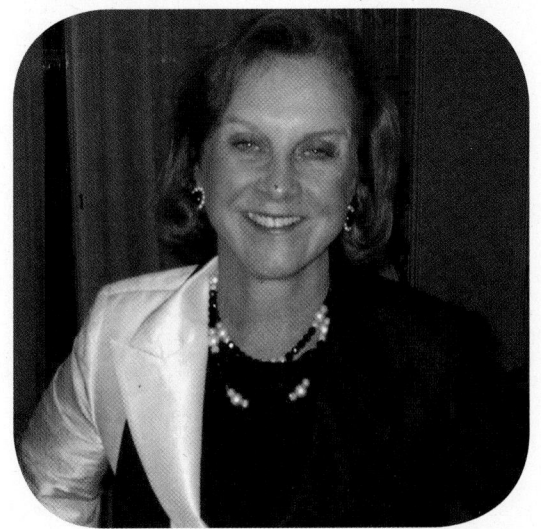

*To my husband, Bob, and my daughter Julia,*

*who make every day an invitation to joy.*

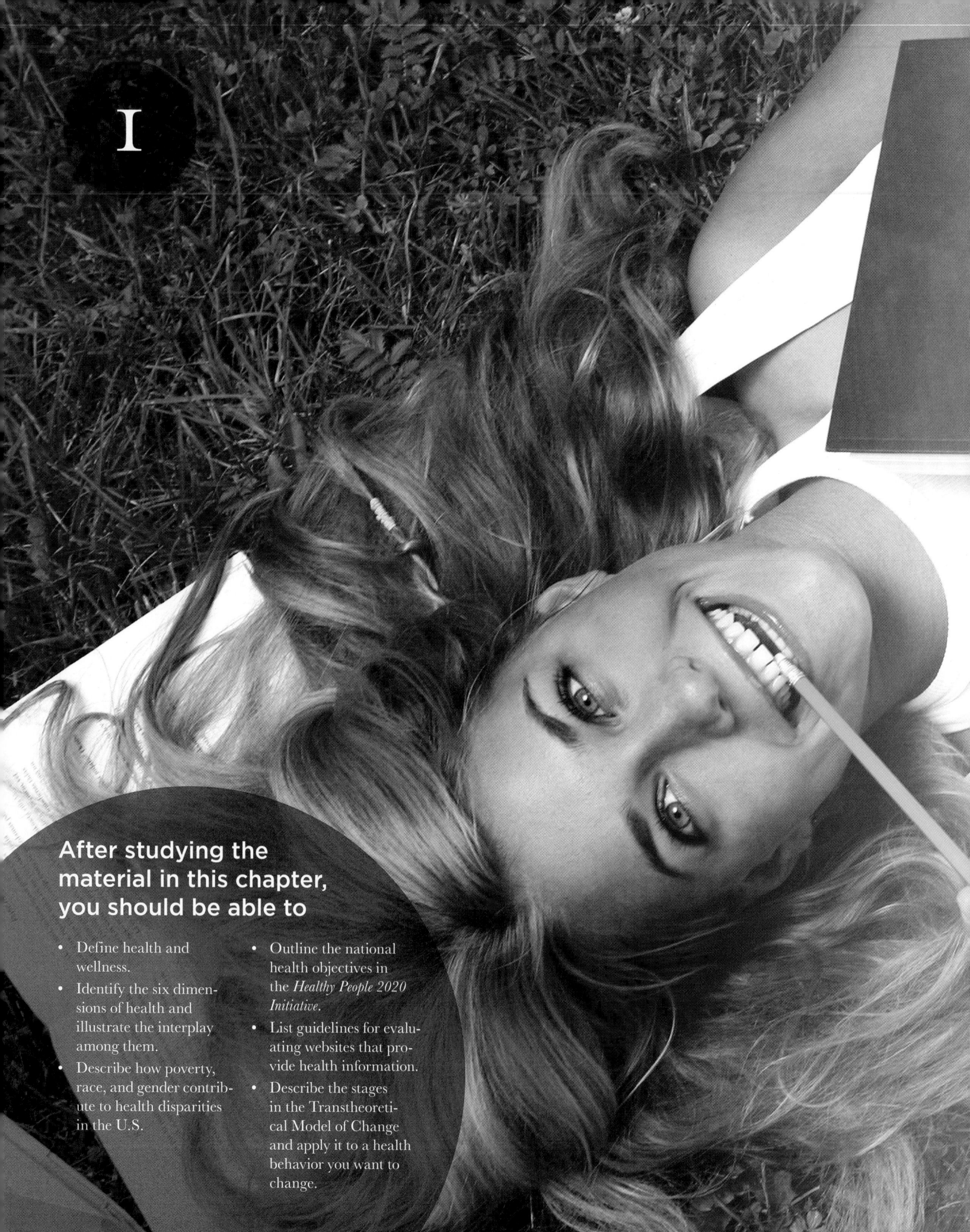

# I

## After studying the material in this chapter, you should be able to

- Define health and wellness.
- Identify the six dimensions of health and illustrate the interplay among them.
- Describe how poverty, race, and gender contribute to health disparities in the U.S.
- Outline the national health objectives in the *Healthy People 2020 Initiative*.
- List guidelines for evaluating websites that provide health information.
- Describe the stages in the Transtheoretical Model of Change and apply it to a health behavior you want to change.

Corinna always thought of health as something you worry about when you get older. Then her twin brother developed a health problem she'd never heard of: prediabetes (discussed in Chapter 15), which increased his risk of diabetes and heart disease. At a health fair on campus, she learned that her blood pressure was higher than normal. "Maybe I'm not too young to start thinking about my health," she concluded. Neither are you—

# Your Invitation to a Healthy Future

whether you're a traditional-age college student or older, like an ever-increasing number of undergraduates.

*An Invitation to Health* asks you to go beyond thinking about your health to taking charge and making healthy choices for yourself and your future. This book is both *about* and *for* you: It includes material on your mind and your body, your spirit and your social ties, your needs and your wants, your past and your potential. It will help you explore options, discover possibilities, and find new ways to make your life worthwhile. If you don't make the most of what you are, you risk never discovering what you might become.

You have more control over your life and well-being than anything or anyone else does. Through the decisions you make and the habits you develop, you can influence how well—and perhaps how long—you will live.

Being healthy, as you'll learn in this chapter, means more than not being sick or in pain. Health is a personal choice that you make every day when you decide on everything from what to eat to whether to exercise to how to handle stress. Sometimes making the best choices demands making healthy changes in your life. This chapter will show you how.

This chapter also extends an invitation to live more fully, more happily, and more healthfully. It is an offer that you literally cannot afford to refuse. Your future depends on it.

## Health and Wellness

By simplest definition, **health** means being sound in body, mind, and spirit. The World

Visit www.cengagebrain.com to access course materials for this text, including the Behavior Change Planner, interactive quizzes, tutorials, and more. See the preface on page xv for details.

**health** A state of complete well-being, including physical, psychological, spiritual, social, intellectual, and environmental dimensions.

© Yeko Photo Studio/Shutterstock.com

3

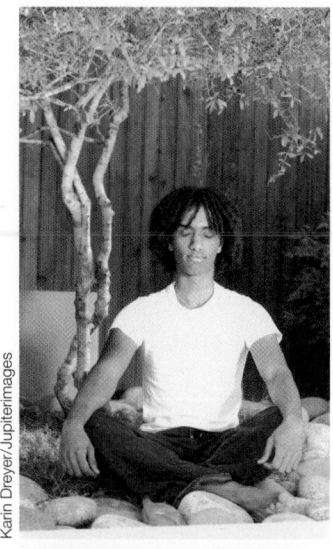

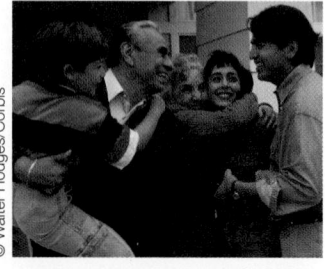

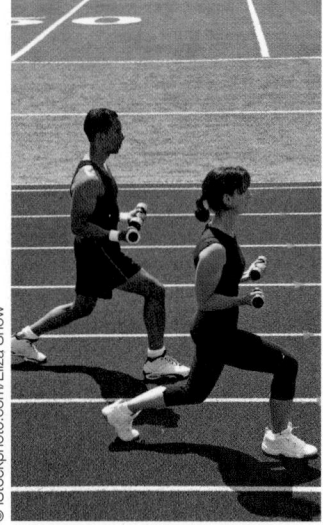

Health is the process of discovering, using, and protecting all the resources within our bodies, minds, spirits, families, communities, and environment.

Health Organization defines health as "not merely the absence of disease or infirmity," but "a state of complete physical, mental, and social well-being."[1] Health is the process of discovering, using, and protecting all the resources within our bodies, minds, spirits, families, communities, and environment.

Health has many dimensions: physical, psychological, spiritual, social, intellectual, and environmental. Some add an "emotional" and a "cultural" dimension. This book integrates these aspects into a *holistic* approach that looks at health and the individual as a whole, rather than part by part.

Your own definition of health may include different elements, but chances are you and your classmates agree that it includes at least some of the following:

- A positive, optimistic outlook.
- A sense of control over stress and worries; time to relax.
- Energy and vitality; freedom from pain or serious illness.
- Supportive friends and family and a nurturing intimate relationship with someone you love.
- A personally satisfying job or intellectual endeavor.
- A clean, healthful environment.

**Wellness** can be defined as purposeful, enjoyable living or, more specifically, a deliberate lifestyle choice characterized by personal responsibility and optimal enhancement of physical, mental, and spiritual health. In the broadest sense, wellness is:

- A decision you make to move toward optimal health.
- A way of life you design to achieve your highest potential.
- A process of developing awareness that health and happiness are possible in the present.
- The integration of body, mind, and spirit.
- The belief that everything you do, think, and feel has an impact on your state of health and the health of the world.

*Health-related quality of life and well-being* is a term that health-care providers and officials use to assess the impact of health status on an individual's quality of life. This multidimensional concept encompasses domains related to physical, mental, emotional, and social functioning. As scientists have shown again and again in recent decades, psychological factors play a major role in enhancing physical well-being and preventing illness, but they also can trigger, worsen, or prolong physical symptoms. Similarly, almost every medical illness affects people psychologically as well as physically.

# The Dimensions of Health

Scientists are discovering that various dimensions and the interplay among them can affect us at a molecular level. For instance, a lack of education—an indicator of poor intellectual health—has long been linked with poor physical health and relatively early death. However, other factors—such as having meaningful relationships with others (part of social health) and a sense of meaning and purpose in life (an indicator of spiritual health)—can overcome the disadvantages associated with poverty or minimal schooling.[2]

By learning more about the six dimensions of health, you gain insight into the complex interplay of factors that determine your level of wellness.

## Physical Health

Webster's 1913 dictionary defined health as "the state of being hale, sound, or whole, in body, mind, or soul, especially the state of being free from physical disease or pain." According to a contemporary medical dictionary, health is "an optimal state of physical, mental, and social well-being, not merely the absence of disease or infirmity."

Health is not a static state, but a process that depends on the decisions we make and the behaviors we practice every day. To assure optimal physical health, we must feed our bodies nutritiously, exercise them regularly, avoid harmful behaviors and substances, watch for early signs of sickness, and protect ourselves from accidents.

## Psychological Health

Like physical well-being, psychological health, discussed in the following chapters, is more than the absence of problems or illness. Psychological health refers to both our emotional and mental states—that is, to our feelings and our thoughts. It involves awareness and acceptance of a wide range of feelings in oneself and others, as well as the ability to express emotions, to function independently, and to cope with the challenges of daily stressors.

## Spiritual Health

Spiritually healthy individuals identify their own basic purpose in life; learn how to experience love, joy, peace, and fulfillment; and help themselves and others achieve their full potential. As they devote themselves to others' needs more than their own, their spiritual development produces a sense of greater meaning in their lives. (See Chapter 2 for an in-depth discussion of spiritual and emotional well-being.)

## Social Health

Social health refers to the ability to interact effectively with other people and the social environment, to develop satisfying interpersonal relationships, and to fulfill social roles. It involves participating in and contributing to your community, living in harmony with fellow human beings, developing positive interdependent relationships, and practicing healthy sexual behaviors. (See Chapter 5, "Your Social Health.")

Health educators are placing greater emphasis on social health in its broadest sense as they expand the traditional individualistic concept of health to include the complex interrelationships between one person's health and the health of the community and environment. This change in perspective has given rise to a new emphasis on **health promotion**, which educators define as "any planned combination of educational,

political, regulatory, and organizational supports for actions and conditions of living conducive to the health of individuals, groups, or communities." Examples on campus include establishing smoke-free policies for all college buildings, residences, and dining areas; prohibiting tobacco advertising and sponsorship of campus social events; promoting safety at parties; and enforcing alcohol laws and policies.

## Intellectual Health

Your brain is the only one of your organs capable of self-awareness. Every day you use your mind to gather, process, and act on information; to think through your values; to make decisions, set goals, and figure out how to handle a problem or challenge. Intellectual health refers to your ability to think and learn from life experience, your openness to new ideas, and your capacity to question and evaluate information. Throughout your life, you'll use your critical thinking skills, including your ability to evaluate health information, to safeguard your well-being.

## Environmental Health

You live in a physical and social setting that can affect every aspect of your health. Environmental health refers to the impact your world has on your well-being. It means protecting yourself from dangers in the air, water, and soil, and in products you use—and working to preserve the environment itself. (Chapter 19 offers a thorough discussion of environmental health.)

# A Report Card on the Health of Americans

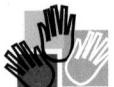 The United States spends more than any other nation on health care: a whopping $2.26 trillion total, or $7,400 per person per year. However, Americans rank twenty-third in life expectancy for men and twenty-fifth for women. Life expectancy has increased more slowly in the United

**wellness** A deliberate lifestyle choice characterized by personal responsibility and optimal enhancement of physical, mental, and spiritual health.

**health promotion** Any planned combination of educational, political, regulatory, and organizational supports for actions and conditions of living conducive to the health of individuals, groups, or communities.

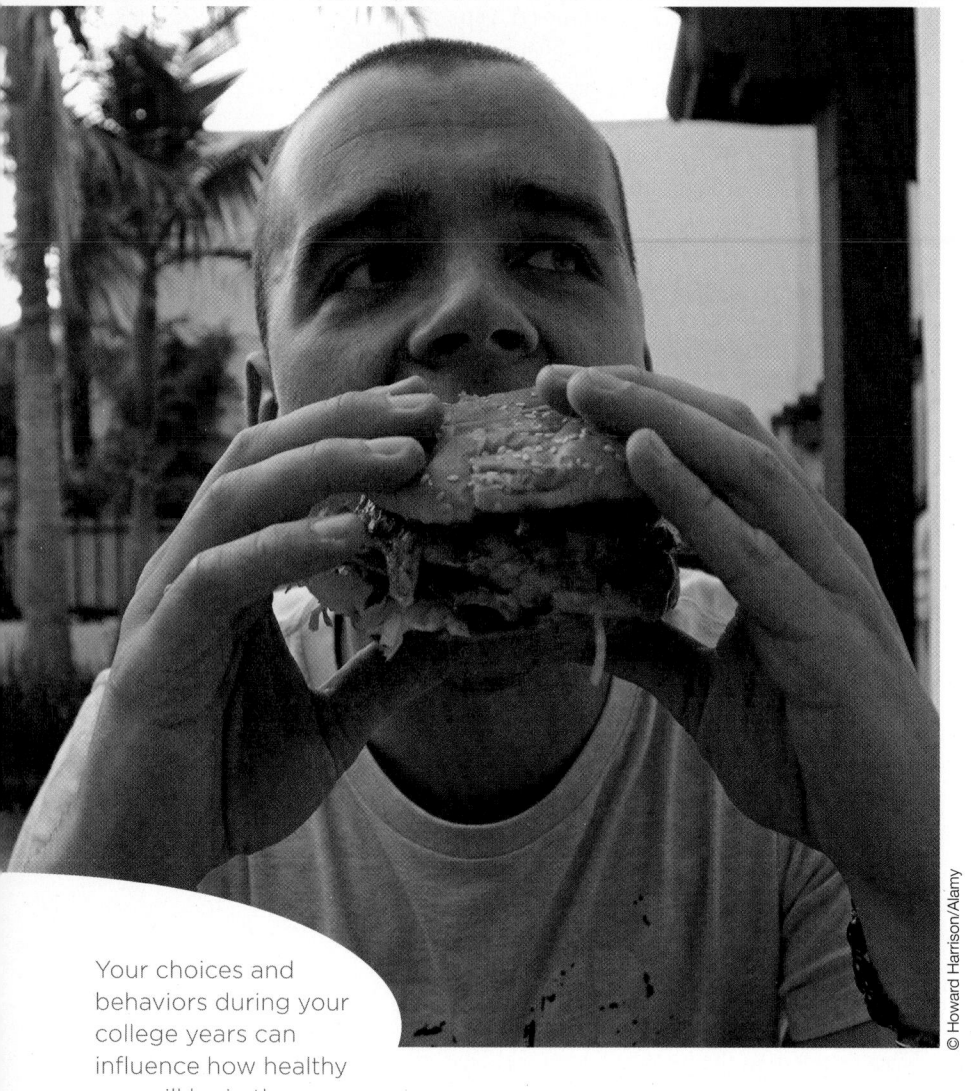

Your choices and behaviors during your college years can influence how healthy you will be in the future.

a minority of Americans at every age have adapted healthy behaviors. Here are the latest findings on our health and habits from the Centers for Disease Control and Prevention (CDC):[5]

- **Fitness**. Americans have become more active but fewer than 20 percent of men and women exercise regularly.

- **Weight**. The percentage of obese Americans has risen from 30 percent in 2000 to 34 percent. Two-thirds of the population are either overweight or obese.

- **Overall health**. Ten percent of Americans overall describe their health as fair or poor. This percentage increases to 18 percent of those over age 65.

- **Medical conditions**. Almost a third (33 percent) of Americans over age 20 have hypertension; 15 percent have high cholesterol; 12 percent have diabetes. About 18 percent of Americans over age 65 have had cancer.

- **Health care**. Almost a quarter (23 percent) of men and women between ages 18 and 44 did not see a health-care professional in the previous year. A similar percentage (22 percent) in this age group reported at least one emergency room visit. About four in ten Americans (38 percent) between ages 18 and 44 took at least one prescription medication.

- **Mortality.** The number of Americans who die every year—the national mortality rate—has fallen to an all-time low. Death rates declined for 10 of the leading 15 causes of death, including heart disease, cancer, stroke, accidents, Alzheimer's disease, homicide, influenza, and pneumonia.

## Healthy People 2020

Every decade since 1980, the U.S. Department of Health and Human Services (HHS) has published a comprehensive set of national public health objectives as part of the Healthy People Initiative. The department's vision is to create a society in which all people can live long, healthy lives. Its mission includes identifying nationwide health improvement priorities, increasing public awareness of health issues, and providing measurable objectives and goals.[6]

States than in other developed countries such as Japan, Australia, Sweden, and Switzerland. The primary reasons, according to researchers, are smoking, particularly by women, and obesity.[3]

Yet Americans are living longer. According to the latest statistics from the Centers for Disease Control (CDC), life expectancy at birth is now 77.9 years, up from 75.4 years in 1990. This represents an increase of 3.5 years for men and 1.6 years for women. The gender gap in longevity has narrowed to 4.9 years, with female life expectancy at 80.6 years and male at 75.7 years. The racial longevity gap also has shrunk, from a difference of 7 years between whites and blacks in 1990 to 4.3 years.

Americans could be living both longer and healthier lives. A healthy lifestyle, recent research has confirmed, can cut the death rate for nonsmokers by about half.[4] However, only

Drawing on the lessons learned and needs identified in *Healthy People 2010*, HHS has set the following overarching goals for *Healthy People 2020*:

- Eliminate preventable disease, disability, injury, and premature death.
- Achieve health equity, eliminate disparities, and improve the health of all groups.
- Create social and physical environments that promote good health for all.
- Promote healthy development and healthy behaviors across every stage of life.[7]

Here are examples of specific new recommendations that have been added to the national health agenda for 2020:

- **Nutrition and Weight Status:** prevent inappropriate weight gain in youth and adults.
- **Tobacco Use:** increase recent smoking-cessation success by adult smokers.
- **Sexually Transmitted Disease:** increase the proportion of adolescents who abstain from sexual intercourse or use condoms if sexually active.
- **Substance Abuse:** reduce misuse of prescription drugs.
- **Heart Disease and Stroke:** increase overall cardiovascular health in the U.S. population.
- **Injury and Violence Prevention:** reduce sports and recreation injuries.

If you were setting personal health objectives for yourself to obtain by 2020, what would they be? What would be your goals for your family, community, and the entire nation?

## Health Disparities

*The Toll of Poverty* The primary reason for the health problems faced by minorities in the United States is poverty. Without adequate insurance or the ability to pay, many cannot afford the tests and treatments that could prevent illness or overcome it at the earliest possible stages. According to public health experts, low income may account for one-third of the racial differences in death rates for middle-aged African American adults.

In some cases, both genetic and environmental factors may play a role. Take, for example, the

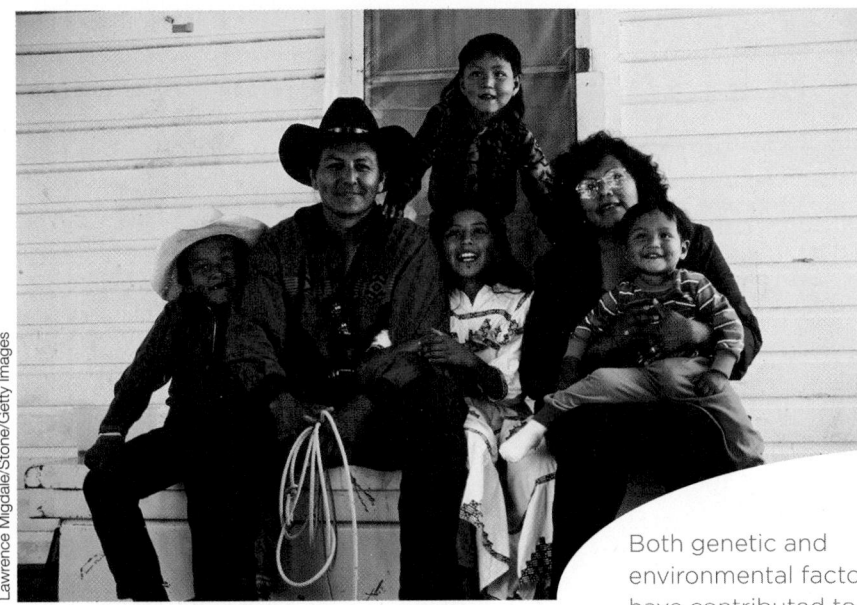

Both genetic and environmental factors have contributed to the increase in diabetes among the Pima tribe. Half of all Pima adults in the United States have diabetes.

high rates of diabetes among the Pima Indians. Until 50 years ago, these American Indians were not notably obese or prone to diabetes. After World War II, the tribe started trading handmade baskets for lard and flour. Their lifestyle became more sedentary and their diet higher in fats. In addition, researchers have discovered that many Pima Indians have an inherited resistance to insulin that increases their susceptibility to diabetes. The combination of a hereditary predisposition and environmental factors may explain why the Pimas now have epidemic levels of diabetes.

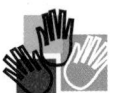 Despite great improvements in the overall health of the nation, Americans who are members of racial and ethnic groups—including black or African Americans, American Indians, Alaska Natives, Asian Americans, Hispanics, Latinos, and Pacific Islanders—are more likely than whites to suffer poor health and die prematurely. The longevity gap between white and black women is 4 years; for white and black men it is 6 years.[8] Many factors, including genetic variations, environmental influences, and specific health behaviors, contribute to these disparities.

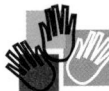 Quality of health care has been slowly improving for all Americans, but a recent government analysis found that poor people receive worse care than high-income people for about 80 percent of

measures such as health screenings and immunizations. Hispanics receive worse care than whites for about 60 percent of these measures; blacks, American Indians, and Alaska Natives, for 40 percent; and Asians, for 20 percent.[9]

*Why Race Matters*   We live in the most diverse nation on Earth, one that is becoming increasingly diverse. For society, this variety can be both enriching and divisive. Tolerance and acceptance of others have always been part of the American creed. By working together, Americans have created a country that remains, to those outside our borders, a symbol of opportunity.

This racial diversity also means varying susceptibility to disease. However, in defining race as a risk factor for certain health conditions, classifications such as "black" or "Hispanic" may be overly broad. Among Hispanics, for instance, Puerto Ricans suffer disproportionately from asthma, HIV/AIDS, and high infant mortality, while Mexican Americans have higher rates for diabetes. If, like many Americans, you come from a racially mixed background, your health profile may be complex.

Black Americans lose substantially more years of potential life to homicide (nine times as many), stroke (three times as many), and diabetes (three times as many) as whites. Hispanics suffer more fatal injuries, chronic liver disease, and cirrhosis of the liver. Compared with whites, blacks have more new AIDS cases. American Indian and Alaska Native women are less likely to receive prenatal care, and Asian American women have significantly lower rates of mammography.

Caucasians are prone to osteoporosis (progressive weakening of bone tissue); cystic fibrosis; skin cancer; and phenylketonuria (PKU), a metabolic disorder that can lead to mental retardation.

Native Americans, including those indigenous to Alaska, are more likely to die young than the population as a whole, primarily as a result of accidental injuries, cirrhosis of the liver, homicide, pneumonia, and the complications of diabetes. The suicide rate among American Indians and Alaska Natives is 50 percent higher than the national rate. The rates of co-occurring mental illness and substance abuse (especially alcohol) are also higher among Native American youth and adults.

If you do face greater health threats because of your race or ethnicity, it is up to you to educate yourself, take responsibility for the risks within your control, and become a savvy, assertive consumer of health-care services. The federal Office of Minority Health (www.cdc.gov/omh), which provides general information and the latest research and recommendations, is a good place to start.

**Cancer Screening and Management**   Overall, black Americans are more likely to develop cancer than persons of any other racial or ethnic group. Black women have higher rates of colon, pancreatic, and stomach cancer. Black men have higher rates of prostate, colon, and stomach cancer.

African Americans have the highest death rates for lung cancer of any racial or ethnic group in the United States. Medical scientists have debated whether the reason might be that treatments are less effective in blacks or whether many are not diagnosed early enough nor treated rigorously enough.

African American women are more than twice as likely to die of cervical cancer than are white women and are more likely to die of breast cancer than are women of any other racial or ethnic group. Native Hawaiian women have the highest rates of breast cancer. Women from many racial minorities, including those of Filipino, Pakistani, Mexican, and Puerto Rican descent, are more likely to be diagnosed with late-stage breast cancer than white women.

**Cardiovascular Disease**   Heart disease and stroke are the leading causes of death for all racial and ethnic groups in the United States, but rates of death from heart disease and from stroke are higher among African American adults than among white adults. African Americans also have higher rates of high blood pressure (hypertension), develop this problem earlier in life, suffer more severe hypertension, and have higher rates of stroke.

**Diabetes**   American Indians and Alaska Natives, African Americans, and Hispanics are twice as likely to be diagnosed with diabetes compared with non-Hispanic whites. American Indians have the highest rate of diabetes in the world.

## If You Are at Risk

Certain health risks may be genetic, but behavior influences their impact. Here are specific steps you can take to protect your health:

- Ask if you are at risk for any medical conditions or disorders based on your family history or racial or ethnic background.

- Find out if there are tests that could determine your risks. Discuss the advantages and disadvantages of such testing.

- If you or a family member require treatment for a chronic illness, ask your doctor whether any medications have proved particularly effective for your racial or ethnic background.

- If you are African American, you are significantly more likely to develop high blood pressure, diabetes, and kidney disease. Being overweight or obese adds to the danger. The information in Chapters 6, 7, and 8 can help you lower your risk by keeping in shape, making healthy food choices, and managing your weight.

- Hispanics and Latinos have disproportionately high rates of respiratory problems, such as asthma, chronic obstructive lung disease, and tuberculosis. To protect your lungs, stop smoking and avoid secondary smoke. Learn as much as you can about the factors that can trigger or worsen lung diseases.

**Infant Mortality**  African American, American Indian, and Puerto Rican infants have higher death rates than white infants.

**Mental Health**  American Indians and Alaska Natives suffer disproportionately from depression and substance abuse. Minorities have less access to mental health services and are less likely to receive needed high-quality mental health services.

**Infectious Disease**  Asian Americans and Pacific Islanders have much higher rates of hepatitis B. Black teenagers and young adults become infected with hepatitis B three to four times more often than those who are white. Black people also have a higher incidence of hepatitis C infection than white people. Almost 80 percent of reported cases affect racial and ethnic minorities.

**HIV and Sexually Transmitted Infections**
Although African Americans and Hispanics represent only about a quarter of the U.S. population, they account for about two-thirds of adult AIDS cases and more than 80 percent of pediatric AIDS cases. The rate of syphilis infection for African Americans is nearly 30 times the rate for whites.

*Why Sex and Gender Matter*  Medical scientists define *sex* as a classification, generally as male or female, according to the reproductive organs and functions that derive from the chromosomal complement. *Gender* refers to a person's self-representation as male or female or how that person is responded to by social institutions on the basis of the individual's gender presentation. Rooted in biology, gender is shaped by environment and experience.

The experience of being male or female in a particular culture and society can and does have an effect on physical and psychological well-being. In fact, sex and gender may have a greater impact than any other variable on how our bodies function, how long we live, and the symptoms, course, and treatment of the diseases that strike us. (See Figure 1.1.)

As you will see throughout this text, gender affects many aspects of health. Although many assume that men are the stronger sex, they die at a faster rate than women. About 115 males are conceived for every 100 females, but males die more often before birth. Boys are more likely to be born prematurely, to suffer birth-related injuries, and to die before their first birthdays than girls.

Men's overall mortality rate is 41 percent higher than women's. They have higher rates of cancer, heart disease, stroke, lung disease, kidney disease, liver disease, and HIV/AIDS. They are four times more likely to take their own lives or to be murdered than women. By age 65, there are only 77 men for every 100 women. At age 85 women outnumber men by 2.6 to 1. More than half of all women older than age 65 are

Figure 1.1 **Some of the Many Ways Men and Women Are Different**

## He:

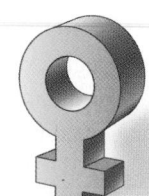

- averages 12 breaths a minute
- has lower core body temperature
- has a slower heart rate
- has more oxygen-rich hemoglobin in his blood
- is more sensitive to sound
- produces twice as much saliva
- has a 10 percent larger brain
- is 10 times more likely to have attention deficit disorder
- as a teen, has an attention span of 5 minutes
- is more likely to be physically active
- is more prone to lethal diseases, including heart attacks, cancer, and liver failure
- is five times more likely to become an alcoholic
- has a life expectancy of 75.2 years

## She:

- averages 9 breaths a minute
- has higher core body temperature
- has a faster heart rate
- has higher levels of protective immunoglobulin in her blood
- is more sensitive to light
- takes twice as long to process food
- has more neurons in certain brain regions
- is twice as likely to have an eating disorder
- as a teen, has an attention span of 20 minutes
- is more likely to be overweight
- is more vulnerable to chronic diseases, like arthritis and autoimmune disorders, and age-related conditions like osteoporosis
- is twice as likely to develop depression
- has a life expectancy of 80.4 years

widows. Among centenarians, there are four females for every male.

Among the reasons that may contribute to the health and longevity gap between the sexes are:

- **Biological factors**, such as the fact that women have two X chromosomes and men only one, different levels of sex hormones (particularly testosterone and estrogen), and metabolic variations.

- **Social factors**, including work stress, hostility levels, and social networks and supports.

- **Behavioral factors**, such as risky behavior, aggression, violence, smoking, and substance abuse.

- **Health habits**, including regular screenings, preventive care, and minimizing of symptoms.

Sexual orientation also can affect health. Lesbian, gay, bisexual, and transgender (LGBT) individuals are more likely to encounter health disparities linked to social stigma, discrimination, and denial of their human and civil rights. Such discrimination has been implicated as a cause of high rates of psychiatric disorders, substance abuse, and suicide. The *Healthy People 2020* initiative has made improvements in LGBT health one of its new goals.[10]

# A Report Card on the Health of College Students

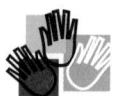  As one of an estimated 18 million college students in the United States, you are part of a remarkably diverse group. Today's undergraduates come from every age group and social, racial, ethnic, economic, political, and religious background. You may have served in the military, started a family, or immigrated from another country. You might be enrolled in a two-year college, a four-year university, or a technical school. Your classrooms might be in a busy city or a small town—or exist solely as a virtual campus. Although most undergraduates are "traditional" age—between 18 and 24 years old—more and more of you are over age 25.

The health of college students is as varied as their demographic makeup. In the American College Health Association National College Health Assessment, based on surveys of more than 30,000 students, 91.7 percent (92.8 percent of men and 91.1 percent of women) rated their health as good, very good, or excellent. The most common health problems students experienced in the previous 12 months were allergies (20 percent) and sinus infection (18 percent). The most common impediments to academic performance were stress (27 percent), sleep difficulties (20 percent), and cold/flu/sore throat (18 percent). Eighty percent said they had felt exhausted (not from physical activity) within the last 12 months.[11]

The health habits of college students also vary. Sixteen percent reported smoking at least once in the last month; 65 percent drank alcohol at least once. About half said they had used a condom (mostly or always) during vaginal intercourse in the last 30 days. More than three in four reported at least some moderate exercise in the prior week.[12]

Many students simply don't get enough sleep or keep irregular schedules that throw their sleep patterns off. Only 12 percent report getting enough sleep to feel rested in the morning six or more days a week; 9 percent report never feeling rested in the morning. More than nine in ten students say they feel tired, dragged out, or sleepy at least one morning a week. About four in ten describe daytime sleepiness as "more than a little problem," "a big problem," or "a very big problem." Sleeping less and juggling responsibilities more, students can quickly end up exhausted—and at greater risk for colds, flus, digestive problems, and other maladies.[13]

Students also become more sedentary in college, as they log more hours in classes and in front of computers. Fewer than half of college students meet recommended levels for moderate or vigorous aerobic exercise. The combination of a high-fat diet and a sedentary lifestyle in college can set the stage for the development of health problems that include obesity, diabetes, metabolic syndrome, heart disease, and certain cancers.

## The Perils of Young Adulthood

Your personal health depends on many factors, including your age, gender, race, and ethnic background. If you're in your late teens or early twenties, you are in a potentially risky transition phase.

Nine in ten Americans between ages 18 and 24 believe they're living healthy lifestyles, according to a recent poll by the American Stroke Association. However, most eat too much fast food, drink too many alcoholic and sugar-sweetened beverages, and engage in other behaviors that could put them at risk of cardiovascular disease, including stroke.[14] (See "How Do You Compare?")

Most of the 18–24-year-olds surveyed said they want to live long (to age 98) and maintain quality health throughout their life. However, one-third don't believe engaging in healthy behaviors *now* could affect their risk of stroke in the future. Eight in ten people between ages 25 and 44 also believe they are living healthy lifestyles, but they are more likely to engage in healthy behaviors than the younger cohort.[15]

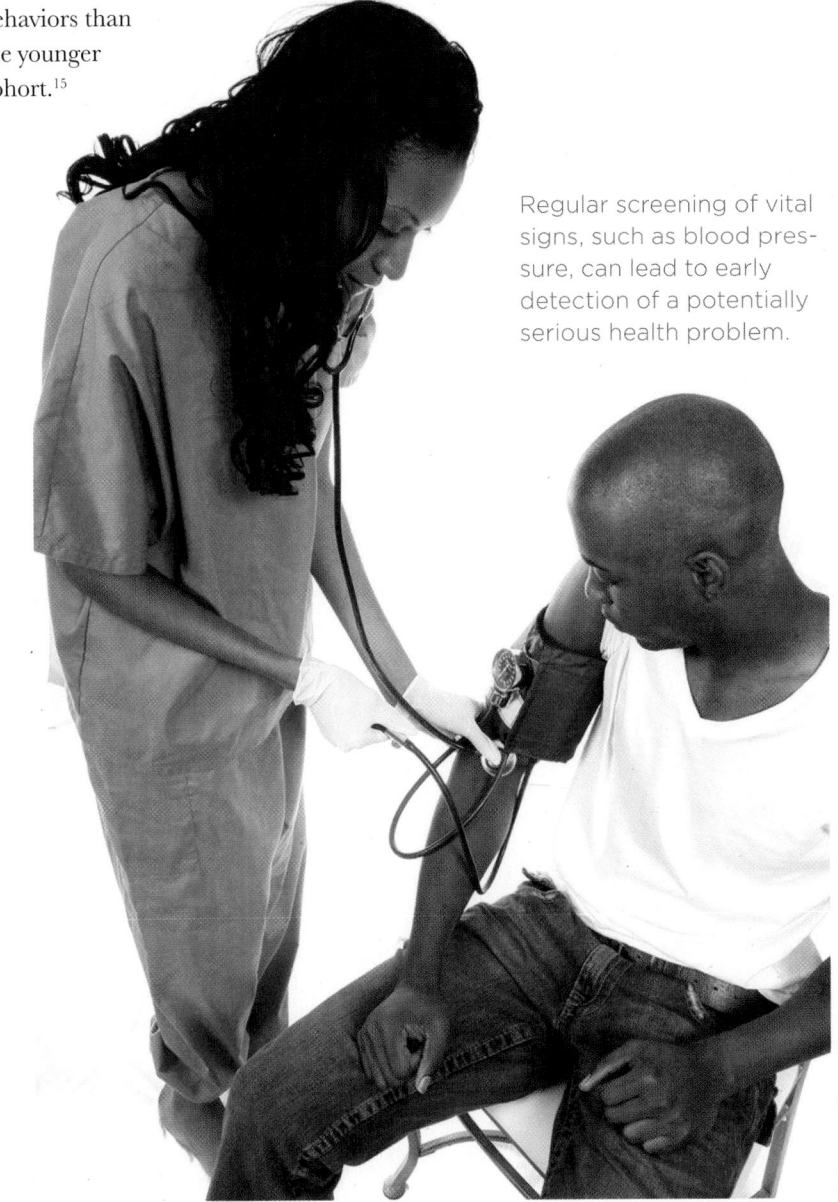

Regular screening of vital signs, such as blood pressure, can lead to early detection of a potentially serious health problem.

© Dewayne Flowers/Shutterstock.com

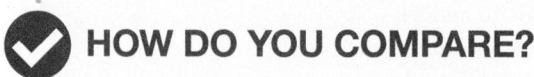

# DO YOUNG ADULTS PRACTICE HEALTHY HABITS?

**Percentage who say they**

- engage in healthy behaviors
  - 18- to 24-year-olds — 43
  - 25- to 34-year-olds — 34

- engage in regular physical activity
  - 18- to 24-year-olds — 48
  - 25- to 34-year-olds — 39

- are likely to achieve or maintain a healthy weight
  - 18- to 24-year-olds — 55
  - 25- to 34-year-olds — 53

- are likely to eat fast food
  - 18- to 24-year-olds — 29
  - 25- to 34-year-olds — 25

- are likely to eat recommended servings of fruits and vegetables
  - 18- to 24-year-olds — 26
  - 25- to 34-year-olds — 33

- are likely to limit alcohol consumption
  - 18- to 24-year-olds — 76
  - 25- to 34-year-olds — 77
  - men — 60
  - women — 72

- are likely to smoke
  - 18- to 24-year-olds — 15
  - 25- to 34-year-olds — 23

## HOW DO YOU COMPARE?

Rate yourself in each of the categories above. Are you more or less likely than other young Americans to practice healthy behaviors? Do you do better in some areas than others? What changes do you think would benefit you most? Record your thoughts in your online journal.

Source: American Heart Association, www.newsroom.heart.org/index.php?s=43.

According to a longitudinal study that followed 10,000 young Americans from adolescence into adulthood, health risks increase significantly as they come of age. Young men and women of every race and ethnic group are more likely to eat fast food, not exercise, be obese, and smoke cigarettes. Many do not get regular physical or dental examinations and do not receive health care when they need it. (See Health on a Budget.) Drug abuse and sexually transmitted infections (STIs) are widespread in this age group.

Certain serious health threats—substance abuse, sexually transmitted infections, homicide, and motor vehicle crashes—peak in young adulthood. As they leave their teens, young adults are less likely to seek preventive care or regular treatment for chronic conditions. Young men, especially black and Hispanic males, have less than one-fourth the rate of preventive care visits as young women. On average they see doctors less than once every nine years and even less often if they lack health insurance.

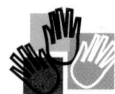 No single race or ethnic group leads or falters in health across all the health indicators studied. White Americans, who have the best health in adolescence, experience the greatest decline in early adulthood. American Indians face higher health risks both as teens and adults. Individuals in minority groups are most likely to need care but to be unable to pay for it.

In the past, young adults were the least likely to have health insurance and represented one in five uninsured Americans. With passage of the Affordable Care Act, adult children can remain on their parents' health insurance policies until age 26, even if they no longer live at home and are not students. Young adults who obtain their own policies must be offered the same benefits available to others.[16]

## Preventing Health Problems

College students often think they are too young to worry about serious health conditions. Yet many chronic problems begin early in life. Two percent of college-age women already have osteoporosis, a bone-weakening disease; another 15 percent have osteopenia, low bone densities that put them at risk of osteoporosis. Many college students have several risk factors for heart disease, including high blood pressure and high cholesterol. Others increase their risk by eating a high-fat diet and not exercising regularly. The time to change is now.

No medical treatment, however successful or sophisticated, can compare with the power of **prevention**. Two out of every three deaths and one in three hospitalizations in the United States could be prevented by changes in six main risk factors: tobacco use, alcohol abuse, accidents, high blood pressure, obesity, and gaps in screening and primary health care. Prevention remains the best weapon against cancer and heart disease.

Prevention can take many forms. Primary, or before-the-fact, prevention efforts might seek to reduce stressors and increase support to prevent problems in healthy people. Consumer education, for instance, provides guidance about how to change our lifestyles to prevent problems and enhance well-being. Other preventive programs identify people at risk and empower them with information and support so they can avoid potential problems. Prevention efforts may target an entire community and try to educate all of its members about the dangers of alcohol abuse or environmental hazards, or they may zero in on a particular group (for instance, seminars on safer sex practices offered to teens) or an individual (such as one-on-one counseling about substance abuse).

## Protecting Yourself

There is a great deal of overlap between prevention and **protection**. Some people might think of immunizations (discussed in Chapter 16) as a way of preventing illness; others see them as a form of protection against dangerous diseases. In many ways, protection picks up where prevention leaves off. You can prevent STIs or

---

# Invest in Your Future

As the economy has declined, visits to doctors have dropped, and millions of people are not taking prescribed medications. However, trying to save money in the short term by doing without needed health care can cost you a great deal—financially and physically—in the long term. Here are some ways to keep medical costs down without sacrificing your good health:

- **Stay healthy.** Use this book to learn the basics of a healthy lifestyle, then live accordingly. By eating nutritiously, exercising, getting enough sleep, not smoking, and getting regular immunizations you'll reduce your risk of conditions that require expensive treatments.

- **Build a good relationship with a primary care physician.** Although your choices may be limited, try to schedule appointments with the same doctor. A physician who knows you, your history, and your concerns can give the best advice on staying healthy.

- **Don't go to a specialist without consulting your primary care provider,** who can help you avoid overtesting and duplicate treatments.

- **If you need a prescription, ask if a generic form is available.** Brand names cost more, and most insurers charge higher co-payments for them.

- **Take medications as prescribed.** Skipping doses or cutting pills in two may seem an easy way to save money, but you may end up spending more for additional care because the treatment won't be as effective.

- **Don't go to an emergency department unless absolutely necessary.** Call your doctor for advice, or go to the student health service. Emergency departments are overburdened with caring for the very ill and injured, and their services are expensive.

---

unwanted pregnancy by abstaining from sex. But if you decide to engage in sexual activities, you can protect yourself with condoms and spermicides (discussed in Chapter 10). Similarly, you can prevent many automobile accidents by not driving when road conditions are hazardous. But if you do have to drive, you can protect yourself by wearing a seat belt and using defensive driving techniques (discussed in Chapter 18). (See Health in Action.)

The very concept of protection implies some degree of risk—immediate and direct (for instance, the risk of intentional injury from an assailant or unintentional harm from a fire) or

**prevention** Information and support offered to help healthy people identify their health risks, reduce stressors, prevent potential medical problems, and enhance their well-being.

**protection** Measures that an individual can take when participating in risky behavior to prevent injury or unwanted risks.

- To lower your risk of heart disease, get your blood pressure and cholesterol checked. Don't smoke. Stay at a healthy weight. Exercise regularly.

- To lower your risks of major diseases, get regular checkups. Make sure you are immunized against infectious illnesses.

- To lower your risks of substance abuse and related illnesses and injuries, don't drink, or limit how much you drink. Avoid illegal drugs.

- To lower your risk of sexually transmitted infections (STIs) or unwanted pregnancy, abstain from sex. If you engage in sexual activities, protect yourself with contraceptives, condoms, and spermicides.

- To prevent car accidents, stay off the road in hazardous circumstances, such as bad weather. Wear a seat belt when you drive, and use defensive driving techniques.

Identify your top preventive health priority—lowering your risk of heart disease, for instance, or avoiding accidents. Write down a single action you can take this week that will reduce your health risks. As soon as you take this step, write a brief reflection in your online journal.

**social norm** A behavior or attitude that a particular group expects, values, and enforces.

long-term and indirect (such as the risk of heart disease and cancer as a result of smoking). To know how best to protect yourself, you have to be able to realistically assess risks.

## Understanding Risky Behaviors

Risky behaviors are not new or unusual on campus, but today's students face different—and potentially deadlier—risks than undergraduates did a generation or two ago. The problem is not that students who engage in risky behavior do not know the danger or feel invulnerable. Young people, according to recent research, actually overestimate the risk of some outcomes. However, they also overestimate the benefit of immediate pleasure when, for instance, engaging in unsafe sex, and underestimate the negative consequences, such as a sexually transmitted infection.

College-age men are more likely than women to engage in risky behaviors—to use drugs and alcohol, to have unprotected sex, and to drive dangerously. Men also are more likely to be hospitalized for injuries and to commit suicide. Three-fourths of the deaths in the 15- to 24-year age range are men.

Drinking has long been part of college life and, despite the efforts across U.S. college campuses to curb alcohol abuse, two out of five students engage in binge drinking—consumption of five or more drinks at a single session for men, four for women. Heavy drinking increases the likelihood of other risky behaviors, such as smoking cigarettes, using drugs, or having multiple sexual partners. (See "Don't Go There" in *Labs for IPC*.) New trends, such as drinking caffeinated alcoholic beverages (discussed in Chapter 13), smoking tobacco from a hookah or water pipe (see Chapter 14), and using the dangerous stimulants called "bath salts" (see Chapter 12), present new risks.

## Student Health Norms

Psychologists use the term *norm*, or **social norm**, to refer to a behavior or attitude that a particular group expects, values, and enforces. Norms influence a wide variety of human activities, including health habits. However, perceptions of social norms are often inaccurate.

Only anonymous responses to a scientifically designed questionnaire can reveal what individuals really do—the actual social norms—as compared to what they may say they do to gain social approval.

Undergraduates are particularly likely to misjudge what their peers are—and aren't—doing. In recent years colleges have found that publicizing research data on behaviors such as drinking, smoking, and drug use helps students get a more accurate sense of the real health norms on campus.

The gap between students' misperceptions and accurate health norms can be enormous. For example, undergraduates in the ACHA-NCHA survey estimated that only 9 percent of students had never smoked cigarettes. In fact, 66 percent never had. Students guessed that only 4 percent of their peers never drank alcohol. In reality, 21 percent never did.[17] Providing accurate information on drinking norms on campus has proven effective in changing students' perceptions and in reducing alcohol consumption by both men and women.

The "How Do You Compare?" feature in every chapter allows you to test the accuracy of your perceptions of students' health behaviors.

# Making Quality Health-Care Decisions

Although you may not realize it, you make crucial decisions that affect your health every day. You choose what you eat, whether you exercise, if you smoke or drink, when to fasten your seat belt. You determine when to see a doctor, what kind of doctor, and with what sense of urgency. You decide what to tell the physician and whether to follow his or her advice, take a prescribed medication as directed, or seek further help or a second opinion. The entire process of maintaining or restoring health depends on your decisions. It cannot start or continue without them. The following sections can help you make better choices about your health and health care.

## How to Boost Health Understanding

Always ask these three questions of your doctor, nurse, or pharmacist:

- **What is my main problem?**

- **What do I need to do?**

- **Why is it important for me to do this?**

- **If you don't understand, say, "This is new to me.** Can you explain it one more time?"

- **If you don't know the meaning of a medical term, don't hesitate to ask what it means.** Health professionals sometimes forget they're using technical terms, such as "myocardial infarction" for heart attack.

- **Write down a list of your health concerns,** and bring it with you whenever you seek health care.

See "Health Assurance" in *Labs for IPC* and *Your Personal Wellness Guide* for more advice on taking charge of your health care.

## Improving Your Health Literacy

According to federal estimates, about one-third of the population in the United States has limited ability to understand health information and to use that information to make good decisions about health and medical care. Because of poor **health literacy**, more than 90 million Americans may not understand how to take medication, monitor cholesterol levels or blood sugar, manage a chronic disease, find health providers and services, or fill out necessary forms. According to research studies, people with limited health literacy are more likely to report poor health, to skip important preventive measures such as regular Pap smears, to have chronic conditions such as diabetes or asthma, and to have higher rates of preventable hospitalizations.[18] In patients with life-threatening conditions such as heart failure, low health literacy has been associated with higher mortality rates.[19]

 Regardless of their literacy skills, college students often do not seek out information on health concerns. In one study that tracked college students' communications for a two-week period, they sought health-related advice and information in a little more than one-fourth of their communications about health. When they did seek help, they were most likely to turn to family and friends. About half of students also turn to health educators for information, and most rank them and health center medical staff as believable. Although students regularly get information from flyers, pamphlets, magazines, and television, they are less likely to consider these as authoritative, believable sources. (See Health in the Headlines: Patient Education.)

## Finding Good Advice Online

Three in four Internet users are "e-health" consumers who seek information or support, communicate with health-care providers, or buy medical products online. "They use the Internet as an adjunct to physicians, who remain their primary source of health advice," says Mark Bard, president of Manhattan Research, a health-care marketing firm. About three in four college students have used the Internet to get health information, but many are skeptical of what they find.

If you go to websites for medical information, here are some guidelines for evaluating them:

- **Check the creator**. Websites are produced by health agencies, health support groups, school health programs, health-product advertisers, health educators, and health-education organizations. Read site headers and footers carefully to distinguish biased commercial advertisements from unbiased sites created by scientists and health agencies.

- **If you are looking for the most recent research,** check the date the page was created and last updated as well as the links. Several nonworking links signal that the site isn't carefully maintained or updated.

- **Check the references**. As with other health-education materials, web documents should provide the reader with references.

## Patient Education

Knowledge and understanding are critical to making good decisions about your health, and health-care professionals are placing more emphasis on educating consumers about their health. To find out more, go to Global Health Watch and click on "Health and Wellness." Scan down to "Consumer Health" and click on "Patient Education." Scan the headlines that appear on the right of your screen, and select an article that reports on the importance of health literacy or the impact of informed decision making by patients. Write a brief summary in your online journal.

**health literacy** Ability to understand health information and use it to make good decisions about health and medical care.

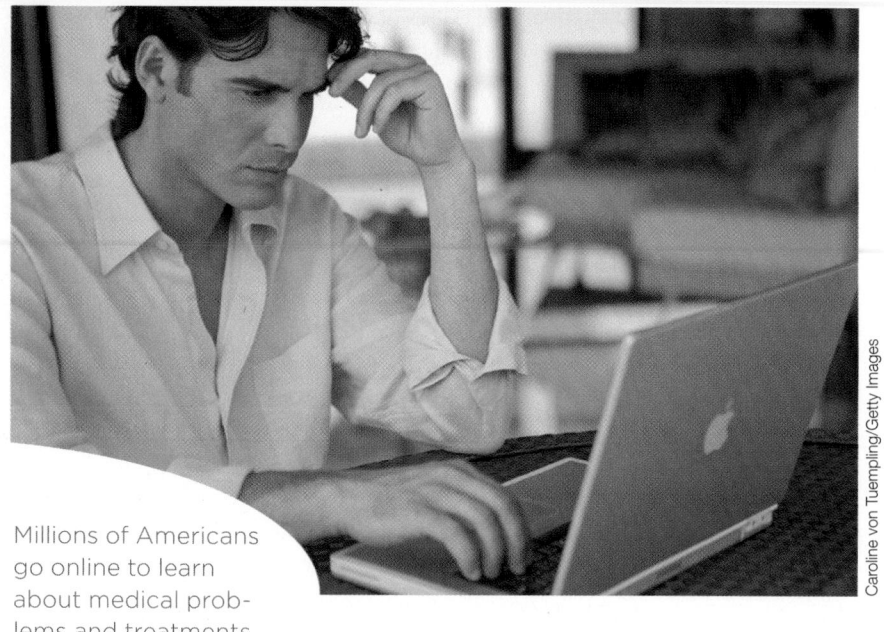

Millions of Americans go online to learn about medical problems and treatments and to chat with others who have similar conditions.

Caroline von Tuempling/Getty Images

Unreferenced suggestions may be scientifically unsound and possibly unsafe.

- **Consider the author**. Is he or she recognized in the field of health education or otherwise qualified to publish a

health-information web document? Does the author list his or her occupation, experience, and education?

- **Look for possible bias**. Websites may be attempting to provide health information to consumers, but they also may be attempting to sell a product. Many sites are merely disguised advertisements. (See Table 1.1 for some doctor-endorsed websites.)

## Getting Medical Facts Straight

Cure! Breakthrough! Medical miracle! These words make headlines. Remember that although medical breakthroughs and cures do occur, most scientific progress is made one small step at a time. Rather than putting your faith in the most recent report or the hottest trend, try to gather as much background information and as many opinions as you can. (See Consumer Alert, p. 19.)

When reading a newspaper or magazine story or listening to a radio or television report about a medical advance, look for answers to the following questions:

- **Who are the scientists involved?** Are they recognized, legitimate health professionals? What are their credentials? Are they affiliated with respected medical or scientific institutions? Be wary of individuals whose degrees or affiliations are from institutions you've never heard of, and be sure that the person's educational background is in a discipline related to the area of research reported.

- **Where did the scientists report their findings?** The best research is published in peer-reviewed professional journals, such as the *New England Journal of Medicine*. Research developments also may be reported at meetings of professional societies.

- **Is the information based on personal observations?** Does the report include testimonials from cured patients or satisfied customers? If the answer to either question is yes, be wary.

- **Does the article, report, or advertisement include words like *amazing*, *secret*, or *quick*?** Does it claim to be something the public has never seen or been offered before? Such sensationalized

Table 1.1 **Doctor Recommended Websites**

**National Library of Medicine: MedlinePlus**     http://medlineplus.gov

MedlinePlus contains links to information on hundreds of health conditions and issues. The site also includes a medical dictionary, an encyclopedia with pictures and diagrams, and links to physician directories.

**FDA Center for Drug Evaluation and Research**     www.fda.gov

Click on Drugs@FDA for information on approved prescription drugs and some over-the-counter medications.

**WebMD**     www.webmd.com

WebMD is full of information to help you manage your health. The site's quizzes and calculators are a fun way to test your medical knowledge. Get diet tips, find information on drugs and herbs, and check out special sections on men's and women's health.

**Mayo Clinic**     http://mayoclinic.com

The renowned Mayo Clinic offers a one-stop health resource website. Use the site's Health Decision Guides to make decisions about prevention and treatment. Learn more about complementary and alternative medicine, sports medicine, and senior health in the Healthy Living Centers.

**Centers for Disease Control and Prevention**     www.cdc.gov

Stay up to date on the latest public health news and get the CDC's recommendations on travelers' health, vaccines and immunizations, and protecting your health in case of a disaster.

**Medscape**     www.medscape.com

Medscape delivers news and research specifically tailored to your medical interests. The site requires (free) registration.

language is often a tip-off to a dubious treatment.

- **Is someone trying to sell you something?** Manufacturers who cite studies to sell a product have been known to embellish the truth.

- **Does the information defy all common sense?** Be skeptical. If something sounds too good to be true, it probably is.

## Evidence-Based Medicine

Large randomized controlled trials and large prospective studies provide the best evidence, or scientific proof, that a particular treatment is effective. **Evidence-based medicine** is a way of improving and evaluating patient care by combining the best research evidence with the patient's personal values.

Reviewing all available medical studies pertaining to an individual patient or group of patients helps doctors to diagnose illnesses more precisely, to choose the best tests, and to select the best treatments or methods of disease prevention. By using evidence-based medical techniques for large groups of patients with the same illness, doctors can develop **practice guidelines** for evaluating and treating particular illnesses.

## Outcomes Research

Evidence-based medicine pays particular attention to **outcomes**—that is, the impact that a specific medication or treatment has on a patient's condition, overall health, and quality of life.

Outcomes research is designed to answer questions such as: Is treatment better or worse than no treatment? Is one treatment better than another? If a treatment is effective, is a little just as good as a lot? Does quality of life change because of treatment? Are the benefits of treatment worth the cost or the risks to the patient?

Studies of outcomes look at how patients fared with or without a specific treatment, the costs involved, and the impact of undergoing or not undergoing treatment in terms of the patients' quality of life. Outcomes research can help determine which of several therapies or approaches provides the best results at the most reasonable costs.

When you are diagnosed with a health problem, ask your doctor if your treatment is based on the latest evidence and clinical guidelines. The National Guideline Clearinghouse provides a comprehensive database of evidence-based clinical practice guidelines for many common health problems, available at www.guideline.gov.

# Making Healthy Changes

In terms of human health, the 1800s were the century of hygiene, with life-saving advances in sanitation and clean drinking water. The 1900s were the century of medicine, with breakthroughs in diagnosing and treating major illnesses. The 2000s, medical experts predict, will be the century of behavioral change, when individuals take charge of their health by breaking unhealthy habits and creating new, healthier ones.

The stakes for modifying student behavior are high. Four in ten students are binge drinkers; one in four smokes. Among those who are sexually active, almost three in four say they've engaged in unprotected sex. Only about a third of undergraduates exercise regularly. Their nutrition is notoriously poor. Weights—and weight problems—are rising on campus. By graduation, one in four students has at least one major risk factor for diabetes, metabolic syndrome, or heart disease. Yet even students who recognize the risks and want to change their behavior often have no idea how to begin.

If you would like to improve your health behavior, you have to realize that change isn't easy. Between 40 and 80 percent of those who try to kick bad health habits lapse back into their unhealthy ways within six weeks.

Yet even simple behavioral changes could have a significant impact. A study that tracked about 20,000 adults in the United Kingdom found that those who adopted just four healthy habits lived an average of 14 years longer than the others. These life-extending behaviors are:

- Not smoking.

- Eating lots of fruits and vegetables.

**evidence-based medicine** The choice of a medical treatment on the basis of large randomized controlled research trials and large prospective studies.

**practice guidelines** Recommendations for diagnosis and treatment of various health problems based on evidence from scientific research.

**outcomes** The ultimate impacts of particular treatments or absence of treatment.

Figure 1.2  **Factors That Shape Positive Behavior**

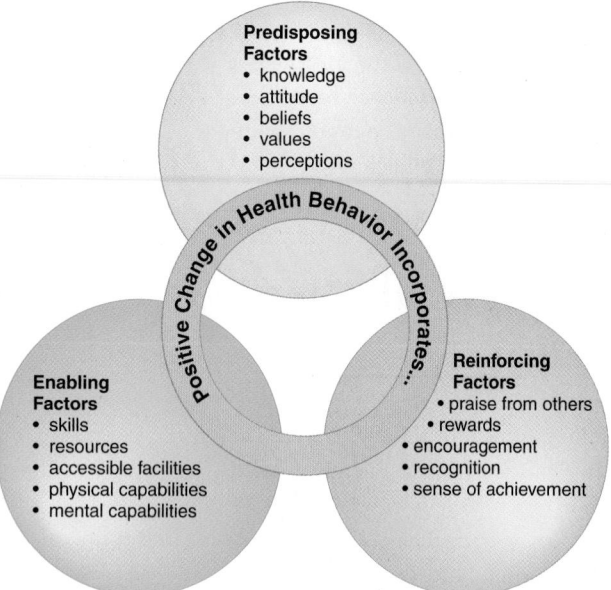

continue to puff away. Nor is attitude—one's likes and dislikes—sufficient; an individual may dislike the smell and taste of cigarettes but continue to smoke regardless.

Beliefs are more powerful than knowledge and attitudes, and researchers report that people are most likely to change health behavior if they hold three beliefs:

- **Susceptibility**. They acknowledge that they are at risk for the negative consequences of their behavior.

- **Severity**. They believe that they may pay a very high price if they don't make a change.

- **Benefits**. They believe that the proposed change will be advantageous to their health.

There can be a gap between stated and actual beliefs, however. Young adults may say they recognize the very real dangers of casual, careless sex in this day and age. Yet, rather than act in accordance with these statements, they may impulsively engage in unprotected sex with individuals whose health status and histories they do not know. The reason: Like young people everywhere and in every time, they feel invulnerable, that nothing bad can or will happen to them, that if there were a real danger, they would somehow know it. Often it's not until something happens—a former lover may admit to having a sexually transmitted infection—that their behaviors become consistent with their stated beliefs.

**Enabling Factors**  **Enabling factors** include skills, resources, accessible facilities, and physical and mental capacities. Before you initiate a change, assess the means available to reach your goal. No matter how motivated you are, you'll become frustrated if you keep encountering obstacles. That's why breaking a task or goal down into step-by-step strategies is so important in behavioral change.

**Reinforcing Factors**  **Reinforcing factors** may be praise from family and friends, rewards from teachers or parents, or encouragement and recognition for meeting a goal. Although these help a great deal in the short run, lasting change depends not on external rewards but on an internal commitment and sense of achievement. To make a difference, reinforcement must come from within.

- Exercising regularly.

- Drinking alcohol in moderation.[20]

Participants got a point for each of these healthy habits, and those who scored four points were four times less likely to die than those who scored zero.

Fortunately, our understanding of change has itself changed. Thanks to decades of research, we now know what sets the stage for change, the way change progresses, and the keys to lasting change. We also know that personal change is neither mysterious nor magical but a methodical science that anyone can master. (See "Part I: The New Science of Personal Change" in *IPC* for a comprehensive review.)[21]

## Understanding Health Behavior

Three types of influences shape behavior: predisposing, enabling, and reinforcing factors (Figure 1.2).

**Predisposing Factors**  **Predisposing factors** include knowledge, attitudes, beliefs, values, and perceptions. Unfortunately, knowledge isn't enough to cause most people to change their behavior; for example, people fully aware of the grim consequences of smoking often

**predisposing factors** The beliefs, values, attitudes, knowledge, and perceptions that influence our behavior.

**enabling factors** The skills, resources, and physical and mental capabilities that shape our behavior.

**reinforcing factors** Rewards, encouragement, and recognition that influence our behavior in the short run.

## Too Good to Be True?

Almost every week you're likely to see a commercial or an ad for a new health product that promises better sleep, more energy, clearer skin, firmer muscles, lower weight, brighter moods, longer life—or all of these combined. As the Consumer Alerts throughout this book point out, you can't believe every promise you read or hear. Keep these general guidelines in mind the next time you come across a health claim.

### Facts to Know

- **Do your own research.** Check with your doctor or with the student health center. Go to the library or do some online research to gather as much information as you can.

- **Check credentials.** Anyone can claim to be a scientist or a health expert. Find out if advocates of any type of therapy have legitimate degrees from recognized institutions and are fully licensed in their fields.

### Steps to Take

- **Look for objective evaluations.** If you're watching an infomercial for a treatment or technique, you can be sure that the enthusiastic endorsements have been skillfully scripted and rehearsed. Even ads that claim to be presenting the science behind a new breakthrough are really sales pitches in disguise.

- **Consider the sources.** Research findings from carefully controlled scientific studies are reviewed by leading experts in the field and published in scholarly journals. Just because someone has conducted a study doesn't mean it was a valid scientific investigation.

- **If it sounds too good to be true, it probably is.** If a magic pill could really trim off excess pounds or banish wrinkles, the world would be filled with thin people with unlined skin. Look around and you'll realize that's not the case.

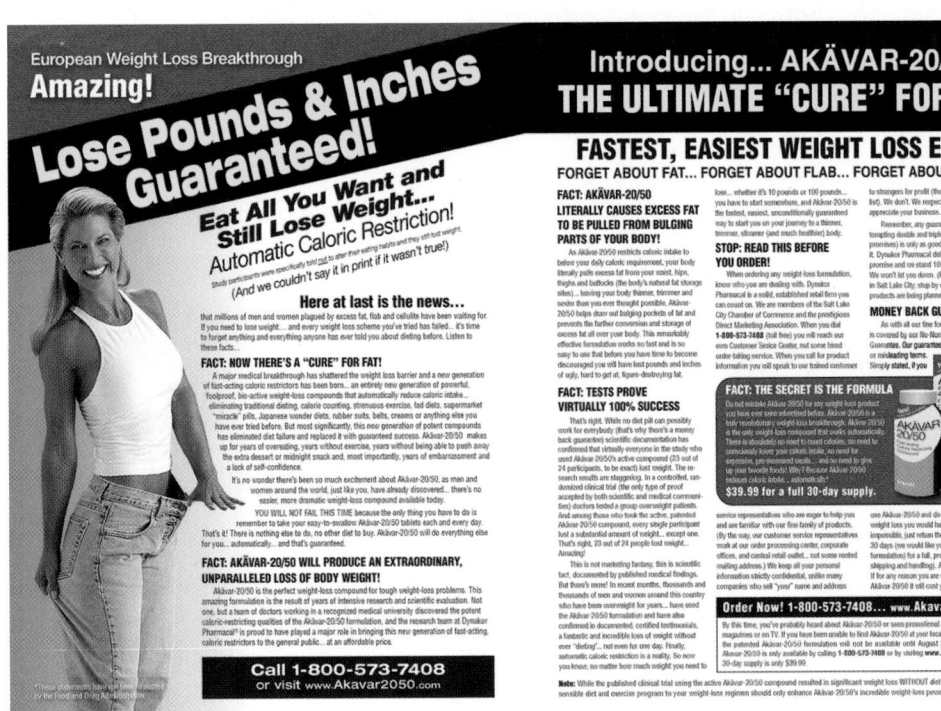

PR Newswire/AP Images

A decision to change a health behavior should stem from a permanent, personal goal, not from a desire to please or impress someone else. If you lose weight for the homecoming dance, you're almost sure to regain pounds afterward. But if you shed extra pounds because you want to feel better about yourself or get into shape, you're far more likely to keep off the weight.

# How and Why People Change

Change can simply happen. You get older. You put on or lose weight. You have an accident. Intentional change is different: A person consciously, deliberately sets out either to change a negative behavior, such as chronic procrastination, or to initiate a healthy behavior, such as daily exercise. For decades psychologists have studied how people intentionally change and have developed various models that reveal the anatomy of change.

In the *moral model*, you take responsibility for a problem (such as smoking) and its solution; success depends on adequate motivation, while failure is seen as a sign of character weakness. In the *enlightenment model*, you submit to strict discipline to correct a problem; this is the approach used in Alcoholics Anonymous. The *behavioral model* involves rewarding yourself when you make positive changes. The *medical model* sees the behavior as caused by forces beyond your control (a genetic predisposition to being overweight, for example) and employs an expert to provide advice or treatment. For many people, the most effective approach is the *compensatory model*, which doesn't assign blame but puts responsibility on individuals to acquire whatever skills or power they need to overcome their problems.

## The Health Belief Model

Psychologists developed the **health belief model (HBM)** about 50 years ago to explain and predict health behaviors by focusing on the attitudes and beliefs of individuals. (Remember that your attitudes and beliefs are predisposing influences on your capacity for change.)

According to this model, people will take a health-related action (e.g., use condoms) if they:

- **Feel that they can avoid a negative consequence**, such as a sexually transmitted infection (STI).
- **Expect a positive outcome** if they take the recommended advice—for instance, that condoms will protect them from STIs.
- **Believe that they can successfully take action**—for example, use condoms comfortably and confidently.

Readiness to act on health beliefs, in this model, depends on how vulnerable individuals feel, how severe they perceive the danger to be, the benefits they expect to gain, and the barriers they think they will encounter. Another key factor is self-efficacy, their confidence in their ability to take action.

Over the years the health belief model has been used to help people change unhealthy behaviors, such as smoking, overeating, and inactivity, or to encourage them to take positive health actions, such as using condoms and getting needed vaccinations and medical checkups.

## Self-Determination Theory

This approach, developed several decades ago by psychologists Edward Deci and Richard Ryan, focuses on whether an individual lacks motivation, is externally motivated, or is intrinsically motivated. Someone who is "amotivated" does not value an activity, such as exercise, or does not believe it will lead to a desired outcome, such as more energy or lower weight. Individuals who are externally motivated may engage in an activity like exercise to gain a reward or avoid a negative consequence (such as a loved one's nagging). Some people are motivated by a desired outcome; for instance, they might exercise for the sake of better health or longer life. Behavior becomes self-determined when someone engages in it for its own sake, such as exercising because it's fun.

Numerous studies have evaluated self-determination as it relates to health behavior. In research on exercise, individuals with greater self-determined motivation are less likely to stop exercising and have stronger intentions to continue exercise, higher physical self-worth, and lower social anxiety related to their physique.

**health belief model (HBM)**
A model of behavioral change that focuses on the individual's attitudes and beliefs.

## Motivational Interviewing

Health professionals, counselors, and coaches use motivational interviewing, developed by psychologists William Miller and Stephen Rollnick, to inspire individuals, regardless of their enthusiasm for change, to move toward improvements that could make their lives better. Building a collaborative partnership, the therapist does not persuade directly but uses empathy and respect for the patient's perspective to evoke recognition of the desirability of change.

## The Transtheoretical Model

Psychologist James Prochaska and his colleagues, by tracking what they considered to be universal stages in the successful recovery of drug addicts and alcoholics, developed a way of thinking about change that cuts across psychological theories. Their **transtheoretical model** focuses on universal aspects of an individual's decision-making process rather than on social or biological influences on behavior.

The transtheoretical model has become the foundation of programs for smoking cessation, exercise, healthy food choices, alcohol cessation, weight control, condom use, drug use cessation, mammography screening, and stress management. Recent studies have demonstrated its usefulness in helping adolescents quit smoking[22] and in increasing fruit and vegetable intake.[23]

The following sections describe these key components of the transtheoretical model:

- **Stages of change.**
- **Processes of change**—cognitive and behavioral activities that facilitate change.
- **Self-efficacy**—the confidence people have in their ability to cope with challenge.

*The Stages of Change*  According to the transtheoretical model of change, individuals progress through a sequence of stages as they make a change (Figure 1.3). No one stage is more important than another, and people often move back and forth between them. Most "spiral" from stage to stage, slipping from maintenance to contemplation or from action to precontemplation before moving forward again.

People usually cycle and recycle through the stages several times. Smokers, for instance,

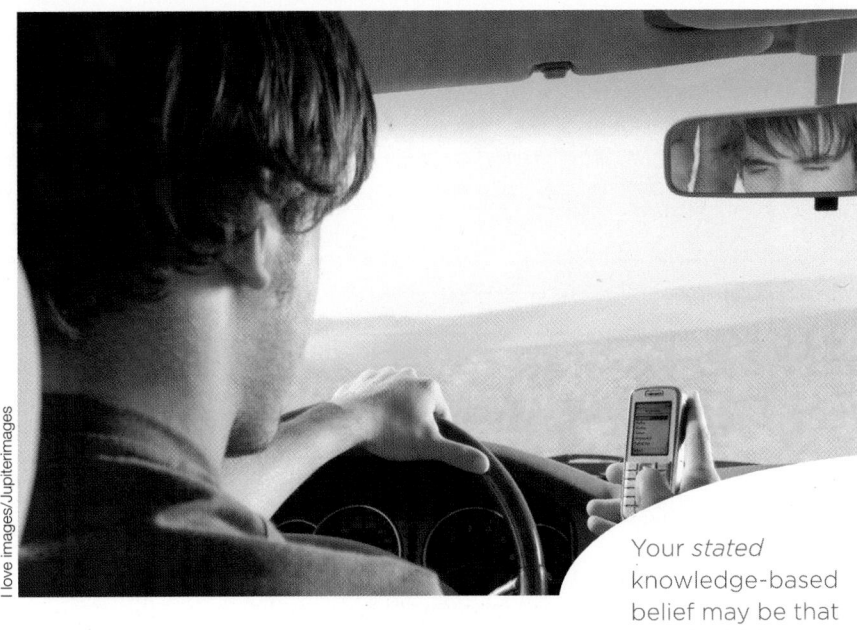

I love images/JupiterImages

Your *stated* knowledge-based belief may be that unsafe driving can cause accidents. Your *actual* belief is that it won't happen to you.

report making three or four serious efforts to quit before they succeed.

The six stages of change are:

1. **Precontemplation.** You are at this stage if you, as yet, have no intention of making a change. You are vaguely uncomfortable, but this is where your grasp of what is going on ends. If you feel healthy and are busy with your classes and activities, for instance, you may never think about exercise. Then you notice that it's harder to zip your jeans or that you get winded walking up stairs. Still you don't quite register the need to do anything about it.

   During precontemplation, change remains hypothetical, distant, and vague. Yet you may speak of something bugging you and wish that things were somehow different.

2. **Contemplation.** In this stage you begin to get it. You acknowledge that something is amiss and begin to consider what it is and whether you can do anything about it. You still prefer not to have to change, but you start to realize that you can't avoid reality. Maybe none of your jeans fit anymore, or you feel sluggish and listless. As you begin to weigh the trade-offs of standing pat versus acting, you may alternate between wanting to take action and resisting it.

   The way you talk to yourself expresses your feeling that change is necessary but

**transtheoretical model**  A model of behavioral change that focuses on the individual's decision making; it states that an individual progresses through a sequence of six stages as he or she makes a change in behavior.

Figure 1.3 **The Stages of Change and Some Change Processes**
These change processes can help you progress through the stages of change. Each may be most useful at particular stages.

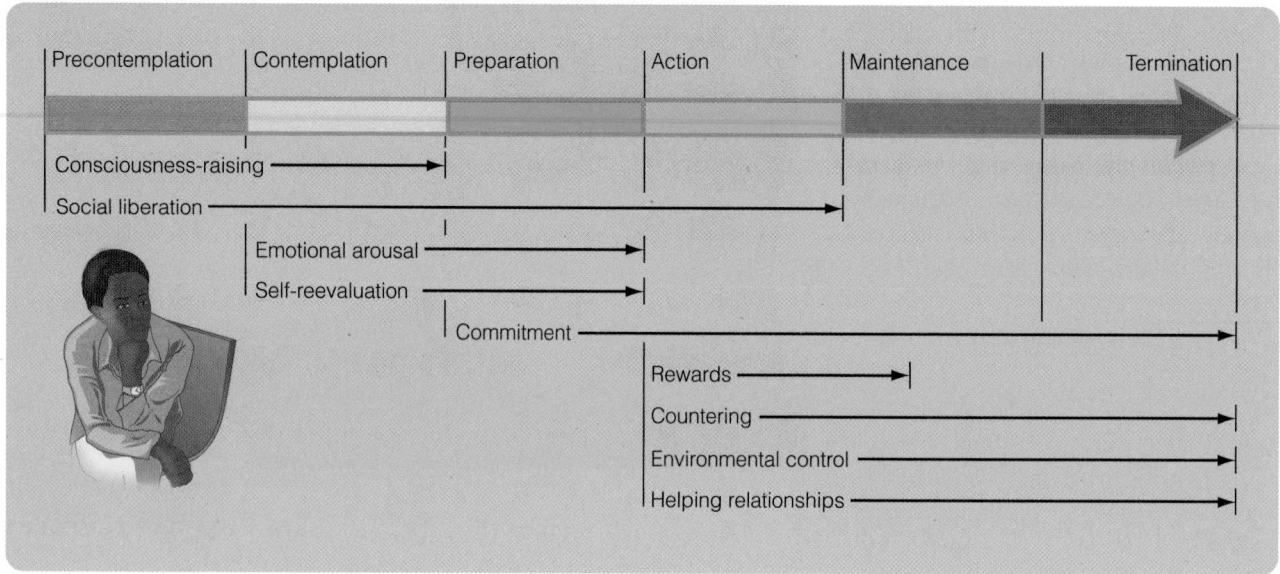

demonstrates your lack of commitment to taking action. Here are some examples of how the contemplation stage sounds:

- "I hate it that I keep . . . "
- "I should . . . "
- "Maybe I'll do it someday—not tomorrow, but someday."

3. **Preparation.** At some point you stop waffling, make a clear decision, and feel a burst of energy. This decision heralds the preparation stage. You gather information, make phone calls, do research online, and look into exercise classes at the gym. You begin to think and act with change specifically in mind even if you hold something back.

   If you eavesdrop on what you're saying to yourself, you would hear statements such as, "I am going to do this," and you set a date, such as "I will begin on New Year's Day." Yet you may not share your plans with others, despite all the internal progress you've made.

4. **Action.** This is the stage of actively modifying your behavior according to your plan. Your resolve is strong, and you know you're on your way to a better you. You no longer keep your plan under wraps—not that you could. Change produces signs that are

visible to others. You may be getting up 15 minutes earlier to make time for a healthy breakfast or to walk to class rather than taking the shuttle. In a relatively short time you acquire a sense of comfort and ease with the change in your life.

5. **Maintenance.** Maintenance is about locking in and consolidating gains. This stabilizing stage, which follows the flurry of specific steps taken in the action stage, is absolutely necessary to retain what you've worked for and to make change permanent. In this stage, you strengthen, enhance, and extend the changes you've initiated. You bring the rest of what you do into line with the change to support it. By securing the progress you've made, even if you hit a plateau or slip backward, you can regain your footing and keep moving forward.

6. **Termination.** At this stage, your "change" has become status quo. While it may take two to five years, the behavior has become so deeply ingrained that you can't imagine abandoning it. More than eight in ten college seniors who exercised regularly remain as active, or even more active, after graduation.

As research on college students has shown, attitudes and feelings are related to stages of change. Smokers who believe that continuing to smoke would have only a minor or no impact on their health remain in the precontemplation stage; those with respiratory symptoms move on to contemplation and preparation.

*The Processes of Change*   Anything you do to modify your thinking, feeling, or behavior can be called a change process. The nine included in the transtheoretical model are shown in Figure 1.3 in their corresponding stages.

- **Consciousness-raising.** The most widely used change process involves increasing knowledge about yourself or the nature of your problem. As you learn more, you gain understanding and feedback about your behavior.

  **Example:** Reading Chapter 6 on making healthy food choices.

- **Social liberation.** This process takes advantage of alternatives in the external environment that can help you begin or continue your efforts to change.

  **Example:** Spending as much time as possible in nonsmoking areas.

- **Emotional arousal.** This process, also known as dramatic relief, works on a deeper level than consciousness-raising and is equally important in the early stages of change. Emotional arousal means experiencing and expressing feelings about a problem behavior and its potential solutions.

  **Example:** Resolving never to drink and drive after the death of a friend in a car accident.

- **Self-reevaluation.** This process requires a thoughtful reappraisal of your problem, including an assessment of the person you might be once you have changed the behavior.

  **Example:** Recognizing that you have a gambling problem and imagining yourself as a nongambler.

- **Commitment.** This process acknowledges—first privately and then publicly—that you are responsible for your behavior and the only one who can change it.

  **Example:** Joining a self-help or support group.

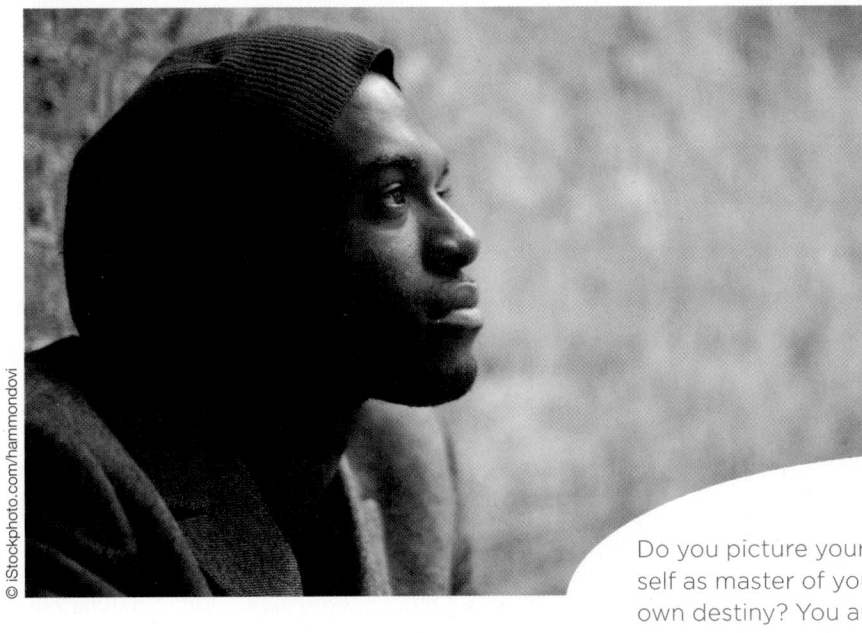

© iStockphoto.com/hammondovi

Do you picture yourself as master of your own destiny? You are more likely to achieve your health goals if you do.

- **Rewards.** This process reinforces positive behavioral changes with self-praise or small gifts.

  **Example:** Getting a massage after a month of consistent exercise.

- **Countering.** Countering, or counterconditioning, substitutes healthy behaviors for unhealthy ones.

  **Example:** Chewing gum rather than smoking.

- **Environmental control.** This action-oriented process restructures your environment so you are less likely to engage in a problem behavior.

  **Example:** Getting rid of your stash of sweets.

- **Helping relationships.** This process recruits individuals—family, friends, therapist, coach—to provide support, caring, understanding, and acceptance.

  **Example:** Finding an exercise buddy.

Researchers are zeroing in on the optimal stages to address certain behaviors. A study of college students, for instance, indicated that precontemplation might be the best time to address alcohol consumption, healthy eating, and managing depression (by means of Prochaska's recommended processes of consciousness-raising, dramatic relief, and environmental reevaluation). The contemplation stage might be a better time to address smoking by helping students minimize what they see as the drawbacks of quitting (such as awkwardness around friends who smoke).

### Self-Efficacy and Locus of Control

Do you see yourself as master of your fate, asserting control over your destiny? Or do so many things happen in your life that you just hang on and hope for the best? The answers to these questions reveal two important characteristics that affect your health: your sense of **self-efficacy** (the belief in your ability to change and to reach a goal) and your **locus of control** (the sense of being in control of your life).

Your confidence in your ability to cope with challenge can determine whether you can and will succeed in making a change. In his research on self-efficacy, psychologist Albert Bandura of Stanford University found that the individuals most likely to reach a goal are those who believe that they can. The stronger their faith in them-selves, the more energy and persistence they put into making a change. The opposite is also true, especially for health behaviors. Among people who begin an exercise program, those with lower self-efficacy are more likely to drop out.

If you believe that your actions will make a difference in your health, your locus of control is internal. If you believe that external forces or factors play a greater role, your locus of control is external. Hundreds of studies have compared people who have these different perceptions of control. "Internals," who believe that their actions largely determine what happens to them, act more independently, enjoy better health, and are more optimistic about their future. "Externals," who perceive that chance or outside forces determine their fate, find it harder to cope with stress and feel increasingly helpless over time. When it comes to weight, for instance, they see themselves as destined to be fat.

**self-efficacy** Belief in one's ability to accomplish a goal or change a behavior.

**locus of control** An individual's belief about the sources of power and influence over his or her life.

**Build Your Future**

## Making Healthy Changes

Ultimately you have more control over your health than anyone else. Use this course as an opportunity to zero in on at least one less-than-healthful behavior and improve it. Here are some suggestions for small steps that can have a big payoff. Check those that you commit to making today, this week, this month, or this term. Indicate "t," "w," "m," or term, and repeat this self-evaluation throughout the course.

_____ **Use seat belts.** In the last decade, seat belts have saved more than 40,000 lives and prevented millions of injuries.

_____ **Eat an extra fruit or vegetable every day.** Adding more fruit and vegetables to your diet can improve your digestion and lower your risk of several cancers.

_____ **Get enough sleep.** A good night's rest provides the energy you need to make it through the following day.

_____ **Take regular stress breaks.** A few quiet minutes spent stretching, looking out the window, or simply letting yourself unwind are good for body and soul.

_____ **Lose a pound.** If you're overweight, you may not think a pound will make a difference, but it's a step in the right direction.

_____ **If you're a woman, examine your breasts regularly.** Get in the habit of performing a breast self-examination every month after your period (when breasts are least swollen or tender).

_____ **If you're a man, examine your testicles regularly.** These simple self-exams can spot the signs of cancer early, when it is most likely to be cured.

_____ **Get physical.** Just a little exercise will do some good. A regular workout schedule will be good for your heart, lungs, muscles, bones—even your mood.

_____ **Drink more water.** Eight glasses a day are what you need to replenish lost fluids, prevent constipation, and keep your digestive system working efficiently.

_____ **Do a good deed.** Caring for others is a wonderful way to care for your own soul and connect with others.

# Are You in Control of Your Health?

To test whether you are the master of your fate, asserting control over your destiny or just hanging on, hoping for the best, take the test below. Depending on which statement you agree with, check either a or b for each of the following.

1. (a) Many of the unhappy things in people's lives are partly due to bad luck. ____

   (b) People's misfortunes result from mistakes they make. ____

2. (a) One of the major reasons why we have wars is that people don't take enough interest in politics. ____

   (b) There will always be wars, no matter how hard people try to prevent them. ____

3. (a) In the long run, people get the respect they deserve in this world. ____

   (b) Unfortunately, an individual's worth often passes unrecognized no matter how hard he tries. ____

4. (a) The idea that teachers are unfair to students is nonsense. ____

   (b) Most students don't realize the extent to which their grades are influenced by accidental happenings. ____

5. (a) Without the right breaks, one cannot be an effective leader. ____

   (b) Capable people who fail to become leaders have not taken advantage of their opportunities. ____

6. (a) No matter how hard you try, some people just don't like you. ____

   (b) People who can't get others to like them don't understand how to get along with others. ____

7. (a) I have often found that what is going to happen will happen. ____

   (b) Trusting to fate has never turned out as well for me as making a decision to take a definite course of action. ____

8. (a) In the case of the well-prepared student, there is rarely, if ever, such a thing as an unfair test. ____

   (b) Many times exam questions tend to be so unrelated to course work that studying is really useless. ____

9. (a) Becoming a success is a matter of hard work; luck has little or nothing to do with it. ____

   (b) Getting a good job depends mainly on being in the right place at the right time. ____

10. (a) The average citizen can have influence in government decisions. ____

    (b) This world is run by the few people in power, and there is not much the little guy can do about it. ____

11. (a) When I make plans, I am almost certain that I can make them work. ____

    (b) It is not always wise to plan too far ahead because many things turn out to be a matter of luck anyway. ____

12. (a) In my case, getting what I want has little or nothing to do with luck. ____

    (b) Many times we might just as well decide what to do by flipping a coin. ____

13. (a) What happens to me is my own doing. ____

    (b) Sometimes I feel that I don't have enough control over the direction my life is taking. ____

**Scoring:** Give yourself one point for each of the following answers:

1a, 2b, 3b, 4b, 5a, 6a, 7a, 8b, 9b, 10b, 11b, 12b, 13b

You do not get any points for other choices.

**Add up the totals.** Scores can range from 0 to 13. A high score indicates an external locus of control, the belief that forces outside yourself control your destiny. A low score indicates an internal locus of control, a belief in your ability to take charge of your life.

*Source: Based on J. B. Rotter, "Generalized Expectancies for Internal versus External Control of Reinforcement," Psychological Monographs, Vol. 80, Whole No. 609 (1966).*

If you turned out to be external on this self-assessment quiz, don't accept your current score as a given for life. If you want to shift your perspective, you can. People are not internal or external in every situation. At home you may go along with your parents' or roommates' preferences and let them call the shots. In class you might feel confident and participate without hesitation.

Take inventory of the situations in which you feel most and least in control. Are you bold on the basketball court but hesitant on a date? Do you feel confident that you can resolve a dispute with your friends but throw up your hands when a landlord refuses to refund your security deposit? Look for ways to exert more influence in situations in which you once yielded to external influences. See what a difference you can make.

# Making Change Happen

## Take Charge of Your Future

You—your resources, your common sense, your choices, your feelings of self-efficacy and self-worth—determine how long and how well you live. Nothing and no one else has a greater impact on your health than you. Knowledge about health and health care is indeed power, but information alone isn't enough. Action is the key. The habits you form now, the decisions you make while in college, will affect you for decades to come.

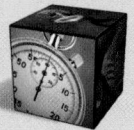

### Get Real

1. **Are you taking good care of yourself?** Your body belongs to you. The most sophisticated health-care delivery system or the newest breakthrough cannot do as much good for you as you can. Modern medicine's finest hours generally come when the body is in crisis. Only you can prevent such crises. To evaluate how you are doing, answer the following questions:

- Do you know your Body Mass Index (BMI)?
- Have you had your blood pressure checked in the last year?
- Have you had a lipoprotein profile—tests of your lipids, or blood fats—done in the last two years? Do you know your LDL level (the bad form of cholesterol)? Do you know your HDL (the good form of cholesterol)?
- Have you had your blood glucose checked? (This is a test for prediabetes and diabetes.)
- If you're a woman, do you examine your breasts every month?
- If you're a man, do you examine your testicles?
- Do you check your entire body for changes in moles and other early signs of skin cancer at least once a year?
- How often do you see a doctor for a medical checkup?
- How often do you go to the dentist?
- How often do you have your vision checked?
- Are your immunizations current? Have you been vaccinated against meningitis? hepatitis B? human papillomavirus (HPV)? influenza?
- Do you get an annual flu shot?
- Do you know if your family history puts you at risk for any serious health problem or condition?
- Do you always wear a seat belt when you're in a car?
- Do you wear a helmet when you ride a bicycle or motorcycle?
- Do you commit "self-malpractice" by engaging in any of the following?
  - cigarette smoking
  - excess drinking
  - abuse of prescription drugs
  - use of illegal drugs
  - careless driving or failure to wear a seat belt
  - carelessness in sexual relationships

2. **Assess yourself.** Based on your answers, rate your well-being on a scale from 1 (barely breathing) to 10 (potential Olympian). Then rate your conscientiousness in taking care of your health on a scale of 1 (whatever happens happens) to 10 (ever vigilant).

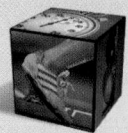

### Get Ready

1. **Request information.** To ensure quality medical care throughout your life, you will need information on your health history and your family history. If you do not have such information with you, your parents or partner may be able to provide it. However, you may need to contact your doctors' offices. Ask if your records are in an electronic format that you can access yourself, or if you need to request that they make copies for you. Also, ask for help in determining which parts of your record will be useful. You may need to fill out a form to authorize the release of information. Most facilities charge for copies of medical records. Allow time for this transfer.

2. **Contact family members.** In order to prepare a complete family history, you may need to interview your parents, uncles and aunts, grandparents, cousins, and so on. Let them know in advance of your project and your interests. Build time for these interviews in your schedule.

3. **Schedule medical appointments.** If you are due for a routine checkup, need an immunization or allergy shot, or want your doctor's advice on a non-urgent health problem, schedule an appointment toward the end of the term. You may have to call several weeks or even months in advance.

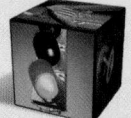

### Get Going

1. **Create your personal health record.** The best way to be sure that you have immediate access to medical information when you need it is to keep your own version of a medical "chart." We suggest that you create both a computer file as well as an actual file for hard copies of lab results, notes, and other information.

Here is what your personal health record should contain.

- Your name, birth date, blood type, and emergency contact.
- Date of last physical.
- Dates and results of tests and screenings.
- Major illnesses and surgeries, with dates.
- A list of your medicines, dosages, and how long you've taken them.
- Any allergies.
- Any chronic diseases.

2. **Assemble your family health history.** Family history is the single greatest risk factor for disease. Collect information about your grandparents, parents, aunts and uncles, nieces and nephews, siblings, and children. You can interview your relatives online, on the phone, or in person. Questions to ask include the following:

- What major diseases has the family experienced? Examples are hypertension, heart disease, stroke, cancer, depression, diabetes, Alzheimer's disease, obesity, blindness, and deafness. At what age were these diseases or conditions diagnosed? Was treatment successful?
- Have family members had a tendency toward other conditions, such as allergies, asthma, migraines, or frequent colds?
- Is there any family history of infertility, miscarriages, stillbirths, birth defects, or infant deaths?
- What is the family's dominant racial and ethnic background? Some diseases are more common among members of certain races and ethnicities.

For more guidance on creating a family history, check the CDC's family history website at http://www.cdc.gov/genomics/public/famhist.htm.

3. **Create your health history summary.** Based on the first two exercises, put together a summary that includes the following:

- Major injuries/conditions/illnesses and the dates when they occurred or were diagnosed.
- Allergies, specifying the type (food, medicine, etc.) and reaction.
- Any hospitalizations, the reasons for them, and the dates.
- Immunizations and dates, including tetanus, hepatitis B, meningitis, human papillomavirus (for women), and influenza.

- Any medicines/supplements that you take.
- Family members with serious health conditions.
- All the health-care providers you see, including nontraditional ones.

4. **Inform yourself.** Select a personally relevant topic, such as high blood pressure or diabetes, based on your personal or family medical history, and research it. The best place to turn is the Internet—if you know how to evaluate what you find. Start with these top health websites:

www.medlineplus.gov
www.cdc.gov
www.fda.gov
www.mayoclinic.com
www.webmd.com
www.medscape.com

With other sites, always look for the sponsor (is it commercial or a university or federal agency?), the authors' credentials, references, currency, and possible biases.

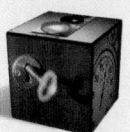

## Lock It In

1. **Check your health every week.** Record any new health problems, such as a headache, rash, or backache. Make note of the date, describe the symptoms, and record what treatments you use and when you get better. Review your observations before your next doctor's visit, and call attention to any troubling pattern or recurring symptoms.

2. **Keep up with health news,** particularly any conditions that affect you or your family. The government website www.medlineplus.gov includes news stories as well as background information on a host of health topics.

# Making This Chapter Work for You

## Review Questions

1. The development of health behaviors is influenced by all of the following *except*
   a. reinforcing factors, which involve external recognition for achieving a goal.
   b. preexisting health factors, which take into account the individual's current position on the wellness continuum.
   c. predisposing factors, which include knowledge, attitudes, and beliefs.
   d. enabling factors, which are related to an individual's skills and capabilities for making behavioral changes.

2. A group of students is discussing the differences between the sexes. Whose statement is *incorrect*?
   a. Matt: "Men breathe faster but have a slower heart rate—and have a larger brain."
   b. Elena: "But women have more neurons in certain brain regions."
   c. Kristin: "And women *are* less likely to get arthritis."
   d. Rick: "Got me there—Men *are* more likely to have heart attacks and to get cancer."

3. Which of the following statements about health information on the Internet is true?
   a. Chat rooms are the most reliable source of accurate medical information.
   b. Physicians who have websites must adhere to a strict set of standards set by the American Medical Association.
   c. Government-sponsored sites such as that of the Centers for Disease Control and Prevention are excellent sources of accurate health-care information.
   d. The Internet is a safe and cost-effective source of prescription drugs.

4. The term for a behavior or attitude that a particular group expects is
   a. social health.
   b. self-efficacy.
   c. social norm.
   d. reinforcement.

5. Which of the following is *not* a question you must ask your doctor to understand your health condition and what to do about it?
   a. What is my main problem?
   b. Why do I have this problem?
   c. What do I need to do?
   d. Why is it important for me to do this?

6. According to the stages of change in the transtheoretical model of change, which statement is *incorrect*?
   a. In the maintenance stage, individuals have avoided relapse for six months.
   b. In the contemplation stage, individuals are considering changing a problem behavior in the next six months.
   c. In the action stage, individuals are actually modifying their behavior according to their plan.
   d. In the preparation stage, individuals intend to change a problem behavior in the next six months.

7. Relapses are common (you're human, aren't you?), but don't let them keep you from your goal. Which of these strategies might help you recover from a relapse?
   a. Have a hot fudge sundae.
   b. Decide to think about it after finals.
   c. Analyze what went wrong and why.
   d. Put yourself back into contemplation stage.

8. Which of the following statements about the dimensions of health is true?
   a. Spirituality provides solace and comfort for those who are severely ill, but it has no health benefits.
   b. The people who reflect the highest levels of social health are usually among the most popular individuals in a group and are often thought of as the life of the party.
   c. Intellectual health refers to one's academic abilities.
   d. Optimal physical health requires a nutritious diet, regular exercise, avoidance of harmful behaviors and substances, and self-protection from accidents.

9. Change processes—cognitive and behavioral activities that facilitate change—include all of these *except*
   a. consciousness-raising.
   b. health awareness.
   c. countering.
   d. helping relationships.

10. If you want to change unhealthy behavior, which of the following strategies is *least* likely to promote success?
    a. Believe that you can make the change.
    b. Reward yourself regularly.
    c. Remind yourself about all your faults.
    d. Accept that you are in control of your health.

*Answers to these questions can be found on page 672.*

## Critical Thinking

1. Where are you on the wellness–illness continuum? What variables might affect your place on the scale? What do you consider your optimum state of health to be?

2. Talk to classmates from different racial or ethnic backgrounds than yours about their culture's health attitudes. Ask them what is considered healthy behavior in their cultures. For example, is having a good appetite a sign of health? What kinds of self-care practices did their parents and grandparents use to treat colds, fevers, rashes, and other health problems? What are their attitudes about the health-care system?

3. Jocelyn has been experiencing a great deal of fatigue and frequent headaches for the past couple of months. She doesn't have health insurance and doesn't want to spend money on a doctor visit. So she did some research on the Internet about ways to relieve her symptoms and was considering taking a couple of herbal supplements that were touted as potential treatments. If she asked you for your advice, what would you tell her? Do you think that self-care is appropriate in this situation?

## Media Menu

Visit www.cengagebrain.com to access course materials and companion resources for this text that will:

- Help you evaluate your knowledge of the material.

- Allow you to prepare for exams with interactive quizzing.

- Use the CengageNOW product to develop a Personalized Learning Plan targeting resources that address areas you should study.

- Coach you through identifying target goals for behavioral change and creating and monitoring your personal change plan throughout the semester using the Behavior Change Planner available in the CengageNOW resource.

## Key Terms

The terms listed are used on the page indicated. Definitions of the terms are in the Glossary at the end of the book.

enabling factors   18

evidence-based medicine   17

health   4

health belief model (HBM)   20

health literacy   15

health promotion   5

locus of control   24

outcomes   17

practice guidelines   17

predisposing factors   18

prevention   13

protection   13

reinforcing factors   18

self-efficacy   24

social norms   14

transtheoretical model   21

wellness   4

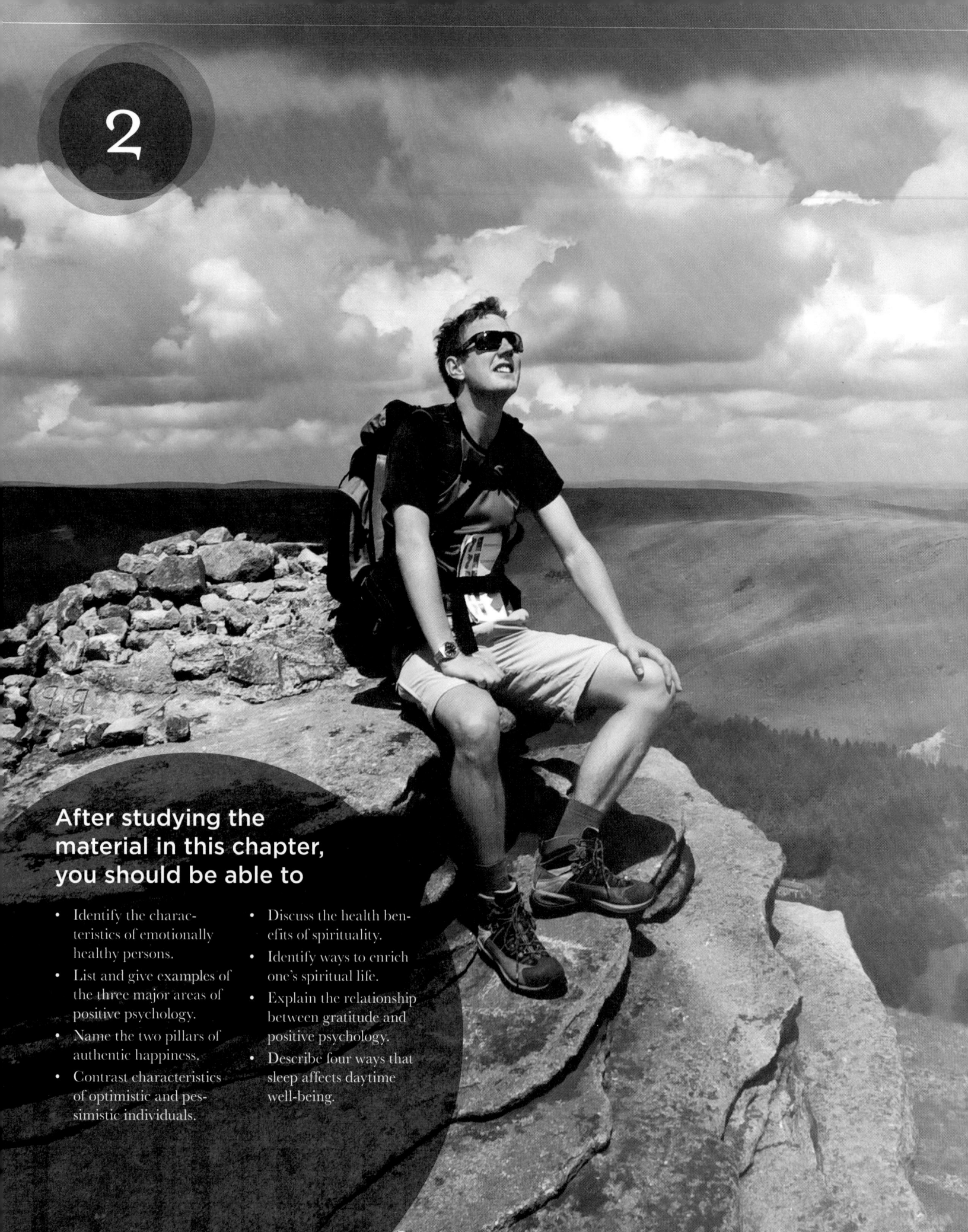

**2**

## After studying the material in this chapter, you should be able to

- Identify the characteristics of emotionally healthy persons.
- List and give examples of the three major areas of positive psychology.
- Name the two pillars of authentic happiness.
- Contrast characteristics of optimistic and pessimistic individuals.
- Discuss the health benefits of spirituality.
- Identify ways to enrich one's spiritual life.
- Explain the relationship between gratitude and positive psychology.
- Describe four ways that sleep affects daytime well-being.

Adam never considered himself a spiritual person until he enrolled in a class on the science of personal well-being. For a homework assignment he had to pursue different paths to happiness. As part of his experiment, he went to a Mardi Gras celebration and partied all night to see if having fun made him happier. To test whether doing good makes a person happy, Adam volunteered to help build a house for a homeless family. "I can't

# Your Psychological and Spiritual Well-Being

remember the name of a single person I met at the party," he says. "But I'll never forget the look on the family's faces when we handed them the keys to their new home."

For his final project, Adam, who did not have a religious upbringing, focused on developing a richer spiritual life. "The spirituality didn't end with the term," he says. "I continue to meditate, do yoga, and read religious texts because I believe a more spiritual life will help me in the long run with happiness and health."

The quest for a more fulfilling and meaningful life is attracting more people of all ages. The reason? As the burgeoning field of positive psychology has resoundingly proved, people who achieve emotional and spiritual health are more creative and productive, earn more money, attract more friends, enjoy better marriages, develop fewer illnesses, and live longer.

This chapter reports the latest findings on making the most of psychological strengths,

enhancing happiness, and developing the spiritual dimension of your health and your life. It also explores an often overlooked dimension of physical and emotional well-being: sleep.

## Emotional and Mental Health

"A sound mind in a sound body" was, according to the ancient Roman poet Juvenal, something all should strive for. This timeless advice still holds. Almost 2,000 years later we understand on a much more scientific level that physical and mental health are interconnected in complex and vital ways. One does not guarantee the other, but recent research has found that individuals who practice four fundamental behaviors—regular exercise, a healthful diet, moderate alcohol use, and no tobacco—are less

Visit www.cengagebrain.com to access course materials for this text, including the Behavior Change Planner, interactive quizzes, tutorials, and more. See the preface on page xv for details.

likely to become depressed, be overwhelmed by stress, or suffer poor mental health.[1]

Unlike physical health, psychological well-being cannot be measured, tested, X-rayed, or dissected. Yet psychologically healthy men and women generally share certain characteristics: They value themselves and strive toward happiness and fulfillment. They establish and maintain close relationships with others. They accept the limitations as well as the possibilities that life has to offer. And they feel a sense of meaning and purpose that makes the gestures of living worth the effort required.

Psychological health encompasses both our emotional and mental states—that is, our feelings and our thoughts. **Emotional health** generally refers to feelings and moods, both of which are discussed later in this chapter. Characteristics of emotionally healthy persons, identified in an analysis of major studies of emotional wellness, include the following:

- Determination and effort to be healthy.
- Flexibility and adaptability to a variety of circumstances.
- Development of a sense of meaning and affirmation of life.
- An understanding that the self is not the center of the universe.
- Compassion for others.
- The ability to be unselfish in serving or relating to others.
- Increased depth and satisfaction in intimate relationships.
- A sense of control over the mind and body that enables the person to make health-enhancing choices and decisions.

"Emotional vitality," a sense of positive energy and engagement in life, correlates with physical vitality. In a recent study the individuals who ranked highest in this state of heightened emotional well-being had the lowest risk of cardiovascular disease.

**Mental health** describes our ability to perceive reality as it is, to respond to its challenges, and to develop rational strategies for living. The mentally healthy person doesn't try to avoid conflicts and distress but can cope with life's transitions, traumas, and losses in a way that allows for emotional stability and growth. The characteristics of mental health include:

- The ability to function and carry out responsibilities.
- The ability to form relationships.
- Realistic perceptions of the motivations of others.
- Rational, logical thought processes.
- The ability to adapt to change and to cope with adversity.

**Culture** also helps to define psychological health. In one culture, men and women may express feelings with great intensity, shouting in joy or wailing in grief, while in another culture such behavior might be considered abnormal or unhealthy. In our diverse society, many cultural influences affect Americans' sense of who they are, where they came from, and what they believe. Cultural rituals help bring people together, strengthen their bonds, reinforce the values and beliefs they share, and provide a sense of belonging, meaning, and purpose.

To find out where you are on the psychological well-being scale, take the Self Survey: "Well-Being Scale" on page 51.

# The Lessons of Positive Psychology

Positive psychology has been defined as "the scientific study of ordinary human strengths and virtues." Rather than concentrating on what goes wrong in our lives and in our minds, it focuses on "the aspects of the human condition that lead to happiness, fulfillment, and flourishing"—in other words, on what makes life worth living.[2] The three major areas of positive psychology are the study of positive emotions, such as hope and trust; positive traits, such as wisdom and courage; and positive institutions, such as strong families and democracy.

According to psychologist Martin Seligman, Ph.D., author of *Flourish: A Visionary New Understanding of Happiness and Well-Being*, who popularized the positive psychology movement,

**emotional health** The ability to express and acknowledge one's feelings and moods and exhibit adaptability and compassion for others.

**mental health** The ability to perceive reality as it is, respond to its challenges, and develop rational strategies for living.

**culture** The set of shared attitudes, values, goals, and practices of a group that are internalized by an individual within the group.

**self-compassion** A healthy form of self-acceptance in the face of perceived inadequacy or failure.

everyone, regardless of genes or fate, can achieve a happy, gratifying, meaningful life. The goal is not simply to feel good momentarily or to avoid bad experiences, but to build positive strengths and virtues that enable us to find meaning and purpose in life. The core philosophy is to add a "build what's strong" approach to the "fix what's wrong" focus of traditional psychotherapy.

Some researchers categorize the spectrum of positive traits as those related to knowledge (creativity, curiosity, open-mindedness, love of learning, perspective); humanity (love, kindness, social intelligence); justice (citizenship, fairness, leadership); transcendence (appreciation of beauty and excellence, gratitude, hope, humor, spirituality); and temperance (humility, prudence, self-regulation, forgiveness).[3]

According to the "broaden-and-build" theory of positive emotions, such emotions expand our ways of thinking and acting. Joy, for instance, sparks an urge to play; contentment, an urge to appreciate and be grateful. In contrast, negative emotions narrow our behavioral range. When frightened, for instance, we may think only of fleeing from danger. As more than a decade of research has shown, broadening and building can produce significant positive effects, including buffering us against negative life events, promoting resilience, lowering the risk of psychological disorders, and enhancing physical well-being.[4]

Individuals vary in the ways they respond to and regulate positive emotions. Those with high self-esteem (discussed later in this chapter) are more likely to savor positive emotions, while those with low self-esteem tend to dampen them. ("Health in Action" offers ways of making the most of positive experiences and emotions.)

Clinical psychologists have developed and tested various interventions that bolster positive emotions, such as recalling positive memories from one's life, using one's unique or signature strengths in new ways, and cultivating gratitude and acceptance. These approaches have proven effective in enhancing well-being and decreasing negative feelings in individuals with and without psychological symptoms.[5]

The labs in *An Invitation to Personal Change (IPC)* apply the principles of positive psychology.

You can start practicing positive psychology right away. The next time you think, "I've never tried that before," also say to yourself, "This is an opportunity to learn something new." When something seems too complicated, remind yourself to tackle it from another angle. If you get discouraged and feel that you're never going to get better at some new skill, tell yourself to give it another try.

## Develop Self-Compassion

"College life is notorious for challenging students' sense of well-being," a team of educational psychologists at the University of Texas wrote in a recent paper, noting that students must "manage competing academic and social goals as well as their emotional reactions to both success and disappointment."[6]

One of the best ways to maintain well-being, they found, is **self-compassion**, a healthy form of self-acceptance that includes three components:

- Treating oneself kindly in the face of perceived inadequacy by engaging in self-soothing and positive self-talk.

- Recognizing that such discomfort is an unavoidable part of the human experience. This recognition of "common humanity" promotes a sense of connection to others even in the face of isolation and disappointment.

- Facing painful thoughts without avoiding or exaggerating them and managing disappointment and frustration by quelling self-pity and melodrama.

In their research, the ability to respond to life's disappointments, daily hassles, and stressful life events with self-compassion was a strong predictor of students' well-being. (See "Your Psychological Self-Care Pyramid" in Making Change Happen, p. 53, and in *Labs for IPC* to learn specific methods for being kinder to yourself.)

## Boost Emotional Intelligence

A person's "IQ"—or intelligence quotient—was once considered the leading predictor of achievement. However, psychologists have determined that another "way of knowing,"

### Accentuate the Positive

Try some of these strategies from positive psychology and comment on your experience in your online journal.

#### Do

✓ **Smile.** Putting on a happy face makes for a happy spirit.

✓ **Focus.** By being fully present in the moment, you'll experience it more intensely.

✓ **Share your joy.** Talking about and celebrating good experiences extends positive feelings over and above the positive event.

✓ **Travel through time.** Vividly remembering or anticipating positive events—a technique psychologists call "Positive Mental Time Travel"—boosts levels of happiness and life satisfaction.

#### Don't

✗ **Don't hide your feelings.** Suppressing positive feelings—because of shyness or a sense of modesty, for instance—diminishes them and may have physiological consequences on your health.

✗ **Don't get distracted.** Unrelated worries and thoughts detract from the here-and-now of a positive experience.

✗ **Don't find fault.** Paying attention to negative aspects of otherwise positive experiences sabotages levels of happiness, optimism, self-esteem, and life satisfaction.

✗ **Don't go there.** "Negative Mental Time Travel"—reflecting on what went wrong or what may go wrong—can lower self-esteem and foster depressive symptoms.

dubbed **emotional intelligence**, makes an even greater difference in a person's personal and professional success.

"EQ" (for emotional quotient) is the ability to monitor and use emotions to guide thinking and actions. Strong social or interpersonal skills are one measure of EQ. As more than a decade of research has shown, people with high EQ are more productive at work and happier at home. They're also less prone to stress, depression, and anxiety and bounce back more quickly from serious illnesses. Individuals with high EQ also seem more likely to have good mental and physical health.[7]

According to recent research, females score slightly higher in emotional intelligence than males, but in both sexes, individuals who are outgoing, dependable, and independent-minded tend to have higher EQs. Both sexes are equally capable of cultivating greater emotional intelligence. Emotional intelligence isn't fixed at birth, nor is it the same as intuition. Among the emotional competencies that most benefit students are focusing on clear, manageable goals and identifying and understanding emotions rather than relying on "gut" feelings.

## Know Yourself

Why do some students consistently invest in taking the best possible care of themselves while others repeatedly put their well-being at risk? The answers may lie within their personalities. According to recent research, two personality traits—conscientiousness (striving for competence and achievement, self-discipline, orderliness, reliability, deliberativeness) and extraversion (being active, talkative, assertive, social, stimulation-seeking)—correlate with very different health behaviors.[8]

College students who rate high in conscientiousness tend to wear seat belts, get enough sleep, drive safely, use safer sex practices, exercise, not smoke, drink less, and eat fruits and vegetables. The reason may be that they are thorough in their decision making and carefully weigh the risks and benefits of their behavior. They also can delay immediate gratification for the sake of long-term benefits, such as preventing cardiovascular disease or sexually transmitted infections.

Although they're more likely to participate in vigorous exercise, students who score high in extraversion are more likely to put their health at risk. They often drink more alcohol, binge-drink, smoke, engage in risky sexual behaviors, and don't get enough sleep. The reasons may involve brain chemistry. Individuals with low levels of neurochemical arousal may pursue highly stimulating (though risky) behaviors to feel more alert and excited.

Personality is not destiny. If you see yourself as low in conscientiousness or high in extraversion, you can take deliberate steps that will safeguard your health. For instance, you might fulfill your need for stimulation and excitement with less risky alternatives, such as X-Game competitions, rock-climbing, or volunteering with student-led emergency response services.[9]

## Meet Your Needs

Newborns are unable to survive on their own. They depend on others for the satisfaction of their physical needs for food, shelter, warmth, and protection, as well as their less tangible emotional needs. In growing to maturity, children take on more responsibility and become more independent. No one, however, becomes totally self-sufficient. As adults, we easily recognize our basic physical needs, but we often fail to acknowledge our emotional needs. Yet they, too, must be met if we are to be as fulfilled as possible.

The humanist theorist Abraham Maslow believed that human needs are the motivating factors in personality development. First, we must satisfy basic physiological needs, such as those for food, shelter, and sleep. Only then can we pursue fulfillment of our higher needs—for safety and security, love and affection, and self-esteem. Few individuals reach the state of **self-actualization**, in which one functions at the

**emotional intelligence** A term used by some psychologists to evaluate the capacity of people to understand themselves and relate well with others.

**self-actualization** A state of wellness and fulfillment that can be achieved once certain human needs are satisfied; living to one's full potential.

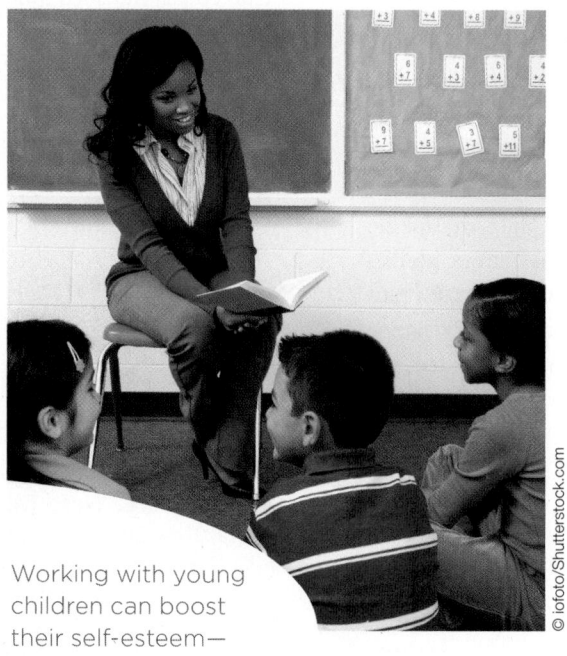

© iofoto/Shutterstock.com

Working with young children can boost their self-esteem—and yours.

highest possible level and derives the greatest possible satisfaction from life (Figure 2.1).

## Boost Self-Esteem

Each of us wants and needs to feel significant as a human being with unique talents, abilities, and roles in life. A sense of **self-esteem**, of belief or pride in ourselves, gives us confidence to dare to attempt to achieve at school or work and to reach out to others to form friendships and close relationships. Self-esteem is the little voice that whispers, "You're worth it. You can do it. You're okay."

Self-esteem is based not on external factors like wealth or beauty, but on what you believe about yourself. It's not something you're born with; self-esteem develops over time. It's also not something anyone else can give to you, although those around you can either help boost or diminish your self-esteem.

The seeds of self-esteem are planted in childhood when parents provide the assurance and appreciation youngsters need to push themselves toward new accomplishments: crawling, walking, forming words and sentences, learning control over their bladder and bowels.

Adults, too, must consider themselves worthy of love, friendship, and success if they are to be loved, to make friends, and to achieve their goals. Low self-esteem is more common in people who have been abused as children and in those with psychiatric disorders, including depression, anxiety, alcoholism, and drug dependence. Feeling a lack of love and encouragement as a child can also lead to poor self-esteem. Adults with poor self-esteem may unconsciously enter relationships that reinforce their self-perceptions and may prefer and even seek out people who think poorly of them.

One of the most useful techniques for bolstering self-esteem and achieving your goals is developing the habit of positive thinking and talking. While negative observations—such as constant criticisms or reminders of the most minor faults—can undermine self-image, positive affirmations—compliments, kudos, encouragements—have proved effective in enhancing self-esteem and psychological well-being. Individuals who fight off negative thoughts fare

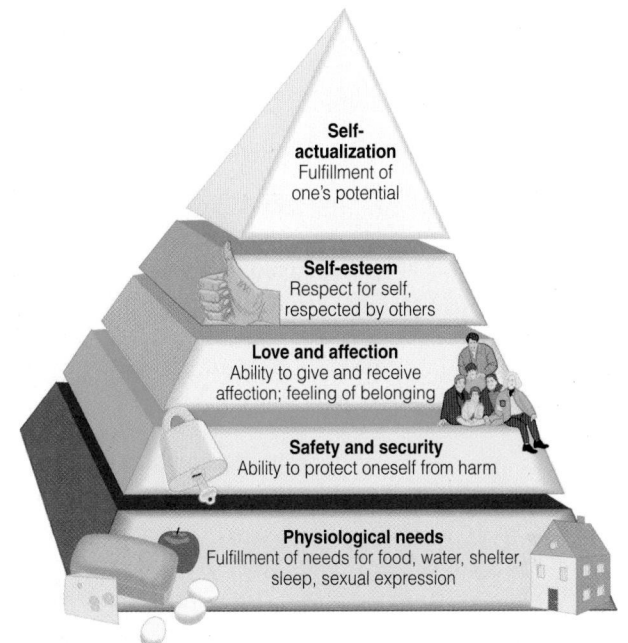

Figure 2.1 **The Maslow Pyramid**
To attain the highest level of psychological health, you must first satisfy your needs for safety and security, love and affection, and self-esteem.

Source: From Maslow, Abraham H.; Frager, Robert D. (Editor); Fadiman, James (Editor), *Motivation and Personality,* 3/e. Copyright © 1987. Reproduced by permission of Pearson Education, Inc., Upper Saddle River, New Jersey.

better psychologically than those who collapse when a setback occurs or who rely on others to make them feel better.

Self-esteem has proved to be one of the best predictors of college adjustment. Students with high self-esteem report better personal, emotional, social, and academic adjustment.

## Pursue Happiness

"Imagine a drug that causes you to live eight or nine years longer, to make $15,000 more a year, to be less likely to get divorced," says Martin Seligman, the "father" of positive psychology. "Happiness seems to be that drug."[10] But even if just about everyone might benefit by smiling more and scowling less, can almost anyone learn to live on the brighter side of life?

Skeptics who dismiss "happichondria" as the latest feel-good fad are dubious. However, happiness researchers, now backed by thousands of scientific studies, cite mounting evidence suggesting that happiness is a learned behavior. "Happiness is measurable, and it's buildable,"

**self-esteem** Confidence and satisfaction in oneself.

## Health on a Budget

# Happiness for Free!

Money can't buy happiness. As long as you have enough money to cover the basics, you don't need more wealth or more possessions for greater joy. Even people who win a fortune in a lottery return to their baseline of happiness within months. So rather than spending money on lottery tickets, try these ways to put a smile on your face:

- **Make time for yourself.** It's impossible to meet the needs of others without recognizing and fulfilling your own.

- **Up your appreciation quotient.** Regularly take stock of all the things for which you are grateful. To deepen the impact, write a letter of gratitude to someone who's helped you along the way.

- **String beads.** Think of every positive experience during the day as a bead on a necklace. This simple exercise focuses you on positive experiences, such as a cheery greeting from a cashier or a funny e-mail from a friend, and encourages you to act more kindly toward others.

- **Create a virtual DVD.** Visualize several of your happiest memories with as much detail as possible. Smell the air. Feel the sun. Hear the sea. Play this video in your mind when your spirits slump.

- **Fortify optimism.** Whenever possible, see the glass as half-full. Keep track of what's going right in your life. Imagine and write down your vision for your best possible future and track your progress toward it.

- **Immerse yourself.** Find activities that delight and engage you so much that you lose track of time. Experiment with creative outlets. Look for ways to build these passions into your life.

- **Seize the moment.** Rather than waiting to celebrate big birthday-cake moments, savor a bite of cupcake every day. Delight in a child's cuddle, a glorious sunset, a lively conversation. Cry at the movies. Cheer at football games. This life is your gift to yourself. Open it!

says Seligman. "We're not talking about just feeling good but about something more substantial and durable. The newest finding of positive psychology is that simple, proven strategies can make you lastingly happier. However, it's not easy, and it's not obvious how to go about it."

As researchers and therapists agree, happiness is more than a smiley face. Rather than a superficial sense of glee, true happiness "has depth and deliberation to it," as one writer put it. "It encompasses living a meaningful life, utilizing your gifts and your time, living with thought and purpose. It's maximized when you also feel

part of a community and when you confront annoyances and crises with grace. It involves a willingness to learn and stretch and grow, which sometimes involves discomfort. It requires acting on life, not merely taking it in. It's not joy, a temporary exhilaration, or even pleasure, that sensual rush—although a steady supply of those feelings course[s] through those who seize the day."[11]

Why pursue happiness? The answer goes beyond the psychological benefits. As a meta-analysis of long-term studies has shown, happiness reduces the risk of dying—both in healthy people and in those with diagnosed diseases. "Happiness is beneficial over and above the absence of misery," researchers have concluded. The reason may be that happiness induces changes in the brain or encourages stronger social connections.[12]

*Happiness 101* Genetics, as research on thousands of sets of twins has demonstrated, accounts for about 50 percent of your happiness quotient and for related personality traits, such as extraversion and conscientiousness. But even if you inherited the family frown rather than its joy genes, you're not fated to a life of gloom. Just don't pin your hopes on advantages like fitness, fortune, education, or good looks. The healthy, the wealthy, the bookish, and the beautiful report only somewhat greater happiness than those who are less blessed. Unless you're extremely poor or gravely ill, life circumstances account for only about 10 percent of happiness. The other 40 percent depends on what you do to make yourself happy. (See Health on a Budget.)

Unfortunately, most of us look for happiness in all the wrong places. We assume that external things—a bigger house, a better job, a winning lottery ticket—will gladden our lives. While they do bring temporary delight, the thrill invariably fades.

 In one study, more than 150 older college students rated a recent purchase—either of an object or of a life experience—that they invested in to make themselves happy. Those who spent their money on a pleasurable experience reported feeling more alive and invigorated than those who bought material things. The reason, according to the researchers, is that life experiences bring people closer, satisfy a natural human need for connection, and create memories that can be savored again and again.[13]

"After 18 years studying happiness, I fell into the same trap as everyone else," says psychologist Sonja Lyubomirsky, Ph.D., author of *The How of Happiness: A Scientific Approach to Getting the Life You Want*. "I was so excited to get a new car, a hybrid I'd wanted for a long time, but within two months driving it became routine. Happiness is like weight loss. We all know how to take off a few pounds but the trick is maintaining it."[14]

Lyubomirsky and her colleagues have fine-tuned proven strategies into practical prescriptions to enhance happiness. "Different methods are a better 'fit' for different people," she explains. "Keeping a daily gratitude journal seems hokey to some people, but writing a letter of gratitude may be very meaningful." Timing and "doses" also matter. Performing five acts of kindness on a single day, she's found, yields a greater halo effect than a single daily altruistic gesture. "But to sustain happiness you have to make the effort and commitment every day for the rest of your life," she emphasizes. For enduring joy, the key is looking beyond fleeting pleasures to the two pillars of "authentic" happiness: engagement with family, work, or a passionate pursuit and finding meaning from some higher purpose.

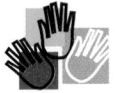 Education, intelligence, gender, and race do not matter much for happiness. African Americans and Hispanics have lower rates of depression than white Americans, but they do not report greater happiness. Neither gender is clearly happier, but in different studies women are both happier and sadder than men.

 In a recent study of college students, possessions mattered less to their personal satisfaction than how much they valued them. "The American undergraduates who are happiest in this life are not necessarily those who amass great numbers of things," the researchers concluded. "Rather they are those who both have the things they want and want the things they have."

In another survey of 222 college students, psychologists found that the "happiest" 10 percent, as determined by six different rating scales,

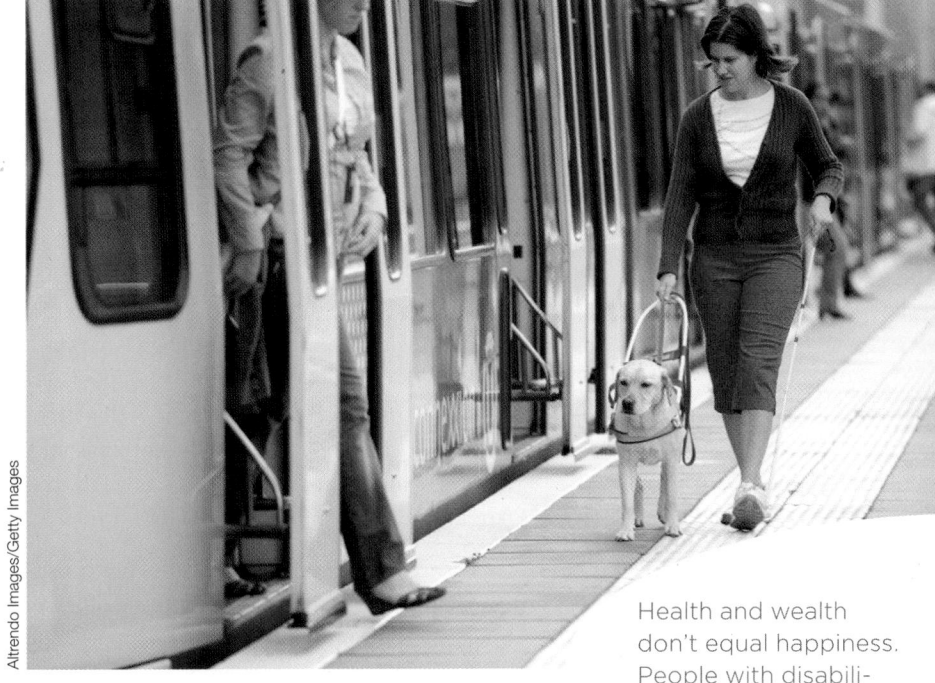

Altrendo Images/Getty Images

shared one distinctive characteristic: a rich and fulfilling social life. Almost all were involved in a romantic relationship as well as in rewarding friendships. The happiest students spent the least time alone, and their friends rated them as highest on good relationships.

Even people we don't know may make us happy. By analyzing 20 years of data on the social ties of almost 5,000 participants in the Framingham Heart Study, researchers found that happy people spread happiness to others. Spouses, neighbors, relatives, and friends benefit most, but so did more distant contacts. The more happy people you surround yourself with, the happier you—and your social network—are likely to be in the future.

 This may also be true online—at least to a certain extent. According to a recent study of college students, their feelings of well-being increase along with the number of their Facebook friends—perhaps because seeing friends' photos reminds them of their social connections and enhances their feelings of self-worth. However, the Facebook users who presented themselves honestly were more likely to receive meaningful social support from their online friends than those who, as the researchers put it, were always "hiding behind a smiling Facebook mask."[15] (See Chapter 5 for more on social networking.)

Health and wealth don't equal happiness. People with disabilities report almost the same level of life satisfaction as others.

## Become Optimistic

The dictionary defines **optimism** as "an inclination to anticipate the best possible outcome." For various reasons—because they believe in themselves, because they trust in a higher power, because they feel lucky—optimists expect positive experiences from life. When bad things happen, they tend to see setbacks or losses as specific, temporary incidents. In their eyes, a disappointment is "one of those things" that happens every once in a while, rather than the latest in a long string of disasters. And rather than blaming themselves ("I always mess things up," pessimists might say), optimists look at all the different factors that may have caused the problem.

As research over the last few decades has consistently shown, optimists and pessimists differ in how they confront problems and how they cope with adversity. These differences affect their physical and psychological well-being. People who expect good things respond to difficulty and adversity in more adaptive ways than those who expect bad things.

In terms of health, optimists not only expect good outcomes—for instance, that a surgery will be successful—but take steps to increase this likelihood. Pessimists, expecting the worst, are more likely to deny or avoid a problem, sometimes by drinking or other destructive behaviors. Optimism itself may protect against disease. In the large-scale Women's Health Initiative, which studied 95,000 women over an eight-year period, optimists were significantly less likely to develop coronary heart disease or to die of heart disease or any other cause.[16]

 Individuals aren't born optimistic or pessimistic; in fact, researchers have documented changes over time in the ways that individuals view the world and what they expect to experience in the future. Cognitive-behavioral techniques (discussed in Chapter 3) have proven effective in helping pessimists become more optimistic. In a study with college students, learning to decrease automatic negative thoughts and increase more constructive ones reduced episodes of moderate depression.[17]

## Manage Your Moods

Feelings come and go within minutes. A **mood** is a more sustained emotional state that colors

our view of the world for hours or days. According to surveys by psychologist Randy Larsen of the University of Michigan, bad moods descend upon us an average of three out of every ten days. "A few people—about 2 percent—are happy just about every day," he says. "About 5 percent report bad moods four out of every five days."[18]

There are gender differences in mood management: Men typically try to distract themselves (a partially successful strategy) or use alcohol or drugs (an ineffective tactic). Women are more likely to talk to someone (which can help) or to ruminate on why they feel bad (which doesn't help). Learning effective mood-boosting, mood-regulating strategies can help both men and women pull themselves up and out of an emotional slump.

The most effective way to banish a sad or bad mood is by changing what caused it in the first place—if you can figure out what made you upset and why. "Most bad moods are caused by loss or failure in work or intimate relationships," says Larsen. "The questions to ask are: What can I do to fix the failure? What can I do to remedy the loss? Is there anything under my control that I can change? If there is, take action and solve it." Rewrite the report. Ask to take a makeup exam. Apologize to the friend whose feelings you hurt. Tell your parents you feel bad about the argument you had.

If there's nothing you can do, accept what happened and focus on doing things differently next time. "In our studies, resolving to try harder actually was as effective in improving mood as taking action in the present," says Larsen. You also can try to think about what happened in a different way and put a positive spin on it. This technique, known as *cognitive reappraisal, or reframing,* helps you look at a setback in a new light: What lessons did it teach you? What would you have done differently? Could there be a silver lining or hidden benefit?

If you can't identify or resolve the problem responsible for your emotional funk, the next-best solution is to concentrate on altering your negative feelings. For example, try setting a quick, achievable goal that can boost your spirits with a small success. Clean out a drawer; sort through the piles of paper on your desk; send an e-mail or text message to an old friend.

**optimism** The tendency to seek out, remember, and expect pleasurable experiences.

**mood** A sustained emotional state that colors one's view of the world for hours or days.

Another good option is to get moving. In studies of mood regulation, exercise consistently ranks as the single most effective strategy for banishing bad feelings. Numerous studies have confirmed that aerobic workouts, such as walking or jogging, significantly improve mood. Even nonaerobic exercise, such as weight lifting, can boost spirits; improve sleep and appetite; reduce anxiety, irritability, and anger; and produce feelings of mastery and accomplishment.

## Look on the Light Side

Humor, which enables us to express fears and negative feelings without causing distress to ourselves or others, is one of the healthiest ways of coping with life's ups and downs. Laughter stimulates the heart, alters brain wave patterns and breathing rhythms, reduces perceptions of pain, decreases stress-related hormones, and strengthens the immune system.

Joking and laughing are ways of expressing honest emotions, of overcoming dread and doubt, and of connecting with others. They also can defuse rage. After all, it's almost impossible to stay angry when you're laughing. To tickle your funny bone, try keeping a file of favorite cartoons or jokes. Go to a comedy club instead of a movie. If you get an e-mail joke that makes you laugh out loud, don't keep it to yourself—multiply the mirth by sharing it with a friend.

## Develop Autonomy

One goal that many people strive for is **autonomy**, or independence. Both family and society influence our ability to grow toward independence. Autonomous individuals are true to themselves. As they weigh the pros and cons of any decision, whether it's using or refusing drugs or choosing a major or career, they base their judgment on their own values, not those of others. Their ability to draw on internal resources and cope with challenges has a positive impact on both their psychological well-being and their physical health, including recovery from illness.

Those who've achieved autonomy may seek the opinions of others, but they do not allow their decisions to be dictated by external influences. For autonomous individuals, their **locus of control**—that is, where they view control as

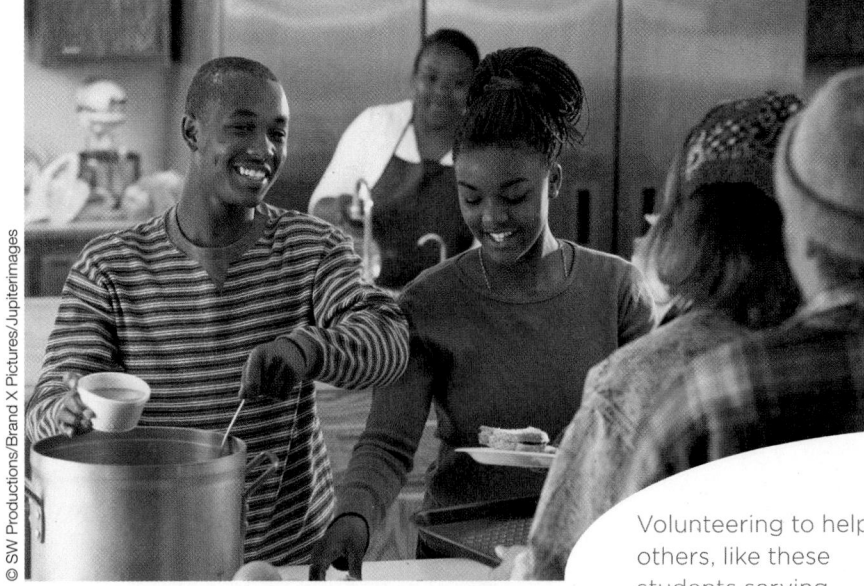

originating—is *internal* (from within themselves) rather than *external* (from others).

Volunteering to help others, like these students serving meals to the homeless, can contribute to a profound sense of life satisfaction.

# Spiritual Health

Whatever your faith, whether or not you belong to any formal religion, you are more than a body of a certain height and weight occupying space on the planet. You have a mind that equips you to learn and question. And you have a spirit that animates everything you say and do. **Spiritual health** refers to this breath of life and to our ability to identify our basic purpose in life and to experience the fulfillment of achieving our full potential. Spiritual readings or practices can increase calmness, inner strength, and meaning; improve self-awareness; and enhance your sense of well-being. Religious support has also been shown to help lower depression and increase life satisfaction beyond the benefits of social support from friends and family.

**Spirituality** is a belief in what some call a higher power, in someone or something that transcends the boundaries of self. It gives rise to a strong sense of purpose, values, morals, and ethics. Throughout life you make choices and decide to behave in one way rather than another because your spirituality serves as both a compass and a guide.

The term *religiosity* refers to various spiritual practices. That definition may seem vague, but

**autonomy** The ability to draw on internal resources; independence from familial and societal influences.

**locus of control** An individual's belief about the sources of power and influence over his or her life.

**spiritual health** The ability to identify one's basic purpose in life and to achieve one's full potential.

**spirituality** A belief in someone or something that transcends the boundaries of self.

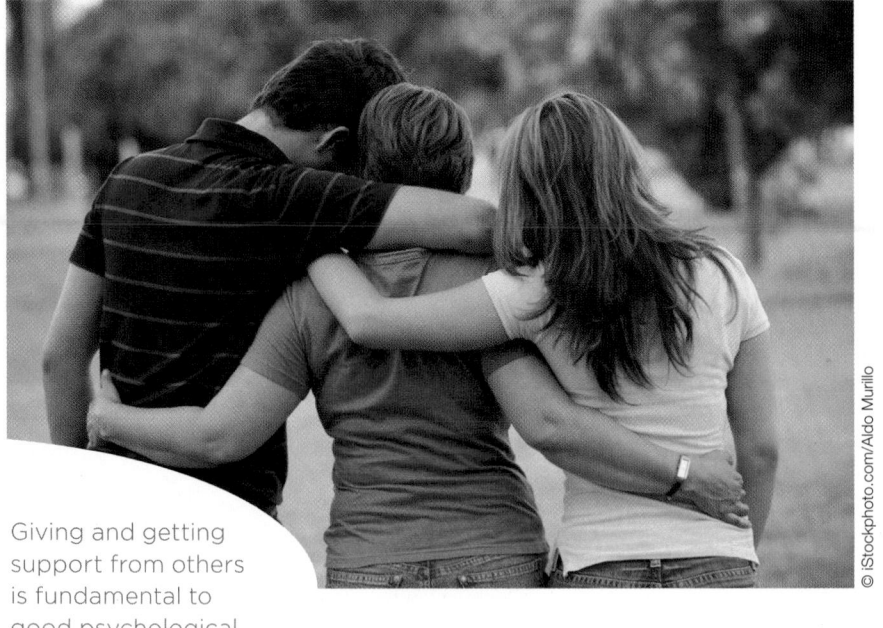

Giving and getting support from others is fundamental to good psychological health and emotional well-being.

going to church add years to a life? Researchers speculate that the reason may be the sense of community or support or that people feel less depressed when they join in religious services.[21]

Prayer and other religious experiences, including meditation, may actually change the brain—for the better. Using neuroimaging techniques, scientists have documented alterations in various parts of the brain that are associated with stress and anxiety. This effect may slow down the aging process, reduce psychological symptoms, and increase feelings of security, compassion, and love.[22]

In a recent study, undergraduates with higher levels of spirituality coped with challenges by "turning to religion" along with other practical problem-solving strategies, such as positive reframing, acceptance, and humor. This implies that students who are already religious use their spirituality to bolster resources to focus on the problem at hand. Those who did not score high in spirituality but turned to religion in a crisis were more likely to do so as a way of avoiding or denying the problem, along with such maladaptive strategies as trying to distract themselves from it.[23]

## Deepen Your Spiritual Intelligence

Mental health professionals have recognized the power of **spiritual intelligence**, which some define as "the capacity to sense, understand, and tap into the highest parts of ourselves, others, and the world around us." Spiritual intelligence, unlike spirituality, does not center on the worship of a God above, but on the discovery of a wisdom within.

All of us are born with the potential to develop spiritual intelligence, but most of us aren't even aware of it—and do little or nothing to nurture it. Part of the reason is that we confuse spiritual intelligence with religion, dogma, or old-fashioned morality. "You don't have to go to church to be spiritually intelligent; you don't even have to believe in God," says Reverend Paul Edwards, a retired Episcopalian minister and therapist in Fullerton, California. "It is a scientific fact that when you are feeling secure, at peace, loved, and happy, you see, hear, and act differently than when you're feeling

one thing is clear. According to thousands of studies on the relationship between religious beliefs and practices and health, religious individuals are less depressed, less anxious, and better able to cope with crises such as illness or divorce than are nonreligious ones. The more that a believer incorporates spiritual practices—such as prayer, meditation, or attending services—into daily life, the greater his or her sense of satisfaction with life. Individuals with religious affiliations are less likely to attempt suicide than others.[19]

## Spirituality and Physical Health

A growing body of scientific evidence indicates that faith and spirituality can enhance health—and perhaps even extend life. Individuals who pray and report greater spiritual well-being consistently describe themselves as enjoying greater psychological and overall well-being.[20]

Church attendance may account for an additional two to three years of life (by comparison, exercise may add three to five extra years), according to researchers' calculations. According to data on nearly 95,000 participants in the landmark Women's Health Initiative, attending a weekly church service, regardless of an individual's faith, lowers the risk of death by 20 percent, compared with those who don't attend at all. Attending less frequently also reduces the risk, but by a smaller percentage. How does

**spiritual intelligence** The capacity to sense, understand, and tap into ourselves, others, and the world around us.

insecure, unhappy, and unloved. Spiritual intelligence allows you to use the wisdom you have when you're in a state of inner peace. And you get there by changing the way you think, basically by listening less to what's in your head and more to what's in your heart."[24]

## Clarify Your Values

Your **values** are the criteria by which you evaluate things, people, events, and yourself; they represent what's most important to you. In a world of almost dizzying complexity, values can provide guidelines for making decisions that are right for you. If understood and applied, they help give life meaning and structure.

There can be a large discrepancy between what people say they value and what their actions indicate about their values. That's why it's important to clarify your own values, making sure you understand what you believe so that you can live in accordance with your beliefs.

When you confront a situation in which you must choose different paths or behaviors, follow these steps:

1. Carefully consider the consequences of each choice.

2. Choose freely from among all the options.

3. Publicly affirm your values by sharing them with others.

4. Act out your values.

Values clarification is not a once-in-a-lifetime task, but an ongoing process of sorting out what matters most to you. If you believe in protecting the environment, do you shut off lights, or walk rather than drive, in order to conserve energy? Do you vote for political candidates who support environmental protection? Do you recycle newspapers, bottles, and cans? Values are more than ideals we'd like to attain; they should be reflected in the way we live day by day.

## Enrich Your Spiritual Life

Do you attend religious services? Pray or meditate on a weekly basis? In a national survey, a majority of the members of the Class of 2011 answered yes: Eight in ten went to religious services frequently or occasionally, while a third prayed or meditated every week. These percentages are somewhat lower than in the past, but a growing number of students report frequent discussions of religion.

Whatever role religion plays in your life, you have the capacity for deep, meaningful spiritual experiences that can add great meaning to everyday existence. You don't need to enroll in theology classes or commit to a certain religious preference. The following simple steps can start you on an inner journey to a new level of understanding:

- **Sit quietly**. The process of cultivating spiritual intelligence begins in solitude and silence. "There is an inner wisdom," says Dr. Dean Ornish, the pioneering cardiologist who incorporates spiritual health into his mind-body therapies, "but it speaks very, very softly." To tune into its whisper, you have to turn down the volume in your busy, noisy, complicated life and force yourself to do nothing at all. This may sound easy; it's anything but.

- **Start small**. Create islands of silence in your day. Don't reach for the radio dial as soon as you get in the car. Leave your earbuds on as you walk across campus but turn off the music. Shut the door to your room, take a few huge deep breaths, and let them out very, very slowly. Don't worry if you're too busy to carve out half an hour for quiet contemplation. Even ten minutes every day can make a difference.

- **Step outside**. For many people, nature sets their spirit free. Being outdoors, walking by the ocean, or looking at the hills gives us a sense of timelessness and puts the little hassles of daily living into perspective. As you wait for the bus or for a traffic light to change, let your gaze linger on silvery ice glazing a branch or an azalea bush in wild bloom. Follow the flight of a bird; watch clouds float overhead. Gaze into the night sky and think of the stars as holes in the darkness letting the light of heaven shine through.

- **Use activity to tune into your spirit**. Spirituality exists in every cell of the body, not just in the brain. As a student, you devote much of your day to mental labor. To tap into your spirit, try a less cerebral activity, such as singing, chanting, dancing, or drumming. Alternative ways of quieting

**values** The criteria by which one makes choices about one's thoughts, actions, goals, and ideals.

your mind and tuning into your spirit include gardening, walking, arranging flowers, listening to music that touches your soul, or immersing yourself in a simple process like preparing a meal.

- **Ask questions of yourself**. Some people use their contemplative time to focus on a line of scripture or poetry. Others ask open-ended questions, such as What am I feeling? What are my choices? Where am I heading? Dr. Ornish ends his own daily meditations by asking, "What am I not paying attention to that's important?"

  In her meditations, one minister often paints a lush scene with a golden meadow, a shade tree, and a gentle brook and invites the divine spirit to enter. "Rarely do I get an immediate answer or solution, but later that day something may happen—often just a random conversation—and I suddenly find myself thinking about a problem from a perspective I never considered before."

- **Trust your spirit**. While most of us rely on gut feelings to alert us to danger, our inner spirit usually nudges us, not away from, but toward some action that will somehow lead to a greater good—even if we can't see it at the time. You may suddenly feel the urge to call or e-mail a friend you've lost touch with—only to discover that he just lost a loved one and needed the comfort of your caring. If you ignore such silent signals, you may look back and regret the consequences. Pay a little more attention the next time you feel an unexpected need to say or do something for someone.

- **Develop a spiritual practice**.

  - **If you are religious**: Deepen your spiritual commitment through prayer, more frequent church attendance, or joining a prayer group.

  - **If you are not religious**: Keep an open mind about the value of religion or spirituality. Consider visiting a church or synagogue. Read the writings of inspired people of deep faith, such as Rabbi Harold Kushner and Rev. Martin Luther King, Jr.

  - **If you are not ready to consider religion**: Try nonreligious meditation or relaxation training. Research has shown that focusing the mind on a single sound or image can slow heart rate, respiration, and brain waves; relax muscles; and lower stress-related hormones—responses similar to those induced by prayer.

## Consider the Power of Prayer

Prayer, a spiritual practice of millions, is the most commonly used form of complementary and alternative medicine. However, only in recent years has science launched rigorous investigations of the healing power of prayer.

Petitionary prayer—praying directly to a higher power—affects both the quality and quantity of life, says Dr. Harold Koenig, director of Duke University's Center for the Study of Religion/Spirituality and Health. "It boosts morale; lowers agitation, loneliness, and life dissatisfaction; and enhances ability to cope in men, women, the elderly, the young, the healthy, and the sick."[25]

People who pray regularly have significantly lower blood pressure and stronger immune systems than the less religious, says Dr. Koenig. They're also less prone to alcoholism and less likely to smoke heavily, and are hospitalized less often. Science cannot explain the physiological mechanisms for what happens in human beings when they pray, but in cultures around the world throughout recorded history when people or their loved ones are sick, they pray.

Some scientists speculate that prayer may foster a state of peace and calm that could lead to beneficial changes in the cardiovascular and immune systems. Sophisticated brain imaging techniques have shown that prayer and meditation cause changes in blood flow in particular regions of the brain that may lead to lower blood pressure, slower heart rate, decreased anxiety, and an enhanced sense of well-being. Membership in a faith community provides an identity as well as support, although individuals vary in their religious practices and observances.

In recent research, praying for others has not improved their symptoms or recovery. In a study of patients undergoing heart procedures, prayers (whether by Christian, Muslim, Jewish, or Buddhist groups) and other complementary bedside therapies, such as imaging and therapeutic touching, did not measurably improve their outcome.

## Be True to Yourself

- **Take the tombstone test: What would you like to have written on your tombstone?** In other words, how would you like to be remembered? Your honest answer should tell you, very succinctly, what you value most.

- **Describe yourself, as you are today, in a brief sentence.** Ask friends or family members for their descriptions of you. How would you have to change to become the person you want to be remembered as?

- **Try the adjective test: Choose three adjectives that you'd like to see associated with your reputation.** Then list what you've done or can do to earn such descriptions.

---

Will science ever be able to prove the power of prayer? No one is certain. "While I personally believe that God heals people in supernatural ways, I don't think science can shape a study to prove it," says Duke's Dr. Koenig. "But we now know enough, based on solid scientific research, to recommend prayer, much like exercise and diet, as one of the best and most cost-effective ways of protecting and enhancing health."

## Cultivate Gratitude

A grateful spirit brightens mood, boosts energy, and infuses daily living with a sense of glad abundance. Although giving thanks is an ancient virtue, only recently have researchers focused on the "trait" of gratitude—appreciation, not just for a special gift, but for everything that makes life a bit better.

Gratitude is what researchers call "the quintessential positive personality trait, being an indicator of a worldview orientated toward noticing and appreciating the positive in life." Grateful people feel more frequent and intense positive emotions, have more positive views of their social environment, use more productive coping strategies, sleep better, and appreciate their lives and possessions more.[26] College students who keep gratitude journals report higher levels of optimism,

feel better about their lives as a whole, are more likely to have made progress toward important personal goals, exercise more regularly, and report fewer negative health symptoms.[27]

Men and women differ in the ways they perceive, experience, and express gratitude. In general women view gratitude as less complex, uncertain, and conflicting and as more interesting and exciting than men do. In research with college students, women responded to a gift with more gratitude and less sense of burden and obligation than men.[28]

The reasons may be that women are more emotionally expressive and, with the exception of anger, experience emotions more intensely and frequently than men. In cross-cultural studies women's most important values were understanding and improving relationships, while men rated power and achievement as higher priorities. Because they express more gratitude, women are more likely to receive additional benefits, whether in the form of nurturing or material possessions, from their benefactors.[29]

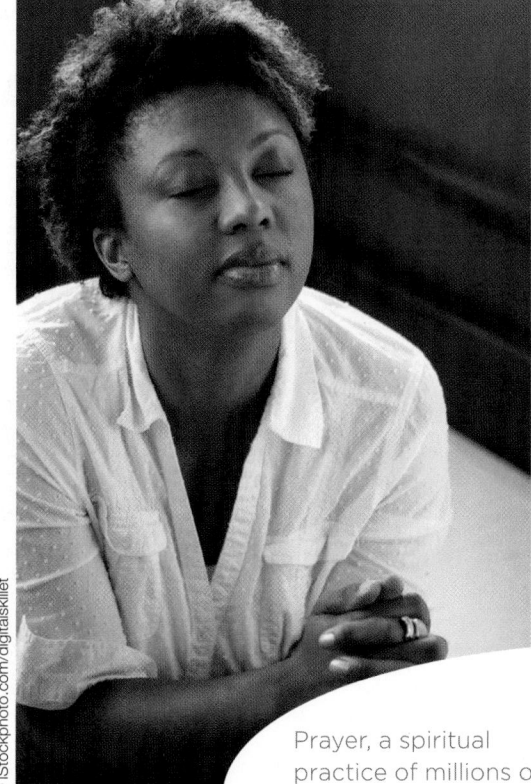

Prayer, a spiritual practice of millions of people, is the most widely used form of complementary and alternative medicine.

In the last two decades gratitude has emerged as one of the most significant dimensions of positive psychology. Traditionally gratitude has been defined as appreciation for the helpful actions of others. However, psychologists have broadened this definition to include "a habitual focusing on and appreciating the positive aspects of life."[30] The "lifestyle orientation" of feeling grateful has been shown to reduce levels of stress over time and may be especially effective in promoting good sleep (discussed later in this chapter).

Among the most effective "gratitude interventions"—proven techniques for increasing appreciation—is keeping a diary and recording three things you are grateful for every day. In clinical studies, this

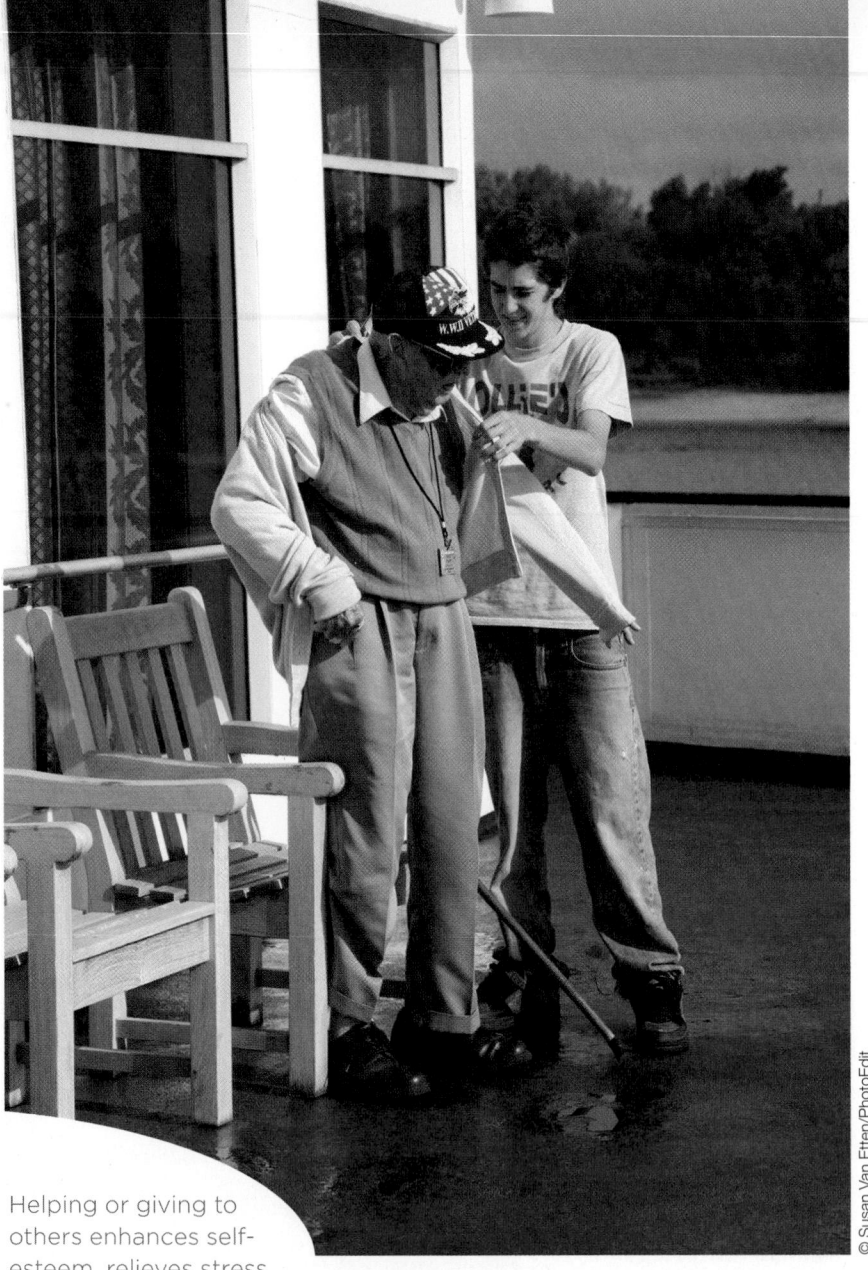

Helping or giving to others enhances self-esteem, relieves stress, and protects psychological well-being.

© Susan Van Etten/PhotoEdit

from the Greek for letting go, and that's what happens when you forgive: You let go of all the anger and pain that have been demanding your time and wasting your energy.

To some people, forgiveness seems a sign of weakness or submission. People may feel more in control, more powerful, when they're filled with anger, but forgiving instills a much greater sense of power. Forgiving a friend or family member may be more difficult than forgiving a stranger because the hurt occurs in a context in which people deliberately make themselves vulnerable.[33]

When you forgive, you reclaim your power to choose. It doesn't matter whether someone deserves to be forgiven; you deserve to be free. However, forgiveness isn't easy. It's not a one-time thing but a process that takes a lot of time and work involving both the conscious and unconscious mind.[34] Most people pass through

*Your Strategies for Change*

## How to Forgive

- **Compose an apology letter.** Address it to yourself, and write it from someone who's hurt you. This simple task enables you to get a new perspective on a painful experience.

- **Leap forward in time.** In a visualization exercise imagine that you are very old, meet a person who hurt you long ago, and sit down together on a park bench on a beautiful spring day. You both talk until everything that needs to be said finally is. This allows you to benefit from the perspective time brings without having to wait for years to achieve it.

- **Talk with "safe" people.** Vent your anger or disappointment with a trusted friend or a counselor without the danger of saying or doing anything you'll regret later. And if you can laugh about what happened with a friend, the laughter helps dissolve the rage.

- **Forgive the person, not the deed.** In themselves, abuse, rape, murder, and betrayal are beyond forgiveness. But you can forgive people who couldn't manage to handle their own suffering, misery, confusion, and desperation.

approach has proven as effective as the rigorously developed and tested techniques used in psychotherapy.[31] (See further discussion of this in Chapter 3.) In experiments with students, expressions and displays of gratitude not only increased the helpers' sense of self-worth by making them feel valued but also spurred them to do more to help others.[32]

## Forgive

While "I forgive you" may be three of the most difficult words to say, they are also three of the most powerful—and the most beneficial for the body as well as the soul. Being angry, harboring resentments, or reliving hurts over and over again is bad for your health in general and your heart in particular. The word *forgive* comes

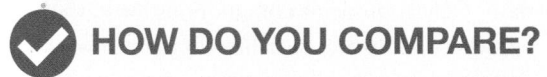
several stages in their journey to forgiveness. The initial response may involve anger, sadness, shame, or other negative feelings. Later, there's a reevaluation of what happened, then reframing to try to make sense of it or to take mitigating circumstances into account. This may lead to a reduction in negative feelings, especially if the initial hurt turns out to be accidental rather than intentional.

# Sleepless on Campus

You stay up late cramming for a final. You drive through the night to visit a friend at another campus. You get up for an early class during the week but stay in bed until noon on weekends. And you wonder: "Why am I so tired?" The answer: You're not getting enough sleep.

You're hardly alone. According to a recent report by the Centers for Disease Control and Prevention, only one-third of Americans say they get enough sleep. An estimated 50 to 70 million American adults suffer from sleep and wakefulness disorders. Women are more likely than men to report not getting enough sleep. African Americans reported getting less sleep compared with all other ethnic groups.[35]

In a national survey, 43 percent of respondents reported sleeping less than 7 hours a night during the week, with 20 percent of these sleeping less than 6 hours a night.[36]

Inadequate sleep has been linked to a host of problems, including mental distress, depression, anxiety, obesity, hypertension, diabetes, high cholesterol, and risky behaviors such as smoking, physical inactivity, and heavy drinking. Drowsy drivers are responsible for almost 20 percent of all serious car crash injuries.

## Sleepy Students

 College students, notorious for erratic sleep patterns, may be sleepier than ever. In the last decade the average sleep time of an undergraduate decreased from 7 hours 45 minutes to 7 hours. In a recent study, students reported sleeping an hour less than their ideal total sleep time; 43 percent slept less than five hours a night at least once a week.[37] Cadets at the U.S. Military Academy average less than 5.5 hours of sleep on all school nights.[38] (To see how you compare, see "How Do You Compare?: Student Night Life.")

The most common sleep problems on campus are sleep deprivation and excessive daytime sleepiness, which can stem from many causes. Like other adolescents, undergraduates still in their teens may have what scientists call "delayed sleep phase" and not feel sleepy in the late evening. An estimated 59 percent of young adults between ages 18 and 29 describe themselves as

## Sleep Problems

Sleep problems have become an epidemic on college campuses and throughout the country. Research is revealing new insights into sleep and sleep disorders. Access the "Sleep Disorders" portal of Global Health Watch (found under Health & Wellness then Mental Health & Wellness) and scan the latest news. Then go to your online journal and comment about what you learned. Do you think sleep problems impact your health?

"night owls" who stay up late and have difficulty getting up early in the morning.[39]

Students also may not get adequate sleep because of late-night studying or socializing, a noisy residence hall or apartment, or an underlying sleep disorder (discussed later in this chapter). Many try to make up for sleep loss during the week by sleeping more on weekends—an average of 2.6 hours in a recent survey.[40]

In a recent study of 1,845 undergraduates, 86 percent reported waking up tired at least some of the time, and 27 percent had some type of sleep disorder. The most common was insomnia, which affected 15 percent of undergraduates.[41] Too little sleep can affect every aspect of a student's life, including moods, physical well-being, performance in class and on tests, and grades. Students with sleep disorders are more likely to have lower GPAs and poorer academic performance, possibly because of daytime sleepiness, lower levels of attention, and impaired memory and decision making.

Some students turn to medications and other substances either to sleep at night or to feel more alert in the day. About 5 percent of students use prescription sleep aids an average of two nights a week. Two percent use over-the-counter sleep aids, while 11 percent of those who use alcohol have a drink to help fall asleep. To boost alertness, 60 percent of undergraduates use some form of stimulant, including caffeinated beverages.[42]

 Sleep problems start young. Nearly one-half of adolescents sleep less than eight hours on school nights; more than half report feeling sleepy during the day.[43] College students are notorious for staying up late to study and socialize during the week and sleeping in on weekends.

In a national survey, three-quarters of undergraduates reported occasional sleep problems while 12 percent experienced poor sleep quality. The most common complaints are general morning tiredness and insomnia (Table 2.1). Risk behaviors linked with poor sleep include fighting, suicidal thoughts, smoking, and alcohol use.[44]

On average college students go to bed 1 to 2 hours later and sleep 1 to 1.6 hours less than students of a generation ago. When compared to exhaustion levels reported by workers in various occupations, college students score extremely high.

Sleep affects academic performance. In a recent study of undergraduates, the students reporting the poorest sleep quality had lower grades than those who slept better.[45]

Fortunately, college students can learn to sleep better. In an experiment with introductory psychology students—mostly freshmen—those who learned basic sleep skills significantly improved their overall sleep quality compared with students who did not receive such training.

## Sleep's Impact on Health

Sleep is essential for functioning at your best—physically and psychologically. The following are some of the key ways in which your nighttime sleep affects your daytime well-being.

- **Learning and memory**. When you sleep, your brain helps "consolidate" new information so you are more likely to retain it in your memory.

- **Metabolism and weight.** The less you sleep, the more weight you may gain. Chronic sleep deprivation may cause weight gain by altering metabolism (for example, changing the way individuals process and store carbohydrates) and by stimulating excess stress hormones. Loss of sleep also reduces levels of the hormones that regulate appetite (discussed in Chapter 6), which may encourage eating.

- **Safety**. People who don't get adequate nighttime sleep are more likely to fall asleep

Table 2.1 **Sleepy Students**

| | |
|---|---|
| • Took more than 30 minutes to fall asleep | 18% |
| • Had insomnia in the last three months | 28% |
| • Have difficulty falling asleep three or more days a week | 11% |
| • Have disturbed sleep three or more days a week | 11% |
| • Have nocturnal wakings three or more times a week | 13% |
| • Awakened too early three or more days a week | 11% |
| • Have general morning tiredness | 82% |
| • Used sleep medication at least once a week in past three weeks | 2% |

Source of data: Vail-Smith, Karen, et al. "Relationship between Sleep Quality and Health Risk Behaviors in Undergraduate College Students." *College Student Journal*, Vol. 43, No. 3, 2009.

## How to Sleep Better

- **Keep regular hours** for going to bed and getting up in the morning. Stay as close as possible to this schedule on weekends as well as weekdays.

- **Develop a sleep ritual**—such as stretching, meditation, yoga, prayer, or reading a not-too-thrilling novel—to ease the transition from wakefulness to sleep.

- **Don't drink coffee late in the day.** The effects of caffeine can linger for up to eight hours. And don't smoke. Nicotine is an even more powerful stimulant—and sleep saboteur—than caffeine.

- **Don't rely on alcohol to get to sleep.** Alcohol disrupts normal sleep stages, so you won't sleep as deeply or as restfully as you normally would.

- **Although experts generally advise against daytime napping for people who have problems sleeping at night,** a recent study of college students found that a 30-minute "power nap" lowers stress and refreshes energy with no disruption in nighttime sleep. (See "Sleep Power" in Labs for IPC.)

during the daytime. Daytime sleepiness can cause falls, medical errors, air traffic mishaps, and road accidents.

- **Mood/quality of life.** Too little sleep—whether just for a night or two or for longer periods—can cause psychological symptoms, such as irritability, impatience, inability to concentrate, moodiness, and lowered long-term life satisfaction.[46] Poor sleep also affects motivation and ability to work effectively. Growing evidence suggests that disturbed sleep is associated with increased risk of psychiatric disorders.

- **Life satisfaction.** Sleep-deprived university students score lower on life-satisfaction scales. Students who get eight hours of sleep but shift their sleep schedules by as little as two hours suffer more depressive symptoms, lower sociability, and more frequent attention and concentration problems. They even get lower grades.

- **Cardiovascular health.** In a five-year study of middle-aged men and women, an extra hour of shut-eye was linked with healthier arteries and less build-up of calcium. Serious sleep disorders such as insomnia and sleep apnea have been linked to hypertension, increased stress hormone levels, irregular heartbeats, and increased inflammation (which, as discussed in Chapter 9, may play a role in heart attacks).

- **Immunity/cancer prevention.** If you get less than seven hours of sleep a night, you're three times more likely to catch a cold. And if you sleep poorly, you're five times more susceptible.[47] Sleep deprivation alters immune function, including the activity of the body's killer cells. For example, inadequate sleep at the time of a flu vaccination can reduce the production of flu-fighting antibodies. Keeping up with sleep may also help fight cancer. Harvard researchers have shown that women who work at night are at increased risk for breast and colon cancer, possibly because light at night alters production of melatonin, a hormone that helps put us to sleep.[48]

## What Happens When We Sleep?

A normal night of sleep consists of several distinct stages of sleep, divided into two major types: an active state, characterized by **rapid eye movement (REM)** and called **REM sleep** (or dream sleep), and a quiet state, referred to as non-REM or NREM sleep, that consists of four stages:

- In **Stage 1**, a twilight zone between full wakefulness and sleep, the brain produces small, irregular, rapid electrical waves. The muscles of the body relax, and breathing is smooth and even.

- In **Stage 2,** brain waves are larger and punctuated with occasional sudden bursts of electrical activity. The eyes are no longer responsive to light. Bodily functions slow still more.

- **Stages 3 and 4** constitute the most profound state of unconsciousness. The brain produces slower, larger waves, and this is sometimes referred to as "delta" or slow-wave sleep (Figure 2.2).

**rapid eye movement (REM) sleep** Regularly occurring periods of sleep during which the most active dreaming takes place.

## Figure 2.2 **Stages of Sleep**
Differences in brain wave patterns characterize the various stages of sleep.

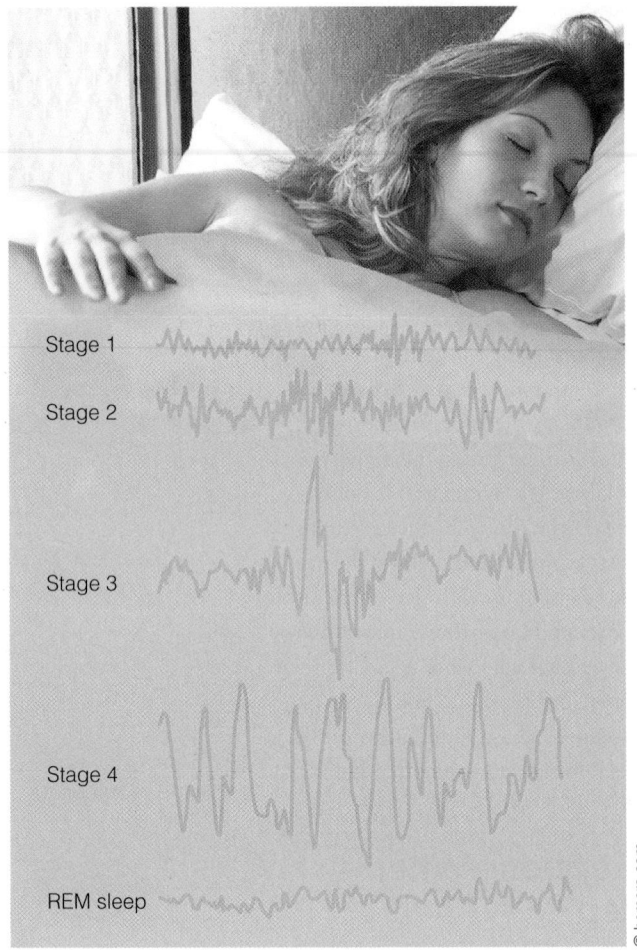

Stage 1

Stage 2

Stage 3

Stage 4

REM sleep

© hemera.com

After about an hour in the four stages of non-REM sleep, sleepers enter the time of vivid dreaming called **REM** sleep, when brain waves resemble those of waking more than those of quiet sleep. The large muscles of the torso, arms, and legs are paralyzed and cannot move—possibly to prevent sleepers from acting out their dreams. The fingers and toes may twitch; breathing is quick and shallow; blood flow through the brain speeds up; men may have partial or full erections.

## Sleep Disorders

Three of four Americans struggle to get a good night's sleep at least a few nights a week. According to the National Commission on Sleep Disorders Research, 40 million adults suffer from a specific sleep disorder, such as chronic insomnia or sleep apnea; an additional 20 to 30 million have occasional sleep difficulties. The estimated economic cost of sleeplessness may be higher than $300 million a year.

*Insomnia* Individuals with insomnia—a lack of sleep so severe that it interferes with functioning during the day—may toss and turn for an hour or more when they get into bed, wake frequently in the night, wake up too early, or not be able to sleep long enough to feel alert and energetic the next day. Most often insomnia is transient, typically occurring before or after a major life event (such as a job interview) and lasting for three or four nights. During periods of prolonged stress (such as a marriage breakup), short-term insomnia may continue for several weeks. Chronic or long-term insomnia, which can begin at any age, may persist for long periods. About three-fourths of insomniacs struggle to sleep more for at least a year; almost half, for three years.[49]

For about a third of those with chronic insomnia, the underlying problem is a mental disorder, most often depression or an anxiety disorder. Many substances, including alcohol, medications, and drugs of abuse, often disrupt sleep. About 15 percent of those seeking help for chronic insomnia suffer from "learned" or "behavioral" insomnia. While a life crisis may trigger their initial sleep problems, each night they try harder and harder to get to sleep, but they cannot—although they often doze off while reading or watching a movie.

Sleeping pills may be used for a specific, time-limited problem—always with a physician's supervision. (See Consumer Alert, p. 50.) In the long term, behavioral approaches, including the following, have proved more effective:

- **Relaxation therapy,** which may involve progressive muscle relaxation, diaphragmatic breathing, hypnosis, or meditation.

- **Cognitive therapy,** which challenges misconceptions about sleep and helps shift a poor sleeper's mind away from anxiety-inducing thoughts.

- **Stimulus control therapy,** in which individuals who do not fall asleep quickly must get up and leave their beds until they are very sleepy.

- **Sleep restriction therapy,** in which sleep times are sharply curtailed in order to improve the quality of sleep.

***Breathing Disorders (Snoring and Sleep Apnea)*** Although most people snore in certain positions or when they have stuffed-up noses, snoring can be a sign of a serious problem and increases the likelihood of health problems and of accidents.[50] Caused by the vibration in tissues in the mouth and throat as a sleeper tries to suck air into the lungs, snoring can be so loud that it disrupts a bed partner or others in the same house. In young people, the cause is most likely to be enlarged tonsils or adenoids. In adults, extreme snoring may be a symptom of sleep apnea, which may itself be harmful to health.

Translated from the Greek words meaning "no" and "breath," apnea is exactly that: the absence of breathing for a brief period. People with sleep apnea may briefly stop breathing dozens or even hundreds of times during the night. As they struggle for breath, they may gasp for air, snore extremely loudly, or thrash about.

Although apnea, which can lead to high blood pressure, stroke, and cardiovascular disease, may affect as many as 10 million Americans, most are unaware of the problem. More physical activity and fewer hours sitting can lead to improvements.[51] Effective treatments include weight loss (if obesity is contributing to the problem), a nasal mask that provides continuous positive airway pressure (CPAP) to ensure a steady flow of air into the lungs, and, in severe cases, surgery to enlarge the upper airway.

***Movement Disorders*** Restless legs syndrome, which may affect 12 million Americans, is a movement disorder characterized by symptoms that patients describe as pulling, burning, tingling, creepy-crawly, grabbing, buzzing, jitteriness, or gnawing. Many people with these symptoms have difficulty falling or staying asleep but do not realize that the cause is a medical disorder that can be treated with regular physical activity. Medications also are available.

***Circadian Rhythm Sleep Disorders*** Problems involving the timing of sleep are called circadian rhythm disorders because they affect the basic circadian ("about a day") rhythm that influences many biological processes. The most common causes are jet lag and shift work. Jet lag generally improves on its own within two to seven days, depending on the length of the trip and the individual's response. Avoiding caffeine and alcohol and immediately switching to the new time zone's schedule can help in overcoming jet lag.

A "shift work" circadian rhythm disorder consists of any inability to sleep when one wants or to stay alert when needed because of frequently changing work shifts. Behavioral strategies and good sleep habits can help. In addition, phototherapy—exposure to bright light for periods ranging from 30 minutes to two hours—has shown promise as an experimental treatment to help shift workers adjust to their changing schedules.

## How Much Sleep Do You Need?

Over the last century, we have cut our average nightly sleep time by 20 percent. More than half of us try to get by with less than seven hours of shut-eye a night. College students are no exception, with an average sleep time slightly less than seven hours, with little difference between men and women.

No formula can say how long a good night's sleep should be. Normal sleep times range from five to ten hours; the average is seven and a half. About one or two people in a hundred can get by with just five hours; another small minority needs twice that amount. Each of us seems to have an innate sleep *appetite* that is as much a part of our genetic programming as hair color and skin tone.

To figure out your sleep needs, keep your wake-up time the same every morning and vary your bedtime. Are you groggy after six hours of shut-eye? Does an extra hour give you more stamina? What about an extra two hours? Since too much sleep can make you feel sluggish, don't assume that more is always better. Listen to your body's signals, and adjust your sleep schedule to suit them.

Are you better off pulling an all-nighter before a big test or closing the books and getting a good night's sleep? According to researchers, that depends on the nature of the exam. If it's a test of facts—Civil War battles, for instance—cramming all night works. However, if you will have to write analytical essays in which you compare, contrast, and make connections, you need to sleep to make the most of your reasoning abilities.

## Sleeping Pill Precautions

Chances are you've taken some form of sleep medication. After aspirin, they are the most widely used drugs in the United States. If sleeping pills seem the best option at a certain time in your life, use them with caution.

### Facts to Know

- **Sleeping pills** are not a long-term solution to a sleep problem, but they can be helpful if travel, injury, or illness interfere with your nightly rest.
- **Prescription and over-the-counter sleep aids** can interact with other medications or a medical condition, so always check with your doctor before taking them.
- **If taken too often** or for more than several nights, some sleeping pills may cause rebound insomnia—sleeplessness that returns in full force when you stop taking the medication.

### Steps to Take

- **Read carefully.** Take time to read through the informational materials and warnings on pill containers. Make sure you understand the potential risks and the behaviors to avoid.
- **Avoid alcohol.** Never mix alcohol and sleeping pills. Alcohol increases the sedative effects of the pills. Even a small amount of alcohol combined with sleeping pills can make you feel dizzy, confused, or faint.
- **Quit carefully.** When you're ready to stop taking sleeping pills, follow your doctor's instructions or the directions on the label. Some medications must be stopped gradually.
- **Watch for side effects.** If you feel sleepy or dizzy during the day, talk to your doctor about changing the dosage or discontinuing the pills.

## Sleeping Pills

The use of prescription sleeping pills has more than doubled since 2000, and increasing numbers of teenagers and young adults use these medications either occasionally or regularly. (See Consumer Alert.) An even greater number buy nonprescription or over-the-counter (OTC) sleep inducers. Others rely on herbal remedies, antihistamines, and other medications to get to sleep.

In the long run, good sleep habits, regular exercise, and a tranquil sleep environment are the cornerstones of high-quality sleep. But if circumstances, travel, injury, or illness have disrupted your sleep, you may consider sleep medications. Here is what you need to know about them.

- **Over-the-counter medications**. Various over-the-counter sleeping pills, sold in any pharmacy or supermarket, contain antihistamines, which induce drowsiness by working against the central nervous system chemical histamine. They may help for an occasional sleepless night, but the more often you take them, the less effective they become.

- **Dietary supplements**. The most widely publicized dietary supplement is the hormone melatonin, which may help control your body's internal clock. The melatonin supplements most often found in health food stores and pharmacies are synthetic versions of the natural hormone. Although these supplements may help some people fall asleep or stay asleep and may sometimes help prevent jet lag, there are many unanswered questions about melatonin. Reported side effects include drowsiness, headaches, stomach discomfort, confusion, decreased body temperature, seizures, and drug interactions. The optimal dose isn't certain, and the long-term effects are unknown. Other supplements—such as valerian, chamomile, and kava—have yet to be fully studied for safety or effectiveness in relieving insomnia.

- **Prescription medications**. The newest sleep drugs—nonbenzodiazepine hypnotic medications such as Lunesta (eszopiclone), Ambien/Ambien CR (zolpidem), and Sonata (zaleplon)—quiet the nervous system, which helps induce sleep. They're metabolized quickly, which helps reduce the risk of side effects the next day. These medications are mainly intended for short-term or intermittent use.

- **Benzodiazepines**, such as Halcion (triazolam) and Restoril (temazepam), belong to an older class of sleeping pills that are more likely to cause drowsiness or headaches the next morning. They also may become habit forming.

The FDA has required stronger language about the potential risks of both nonbenzodiazepine and benzodiazepine sleeping pills. These include severe allergic reactions and complex sleep-related behaviors, including sleep-driving (driving while not fully awake after taking a sleeping pill with no memory of the driving).

## Keys to a Fulfilling Life

*Build Your Future*

Just like physical health, psychological well-being involves more than an absence of problems. By developing your inner strengths and resources, you become the author of your life, capable of confronting challenges and learning from them. As positive psychologists have discovered, you have greater control over how happy, optimistic, upbeat, and lovable you are than anyone or anything else. But only by consciously taking charge of your life can you find happiness and fulfillment. (See "Your Perfect Balance Point" in *IPC*.)

Here are some suggestions to enhance your emotional health now and in the future. Check the ones that you already practice and then work on adding others.

_____ **Recognize and express your feelings.** Pent-up emotions tend to fester inside, building into anger or depression.

_____ **Don't brood.** Rather than merely mulling over a problem, try to find solutions that are positive and useful.

_____ **Take one step at a time.** As long as you're taking some action to solve a problem, you can take pride in your ability to cope.

_____ **Spend more time doing those activities you know you do best.** For example, if you are a good cook, prepare a meal for someone.

_____ **Separate what you do, especially any mistakes you make, from who you are.** Instead of saying, "I'm so stupid," tell yourself, "That wasn't the smartest move I ever made, but I'll learn from it."

_____ **Use affirmations,** positive statements that help reinforce the most positive aspects of your personality and experience. Every day, you might say, "I am a loving, caring person," or "I am honest and open in expressing my feelings." Write some affirmations of your own on index cards and flip through them occasionally.

_____ **List the things you would like to have or experience.** Construct the statements as if you were already enjoying the situations you list, beginning each sentence with "I am." For example, "I am feeling great about doing well in my classes."

## Well-Being Scale

*Self Survey*

### Part I

The following questions contain statements and their opposites. Notice that the statements extend from one extreme to the other. Where would you place yourself on this scale? Place a circle on the number that is most true for you at this time. Do not put your circles between numbers.

**Life Purpose and Satisfaction**

1. During most of the day, my energy level is — very low 1 2 3 4 5 6 7 very high
2. As a whole, my life seems — dull 1 2 3 4 5 6 7 vibrant
3. My daily activities are — not a source of satisfaction 1 2 3 4 5 6 7 a source of satisfaction
4. I have come to expect that every day will be — exactly the same 1 2 3 4 5 6 7 new and different
5. When I think deeply about life — I do not feel there is any purpose to it 1 2 3 4 5 6 7 I feel there is a purpose to it
6. I feel that my life so far has — not been productive 1 2 3 4 5 6 7 been productive
7. I feel that the work* I am doing — is of no value 1 2 3 4 5 6 7 is of great value
8. I wish I were different than who I am. — agree strongly 1 2 3 4 5 6 7 disagree strongly

*The definition of work is not limited to income-producing jobs. It includes childcare, housework, studies, and volunteer services

| | | | |
|---|---|---|---|
| 9. At this time, I have | no clearly defined goals for my life | 1 2 3 4 5 6 7 | clearly defined goals for my life |
| 10. When sad things happen to me or other people | I cannot feel positive about life | 1 2 3 4 5 6 7 | I continue to feel positive about life |
| 11. When I think about what I have done with my life, I feel | worthless | 1 2 3 4 5 6 7 | worthwhile |
| 12. My present life | does not satisfy me | 1 2 3 4 5 6 7 | satisfies me |
| 13. I feel joy in my heart | never | 1 2 3 4 5 6 7 | all the time |
| 14. I feel trapped by the circumstances of my life. | agree strongly | 1 2 3 4 5 6 7 | disagree strongly |
| 15. When I think about my past | I feel many regrets | 1 2 3 4 5 6 7 | I feel no regrets |
| 16. Deep inside myself | I do not feel loved | 1 2 3 4 5 6 7 | I feel loved |
| 17. When I think about the problems that I have | I do not feel hopeful about solving them | 1 2 3 4 5 6 7 | I feel very hopeful about solving them |

*Part II*

**Self-Confidence during Stress** (Answer according to how you feel during stressful times.)

| | | | |
|---|---|---|---|
| 1. When there is a great deal of pressure being placed on me | I get tense | 1 2 3 4 5 6 7 | I remain calm |
| 2. I react to problems and difficulties | with a great deal of frustration | 1 2 3 4 5 6 7 | with no frustration |
| 3. In a difficult situation, I am confident that I will receive the help that I need. | disagree strongly | 1 2 3 4 5 6 7 | agree strongly |
| 4. I experience anxiety | all the time | 1 2 3 4 5 6 7 | never |
| 5. When I have made a mistake | I feel extreme dislike for myself | 1 2 3 4 5 6 7 | I continue to like myself |
| 6. I find myself worrying that something bad is going to happen to me or those I love | all the time | 1 2 3 4 5 6 7 | never |
| 7. In a stressful situation | I cannot concentrate easily | 1 2 3 4 5 6 7 | I can concentrate easily |
| 8. I am fearful | all the time | 1 2 3 4 5 6 7 | never |
| 9. When I need to stand up for myself | I cannot do it | 1 2 3 4 5 6 7 | I can do it easily |
| 10. I feel less than adequate in most situations. | agree strongly | 1 2 3 4 5 6 7 | disagree strongly |
| 11. During times of stress, I feel isolated and alone. | agree strongly | 1 2 3 4 5 6 7 | disagree strongly |
| 12. In really difficult situations | I feel unable to respond in positive ways | 1 2 3 4 5 6 7 | I feel able to respond in positive ways |
| 13. When I need to relax | I experience no peace—only thoughts and worries | 1 2 3 4 5 6 7 | I experience a peacefulness—free of thoughts and worries |
| 14. When I am frightened | I panic | 1 2 3 4 5 6 7 | I remain calm |
| 15. I worry about the future | all the time | 1 2 3 4 5 6 7 | never |

*Scoring*

The number you circled is your score for that question. Add your scores in each of the two sections and divide each sum by the number of questions in the section.

- Life Purpose and Satisfaction: _____ x 17 = _____.____
- Self-Confidence during Stress: _____ x 15 = _____.____
- Combined Well-Being:
  (add scores for both) _____ x 32 = _____.____

Each score should range between 1.00 and 7.00 and may include decimals (for example, 5.15).

**Interpretation**

VERY LOW: 1.00 TO 2.49

MEDIUM LOW: 2.50 TO 3.99

MEDIUM HIGH: 4.00 TO 5.49

VERY HIGH: 5.50 TO 7.00

These scores reflect the strength with which you feel these positive emotions. Do they make sense to you? Review each scale and each question in each scale. Your score on each item gives you information about the emotions and areas in your life where your psychological resources are strong, as well as the areas where strength needs to be developed.

If you notice a large difference between the LPS and SCDS scores, use this information to recognize which central attitudes and aspects of your life most need strengthening. If your scores on both scales are very low, talk with a counselor or a friend about how you are feeling about yourself and your life.

# *Making Change Happen*

## Soul Food

There is more to you than intellect and passion, more than what resides between your ears or below your waist. Sometimes overshadowed by the speed and loud talk that surround you is the quieter, feeling part of you. Although immaterial, it is no less real. Tied to your spiritual self, it can be seen as your essence—what is always there and what is most essentially you.

If you feel you have been running too hard, need more down time, are close to burnout, or are in some way seeking to make better contact with your deeper self, "Soul Food" in *Labs for IPC* will help you provide the nourishment that your spirit needs. Here is a preview:

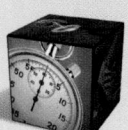

### Get Real
To provide sound nutrition for the soul, you need to know what makes up such a diet. Here is the first step:

**Assess your soul food diet.**

For each of thirteen items, you will put a + (if you meet this daily requirement) or a − (if you don't) in the space provided. Here are three examples:

- **Movement:** _____
  You consciously and intentionally pay disciplined attention to the movement of your body, be it in some slow, mindful exercise like yoga or tai chi, or in dance, or in stretching or walking.

- **Being:** _____
  You set aside a time when you are not multitasking—or tasking at all. It is one thing to *do,* and there is much to do. It is another thing to focus on *being.* Being there, being you—not working, worrying, or calculating. In this sitting-on-the-stoop or front-porch mode, you attune yourself to being alive in the moment.

- **Creating:** _____
  You daily take time to express your creative nature through painting, drawing, writing, composing music, choreographing dance, solving a problem, cooking—the possibilities are inexhaustible.

If you did not mark a plus by many activities listed in the lab, your soul food diet is insufficient. Progressing through the stages of change by completing the lab will help you correct this. We guarantee you are going to love the results.

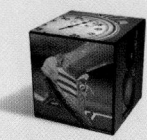

### Get Ready
We know that as a college student you are busy. You may need to cut or trim activities or reclaim time that currently goes to activities that do not feed your deeper, quieter self. Start with this step:

- **Examine your schedule.** When are you going to fit in, on a daily basis, time for soul food? Will your schedule require fine-tuning?

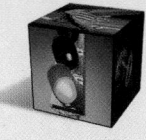

### Get Going
In this stage your task is to provide yourself with soul food by completing each of thirteen activities a minimum of four times per week. Here are three examples of the minimum dietary requirements for feeding your soul:

- Movement: 5 minutes

- Being: 10 minutes

- Creating: 10 minutes

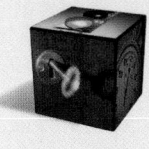

### Lock It In
It will take time and practice to lock in the habit of feeding your soul on a regular basis. This is why we offer the following advice:

- Regardless of how often you have or have not done the activities in this lab, most of them are likely to seem completely natural. But some may present a challenge. Do not be concerned about whether you are moving, being, creating, or doing any of the other activities correctly. Just relax . . .

# Making This Chapter Work for You

## Review Questions

1. Lack of sleep
   a. improves memory and concentration.
   b. may cause irritability.
   c. may cause weight loss.
   d. enhances the immune system.

2. Which statement about sleep is correct?
   a. People cannot learn to sleep better.
   b. People dream during REM sleep.
   c. Drinking alcohol helps most people sleep better.
   d. Snoring may be a symptom of insomnia.

3. Normal shyness can usually be overcome by
   a. medication.
   b. psychotherapy.
   c. retail therapy.
   d. working at improving social skills.

4. Psychological health is influenced by all of the following *except*
   a. emotional health.
   b. physical agility.
   c. culture.
   d. a firm grasp on reality.

5. Which of the following activities can contribute to fulfillment?
   a. being a Big Sister or Big Brother to a child from a single-parent home
   b. being accepted by your first choice sorority or fraternity
   c. being a regular participant in an Internet chat room
   d. negotiating the price on a new car

6. Enduring happiness is most likely to come from
   a. winning a sweepstakes.
   b. work you love.
   c. a trip to the place of your dreams.
   d. having more money than your friends and neighbors.

7. Which activity is probably enriching the student's spiritual life?
   a. Claire goes dancing with her friends.
   b. James takes a 15-minute walk along the river trail with a group of friends every day.
   c. Kate keeps a gratitude journal.
   d. Charlie goes to a taize music group with friends.

8. Which of these statements about self-esteem is *true*?
   a. Self-esteem is determined by genetics.
   b. Parents have little influence on a child's self-esteem.
   c. A person's sense of self-esteem can change over time.
   d. Self-esteem is seldom boosted by achievement.

9. People who pray regularly
   a. are less likely to get cancer.
   b. never get sick.
   c. recover from heart attacks more quickly.
   d. get better grades.

10. Individuals who have developed a sense of mastery over their lives are
    a. aware that their locus of control is internal, not external.
    b. skilled at controlling the actions of others.
    c. usually passive and silent when faced with a situation they don't like.
    d. aware that their locus of control is external, not internal.

*Answers to these questions can be found on page 672.*

## Critical Thinking

1. Would you say that you view life positively or negatively? Would your friends and family agree with your assessment? Ask two of your closest friends for feedback about what they perceive are your typical responses to a problematic situation. Are these indicative of positive attitudes? If not, what could you do to become more psychologically positive?

2. Were you raised in a religious family? If yes, have you continued the same religious practices from your childhood? Why or why not? If no, have you been to places of worship to explore religious practices? Why or why not?

3. What is your personal experience with lack of sleep? Have you suffered effects described in the text? Has cramming all night ever worked for you? Why or why not?

## Media Menu

Visit www.cengagebrain.com to access course materials and companion resources for this text that will:

- Help you evaluate your knowledge of the material.

- Allow you to prepare for exams with interactive quizzing.

- Use the CengageNOW product to develop a Personalized Learning Plan targeting resources that address areas you should study.

- Coach you through identifying target goals for behavioral change and creating and monitoring your personal change plan throughout the semester using the Behavior Change Planner available in the CengageNOW resource.

## Internet Connections

**www.ppc.sas.upenn.edu**
This positive psychology website at the University of Pennsylvania has questionnaires on authentic happiness and gratitude.

**www.apa.org**
The APA is the scientific and professional organization for psychology in the United States. Its website provides up-to-date information on psychological issues.

**www.spiritualityhealth.com**
Developed by the Publishing Group of Trinity Church, Wall Street in New York City, this website offers self-tests,

guidance on spiritual practices, resources for people on spiritual journeys, and subscriptions to a bimonthly print magazine.

**www.newvision-psychic.com/bookshelf/womenspirit.html**
A comprehensive list of books dealing with women and spirituality.

**www.beliefnet.com**
An eclectic, informative guide to different forms of religion and spirituality.

## Key Terms

The terms listed are used on the page indicated. Definitions of the terms are in the Glossary at the end of the book.

autonomy  39

culture  32

emotional health  32

emotional intelligence  33

locus of control  39

mental health  32

mood  38

optimism  38

rapid eye movement (REM) sleep  47

self-actualization  34

self-compassion  33

self-esteem  35

spiritual health  39

spiritual intelligence  40

spirituality  39

values  41

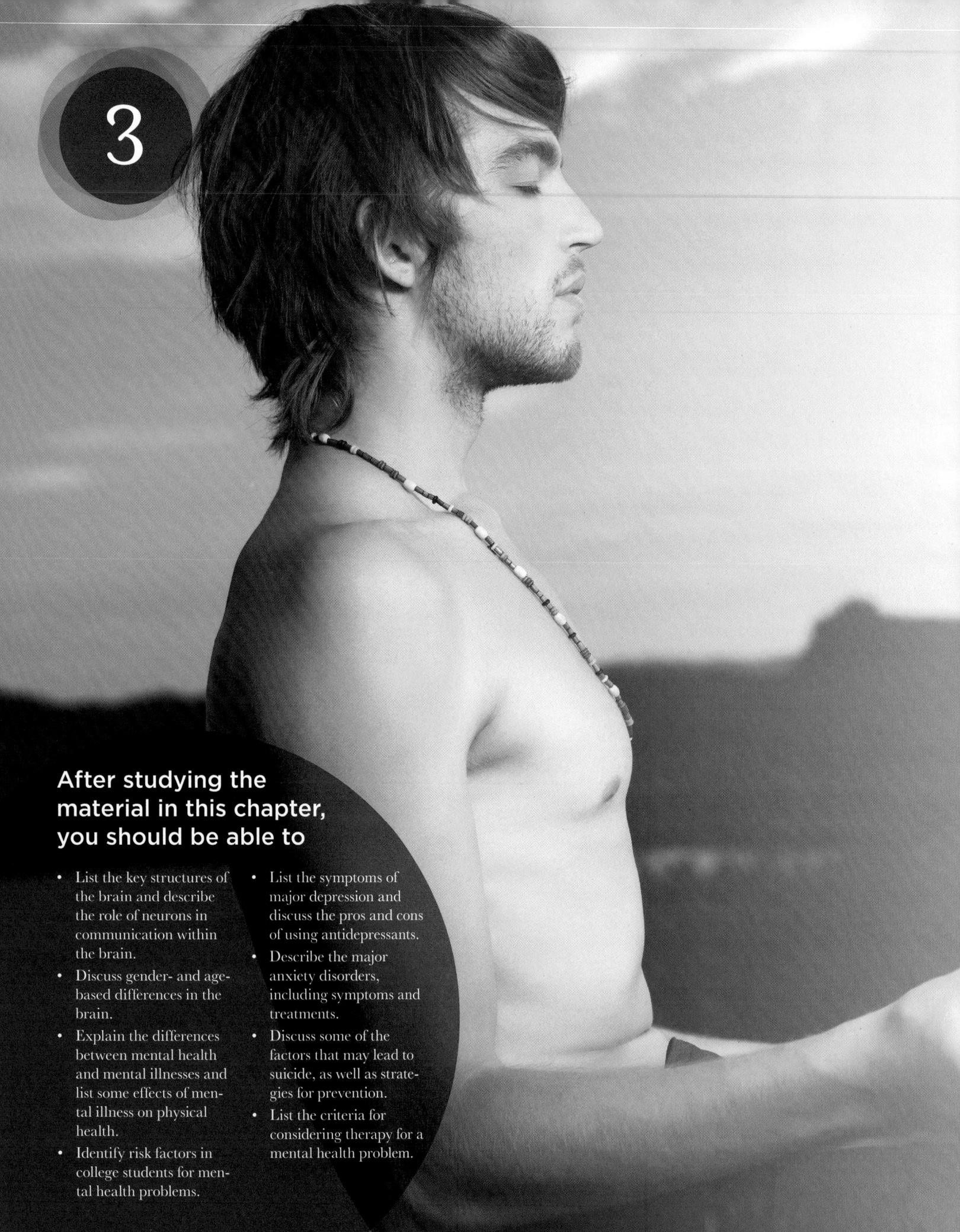

# 3

## After studying the material in this chapter, you should be able to

- List the key structures of the brain and describe the role of neurons in communication within the brain.
- Discuss gender- and age-based differences in the brain.
- Explain the differences between mental health and mental illnesses and list some effects of mental illness on physical health.
- Identify risk factors in college students for mental health problems.
- List the symptoms of major depression and discuss the pros and cons of using antidepressants.
- Describe the major anxiety disorders, including symptoms and treatments.
- Discuss some of the factors that may lead to suicide, as well as strategies for prevention.
- List the criteria for considering therapy for a mental health problem.

For years, Travis put on his "happy face" around his friends and family. Popular and athletic in high school, he never let anyone know how desperately unhappy he actually felt. "Whatever I was doing during the day, nothing was on my mind more than wanting to die," he recalls. On a perfectly ordinary day in his senior year, Travis tried to kill himself with an overdose of pills. Rushed to a hospital, Travis recovered, resumed his studies, and

# Caring for Your Mind

entered college. By the middle of his freshman year, he was struggling once more with feelings of hopelessness. This time he realized what was happening and sought help from a therapist. "I thought college was supposed to be the happiest time of your life," he said. "What went wrong?"

This is a question many young people might ask. Although youth can seem a golden time, when body and mind glow with potential, the process of becoming an adult is a challenging one in every culture and country. Psychological health can make the difference between facing this challenge with optimism and confidence or feeling overwhelmed by expectations and responsibilities.

This isn't always easy. At some point in life almost half of Americans develop an emotional disorder. Young adulthood—the years from the late teens to the midtwenties—is a time when many serious disorders, including bipolar illness (manic depression) and schizophrenia, often develop. The saddest fact is not that so many feel so bad, but that so few realize they can feel better. Only a third of those with a mental disorder receive any treatment at all. Yet 80 to 90 percent of those treated for psychological problems recover, most within a few months.

By learning about psychological disorders covered in this chapter, you may be able to recognize early warning signals in yourself or your loved ones so you can deal with potential difficulties or seek professional help for more serious problems.

## The Brain: The Last Frontier

The brain has intrigued scientists for centuries, but only recently have its explorers made dramatic progress in unraveling its mysteries. Leaders in **neuropsychiatry**—the field that brings together the study of the brain and the mind—remind us that 95 percent of what is known about brain anatomy, chemistry, and physiology has been learned in the last 25 years. These discoveries have reshaped our understanding of the organ that is central to our identity and

**neuropsychiatry** The study of the brain and mind.

Visit www.cengagebrain.com to access course materials for this text, including the Behavior Change Planner, interactive quizzes, tutorials, and more. See the preface on page xv for details.

© Kiselev Andrey Valerevich/Shutterstock.com

well-being and have fostered great hope for more effective therapies for the more than 1,000 disorders—psychiatric and neurologic—that affect the brain and nervous system.

## Inside the Brain

The human brain, the most complex organ in the body, controls the central nervous system (CNS) and regulates virtually all our activities, including involuntary, or "lower," actions like heart rate, respiration, and digestion, and conscious, or "higher," mental activity like thought, reason, and abstraction. More than one hundred billion **neurons**, or nerve cells, within the brain are capable of electrical and chemical communication with tens of thousands of other nerve cells. (The basic anatomy of the brain is shown in Figure 3.1.)

The neurons are the basic working units of the brain. Like snowflakes, no two are exactly the same. Each consists of a cell body containing the **nucleus**; a long fiber called the **axon**, which can range from less than an inch to several feet in length; an **axon terminal**, or ending; and multiple branching fibers called **dendrites** (Figure 3.2). The **glia** serve as the scaffolding for the brain, separate the brain from the bloodstream, assist in the growth of neurons, speed up the transmission of nerve impulses, and engulf and digest damaged neurons.

Until quite recently scientists believed no new neurons or synapses formed in the brain after birth. This theory has been soundly disproved. The brain and spinal cord contain stem cells, which turn into thousands of new neurons a day. The process of creating new brain cells and synapses occurs most rapidly in childhood but continues throughout life, even into old age. Whenever you learn and change, you establish new neural networks.

Anatomically, the brain consists of three parts: the forebrain, midbrain, and hindbrain. The forebrain includes the several lobes of the cere-

**neuron** A nerve cell; the basic working unit of the brain, which transmits information from the senses to the brain and from the brain to specific body parts; each neuron consists of a cell body, an axon terminal, and dendrites.

**nucleus** The central part of a cell, contained in the cell body of a neuron.

**axon** The long fiber that conducts impulses from the neuron's nucleus to its dendrites.

**axon terminal** The ending of an axon, from which impulses are transmitted to a dendrite of another neuron.

**dendrites** Branching fibers of a neuron that receive impulses from axon terminals of other neurons and conduct these impulses toward the nucleus.

**glia** Support cells for neurons in the brain and spinal cord that separate the brain from the bloodstream, assist in the growth of neurons, speed transmission of nerve impulses, and eliminate damaged neurons.

Figure 3.1  **The Brain**
The three major parts of the brain are the cerebrum, cerebellum, and brainstem (medulla). The cerebrum is divided into two hemispheres—the left, which regulates the right side of the body, and the right, which regulates the left side of the body. The cerebellum plays the major role in coordinating movement, balance, and posture. The brainstem contains centers that control breathing, blood pressure, heart rate, and other physiological functions.

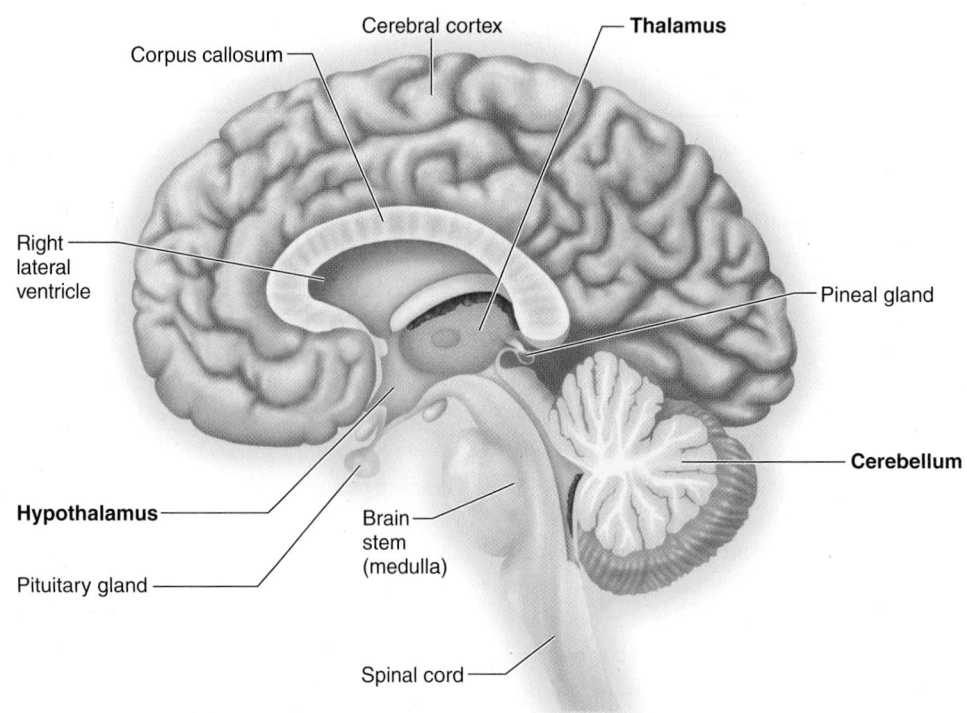

Section I  Building Your Future

Figure 3.2 **Brain Messaging: Anatomy of a Neuron**
This figure shows how nerve impulses are transmitted from one neuron to another within the brain.

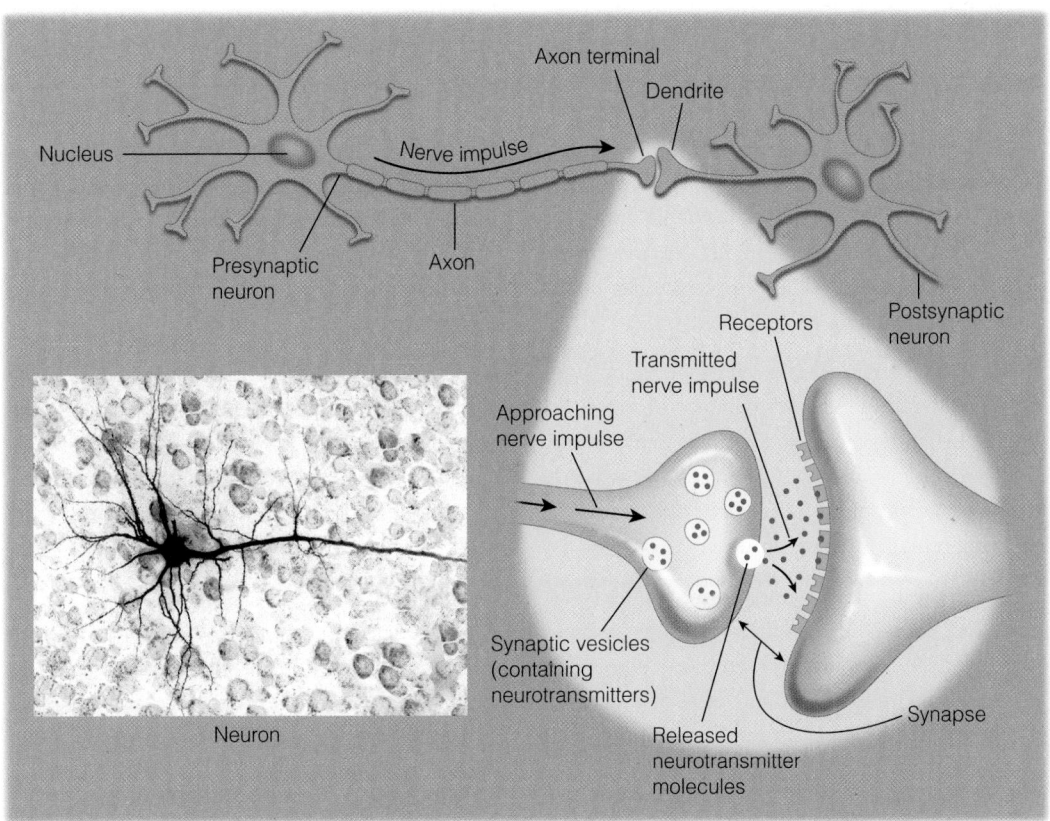

## Communication within the Brain

Neurons "talk" with each other by means of electrical and chemical processes (see Figure 3.2). An electric charge, or impulse, travels along an axon to the terminal, where packets of chemicals called **neurotransmitters** are stored. When released, these messengers flow out of the axon terminal and cross a **synapse**, a specialized site at which the axon terminal of one neuron comes extremely close to a dendrite from another neuron.

On the surface of the dendrite are **receptors**, protein molecules designed to bind with neurotransmitters. It takes only about a ten-thousandth of a second for a neurotransmitter

bral cortex that control higher functions, while the mid- and hindbrain are more involved with unconscious, autonomic functions. The normal adult human brain typically weighs about three pounds.

and a receptor to come together. Neurotransmitters that do not connect with receptors may remain in the synapse until they are reabsorbed by the cell that produced them—a process called **reuptake**—or broken down by enzymes.

A malfunction in the release of a neurotransmitter, in its reuptake or elimination, or in the receptors or secondary messengers may result in abnormalities in thinking, feeling, or behavior. Some of the most promising and exciting research in neuropsychiatry is focusing on correcting such malfunctions.

The neurotransmitter serotonin and its receptors have been shown to affect mood, sleep, behavior, appetite, memory, learning, sexuality, and aggression and to play a role in several mental disorders. The discovery of a possible link between low levels of serotonin and some cases of major depression has led to the development of more precisely targeted **antidepressant** medications that boost serotonin to normal levels. (See "Psychiatric Drugs" later in the chapter.)

**neurotransmitters** Chemicals released by neurons that stimulate or inhibit the action of other neurons.

**synapse** A specialized site at which electrical impulses are transmitted from the axon terminal of one neuron to a dendrite of another.

**receptors** Molecules on the surface of neurons on which neurotransmitters bind after their release from other neurons.

**reuptake** Reabsorption by the originating cell of neurotransmitters that have not connected with receptors and have been left in synapses.

**antidepressant** A drug used primarily to treat symptoms of depression.

## Sex Differences in the Brain

From birth, male and female brains differ in a variety of ways. Overall, a woman's brain, like her body, is 10 to 15 percent smaller than a man's, yet the regions dedicated to higher cognitive functions such as language are more densely packed with neurons—and women use more of them. When a male puts his mind to work, neurons turn on in highly specific areas. When females set their minds on similar tasks, cells light up all over the brain.

Male and female brains perceive light and sound differently. A man's eyes are more sensitive to bright light and retain their ability to see well at long distances longer in life. A woman hears a much broader range of sounds, and her hearing remains sharper longer.

The female brain responds more intensely to emotion. According to neuroimaging studies, the genders respond differently to emotions, especially sadness, which activates, or turns on, neurons in an area eight times larger in women than men.

Neither gender's brain is "better." Intelligence per se appears equal in both. The greatest gender differences appear both at the top and bottom of the intelligence scales. Nevertheless, more than half the time, regardless of the type of test, most women and men perform more or less equally—even though they may well take different routes to arrive at the same answers.

Cognitive skills show greater variability both among women and among men than between the genders. The best evaluation may have come from essayist Samuel Johnson. When asked whether women or men are more intelligent, he responded, "Which man? Which woman?"

## The Teenage and Twenty-Something Brain

If you are under the age of 25, your brain is a work in progress. As neuroimaging techniques such as PET scans (positron-emission tomography) and fMRIs (functional magnetic resonance imaging) have revealed, the brain continues to develop throughout the first quarter-century of life.

The number of synapses surges in the "tween" years before adolescence, followed by a "pruning" of nonessential connections. In a sense, each individual determines which synapses stay and which are deleted. If you started to play the piano as a child and continue as an adolescent, for instance, you retain the synapses involved in this skill. If you don't practice regularly, your brain will prune the unused synapses, and your piano-playing ability will diminish. Inadequate pruning of synapses may contribute to mental disorders such as schizophrenia, which usually first occur in late adolescence.

Brain areas responsible for tasks such as organizing, controlling impulses, planning, and strategizing do not fully develop until the mid-twenties. Brain chemicals such as dopamine that help distinguish between what is worthy of attention and what is mere distraction also do not reach optimal levels until then.

The brains of teens and young adults function differently than those of older individuals. In dealing with daily life, they rely more on the amygdala, a small almond-shaped region in the medial and temporal lobes that processes emotions and memories. This is one reason why any setback—a poor grade or a friend's snub—can feel like a major crisis. As individuals age, the frontal cortex, which governs reason and forethought, plays a greater role and helps put challenges into perspective.

A young, "maturing" brain does not necessarily lead to poor judgments and risky behaviors. However, if you are under 25, you should be aware that your brain may not always grasp the long-term consequences of your actions, set realistic priorities, or restrain potentially harmful impulses. You can learn to center yourself, seek the counsel of others, and not fly off the handle. Be cautious of drugs and alcohol, which are especially toxic to the developing brain and increase the risk of acts you may later regret.[1]

## Understanding Mental Health

Mentally healthy individuals value themselves, perceive reality as it is, accept their limitations and possibilities, carry out their responsibilities, establish and maintain close relationships, pursue work that suits their talent and training, and feel a sense of fulfillment that makes the efforts of daily living worthwhile (Figure 3.3).

The state of mental health around the world is far from ideal. Psychiatric illness and substance abuse cause more premature deaths than any other factor, according to a recent report by the World Health Organization (WHO). These conditions also account for about a third of years lost to disability among people older than 14. The most common psychiatric conditions worldwide are depression, alcohol dependence and abuse, bipolar disorder, schizophrenia, Alzheimer's and other forms of dementia, panic disorder, and drug dependence and abuse.

Across the globe, depression is the leading cause of years of health lost to disease in both men and women. The worldwide rate of depression among women is 50 percent higher than in men, and women and girls have higher rates of anxiety disorders, migraine, and Alzheimer's disease. Men's rates of alcohol and substance abuse are nearly seven times higher than women's.

Preventive steps can help maintain and enhance your psychological health, just as similar actions boost physical health. (See Making Change Happen, p. 84.)

Despite public education campaigns, the level of prejudice and discrimination against people with a serious mental illness has changed little over the last ten years. More people now attribute problems like depression and substance abuse to neurobiological causes—and are more likely to favor providing treatment. Yet even these individuals are no less likely to stigmatize patients with mental illness.[2]

## What Is a Mental Disorder?

While laypeople may speak of "nervous breakdowns" or "insanity," these are not scientific terms. The U.S. government's official definition states that a serious mental illness is "a diagnosable mental, behavioral, or emotional disorder that interferes with one or more major activities in life, like dressing, eating, or working."

The mental health profession's standard for diagnosing a mental disorder is the pattern of symptoms, or diagnostic criteria, spelled out

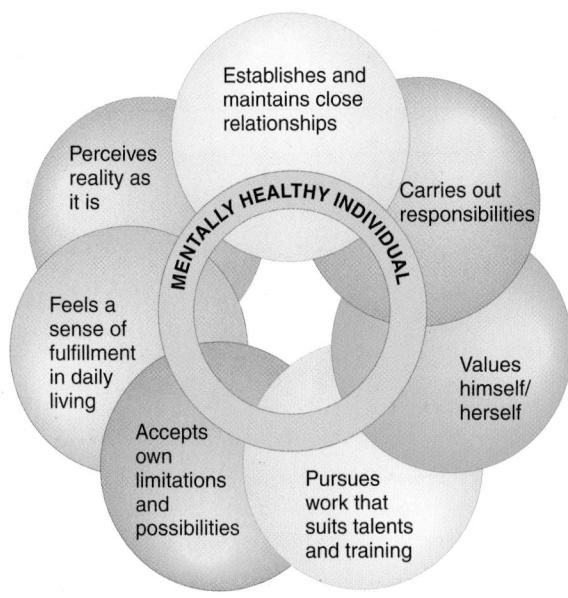

Figure 3.3  **The Mentally Healthy Individual**
Mental well-being is a combination of many factors.

MENTALLY HEALTHY INDIVIDUAL

Establishes and maintains close relationships

Perceives reality as it is

Carries out responsibilities

Feels a sense of fulfillment in daily living

Values himself/ herself

Accepts own limitations and possibilities

Pursues work that suits talents and training

for the almost 300 disorders in the American Psychiatric Association's *Diagnostic and Statistical Manual*, 4th edition (DSM-IV). Psychiatrists define a **mental disorder** as a clinically significant behavioral or psychological syndrome or pattern that is associated with present distress (a painful symptom) or disability (impairment in one or more important areas of functioning) or with a significantly increased risk of suffering death, pain, disability, or an important loss of freedom.[3]

## Who Develops Mental Disorders?

In the course of their lifetime, almost half of all Americans experience a diagnosable psychological problem. The most common mental disorders are substance abuse (discussed in Chapters 11 and 12), mood disorders such as depression and bipolar disorder, and anxiety disorders such as phobias and panic disorder.

Unlike most disabling physical diseases, mental illness starts early in life. Anxiety disorders often begin in late childhood, mood disorders in late adolescence, and substance abuse in the early twenties. Researchers describe such problems as "the chronic diseases of the young," striking when men and women are in their prime.

**mental disorder** Behavioral or psychological syndrome associated with distress or disability or with a significantly increased risk of suffering death, pain, disability, or loss of freedom.

# The Exercise Prescription

Imagine a drug so powerful it can alter brain chemistry, so versatile it can help prevent or treat many common mental disorders, so safe that moderate doses cause few, if any, side effects, and so inexpensive that anyone can afford it. This wonder drug, proved in years of research, is exercise.

Chapter 8 provides detailed information on improving your fitness. To make a difference in the way you look and feel, follow these simple guidelines:

- **Work in short bouts.** Three 10-minute intervals of exercise can be just as effective as exercising for 30 minutes straight.

- **Mix it up.** Combine moderate and vigorous intensity exercises to meet the guidelines. For instance, you can walk briskly two days a week and jog at a faster pace on the other days.

- **Set aside exercise times.** Schedule exercise in advance so you can plan your day around it.

- **Find exercise buddies.** Recruit roommates, friends, family, coworkers. You'll have more fun on your way to getting fit.

The prevalence of mental disorders increases from early adulthood (ages 18 to 29) to the next-oldest age group (ages 30 to 44) and then declines. Women have higher rates of depressive and anxiety disorders; men have higher rates of substance abuse and impulse disorders.

About 6 percent of Americans have a "severe" mental disorder, one that significantly limits their ability to work or carry out daily activities or that has led to a suicide attempt or psychosis (a gross impairment of a person's perception of reality). On average, they are unable to function for nearly three months of the year.

## The Mind-Body Connection

According to a growing number of studies, mental attitude may be just as important a risk factor for certain diseases as age, race, gender, education, habits, and health history. Positive states like happiness and optimism have been linked with longer lifespans as well as lower risk of cardiovascular and lung disease, stroke, diabetes, colds, and upper respiratory infections. Gratitude, in particular, has proven health benefits. (See "Health in Action: Count Your Blessings," p. 63.)

In addition to its head-to-toe physical benefits, discussed in Chapter 8, exercise may be, as one therapist puts it, the single most effective way to lift a person's spirits and to restore feelings of potency about all aspects of life. People who exercise regularly report a more cheerful mood, higher self-esteem, and less stress. Their sleep and appetite also tend to improve. In clinical studies, exercise has proved effective as a treatment for depression and anxiety disorders. But remember: Although exercise can help prevent and ease problems for many people, it's no substitute for professional treatment of serious psychiatric disorders.

*Disease Risks* Mental disorders, on the other hand, can undermine physical well-being. Anxiety can lead to intensified asthmatic reactions, skin conditions, and digestive disorders. Stress can play a role in hypertension, heart attacks, sudden cardiac death, and immune disorders in the young as well as in older individuals. People who suffer from migraine headaches are at increased risk of depression, anxiety, and neurological disorders.

The brain and the heart—and the health of each—are linked in complex ways. Heart disease increases the likelihood of depression, and depression increases the likelihood of heart disease. For people with heart disease, depression can be fatal. It may contribute to sudden cardiac death and increase all causes of cardiac mortality.

Large-scale, longitudinal studies have found complex links between depression and diabetes. Individuals who are depressed are at much higher risk of developing diabetes, and those with diabetes are much more likely to become depressed. Preventing diabetes, which affects about 10 percent of Americans, may prevent depression—and preventing depression, which affects about 7 percent of adults over age 18, could prevent diabetes.[4]

Major depression is associated with lower bone density in young men and in adolescent girls. A history of depression increases the risk of physi-

## MENTAL HEALTH PROBLEMS ON CAMPUS

**Students reporting the following feelings at any time with the last 12 months:**

| | |
|---|---|
| _____ Exhausted (not from physical activity) | **80 percent** |
| _____ Very sad | **61 percent** |
| _____ Overwhelmingly anxious | **48 percent** |
| _____ Hopeless | **46 percent** |
| _____ So depressed it was difficult to function | **31 percent** |

**Students reporting a diagnosis of a mental disorder by a professional in the last 12 months.**

| | |
|---|---|
| _____ Anxiety | **10 percent** |
| _____ Depression | **10 percent** |
| _____ Both anxiety and depression | **6 percent** |
| _____ Panic attacks | **5 percent** |
| _____ Attention disorder | **4 percent** |
| _____ Insomnia | **4 percent** |

### HOW DO YOU COMPARE?

Check any of the feelings or diagnoses that apply to you. To tune into your current moods, track your feelings over a three-day period. Several times a day, jot down a few words about how you're feeling: blue, worried, excited, frustrated, happy, content. Think of it as taking your emotional temperature. Record your reflections on your feelings in your online journal.

Source: American College Health Association. *National College Health Assessment Reference Group Executive Summary*, Spring 2010.

cal problems such as headache and shoulder and neck pain in women as they reach middle age.

*Personality and Health*    Various personality types and behaviors have also been linked to certain illnesses. Aggressive, impatient, Type A people may be more prone to heart disease, high blood pressure, high cholesterol levels, and increased stomach acid secretion than more relaxed Type B people.

Individuals with a Type C personality—hardworking, highly responsible, quiet, courteous—tend to suppress negative emotions (especially anger), avoid conflicts, never retaliate, and rarely pursue their own desires. These behavioral and emotional characteristics are frequently seen in patients with cancer and may be associated with a suppressed immunity in patients with AIDS.

The Type D (for distressed) personality, characterized by tendencies both to experience negative emotions and to inhibit these emotions while avoiding contact with others, has emerged as an independent risk factor for heart disease, a poor prognosis if cardiovascular problems develop, and increased mortality.

# Mental Health on Campus

Young people in their late teens and early twenties are at risk of mental health problems simply because of their age. In three of four cases, the first episodes of mental and substance abuse disorders occur before age 24.[5] Nearly half of all young adults have suffered some form of a psychological disorder. The rates of such problems are lower among students than among those not enrolled in higher education, but undergraduates are far from immune.

Among entering freshmen, self-reported emotional health is at the lowest point in the last quarter-century. The percentage of students describing their mental state as above average or in the top 10 percent dropped to 52 percent, with much fewer women (46 percent) than men (59 percent) rating their mental health highly.[6]

In the American College Health Association National College Health Assessment, almost half (46 percent) of the more than 95,000

## Health in Action

### Count Your Blessings

As discussed in Chapter 2, gratitude has proven as effective in brightening mood and boosting energy as the standard, well-studied techniques used in psychotherapy. Below are some simple steps to cultivating and expressing gratitude. See "The Grateful Thread" in *Labs for IPC* for more suggestions:

- Every day write down ten new things for which you are grateful. You can start with this list and keep adding to it: your bed, your cell phone and every person whose efforts led to its development, every road you take, loyalty, your toothbrush, your toes, the sky, ice cream, etc.

- Record the ways you express gratitude. How do you feel when doing so?

- Create a daily practice of appreciation. This may be as simple as saying a few words of thanks before each meal (if only to yourself) or writing down your feelings of gratitude.

- Make a list of ten people to whom you owe a debt of gratitude. Write a one- to two-page letter to each of them, stating your appreciation of what he or she has contributed to you and your well-being. These people could include schoolteachers, music or dance instructors, coaches, doctors, neighbors, and, of course, family members. It is not important that you send the letters. What is important is that you focus deeply on the contribution of each person and allow feelings of gratitude to come as they may.

undergraduates surveyed reported feeling that things were hopeless within the last 12 months. About 61 percent felt very sad at least once, while 48 percent reported overwhelming anxiety and 31 percent reported being so depressed that it was difficult for them to function.[7] (See table in "How Do You Compare?: Mental Health Problems on Campus.)

According to the American College Counseling Association (ACCA), which surveyed 28,000 students from 66 colleges and universities, more students are seeking counseling—and with more serious problems than in the past. Here are some of the survey findings:[8]

- Forty-four percent of students treated—up from 16 percent in 2000—suffer from a severe psychological disorder, such as depression, anxiety, attention disorders, alcohol or drug abuse, or eating disorders.

- About one in four undergraduates (24 percent) takes a psychiatric medication, up from 17 percent a decade ago.

- A quarter (25 percent) of students have seriously considered suicide prior to college, after starting college, or both; 21 percent have engaged in "nonsuicidal self-injury."

- Five percent have intentionally harmed another person. (See Chapter 18 for a discussion of violence on campus.)

## Students at Risk

Why are so many students feeling so distressed? Many arrive on campus with a history of psychological problems. Medications for common disorders such as depression and attention disorder have made it possible for young people who might otherwise not have been able to function in a college setting to pursue higher education. Some are dealing with ongoing issues such as bulimia, self-cutting, and childhood sexual abuse. Others become depressed in college or begin abusing alcohol or drugs.

Among the strongest factors that put college students at risk for mental problems is a romantic breakup or loss. In the survey, about one in eight individuals reported a breakup in the previous year. Their odds of having a psychiatric disorder are significantly higher than those who hadn't been through a breakup.

Some psychiatric symptoms increase the risk of developing other disorders. College women who reported symptoms of depression, for example, are at higher risk for alcohol problems.

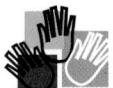 The few studies that have looked into ethnic differences in psychological health have yielded conflicting or inconclusive results: Some found no differences; others suggested higher rates of depression among Indian, Korean, and South Asian students.[9] Various ethnic groups report less of a sense of belonging and a lack of mentoring and peer support. A recent survey of Latino/a college students found that they did not differ from other students in overall mental health, but showed subtle signs of low-level psychological problems, such as a past history of depression and feeling "worried" or "sad."

## The Toll on Students

Psychological and emotional problems can affect every aspect of a student's life, including physical health, overall satisfaction, and relationships. Students who struggle with symptoms of anxiety or depression, which can interfere with concentration, study habits, classroom participation, and testing, commonly report struggling with academics.

In the ACHA's national assessment, 18 percent of students reported that anxiety had impaired their ability to learn and earn higher grades; 12 percent said that depression had affected their academic performance.[10] Some estimate that 5 percent of undergraduates may not complete their degrees because of psychological problems.

The impact of mental health problems extends beyond an individual student to roommates, friends, classmates, family, and instructors. Suicides or suicide attempts affect all members of the campus community, who may experience profound sadness and grief. (See the discussion of suicide later in this chapter.)

Many schools are setting up programs, such as depression screening days, to identify students at risk and refer them for follow-up and, when needed, professional treatment. Others have set up peer-counseling networks and are using social networking to raise awareness of problems like depression. However, there is only limited evidence that interventions like these might prevent a psychological disorder or lead to earlier recognition and treatment.[11]

Why don't distressed students seek professional care? Many feel they don't need help. Others worry about the stigma of admitting there's something wrong or of seeing a therapist. Although they are as likely to suffer psychological problems as others, African American students are much less likely to seek help. Their families' negative views about seeking help are a common deterrent.

Without help, many students' problems remain unresolved. When researchers assessed students' mental health and then checked back in two years later, more than a third of those surveyed had a mental health problem.

# Depressive Disorders

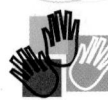

Depression, the world's most common mental ailment, affects more than 13 million adults in the United States every year and costs billions of dollars for treatment and lost productivity and lives. In a Centers for Disease Control and Prevention (CDC) survey of more than 235,000 people, 9 percent met the criteria for clinical depression, including 3 percent who could be diagnosed with major depression.[12] The prevalence of major depression increased with age, from about 3 percent among those ages 18 to 24 to almost 5 percent among persons ages 45 to 64. It declined to less than 2 percent among those older than age 65.

Those most likely to have major depression include:

- women
- racial and ethnic minorities
- those without a high school education
- divorced or never-married individuals
- the jobless
- those without health insurance[13]

# Depression in Children and Teens

An estimated 5 to 10 percent of American teenagers suffer from a serious depressive disorder; girls are twice as susceptible as boys. Prior to puberty, girls and boys are equally likely to develop depression.

The risks of depression in the young are high. Four in ten depressed adolescents think about killing themselves; two in ten actually try to do so. Every year an estimated 11 to 13 in every 100,000 teens take their own lives, twice as many as the number who die from all natural causes combined.

No one knows the reason for this steady surge in sadness, but experts point to the breakdown of families, the pressures of the information age, and increased isolation. A family history of depression greatly increases a young person's vulnerability. A mother's anxiety and depression during early childhood can increase the risk that adolescents will develop symptoms of anxiety and depression. Racial and ethnic factors also contribute. Among Asian American college students, for instance, perfectionism has been linked to depressive symptoms.

Teens who spend many hours watching television are at higher risk of depression as adults. However, the strongest predictor of depression is cigarette smoking. Depressed teens may smoke because they think smoking will make them feel better, but nicotine alters brain chemistry and actually worsens symptoms of depression.

Treatment with antidepressants and cognitive behavioral therapy helps most adolescents recover from major depression, but the risk of relapse is high, especially in girls. In one recent study, nearly half of adolescents developed a second episode of major depression.[14]

## Depression in Students

An estimated 15 to 40 percent of college-age men and women (18- to 24-year-olds) may develop depression. Among the most vulnerable students are those being treated for mental disorders. (See the Self Survey: "Recognizing Depression," p. 83.)

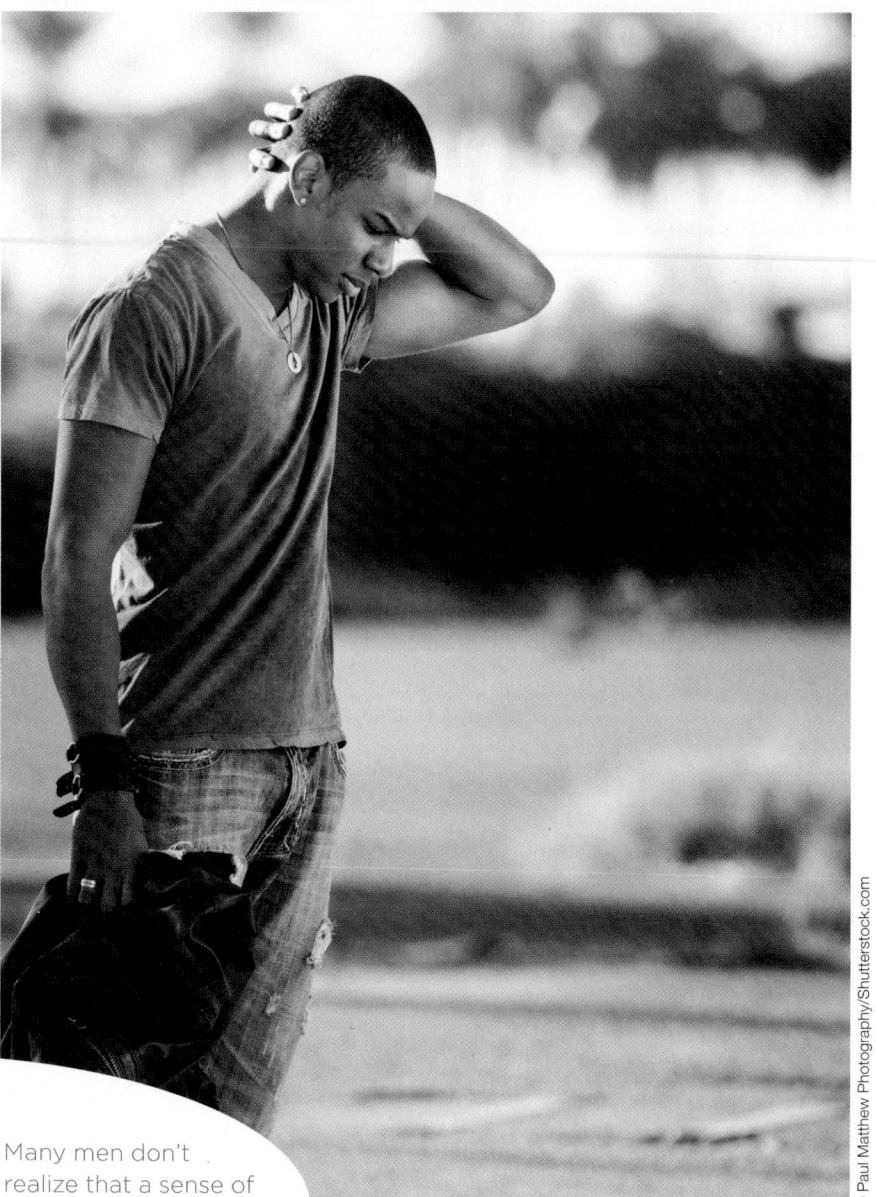

Many men don't realize that a sense of hopelessness, worthlessness, helplessness, or feeling dead inside can be a symptom of depression.

© Paul Matthew Photography/Shutterstock.com

around-the-clock television, and the college tradition of pulling all-nighters can conspire to sabotage rest and increase vulnerability to depression.

## Gender and Depression

*Female Depression* Depression is twice as common in women as men. However, this gender gap decreases or disappears in studies of men and women in similar socioeconomic situations, such as college students, civil servants, and the Amish community. Women may not necessarily be more likely to develop depression, this research suggests, but may have an underlying predisposition that puts them at greater risk under various social stressors.[15]

Brain chemistry and sex hormones may play a role. Women produce less of certain metabolites of serotonin, a messenger chemical that helps regulate mood. Their brains also register sadness much more intensely than men's, and they are more sensitive to changes in light and temperature. Women are at least four times more likely than men to develop seasonal affective disorder (SAD) and to become depressed in the dark winter months.

Some women also seem more sensitive to their own hormones or to the changes in them that occur at puberty, during the menstrual cycle, after childbirth, or during perimenopause and menopause. Primary ovarian insufficiency, a condition that causes menopause-like symptoms and that can develop as early as the teens or twenties, greatly increases a woman's risk of depression.[16] Pregnancy, contrary to what many people assume, does not "protect" a woman from depression, and women who discontinue treatment when they become pregnant are at risk of a relapse. Women and their psychiatrists must carefully weigh the risks and benefits of psychiatric medications during pregnancy.

Childhood abuse also contributes to female vulnerability. In epidemiological studies, 60 percent of women diagnosed with depression—compared with 39 percent of men—were abused as children. In adulthood, relationships may protect women from depression, while a lack of social support increases vulnerability to depression. Women with at least one "confiding relationship," as researchers put it, are physically and psychologically more resilient.

Researchers at the University of Michigan have identified three key contributors to depression in college students: stress, substance abuse, and sleep loss.

As they adjust to campus life, undergraduates face the ongoing stress of forging a new identity and finding a place for themselves in various social hierarchies. This triggers the release of the so-called stress hormones (discussed in Chapter 4), which can change brain activity. Drugs and alcohol, widely used on campus, also affect the brain in ways that make stress even harder to manage.

Too little sleep adds another ingredient to this dangerous brew. Computers, the Internet,

*Male Depression*  More than 6 million men in the United States—1 in every 14—suffer from this insidious disorder, many without recognizing what's wrong. Experts describe male depression as an "under" disease: under-discussed, underrecognized, underdiagnosed, and undertreated.

Depression "looks" different in men than women. Rather than becoming sad, men may be irritable or tremendously fatigued. They feel a sense of being dead inside, of worthlessness, hopelessness, helplessness, of losing their life force. Physical symptoms, such as headaches, pain, and insomnia, are common, as are attempts to "self-medicate" with alcohol or drugs.

Genes may make some men more vulnerable, but chronic stress of any sort plays a major role in male depression, possibly by raising levels of the stress hormone cortisol and lowering testosterone. Men also are more likely than women to become depressed following divorce, job loss, or a career setback. Whatever its roots, depression alters brain chemistry in potentially deadly ways. Four times as many men as women kill themselves; depressed men are two to four times more likely to take their own lives than depressed women.

## Dysthymic Disorder

**Dysthymia** is a depressive disorder characterized by a chronically depressed mood. Symptoms include feelings of inadequacy, hopelessness, and guilt; low self-esteem; low energy; fatigue; indecisiveness; and an inability to enjoy pleasurable activities.

## Minor Depression

Minor depression is a common disorder that is often unrecognized and untreated, affecting about 7.5 percent of Americans during their lifetime. Its symptoms are the same as those of major depression, but less severe and fewer in number. They include either a depressed mood most of the day, nearly every day, or diminished interest or pleasure in daily activities.

Psychotherapy is remarkably effective for mild depression. In more serious cases, antidepressant medication can lead to dramatic improvement in 40 to 80 percent of depressed patients.

## How to Help Someone Who Is Depressed

- **Express your concern, but don't nag.** You might say: "I'm concerned about you. You are struggling right now. We need to find some help."

- **Don't be distracted by behaviors like drinking or gambling, which can disguise depression in men.**

- **Encourage the individual to remain in treatment until symptoms begin to lift (which takes several weeks).**

- **Provide emotional support.** Listen carefully. Offer hope and reassurance that with time and treatment, things will get better.

- **Do not ignore remarks about suicide.** Report them to his or her doctor or, in an emergency, call 911.

Exercise also works. Several studies have shown that exercise effectively lifts mild to moderate depression.

## Major Depression

The simplest definition of **major depression** is sadness that does not end. The incidence of major depression has soared over the last two decades, especially among young adults. Major depression can destroy a person's joy for living. Food, friends, sex, or any form of pleasure no longer appeals. It is impossible to concentrate on work and responsibilities. Unable to escape a sense of utter hopelessness, depressed individuals may fight back tears throughout the day and toss and turn through long, empty nights. Thoughts of death or suicide may push into their minds.

The characteristic symptoms of major depression include:

- **Feeling depressed,** sad, empty, discouraged, tearful.

- **Loss of interest** or pleasure in once-enjoyable activities.

- **Eating more or less** than usual and either gaining or losing weight.

**dysthymia** Frequent, prolonged mild depression.

**major depression** Sadness that does not end; ongoing feelings of utter helplessness.

- **Having trouble sleeping** or sleeping much more than usual.
- **Feeling slowed down** or restless and unable to sit still.
- **Lack of energy**.
- **Feeling helpless,** hopeless, worthless, inadequate.
- **Difficulty concentrating**, forgetfulness.
- **Difficulty thinking clearly** or making decisions.
- **Persistent thoughts of death** or suicide.
- **Withdrawal from others**, lack of interest in sex.
- **Physical symptoms** (headaches, digestive problems, aches and pains).

As many as half of major depressive episodes are not recognized because the symptoms are "masked." Rather than feeling sad or depressed, individuals may experience low energy, insomnia, difficulty concentrating, and physical symptoms.

## Treating Depression

The most recent guidelines for treating depression, developed by the American Psychiatric Association, call for an individualized approach tailored to each patient's symptoms. Specific treatments might include medication, healthy behaviors, exercise (proven to reduce depressive symptoms, especially in older adults and those with chronic medical problems), and psychotherapy.[17]

The rate of depression treatment, particularly with antidepressants, has increased in the last decade. Medication has become the most common approach, while fewer patients receive psy-

## ❶ CONSUMER ALERT

### The Pros and Cons of Antidepressants

Millions of individuals have benefited from the category of antidepressant drugs called selective serotonin reuptake inhibitors (SSRIs). However, like all drugs, they can cause side effects that range from temporary physical symptoms, such as stomach upset and headaches, to more persistent problems, such as sexual dysfunction. The most serious—and controversial—risk is suicide.

### Facts to Know

- The FDA has issued a "black box" warning about the risk of suicidal thoughts, hostility, and aggression in both children and young adults. The danger is greatest just after pill use begins.
- This risk of suicide while taking an antidepressant is about 1 in 3,000; the risk of a serious attempt is 1 in 1,000.
- Recent reviews of antidepressant use have found that the risk of suicide for both children and adults was *higher* in the month *before* starting treatment, dropped sharply in the month after it began, and tapered off in the following months.

### Steps to Take

- If you are younger than age 20, be aware of the increased suicide risk with the use of SSRIs. Talk these over carefully with a psychiatrist. Discuss alternative treatments, such as psychotherapy.
- For individuals older than age 20, the benefits of antidepressants have proved to outweigh their risks in most cases. Adults treated with SSRIs are 40 percent less likely to commit suicide than depressed individuals who do not receive this therapy.
- In patients initially treated with antidepressants, two approaches based on mindfulness (discussed in Chapter 4)—mindfulness-based cognitive therapy and mindfulness meditation—have proven as effective as continuing drug therapy in preventing a return of depression symptoms.[19]
- Whatever your age, arrange for careful monitoring and follow-up with a psychiatrist when you start taking an antidepressant. Familiarize yourself with possible side effects, and seek help immediately if you begin to think about taking your own life.

chotherapy than in the past, possibly because of limited insurance coverage. A combination of psychotherapy and medication is considered the most effective approach for most patients.[18]

Psychotherapy helps individuals pinpoint the life problems that contribute to their depression, identify negative or distorted thinking patterns, explore behaviors that contribute to depression, and regain a sense of control and pleasure in life. Two specific psychotherapies—cognitive-behavioral therapy and interpersonal therapy (described later in this chapter)—have proved as helpful as antidepressant drugs, although they take longer than medication to achieve results.

Antidepressants have proven most effective in individuals with severe depression, with minimal or nonexistent benefits for those with mild or moderate symptoms. (See "Consumer Alert: The Pros and Cons of Antidepressants.")

For individuals who cannot take antidepressant medications because of medical problems, or who do not improve with psychotherapy or drugs, *electroconvulsive therapy* (ECT)—the administration of a controlled electrical current through electrodes attached to the scalp—remains the safest and most effective treatment. About 70 to 90 percent of depressed individuals improve after ECT. Newer options include transcranial magnetic stimulation, which uses highly focused, pulsed magnetic fields to stimulate brain regions linked with depression, and vagus nerve stimulation, which delivers electrical stimulation to a major nerve linking the brain to internal organs.

Even without treatment, depression generally lifts after six to nine months. However, in more than 80 percent of people, it recurs, with each episode lasting longer and becoming more severe and difficult to treat.

"All the while the depression goes untreated, it is causing ongoing damage that shrivels important regions of the brain," says John Greden, M.D., director of the University of Michigan Depression Center. "The exciting news is that, as brain scans show, treatment turns the destructive process around and stops depression in its tracks."[20]

## Bipolar Disorder

**Bipolar disorder**, known as manic depression in the past, consists of mood swings that may take individuals from manic states of feeling euphoric and energetic to depressive states of utter despair. In episodes of full mania, they may become so impulsive and out of touch with reality that they endanger their careers, relationships, health, or even survival. Psychiatrists view bipolar symptoms on a spectrum that includes depression and states of acute irritability and distress.[21]

One percent of the population—about 2 million American adults—suffer from this serious but treatable disorder. Men tend to develop bipolar disorder earlier in life (between ages 16 and 25), but women have higher rates overall. About 50 percent of patients with bipolar illness have a family history of the disorder.

The characteristic symptoms of bipolar disorder include:

- **Mood swings** (from happy to miserable, optimistic to despairing, and so on).
- **Changes in thinking** (thoughts speeding through one's mind, unrealistic self-confidence, difficulty concentrating, delusions, hallucinations).
- **Changes in behavio**r (sudden immersion in plans and projects, talking very rapidly and much more than usual, excessive spending, impaired judgment, impulsive sexual involvement).
- **Changes in physical condition** (less need for sleep, increased energy, fewer health complaints than usual).

During manic periods, individuals may make grandiose plans or take dangerous risks. But they often plunge from this highest of highs to a horrible, low depressive episode, in which they may feel sad, hopeless, and helpless and develop other symptoms of major depression.

Professional therapy is essential in treating bipolar disorders. An estimated 25 to 50 percent of bipolar patients attempt suicide at least once. About 1 percent take their own lives every year.[22] Mood-stabilizing medications are the keystone of treatment, although psychotherapy plays a critical role in helping individuals understand their illness and rebuild their lives. Most individuals continue taking medication indefinitely after remission of their symptoms because the risk of recurrence is high.

## Health in the Headlines

### Depression

Depression is the most common ailment in the world. Every month brings new insights, new studies, and new understanding of its effects on physical and mental health. Use the "Depression" portal on Global Health Watch to explore the latest information about depression (located under Health and Wellness → Mental Health and Wellness). Using the latest research about depression as a starting point, reflect on how depression affects your everyday life. Are there steps you can take that would have a positive impact?

**bipolar disorder** Severe depression alternating with periods of manic activity and elation.

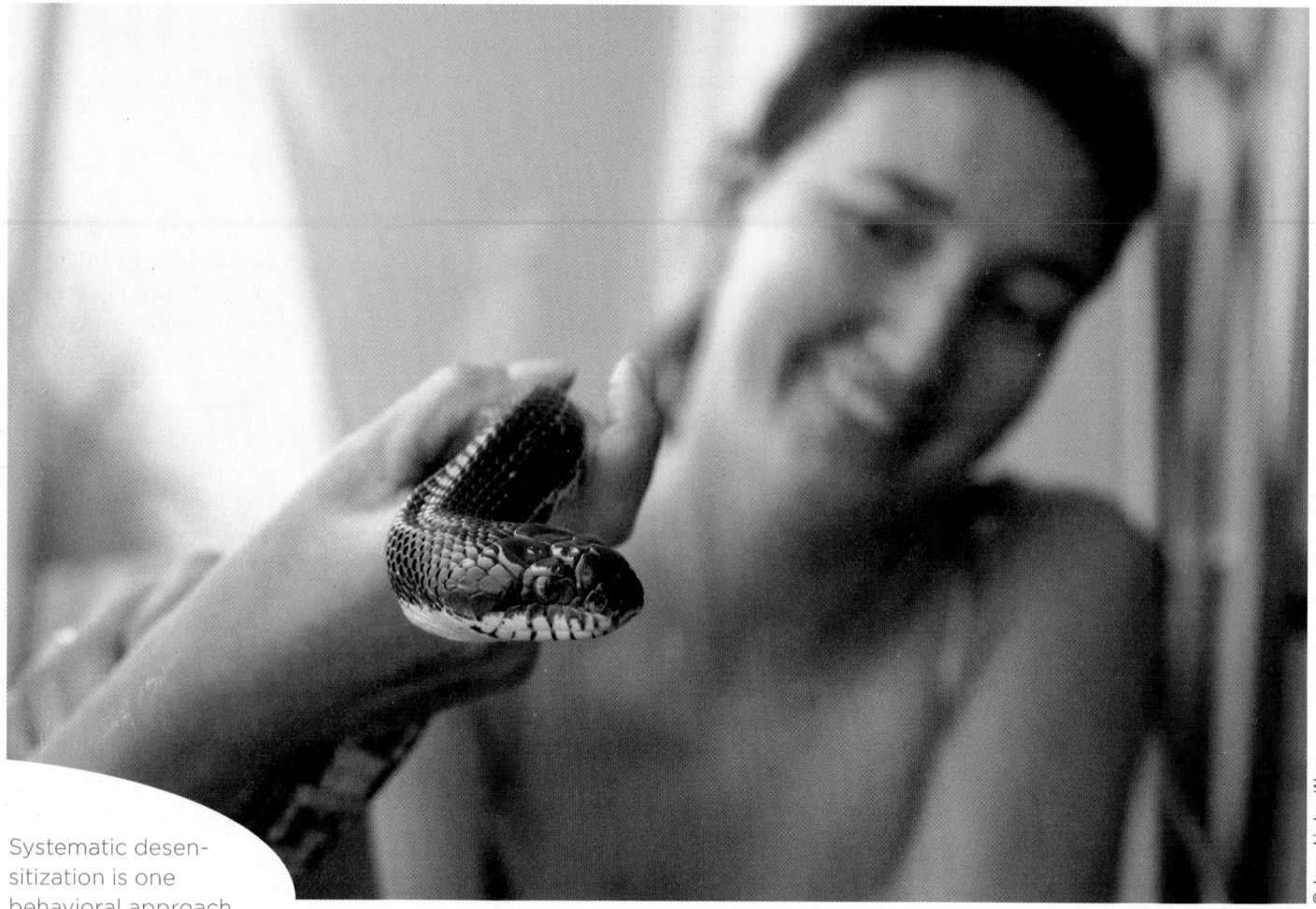

© Jason Lindsey/Alamy

Systematic desensitization is one behavioral approach to treating a fear of snakes and other phobias.

**anxiety disorders** A group of psychological disorders involving episodes of apprehension, tension, or uneasiness, stemming from the anticipation of danger and sometimes accompanied by physical symptoms, which cause significant distress and impairment to an individual.

**phobia** An anxiety disorder marked by an inordinate fear of an object, a class of objects, or a situation, resulting in extreme avoidance behaviors.

**panic attack** A short episode characterized by physical sensations of light-headedness, dizziness, hyperventilation, and numbness of extremities, accompanied by an inexplicable terror, usually of a physical disaster such as death.

# Anxiety Disorders

**Anxiety disorders** are as common as depression but are often undetected and untreated.[23] They may involve inordinate fears of certain objects or situations (**phobias**), episodes of sudden, inexplicable terror (**panic attacks**), chronic distress (**generalized anxiety disorder**, or **GAD**), or persistent, disturbing thoughts and behaviors (**obsessive–compulsive disorder**, or **OCD**). These disorders can increase the risk of developing depression. Over a lifetime, as many as one in four Americans may experience an anxiety disorder. More than 40 percent are never correctly diagnosed and treated. Yet most individuals who do get treatment, even for severe and disabling problems, improve dramatically.

## Phobias

Phobias—the most prevalent type of anxiety disorder—are out-of-the-ordinary, irrational, intense, persistent fears of certain objects or situations. About 2 million Americans develop such acute terror that they go to extremes to avoid whatever it is that they fear, even though they realize that these feelings are excessive or unreasonable. The most common phobias involve animals, particularly dogs, snakes, insects, and mice; the sight of blood; closed spaces (claustrophobia); heights (acrophobia); air travel and being in open or public places or situations from which one perceives it would be difficult or embarrassing to escape (agoraphobia).

Although various medications have been tried, none is effective by itself in relieving phobias. The best approach is behavioral therapy, which consists of gradual, systematic exposure to the feared object (a process called systematic desensitization). Numerous studies have proved that exposure—especially in vivo exposure, in which individuals are exposed to the actual source of their fear rather than simply imagining it—is highly effective. Medical hypnosis—the use of induction of an altered state of consciousness—also can help.

## Panic Attacks and Panic Disorder

Individuals who have had panic attacks describe them as the most frightening experiences of their lives. Without reason or warning, their hearts race wildly. They may become light-headed or dizzy. Because they can't catch their breath, they may start breathing rapidly and hyperventilate. Parts of their bodies, such as their fingers or toes, may tingle or feel numb. Worst of all is the terrible sense that something horrible is about to happen: that they will die, lose their minds, or have a heart attack.

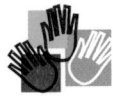 Individuals of different ethnic and racial backgrounds may experience panic symptoms differently. In one cross-cultural study of undergraduates, Asians tended to report symptoms such as dizziness, unsteadiness, choking, and feeling terrified more frequently than did Caucasians. African Americans reported feeling less nervous than Caucasians. However, panic symptoms were equally severe across all racial and ethnic groups.[24]

Most attacks reach peak intensity within ten minutes. Afterward, individuals live in dread of another one. In the course of a lifetime, your risk of having a single panic attack is 7 percent.

**Panic disorder** develops when attacks recur or apprehension about them becomes so intense that individuals cannot function normally. Full-blown panic disorder occurs in about 2 percent of all adults in the course of a lifetime and usually develops before age 30. Women are more than twice as likely as men to experience panic attacks, although no one knows why. Parents, siblings, and children of individuals with panic disorders also are more likely to develop them than are others.

The two primary treatments for panic disorder are (1) cognitive-behavioral therapy (CBT), which teaches specific strategies for coping with symptoms like rapid breathing, and (2) medication. Treatment helps as many as 90 percent of

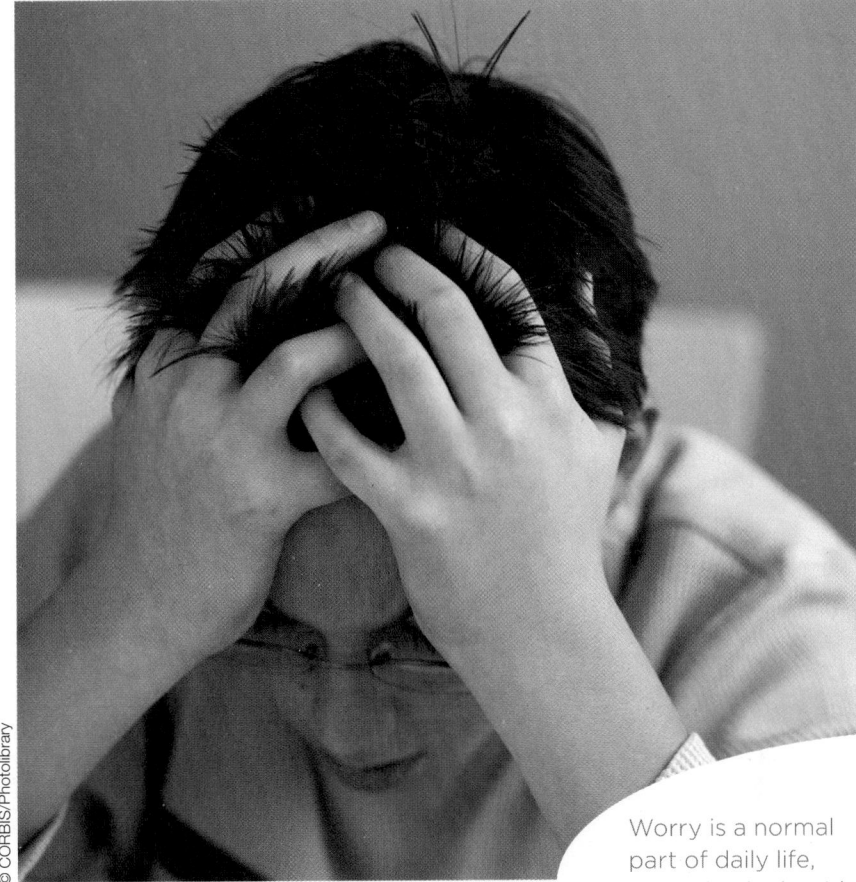

Worry is a normal part of daily life, but individuals with generalized anxiety disorder worry constantly about everything that might go wrong.

those with panic disorder either improve significantly or recover completely, usually within six to eight weeks. Individuals with a greater internal locus of control (discussed in Chapter 1) may respond better to CBT.

## Generalized Anxiety Disorder

About 10 million adults in the United States suffer from a generalized anxiety disorder (GAD), excessive or unrealistic apprehension that causes physical symptoms and lasts for six months or longer. It usually starts when people are in their twenties. Unlike fear, which helps us recognize and avoid real danger, GAD is an irrational or unwarranted response to harmless objects or situations of exaggerated danger. The most common symptoms are faster heart rate, sweating, increased blood pressure, muscle aches, intestinal pains, irritability, sleep problems, and difficulty concentrating.

**generalized anxiety disorder (GAD)** An anxiety disorder characterized as chronic distress.

**obsessive-compulsive disorder (OCD)** An anxiety disorder characterized by obsessions and/or compulsions that impair one's ability to function and form relationships.

**panic disorder** An anxiety disorder in which the apprehension or experience of recurring panic attacks is so intense that normal functioning is impaired.

Chronically anxious individuals worry—not just some of the time, and not just about the stresses and strains of ordinary life—but constantly, about almost everything: their health, families, finances, marriages, potential dangers. Treatment for GAD may consist of a combination of psychotherapy, behavioral therapy, and antianxiety drugs.

## Obsessive-Compulsive Disorder

As many as 1 in 40 Americans has a type of anxiety called obsessive-compulsive disorder (OCD). Some of these individuals suffer only from an *obsession*, a recurring idea, thought, or image that they realize, at least initially, is senseless. The most common obsessions are repetitive thoughts of violence (for example, killing a child), contamination (becoming infected by shaking hands), and doubt (wondering whether one has performed some act, such as having hurt someone in a traffic accident).

Most people with OCD also suffer from a *compulsion*, a repetitive behavior performed according to certain rules or in a stereotyped fashion. The most common compulsions involve handwashing, cleaning, hoarding useless items, counting, or checking (for example, making sure dozens of times that a door is locked).

Individuals with OCD realize that their thoughts or behaviors are bizarre, but they cannot resist or control them. Eventually, the obsessions or compulsions consume a great deal of time and significantly interfere with normal routines, job functioning, or usual social activities or relationships with others. A young woman who must follow a very rigid dressing routine may always be late for class, for example; a student who must count each letter of the alphabet as he types may not be able to complete a term paper.

Treatment may consist of cognitive therapy to correct irrational assumptions, behavioral techniques such as progressively limiting the amount of time someone obsessed with cleanliness can spend washing and scrubbing, and medication. Using neuroimaging techniques, researchers have found significant changes in activity in certain regions of the brain after four weeks of daily therapy in patients with obsessive-compulsive disorder.

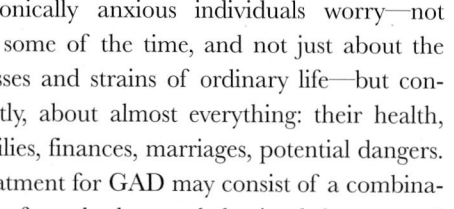

# Attention Disorders

**Attention-deficit/hyperactivity disorder (ADHD)** is the most common mental disorder in childhood. About one in ten school-age children suffer from ADHD and show marked differences in their brain chemistry.[25] Contrary to previous beliefs, most children do not outgrow it. For as many as two-thirds of youngsters, ADHD persists into adolescence and young adulthood. About 4 percent of college students have ADHD and another 11 percent have ADHD symptoms.[26]

 ADHD looks and feels different in adults. Hyperactivity is more subtle, an internal fidgety feeling rather than a physical restlessness. As youngsters with ADHD mature, academic difficulties become much more of a problem. Students with ADHD may find it hard to concentrate, read, make decisions, complete complex projects, and meet deadlines. The academic performance and standardized test scores of college students with ADHD are significantly lower than those of their peers.

Relationships with peers also can become more challenging. Young people with ADHD may become frustrated easily, have a short fuse, and erupt into angry outbursts. Some become more argumentative, negative, and defiant than most other teens. Sleep problems, including sleeping much more or less than normal, are common. The likelihood of developing other emotional problems, including depression and anxiety disorders, is higher. As many as 20 percent of those diagnosed with depression, anxiety, or substance abuse also have ADHD.

The risk of substance use disorders for individuals with ADHD is twice that of the general population. According to several reports, between 15 and 25 percent of adults with substance use disorders have ADHD. In addition, individuals with ADHD start smoking at a younger age and have higher rates of smoking and drinking. (The use of stimulant medication to treat ADHD does not increase the risk of substance abuse.)

**attention-deficit/hyperactivity disorder (ADHD)** A spectrum of difficulties in controlling motion and sustaining attention, including hyperactivity, impulsivity, and distractibility.

The medications used for this disorder include stimulants (such as Ritalin), which improve behavior and cognition for about 70 percent of adolescents. Extended-release preparations (including a skin patch) are longer acting, so individuals do not have to take these medications as often as in the past. As discussed in Chapter 12, misuse of prescription stimulants by students without ADHD is a growing problem on college campuses.

 According to recent research, college students who have not been diagnosed with ADHD but use prescription stimulants may be self-medicating themselves for attention problems. In one survey, 10 percent of those who had never been diagnosed with ADHD had high levels of ADHD symptoms. However, it's not clear whether they suffer from true ADHD or are using medication to deal with short-term academic challenges. The dangers of doing so include drug abuse and addiction (discussed in Chapter 12).[27]

Although many students take stimulants to improve performance, they generally get poorer grades, perhaps because they fall behind and then take stimulants in order to cram and catch up.

An alternative nonstimulant treatment is Strattera (atomoxetine), which treats ADHD and coexisting problems such as depression and anxiety. Its effects are more gradual, and it does not seem to have any known potential for abuse. Adverse effects include drowsiness, loss of appetite, nausea, vomiting, and headaches. Its long-term effects are not known. A promising new approach is transcendental meditation (TM), which may calm anxiety and improve ability to concentrate.[28]

 In the ACHA survey, 5 percent of students reported that ADHD had affected their academic performance.[29] Undergraduates with ADHD are at higher risk of becoming smokers, abusing alcohol and drugs, and having automobile accidents. The normal challenges of college—navigating the complexities of scheduling, planning courses, and honing study skills—may be especially daunting.

Psychological therapies have not been studied extensively in adolescents and young adults with ADHD. However, if you have ADHD, check with your student health or counseling center to see if any special services are available.

Many students with ADHD benefit from strategies such as sitting in the front row to avoid distraction, recording lectures if they have difficulty listening and taking notes at the same time, being allowed extended time for tests, and taking oral rather than written exams.[30] Some students have tried to feign ADHD to qualify for such special treatment or to obtain prescriptions for stimulants. However, a thorough examination by an experienced therapist can usually determine whether a student actually suffers from ADHD.[31]

# Autism and Autism Spectrum Disorders

Autism, a complex neurodevelopmental disability that causes social and communication impairments, is a "spectrum" disorder that includes several disorders with similar features. These problems affect all racial, ethnic, and socioeconomic groups but are four times more likely to occur in boys than girls.

The CDC estimates that between about 1 in 80 and 1 in 240, with an average of 1 in 110, children in the United States have an autism spectrum disorder. Autism rates have risen steadily in recent decades, but the reasons why are not clear. There is no scientific evidence that any part of a vaccine or combination of vaccines causes autism, nor is there proof that any material used to produce the vaccine, such as thimerosal, a mercury-containing preservative, plays a role in causing autism. Although past studies linked vaccines to autism, further investigations have refuted these findings.[32]

Symptoms, which include repetitive patterns of thoughts and behavior and inability to communicate verbally, usually start before age three and can create delays or problems in many different skills that develop from infancy to adulthood. The earlier that interventions begin, the more effective they have proved to be.[33]

Individuals with **Asperger syndrome**, the mildest of the autism spectrum disorders, have autism-like problems in social interaction and communication but normal to above-average intelligence. However, they usually are very rigid and literal and may have trouble understanding nonverbal communications, such as body language. One of their most distinctive symptoms is having such an obsessive interest in a single object or topic that they ignore other objects, topics, or thoughts.

Treatments for managing autism spectrum disorders include behavioral therapy to reinforce wanted behaviors and reduce unwanted behaviors; speech–language therapy to improve ability to communicate and interact with others; physical therapy to build motor control and improve posture and balance; and school-based educational programs. There are no medications specifically for the treatment of autism, but various medicines can help manage associated symptoms.

# Schizophrenia

**Schizophrenia**, one of the most debilitating mental disorders, profoundly impairs an individual's sense of reality. As the National Institute of Mental Health (NIMH) puts it, schizophrenia, which is characterized by abnormalities in brain structure and chemistry, destroys "the inner unity of the mind" and weakens "the will and drive that constitute our essential character." It affects every aspect of psychological functioning, including the ways in which people think, feel, view themselves, and relate to others.

The symptoms of schizophrenia include:

- **Hallucinations.**
- **Delusions.**
- **Inability to think** in a logical manner.
- **Talking** in rambling or incoherent ways.
- **Making odd or purposeless movements** or not moving at all.
- **Repeating others' words** or mimicking their gestures.
- **Showing few, if any, feelings;** responding with inappropriate emotions.

- **Lacking will or motivation** to complete a task or accomplish something.
- **Functioning at a much lower level** than in the past at work, in interpersonal relations, or in taking care of themselves.

Schizophrenia is one of the leading causes of disability among young adults. The mean age for schizophrenia to develop is 21.4 years for men and 26.8 years for women. Although symptoms do not occur until then, they are almost certainly the result of a failure in brain development that occurs very early in life. The underlying defect is probably present before birth. The risk increases along with the age of a father at the birth of his first child.[34] Schizophrenia has a strong genetic basis and is not the result of upbringing, social conditions, or traumatic experiences.

For the vast majority of individuals with schizophrenia, antipsychotic drugs are the foundation of treatment. Newer agents are more effective in making most people with schizophrenia feel more comfortable and in control of themselves, helping organize chaotic thinking, and reducing or eliminating delusions or hallucinations, allowing fuller participation in normal activities.

# Suicide

Suicide is not in itself a psychiatric disorder, but it is often the tragic consequence of emotional and psychological problems. Every year 30,000 Americans—among them many young people who seem to have "everything to live for"—commit suicide, and an estimated 811,000 attempt to take their own lives. There may be 4.5 million suicide "survivors" in the United States.

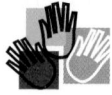 The suicide rate for African American and Caucasian men peaks between ages 20 and 40. It rises again after age 65 among white men and after age 75 among blacks. In general, whites are at highest risk for suicide, followed by American Indians, African Americans, Hispanic Americans, and Asian Americans. Internationally, suicide rates are highest in Germany, Scandinavia, Eastern Europe, and Japan; average in the United States, Canada, and Great Britain; and low in Italy, Spain, and Ireland.

**Asperger syndrome** is a high-functioning form of autism characterized by difficulty interacting socially, repetitive behaviors, clumsiness, and delays in motor development.

**schizophrenia** A general term for a group of mental disorders with characteristic psychotic symptoms, such as delusions, hallucinations, and disordered thought patterns during the active phase of the illness, and a duration of at least six months.

At all ages, men *commit* suicide three to four times more frequently than women, but women *attempt* suicide much more often than men (Table 3.1). Elderly men are ten times more likely to take their own lives than elderly women. (See Chapter 20 for more on depression and suicide in older men and women.

## Suicide in the Young

Suicide rates among youths between ages 10 and 19 in the United States have risen after a decade-long decline. In a national survey, an estimated 15 percent of high school students seriously considered suicide, and 7 percent attempted suicide at least once. Girls and black and Hispanic students were most likely to attempt suicide. Up to 50 percent of adolescents who attempt suicide try again to take their own lives. An estimated 11 percent of those who attempt suicide eventually die by suicide.

The controversy about the use of antidepressants in children and teens may play a role in the spike in youth suicide. Although several re-analyses and reviews have confirmed that these medications can themselves increase the likelihood of suicide in individuals younger than age 20, this risk is small. In many cases, the benefits may well outweigh the risk, but there is a need for careful monitoring for warning signs of suicide whenever a child or teen begins antidepressant therapy.

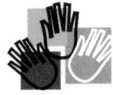 Native American communities have especially high rates of suicide among both young men and women. Young African American men, historically at low suicide risk, are narrowing the gap with their white peers, while suicide by Hispanic young men has declined. The lowest rates are for Asian Pacific males and African American females.

Firearms and suffocation (mainly by hanging) are the most common methods of suicide among young people. In recent years, deaths with firearms have decreased, in part because of laws restricting access to guns by youngsters.

Researchers also have identified factors that protect young people from suicide. Number one for both boys and girls was feeling connected to their parents and family. For girls, emotional well-being was also protective; grade-point average was an additional protective factor for boys.

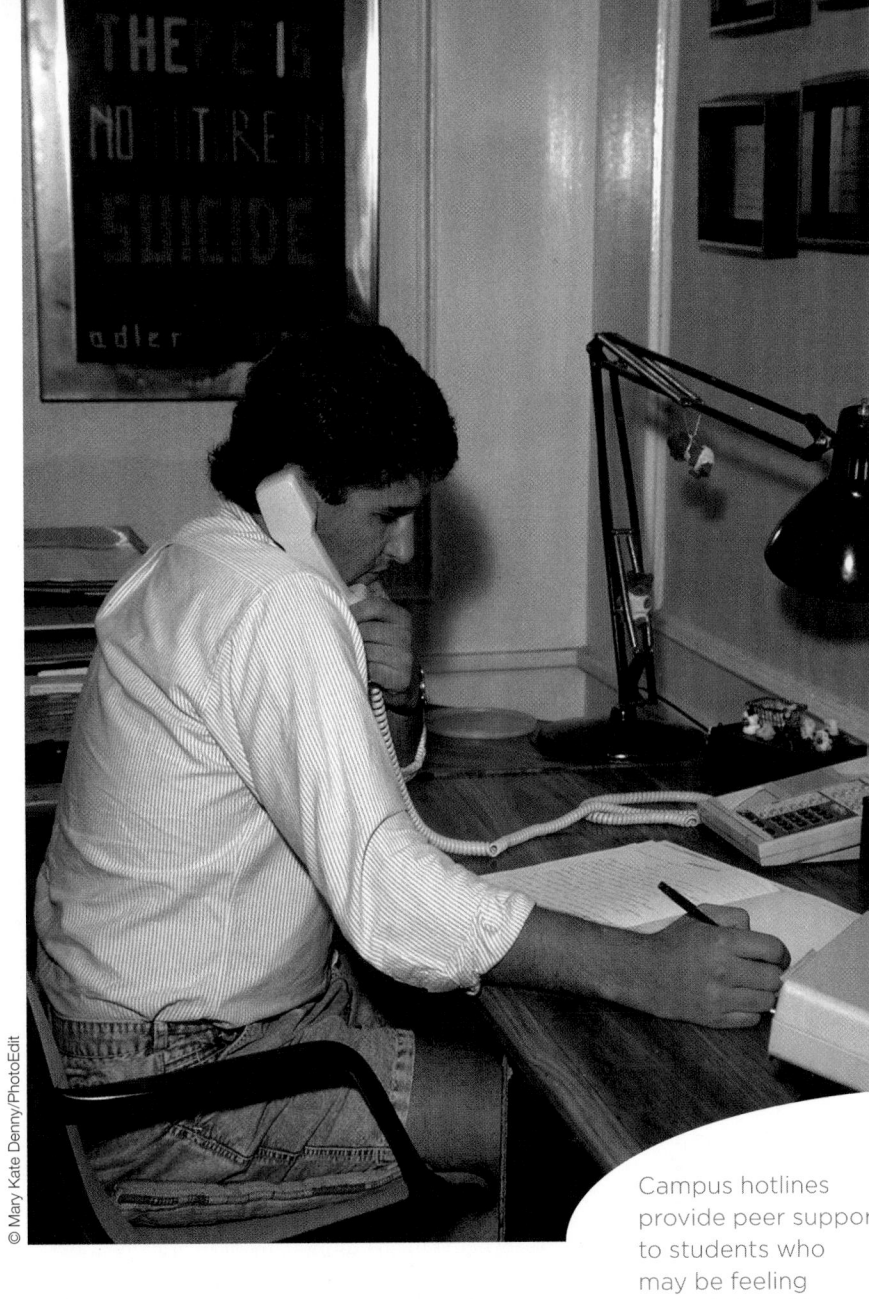

Campus hotlines provide peer support to students who may be feeling overwhelmed but don't know where to turn for help.

Table 3.1 **Suicide Risk**

|  | **Who Attempts Suicide?** | **Who Commits Suicide?** |
|---|---|---|
| Sex | Female | Male |
| Age | Under 35 | Under 20 or over 60 |
| Means | Less deadly, such as a wrist slashing | More deadly, such as a gun |
| Circumstances | High chance of rescue | Low chance of rescue |

## Suicide on Campus

More than 1,100 college students take their own lives every year; 1.5 percent attempt to do so. In a recent survey, 12 percent of students reported suicidal thoughts; 25 percent of these had more than one episode.[35] The rates of self-harm without intent to die are even higher.[36]

The reasons that students consider or attempt suicide vary, but the most significant is untreated depression. Two-thirds of individuals who kill themselves experienced depressive symptoms at the time of their deaths. However, rates of suicide attempts and completions are consistently lower than among college-age peers who are not in college.

Suicide rarely stems from a single cause. Researchers have identified several common ones for college students, including the following:

- Depression or depressive symptoms.
- Family history of mental illness.
- Personality traits, such as hopelessness, helplessness, impulsivity, and aggression.
- Alcohol use and binge drinking. Among college students, binge drinkers are significantly more likely to contemplate suicide, to have attempted suicide in the past, and to believe they would make a future suicide attempt than non-binge drinkers.
- Ineffective problem solving and coping skills.
- Recent sexual or physical victimization; being in an emotionally or physically abusive relationship;
- Family problems.
- Exposure to trauma or stress.
- Feelings of loneliness or social isolation.
- Harassment because of sexual orientation.

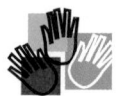 The stress of acculturation (the psychosocial adjustments that occur when an ethnic minority interacts with the ethnic majority, discussed in Chapter 4) may also play a role. Blacks who take their own lives tend to be younger, less likely to have been depressed, and less likely to have financial problems, chronic illness, or substance abuse problems. While alcohol and cocaine play a role in more than 40 percent of suicides by European American youths, they are involved in less than 18 percent of suicides of African Americans.

Although many schools offer counseling and crisis services, students often don't know where to turn when they feel hopeless or are thinking about suicide. In a study of undergraduates, as suicidal thoughts increased, students' help-seeking decreased. Negative feelings or stigma, both about themselves and about getting mental health care, contributed to the inability or unwillingness to reach out for professional help.[37]

## Factors That Lead to Suicide

Researchers have looked for explanations for suicide by studying everything from phases of the moon to seasons (suicides peak in the spring and early summer) to birth order in the family. They have found no conclusive answers. However, the most important risk factors for suicide appear to be impulsivity, high levels of arousal and aggression, and past suicidal behavior.[38] (See Table 3.2 on page 78.)

***Mental Disorders*** More than 95 percent of those who commit suicide have a mental disorder. Two in particular—depression and alcoholism—account for two-thirds of all suicides. Suicide also is a risk for those with other disorders, including schizophrenia, posttraumatic stress disorder, personality disorders, and untreated depression. The lifetime suicide rate for people with major depression is 15 percent.

***Substance Abuse*** Many of those who commit suicide drink beforehand, and their use of alcohol may lower their inhibitions. Since alcohol itself is a depressant, it can intensify the despondency suicidal individuals are already feeling. Alcoholics who attempt suicide often have other risk factors, including major depression, poor social support, serious medical illness, and unemployment. Drugs of abuse also can alter thinking and lower inhibitions against suicide.

***Hopelessness*** The sense of utter hopelessness and helplessness may be the most common contributing factor in suicide. When hope dies, individuals view every experience in negative terms and come to expect the worst possible outcomes for their problems. Given this way of thinking, suicide often seems a reasonable response to a life seen as not worth living. Optimism, on the other hand, correlates with fewer thoughts of suicide by college students.

**Combat Stress** According to a congressional report, veterans who have been exposed to the violence and trauma of combat or deployment in a war zone may account for as many as 20 percent of suicides. Conditions that may increase a veteran's risk of suicide include depression, PTSD, traumatic brain injury, and lack of social support.[39] In response to this, the Veterans Administration has set up a Suicide Prevention Hotline number: 1-800-274-TALK.

**Family History** One of every four people who attempt suicide has a family member who also tried to commit suicide. While a family history of suicide is not in itself considered a predictor of suicide, two mental disorders that can lead to suicide—depression and bipolar disorder (manic depression)—do run in families.

**Physical Illness** People who commit suicide are likely to be ill or to believe that they are. About 5 percent actually have a serious physical disorder, such as AIDS or cancer. While suicide may seem to be a decision rationally arrived at in persons with serious or fatal illness, this may not be the case. Depression, not uncommon in such instances, can warp judgment. When the depression is treated, the person may no longer have suicidal intentions.

**Brain Chemistry** Investigators have found abnormalities in the brain chemistry of individuals who complete suicide, especially low levels of a metabolite of the neurotransmitter serotonin. There are indications that individuals with a deficiency in this substance may have as much as a ten times greater risk of committing suicide than those with higher levels.

**Access to Guns** For individuals already facing a combination of predisposing factors, access to a means of committing suicide, particularly to guns, can add to the risk. Unlike other methods of suicide, guns almost always work. Suicide rates among children, women, and men of all ages are higher in states where more households have guns. Although only 5 percent of suicide attempts involve firearms, more than 90 percent of these attempts are fatal. States with stricter gun-control laws have much lower rates of suicide than states with more lenient laws.

**Other Factors** Individuals who kill themselves have often gone through more major life crises—job changes, births, financial reversals, divorce, retirement—in the previous six months,

## Steps to Prevent Suicide

If you worry that someone you know may be contemplating suicide, express your concern. Here are some specific guidelines:

- **Ask concerned questions.** Listen attentively. Show that you take the person's feelings seriously and truly care.

- **Don't offer trite reassurances.** Don't list reasons to go on living, try to analyze the person's motives, or try to shock or challenge him or her.

- **Suggest solutions or alternatives to problems.** Make plans. Encourage positive action, such as getting away for a while to gain a better perspective on a problem.

- **Don't be afraid to ask whether your friend has considered suicide.** The opportunity to talk about thoughts of suicide may be an enormous relief and—contrary to a long-standing myth—will not fix the idea of suicide more firmly in a person's mind.

- **Don't think that people who talk about killing themselves never carry out their threat.** Most individuals who commit suicide give definite indications of their intent to die.

- **Watch out for behavioral clues.** If your friend begins to behave unpredictably or suddenly emerges from a severe depression into a calm, settled state of mind, these could signal increased danger of suicide. Don't leave your friend alone. Call a suicide hotline, or get in touch with a mental health professional.

## If you are thinking about suicide . . .

- **Talk to a mental health professional.** If you have a therapist, call immediately. If not, call a suicide hotline.

- **Find someone you can trust and talk honestly about what you're feeling.** If you suffer from depression or another mental disorder, educate trusted friends or relatives about your condition so they are prepared if called upon to help.

- **Write down your more uplifting thoughts.** Even if you are despondent, you can help yourself by taking the time to retrieve some more positive thoughts or memories. A simple record of your hopes for the future and the people you value in your life can remind you of why your own life is worth continuing.

- **Avoid drugs and alcohol.** Most suicides are the results of sudden, uncontrolled impulses, and drugs and alcohol can make it harder to resist these destructive urges.

- **Go to the hospital.** Hospitalization can sometimes be the best way to protect your health and safety.

## Table 3.2 **Risk Factors for Suicide**

### Biopsychosocial Risk Factors

- Mental disorders, particularly depressive disorders, schizophrenia, and anxiety disorders
- Alcohol and other substance use disorders
- Hopelessness
- Impulsive and/or aggressive tendencies
- History of trauma or abuse
- Some major physical illness
- Previous suicide attempt
- Family history of suicide

### Environmental Risk Factors

- Job or financial loss
- Relational or social loss
- Easy access to lethal means
- Local clusters of suicide that have a contagious influence

### Sociocultural Risk Factors

- Lack of social support and sense of isolation
- Stigma associated with help-seeking behavior
- Barriers to accessing health care, especially mental health and substance abuse treatment
- Certain cultural and religious beliefs (for instance, the belief that suicide is a noble resolution of a personal dilemma)
- Exposure to suicide, including through the media, and the influence of others who have died by suicide

Source: Suicide Prevention Resource Center: http://www.sprc.org/

compared with others. Long-standing, intense conflict with family members or other important people may add to the danger. In some cases, suicide may be an act of revenge that offers the person a sense of control—however temporary or illusory. For example, some may feel that, by rejecting life, they are rejecting a partner or parent who abandoned or betrayed them.

# Overcoming Problems of the Mind

About 80 percent of those with mental disorders eventually seek treatment, but many suffer for years, even decades. As discussed earlier in this chapter, college students are especially likely to delay getting help for a psychological problem.

The median delay for all disorders is nearly ten years. Those with social phobia and separation anxiety disorders may not get help for more than 20 years. The earlier in life that a disorder begins, the longer that individuals tend to delay treatment.

Without treatment, mental disorders take a toll on every aspect of life, including academics, relationships, careers, and risk-taking. Symptoms or episodes of a disorder typically become more frequent or severe. Individuals with one mental disorder are at high risk of having a second one (this is called comorbidity).

## Getting Help for a Psychological Problem

Sometimes we all need outside help from a trained, licensed professional to work through personal problems. Here is what you need to know if you are experiencing psychological difficulties.

Consider therapy if you

- Feel an overwhelming and prolonged sense of helplessness and sadness, which does not lift despite your efforts and help from family and friends.
- Find it difficult to carry out everyday activities such as homework, and your academic performance is suffering.
- Worry excessively, expect the worst, or are constantly on edge.
- Are finding it hard to resist or are engaging in behaviors that are harmful to you or others, such as drinking too much alcohol, abusing drugs, or becoming aggressive or violent.
- Have persistent thoughts or fantasies of harming yourself or others.

Most people who have at least several sessions of psychotherapy are far better off than individuals with emotional difficulties who do not get treatment. According to the American Psychological Association, 50 percent of patients noticeably improve after eight sessions, while 75 percent of individuals in therapy improved by the end of six months.

## Where to Turn for Help

As a student, your best contact for identifying local services may be your health education instructor or department. The health instructors can tell you about general and mental health counseling available on campus, school-based support groups, community-based programs, and special emergency services. On campus, you can also turn to the student health services or the office of the dean of student services or student affairs. (See "Help Yourself" in *Labs for IPC*.)

Within the community, you may be able to get help through the city or county health department and neighborhood health centers. Local hospitals often have special clinics and services; and there are usually local branches of national service organizations, such as United Way or Alcoholics Anonymous, other 12-step programs, and various support groups. You can call the psychiatric or psychological association in your city or state for the names of licensed professionals. (Check the telephone directory for listings.) Your primary physician may also be able to help.

Search the Internet for special programs, found either by the nature of the service, by the name of the neighborhood or city, or by the name of the sponsoring group. In addition to suicide-prevention programs, look for crisis intervention, violence prevention, and child-abuse prevention programs; drug-treatment information; shelters for battered women; senior citizen centers; and self-help and counseling services. Many services have special hotlines for coping with emergencies. Others provide information as well as counseling over the phone.

*Types of Therapists*   Only professionally trained individuals who have met state licensing requirements are certified as psychiatrists, psychologists, or social workers. Before selecting any of these mental health professionals, be sure to check the person's background and credentials.

**Psychiatrists** are licensed medical doctors (M.D.) who complete medical school; a year-long internship; and a three-year residency that provides training in various forms of psychotherapy, psychopharmacology, and both

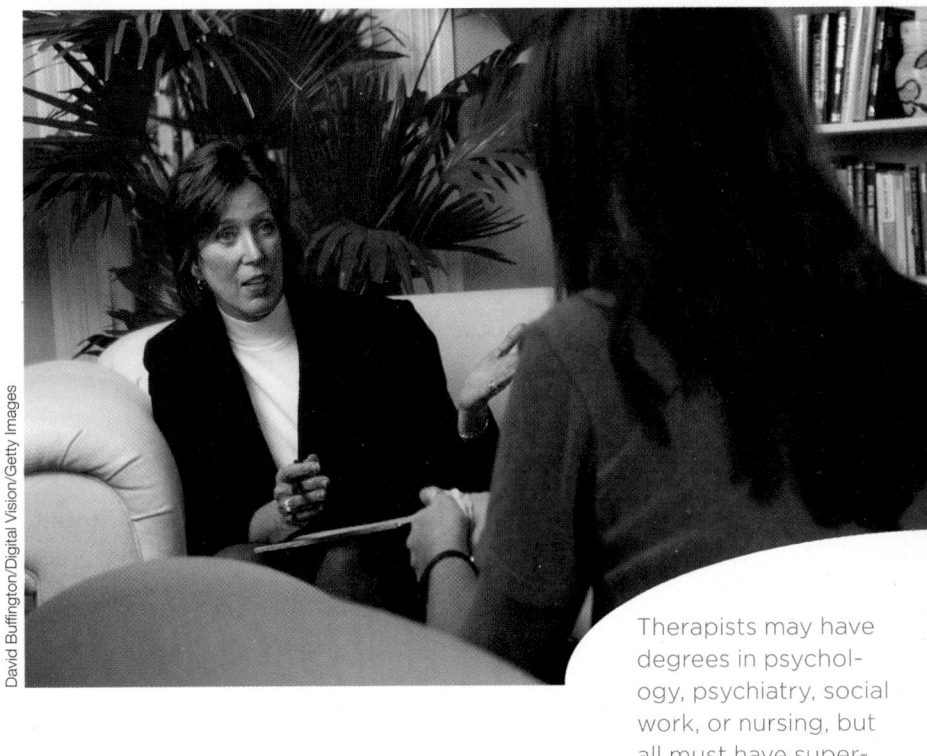

David Buffington/Digital Vision/Getty Images

Therapists may have degrees in psychology, psychiatry, social work, or nursing, but all must have supervised clinical training and meet state licensing requirements.

outpatient and inpatient treatment of mental disorders. They can prescribe medications and make medical decisions. *Board-certified* psychiatrists have passed oral and written examinations following completion of residency training.

**Psychologists** complete a graduate program (including clinical training and internships) in human psychology but do not study medicine and cannot prescribe medication. They must be licensed in most states in order to practice independently.

**Certified social workers** or **licensed clinical social workers** (**LCSWs**) usually complete a two-year graduate program and have specialized training in helping people with mental problems in addition to conventional social work.

**Psychiatric nurses** have nursing degrees and have passed a state examination. They usually have special training and experience in mental health care, although no specialty licensing or certification is required.

**Marriage and family therapists**, licensed in some but not all states, usually have a graduate degree, often in psychology, and at least two years of supervised clinical training in dealing with relationship problems.

**psychiatrist** Licensed medical doctor with additional training in psychotherapy, psychopharmacology, and treatment of mental disorders.

**psychologist** Mental health care professional who has completed doctoral or graduate program in psychology and is trained in psychotherapeutic techniques, but who is not medically trained and does not prescribe medications.

**certified social worker or licensed clinical social worker (LCSW)** A person who has completed a two-year graduate program in counseling people with mental problems.

**psychiatric nurse** A nurse with special training and experience in mental health care.

**marriage and family therapist** A psychiatrist, psychologist, or social worker who specializes in marriage and family counseling.

Other therapists include pastoral counselors, members of the clergy who offer psychological counseling; hypnotherapists, who use hypnosis for problems such as smoking and obesity; stress-management counselors, who teach relaxation methods; and alcohol and drug counselors, who help individuals with substance abuse problems. Anyone can use these terms to describe themselves professionally, and there are no licensing requirements.

*Choosing a Therapist* Ask your physician or another health professional. Call your local or state psychological association. Consult your university or college department of psychology or health center. Contact your area community mental health center. Inquire at your church or synagogue.

- A good rapport with your psychotherapist is critical. Choose someone with whom you feel comfortable and at ease.
- Ask the following questions:
  - Are you licensed?
  - How long have you been practicing?
  - I have been feeling (anxious, tense, depressed, etc.), and I'm having problems (with school, relationships, eating, sleeping, etc.). What experience do you have helping people with these types of problems?
  - What are your areas of expertise— phobias? ADHD? depression?
  - What kinds of treatments do you use? Have they proved effective for dealing with my kind of problem or issue?
  - What are your fees? (Fees are usually based on a 45-minute to 50-minute session.) Do you have a sliding-scale fee policy?
  - How much therapy would you recommend?
  - What types of insurance do you accept?

As you begin therapy, establish clear goals with your therapist. Some goals require more time to reach than others. You and your therapist should decide at what point you might expect to begin to see progress.

As they begin therapy, some people may have difficulty discussing painful and troubling experiences. Feelings of relief or hope are positive signs indicating that you are starting to explore your thoughts and behaviors.

## Types of Therapy

The term **psychotherapy** refers to any type of counseling based on the exchange of words in the context of the unique relationship that develops between a mental health professional and a person seeking help. The process of talking and listening can lead to new insight, relief from distressing psychological symptoms, changes in unhealthy or maladaptive behaviors, and more effective ways of dealing with the world. "Spirituality oriented" psychotherapy pays particular attention to the roles that religion and spiritual and religious beliefs play in an individual's psychological life.[40]

Landmark research has shown that psychotherapy does not just benefit the mind but actually changes the brain. In studies comparing psychotherapy and psychiatric medications as treatments for depression, both proved about equally effective. But a particular group of patients— those who had lost a parent at an early age or had experienced childhood trauma, including physical or sexual abuse—gained greater benefits with talk therapy.

The most common goal of psychotherapy is to improve quality of life. Most mental health professionals today are trained in a variety of psychotherapeutic techniques and tailor their approach to the problem, personality, and needs of each person seeking their help. Because skilled therapists may combine different techniques in the course of therapy, the lines between the various approaches often blur.

Brief or short-term psychotherapy typically focuses on a central theme, problem, or topic and may continue for several weeks to several months. The individuals most likely to benefit are those who are interested in solving immediate problems rather than changing their characters, who can think in psychological terms, and who are motivated to change.

*Psychodynamic Psychotherapy* For the most part, today's mental health professionals base their assessment of individuals on a **psychodynamic** understanding that takes into account the role of early experiences and unconscious influences in *actively* shaping behavior. (This is the *dynamic* in psychodynamic.) Psychodynamic treatments work toward the goal

**psychotherapy** Treatment designed to produce a response by psychological rather than physical means, such as suggestion, persuasion, reassurance, and support.

**psychodynamic** Interpreting behaviors in terms of early experiences and unconscious influences.

of providing greater insight into problems and bringing about behavioral change. Therapy may be brief, consisting of 12 to 25 sessions, or may continue for several years.

### Cognitive-Behavioral Therapy (CBT)

Cognitive-behavioral therapy (CBT) focuses on inappropriate or inaccurate thoughts or beliefs to help individuals break out of a distorted way of thinking. The techniques of **cognitive therapy** include identification of an individual's beliefs and attitudes, recognition of negative thought patterns, and education in alternative ways of thinking. Individuals with major depression or anxiety disorders are most likely to benefit, usually in 15 to 25 sessions. However, many of the positive messages used in cognitive therapy can help anyone improve a bad mood or negative outlook.

**Behavioral therapy** strives to substitute healthier ways of behaving for maladaptive patterns used in the past. Its premise is that distressing psychological symptoms, like all behaviors, are learned responses that can be modified or unlearned. Some therapists believe that changing behavior also changes how people think and feel. As they put it, "Change the behavior, and the feelings will follow." Behavioral therapies work best for disorders characterized by specific, abnormal patterns of acting—such as alcohol and drug abuse, anxiety disorders, and phobias—and for individuals who want to change bad habits.

### Interpersonal Therapy (IPT)

**Interpersonal therapy** (**IPT**), originally developed for research into the treatment of major depression, focuses on relationships in order to help individuals deal with unrecognized feelings and needs and improve their communication skills. IPT does not deal with the psychological origins of symptoms but rather concentrates on current problems of getting along with others. The supportive, empathic relationship that is developed with the therapist, who takes an even more active role than in psychodynamic psychotherapy, is the most crucial component of this therapy. The emphasis is on the here and now and on interpersonal—rather than intrapsychic—issues. Individuals with major depression, chronic difficulties developing relationships, and chronic mild depression are most likely to benefit. IPT usually consists of 12 to 16 sessions.

## Other Treatment Options

*Psychiatric Drugs* Medications that alter brain chemistry and relieve psychiatric symptoms have brought great hope and help to millions of people. Thanks to the recent development of a new generation of more precise and effective **psychiatric drugs**, success rates for treating many common and disabling disorders—depression, panic disorder, schizophrenia, and others—have soared. Often used in conjunction with psychotherapy, sometimes used as the primary treatment, these medications have revolutionized mental health care.

At some point in their lives, about half of all Americans will take a psychiatric drug. The reason may be depression, anxiety, a sleep difficulty, an eating disorder, alcohol or drug dependence, impaired memory, or another disorder that disrupts the intricate chemistry of the brain.

Psychiatric drugs are now among the most widely prescribed drugs in the United States. Serotonin-boosting medications (SSRIs) have become the drugs of choice in treating depression. They also are effective in treating obsessive-compulsive disorder, panic disorder, social phobia, posttraumatic stress disorder, premenstrual dysphoric disorder, and generalized anxiety disorder. In patients who don't respond, psychiatrists may add another drug to boost the efficacy of the treatment.

 According to various studies, 5 to 7 percent of college students take antidepressant medications. Direct-to-consumer advertisements for antidepressant drugs can influence students' perceptions of what is wrong with them. In one study, college women were more likely to rate themselves as having mild-to-moderate depression as a result of reading pharmaceutical company information for popular antidepressants.

*Alternative Mind-Mood Products* People with serious mental illnesses, including depression and bipolar disorder, often use at least one alternative health-care practice, such as yoga or meditation. In a recent survey of women with depression, about half (54 percent) reported trying herbs, vitamins, and manual therapies such as massage and acupressure. Some "natural"

**cognitive therapy** A technique used to identify an individual's beliefs and attitudes, recognize negative thought patterns, and educate in alternative ways of thinking.

**behavioral therapy** A technique that emphasizes application of the principles of learning to substitute desirable responses and behavior patterns for undesirable ones.

**interpersonal therapy (IPT)** A technique used to develop communication skills and relationships.

**psychiatric drugs** Medications that regulate a person's mental, emotional, and physical functions to facilitate normal functioning.

## Before Taking a Psychiatric Drug

Before taking any psychoactive drug (one that affects the brain), talk to a qualified health professional. Here are some points to raise:

- **What can this medication do for me?** What specific symptoms will it relieve? Are there other possible benefits?

- **When will I notice a difference?** How long does it take for the medicine to have an effect?

- **Are there any risks?** What about side effects? Do I have to take it before or after eating? Will it affect my ability to study, work, drive, or operate machinery?

- **Is there a risk of suicide or increased aggression?** What should I do if I start thinking about taking my own life or of harming others?

products, such as herbs and enzymes, claim to have psychological effects. However, they have not undergone rigorous scientific testing.

St. John's wort has been used to treat anxiety and depression in Europe for many years. Data from clinical studies in the United States do not support the efficacy of St. John's wort for moderate to severe depression. In ten carefully controlled studies, the herb did not prove more effective than a placebo. However, more than two dozen studies have found that St. John's wort was similar in efficacy to standard antidepressants. Side effects include dizziness, abdominal pain and bloating, constipation, nausea, fatigue, and dry mouth. St. John's wort should not be taken in combination with other prescription antidepressants. St. John's wort can lower the efficacy of oral contraceptives and increase the risk of an unwanted pregnancy.

## Build Your Future

# Taking Care of Your Mental Health

Like physical health, psychological well-being is not a fixed state of being, but a process. The way you live every day affects how you feel about yourself and your world. Here are some basic guidelines that you can rely on to make the most of the process of living. Check those that you commit to making part of your mental and psychological self-care:

____ **Accept yourself.** As a human being, you are, by definition, imperfect. Come to terms with the fact that you are a worthwhile person despite your mistakes.

____ **Respect yourself.** Recognize your abilities and talents. Acknowledge your competence and achievements, and take pride in them.

____ **Trust yourself.** Learn to listen to the voice within you, and let your intuition be your guide.

____ **Love yourself.** Be happy to spend time by yourself. Learn to appreciate your own company and to be glad you're you.

____ **Stretch yourself.** Be willing to change and grow, to try something new and dare to be vulnerable.

____ **Look at challenges as opportunities for personal growth.** "Every problem brings the possibility of a widening of consciousness," psychologist Carl Jung once noted. Put his words to the test.

____ **When your internal critic**—the negative inner voice we all have—starts putting you down, force yourself to think of a situation that you handled well.

____ **Set a limit on self-pity.** Tell yourself, "I'm going to feel sorry for myself this morning, but this afternoon, I've got to get on with my life."

____ **Think of not only where but also who you want to be a decade from now.** The goals you set, the decisions you make, the values you adopt now will determine how you feel about yourself and your life in the future.

# Recognizing Depression

Depression comes in different forms, just like other illnesses such as heart disease. Not everyone with a depressive disorder experiences every symptom. The number and severity of symptoms may vary among individuals and also over time.

Read through the following list, and check all the descriptions that apply.

- ☐ I am often restless and irritable.
- ☐ I am having irregular sleep patterns—either too much or not enough.
- ☐ I don't enjoy hobbies, my friends, family, or leisure activities any more.
- ☐ I am having trouble managing my diabetes, hypertension, or other chronic illness.
- ☐ I have nagging aches and pains that do not get better no matter what I do.
- ☐ Specifically, I often experience:
  - ☐ Digestive problems
  - ☐ Headache or backache
  - ☐ Vague aches and pains like joint or muscle pains
  - ☐ Chest pains
  - ☐ Dizziness
- ☐ I have trouble concentrating or making simple decisions.
- ☐ Others have commented on my mood or attitude lately.
- ☐ My weight has changed a considerable amount.
- ☐ I have had several of the symptoms I checked above for more than two weeks.
- ☐ I feel that my functioning in my everyday life (work, family, friends) is suffering because of these problems.
- ☐ I have a family history of depression.
- ☐ I have thought about suicide.*

Checking several items on this list does not mean that you have a depressive disorder because many conditions can cause similar symptoms. However, you should take this list with you to discuss with your health-care provider or mental health therapist. Even though it can be difficult to talk about certain things, your health-care provider is knowledgeable, trained, and committed to helping you.

If you can't think of what to say, try these conversation starters:

"I just don't feel like myself lately."

"My friend (parent, roommate, spouse) thinks I might be depressed."

"I haven't been sleeping well lately."

"Everything seems harder than before."

"Nothing's fun anymore."

If you are diagnosed with depression, remember that it is a common and highly treatable illness with medical causes. Your habits or personality did not cause your depression, and you do not have to face it alone.

*University of Michigan Depression Center, 800-475-MICH, www.med.umich.edu/depression

# Making Change Happen

## Your Psychological Self-Care Pyramid

Your physical well-being and psychological health are so intimately related that to a significant degree they are expressions of each other. Yes, grave diseases can occur despite a healthy mental outlook, and physically healthy people can experience psychological difficulties. But overwhelming evidence demonstrates that physical health affects mood and thoughts, and mood and thoughts affect physical health.

"Your Psychological Self-Care Pyramid" from *Labs for IPC* deals with optimizing your psychological health to benefit body, mind, and spirit. It will teach you how to infuse your life with mentally rewarding and stimulating activities that not only provide balance, prevent the blahs, and add zest but also, if continued, form a lifelong foundation for optimal mental health. Here's a preview.

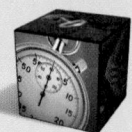

### Get Real

In this stage you rate yourself from 0 to 10, with 0 being the low end and 10 the high end, on the degree to which you now include or exhibit in your weekly life the 13 elements of Your Psychological Self-Care Pyramid shown in *Labs for IPC*. Here are three examples:

- **Self-knowledge and self-control.** \_\_\_\_
  You make your inner world of feelings and thoughts and your relationship to the outer world a source of ongoing contemplation. You seek self-understanding and systematically develop your ability to consider and weigh actions before taking them.

- **Community.** \_\_\_\_
  You have a circle of trusted friends and participate in a larger social milieu. You look out for and assist the interests of the community as a whole, not merely those of your circle of immediate friends.

- **Generosity.** \_\_\_\_
  You are giving of your time and your self both toward others and toward yourself. You give materially when this is advisable but more than that when asked you give that which is most precious—that is, who you are.

You will then examine your self-ratings. Are some unacceptably lower than you would like them to be? Completing this lab will address this concern for the short run and, if you continue the activities, for the future.

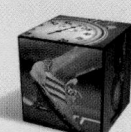

### Get Ready

In this stage you examine your schedule and create pockets of time for the activities that serve as building blocks of Your Psychological Self-Care Pyramid and for journaling about your experiences doing so.

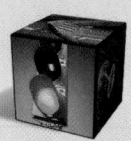

### Get Going

In this stage you begin the exercises related to each of the areas you want to bolster by engaging in related activities for at least five minutes four times per week. *Immediately after* completing the exercise or at some other point the *same* day, you will make an entry of at least five lines in your *IPC Journal* and reflect on your experiences . . .

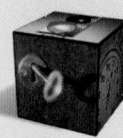

### Lock It In

Just as you can use the USDA Food Pyramid to guide your eating choices every day, pay attention to Your Psychological Self-Care Pyramid. Here is one of the steps that can ensure that you are providing adequate daily nourishment for your mind and spirit.

- **Rate yourself.** Every four weeks rate yourself between 0 and 10, with 0 being the low end and 10 the high end, on each element of Your Psychological Self-Care Pyramid. Record your scores.

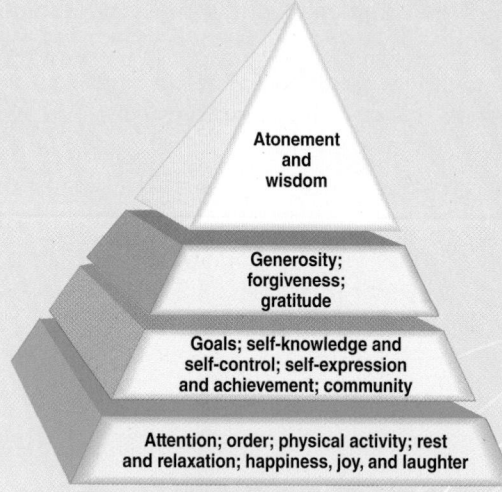

Atonement and wisdom

Generosity; forgiveness; gratitude

Goals; self-knowledge and self-control; self-expression and achievement; community

Attention; order; physical activity; rest and relaxation; happiness, joy, and laughter

## Review Questions

1. Depression
   a. is not likely to occur in young adults.
   b. is twice as common in men as women.
   c. has the same symptoms in men and women.
   d. is more likely to occur again in those who suffer a first episode.

2. Which statement about depression treatment is true?
   a. Psychotherapy and drug therapy are effective in treating depression, but only about 50 percent of people seek treatment.
   b. Antidepressants help about 90 percent of individuals feel better within four weeks.
   c. Jogging has only a small benefit for most depressed individuals.
   d. With the right therapy, depression will not reoccur.

3. Neurons
   a. transmit information within the brain and throughout the body by means of electrical impulses and chemical messengers.
   b. are specialized support cells that travel through the spinal cord, carrying signals related to movement.
   c. are protein molecules designed to bind with neurotransmitters.
   d. cross a synapse before reuptake.

4. Students with attention-deficit/hyperactivity disorder
   a. perform as well on standardized tests as students without ADHD.
   b. have an increased risk of substance use disorders.
   c. have a decreased risk of developing depression or anxiety disorders.
   d. constitute 10 percent of the student population.

5. Some characteristic symptoms of major depression are
   a. difficulty concentrating, lack of energy, and eating more than usual.
   b. exaggerated sense of euphoria and energy.
   c. palpitations, sweating, numbness, and tingling sensations.
   d. talking in rambling ways, inability to think in a logical manner, and delusions.

6. Which of the following statements is true?
   a. Individuals with phobias are most likely to benefit from psychiatric medications.
   b. Antidepressant medications now require a warning label about the increased risk of suicidal thoughts.
   c. Only children have attention disorders.
   d. Interpersonal therapy focuses on the role of early experiences and unconscious influences in shaping patterns of behavior, such as repeated failed relationships.

7. Which of the following statements about anxiety disorders is true?
   a. Anxiety disorders are the least prevalent type of mental illness.
   b. An individual suffering from a panic attack may mistake her symptoms for a heart attack.
   c. The primary symptom of obsessive-compulsive disorder is irrational, intense, and persistent fear of a specific object or situation.
   d. Generalized anxiety disorders respond to systematic desensitization behavior therapy.

8. A mental disorder can be described as
   a. a condition associated with migraine headaches and narcolepsy.
   b. a condition that is usually caused by severe trauma to the brain.
   c. a behavioral or psychological disorder that impairs an individual's ability to conduct one or more important activities of daily life.
   d. a psychological disorder that is easily controlled with medication and a change in diet.

9. A person may be at higher risk of committing suicide if
   a. he is taking blood pressure medication.
   b. he lives in a rural environment and is married.
   c. he has been diagnosed with hyperactivity disorder.
   d. he has lost his job because of alcoholism.

10. Which of these therapies focuses on recognizing negative thought patterns and changing those patterns?
    a. psychodynamic psychotherapy
    b. behavioral activation
    c. interpersonal therapy
    d. cognitive therapy

*Answers to these questions can be found on page 672.*

## Critical Thinking

1. Jake, who took antidepressants to recover from depression in high school, began feeling the same troubling symptoms. A physician at the student health center prescribed the same medication that had helped him in the past, but this time Jake noticed the warning about an increased risk of suicide. He has had thoughts of killing himself, and he worries whether or not to start the medication. When he did some online research, he learned that the risk of suicide is greater if depression is untreated than it is with medication. How would you counsel Jake? How would you weigh the risks and benefits of taking an antidepressant? Do you know someone who might benefit from taking antidepressants but is afraid to take them because of the possible risk of suicide? What might you say to this person based on what you have read in this chapter?

2. Research has indicated that many homeless men and women are in need of outpatient psychiatric care, often because they suffer from chronic mental illnesses or alcoholism. Yet government funding for the mentally ill is inadequate, and homelessness itself can make it difficult, if not impossible, for people to gain access to the care they need. How do you feel when you pass homeless individuals who seem disoriented or out of touch with reality? Who should take responsibility for their welfare? Should they be forced to undergo treatment at psychiatric institutions?

## Media Menu

Visit www.cengagebrain.com to access course materials and companion resources for this text that will:

- Help you evaluate your knowledge of the material.

- Allow you to prepare for exams with interactive quizzing.

- Use the CengageNOW product to develop a Personalized Learning Plan targeting resources that address areas you should study.

- Coach you through identifying target goals for behavioral change and creating and monitoring your personal change plan throughout the semester using the Behavior Change Planner available in the CengageNOW resource.

## Internet Connections

**www.save.org**
This site (formerly American Foundation for Suicide Prevention) offers research, facts, survivor support, and more.

**www.nimh.nih.gov**
The National Institute of Mental Health is a federally sponsored organization that provides useful information on a variety of mental health topics including current mental health research.

**www.apa.org**
The APA is the scientific and professional organization for psychology in the United States. Its website provides up-to-date information on psychological issues and disorders.

**www.nmha.org**
This site features fact sheets on a variety of mental health topics, including depression screening, college initiative, substance abuse prevention, and information for families. Also available are current mental health articles, an e-mail newsletter, and a bookstore.

**www.afsp.org**
This site provides facts and statistics about suicide and depression, as well as information about current research and educational projects. It also provides support information for survivors.

**www.activeminds.org**
This site provides fact sheets on mental illness and information about starting an Active Minds chapter and planning events at your campus to create awareness about mental health.

## Key Terms

The terms listed are used on the page indicated. Definitions
of the terms are in the Glossary at the end of the book.

antidepressant  59

anxiety disorders  70

Asperger syndrome  74

attention-deficit/hyperactivity
disorder (ADHD)  72

axon  58

axon terminal  58

behavioral therapy  81

bipolar disorder  69

certified social worker or licensed
clinical social worker  79

cognitive therapy  81

dendrites  58

dysthymia  67

generalized anxiety disorder
(GAD)  70

glia  58

interpersonal therapy (IPT)  81

major depression  67

marriage and family therapist  79

mental disorder  61

neuron  58

neuropsychiatry  57

neurotransmitters  59

nucleus  58

obsessive-compulsive disorder
(OCD)  70

panic attack  70

panic disorder  71

phobia  70

psychiatric drugs  81

psychiatric nurse  79

psychiatrist  79

psychodynamic  80

psychologist  79

psychotherapy  80

receptors  59

reuptake  59

schizophrenia  74

synapse  59

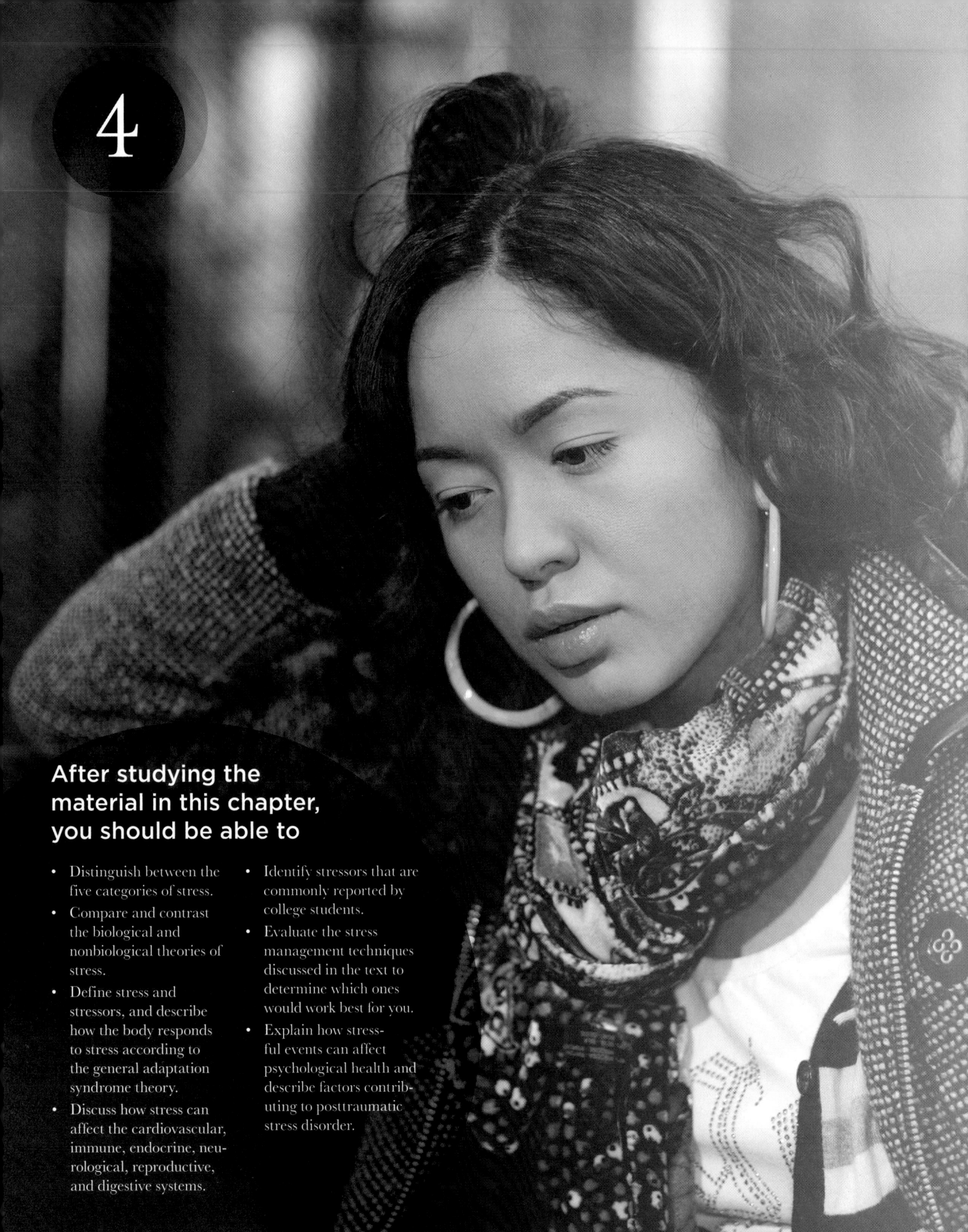

# 4

## After studying the material in this chapter, you should be able to

- Distinguish between the five categories of stress.
- Compare and contrast the biological and nonbiological theories of stress.
- Define stress and stressors, and describe how the body responds to stress according to the general adaptation syndrome theory.
- Discuss how stress can affect the cardiovascular, immune, endocrine, neurological, reproductive, and digestive systems.

- Identify stressors that are commonly reported by college students.
- Evaluate the stress management techniques discussed in the text to determine which ones would work best for you.
- Explain how stressful events can affect psychological health and describe factors contributing to posttraumatic stress disorder.

Getting laid off felt like a punch in the stomach. Chayla had heard the rumors about all part-time positions being eliminated. But her boss always said she was the best assistant they had ever hired. And now she was fired—with tuition, rent, and insurance bills all due in a month. And so in between writing papers and preparing for finals, Chayla would have to look for another job. Just thinking about all she had to do made her head throb.

# Personal Stress Management

Like Chayla, you live with stress every day, whether you're studying for exams, meeting people, facing new experiences, or figuring out how to live on a budget. You're not alone. College students rank stress as the top impediment to their academic performance. Everyone, regardless of age, gender, race, or income, has to deal with stress—as an individual and as a member of society.

As researchers have demonstrated time and again, stress has profound effects, both immediate and long-term, on our bodies and minds. While stress alone doesn't cause disease, it triggers molecular changes throughout the body that make us more susceptible to many illnesses. Its impact on the mind is no less significant. The burden of chronic stress can undermine one's ability to cope with day-to-day hassles and can exacerbate psychological problems like depression and anxiety disorders.

Yet stress in itself isn't necessarily bad. What matters most is not the stressful situation itself, but an individual's response to it. This chapter will help you learn to anticipate stressful events,

to manage day-to-day hassles, to prevent stress overload, and to find alternatives to running endlessly on a treadmill of alarm, panic, and exhaustion. As you organize your schedule, find ways to release tension, and build up coping skills, you will begin to experience the sense of control and confidence that makes stress a challenge rather than an ordeal.

## What Is Stress?

People use the word *stress* in different ways: as an external force that causes a person to become tense or upset, as the internal state of arousal, and as the physical response of the body to various demands. Dr. Hans Selye, a pioneer in studying physiological responses to challenge, defined **stress** as "the nonspecific response of the body to any demand made upon it." In other words, the body reacts to **stressors**—the things that upset or excite us—in the same way, regardless of whether they are positive or negative.

**stress** The nonspecific response of the body to any demands made upon it; may be characterized by muscle tension and acute anxiety, or may be a positive force for action.

**stressors** Specific or nonspecific agents or situations that cause the stress response in a body.

Visit www.cengagebrain.com to access course materials for this text, including the Behavior Change Planner, interactive quizzes, tutorials, and more. See the preface on page xv for details.

© clokr/Shutterstock.com

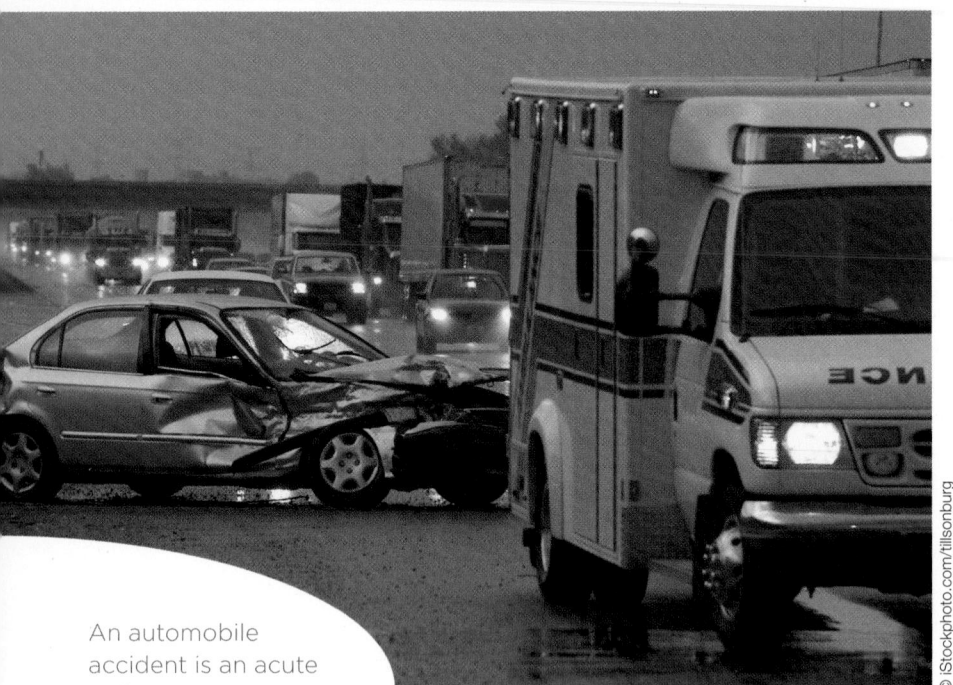

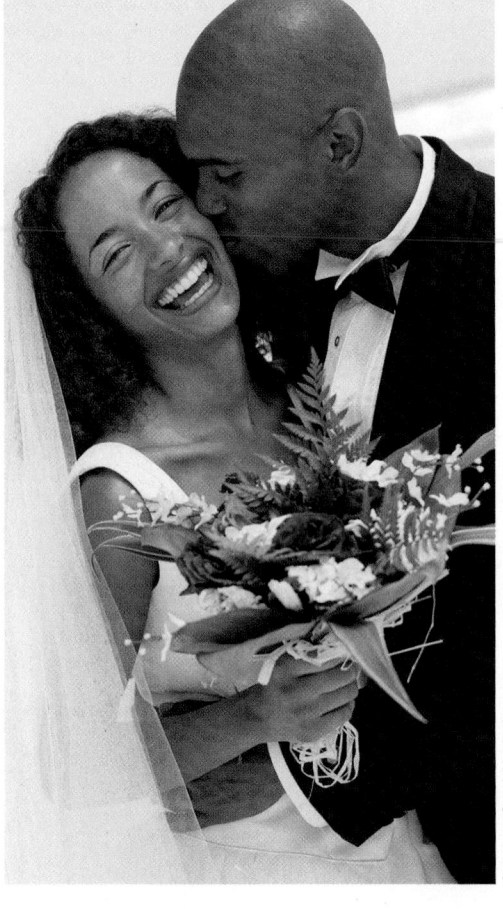

An automobile accident is an acute negative stressor. A wedding is an example of a positive stressor that triggers both joy and anxiety.

Based on nearly 300 studies over four decades, researchers have distinguished five categories of stressors:

- **Acute time-limited stressors** include anxiety-provoking situations such as having to give a talk in public or work out a math problem, such as calculating a tip or dividing a bill, under pressure.

- **Brief naturalistic stressors** are more serious challenges such as taking SATs or meeting a deadline for a big project.

- **Stressful event sequences** are the difficult consequences of a natural disaster or another traumatic occurrence, such as the death of a spouse. The individuals involved recognize that these difficulties will end at some point in the future.

- **Chronic stressors** are ongoing demands caused by life-changing circumstances, such as permanent disability following an accident or caregiving for a parent with dementia, that do not have any clear end point.

- **Distant stressors** are traumatic experiences that occurred long ago, such as child abuse or combat, yet continue to have an emotional and psychological impact.

Not all stressors are negative. Some of life's happiest moments—births, reunions, weddings—are enormously stressful. We weep with the stress of frustration or loss; we weep, too, with the stress of love and joy. Selye coined the term **eustress** for positive stress in our lives (*eu* is a Greek prefix meaning "good"). Eustress challenges us to grow, adapt, and find creative solutions in our lives. **Distress** refers to the negative effects of stress that can deplete or even destroy life energy. Ideally, the level of stress in our lives should be just high enough to motivate us to satisfy our needs and not so high that it interferes with our ability to reach our fullest potential.

## What Causes Stress?

The scientific study of stress began more than a century ago. Over the years scientists have formulated various theories about the nature of stress. Some place greater emphasis on physiological aspects; others, on psychological and social dimensions. The following are among the most influential.

**eustress** Positive stress, which stimulates a person to function properly.

**distress** A negative stress that may result in illness.

## The General Adaptation Syndrome

Of the many biological theories of stress, the best known may be the **general adaptation syndrome (GAS)**, developed by Hans Selye. He postulated that our bodies constantly strive to maintain a stable and consistent physiological state, called **homeostasis**. Stressors, whether in the form of physical illness or a demanding job, disturb this state and trigger a nonspecific physiological response. The body attempts to restore homeostasis by means of an **adaptive response**.

Selye's general adaptation syndrome, which describes the body's response to a stressor—whether threatening or exhilarating—consists of three distinct stages:

1. **Alarm.** When a stressor first occurs, the body responds with changes that temporarily lower resistance. Levels of certain hormones may rise; blood pressure may increase (Figure 4.1). The body quickly makes internal adjustments to cope with the stressor and return to normal activity.

2. **Resistance.** If the stressor continues, the body mobilizes its internal resources to try to sustain homeostasis. For example, if a loved one is seriously hurt in an accident, we initially respond intensely and feel great anxiety. During the subsequent stressful period of recuperation, we struggle to carry on as normally as possible, but this requires considerable effort.

3. **Exhaustion.** If the stress continues long enough, we cannot keep up our normal functioning. Even a small amount of additional stress at this point can cause a breakdown.

## Cognitive-Transactional Model

Among the nonbiological theories is the cognitive-transactional model of stress, developed by Richard Lazarus, which looks at the relation between stress and health. As he sees it, stress can have a powerful impact on health. Conversely, health can affect a person's resistance or coping ability. Stress, according to Lazarus, is "neither an environmental stimulus, a characteristic of the person, nor a response, but a

**Figure 4.1 General Adaptation Syndrome (GAS)**
The three stages of Selye's GAS are alarm, resistance, and exhaustion.

Source: From A. Maslow, R. Frager (ed.), J. Fadiman (ed.), *Motivation and Personality*, 3rd ed. 1987. Electronically reproduced by permission of Pearson Education, Inc., Upper Saddle River, NJ.

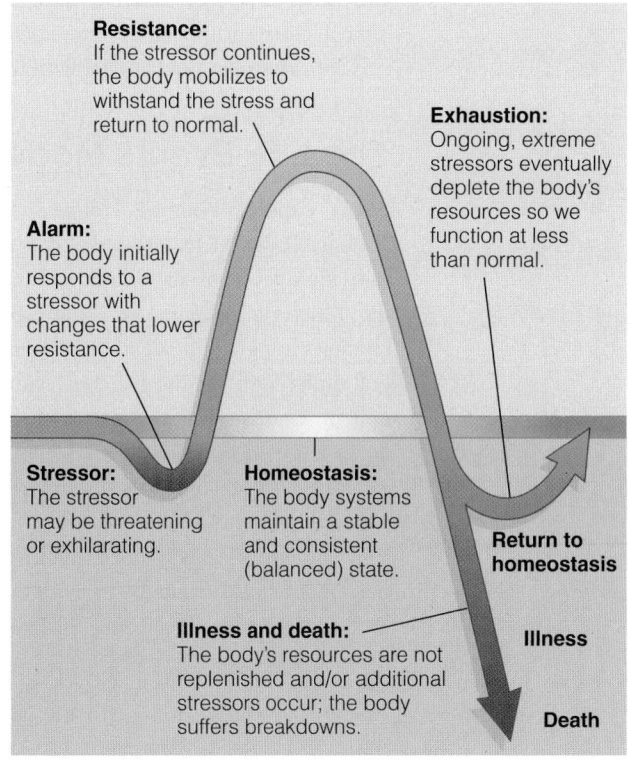

**Resistance:** If the stressor continues, the body mobilizes to withstand the stress and return to normal.

**Alarm:** The body initially responds to a stressor with changes that lower resistance.

**Exhaustion:** Ongoing, extreme stressors eventually deplete the body's resources so we function at less than normal.

**Stressor:** The stressor may be threatening or exhilarating.

**Homeostasis:** The body systems maintain a stable and consistent (balanced) state.

**Return to homeostasis**

**Illness and death:** The body's resources are not replenished and/or additional stressors occur; the body suffers breakdowns.

**Illness**

**Death**

relationship between demands and the power to deal with them without unreasonable or destructive costs."[1] Thus, an event may be stressful for one person but not for another, or it may seem stressful on one occasion but not on another. For instance, one student may think of speaking in front of the class as extremely stressful, while another relishes the chance to do so—except on days when he's not well prepared.

At any age, some of us are more vulnerable to life changes and crises than are others. The stress of growing up in families troubled by alcoholism, drug dependence, or physical, sexual, or psychological abuse may have a lifelong impact and make people more vulnerable to disease and premature death.[2] Other early experiences, positive and negative, also can affect our attitude toward stress—and our resilience to it.

"Perceived" stress—an individual's view of how challenging life is—undermines a sense of well-being in people of all ages and circumstances. However, good self-esteem, social support, and internal resources buffer the impact of perceived stress.

**general adaptation syndrome (GAS)** An anxiety disorder characterized as chronic distress.

**homeostasis** The body's natural state of balance or stability.

**adaptive response** The body's attempt to reestablish homeostasis or stability.

Our level of ongoing stress affects our ability to respond to a new day's stressors. Each of us has a breaking point for dealing with stress. A series of too-intense pressures or too-rapid changes can push us closer and closer to that point. That's why it's important to anticipate potential stressors and plan how to deal with them.

## The Life Events Model

Stress experts Thomas Holmes, M.D., and Richard Rahe, M.D., devised a scale to evaluate individual levels of stress and potential for coping, based on *life-change units* that estimate each change's impact. The death of a partner or parent ranks high on the list, but even changing apartments is considered a stressor. People who accumulate more than 300 life-change units in a year are more likely to suffer serious health problems. Scores on the scale, however, represent "potential stress"; the actual impact of the life change depends on the individual's response and coping skills.[3] (See Self Survey: "Student Stress Scale," on page 112.)

If you score high on the Student Stress Scale, think about the reasons your life has been in such turmoil. Of course, some events, such as your or your parents' divorce or a friend's accident, are beyond your control. Even then, you can respond in ways that may protect you from disease.

## The Diathesis Stress Model

The **diathesis stress model** is a psychological theory that explains behavior as a result of both nature (biological factors such as genetics) and nurture (early life experiences). Originally developed to explain the causes of psychiatric disorders such as schizophrenia, this model has stimulated research on the impact of many common stressors.

According to this model, particular stressors have different effects on different people because individuals vary in their vulnerabilities or predispositions—called diatheses—to psychological problems and mental disorders. Biological and psychological factors, including genetics, put certain people at greater risk but do not in themselves trigger illness. Interaction with stressful life events (whether social, psychological, or biological) must occur to precipitate symptoms.

The greater one's inherent vulnerability, the less environmental stress is required to cause problems. In someone with a diathesis for depression, for instance, a job layoff, a breakup, or even normal milestones such as puberty can be powerful enough to create depressive symptoms. Similar events might not faze other individuals that much. Research is continuing on identifying hidden or latent diatheses and developing protective strategies in times of stress.

# Stress and Physical Health

These days we've grown accustomed to warning labels advising us of the health risks of substances like alcohol and cigarettes. Medical researchers speculate that another component of twenty-first-century living also warrants a warning: stress. In recent years, an ever-growing number of studies has implicated stress as a culprit in a range of medical problems. While stress itself may not kill, it clearly undermines our ability to stay well.

While stress alone doesn't cause disease, it triggers molecular changes throughout the body that make us more susceptible to many illnesses. Severe emotional distress—whether caused by a divorce, the loss of a job, or caring for an ill child or parent—can have such a powerful effect on the DNA in body cells that it speeds up aging, adding the equivalent of a decade to biological age.

This occurs because of a shortening of structures called telomeres in the chromosomes of cells. An enzyme called telomerase maintains these structures but declines with age. Every time a cell divides, which is a continuous process, the telomeres shorten. The shorter your telomeres, the more likely you are to die.[4]

Stress also triggers complex changes in the body's endocrine, or hormone-secreting, system. When you confront a stressor, the adrenal glands, two triangle-shaped glands that sit atop the kidneys, respond by producing stress hormones, including catecholamines, cortisol (hydrocortisone), and epinephrine (adrenaline), that speed up heart rate and raise blood pressure and prepare the body to deal with the threat.

**diathesis stress model** A psychological theory that explains behavior as a result of both nature and nurture.

This "fight-or-flight" response prepares you for quick action: Your heart works harder to pump more blood to your legs and arms. Your muscles tense, your breathing quickens, and your brain becomes extra alert. Because it's nonessential in a crisis, your digestive system practically shuts down.

Figure 4.2 illustrates how persistent or repeated increases in the stress hormones can be hazardous throughout the body. Prolonged or severe stress can damage the brain's ability to remember and can actually cause brain cells, or neurons, to atrophy and die. Recent research has implicated stress in both contributing to the development of cancer and reducing the effectiveness of cancer treatment.

## The Impact of Cortisol

Psychosocial stress is a recognized risk factor for cardiorespiratory disease. In particular, three negative emotions—anxiety, anger, and depression—increase the risk of heart problems, and chronic exposure to stress hormones, including cortisol and aldosterone, may be the reason why.[5]

Cortisol speeds the conversion of proteins and fats into carbohydrates, the body's basic fuel, so we have the energy to fight or flee from a threat. However, stress increases the amount of time required to clear triglycerides, a type of fat linked to heart disease, from the bloodstream.

Cortisol can cause excessive central or abdominal fat, which heightens the risk of diseases such as diabetes, high blood pressure, and stroke. Even slender, premenopausal women faced with increased stress and lacking good coping skills are more likely to accumulate excess weight around their waists, thereby increasing their risk of heart disease and other health problems.

Numerous studies have linked cortisol, which seems to increase most in the face of uncontrollable and socially threatening stressors, with harmful changes in the heart, liver, and kidney. Cortisol also has been tied to the development

Figure 4.2  **The Effects of Stress on the Body**

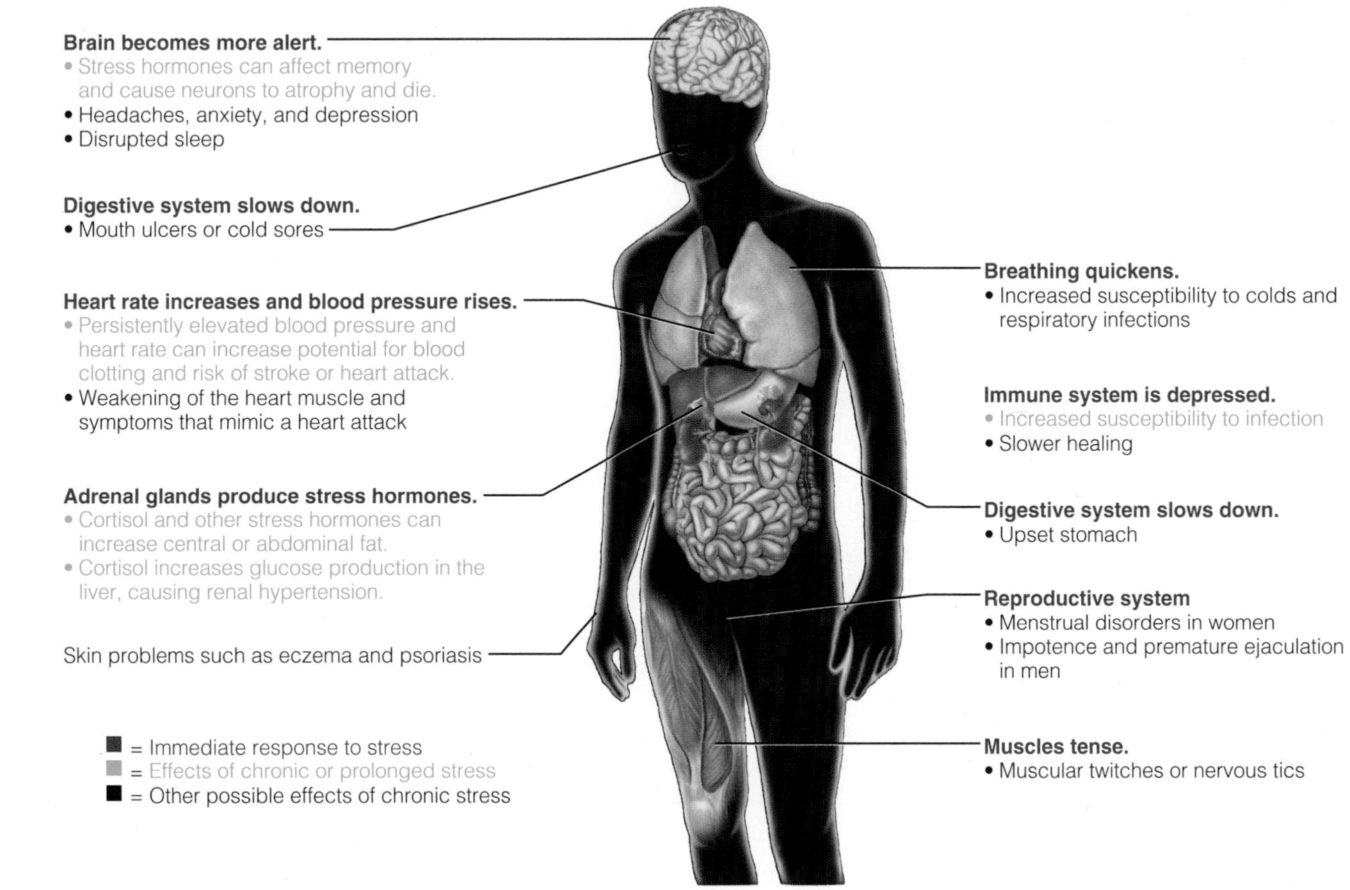

**Brain becomes more alert.**
• Stress hormones can affect memory and cause neurons to atrophy and die.
• Headaches, anxiety, and depression
• Disrupted sleep

**Digestive system slows down.**
• Mouth ulcers or cold sores

**Heart rate increases and blood pressure rises.**
• Persistently elevated blood pressure and heart rate can increase potential for blood clotting and risk of stroke or heart attack.
• Weakening of the heart muscle and symptoms that mimic a heart attack

**Adrenal glands produce stress hormones.**
• Cortisol and other stress hormones can increase central or abdominal fat.
• Cortisol increases glucose production in the liver, causing renal hypertension.

Skin problems such as eczema and psoriasis

**Breathing quickens.**
• Increased susceptibility to colds and respiratory infections

**Immune system is depressed.**
• Increased susceptibility to infection
• Slower healing

**Digestive system slows down.**
• Upset stomach

**Reproductive system**
• Menstrual disorders in women
• Impotence and premature ejaculation in men

**Muscles tense.**
• Muscular twitches or nervous tics

■ = Immediate response to stress
■ = Effects of chronic or prolonged stress
■ = Other possible effects of chronic stress

of metabolic syndrome and diabetes (both discussed in Chapter 9).

## Stress and the Heart

The links between stress, behavior, and the heart are complex. Scientists continue to explore the impact of acute and chronic stress, gender, race, and socioeconomic status.[6] One way in which stress increases the risk of heart attack and other cardiovascular problems is by pushing people toward bad habits. In a study that followed about 6,500 men and women for seven years, those with the highest stress levels smoked more and exercised less—and had a 50 percent higher rate of heart attacks, strokes, and bypass surgeries.[7]

Chronic stress, whether because of finances, a demanding job, racial discrimination, or marital problems, can contribute to hypertension (discussed in depth in Chapter 15). Ruminating—mulling over stressful events or upsetting thoughts—may be the mechanism that elevates blood pressure even hours or days after a stressful occurrence. The relaxation technique that has proven most effective in reducing blood pressure is meditation (discussed later in this chapter).[8]

Stressed individuals may be at increased risk because of overeating, coelevation of cortisol and insulin, and suppression of other hormones, all of which contribute to greater abdominal or visceral fat. As discussed in Chapter 7, "belly" fat is particularly dangerous because of its role in systemic inflammation, which can contribute to cardiovascular disease.[9]

Stress may be the most significant inherited risk factor in people who develop heart disease at a young age. According to behavioral researchers, family transmission of emotional and psychosocial stress, specifically anger in males, greatly increases the likelihood of early heart disease.[10]

In the 1970s, cardiologists Meyer Friedman, M.D., and Ray Rosenman, M.D., compared their patients to individuals of the same age with healthy hearts and developed two general categories of personality: Type A and Type B. Hardworking, aggressive, and competitive, Type As never have time for all they want to accomplish, even though they usually try to do several tasks at once. Type Bs are more relaxed, though not necessarily less ambitious or successful.

The degree of danger associated with Type-A behavior remains controversial. Of all the personality traits linked with Type-A behavior, the most sinister are anger and chronic hostility. People who are always mistrustful, cynical, and suspicious are twice as likely to suffer blockages of their coronary arteries. Social isolation, depression, and stress may be even stronger risk factors for men.

## Stress and Immunity

The immune system is the network of organs, tissues, and white blood cells that defend against disease. Impaired immunity makes the body more susceptible to many diseases, including infections (from the common cold to tuberculosis) and disorders of the immune system itself. In the short term, stress "revs up" the immune system, a way of preparing for injury or infection. Acute time-limited stressors, the type that produce a fight-or-flight response, prompt the immune system to ready itself for the possibility of infections resulting from bites, punctures, or other wounds.

However, long-term, or chronic, stress creates excessive wear and tear, and the system breaks down. Chronic stressors, so profound and persistent that they seem endless and beyond a person's control, suppress immune responses the most.[11] The longer the stress, the more the immune system shifts from potentially adaptive changes to potentially harmful ones, first in cellular immunity and then in broader immune function. Traumatic stress, such as losing a loved one through death or divorce, can impair immunity for as long as a year.

 Even minor hassles that aren't related to trauma take a toll. Under exam stress, students experience a dip in immune function and a higher rate of infections. Researchers have documented a significant drop in the immune cells that normally ward off infection and cancer in medical students during exams.

Because of sex-linked differences in the immune system, women may have a more potent response to stressors, which increases their risk of stress-related disorders, such as anxiety and depression, and of autoimmune or allergic disorders, such as rheumatoid arthritis, multiple sclerosis, and asthma.[12] (See Chapter 16 for a discussion of immune disorders.)

Age and overall health also affect immune response. The immune systems of individuals who are elderly or ill are more vulnerable to acute and chronic stressors, possibly because their bodies find it more difficult to regulate their reactions.[13] However, stress intensifies the symptoms and lowers the quality of life even for young adults with asthma and other chronic conditions.

## Stress and Digestion

Do you ever get butterflies in your stomach before giving a speech in class or before a big game? The digestive system is, as one psychologist quips, "an important stop on the tension trail."

Stress can lead to poor food choices, and can affect the way the body responds to unhealthy foods, which might lead to weight gain.[14] No studies have ever demonstrated that stress alone causes ulcers, but it may make people more vulnerable to infection with *Helicobacter pylori* bacteria, a known culprit in many cases. To avoid problems, pay attention to how you eat. Eating on the run, gulping food, or overeating results in poorly chewed foods, an overworked stomach, and increased abdominal pressure.

Some simple strategies can help you avoid stress-related stomachaches. Many people experience dry mouth or sweat more under stress. By drinking plenty of water, you replenish lost fluids and prevent dehydration. Fiber-rich foods counteract common stress-related problems, such as cramps and constipation. Do not skip meals. If you do, you're more likely to feel fatigued and irritable.

Be wary of overeating under stress. Some people eat more because they scarf down meals too quickly. Others reach for snacks to calm their nerves or comfort themselves. Watch out for caffeine. Coffee, tea, and cola drinks can make your strained nerves jangle even more. Research on laboratory animals suggests that eating sweets and other "comfort foods," even in small amounts, may alter brain chemistry and reduce stress.[15] However, don't have more than a few bites. Sugary snacks will send your blood sugar levels on a roller coaster ride—up one minute, down the next.

## Other Stress Symptoms

The first signs of stress include muscle tightness, tension headaches, backaches, upset stomach, and sleep disruptions (caused by stress-altered brain-wave activity). Some people feel fatigued, their hearts may race or beat faster than usual at rest, and they may feel tense all the time, easily frustrated, and often irritable. Others feel sad; lose their energy, appetite, or sex drive; and develop psychological problems, including depression, anxiety, and panic attacks.

Stress also is closely linked to skin conditions. If you break out the week before an exam, you know firsthand that skin can be extremely sensitive to stress. Skin conditions worsened by stress include acne, psoriasis, herpes, hives, and eczema. With acne, increased touching of the face, perhaps while cramming for a test, may be partly responsible. Other factors, such as temperature, humidity, and cosmetics and toiletries, may also play a role.

# Stress on Campus

 Being a student—full-time or part-time, in your late teens, early twenties, or later in life—can be extremely stressful. You may feel pressure to perform well to qualify for a good job or graduate school. To meet steep tuition payments, you may have to juggle part-time work and coursework. You may feel stressed about choosing a major, getting along with a difficult roommate, passing a particularly hard course, or living up to your parents' and teachers' expectations. If you're an older student, you may have children, jobs, housework, and homework to balance. Your days may seem so busy and your life so full that you worry about coming apart at the seams.

In the American College Health Association's national survey, about nine in ten students rate the overall level of stress they experienced in the previous 12 months as "average," "more than average," or "tremendous."[16] (See "How Do You Compare? Stressed Out on Campus.") Common stressors reported by students around the world include test pressures; financial problems; frustrations, such as delays in reaching

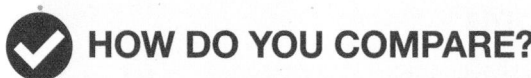

# HOW DO YOU COMPARE?

## STRESSED OUT ON CAMPUS

**Students reporting that**

| | |
|---|---|
| _____ stress has impaired their academic performance | **27 percent** |
| _____ they felt overwhelmed by all they had to do | **85 percent** |

| | |
|---|---|
| _____ they felt overwhelming anger | **38 percent** |
| _____ they felt average stress | **39 percent** |
| _____ they felt more than average stress | **41 percent** |
| _____ they felt tremendous stress | **10 percent** |

### HOW DO YOU COMPARE?

Check any of the statements that apply to you. To track your current stress level, do a "stress check" at least four times a day (on waking, lunch time, dinner time, before bed) and rate yourself on a 1 to 10 scale, with 1 signifying completely relaxed and 10 stressed to the max. Record your ratings and your reflections on them in your online journal.

Source: American College Health Association-National College Health Assessment Reference Group Executive Summary, Spring 2010.

goals; problems in friendships and dating relationships; and daily hassles.

In addition to its impact on health, stress can affect students physically, emotionally, academically, and socially. Among its documented effects are difficulty paying attention and concentrating, poor or inadequate sleep, lack of exercise, increased consumption of junk food, greater risk of anxiety and depression, and lessened life satisfaction.[17]

## Students under Stress

College brings growth and change—desirable and necessary but often stressful. The transition from high school to college challenges young adults to live independently, handle finances, maintain academic standards, and adjust to a new life. Their old roles, such as live-in son or daughter, may change while they acquire new roles as roommates and undergraduates. In addition to major negative events, such as being laid off or breaking up, daily hassles contribute to students' stress loads.

During a typical college semester, about half of college students report high levels of stress.[18] (See "How Do You Compare?")

First-generation college students—those whose parents never experienced at least one full year of college—encounter more difficulties with social adjustment than freshmen whose parents attended college. First-generation students also are less likely to disclose or share their experiences with family and friends, who may not be able to relate to and understand college-related stressors. This lack of social support itself adds to their stress levels.[19] Students whose parents and perhaps grandparents attended college may have several advantages: more knowledge of college life, greater social support, more preparation for college in high school, a greater focus on college activities, and more financial resources.

## Coping with Test Stress

For many students, midterms and final exams are the most stressful times of the year. Studies at various colleges and universities found that the incidence of colds and flu soared during finals. Some students feel the impact of test stress in other ways—headaches, upset stomachs, skin flare-ups, or insomnia.

Because of stress's impact on memory, students with advanced skills may perform worse under exam pressure than their less-skilled peers. Sometimes students become so preoccupied with the possibility of failing that they can't concentrate on studying. Others, including many of the best and brightest students, freeze up during tests and can't comprehend multiple-choice

# How to Handle Test Stress

- **Plan ahead.** A month before finals, map out a study schedule for each course. Set aside a small amount of time every day or every other day to review the course materials.

- **Be positive.** Picture yourself taking your final exam. Imagine yourself walking into the exam room feeling confident, opening up the test booklet, and seeing questions for which you know the answers.

- **Take regular breaks.** Get up from your desk, breathe deeply, stretch, and visualize a pleasant scene. You'll feel more refreshed than you would if you chugged another cup of coffee.

- **Practice.** Some teachers are willing to give practice finals to prepare students for test situations, or you and your friends can test each other.

- **Talk to other students.** Chances are that many of them share your fears about test taking and may have discovered some helpful techniques of their own. Sometimes talking to your adviser or a counselor can also help.

- **Be satisfied with doing your best.** You can't expect to ace every test; all you can and should expect is your best effort. Once you've completed the exam, allow yourself the sweet pleasure of relief that it's over.

questions or write essay answers, even if they know the material.

The students most susceptible to exam stress are those who believe they'll do poorly and who see tests as extremely threatening. Unfortunately, such negative thoughts often become a self-fulfilling prophecy. As they study, these students keep wondering: What good will studying do? I never do well on tests. As their fear increases, they try harder, pulling all-nighters. Fueled by caffeine, munching on sugary snacks, they become edgy and find it harder and harder to concentrate. By the time of the test, they're nervous wrecks, scarcely able to sit still and focus on the exam.

Can you do anything to reduce test stress and feel more in control? Absolutely. (See "Defusing Test Stress" in the *Labs for IPC*.) One way is through relaxation. Students taught relaxation techniques—such as controlled breathing, meditation, progressive relaxation, and guided imagery (visualization)—a month before finals tend to have higher levels of immune cells during the exam period and feel in better control during their tests.

## How Students Respond

 Students say they react to stress in various ways: physiologically (by sweating, stuttering, trembling, or developing physical symptoms); emotionally (by becoming anxious, fearful, angry, guilty, or depressed); behaviorally (by crying, eating, smoking, being irritable or abusive); or cognitively (by thinking about and analyzing stressful situations and strategies that might be useful in dealing with them).

Researchers have categorized students' coping strategies as either problem-focused (involving behavioral activities, such as planning and taking action) or emotion-focused (involving expression of feelings). In general, problem-focused strategies are associated with better outcomes, such as better health and greater sense of well-being. Emotion-focused strategies, particularly trying to avoid the problem or difficult situation, are associated with poorer health and more negative feelings. Both female and male undergraduates tend to use more emotion-focused than problem-focused strategies.[20]

Students under stress may engage in behaviors that can harm their health, including smoking, excess drinking, and substance abuse.[21] They're also more prone to night-eating, which can lead to excess weight.[22] Students' stress responses may reflect their personality characteristics and coping styles.

In a recent study, students under stress who typically devote themselves to supporting others often do not reach out to take advantage of the support available to them, while students who focus solely on their own achievements and needs do not have a support network to turn to when stressed. Both are likely to engage in risky sexual behaviors, such as unsafe sex practices or having sex with more partners than usual.[23]

Learning how to cope better with the problems of daily living can reduce student stress and its possible toll. "Problem-solving therapy," a psychological approach that focuses on training in constructive problem-solving attitudes and skills, teaches practical principles, such as reframing a stressful situation as a challenge rather than a difficulty, avoiding impulsive reactions, confronting issues directly, and seeking alternative solutions.[24]

In a national poll, three-quarters of students said they turn to friends when stressed; nearly two-thirds, to their parents; and half to siblings. About a quarter of the survey participants said they had considered talking to a counselor or another professional; just 15 percent had actually done so. Only one in seven undergraduates said they were familiar with the counseling offered at their schools.[25]

## Gender Differences

College women consistently report more stress than college men—at least for some stressors. In a recent study, college women reported greater stress for finances, financial relationships, social relationships, and daily hassle. Among community college students, stress significantly affected the grade point averages of women, although attachment to and support from others moderated its effects.[26]

The immune and hormonal systems of men and women may respond differently to stressors. In psychological experiments men under stress display higher aggression (for example, delivering more shocks to another volunteer) than do women.

Gender differences in lifestyle also may explain why women feel so stressed. College men spend significantly more time doing things that are fun and relaxing: exercising, partying, watching TV, and playing video games. Women, on the other hand, tend to study more, do more volunteer work, and handle more household and childcare chores.

Coping strategies also vary by gender. College men are more likely to disengage by using alcohol. College women report more emotion-focused strategies, such as expressing feelings, seeking emotional support, denial, and positive reframing. They're also more prone to avoid dealing with a problem directly and to taking impulsive measures. Acquiring better problem-solving skills can help in dealing both with daily hassles and with larger stressors.[27]

At all ages, women and men tend to respond to stress differently. While males (human and those of other species) react with the classic fight-or-flight response, females under attack try to protect their children and seek help from other females—a strategy dubbed *tend and befriend*. When exposed to experimental stress (such as a loud, harsh noise), women show more affection for friends and relatives; men show less. When working mothers studied by psychologists had a bad day, they coped by concentrating on their children when they got home. Stressed-out fathers were more likely to withdraw.

## Minority Students under Stress

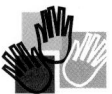 Regardless of your race or ethnic background, college may bring culture shock. You may never have encountered such a degree of diversity in one setting. You probably will meet students with different values, unfamiliar customs, entirely new ways of looking at the world—experiences you may find both stimulating and stressful.

Minority students may face a greater stress burden because of the demands of **acculturation**, a complex psychosocial process in which an ethnic minority changes, both as individuals and as a group, as a consequence of contact with the ethnic majority. Minority students often confront widespread stereotypes—for instance, that Asian Americans are quiet and passive or that Latinos entered the country illegally. Such racist attitudes can affect students' sense of individual and collective self-esteem. In a recent study, both Asian and black undergraduates reported more frequent experiences of discrimination and perceived the campus racial climate as more negative than white students.[28]

Acculturative stress has been linked to various psychological symptoms in African American, Asian, and Hispanic college students. In both African American and European American undergraduates, for instance, acculturative stress

**acculturation** The process of psychosocial change by which an ethnic minority changes as a consequence of contact with the ethnic majority.

contributes to an increase in self-reported symptoms of depression and suicidal thoughts.[29]

***Racism and Discrimination*** Racism has indeed been shown to be a source of stress that can affect health and well-being. In the past, some African American students have described predominantly white campuses as hostile, alienating, and socially isolating and have reported greater estrangement from the campus community and heightened estrangement in interactions with faculty and peers. However, the generalization that all minority students are more stressed may not be valid. Some coping mechanisms, especially spirituality, can buffer the negative effects of racism.[30]

All minority students do share some common stressors. In one study of minority freshmen entering a large, competitive university, Asian, Filipino, African American, and Native American students all felt more sensitive and vulnerable to the college social climate, to interpersonal tensions between themselves and nonminority students and faculty, to experiences of actual or perceived racism, and to racist attitudes and discrimination. Despite scoring above the national average on the SAT, the minority students in this study did not feel accepted as legitimate students and sensed that others viewed them as unworthy beneficiaries of affirmative action initiatives. While most said that overt racism was rare and relatively easy to deal with, they reported subtle pressures that undermined their academic confidence and their ability to bond with the university. Balancing these stressors, however, was a strong sense of ethnic identity, which helped buffer some stressful effects.

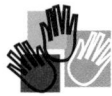 ***Other Stressors*** African American students at historically black colleges identified their top five sources of stress as:

- Important decisions about education.
- Respect of peers for what you have to say.
- Too many things to do at once.
- A lot of responsibilities.
- Financial burdens.

Women scored higher than men in feeling stressed about having too many things to do at once, being separated from people they care

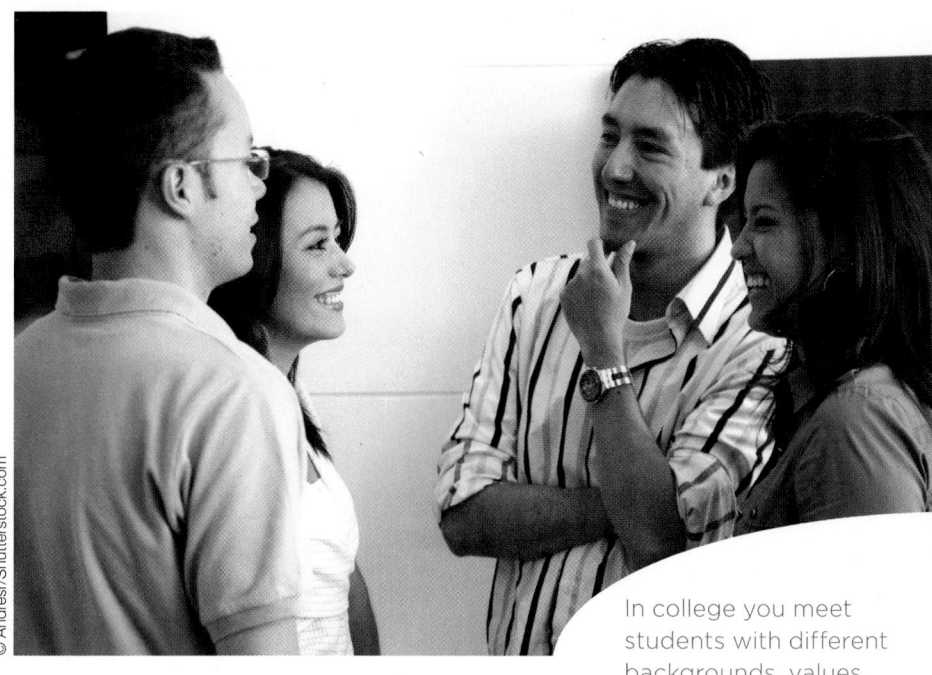

about, financial burdens, and important decisions about their education.[31]

Hispanic students have identified three major types of stressors in their college experiences: academic (related to exam preparation and faculty interaction), social (related to ethnicity and interpersonal competence), and financial (related to their economic situation). Some students who recently immigrated to the United States report feeling ostracized by students of similar ancestry who are second- or third-generation Americans.

African American women may develop chronic illnesses at an earlier age because of their lifetime exposure to social and economic stressors. Chronic powerlessness and anger, researchers speculate, may explain why more African American than white women—47 percent compared with 35 percent—are affected by cardiovascular disease.[32]

## Colleges Respond

Because racism and discrimination can be hard to deal with individually, they are particularly sinister forms of stress. By banding together, however, those who experience discrimination can take action to protect themselves, challenge the ignorance and hateful assumptions that fuel bigotry, and promote a healthier environment for all.

In college you meet students with different backgrounds, values, customs, and entirely new ways of looking at the world—which can be both stimulating and stressful.

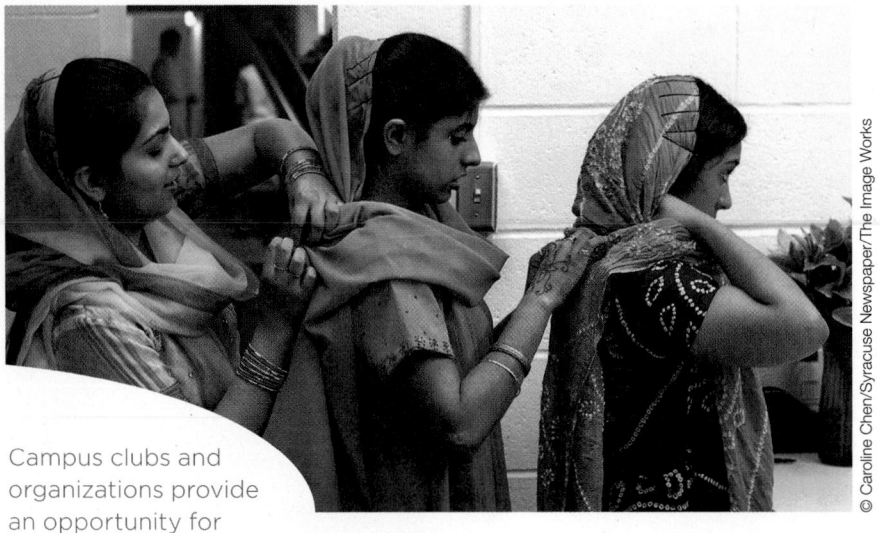

Campus clubs and organizations provide an opportunity for individuals from different ethnic backgrounds to celebrate their culture and educate others about it. These undergraduates are preparing to perform an Indian dance at a special evening sponsored by Asian Students in America.

© Caroline Chen/Syracuse Newspaper/The Image Works

In the last decade, there have been reports of increased intolerance among young people and greater tolerance of expressions and acts of hate on college campuses. To counteract this trend, many schools have set up programs and classes to educate students about each other's backgrounds and to acknowledge and celebrate the richness diversity brings to campus life. Educators have called on universities to make campuses less alienating and more culturally and emotionally accessible, with programs and policies targeted not only at minority students but also at the university as a whole.

Some schools have taken a more lighthearted approach. In addition to extra counseling and extended library hours, they are offering stress-busting experiences, such as laser tag, petting zoos (with bunnies and puppies at California's Claremont University Consortium), karaoke parties, and miniature golf. Does your school or student government offer anything similar? Do you think such activities can reduce stress overload?[33]

## Other Personal Stressors

At every stage of life, you will encounter challenges and stressors. Among the most common are those related to money, anger, work, and illness. (See Health on a Budget, p. 101.)

## Economic Stress

With the recent economic slump, millions of Americans have confronted a serious new stressor: unemployment. Workers who are laid off must deal with multiple losses: the loss of a job; the possible loss of the financial ability to support themselves; the loss of self-respect, security, and a daily routine; and—for some people—the loss of identity.[34]

Even those whose jobs seem secure may feel anxious. As their coworkers depart, many of those who remain feel "survivor's guilt." According to surveys by the American Psychological Association, nearly half of Americans say they are more stressed than a year ago. One-third rate their stress level as "extreme."[35]

In the most recent annual poll of incoming college students, more freshmen expressed concerns about their ability to pay for their education than at any time in the last four decades. Undergraduates also are more likely to have a parent who is unemployed and to have been unable to find a job that would help with tuition and other costs.[36]

## The Anger Epidemic

In recent years, violent aggressive driving—which some dub *road rage*—has exploded. Sideline rage at amateur and professional sporting events has become so widespread that a Pennsylvania midget football game ended in a brawl involving more than 100 coaches, players, parents, and fans.

No one seems immune. Women fly off the handle just as often as men, although they're less likely to get physical. The young and the infamous, including several rappers and musicians sentenced to anger management classes for violent outbursts, may seem more volatile. However, ordinary senior citizens have erupted into "line rage" and pushed ahead of others simply because they feel they've "waited long enough" in their lives.

Experts single out three primary culprits for the anger epidemic: time, technology, and tension. Americans are working longer hours than anyone else in the world. The cell phones and pagers that were supposed to make our lives easier have put us on call 24–7–365. People are tense and low on patience, and the less patience they have, the less they monitor their behavior.

*Getting a Grip*   For years therapists encouraged people to "vent" their anger. However, research now shows that letting anger out only makes it worse. "Catharsis is worse than useless," says psychology professor Brad Bushman of Iowa State University, whose research has shown that letting anger out makes people more aggressive, not less. "Many people think of anger as the psychological equivalent of the steam in a pressure cooker that has to be released or it will explode. That's not true. People who react by hitting, kicking, screaming, and swearing aren't dealing with the underlying cause of their anger. They just feel more angry."[37]

Over time, temper tantrums sabotage physical health as well as psychological equanimity. By churning out stress hormones, chronic anger revs the body into a state of combat readiness, multiplying the risk for stroke and heart attack—even in healthy individuals.

To deal with anger, you have to figure out what's really making you mad. Usually the jammed soda machine is the final straw that unleashes bottled-up fury over a more difficult issue, such as a recent breakup or a domineering parent or boss. Also monitor yourself for early signs of exhaustion and overload. While stress alone doesn't cause a blowup, it makes you more vulnerable to overreacting. (See "Taming a Toxic Temper" in *Labs for IPC*.)

## Job Stress

More so than ever, many people find that they are working more and enjoying it less. Many people, including working parents, spend 55 to 60 hours a week on the job. More people are caught up in an exhausting cycle of overwork, which causes stress, which makes work harder, which leads to more stress. Even the workplace itself can contribute to stress. A noisy, open-office environment can increase levels of stress without workers realizing it.

High job strain—defined as high psychological demands combined with low control or decision-making ability over one's job—may increase blood pressure, particularly among men. People who become obsessed by their

work and careers can turn into workaholics, so caught up in racing toward the top that they forget what they're racing toward and why. In some cases they throw themselves into their work to mask or avoid painful feelings or difficulties in their own lives.

*Burnout*   **Burnout** is a state of physical, emotional, and mental exhaustion brought on by constant or repeated emotional pressure. No one—regardless of age, gender, or job—is immune. Mothers and managers, firefighters and flight attendants, teachers and telemarketers feel the flames of too much stress and not enough satisfaction. Many people, especially those caring for others at work or at home, get to a point where there's an imbalance between their own feelings and dealing with difficult, distressful issues on a day-to-day basis. If they don't recognize what's going on and make some changes, their health and the quality of their work suffer.

**burnout** A state of physical, emotional, and mental exhaustion resulting from constant or repeated emotional pressure.

## How to Deal with an Angry Person

- **Become an impartial observer.** Act as if you were watching someone else's two-year-old have a temper tantrum at the supermarket.

- **Stay calm.** Letting your emotions loose only adds fuel to fury. Talk quietly and slowly; let the person know you understand that he or she is angry.

- **Refuse to engage.** Step back to avoid invading his or her space. Retreat farther if need be until the person is back in control.

- **Find something to agree upon.** Look for common ground, if only to acknowledge that you're both in a difficult situation.

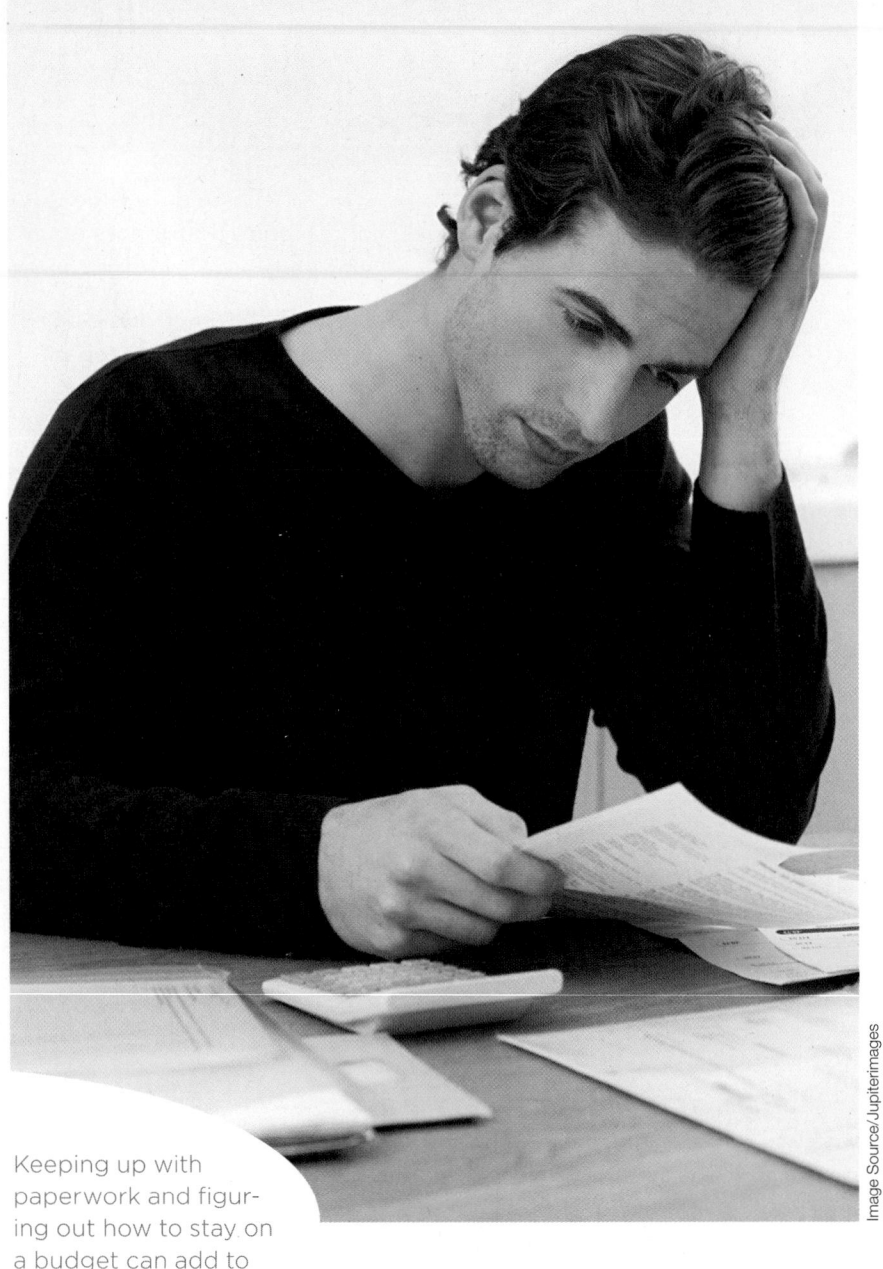

Keeping up with paperwork and figuring out how to stay on a budget can add to a student's stress level.

Image Source/Jupiterimages

Early signs of burnout include exhaustion; sleep problems or nightmares; increased anxiety or nervousness; muscular tension (headaches, backaches, and the like); increased use of alcohol or medication; digestive problems (such as nausea, vomiting, or diarrhea); loss of interest in sex; frequent body aches or pain; quarrels with family or friends; negative feelings about everything; problems concentrating; job mistakes and accidents; and feelings of depression, hopelessness, or helplessness.

## Illness and Disability

Just as the mind can have profound effects on the body, the body can have an enormous impact on our emotions. Whenever we come down with the flu or pull a muscle, we feel under par. When the problem is more serious or persistent—a chronic disease like diabetes, for instance, or a lifelong hearing impairment—the emotional stress of constantly coping with it is even greater.

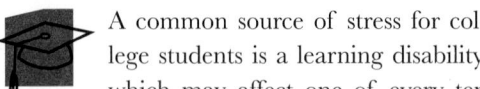 A common source of stress for college students is a learning disability, which may affect one of every ten Americans. Most people with learning disabilities have average or above-average intelligence, but they rarely live up to their ability in school. Some have only one area of difficulty, such as reading or math. Others have problems with attention, writing, communicating, reasoning, coordination, and social skills.

Not all students with learning disabilities experience greater stress. In one in-depth study comparing 34 undergraduates with and without learning disabilities, the students with learning disabilities (LD) reported significantly fewer college stressors and demonstrated a higher need for achievement. The LD students also scored significantly higher in resiliency and initiative in solving problems and working toward goals.

## Societal Stressors

Many college students, faced with ongoing wars in Iraq and continued threat of terrorist attacks, find that they now feel uncertain about a future for which they had just begun to plan. Some may be concerned about parents, relatives, or friends who are in the military or living overseas. Others may wonder how they, themselves, may become directly involved in this crisis. Students who live away from home may have a more difficult time coping without the reassurance of having family nearby.

The deliberate use of physical force to abuse or injure is a leading killer of young people in the United States—and a potential source of stress in all our lives. If you or someone you know has been a victim of a violent crime, a sense of vulnerability may add to the stress of daily living. See Your Strategies for Change on page 108 and "Your Guardian Angel" in *Labs for IPC*.

# Psychological Responses to Stress

It may be tempting to look for a "quick fix" for stress. (See Consumer Alert, p. 105.) Sometimes we respond to stress or challenge with self-destructive behaviors, such as drinking or using drugs. These responses can lead to psychological problems, such as anxiety or depression, and physical problems, including psychosomatic illnesses.

## Defense Mechanisms

**Defense mechanisms**, such as those described in Table 4.1, are another response to stress. These psychological devices are mental processes that help us cope with personal problems. Such responses also are not the answer to stress—and learning to recognize them in yourself will enable you to deal with your stress in a healthier way.

## Cognitive Restructuring

Every day about 60,000 thoughts pass through our brains as we plan, evaluate, judge, interpret, and remember. Some of these thoughts are as precise as a mathematical equation, but others are misleading or inappropriate. These inaccurate or self-defeating thoughts are the target

of cognitive-behavioral therapy (CBT), a highly effective psychological treatment described in Chapter 3.

Cognitive restructuring, one of the techniques of CBT, can reduce stress by helping people examine unhappy, negative thoughts that are making them anxious, challenging these thoughts, and in many cases rewriting the negative thinking that lies behind them. Because thoughts create feelings and drive behavior, this approach enables people to approach stressful situations in a positive frame of mind.

The first step is becoming aware of automatic thoughts that enter your brain, such as "I will never understand this material," "I'm going to flunk this test," or "No one wants to talk with me." Then you challenge these negative assumptions with counterarguments such as "I felt the same way in chemistry class, and eventually I figured it out," "If I focus on the questions I do know, I'll be okay," or "I can try smiling and striking up a conversation." You can also develop specific action techniques to blunt negative thoughts and lessen stress. For instance, you could master some of the relaxation and test-taking techniques described in this chapter and in *Labs for IPC*.

**defense mechanism** A psychological process that alleviates anxiety and eliminates mental conflict; includes denial, displacement, projection, rationalization, reaction formation, and repression.

Table 4.1 **Common Defense Mechanisms Used to Alleviate Anxiety and Eliminate Conflict**

| Defense Mechanism | Example |
| --- | --- |
| Denial: the refusal to accept a painful reality | You don't accept as true the news that a loved one is seriously ill. |
| Displacement: the redirection of feelings from their true object to a more acceptable or safer substitute | Instead of lashing out at a coach or teacher, you snap at your best friend. |
| Projection: the attribution of unacceptable feelings or impulses to someone else | When you want to end a relationship, you project your unhappiness onto your partner. |
| Rationalization: the substitution of "good," acceptable reasons for the real motivations of our behavior | You report a classmate who has been mean for cheating on an exam and explain that cheating is unfair to other students. |
| Reaction formation: adopting attitudes and behaviors that are the opposite of what we feel | You lavishly compliment an acquaintance whom you really despise. |
| Repression: the way we keep threatening impulses, fantasies, memories, feelings, or wishes from becoming conscious | You don't "hear" the alarm after the late night, or you "forget" to take out the trash. |

# Managing Stress

College is a perfect time to learn and practice the art of stress reduction. You can start applying the techniques and concepts outlined in this chapter immediately. You may want to begin by doing some relaxation or awareness exercises. They can give you the peace of mind you need to focus more effectively on larger issues, goals, and decisions.

You needn't see stress as a problem to solve on your own. Reach out to others. As you build friendships and intimate relationships, you may find that some irritating problems are easier to put into perspective. Don't be afraid to laugh at yourself and to look for the comic or absurd aspects of a situation.

If you feel yourself tensing up and don't have time for a longer relaxation technique, try these simple stress-busters:

- **Toe tensing.** Lie down, point your toes back toward your face, and hold for ten seconds. Relax your feet, and repeat several times.
- **Quiet ears.** Stop whatever you're doing. Lie down or sit back, and block your ear canals with your thumbs. Hold this position for 10 to 15 seconds. Close your eyes, and clear your mind.

## Journaling

One of the simplest, yet most effective, ways to work through stress is by putting your feelings into words that only you will read. The more honest and open you are as you write, the better. (See "Health in Action: Write It Out!")

College students who wrote in their journals about traumatic events felt much better afterward than those who wrote about superficial topics. Focus on intense emotional experiences and "autopsy" them to try to understand why they affected you the way they did. Rereading and thinking about your notes may reveal the underlying reasons for your response. See the chapter on "Power Journaling" in *IPC*.

## Exercise

Regular physical activity can relieve stress, boost energy, lift mood, and keep stress under control. Young adults who adopt and continue regular aerobic exercise show less intense cardiovascular responses to stress, which may protect them against coronary heart disease as they age. Strength training may have similar benefits.

 Various studies have examined the correlation between physical activity and stress in college students. Students who report higher levels of leisure-time exercise, along with a good social network and time management skills, generally enjoy better mental health.[38] Other researchers have found that active students report as much stress as inactive ones.[39] Try an experiment with yourself: Keep track of the days when you work out in some way and those you don't. Rate your stress level every day, and see if exercise makes a difference for you.

## Routes to Relaxation

Relaxation is the physical and mental state opposite that of stress. Rather than gearing up for fight or flight, our bodies and minds grow calmer and work more smoothly. We're less likely to become frazzled and more capable of staying in control. A growing number of studies has confirmed the benefits of relaxation techniques. Although they differ in many ways, the various approaches may alter brain chemistry in fundamental ways, such as increasing the levels of pleasure-inducing chemicals in the brain.[40] (See "Rx: Relax" in the *Labs for IPC*.)

**Progressive relaxation** works by intentionally increasing and then decreasing tension in the muscles. While sitting or lying down in a quiet, comfortable setting, you tense and release various muscles, beginning with those of the hand, for instance, and then proceeding to the arms, shoulders, neck, face, scalp, chest, stomach, buttocks, genitals, and so on, down each leg to the toes. Relaxing the muscles can quiet the mind and restore internal balance.[41]

**Visualization**, or **guided imagery**, involves creating mental pictures that calm you down and focus your mind. Some people use this technique to promote healing when they are ill. Visualization skills require practice and, in some cases, instruction by qualified health professionals.

**Biofeedback** is a method of obtaining feedback, or information, about some physiological

**progressive relaxation** A method of reducing muscle tension by contracting, then relaxing, certain areas of the body.

**visualization, or guided imagery** An approach to stress control, self-healing, or motivating life changes by means of seeing oneself in the state of calmness, wellness, or change.

**biofeedback** A technique of becoming aware, with the aid of external monitoring devices, of internal physiological activities in order to develop the capability of altering them.

**meditation** A group of approaches that use quiet sitting, breathing techniques, and/or chanting to relax, improve concentration, and become attuned to one's inner self.

## Stress Scams

Aromatic candles. Gurgling fountains. Squeezable foam balls. Incense burners. Soothing gels. Everywhere you turn you can find something that promises to relieve stress. Do they work? Most don't cause any harm, but they don't necessarily do much good either.

### Facts to Know

- "Natural" products, such as herbs and enzymes, claim to have psychological effects. However, because they are not classified as drugs, these products have not undergone the rigorous scientific testing required of psychiatric medications, and little is known about their safety or efficacy. "Natural" doesn't mean risk-free. Opium and cocaine are "natural" substances that have dramatic and potentially deadly effects on the mind.

- Don't make matters worse by smoking (the chemicals in cigarettes increase heart rate, blood pressure, and stress hormones), consuming too much caffeine (it speeds up your system for hours), eating snacks high in sugar (it produces a quick high followed by a sudden slump), or turning to drugs or alcohol (they can only add to your stress when their effects wear off).

### Steps to Take

- Be wary of instant cures. Regardless of the promises on the label, it's unrealistic to expect any magic ingredient or product to make all your problems disappear.

- Focus on stress-reducing behavior, rather than a product. An aromatic candle may not bring instant serenity, but if you light a candle and meditate, you may indeed feel more at peace.

- Experiment with physical ways to work out stress. Exercise is one of the best ways to lower your stress levels. Try walking, running, swimming, cycling, kickboxing—anything physical that helps you release tension.

activity occurring in the body. An electronic monitoring device attached to the body detects a change in an internal function and communicates it back to the person through a tone, light, or meter. By paying attention to this feedback, most people can gain some control over functions previously thought to be beyond conscious control, such as body temperature, heart rate, muscle tension, and brain waves.

The goal of biofeedback for stress reduction is a state of tranquility, usually associated with the brain's production of alpha waves (which are slower and more regular than normal waking waves).

## Meditation and Mindfulness

**Meditation** has been practiced in many forms over the ages, from the yogic techniques of the Far East to the Quaker silence of more modern times. Brain scans have shown that meditation activates the sections of the brain in charge of the autonomic nervous system, which governs bodily functions, such as digestion and blood pressure, that we cannot consciously control. Research with a group of Tibetan monks and lay practitioners with extensive experience in meditation has demonstrated that meditation produces changes in various regions of the brain and can actually cause people to be more compassionate.[42]

Although many studies have documented the benefits of meditation for overall health, it may be particularly helpful for people dealing with stress-related medical conditions such as high blood pressure and heart problems, and for preventing stress-induced changes in the immune system.[43] (See Figure 4.3.)

Meditation helps a person reach a state of relaxation, but with the goal of achieving inner peace and harmony. There is no one right way to meditate, and many people have discovered how to meditate on their own, without even knowing what it is they are doing.

Increasing numbers of college students are turning to meditation as a way of coping with stress. Most forms of meditation have common elements: sitting quietly for 15 to 20 minutes once or twice a day, concentrating on a word or image, and breathing slowly and rhythmically. If

## Health in Action

### Write It Out!

One of the most effective ways of coping with stress and other psychological challenges is by using a journal to monitor and express your feelings. Try the following stress-reducing exercises, and record your responses and reflections in your online journal:

- Assess your stress. Take a strain inventory of your body every day to determine where things aren't feeling quite right. Ask yourself, "What's keeping me from feeling terrific today?" Focusing on problem spots, such as stomach knots or neck tightness, increases your sense of control over stress.

- Reconstruct stressful situations. Think about a recent episode of distress; then write down three ways it could have gone better and three ways it could have gone worse. This should help you see that the situation wasn't as disastrous as it might have been and help you find ways to cope better in the future.

- Practice self-compassion. As discussed in Chapter 2, treating yourself kindly in the face of stressful circumstances helps turn wisdom and awareness inward and provides a sense of perspective and connectedness.

- List some of the nice things you can do to soothe yourself, and include at least three in your daily routine. Make notes on how you feel after such experiences and which ones seem to have the most lasting impact.

## Figure 4.3 **Benefits of Meditation**

**Meditation**

- Reduces activation of the sympathetic nervous system—which, in turn, dilates the blood vessels and reduces stress hormones, such as adrenaline, noradrenaline, and cortisol.
- Reduces high blood pressure and use of hypertension medications
- Reduces atherosclerosis
- Reduces constriction of blood vessels
- Reduces thickening of coronary arteries
- Reduces mortality rates
- Slows aging
- Reduces hospitalization rates
- Decreases medical care utilization and hospitalization
- Increases creativity
- Improves memory
- Increases intelligence
- Decreases anxiety
- Reduces alcohol abuse
- Increases productivity

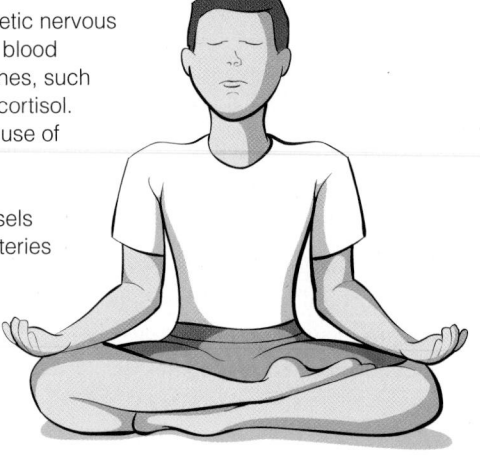

you wish to try meditation, it often helps to have someone guide you through your first sessions. Or try tape recording your own voice (with or without favorite music in the background) and playing it back to yourself, freeing yourself to concentrate on the goal of turning the attention within.

In a recent study, regular practice of Transcendental Meditation reduced sleepiness in college students and improved their alertness and brain functioning. Undergraduates who began meditating during the first week of the term were less tired and more resistant to the stress of finals than others.[44]

**Mindfulness** is a modern form of an ancient Asian technique that involves maintaining awareness in the present moment. Some define it as "paying attention in a particular way, on purpose, in the present moment, and nonjudgmentally."[45]

In mindful meditation, you tune in to each part of your body, scanning from head to toe, noting the slightest sensation. You allow whatever you experience—an itch, an ache, a feeling of warmth—to enter your awareness. Then you open yourself to focus on all the thoughts, sensations, sounds, and feelings that enter your awareness. Mindfulness keeps you in the here and now, thinking about *what is* rather than about *what if* or *if only.*

**mindfulness** A method of stress reduction that involves experiencing the physical and mental sensations of the present moment.

In a study with college students, those who enrolled in movement-based classes, such as Pilates and Gyrokinesis, demonstrated increases in specific aspects of mindfulness, such as acting with awareness and observing sensations and perceptions. These increases were associated with better sleep, improved mood, and lower sense of stress.[46]

Mindfulness-Based Stress Reduction, a group program that focuses on progressive acquisition of mindful awareness, has been used for patients with a wide variety of health problems as well as in healthy people coping with daily stress. Researchers have documented benefits for individuals suffering from chronic pain, fibromyalgia, cancer, anxiety disorders, depression, and the stresses of everything from prison life to medical school.[47]

## Yoga

An estimated 14.9 million Americans practice yoga, which has been defined as a union of mind, body, and spirit (discussed in Chapter 8). In addition to easing conditions such as lower-back pain, migraine, asthma, and hypertension, yoga has proven to reduce anxiety and cortisol levels in those with moderate levels of stress.[48] Compared with other forms of exercise, yoga has a greater positive impact on mood and anxiety, possibly because it increases antidepressant neurotransmitters (messenger chemicals) in the brain.[49]

Yoga practitioners, in a study that compared them with undergraduates, reported engaging in more healthy behaviors, such as exercising regularly, than the students. They also were more likely to express their spirituality and undertake new experiences to enhance their spiritual health.[50]

Yoga may lower harmful compounds associated with stress that increase inflammation. In a recent study, "expert" yoga practitioners, with a year or two of yoga practice, had lower levels of markers of chronic inflammation than novices. Yoga may be beneficial because it increases flexibility and allows relaxation, which can lower stress.[51]

# Traumatic Life Events and Stress

Bad things happen. Cars crash. Close friends and relatives die. Floods, tornadoes, and earthquakes wreak havoc on communities. Armed students shoot senselessly at classmates and professors. According to epidemiological studies, about half of all people experience at least one potentially traumatic event—natural or man-made, large-scale or small—during the course of their lives. As profoundly disturbing as such experiences can be, recent research has shown that after a trauma the vast majority of people, including children, cope well, continue to meet the demands of their daily lives, and recover fully.

Traumatic experiences, as one researcher puts it, are like the common cold, "experienced at some time by nearly all." In a recent study of college women, nine in ten reported having directly experienced at least one traumatic event, usually involving a threat to their own lives or to others. The most frequently reported trauma was a motor vehicle accident.[52]

Many people develop a temporary "acute stress reaction," characterized by symptoms such as reexperiencing the trauma, avoiding certain places or situations, and feeling a sense of arousal or hypersensitivity. But just as the common cold can lead to pneumonia and other serious complications, traumatic experiences can provoke more serious reactions in about 20 to 30 percent of trauma survivors. Of these, about half recover over time even without treatment.[53]

Common responses to crisis include the following:[54]

- Disbelief and shock
- Disorientation; difficulty making decisions or concentrating
- Inability to focus on schoolwork and extracurricular activities
- Apathy and emotional numbing
- Sadness and depression
- Fear and anxiety about the future
- Intrusive thoughts; replaying events in our minds
- Excessive worry about safety and vulnerability; feeling powerless
- Crying for "no apparent reason"
- Irritability and anger
- Headaches and stomach problems
- Difficulty sleeping
- Extreme changes in eating patterns; loss of appetite or overeating
- Excessive use of alcohol or drugs

## Posttraumatic Stress Disorder (PTSD)

In the past, **posttraumatic stress disorder (PTSD)** was viewed as a psychological response to out-of-the-ordinary stressors, such as captivity or combat. However, other experiences can also forever change the way people view themselves and their world. Individuals with PTSD often suffer cognitive impairments, including memory problems.[55]

An estimated 7.7 million American adults have PTSD.[56] PTSD is twice as common in women as in men. Women are most vulnerable between the ages of 44 and 51, while men are more prone to PTSD from ages 41 to 45.[57] Childhood traumas occur equally in both sexes. Adult men encounter more traumas—accidents, violence, combat, terrorism, disasters, injuries—than adult women. Women experience more sexual assaults and abuse. PTSD is especially high in women who have served in the military. Sexual trauma ranks as the most distressing for female veterans, followed by physical assault and war zone experience.

An estimated 4 to 17 percent of veterans of combat in Iraq and Afghanistan develop PTSD, along with other problems such as substance abuse.[58] Many have experienced high-intensity guerilla warfare as well as the chronic threat of roadside bombs and improvised explosive devices; some have suffered traumatic brain injuries.[59] In the long term, veterans with PTSD face an increased chance of developing metabolic syndrome and coronary heart disease and of exhibiting greater risk-taking behavior.[60]

Some people may be especially vulnerable to PTSD. Scientists have identified certain genes that increase susceptibility. Exposure to

**posttraumatic stress disorder (PTSD)** The repeated reliving of a trauma through nightmares or recollection.

traumatic experience in childhood along with poverty, difficult temperament, and low IQ also increase the risk.

PTSD can cause a range of symptoms, including fear, worry, insomnia, and drug and alcohol abuse (particularly in those with a history of alcohol abuse and those who drink to cope with stress).[61] Some individuals reexperience their terror and helplessness again and again in their dreams or intrusive thoughts. To avoid this psychic pain, they may try to avoid anything associated with the trauma. Some enter a state of emotional numbness and no longer can respond to people and experiences the way they once did, especially when it comes to showing tenderness or affection. Those who've been mugged or raped may be afraid to venture out by themselves.

Mental health professionals have found that no single approach to treatment works for all trauma victims. Some approaches, such as immediate "debriefing" to release emotions or treatment with anxiety-reducing medications, may not help and may even hinder long-term recovery.[62] But behavioral, cognitive, and psychodynamic therapy, sometimes along with psychiatric medication (described in Chapter 3), can usually help individuals suffering with PTSD.

## Resilience

Adversity—whether in the form of a traumatic event or chronic stress—has different effects on individuals. Some people never recover and continue on a downward slide that may ultimately prove fatal. Others return, though at different rates, to their prior level of functioning. In recent years researchers have focused their attention on a particularly intriguing group: those people who not only survive stressful experiences but also thrive—that is, who actually surpass their previous level of functioning. See the chapter on "Shock Absorption" in *IPC*.

Resilience can take many forms. A father whose child is kidnapped and killed may become a nationwide advocate for victims' rights. A student whose roommate dies in a car crash after a party may campaign for tougher laws against drunk driving. A couple whose premature baby spends weeks in a neonatal intensive care unit may find that their marriage has grown closer and stronger. Even though their experiences were painful,

*Your Strategies for Change*

## How to Cope with Distress after a Trauma

Senseless acts of violence or terrorism can trigger a variety of emotions, including shock, sorrow, fear, anger, and grief. You may have problems sleeping, concentrating, or going about simple chores. Because the world seems more dangerous, it may take a while for you to regain your sense of equilibrium. The following recommendations from the American Psychological Association can help.

- **Talk about it.** Ask for support from people who will listen to your concerns. It often helps to speak with others who have shared your experience so you do not feel so different or alone.

- **Strive for balance.** Remind yourself of people and events that are meaningful and comforting, even encouraging.

- **Take a break.** While you may want to keep informed, limit your exposure to news on television, the Internet, newspapers, or magazines. Schedule breaks to focus on something you enjoy.

- **Take care of yourself.** Engage in healthy behaviors, such as exercise, that will enhance your ability to cope. Avoid alcohol and drugs because they can suppress your feelings rather than help you to manage your distress.

- **Help others or do something productive.** Try volunteering at your school or within your community. Helping someone else often helps you feel better too.

the individuals often look back at them as bringing positive changes into their lives.[63]

Researchers have studied various factors that enable individuals to thrive in the face of adversity. These include:

- **An optimistic attitude**. Rather than reacting to a stressor simply as a threat, these men and women view stress as a challenge—one they believe they can and will overcome. Researchers have documented that individuals facing various stressors, including serious illness and bereavement, are more likely to report experiencing growth if they have high levels of hope and optimism.

- **Self-efficacy**. A sense of being in control of one's life can boost health, even in times of great stress.

- **Stress inoculation**. People who deal well with adversity often have had previous experiences with stress that toughened them in various ways, such as teaching them skills that enhanced their ability to cope and boosting their confidence in their ability to weather a rough patch.

- **Secure personal relationships**. Individuals who know they can count on the support of their loved ones are more likely to be resilient.

- **Spirituality or religiosity**. Religious coping may be particularly related to growth and resilience. In particular, two types seem most beneficial: spiritually based religious coping (receiving emotional reassurance and guidance from God) and good-deeds coping (living a better, more spiritual life that includes altruistic acts).

Resilience sometimes means developing new skills simply because, in order to get through the stressful experience, people had to learn something they hadn't known how to do before—for instance, wrangling with insurance companies or other bureaucracies. By mastering such skills, they become more fit to deal with an unpredictable world and develop new flexibility in facing the unknown.

Individuals who engage in proactive coping, a concept based on the principles of positive psychology discussed in Chapter 2, perceive stressful situations as challenges instead of threats. In a study of college women who had experienced traumas, those who saw these events as learning experiences and who felt gratitude for what they had learned reported posttraumatic emotional growth, rather than distress, in the form of increased strength, confidence, and maturity.[64]

Along with new abilities comes the psychological sense of mastery. "I survived this," an individual may say. "I'll be able to deal with other hard things in the future." Such confidence keeps people actively engaged in the effort to cope and is itself a predictor of eventual success. Stress also can make individuals more aware of the fulfilling aspects of life, and they may become more interested in spiritual pursuits. Certain kinds of stressful experiences also have social consequences. If a person experiencing a traumatic event finds that the significant others in his or her life can be counted on, the result can be a strengthening of their relationship.

# Organizing Your Time

We live in what some sociologists call hyperculture, a society that moves at warp speed. Information bombards us constantly. The rate of change seems to accelerate every year. Our "time-saving" devices—pagers, cell phones, modems, faxes, palm-size organizers, laptop computers—have simply extended the boundaries of where and how we work.

As a result, more and more people are suffering from "timesickness," a nerve-racking feeling that life has become little more than an endless to-do list. The best antidote is time management, and hundreds of books, seminars, and experts offer training in making the most of the hours in the day. Yet these well-intentioned methods often fail, and sooner or later most of us find ourselves caught in a time trap. (See the chapter on "Time Control" in *IPC*.)

## Are You Running Out of Time?

Every day you make dozens of decisions, and the choices you make about how to use your time directly affect your stress level. If you have a big test on Monday and a term paper due Tuesday, you may plan to study all weekend. Then, when you're invited to a party Saturday night, you go. Although you set the alarm for 7:00 a.m. on Sunday, you don't pull yourself out of bed until noon. By the time you start studying, it's 4:00 p.m., and anxiety is building inside you.

How can you tell if you've lost control of your time? The following are telltale symptoms of poor time management:

- Rushing.
- Chronic inability to make choices or decisions.
- Fatigue or listlessness.

- Constantly missed deadlines.
- Not enough time for rest or personal relationships.
- A sense of being overwhelmed by demands and details and having to do what you don't want to do most of the time.

One of the hard lessons of being on your own is that your choices and your actions have consequences. Stress is just one of them. But by thinking ahead, being realistic about your workload, and sticking to your plans, you can gain better control over your time and your stress levels.

## Time Management

Time management involves skills that anyone can learn, but they require commitment and practice to make a difference in your life. It may help to know the techniques that other students have found most useful:

- **Schedule your time.** Use a calendar or planner. Beginning the first week of class, mark down deadlines for each assignment, paper, project, and test scheduled that semester. Develop a daily schedule, listing very specifically what you will do the next day, along with the times. Block out times for working out, eating dinner, calling home, and talking with friends as well as for studying.
- **Develop a game plan.** Allow at least two nights to study for any major exam. Set aside more time for researching and writing papers. Make sure to allow time to revise and print out a paper—and to deal with emergencies like a computer breakdown. Set daily and weekly goals for every class. When working on a big project, don't neglect your other courses. Whenever possible, try to work ahead in all your classes.
- **Identify time robbers.** For several days keep a log of what you do and how much time you spend doing it. You may discover that disorganization is eating away at your time or that you have a problem getting started. (See the following section on "Overcoming Procrastination.")
- **Make the most of classes.** Read the assignments before class rather than waiting until just before you have a test. By reading ahead of time, you'll make it easier to understand the lectures. Go to class yourself.

Your own notes will be more helpful than a friend's or those from a note-taking service. Read your lecture notes at the end of each day or at least at the end of each week.

- **Develop an efficient study style.** Some experts recommend studying for 50 minutes, then breaking for 10 minutes. Small incentives, such as allowing yourself to call or visit a friend during those 10 minutes, can provide the motivation to keep you at the books longer. When you're reading, don't just highlight passages. Instead, write notes or questions to yourself in the margins, which will help you retain more information. Even if you're racing to start a paper, take a few extra minutes to prepare a workable outline. It will be easier to structure your paper when you start writing.
- **Focus on the task at hand.** Rather than worrying about how you did on yesterday's test or how you'll ever finish next week's project, focus intently on whatever you're doing at any given moment. If your mind starts to wander, use any distraction—the sound of the phone ringing or a noise from the hall—as a reminder to stay in the moment.
- **Turn elephants into hors d'oeuvres.** Cut a huge task into smaller chunks so it seems less enormous. For instance, break down your term paper into a series of steps, such as selecting a topic, identifying sources of research information, taking notes, developing an outline, and so on.
- **Keep your workspace in order.** Even if the rest of your room is a shambles, try to keep your desk clear. Piles of papers are distracting, and you can end up wasting lots of time looking for notes you misplaced or an article you have to read by morning. Try to spend the last ten minutes of the day getting your desk in order so you get a fresh start on the new day.

## Overcoming Procrastination

Putting off until tomorrow what should be done today is a habit that creates a great deal of stress for many students. In various studies, 30 to 60 percent of undergraduates have reported postponing academic tasks, such as studying for exams, writing papers, and reading weekly assignments, so often that their performance and grades suffered.[65] Occasional delay becomes a more serious problem when it triggers internal discomfort, such as anxiety, irritation, regret, despair, and self-blame, as well as external consequences, such as poor performance and lost opportunities.

In studies with students taking a health psychology course, researchers found that although procrastinating provided short-term benefits, including periods of low stress, the tendency to dawdle had long-term costs, including poorer health and lower grades. Early in the semester, the procrastinators reported less stress and fewer health problems than students who scored low on procrastination. However, by the end of the semester, procrastinators reported more health-related symptoms, more stress, and more visits to health-care professionals than did nonprocrastinators. Students who procrastinate also get poorer grades in courses with many deadlines.

In one recent study, older undergraduates were more prone to put off academic tasks than younger ones. The reasons, the researchers speculate, may be that the longer that students remain in school, the less enthusiasm they feel or the more entrenched bad study habits become. They also may have more family and work-related commitments that take priority over their studies.[66]

The three most common types of procrastination are putting off unpleasant things, putting off difficult tasks, and putting off tough decisions. Procrastinators are most likely to delay by wishing they didn't have to do what they must or by telling themselves they "just can't get started," which means they never do.

To get out of the procrastination trap, keep track of the tasks you're most likely to put off, and try to figure out why you don't want to tackle them. Think of alternative ways to get tasks done. If you put off library readings, for instance, is the problem getting to the library or the reading itself? If it's the trip to the library, arrange to walk over with a friend whose company you enjoy.

Do what you like least first. Once you have it out of the way, you can concentrate on the tasks you enjoy. Build time into your schedule for interruptions, unforeseen problems, and unexpected events, so you aren't constantly racing around. Establish ground rules for meeting your own needs (including getting enough sleep and making time for friends) before saying yes to any activity. Learn to live according to a three-word motto: Just do it! (See "Do It Now!" in Making Change Happen and in *Labs for IPC*.)

# Avoiding Stress Overload

Some life stressors are sudden and dramatic. More often, stress builds steadily over time and you may not realize the toll it is taking on your mind and body. Read through the list of warning signs below, and check any that apply to you.

\_\_\_\_ You are experiencing physical symptoms, including chronic fatigue, headaches, indigestion, diarrhea, and sleep problems.

\_\_\_\_ You are having frequent illness or worrying about illness.

\_\_\_\_ You are self-medicating, including nonprescription drugs.

\_\_\_\_ You are having problems concentrating on studies or work.

\_\_\_\_ You are feeling irritable, anxious, or apathetic.

\_\_\_\_ You are working or studying longer and harder than usual.

\_\_\_\_ You are exaggerating, to yourself and others, the importance of what you do.

\_\_\_\_ You are becoming accident-prone.

\_\_\_\_ You are breaking rules, whether it's a curfew at the dorm or a speed limit on the highway.

\_\_\_\_ You are going to extremes, such as drinking too much, overspending, or gambling.

Awareness of stress overload is the first step. For practical help in lowering your stress levels, read through "Rx: Relax," "Your Psychological Self-Care Pyramid," and "Help Yourself" in *Labs for IPC*. Choose one to complete.

If stress continues to be a problem in your life, you may be able to find help through support groups or counseling. Your school may provide counseling services or referrals to mental health professionals; ask your health instructor or the campus health department for this information. Remember that each day of distress robs you of energy, distracts you from life's pleasures, and interferes with achieving your full potential.

Self
Survey

# Student Stress Scale

The Student Stress Scale, an adaptation of Holmes and Rahe's Life Events Scale for college-age adults, provides a rough indication of stress levels and possible health consequences.

In the Student Stress Scale, each event, such as beginning or ending school, is given a score that represents the amount of readjustment a person has to make as a result of the change. In some studies, using similar scales, people with serious illnesses have been found to have high scores.

To determine your stress score, add up the number of points corresponding to the events you have experienced in the past 12 months.

| | | |
|---|---|---|
| 1. | Death of a close family member | 100 |
| 2. | Death of a close friend | 73 |
| 3. | Divorce of parents | 65 |
| 4. | Jail term | 63 |
| 5. | Major personal injury or illness | 63 |
| 6. | Marriage | 58 |
| 7. | Getting fired from a job | 50 |
| 8. | Failing an important course | 47 |
| 9. | Change in the health of a family member | 45 |
| 10. | Pregnancy | 45 |
| 11. | Sex problems | 44 |
| 12. | Serious argument with a close friend | 40 |
| 13. | Change in financial status | 39 |
| 14. | Change of academic major | 39 |
| 15. | Trouble with parents | 39 |
| 16. | New girlfriend or boyfriend | 37 |
| 17. | Increase in workload at school | 37 |
| 18. | Outstanding personal achievement | 36 |
| 19. | First quarter/semester in college | 36 |
| 20. | Change in living conditions | 31 |
| 21. | Serious argument with an instructor | 30 |
| 22. | Getting lower grades than expected | 29 |
| 23. | Change in sleeping habits | 29 |

| | | |
|---|---|---|
| 24. | Change in social activities | 29 |
| 25. | Change in eating habits | 28 |
| 26. | Chronic car trouble | 26 |
| 27. | Change in number of family get-togethers | 26 |
| 28. | Too many missed classes | 25 |
| 29. | Changing colleges | 24 |
| 30. | Dropping more than one class | 23 |
| 31. | Minor traffic violations | 20 |

Total Stress Score _____

Here's how to interpret your score: If your score is 300 or higher, you're at high risk for developing a health problem. If your score is between 150 and 300, you have a 50–50 chance of experiencing a serious health change within two years. If your score is below 150, you have a one in three chance of a serious health change.

Source: *Mullen, Kathleen, and Gerald Costello*. Health Awareness Through Discovery. *Minneapolis: Burgess Publishing Company, 1981.*

## *Making Change Happen*

### Do It Now!

Chronic procrastination can trip you up, slow you down, stress you out, and sabotage your best efforts. You know that. But you may not realize that procrastination isn't a character flaw. All delay stems from a certain degree of fear—fear of failure, fear of success, fear of not being in control. People who procrastinate simply haven't yet developed good habits for getting work done, or they have bad habits they need to unlearn and replace. "Do It Now" in *Labs for IPC* will show you how to do both. Here's a preview.

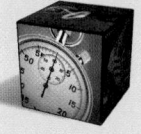

#### Get Real

In this section you get a clear fix on when and how you procrastinate by checking yes for each of ten statements that describe your behavior, including these three examples:

- I put off studying subjects I find difficult.

- I put off studying subjects I find easy because I don't think they will demand much time.

- I wait to have a big block of time before starting a project.

The more checks, the greater your problem with procrastination.

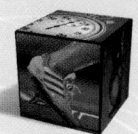

#### Get Ready

At this stage you set aside time for various exercises, including writing refutations of excuses you have used for procrastinating and keeping a simple chart of dates assignments are given and dates they are due for each class.

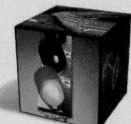

#### Get Going

In this stage you engage in seven exercises, each designed to preempt procrastination. Here are two examples:

- Complete the incompletes. Every day find one thing that you began at some point but have not yet finished. It might be making the bed, replying to an e-mail, buying a birthday card for your grandfather, replacing the bulb in your bedside lamp . . .

- Eavesdrop on your excuses. Every time you balk at writing the first sentence of a report or reading the first page of the assigned novel, stop and listen to what you're telling yourself. Here are three of the excuses you're likely to hear:

  - I'm too tired. I'll rest first.

  - There's no point in starting. I've got to meet my friend Ravi in ten minutes.

  - "Why do it on Friday? The instructor won't get it until Monday."

Write rebuttals to yourself. For instance, you might say, "Yes, I'm tired. I'll just work for half an hour, and then I'll go to bed." Or you might tell yourself, "I'll see how much I can get done in ten minutes."

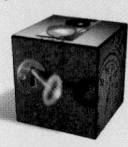

#### Lock It In

Keep doing the exercises, including completing your incompletes. Don't let a day go by when you don't cross something off your to-do list—even if it's making a to-do list.

# Making This Chapter Work for You

## Review Questions

1. In this text we define stress as
   a. a negative emotional state related to fatigue and similar to depression.
   b. the physiological and psychological response to any event or situation that either upsets or excites us.
   c. the end result of the general adaptation syndrome.
   d. a motivational strategy for making life changes.

2. Which of the following illustrates the defense mechanism of displacement?
   a. You have a beer in the evening after a tough day.
   b. You act as if nothing has happened after you have been laid off from your job.
   c. You start an argument with your sister after being laid off from your job.
   d. You argue with your boss after he lays you off from your job.

3. An effective technique for dealing with test stress is
   a. planning ahead.
   b. going on a study blitz the night before the test.
   c. going out for a few beers with friends the night before the test.
   d. talking with friends about everything but the test.

4. A person suffering from posttraumatic stress disorder may experience which of the following symptoms?
   a. procrastination
   b. constant thirst
   c. drowsiness
   d. terror-filled dreams

5. According to the general adaptation syndrome theory, how does the body typically respond to an acute stressor?
   a. The heart rate slows, blood pressure declines, and eye movement increases.
   b. The body enters a physical state called eustress and then moves into the physical state referred to as distress.
   c. If the stressor is viewed as a positive event, there are no physical changes.
   d. The body demonstrates three stages of change: alarm, resistance, and exhaustion.

6. Burnout is
   a. the aftermath of extreme anger triggered by stress.
   b. a feeling of complete defeat.
   c. the feeling that comes after a long evening of partying.
   d. a state of exhaustion brought on by constant or repeated emotional pressure.

7. To develop an efficient studying style:
   a. Schedule your study time on a calendar or planner, have a friend go to class and take notes for you, and join the chess club.
   b. Schedule your study time on a calendar or planner, write notes or questions about the material in the margins of the book, and give yourself a small break after every study hour.
   c. Read assignments before class, call a friend before studying, and plan on working for four continuous hours.
   d. Read assignments before class, skip class when studying for an exam, and have snacks on hand.

8. Over time, increased levels of stress hormones have been shown to increase a person's risk for which of the following conditions?
   a. high blood pressure, memory loss, and skin disorders
   b. stress fractures, male pattern baldness, and hypothyroidism
   c. hemophilia, AIDS, and hay fever
   d. none of the above

9. A relaxed peaceful state of being can be achieved with which of the following activities?
   a. an aerobic exercise class
   b. playing a computer game
   c. meditating for 15 minutes
   d. attending a rap concert

10. Stress levels in college students
    a. may be high due to stressors such as academic pressures, financial concerns, learning disabilities, and relationship problems.
    b. are usually low because students feel empowered living independently of their parents.
    c. are typically highest in seniors because their self-esteem diminishes during the college years.
    d. are lower in minority students because they are used to stressors such as a hostile social climate and actual or perceived discrimination.

*Answers to these questions can be found on page 672.*

## Critical Thinking

1. Identify three stressful situations in your life and determine whether they are examples of eustress or distress. Describe both the positive and negative aspects of each situation.

2. Can you think of any ways in which your behavior or attitudes might create stress for others? What changes could you make to avoid doing so?

3. What advice might you give an incoming freshman at your school about managing stress in college? What techniques have been most helpful for you in dealing with stress? Suppose that this student is from a different ethnic group than you. What additional suggestions would you have for this student?

## Media Menu

Visit www.cengagebrain.com to access course materials and companion resources for this text that will:

- Help you evaluate your knowledge of the material.

- Allow you to prepare for exams with interactive quizzing.

- Use the CengageNOW product to develop a Personalized Learning Plan targeting resources that address areas you should study.

- Coach you through identifying target goals for behavioral change and creating and monitoring your personal change plan throughout the semester using the Behavior Change Planner available in the CengageNOW resource.

## Internet Connections

**www.teachhealth.com**
This comprehensive website is written specifically for college students by Steven Burns, M.D. It features the following topics: signs of how to recognize stress, two stress surveys for adults and college students, information on the pathophysiology of stress, the genetics of stress and stress tolerance, and information on how to best manage and treat stress.

**www.mindtools.com/smpage.html**
This site covers a variety of topics on stress management, including recognizing stress, exercise, time management, coping mechanisms, and more. The site also features a free comprehensive personal self-assessment with questions pertaining to work and home stressors, physical and behavioral signs and symptoms, as well as personal coping skills and resources.

## Key Terms

The terms listed are used on the page indicated. Definitions of the terms are in the Glossary at the end of the book.

acculturation 98

adaptive response 91

biofeedback 104

burnout 101

defense mechanism 103

diathesis stress model 92

distress 90

eustress 90

general adaptation syndrome (GAS) 91

homeostasis 91

meditation 105

mindfulness 106

posttraumatic stress disorder (PTSD) 107

progressive relaxation 104

stress 89

stressors 89

visualization, or guided imagery 104

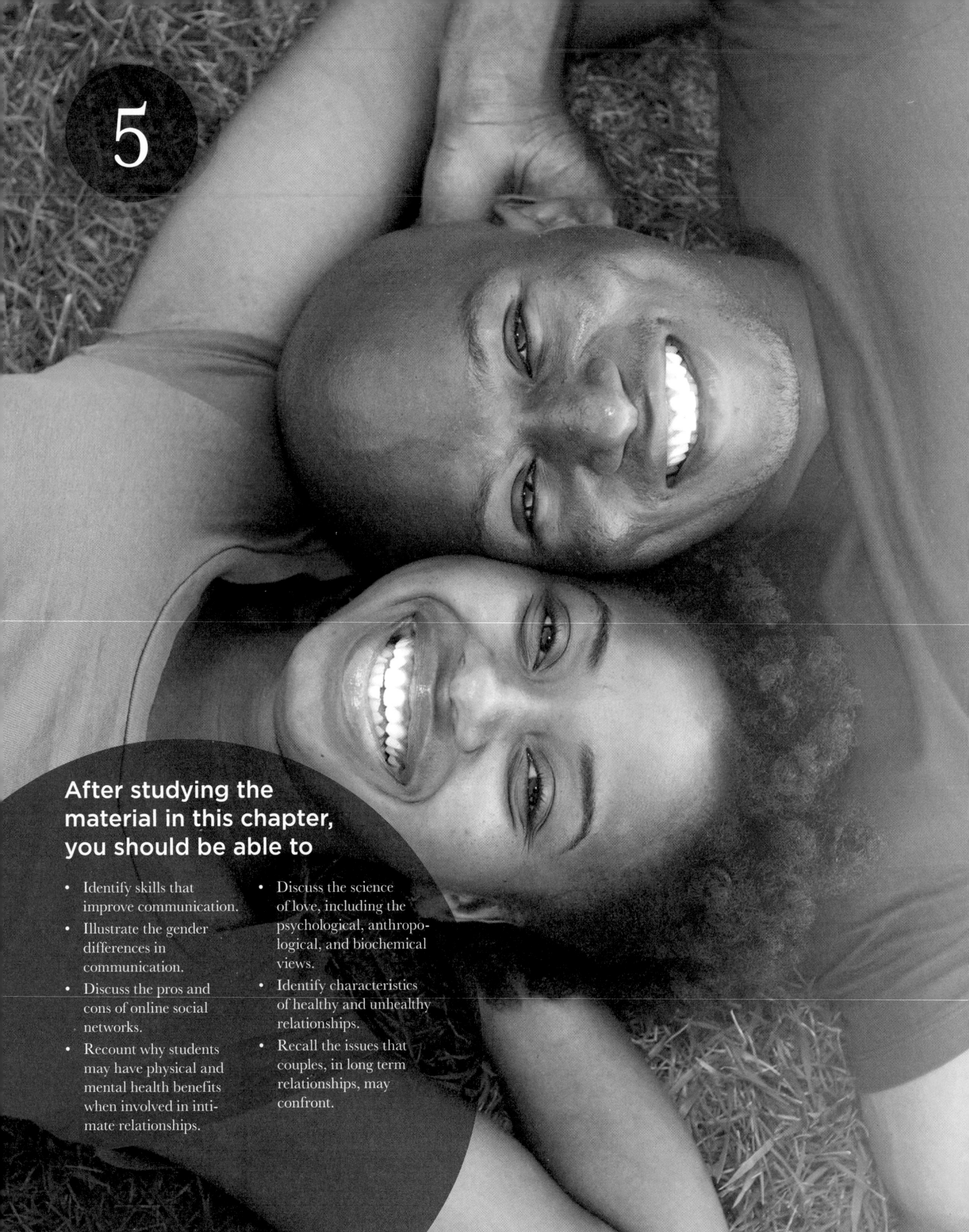

**5**

## After studying the material in this chapter, you should be able to

- Identify skills that improve communication.
- Illustrate the gender differences in communication.
- Discuss the pros and cons of online social networks.
- Recount why students may have physical and mental health benefits when involved in intimate relationships.
- Discuss the science of love, including the psychological, anthropological, and biochemical views.
- Identify characteristics of healthy and unhealthy relationships.
- Recall the issues that couples, in long term relationships, may confront.

Andrea got her first cell phone when she was 8, signed up for e-mail when she was 11, went on Facebook at 13, started tweeting and posting YouTube videos at 16, and joined LinkedIn after getting her first summer job at 17. These days she G-chats, i-Chats, and Facebook chats (often all at the same time) and Skypes with friends.

# Social Health

Wherever she goes, Andrea checks in with Foursquare and posts photos on Flickr. Even in class she texts and sends BBMs (BlackBerry messages) and kik messages. With 800-plus Facebook friends and 500 Twitter followers, Andrea says she can't imagine feeling lonely—as long as she doesn't misplace her cell phone and its battery doesn't die.

Is Andrea the poster child for social health in the twenty-first century? Or is her virtual socializing somehow undermining her overall well-being? Scientists who study relationships are just beginning to explore the impact of our digital world. Will 140-character tweets and "emoticons" replace conversation? Could online social networking make face-to-face friendships obsolete?

No one yet knows, but as much as technology may change our lives, one thing remains constant: We always have craved and always will crave human connection. As individuals and as part of society, we need to care about others and to know that others care about us, to feel for others and have others feel for us, to share what we know and to learn from what others know.

Your relationships with your family, friends, coworkers, and loved ones may amaze, irritate, exhilarate, frustrate, and delight you. They also may affect your health. As noted in Chapter 1,

your ability to communicate, to develop satisfying relationships, and to live in harmony with others is an important dimension of health and wellness.

This chapter discusses the social needs we all share, the ways some of us respond to those needs, healthy and unhealthy relationships, and the possibilities that exist for coming together from our solitude to warm ourselves in each other's glow.

## The Social Dimension of Health

Social health refers to the ability to interact effectively with other people and with the social environment, to develop satisfying interpersonal relationships, and to fulfill social roles. Social health doesn't necessarily mean joining organizations or mingling in large groups, but it does involve participating in your community, living in harmony with others, communicating clearly, and practicing healthy sexual behaviors (discussed in Chapter 9).

Visit www.cengagebrain.com to access course materials for this text, including the Behavior Change Planner, interactive quizzes, tutorials, and more. See the preface on page xv for details.

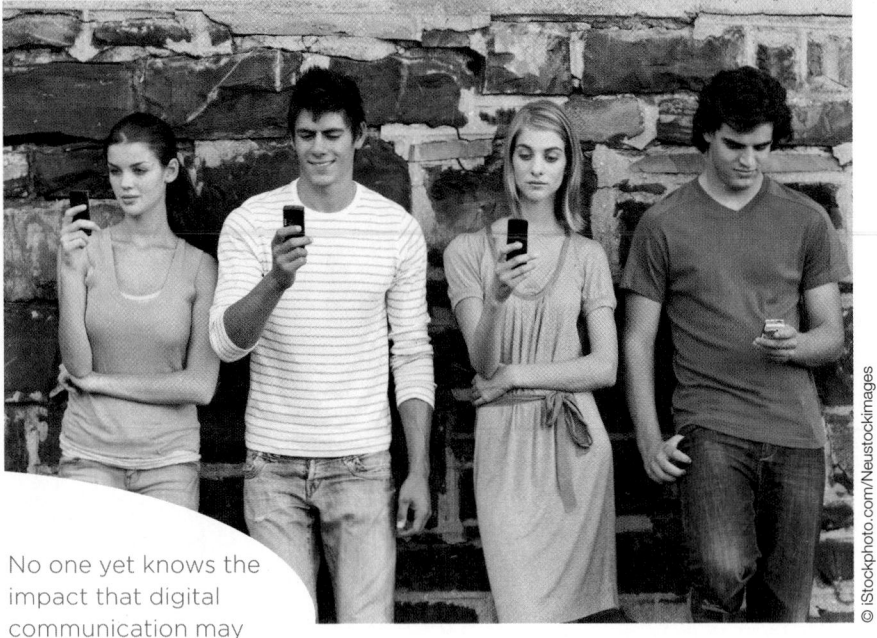

No one yet knows the impact that digital communication may have on relationships. Do you think texting might someday take the place of talking?

Researchers also have been studying the concept of "social contagion," the process by which friends, friends of friends, acquaintances, and others in our social circle influence our behavior and our health—both positively and negatively. By analyzing relationships among the 15,000 people followed over three generations in the Framingham heart study, researchers found that various health-related factors changed, not just individually over time, but among clusters of people.

The effect was most striking for obesity. When one participant became obese, his or her friends were more likely (by 57 percent) to become obese, too. Even if a friend of a friend of a friend gained weight, the risk of obesity rose about 10 percent. Smoking also spread socially. If one participant began smoking, his or her friends were 36 percent more likely to take up the habit. Similar patterns occurred with drinking, happiness, and loneliness.

"People are connected, and their health is connected," the researchers concluded.[1] Some have criticized the methods in this study, but most experts endorse the idea that people not only need but influence people. The reasons may include peer pressure or "mirror neurons" in the brain that automatically mimic what we see in the people around us.

According to social scientists, each of us is connected within three degrees (to a friend, a friend of a friend, and that friend's friend) to more than 1,000 people. Think of this social web as an opportunity. By your good health behaviors you can, in theory, influence 1,000 individuals to become healthier, fitter, and happier.

As huge epidemiological studies have demonstrated beyond any doubt, supportive relationships buffer us from stress, distress, and disease. People with close ties to others have stronger cardiovascular and immune systems, resist colds better, and are less vulnerable to serious illness and premature death.

Specific qualities in a relationship affect physical health, particularly *social support*. This term refers to the ways in which we provide information or assistance, show affection, comfort, and confide in others. As mounting evidence shows, people of all ages function best in socially supportive environments.

This is particularly true of college students, who report more stress and more physical symptoms when they feel a lack of family support. More than any other component of social support, a sense of belonging may have the greatest impact on college students' health. Because college is a transition time, forming new attachments may be especially important—and beneficial to overall health.

Your social support network might consist of people you see almost every day, more casual acquaintances, and friends, followers, and bloggers you get to know online. (Social networking is covered later in this chapter.) Simply staying in touch and sharing each other's lives bolster feelings of self-worth, security, and belonging.

## Communicating and Relating

Healthy, mutually beneficial relationships add joy to our years and maybe even years to our life. Unhealthy or dysfunctional ones can be so toxic that they undermine health as well as happiness. By mastering skills to communicate more clearly and by being responsible and responsive in your interactions with others, you can cultivate what psychologist Daniel Goleman called "social intelligence" and create relationships worth cherishing.

© iStockphoto.com/Neustockimages

## Learning to Listen

Learning to listen and to send clear messages is the essence of good communication. The more effectively we communicate, the more likely we are to create good relationships built on honesty, understanding, and mutual trust. Such relationships can infuse our lives with a richness no solitary pleasure can match.

Communication stems from a desire to know and a decision to tell. The first step is learning how to listen. (See "Listen Up" on page 147 in *Labs for IPC*.) Then you mostly choose what information about yourself to disclose and what to keep private. But in opening up to others, you increase your own self-knowledge and understanding.

A great deal of daily communication focuses on facts: on the who, what, where, when, and how. Information is easy to convey and comprehend. Emotions are not. Some people have great difficulty saying "I appreciate you" or "I care about you," even though they are genuinely appreciative and caring. Others find it hard to know what to say in response and how to accept such expressions of affection.

Some people feel that relationships shouldn't require any effort, that there's no need to talk of responsibility between people who care about each other. Yet responsibility is implicit in our dealings with anyone or anything we value—and what can be more valuable than those with whom we share our lives? Friendships and other intimate relationships always demand an emotional investment, but the rewards they yield are great.

Sometimes people convey strong emotions with a kiss or a hug, a pat or a punch, but such actions aren't precise enough to communicate exact thoughts. Stalking out of a room and slamming the door may be clear signs of anger, but they don't explain what caused the anger or suggest what to do about it. You must learn how to communicate all feelings clearly and appropriately if you hope to become truly close to another person.

As two people build a relationship, they must sharpen their communication skills so that they can discuss all the issues they may confront. They must learn how to communicate anger as well as affection, hurt as well as joy—and they must listen as carefully as they speak.

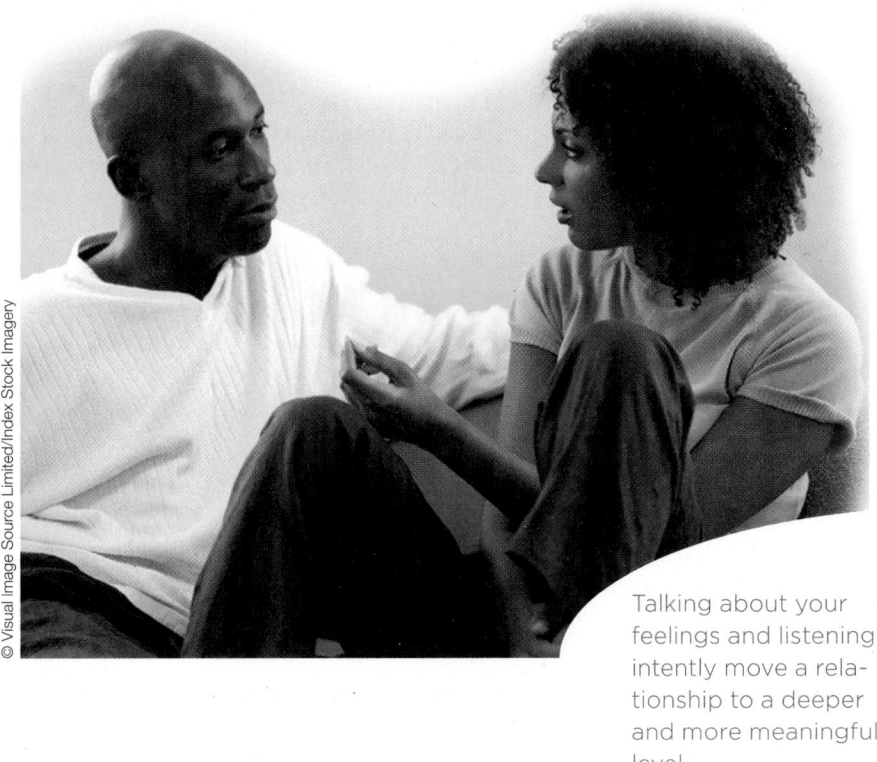

Talking about your feelings and listening intently move a relationship to a deeper and more meaningful level.

Listening involves more than waiting for the other person to stop talking. Listening is an active process of trying to understand the other person's feelings and motivation. Effective listeners ask questions when they're not sure they understand the other person and prompt the other person to continue.

## Being Agreeable But Assertive

There's an old saying that "nice guys finish last," but, according to recent research, that's not the case. Psychologists translate "niceness" into a personality trait called "agreeableness," which includes being helpful, unselfish, generally trusting, considerate, cooperative, sympathetic, warm, and concerned for others. Among the benefits that agreeable people enjoy are strong relationships, less conflict, happy marriages, better job performance, healthier eating habits and behaviors, less stress, and fewer medical complaints.[2]

But agreeable people aren't so "nice" that they are easily influenced or taken advantage of by others. In situations that call for it, they make their needs and desires clear by being assertive—but not aggressive.

© Visual Image Source Limited/Index Stock Imagery

## How to Assert Yourself

- **Use "I" statements to explain your feelings.** This allows you to take ownership of your opinions and feelings without putting down others for how they feel and think.

- **Listen to and acknowledge what the other person says.** After you speak, find out if the other person understands your position. Ask how he or she feels about what you've said.

- **Be direct and specific.** Describe the problem as you see it, using neutral language rather than assigning blame. Also suggest a specific solution, but make it clear that you'd like the lines of communication and negotiation to remain open.

- **Don't think you have to be obnoxious in order to be assertive.** It's most effective to state your needs and preferences without any sarcasm or hostility.

Assertiveness doesn't mean screaming or telling someone off. You can communicate your wishes calmly and clearly. Assertiveness is a behavior that respects your rights and the rights of other people even when you disagree.

You can change a situation you don't like by communicating your feelings and thoughts in nonprovocative words, by focusing on specifics, and by making sure you're talking with the person who is directly responsible.

## How Men and Women Communicate

Gender differences in communication start early.[3] By age 1, boys make less eye contact than girls and pay more attention to moving objects like cars than to human faces. Both mothers and fathers talk less about feelings (except anger) to sons than daughters, and boys' vocabularies include fewer "feeling" words. In the playground, if not at home, boys learn to choke back tears and show no fear. Their faces—once as openly emotional as girls—become less expressive as they move through the elementary years.

As adults, men use fewer words and talk, at least in public, as a means of putting themselves in a one-up situation—unlike women, who talk to draw others closer. Even with friends, men mainly swap information as they talk shop, sports, cars, computers.

In studies of language, Deborah Tannen and other linguists have identified the following gender differences, which may be based on sex or gender roles:

*Men:*

- Speak more often and for longer periods in public.

- Interrupt more, breaking in on another's monologue if they aren't getting the information they need.

- Look into a woman's eyes more often when talking than they would if talking with another man.

- When writing, use more numbers, more prepositions, and more articles such as "an" and "the."

- Write briefer, more utilitarian e-mails.

- Write blogs for the sake of a personal expectation or motive.

- In blogs or chat rooms, are more likely to make strong assertions, disagree with others, and use profanity and sarcasm.

*Women:*

- Speak more in private, usually to build better connections with others.

- Are generally better listeners, facilitating conversation by nodding, asking questions, and signaling interest by saying "uh-huh," or "yes."

- Are more likely to wait for a speaker to finish rather than interrupting.

- Look into another woman's eyes more often than they would if talking with a man.

- When writing, use more words overall, more words related to emotion (positive and negative), more idea words, more hearing, feeling, and sensing words, more causal words (such as *because*), and more modal words (*would, should, could*).

- Write e-mails in much the same way they talk, using words to build a connection with people.

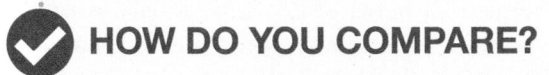
- Write blogs for the sake of self-expression.

- In blogs or chat rooms, are more prone to posing questions, making suggestions, and including polite expressions. Communication researchers studying the differences between "he-mails" and "she-mails" have also found that people who are not generally verbally expressive—mainly but not exclusively men—often convey more feelings in e-mails than they do in face-to-face conversations.

- As students, seek out, forge, and maintain more supportive ties than men, rely on friends more in times of stress, and provide more support than men do.

## Nonverbal Communication

More than 90 percent of communication may be nonverbal. While we speak with our vocal cords, we communicate with our facial expressions, tone of voice, hands, shoulders, legs, torsos, posture. Body language is the building block upon which more advanced verbal forms of communication rest.

In a survey of undergraduates at a large southeastern university, those who saw themselves as "involved" daters were more concerned about nonverbal communication than were "casual" daters.

These individuals were more likely to "work hard" to ensure that their nonverbal behavior backed up the words they said—and to say their partners did the same. Regardless of their dating status, the female students valued nonverbal behavior more than men did. They also engaged in more forms of nonverbal communication, such as looking their partners straight in the eye and nodding their heads as their partners spoke.

Culture has a great deal of influence over body language. In some cultures, for example, establishing eye contact is considered hostile or challenging; in others, it conveys friendliness. A person's sense of personal space—the distance he or she feels most comfortable in keeping from others—also varies in different societies.

## Forming Relationships

We first learn how to relate in our families as children. Our relationships with parents and siblings change dramatically as we grow toward independence. Relationships between friends also change as they move or develop different interests; between lovers, as they come to know

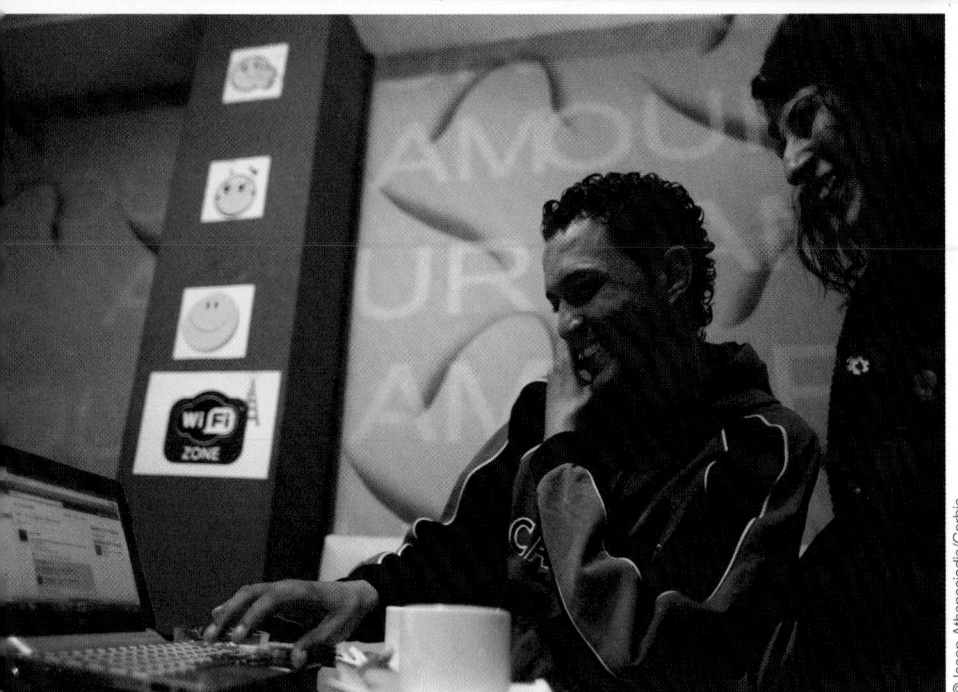

"Computer-mediated communication"—the conveying of written text via the Internet—is changing the ways we relate to others.

more about each other; between spouses, as they pass through life together; and between parents and children, as youngsters develop and mature. But throughout life, close relationships, tested and strengthened by time, allow us to explore the depths of our souls and the heights of our emotions. (See Self Survey, "How Strong Are the Communication and Affection in Your Relationship?" on p. 146.)

## I, Myself, and Me

It is part of our nature as mammals and as human beings to crave relationships. But invariably we end up alone at times. Solitude is not without its own quiet joys—time for introspection, self-assessment, learning from the past, and looking toward the future. Each of us can cultivate the joy of our own company, of being alone without crossing the line and becoming lonely.

The way each of us perceives himself or herself affects all the ways we reach out and relate to others. If we feel unworthy of love, others may share that opinion. Self-esteem (discussed in Chapter 2) provides a positive foundation for our relationships with others. Self-esteem doesn't mean vanity or preoccupation with our own needs; rather, it is a genuine concern and

respect for ourselves so that we remain true to our own feelings and beliefs. We can't know or love or accept others until we know and love and accept ourselves, however imperfect we may be.

## Social Networking

Modern technology is changing our social DNA. Today you can call, text, or video chat with almost anyone almost anywhere with a "smart" cell phone. You also may blog, "tweet," follow Facebook or other networking services, upload photos, and give the world (or selected citizens) front-row seats to your life.

Some experts say humans are only doing what comes naturally—just with twenty-first-century tools. Our brains seem wired to connect. As neuroimaging studies have shown, the amygdala, a brain region involved in processing emotional reactions, is bigger in individuals with large, complex social networks.[4]

These networks are getting bigger than ever—thanks to "computer-mediated communication"—the conveying of written text via the Internet—whether by Facebook, Twitter, or ever-evolving new networks and sites. About one in ten online adults maintains a blog, most often a personal journal or commentary site.[5] College students are blogging and e-mailing less than they did five years ago and communicating more via Facebook and Twitter.[6]

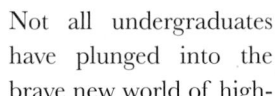 Not all undergraduates have plunged into the brave new world of high-tech communications. Female and white students are more than twice as likely to own cell phones than are male and African American students. Income also matters. Students whose families earn more than $100,000 a year are more than three times as likely to own a cell phone than are those from lower economic brackets.[7]

Computers are more widely used for social networking—and at younger ages. According to recent surveys, seven in ten teens between ages 12 and 17 use social networking sites; eight in ten of those between ages 14 and 17 have a profile page.[8] Young users may face special risks online, including unsuspected contact with pedophiles and perverts, cyber stalking, cyber bullying, and other forms of harassment.[9]

College-age young adults may be the most wired age group. More than 94 percent of college students maintain a social networking profile, with Facebook the most popular choice.[10] In one study undergraduates reported visiting social network profiles 2.4 to 4.2 times a day for an average time of one to two-and-a-half hours.[11] (See How Do You Compare? The Net Generation on p. 121.)

 **The Facebook Phenomenon** The world's most popular website worldwide was created by a college student for college students in 2004. More than 600 million users around the globe have since joined and spend an average of 19 minutes a day on the site. Men and women between ages 18 and 25 make up about a third of Facebook users.[12] However, these days your parents and their friends are as likely to have Facebook pages as your peers.

What draws people, particularly young ones, to social networking sites? According to researchers, the appeal comes from the opportunity such sites offer to:

- Explore users' identities
- Make new friends
- Continue to develop long-standing relationships
- Explore their sexuality
- Voice their opinions
- Be creative

Facebook, users add, is fun and convenient, allowing them to get a peek into the worlds of many acquaintances, not just those they see or interact with regularly.[13] Simply having a certain number of Facebook friends boosts feelings of happiness, researchers have found. Even more meaningful is getting support from online acquaintances—but only if it comes in response to an honest presentation of oneself.[14]

Despite its many benefits and pleasures, social networking also poses risks. At the very least, it can take up time and attention that should be given to studying and other commitments.

Facebook can, deliberately or not, become a tool for humiliating, harassing, bullying, or stalking others. Boyfriends and girlfriends have broken up by "defriending" a partner. Doctors have documented at least one case in which viewing his "ex" in photos with new male friends on Facebook triggered asthma attacks in a rejected suitor.[15]

*Self-Disclosure and Privacy in a Digital Age* A key element of relationships—whether friendships or romantic ones—is **self-disclosure**—that is, how much we reveal about ourselves to another person. What you share about yourself is a critical building block that affects the nature and quality of the bonds you establish with others.

Social networking has transformed the issues of privacy and disclosure. Rather than confiding in a trusted friend, individuals may go online and reveal highly personal information to a stranger—or, if a comment or video makes its way onto a public site, to many strangers.

Previously personal moments now play out in public—sometimes by choice (as in an engagement announced by a change in status on Facebook), sometimes by chance (as when someone uploads a video of drunk beer-pong players).

In surveys of teenagers and young adults with online profiles, a third to a half had posted photos or videos depicting what researchers call "negative health risk behaviors," such as drinking and using drugs. Many viewed the images (of drinking more than drug use) in positive ways.[16] Parents, friends of parents, siblings, coworkers, and employers often have a very different perspective.

Sexual disclosures and references also can have unanticipated consequences. In one recent study, women's sexy pictures or comments increased the sexual expectations of male students. "The sexier the pictures, the wilder you know they are," commented one young man. "Sexual pictures equal sexual activity being around the corner," said another.

Yet at the same time, sexual or suggestive material lessened the guys' interest in a serious relationship with the young women. "I don't want to show my friends a girl I like on Facebook and have them see sexual pictures and her all drunk," a student remarked. Sexual references generate powerful "subconscious impressions," the researchers concluded—and could put female students at risk for unwanted sexual advances.[17]

**self-disclosure** Sharing personal information and experiences with another that he or she would not otherwise discover; self-disclosure involves risk and vulnerability.

# Friendship

Friendship has been described as "the most holy bond of society." Every culture has prized the ties of respect, tolerance, and loyalty that friendship builds and nurtures. An anonymous writer put it well:

*A friend is one who knows you as you are,*
*Understands where you've been,*
*Accepts who you've become,*
*And still gently invites you to grow.*

Friends can be a basic source of happiness, a connection to a larger world, a source of solace in times of trouble. Although we have different friends throughout life, often the friendships of adolescence and young adulthood are the closest we ever form. They ease the normal break from parents and the transition from childhood to independence.

On average we devote 40 percent of our limited social time to the five most important people we know, who represent just 3 percent of our social world.[18] Having more than five best friends is impossible when we interact face-to-face because of time constraints. But thanks to social networking online, it's possible to accumulate hundreds, even thousands, of virtual friends.

Even so, most of us can maintain no more than 150 meaningful relationships online and off—a total called "Dunbar's number" in recognition of the researcher who came up with it.[19] At one time, when almost all humans on earth lived in small, rural, interconnected communities, everyone in a village may have known the same 150 people.

In our modern mobile society, we move time and again, leaving behind old friends. Emotional closeness, Dunbar found, declines by around 15 percent a year in the absence of face-to-face contact. Facebook, at the least, provides us an opportunity to maintain friendships that would otherwise rapidly wither away. Online status reports and, more effectively, everyday images of faraway friends can provide some of the same benefits as real-life friendship, including enhanced self-esteem and happiness.[20]

Campus friends help each other in other ways, including preventing female friends from engaging in risky sexual behavior after heavy drinking. In a recent study of 141 undergraduates, three-quarters said they would persuade a female friend not to go home with a new male acquaintance or that they would make sure she arrived home safely. However, the likelihood of their intervening depended on how well they knew the woman and the man. They would be more likely to step in and protect a friend in what they deemed a risky situation but more willing to do nothing if both they and their friends knew the guy.[21] What would you do?

# Loneliness

More so than many other countries, ours is a nation of loners. Recent trends—longer work hours, busy family schedules, frequent moves, high divorce rates—have created even more lonely people. Only about a quarter of Americans say they're never lonely. Loneliest of all are adolescents and elderly people, those who are divorced, separated, or widowed, and those who live alone or solely with children.[22] Loneliness is most likely to cause emotional distress when it is chronic rather than episodic.

To combat loneliness, people may join groups, fling themselves into projects and activities, or surround themselves with superficial acquaintances. Others avoid the effort of trying to connect, sometimes limiting most of their personal interactions to chat groups on the Internet.

The true keys to overcoming loneliness are developing resources to fulfill our own potential and learning to reach out to others. In this way, loneliness can become a means to personal growth and discovery.

# Shyness and Social Anxiety

Many people are uncomfortable meeting strangers or speaking or performing in public. In some surveys, as many as 40 percent of people describe themselves as shy or socially anxious. Some shy people—an estimated 10 to 15 percent of children—are born with a predisposition to shyness.[23] Others become shy because they don't learn proper social responses or because they experience rejection or shame.

Some people are "fearfully" shy; that is, they withdraw and avoid contact with others and experience a high degree of anxiety and fear in social situations. Others are "self-consciously" shy. They enjoy the company of others but become highly self-aware and anxious in social situations.

In studies of college students, men have reported somewhat more shyness than women. Students may develop symptoms of shyness or social anxiety when they go to a party or are called on in class. Some experience symptoms when they try to perform any sort of action in the presence of others, even such everyday activities as eating in public, using a public restroom, or writing a check.

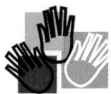 About 7 percent of the population could be diagnosed with a severe form of social anxiety, called **social phobia**, in which individuals typically fear and avoid various social situations. Childhood shyness, emotional abuse, neglect, and chronic illness increase the likelihood of this problem.[24] Asian cultures typically show the lowest rates; Russian and American, the highest.[25]

Adolescents and young adults with severe social anxiety are at increased risk of major depression. The key difference between these problems and normal shyness and self-consciousness is the degree of distress and impairment that individuals experience.

If you're shy, you can overcome much of your social apprehensiveness on your own, in much the same way as you might set out to stop smoking or lose weight. For example, you can improve your social skills by pushing yourself to introduce yourself to a stranger at a party or to chat about the weather or the food selections with the person next to you in a cafeteria line. Gradually, you'll acquire a sense of social timing and a verbal ease that will take the worry out of close encounters with others. Those with more disabling social anxiety may do best with psychotherapy and medication, which have proved highly effective.

## Building a Healthy Community

"No man is an island," the English poet John Donne wrote in 1624. In today's global society, this phrase rings just as true. In addition to our families, friendships, and social networks, we are part of communities—our campus, our neighborhood, our town or city. (Chapter 19 discusses the community we are all citizens of: Planet Earth.)

Contributing to your community can take many forms, from volunteering at a Habitat for Humanity building project to singing in a church choir. By giving to others, you get a great deal in return. As researchers have documented, **altruism**—helping or giving to others—enhances self-esteem, relieves physical and mental stress, and protects psychological well-being.

Hans Selye, the father of stress research, described cooperation with others for the self's sake as altruistic egotism, whereby we satisfy our own needs while helping others satisfy theirs. This concept is essentially an updated version of the golden rule: Do unto others as you would have them do unto you. The important

*Your Strategies for Change*

## Become Involved

- **Evaluate your schedule and current commitments.** Be realistic in assessing how much time you have available to give to others. If you have only an hour or two a week, that's enough to serve a meal at a center for the homeless or read to children at a library.

- **Organize your friends.** If your campus is sponsoring a beach clean-up or your community is organizing a diabetes research walkathon, get your friends to join with you to make an even bigger difference—and have more fun!

- **If your're interested in health, volunteer to assist at screening days on campus or in the community.** Check the schedule of upcoming local events sponsored by groups such as the American Cancer Society, American Heart Association, and American Lung Association.

- **Check out programs like AmeriCorps and the Peace Corps as post-graduation options.** You'll learn a lot about life, the world, and yourself while providing help to people who need it most.

**social phobia** A severe form of social anxiety marked by extreme fears and avoidance of social situations.

**altruism** Acts of helping or giving to others without thought of self-benefit.

difference is that you earn your neighbor's love and help by offering him or her love and help.

 Volunteerism helps those who give as well as those who receive. People involved in community organizations, for instance, consistently report a surge of well-being called *helper's high*, which they describe as a unique sense of calmness, warmth, and enhanced self-worth. College students who provided community service as part of a semester-long course reported changes in attitude (including a decreased tendency to blame people for their misfortunes), self-esteem (primarily a belief that they can make a difference), and behavior (a greater commitment to do more volunteer work).

# Dating on Campus

Dating isn't what it used to be. Many young people socialize in groups until a couple pairs off into a romantic relationship. Rather than the conventional dinner and a movie, college students may just get together to hang out. Is one person interested in something more? Is the other? Often it can take a while for couples to figure out if they are in fact dating.

## Meeting People

With more people remaining single longer, the search for a good date has become more complex. Singles bars have become less popular; cafés, Laundromats, health clubs, and bookstores have become more acceptable as places to meet new people.

Many young people meet or maintain contact online. Facebook, texting, tweeting, and e-mail may be convenient and fun, but virtual encounters can be tricky. Because you can't observe body language or detect the tone in a voice, it can be hard to tell if a person is being sincere or sarcastic, informal or inappropriate.

Flirting in the digital world tends to be bolder and racier than in real life, in part because two people are looking at a screen rather than into each other's eyes. Caught up in the "conversation," they may not reflect on the message

## ❗ CONSUMER ALERT

### Online Flirting and Dating

Virtual flirtations can be fun, but they also entail some risks, particularly if you decide to go off-line and meet in person. Here are some guidelines:

#### Facts to Know

- Remember that you have no way of verifying if a correspondent is telling the truth about anything—sex, age, occupation, marital status. If your online partner seems insincere or strange in any way, stop corresponding.

- Be careful of what you type. Anything you put on the Internet can end up almost anywhere, including with potential employers. To avoid embarrassment, don't say anything you wouldn't want to see in newspaper print.

#### Steps to Take

- Don't give out your address, telephone number, or any other identifying information. The people you meet online are strangers, and you should keep your guard up.

- Don't "date" on an office or university computer. You could end up supplying your professors, classmates, or coworkers with unintentional entertainment. Also, many organizations and institutions consider e-mail messages company property.

- Don't rely on the Internet as your only method of meeting people. Continue to get out in the real world and meet potential dates the old-fashioned way: live and in person.

- If you do decide to meet, make your first face-to-face encounter a double or group date and make it somewhere public, like a café or museum. Don't plan a full-day outing. Coffee or a drink in a crowded place makes the best transition from e-mail.

- Don't let your expectations run wild. Finding Mr. or Ms. Right is no easier in cyberspace than anywhere else, so be realistic about where your relationship might lead.

they're sending—or whether they should be sending it at all. (See Consumer Alert.)

Dating can do more than help you meet people. By dating, you can learn how to make conversation, get to know more about others as well as yourself, and share feelings, opinions, and interests. In adolescence and young adulthood, dating also provides an opportunity for exploring your sexual identity. Some people date for months and never share more than a good-night kiss. Others may fall into bed together before they fall in love or even "like."

Separating your emotional feelings about someone you're dating from your sexual desire is often difficult. The first step to making responsible sexual decisions is respecting your sexual values and those of your partner. If you care about the other person—not just his or her body—and the relationship you're creating, sex will be an important, but not the all-important, factor while you're dating. (See Chapter 9 for more on sexual decision making.)

The Internet may be replacing introductions through mutual friends as the best way to meet potential dates and mates. In a recent survey on "How Couples Meet and Stay Together," 80 percent of those with Internet connections were either married or living with a partner, compared with 63 percent of those without access to the Web. Individuals who traditionally have found it difficult to find a good mate—such as middle-aged heterosexuals and gays and lesbians, as well as those with disabilities—have found online sites particularly useful.[26]

Some young people also engage in sexual activities with friends with whom they are not romantically involved. Many "friends with benefits" may have had a sexual relationship in the past. Others have no expectation of any serious involvement.

## Hooking Up

On some campuses hooking up is as common as or even more common than dating.[27] In various studies, about 75 percent of men and 84 percent of women reported hooking up in college, with a mean of about ten hookups. Fewer—52 percent of men and 36 percent of women—reported a "penetrative" hookup involving oral, vaginal, or anal sex.[28]

Traditional dating and hooking up vary in many ways. In dating, one person (usually the male) asks the other out, picks her up, pays for a meal or a movie, initiates sexual advances, and takes her home. Men may see dating as costly both in terms of responsibility and finances since they are expected to entertain their date and cover the expenses. But they get to decide whom to ask out, what activity to plan, and when to end the date. Women play a passive, reactive role in dating but usually are expected only to be pleasant and look nice. Usually they have the ability to accept or reject a man's sexual advances.[29] (See Table 5.1 on the risks and benefits of dating.)

A college hookup usually involves two people who have met earlier in the evening, often at a bar, fraternity house, club, or party, and agree to engage in some sexual behavior for which there is little or no expectation of future commitment. There is often little or no communication, and the hookup ends when one partner leaves, falls

Table 5.1 **Top Four Perceived Benefits and Costs of Traditional Dating**

| Women ♀ | Men ♂ |
|---|---|
| **Perceived benefits of traditional dating** | |
| 1. Your partner is a friend who you can disclose information/problems/happy moments/tough times with | You have the feeling of being liked/loved |
| 2. You have the feeling of being liked/loved | Dating offers physical intimacy |
| 3. Traditional dating is a more productive/healthy relationship | Your partner is a friend who you can disclose information/problems/happy moments/tough times with |
| 4. You get to share something you enjoy with another person | You get to share something you enjoy with another person |
| **Perceived risks of traditional dating** | |
| 1. Traditional dating is an investment of feelings and there's a potential of getting hurt | Risk of being rejected |
| 2. Risk of broken heart | Traditional dating is an investment of feelings and there's a potential of getting hurt |
| 3. Risk of losing friendship if you cross a line | Risk of broken heart |
| 4. You risk being more interested in your partner than he is in you | Loss of some freedom/independence |

Source: C. Bradshaw et al., "To Hook Up or to Date: Which Gender Benefits?" *Sex Roles,* Vol. 62, No. 9–10, March 2010, pp. 661–669.

asleep, or passes out. For men, there is less risk of rejection, less anxiety, and less financial cost. Women typically experience more negative effects, including being pressured to engage in unwanted sexual activity.

In a recent survey, both men and women preferred traditional dating to hooking up if there was a chance of a long-term relationship. Women preferred dating, with its promise of true intimacy, to hooking up in almost every circumstance while men generally preferred hooking up, with its promise of sexual gratification.[30]

*Why Students Hook Up*  Various factors influence hookup behavior, including gender, alcohol, and a desire to avoid a serious relationship. College men report more sexual partners and are more likely to engage in sex without emotional involvement. In some studies college women engage in just as many hookup experiences as men, but they do so for different reasons. Some, focused on academic and career goals, say they want to interact with interesting or attractive men without compromising their freedom.

Alcohol use and intoxication play a major role, with 65 percent of students in one study reporting drinking before hooking up. Social norms are another influence. Even students who say they've never engaged in any type of casual sex believe that almost everyone else is hooking up. Students who had hooked up in high school are likely to continue this behavior in college. Those who describe themselves as religious or who attend religious services report fewer hookups and less likelihood of intercourse during a hookup.[31]

*Consequences of Hooking Up*  Although hookups imply no conditions and no expectations, they can and do have unanticipated consequences, including unwanted pregnancy, sexually transmitted infections, and sexual assaults. Women, at higher risk for these outcomes, also experience more negative psychological consequences.

Because of the continuing "double standard," men are still lauded and admired for their sexual prowess and experience, while women, who are shamed for them, are more likely to feel guilty or anxious after hooking up. In one study, young women who had engaged in casual sex reported more distress than virgins or women who had engaged in sex only with romantic partners. Such distress increased for women, but not men, with the number of casual sex partners.[32]

In an analysis of self-esteem and casual sex, both men and women reporting hookups had lower self-esteem than those who did not. Depression has been linked with hooking up in women, but not men. Feelings of sexual regret in college women have been associated with sexual intercourse with someone only once and intercourse or oral sex with someone they had known for less than 24 hours.[33]

## Loving and Being Loved

"One can live magnificently in this world if one knows how to work and how to love, to work for the person one loves and to love one's work," Leo Tolstoy wrote. You may not think of love as a basic need like food and rest, but it is essential for both physical and psychological well-being.

Mounting evidence suggests that people who lack love and commitment are at high risk for a host of illnesses, including infections, heart disease, and cancer. "Love and intimacy are at the root of what makes us sick and what makes us well," says cardiologist Dean Ornish, author of

*Your Strategies for Change*

## How to Be Single and Satisfied

- **Fill your life with meaningful work, experiences, and people.**

- **Build a network of supportive friends who care for and about you.**

- **Be open to new experiences** that can expand your feelings about yourself and your world.

- **Don't miss out on a special event** because you don't have someone to accompany you: Go alone.

- **Enjoy your own company.** Allow yourself to be amazed by your own witty or off-the-wall observations.

- **Volunteer to help others less fortunate,** or become involved in church and social organizations.

*Love & Survival: The Scientific Basis for the Healing Power of Intimacy.* "No other factor in medicine—not diet, not smoking, not exercise—has a greater impact."

## Intimate Relationships

Committed romantic relationships may be beneficial for college students' physical and mental health, just as marriage is for spouses. In a study of more than 1,600 undergraduates between ages 18 and 25, those in committed relationships experienced fewer mental health problems, were less likely to be overweight/obese, and engaged in fewer risky behaviors (such as binge drinking).

The reasons may be that these students have less time for risky behavior, that being in a relationship fosters a less impulsive lifestyle, or that partners who use drugs or drink heavily may be unable to keep a romantic partner. Simply having fewer sexual partners lowers general stress as well as the risk of sexual infections or assaults. There was no difference in physical health, possibly because most students are young and healthy to begin with.[34]

In another recent survey of undergraduates between ages 18 and 23, in the long term men received greater emotional benefits than women from the positive aspects of romance and were more likely than women to be emotionally harmed by the stress of a rocky patch.[35]

The term **intimacy**—the open, trusting sharing of close, confidential thoughts and feelings—comes from the Latin word for *within*. Intimacy doesn't happen at first sight, or in a day or a week or a number of weeks. Intimacy requires time and nurturing; it is a process of revealing rather than hiding, of wanting to know another and to be known by that other. Although intimacy doesn't require sex, an intimate relationship often includes a sexual relationship, heterosexual or homosexual.

In an intimate relationship, empathy becomes even more important. You can develop your capacity for empathy by pulling back periodically, particularly in moments of stress or conflict, and asking yourself: "What is my partner or spouse feeling right now? What does he or she need?"

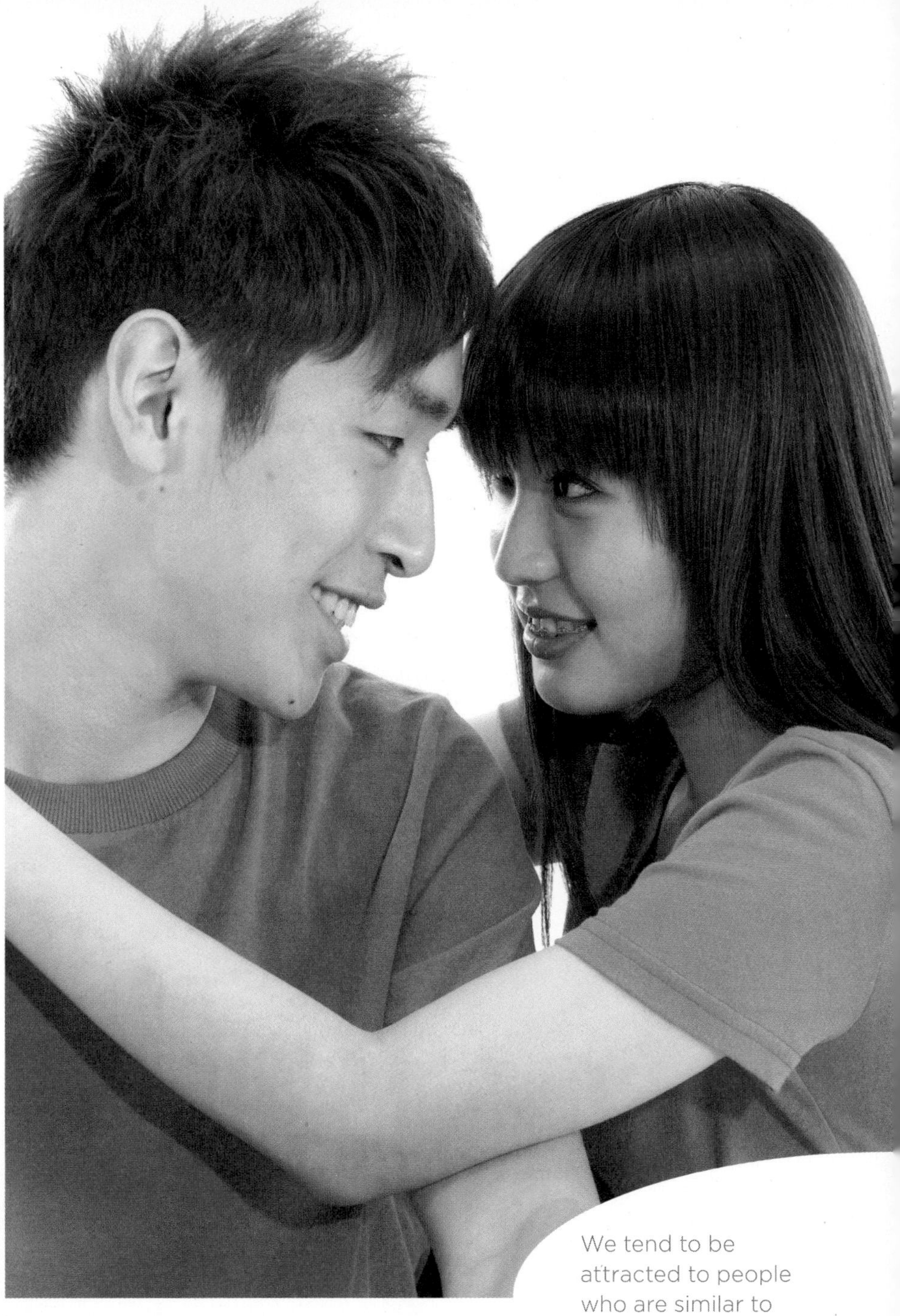

© East/Shutterstock.com

## What Attracts Two People to Each Other?

What draws two people to each other and keeps them together: chemistry or fate, survival instincts or sexual longings? "Probably it's a host of different things," reports sociologist Edward Laumann, coauthor of *Sex in America*, a landmark survey conducted by the National Opinion Research Center at the University of Chicago. "But what's remarkable is that most of us end up with partners much like ourselves—in age, race, ethnicity, socioeconomic class, education."

We tend to be attracted to people who are similar to ourselves in age, race, ethnicity, socio-economic class, and education.

**intimacy** A state of closeness between two people, characterized by the desire and ability to share one's innermost thoughts and feelings with each other either verbally or nonverbally.

Why? "You've got to get close for sexual chemistry to occur," says Laumann. "Sparks may fly when you see someone across a crowded room, but you only see a preselected group of people—people enough like you to be in the same room in the first place. This makes sense because initiating a sexual relationship is very uncertain."

Scientists have tried to analyze the combination of factors that attracts two people to each other. In several studies of college students, four predictors ranked as the most important reasons for attraction: warmth and kindness, desirable personality, something specific about the person, and reciprocal liking. Economic factors, including money or lack thereof, didn't make the list. (See Health on a Budget, p. 131.)

Do opposites attract, or do people find greater happiness with partners who are similar to them? One of the most comprehensive studies ever undertaken on these questions found no evidence that opposites attract. Most people, the researchers found, tend to marry those who are similar in attitudes, religion, and values. However, these similarities have little to do with having a happy marriage. What does matter are similarities in personality, such as being extroverted or conscientious. These take more time to recognize but have a greater impact on how a couple gets along over the long term.

### Figure 5.1 Sternberg's Love Triangle
The three components of love are intimacy, passion, and commitment. The various kinds of love are composed of different combinations of the three components.

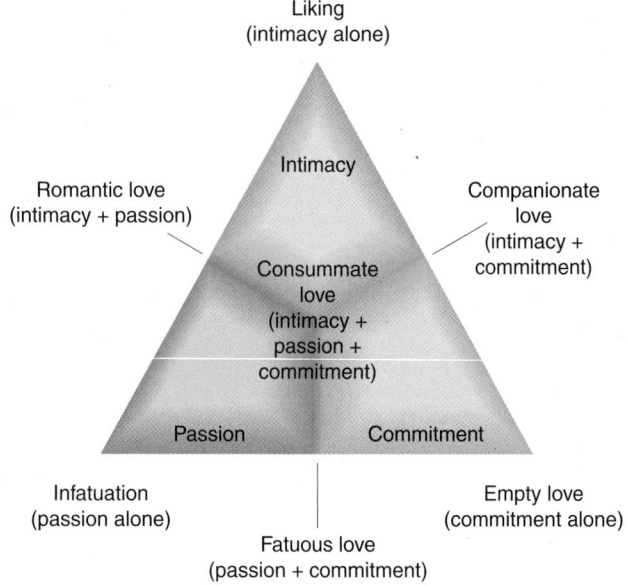

*Infatuation* It is tempting to think of love as scenes from a movie script: blazing sunsets and misty nights, fiery glances and passionate embraces, consuming desire and happy-ever-after endings. However, movies only last for two hours; ideally, love lasts a lifetime. Infatuation falls somewhere in between.

Certainly, falling in love is an intense, dizzying experience. A person not only enters our life but also takes possession. We are intrigued, flattered, captivated, delighted—but is this love or a love of loving?

At the time you're experiencing it, there is no difference between infatuation and lasting love. You feel the same giddy, wonderful way. However, if it's infatuation, it won't last. Infatuation refers only to falling in love. People genuinely in love with each other do more than fall: They start building a relationship together.

Being head over heels in love can have such an impact on the brain that it reduces pain. Stanford University researchers studied 15 undergraduates in the infatuation stage of love and inflicted pain with a handheld thermal probe. Those looking at a photograph of their beloved not only reported less pain but showed the same brain changes as those induced by drugs like cocaine.[36]

Infatuation also can be a disguise for something quite different: a strong sex drive, a fear of loneliness, loneliness itself, or a hunger for approval. Sometimes lovers in love with love may become infatuated with someone who doesn't even exist: the projection of their unmet needs for unconditional love.

## The Science of Romantic Love

We like to think of this powerful force, this source of both danger and delight, as something that defies analysis. However, scientists have provided new perspectives on its true nature.

*A Psychological View* According to psychologist Robert Sternberg, love can be viewed as a triangle with three faces: passion, intimacy, and commitment (Figure 5.1). Each person brings his or her own triangle to a relationship. If they match well, their relationship is likely to be satisfying.

Sternberg also identified six types of love:

- **Liking**, the intimacy friends share.
- **Infatuation**, the passion that stems from physical and emotional attraction.
- **Romantic love**, a combination of intimacy and passion.
- **Companionate love,** a deep emotional bond in a relationship that may have had romantic components.
- **Fatuous love,** a combination of passion and commitment in two people who lack a deep emotional intimacy.
- **Consummate love**, which combines passion, intimacy, and commitment over time.

*An Anthropological View* When you first fall in love, you may be sure that no one else has ever known the same dizzying, wonderful feelings. Yet, while every romance may be unique, romantic love is anything but. Anthropologists have found evidence of romantic love between individuals in most of the cultures they have studied—it seems to be a human universal or, at the least, a near-universal.

Anthropologist Helen Fisher, author of *Anatomy of Love: The Natural History of Monogamy, Adultery and Divorce*, describes romantic love "as a very primitive, basic human emotion, as basic as fear, anger or joy." As she explains, it pulled men and women of prehistoric times into the sort of partnerships that were essential to child rearing. But after about four years—just "long enough to rear one child through infancy," says Fisher—romantic love seemed to wane, and primitive couples tended to break up and find new partners. This "four-year itch" may well have endured through the centuries, contends Fisher, who notes that divorce statistics from most of the 62 cultures she has studied still show a pattern of restlessness four years into a marriage.[37]

*A Biochemical View* The heart is the organ we associate with love, but the brain may be where the action really is. According to research on neurotransmitters (the messenger chemicals within the brain), love sets off a chemical chain reaction that causes our skin to flush, our palms to sweat, and our lungs to breathe more deeply and rapidly. The "love chemicals" within the brain—dopamine, norepinephrine,

and phenylethylamine (PEA)—have effects similar to those of amphetamines, stimulant drugs that intensify physiological reactions (see Chapter 12).

Infatuation may indeed be a natural high, but like other highs, this rush doesn't last—possibly because the body develops tolerance for love-induced chemicals, just as it does with amphetamines. However, as the initial lovers' high fades, other brain chemicals may come into play: the endorphins, morphine-like chemicals that can help produce feelings of well-being, security, and tranquility. These feel-good molecules may increase in partners who develop a deep attachment.

The hormone *oxytocin*, best known for its role in inducing labor during childbirth, seems particularly important in our ability to bond with others. By measuring blood levels of women as they recalled positive and negative relationships, researchers have found that women whose oxytocin levels rose when remembering a positive relationship reported having little difficulty setting appropriate boundaries, being alone, or trying too hard to please others. Women whose oxytocin levels fell in response to remembering a negative emotional relationship reported greater anxiety in close relationships.

## Mature Love

Social scientists have distinguished between *passionate love* (characterized by intense feelings of elation, sexual desire, and ecstasy) and *companionate love* (characterized by friendly affection and deep attachment). Often relationships begin with passionate love and evolve into a more companionate love. Sometimes the opposite happens and two people who know each other well discover that their friendship has "caught fire" and the sparks have flamed an unexpected passion.

Mature love is a complex combination of sexual excitement, tenderness, commitment, and—most of all—an overriding passion that sets it apart from all other love relationships in one's life. This passion isn't simply a matter of orgasm but also entails a crossing of the psychological boundaries between oneself and one's lover. You feel as if you're becoming one with your partner while simultaneously retaining a sense of yourself.

**dysfunctional** Characterized by negative and destructive patterns of behavior between partners or between parents and children.

# Dysfunctional Relationships

Although they enrich and fulfill us in many ways, our relationships with friends, siblings, parents, or colleagues can also sabotage our health. Mental health professionals define a "toxic" relationship as one in which either person is made to feel worthless or incompetent.

Nearly half of all couples experience some form of physical aggression at some point in their relationship. Couples who are cohabiting (see page 137) experience more aggression than married partners and those who are dating but living separately.[38] In teenage couples, dating violence has been linked with higher levels of jealousy, verbal conflict, and cheating.[39] In the most recent ACHA-NCHA survey, about 2 percent of students had been in a physically abusive relationship in the 12 months. One in ten reported being in an emotionally abusive intimate relationship.[40] (See the accompanying table.)

Relationships that don't promote healthy communication, honesty, and intimacy are sometimes called **dysfunctional**. Individuals with addictive behaviors or dependence on drugs or alcohol (see Chapters 12 and 13), and the children or partners of such people, are especially likely to find themselves in such relationships, although they occur in all economic and social groups.

Often partners have magical, unrealistic expectations (e.g., they expect that a relationship with the right person will make their life okay), and one person uses the other almost as if he or she were a mood-altering drug. The partners may compulsively try to get the other to act the way they want. Both persons may distrust or may deceive each other. Often they isolate themselves from others, thus trapping themselves in a recurring cycle of pain.

"Physical symptoms, such as headaches, digestive troubles, tics, and inability to sleep well, can be signs of a destructive relationship," says sociologist Robert Billingham, professor of human development and family studies at Indiana University. Yet, although one person may repeatedly attack, abandon, betray, badger,

| Within the last 12 months, college students reported experiencing: | ♀ | ♂ | Total |
|---|---|---|---|
| An emotionally abusive intimate relationship | 7.4 | 11.4 | 10.0 |
| A physically abusive intimate relationship | 2.4 | 2.4 | 2.4 |
| A sexually abusive intimate relationship | 0.9 | 1.8 | 1.6 |

American College Health Association. *American College Health Association-National College Health Assessment II: Reference Group Executive Summary Spring 2010.* Baltimore: American College Health Association, 2010.

bully, criticize, deceive, dominate, or demean the other, the responsibility for changing the unhealthy dynamic belongs to both.

"The big question is, 'Do I want or have to keep this relationship going?'" says sociologist Jan Yager, author of *When Friendship Hurts.* "If yes, are you willing to invest time and energy to turn it around?"[41]

## Emotional Abuse

Abuse consists of any behavior that uses fear, humiliation, or verbal or physical assaults to control and subjugate another human being. Rather than being physical, emotional abuse often takes the form of constant berating, belittling, and criticism. Aggressive verbal abuse includes calling names, blaming, threatening, accusing, demeaning, and judging. Trivializing, minimizing, or denying what a person says or feels is a more subtle but equally destructive type of abuse. Even if done for the sake of "teaching" or "helping," emotional abuse wears away at self-confidence, sense of self-worth, and trust and belief in oneself. Because it is more than skin deep, emotional abuse can leave deeper, longer-lasting scars.

 In a survey of more than 1,500 never-married undergraduates, 25 percent reported that they had experienced at least two acts of physical abuse in a dating relationship. Far fewer (12 percent) believed that they had ever physically abused their current or most recent dating partner. The majority of students who abuse or are physically abused by a dating partner, the researchers concluded, may not identify themselves as being in an abusive relationship. This may be because of denial, ignorance, or acceptance of physical violence as a norm in a dating relationship.

No one wants to get into an abusive relationship, but often people who were emotionally abused in childhood find themselves in similar circumstances as adults. Dealing with an emotional abuser, regardless of how painful, may feel familiar or even comfortable. Individuals who think very little of themselves also may pick partners who treat them as badly as they believe they deserve.

## Health in Action

### Assessing a Relationship

How do you know if you're in a healthy relationship? Ask yourself the following questions, and jot down your answers in your online journal:

- Do you have a clear sense of who you are, what you believe and value, the goals you want? Such self-knowledge is critical for forming any mature relationship.
- Do you respect the other person and feel respected in return?
- Do you have differences in values, politics, religion, age, or race? Can you accept them?
- Do you still feel like a unique, strong individual within this relationship?
- Do you feel that you can be yourself when you're with this person? Do you feel good about yourself? Do you get—and give—compliments, support, and praise?
- Do you share interests and values? When you have things in common, you have a foundation to expand and build your relationship.

If you're currently involved with someone, read through the following list of positive indicators of a healthy relationship and check all that apply.

___You feel at ease with your new partner.

___You feel good about your new partner when you're together and when you're not.

___Your partner is open with you about his or her life—past, present, and future.

___You can say no to each other without feeling guilty.

___You feel cared for, appreciated, and accepted as you are.

___Your partner really listens to what you have to say.

The more items you've checked, the more reasons you have to keep seeing each other.

Read through the list of negative indicators below and check those that apply. In this case, every check is a red flag warning of dangers ahead.

___You don't feel comfortable together.

___You feel angry or let down when you're together or apart.

___Your partner is very secretive about his or her life.

___You feel your partner isn't attentive to you.

___You don't feel cared for and appreciated.

Reflect on the pluses and minuses of your relationship in your online journal.

## How to Cope with an Unhealthy Relationship

- **Start a dialogue.** Focus on communication, not confrontation. Start with a positive statement, for instance, saying what you really value in the relationship. Volunteer what you might do to make it better, and state what you need from the other person.

- **Distance yourself.** Take a vacation from a toxic friendship. Skip the family reunion or Thanksgiving dinner. When forced into proximity, be polite. If you refuse to engage—not arguing, not getting angry, not trying to make things better—toxic people give up trying to get under your skin.

- **Consult a professional.** A therapist or minister can help people recognize and change toxic behavior patterns. Changes you make in how you act and react may trigger changes in others.

- **Save yourself.** If you can never get what you need in a relationship, you may need to let it go. Nothing is worth compromising your mental or physical health.

Abusers also may have grown up with emotional abuse and view it as a way of coping with feelings of fear, hurt, powerlessness, or anger. They may seek partners who see themselves as helpless and who make them feel more powerful.

Among the signs of emotional abuse are:

- **Attempting to control various aspects of your life,** such as what you say or wear.

- **Frequently humiliating you** or making you feel bad about yourself.

- **Making you feel as if you are to blame** for what your partner does.

- **Wanting to know where you are** and whom you're with at all times.

- **Becoming jealous or angry** when you spend time with friends.

- **Threatening to harm you** if you break up.

- **Trying to coerce you** into unwanted sexual activity with statements such as, "If you loved me, you would . . ."

If you can never get what you need or if you're afraid, you need to get out of the relationship. Take whatever steps necessary to ensure your safety. Find a trusted friend who can help. Don't isolate yourself from family and friends. This is the time when you need their support and often the support of a counselor, minister, or doctor as well.

## Codependency

**Codependency** has expanded its definition to include any maladaptive behaviors learned by family members in order to survive great emotional pain and stress, such as an addiction, chronic mental or physical illness, and abuse. Some therapists refer to codependency as a "relationship addiction" because codependent people often form or maintain relationships that are one-sided, emotionally destructive, or abusive. First identified in studies of the relationships in families of alcoholics, codependent behavior can occur in any dysfunctional family.

Among the characteristics of codependency are:

- **An exaggerated sense of responsibility** for the actions of others.

- **An attraction to people who need rescuing.**

- **Always trying to do more than one's share.**

- **Doing anything to cling to a relationship** and avoid feeling abandoned.

- **An extreme need for approval and recognition.**

- **A sense of guilt** about asserting needs and desires.

- **A compelling need to control others.**

- **Lack of trust in self and/or others.**

- **Fear of being alone.**

- **Difficulty identifying feelings.**

- **Rigidity/difficulty** adjusting to change.

- **Chronic anger.**

- **Lying/dishonesty.**

- **Poor communications.**

- **Difficulty making decisions.**

**codependency** An emotional and psychological behavioral pattern in which the spouses, partners, parents, children, and friends of individuals with addictive behaviors allow or enable their loved ones to continue their self-destructive habits.

Because the roots of codependency run so deep, people don't just "outgrow" this problem or magically find themselves in a healthy relationship. Treatment to resolve childhood hurts and deal with emotional issues may take the form of individual or group therapy, education, or programs such as Codependents Anonymous (www.codependents.org). The goal is to help individuals get in touch with long-buried feelings and build healthier family and relationship dynamics.

*Enabling*   Experts on the subject of addiction first identified traits of codependency in spouses of alcoholics, who followed a predictable pattern of behavior: While intensely trying to control the drinkers, the codependent mates would act in ways that allowed the drinkers to keep drinking. For example, if an alcoholic found it hard to get up in the morning, his wife would wake him up, pull him out of bed and into the shower, and drop him off at work. If he was late, she made excuses to his boss. The husband was the one with the substance-abuse problem, but without realizing it, his wife was **enabling** him to continue drinking. In fact, he might not have been able to keep up his habit without her unintentional cooperation.

Codependency progresses just as an addiction does, and codependents excuse their own behavior with many of the same defense mechanisms used by addicts, such as rationalization ("I cut class so I could catch up on my reading, not to keep an eye on my partner") and denial ("He likes to gamble, but he never loses more than he can afford"). In time, codependents lose sight of everything but their loved one. They feel that if they can only "fix" this person, everything will be fine.

## When Love Ends

As the old song says, breaking up is indeed hard to do. Sometimes two people grow apart gradually, and both of them realize that they must go their separate ways. More often, one person falls out of love first. It hurts to be rejected; it also hurts to inflict pain on someone who once meant a great deal to you.

 In surveys, college students say it's more difficult to initiate a breakup than to be rejected. Those who

*Your Strategies for Change*

## How to Deal with Rejection

- **Remind yourself of your own worth.** You are no less attractive, intelligent, interesting, or lovable because someone ends a relationship with you.

- **Accept the rejection** as a statement of the other person's preference rather than trying to debate or defend yourself.

- **Think of other people who value or have valued you,** who accept and even see as appealing the same characteristics the rejecting person viewed as undesirable.

- **Don't withdraw from others.** Although you may not want to risk further rejection, it's worth the gamble to get involved again. The only individuals who've never been rejected are those who've never reached out to connect with another.

decided to end a relationship report greater feelings of guilt, uncertainty, discomfort, and awkwardness than their girlfriends or boyfriends. However, students with high levels of jealousy are likely to feel a desire for vengeance that can lead to aggressive behavior.

Research suggests that people do not end their relationships because of the disappearance of love. Rather a sense of dissatisfaction or unhappiness develops, which may then cause love to stop growing. The fact that love does not dissipate completely may be why breakups are so painful. While the pain does ease over time, it can help both parties if they end their relationship in a way that shows kindness and respect. Your basic guideline should be to think of how you would like to be treated if someone were breaking up with you. Would it hurt more to find out from someone else? Would it be more painful if the person you cared for lied to you or deceived you, rather than admitted the truth? Saying "I don't feel the way I once did about you; I don't want to continue our relationship" is hard, but it's also honest and direct.

**enabling** Unwittingly contributing to a person's addictive or abusive behavior. Components of enabling include shielding or covering up for an abuser/addict; controlling him or her; taking over responsibilities; rationalizing addictive behavior; or cooperating with him or her.

# Partnering across the Life Span

Even though men and women today may have more sexual partners than in the past, most still yearn for an intense, supportive, exclusive relationship, based on mutual commitment and enduring over time. In our society, most such relationships take the form of heterosexual marriages, but partners of the same sex or heterosexual partners who never marry also may sustain long-lasting, deeply committed relationships.

These couples are much like married people: They make a home, handle daily chores, cope with problems, celebrate special occasions, plan for the future—all the while knowing that they are not alone, that they are part of a pair that adds up to far more than just the sum of two individual souls.

## Relationships in Emerging Adulthood

Growing up is not what it used to be. Social scientists have identified "emerging adulthood" as a unique developmental period that spans the late teens and the twenties, marked by volatility and identity formation. Traditionally the milestones of this life stage were completing school, leaving home, becoming financially independent, marrying, and having a child.

Today more than 95 percent of Americans consider the most important markers of adulthood to be completing school, establishing an independent household, and being employed full-time. Only about half consider it necessary to marry or have children to be regarded as an adult. Unlike their parents and grandparents, young people view these markers as life choices rather than requirements.[42] What do you think?

The changing timetable for adulthood has affected the timing and nature of intimate relationships or, as sociologists describe them, "partnerships." Although just as eager for intimacy—emotional and sexual—younger adults are following a different pattern than past generations. Among a smorgasbord of romantic options, they may enter into casual, short-term relationships, commit to a long-term monogamous relationship, or live with a partner with or without the intent of getting married. Increasingly, marriage has become the final step in a relationship and may take place after sexual involvement, shared living, and even childbearing and parenting.[43]

Nearly half of young people live with their parents. This percentage drops below one in seven by the late twenties and below one in ten by the early thirties. Women are typically younger than men when they leave home because they complete college earlier, form cohabiting unions earlier, and marry about two years earlier.[44]

In 1970, two-thirds of twenty-somethings were married. Now just about a quarter are.[45] "Emerging adults" who want to get married in their twenties generally express greater religiosity and more conservative sexual attitudes, are less sexually active, and engage in fewer risky health behaviors (smoking, drinking, drug use, etc.). Younger adults are more likely than older ones to participate in relationships that cross racial lines, but those in interracial relationships report receiving less social support from family and friends.[46]

Figure 5.2 **Unmarried Couple Households**
The number of unmarried couples living together, both with and without children, has risen dramatically in the last 50 years.

Source: U.S. Census Bureau

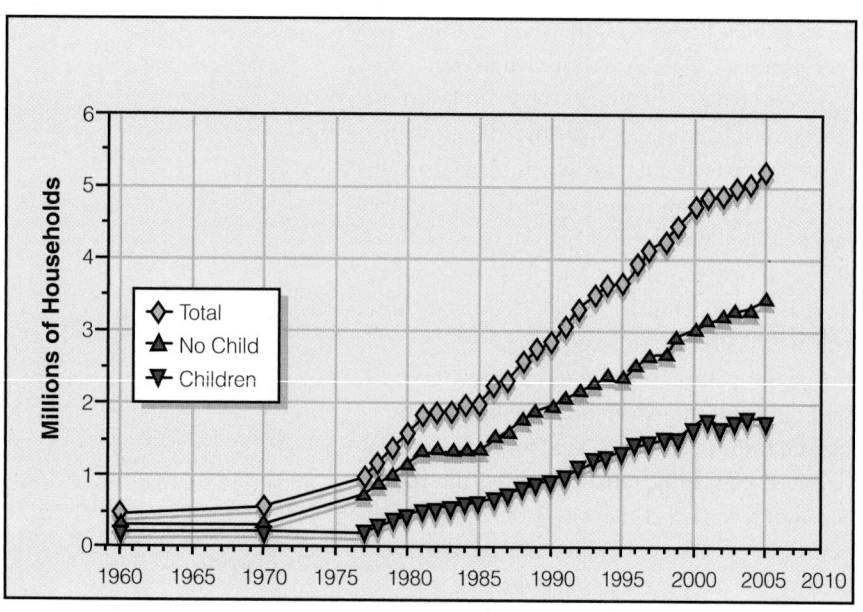

## Cohabitation

Although couples have always shared homes in informal relationships without any official ties, "living together," or **cohabitation**, has become more common (see Figure 5.2).

The majority of young adults have lived with a partner by their midtwenties, but they do not view it as a permanent alternative to marriage. Although cohabitation has been increasing steadily for decades, the number of couples living together has spiked in recent years, increasing by 13 percent from 2009 to 2010.[47]

One reason may be economic. Partners may not have enough money to live alone but don't plan to get married until they have more money—which is harder to get in a bad economy. Social acceptance may also contribute. A few generations ago "shacking up" seemed shocking. Today fewer than half of Americans think living together is a bad idea.

About a quarter of unmarried women ages 25 to 39 are currently living with a partner; an additional quarter lived with a partner in the past. Couples live together before more than half of all marriages, a practice that was practically unknown 50 years ago. In addition, the proportion of cohabiting women between the ages of 20 and 50 has tripled in the last 50 years.

Cohabitation can be a prelude to marriage, an alternative to living alone, or an alternative to marriage. Couples choose to cohabit for different reasons. In one study, spending more time together and convenience were the most common motivations. Couples who move in together to "test" their relationship report more problems—including more negative communication, physical aggression, and symptoms of depression and anxiety—than others. (See Table 5.2.)

The timing of a decision to move in together also matters. Couples who cohabited before getting engaged later reported less marital satisfaction, dedication, and confidence as well as more negative communication and greater potential for divorce than those who lived together after engagement or after getting married.[48]

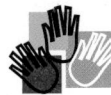 Asians and non-Hispanic white couples are the least likely to cohabit. A higher percentage of Native Ameri-

can, black, and Hispanic couples are unmarried. "Cohabiters" tend to have lower income and education levels. They also are younger—on average, some 12 years younger than married men and women.

Committed couples, both heterosexual and homosexual, can register as domestic partners in certain areas. This may enable them to qualify for benefits such as health insurance.

Employers may require that the couple has lived together for a specified period (generally, at least six months) and are responsible for each other's financial welfare. Recent court rulings have placed domestic partners on the same legal footing as married couples in dealings with businesses.

## Long-Term Same-Sex Relationships

According to recent surveys, 75 percent of lesbians and more than half of gay men are in a relationship with one person. Much like heterosexuals, homosexuals tend to date in their twenties, then settle into a relationship, and maintain

**cohabitation** Two people living together as a couple, without official ties such as marriage.

Table 5.2 **Do you think it's easier to . . .**

Source: www.pewsocialtrends.org/family

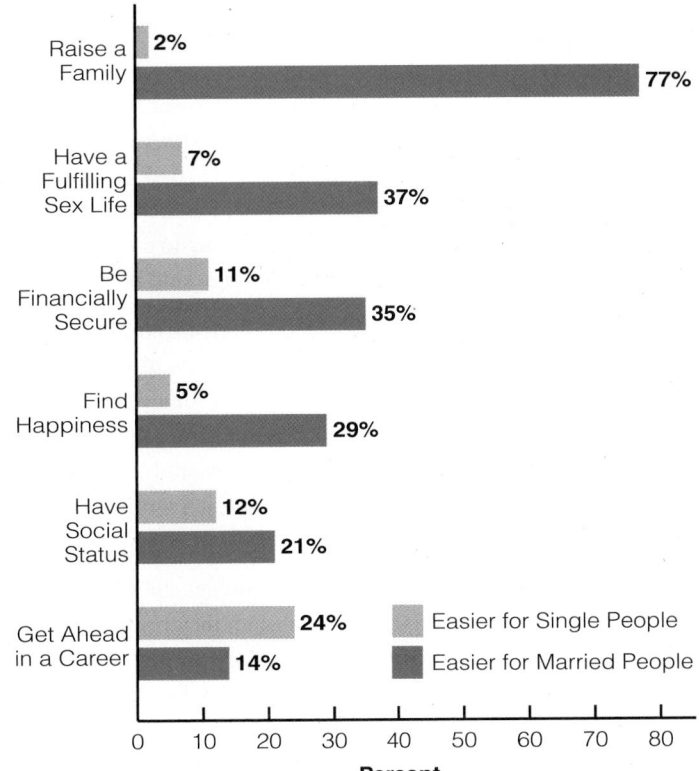

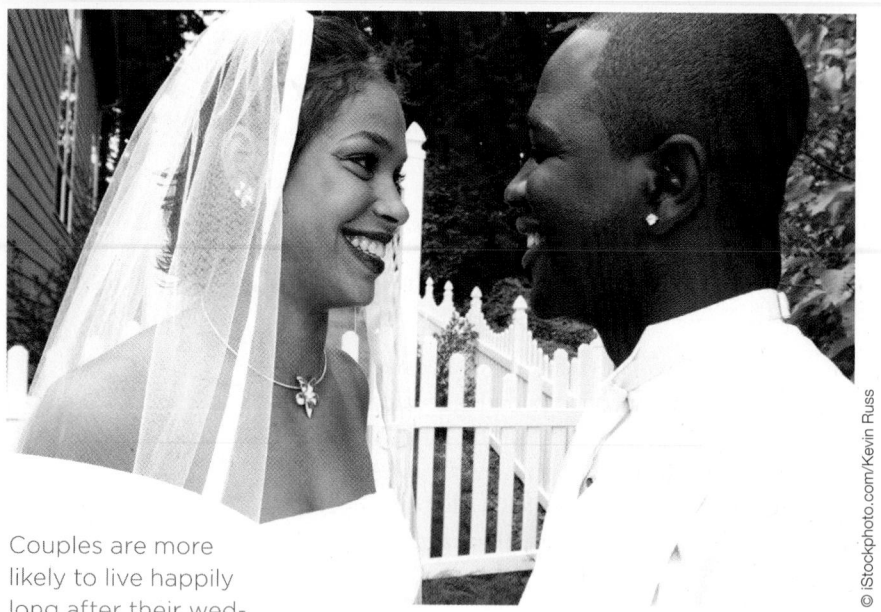

Couples are more likely to live happily long after their wedding day if they share the same values and religious beliefs, tolerate flaws, and communicate effectively.

it long-term. As more states have recognized the legality of same-sex marriage, more gay and lesbian couples have joined together in matrimony (see pages 140–141).[49]

Like heterosexual ("straight") couples, same-sex relationships progress through various stages. The first, blending, is a time of intense passion and romantic love. Gradually the couples move through nesting (starting a home together), to building trust and dependability, to merging assets, to establishing a strong sense of partnership.

Because there are no social norms for same-sex unions, researchers describe these relationships as more egalitarian. Each partner tends to be more self-reliant, and homosexual men and women tend to be more willing to communicate and experiment in terms of sexual behaviors.

Gay and lesbian relationships are comparable to straight relationships in many ways. But same-sex couples have to deal with everyday ups-and-downs in a social context of isolation from family, workplace prejudice, and other social barriers. However, gay and lesbian couples are more upbeat in the face of conflict.

Compared to straight couples, they use more affection and humor when they bring up a disagreement and remain more positive after a disagreement. They also display less belligerence, domineering, and fear with each other than straight couples do. When they argue, they are better able to soothe each other so they show

fewer signs of physiological arousal, such as an elevated heart rate or sweaty palms, than heterosexual couples.

## Marriage

*Like everything which is not the involuntary result of fleeting emotion but the creation of time and will, any marriage, happy or unhappy, is infinitely more interesting and significant than any romance, however passionate.*

*W. H. Auden*

Contemporary marriage has been described as an institution that everyone on the outside wants to enter and everyone on the inside wants to leave. The proportion of married people, especially among younger age groups, has been declining for decades. Across North America and many European countries, the age of first marriage has risen, with both men and women waiting an extra three years before saying "I do," and the rate of first marriages among men has been cut in half.

A generation ago nearly 70 percent of Americans were married; now only about half are (Table 5.3). Yet most young adults view marriage positively, and 95 percent expect to marry in the future—except for young African Americans, who have significantly lower expectations of being wed than their white counterparts, with Hispanics in between.

 If you aren't already married, simply getting a college degree increases your odds of entering into matrimony in the future. According to a recent report, *The Decline of Marriage and Rise of New Families*,[50] college graduates (who make up 30 percent of the adult population) are far more likely to marry (64 percent) than those without a baccalaureate degree (48 percent). Less well educated Americans are not only less likely to marry; if they do, their unions are more likely to end in divorce.[51]

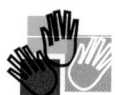 The median age for first marriage, which has gone up about a year every decade since the 1960s, has risen to 28.2 years for men and 26.1 years for women. Men in every age bracket through age 34 are more likely to be single than are women. Black men and women are less likely to be married than whites, with Hispanics between the two.[52]

Table 5.3 **Marriage Statistics, 1960–2008**

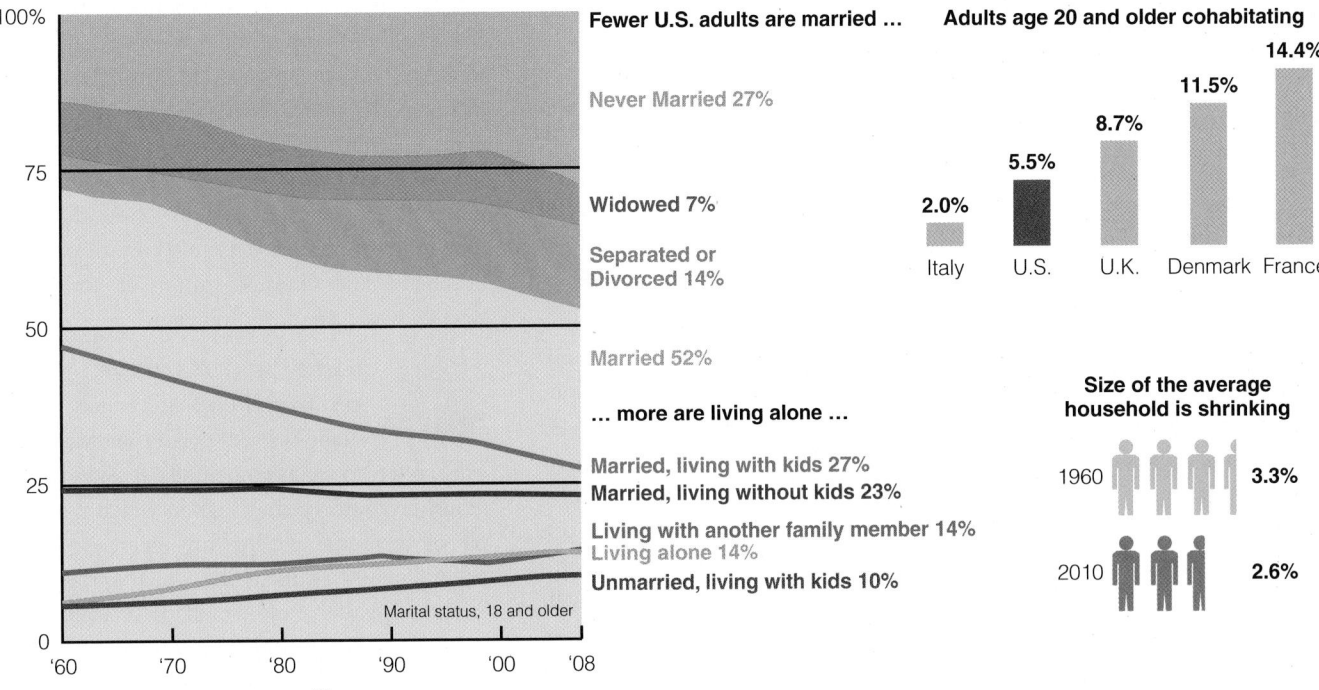

*Preparing for Marriage* Most people say they marry for one far-from-simple reason: love. However, with more than half of all marriages ending in divorce, there's little doubt that modern marriages aren't made in heaven. Are some couples doomed to divorce even before they swap vows? Could counseling before a marriage increase its odds of success? According to recent research findings, the answer to both questions is yes.

There have been government attempts to set requirements for couples who want to marry. Some states, such as Arizona and Louisiana, have established "covenant" marriages in which engaged couples are required to get premarital counseling. Utah allows counties to require counseling before issuing marriage licenses to minors and people who have been divorced. Florida requires high school students to take marriage education classes.

Not too long ago, marriage was often a business deal, a contract made by parents for economic or political reasons when the spouses-to-be were still very young. Today, in some countries, it is still culturally acceptable to arrange marriages in this manner. Even in America, certain ethnic groups, such as Asians who have recently immigrated to the United States, plan marriages for

their children. In such arrangements, the marriage partners are likely to have similar values and expectations. However, the newlyweds also start out as strangers who may not even know whether they like—let alone love—each other. Sometimes arranged marriages trap both partners in loneliness and longing.

**Premarital Assessments** There are scientific ways of predicting marital happiness. Some premarital assessment inventories identify strengths and weaknesses in many aspects of a relationship: realistic expectations, personality issues, communication, conflict resolution, financial management, leisure activities, sex, children, family and friends, egalitarian roles, and religious orientation. Couples who become aware of potential conflicts by means of such inventories may be able to resolve them through professional counseling. In some cases, they may want to reconsider or postpone their wedding.

Other common predictors of marital discord, unhappiness, and separation are:

- **A high level of arousal during a discussion**.
- **Defensive behaviors** such as making excuses and denying responsibility for disagreements.

## Relationships in the Twenty-First Century

As human beings we want to connect with each other. There are many ways to do so right now, from social networking and video chats to phone calls and text messages. In the future, there may be even more ways to interact with people we care about. Knowing how to maintain healthy relationships is an important part of communicating with others. To explore trends in personal relationships, you can search for a topic of interest to you or view the latest news on any of the Healthy Relationships portals (found under Health & Wellness → Healthy Relationships). In looking at how you communicate and relate to others, what is one thing you feel you do well? Is there a change you could make to ensure your relationships stay healthy? Record your answers to these questions and your additional thoughts in your online journal.

**same-sex marriage** Governmentally, socially, or religiously recognized marriage in which two people of the same sex live together as a family.

- **A wife's expressions of contempt**.
- **A husband's stonewalling** (showing no response when a wife expresses her concerns).

By looking for such behaviors, researchers have been able to predict with better than 90 percent accuracy whether a couple will separate within the first few years of marriage.

**The Benefits of Marriage**   Despite its problems, marriage endures because it is a fulfilling way for two people to live. As researchers have proved, saying "I do" can do wonders for your health. Married people are healthier than those who are divorced, widowed, never-married, or living with a partner. They live longer, have lower rates of coronary disease and cancer, are less likely to suffer back pain, headaches, and other common illnesses, and recover faster with a better chance of surviving a serious illness. Three or more marriages and a lower proportion of adult life spent married are each linked with higher mortality after age 50 for both men and women, regardless of their current marital or socioeconomic status.[53]

Married men and women also have lower rates of most mental disorders than single or divorced individuals.

For years researchers thought that marriage was especially beneficial to men. Married men have lower rates of alcohol and drug abuse, depression, and risk-taking behavior than divorced men. They also earn more money—possibly because they have more incentive to do so. However, more recent research indicates that a happy marriage boosts mental health and well-being in both spouses.

Among the theories of why marriage benefits health are:

- **Selection**: People in better physical and psychological health may be more likely to get married in the first place and to remain married.
- **Social support**: Marriage may provide people with emotional satisfaction that buffers them against daily life stressors.
- **Behavioral regulation**: Marriage partners may monitor each other's behaviors, discourage risky behaviors like smoking, and encourage healthier ones such as driving safely.

Marital status affects both weight and fitness. Fitness declines in men who remain single, but declines even more in those who marry. Fitness increases in women who remain single but not in those who marry. Married men who divorce show a small increase in fitness, but their fitness declines if they remarry.[54] Married men are more likely to be overweight or obese. Three in four married men ages 45 to 64 are overweight or obese. The slimmest groups are men and women who have never married.

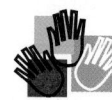

***Same-Sex Marriage***   **Same-sex marriage**, also called gay or single-sex or gender-neutral marriage, refers to a governmentally, socially, or religiously recognized marriage in which two people of the same sex live together as a family. Several countries, including Canada, the Netherlands, Belgium, and Spain, have legitimized same-sex marriages. Several states now recognize same-sex marriages; others recognize domestic partnerships and civil unions that grant some of the legal and economic benefits of marriage.

Same-sex marriages have triggered intense controversy. Some oppose gay unions on religious

## Think Twice about Getting Married If . . .

- You or your partner are constantly asking the other such questions as, "Are you sure you love me?"
- You spend most of your time together disagreeing and quarreling.
- You're both still very young (under the age of 20).
- Your boyfriend or girlfriend has behaviors (such as nonstop talking), traits (such as bossiness), or problems (such as drinking too much) that really bother you and that you're hoping will change after you're married.
- Your partner wants you to stop seeing your friends, quit a job you enjoy, or change your life in some other way that diminishes your overall satisfaction.

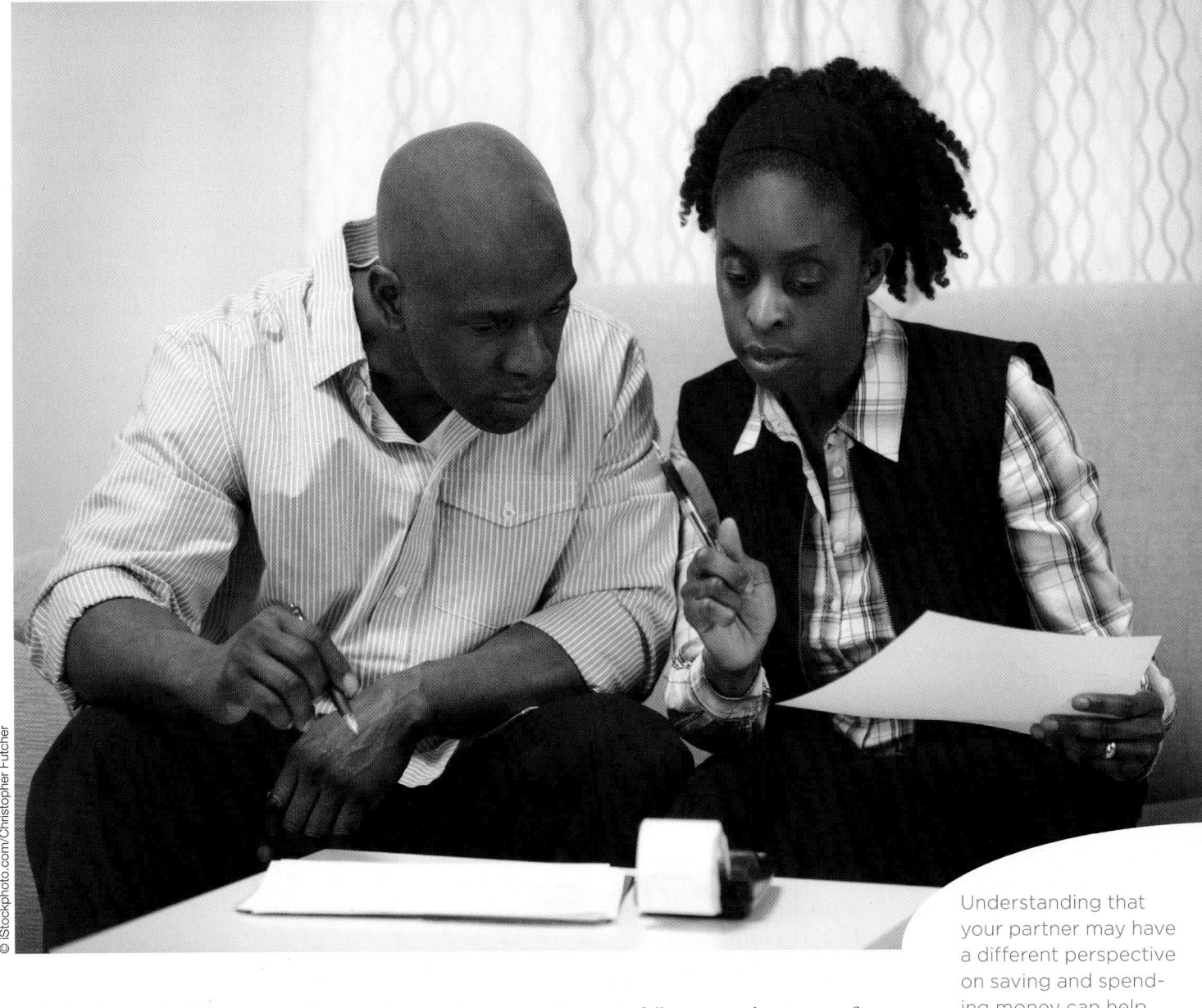

Understanding that your partner may have a different perspective on saving and spending money can help avoid arguments.

and moral grounds. Others argue that marriage is a right based on procreation and designed to protect the children of a man and a woman. Advocates of gay marriage contend that the ban on same-gender unions discriminates against homosexuals and denies them the civil rights and legal protection that heterosexual couples have.

Is marriage as beneficial to the health of same-sex partners as it is for male-female couples? In terms of physical well-being, researchers found no difference between heterosexual and homosexual spouses.

Children adopted into lesbian and gay families appear as well adjusted as those adopted by heterosexual couples, according to recent research. Earlier studies have shown that children born to

homosexual parents follow normal patterns of general development and are virtually indistinguishable from other youngsters.[55]

## Issues Couples Confront

No two people can live together in perfect harmony all the time. Some of the issues that crop up in any long-term relationship include expectations, money, sex, and careers.

*Money*  Money may make the business world go around, but it has the opposite effect on relationships: It knocks them off their tracks, brings them to a halt, twists them upside down. However, even though almost all couples quarrel about money, they rarely fight over how much they have. What matters more—whether they make $10,000 or $100,000 a year—is what money means to both partners. How does each person use money to meet emotional needs? Who decides how the money is spent? Who keeps track? Until they resolve these issues, couples may quarrel over money as long as they're together.

To avoid fighting over money, understand that having different money values or expectations doesn't make one of you right and the other wrong. Recognize the value of unpaid work. A partner who's finishing school or taking care of the children is making an important contribution to the family and its future. It also helps to go over your finances together so that you have a firm basis in reality for what you can and can't afford. Talk about the financial goals you hope to attain five years from now. Set priorities to meet them. Also, set aside money for each of you to spend without asking or answering to the other. Even a small amount can make each partner feel more independent.

**Sex**    Like every other aspect of a relationship, sex evolves and changes over the course of marriage. The redhot sexual chemistry of the early stages of intimacy invariably cools down. Even so, the happiest couples have sex more often than unhappily married pairs do.

What matters most isn't quantity alone, but the quality of sexual activity and intimacy. Are both partners satisfied with their sexual relationship? Does one partner always initiate sex? Do the partners talk about their preferences and pleasures? Sexuality, like personality, is dynamic and changes throughout life. Do the partners acknowledge and adapt to these changes? Do they feel sufficiently at ease with each other to discuss anxieties about sex? The answers to these questions can determine how sexually gratifying a marriage is for both spouses.

**Extramarital Affairs**    How faithful are American mates? The answer depends on the questions researchers ask and who they ask. In face-to-face interviews, University of Chicago researchers found that 25 percent of men and 15 percent of women had had affairs and that 94 percent of the married subjects had been monogamous in the last year. Another survey of Americans found that one out of six Americans had had an extramarital relationship—19

percent of the men and 15 percent of the women.[56]

High or low, numbers are little comfort when affairs do occur. A husband or wife who learns about a spouse's affair typically feels a devastating sense of betrayal as well as deep feelings of shame, fear of abandonment, depression, and anger. Two crucial questions determine whether a marriage can survive: Do the spouses still feel a serious commitment to each other? And do they love each other and want to remain together?

**Two-Career Couples**    More than 75 percent of women with children work—a dramatic increase from the 1960s, when only 30 percent of mothers worked outside the home. Two careers can bring pressure to a relationship: Both individuals may come home tired and irritable; both may have to spend a great deal of time on their jobs; both may have to travel or work on weekends. Two-career couples must be able to discuss their problems openly to resolve these pressures.

Couples pursuing individual careers sometimes face difficult choices. What happens, for example, if one of them is offered a promising job in another city? Does the spouse quit his or her job, pack up, and move? Some couples resolve such dilemmas by working in different cities and spending weekends together. Others try to alternate career and home priorities. However imperfect these arrangements may be, they work for some couples.

**Conflict in Marriage**    While all couples may wish to live happily and peacefully ever after, sooner or later, they argue. In a five-year study of newly married couples, about a third (36 percent) sought some form of help for their relationship, most often from books on relationships and marital therapy.[57] Years of research have shown that while conflict is inevitable, the key difference between happy and unhappy couples is the way they fight.

Happier couples interject positive interactions, like a joke or a smile, into their arguments. As long as the ratio of positive to negative interactions remains at least five to one, the relationship remains intact. By comparison, unhappy couples unfurl a barrage of negative words, gestures, criticisms, and hostility at their mates with hardly any positive interactions. Based on observations of couples in conflict, researchers have been able to predict which would divorce with 94 percent accuracy. Both men and women feel the strain of arguing and being angry because of marital difficulties, but wives are more likely to develop high blood pressure, high cholesterol, high blood sugar, and other markers of metabolic syndrome (discussed in Chapter 14). The reason may be that many women take negativity to heart and become depressed.

**Saving Marriages** Fewer than two-thirds of couples—64 percent of husbands and 60 percent of wives—say their marriages are very happy (down from 70 percent of men and 66 percent of women a generation ago.[58]

According to recent research, happy marriages allow both partners to self-actualize (discussed in Chapter 2) and develop to their fullest potential. Some refer to this mutual benefit as "co-actualization."[59] Others refer to the process of using a relationship to accumulate knowledge and experiences as "self-expansion." The more self-expansion that people experience from their partner, the more committed and satisfied they are in the relationship.[60]

Among the other suggestions therapists offer couples are:

- **Focus on friendship.** If a marriage is not built on a strong friendship, it may be difficult to stay connected over time.

- **Remember what you loved and admired in your partner in the first place.** Focusing on these qualities can foster a much more positive attitude toward him or her.

- **Show respect.** Your spouse deserves the same courtesy and civility that your colleagues do. Without respect, love cannot survive.

- **Compliment what your partner does right.** Noticing the positive can change how both of you feel about each other.

- **Forgive one another.** When your partner hurts your feelings but then reaches out, don't reject his or her attempts to make things better.

Each year, hundreds of thousands of couples go into counseling in an effort to make their unions happier. Among the approaches currently in use are marriage education and various forms of couples therapy.

Marriage education consists of workshops that teach couples practical skills so they get along better. Some studies indicate that graduates of these programs have a lower divorce rate than unhappy couples who do not enroll in them.

Couples therapy, also called marriage counseling or marriage therapy, uses a variety of psychological techniques to help couples understand and overcome their conflicts. These include:

- **Behavioral marital therapy,** which teaches partners to communicate better and to improve their conflict resolution skills.

- **Emotionally focused therapy,** which helps couples identify and break free of destructive emotional cycles.

- **Insight-oriented marital therapy,** which combines behavioral therapy with techniques for understanding negative behaviors, such as power struggles, within the relationship.

## Divorce

According to the most recent government data, the marriage rate now stands at 6.9 per 1,000 Americans. The divorce rate is almost 50 percent: 3.4 per 1,000 Americans.

Your risk of divorce depends on many factors. Simply having some college education improves your odds of a happy marriage.[61] Other factors that do the same are an income higher than $50,000, marrying at age 25 or older, not having a baby during the first seven months after the wedding, coming from an intact family, and having some religious affiliation.

Race also influences marriage and divorce rates. African American couples are more likely to break up than white couples, and black divorcées are less likely to marry again. Researchers have found that African Americans place an equally high value on marriage. However, there is a smaller "marriageable pool" of black men for a variety of reasons, including a higher mortality rate.

Children whose parents divorced are less likely to marry and to stay married. However, their adult relationships aren't doomed to fail. "Divorce isn't in the genes," says child psychologist Judith

Wallerstein, who has studied divorced families for 30 years. "Divorce is an avoidable human error."

# Family Ties

Children have become the exception rather than the rule in American households. A century ago most households contained children under age 18. In 1960, slightly fewer than half did. Only about a third of households now include children.

Attitudes also have changed. While many traditionally viewed having children as the primary purpose for getting married, nearly 70 percent of Americans now cite another reason.

Fertility has declined in the United States since 1960. At that time, the average woman had about three and one-half children over the course of her life. Today's woman has an average of about two children, which is lower than the "replacement level" of 2.1 children per woman. This is the level at which the population would be replaced by births alone. In most European and several Asian countries, fertility has dropped even lower.

## Diversity Within Families

 **Families** have become as diverse as the American population and reflect different traditions, beliefs, and values. Within African American families, for instance, traditional gender roles are often reversed, with women serving as head of the household, a kinship bond uniting several households, and a strong religious commitment or orientation. In Chinese American families, both spouses may work and see themselves as breadwinners, but the wife may not have an equal role in decision making. In Hispanic families, wives and mothers are acknowledged and respected as healers and dispensers of wisdom. At the same time, they are expected to defer to their husbands, who see themselves as the strong, protective, dominant head of the family. As time passes and families from different cultures become more integrated into American life, traditional gender roles and decision-making

patterns often change, particularly among the youngest family members.

American families are diverse in other ways. *Multigenerational families*, with children, parents, and grandparents, make up 3.7 percent of households. They occur most often in areas where new immigrants live with relatives, where housing shortages or high costs force families to double up their living arrangements, or where high rates of out-of-wedlock childbearing force unwed mothers to live with their children in their parents' home.

Three of every ten households consist of **blended families**, formed when one or both of the partners bring children from a previous union. In the future, social scientists predict, American families will become even more diverse, or pluralistic. But as norms or expectations about the configurations of families have changed, values or ideas about the intents and purposes of families have not. American families of every type still support each other and strive toward values such as commitment and caring.

The traditional family with a breadwinner and a homemaker has been replaced by what some call "the juggler family." Two working parents or an unmarried working parent head 70 percent of American families with children. As a result, American parents have fewer hours to spend with their children. Women, balancing multiple roles as parents, spouses, caregivers, and employees often give their own personal needs the lowest priority.

## Unmarried Parents

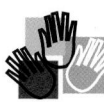 "Fragile families," a term coined by social scientists, refers to those in which the parents are unwed at the time of their child's birth. The proportion of babies born to unmarried parents has grown from about 4 percent in 1940 to about 40 percent. About seven in ten African American babies and half of Hispanic babies are born out of wedlock. Unmarried African American mothers have the lowest rates of marriage and cohabitation and the highest breakup rates. Mexican immigrant mothers have the highest rates of marriage and cohabitation and the lowest breakup rates.[62]

**family** A group of people united by marriage, blood, or adoption; residing in the same household; maintaining a common culture; and interacting with one another on the basis of their roles within the group.

**blended family** A family formed when one or both of the partners bring children from a previous union to the new marriage.

Most unmarried parents are in a romantic relationship when their baby is born, with about half cohabiting and the others living apart. The majority are not able to establish stable unions. A third of fathers virtually disappear from their children's lives within five years.[63]

The percentage of undergraduates who are unmarried parents nearly doubled over the last 20 years, from 7 percent to just over 13 percent. Overall 8 percent of male undergraduates and 17 percent of female undergraduates are unmarried parents.[64]

More than a third of African American college women and 15 percent of African American college men are unmarried parents, as are 20 percent of Native American undergraduates, 16 percent of all Latino undergraduates, and 10 percent of whites.[65]

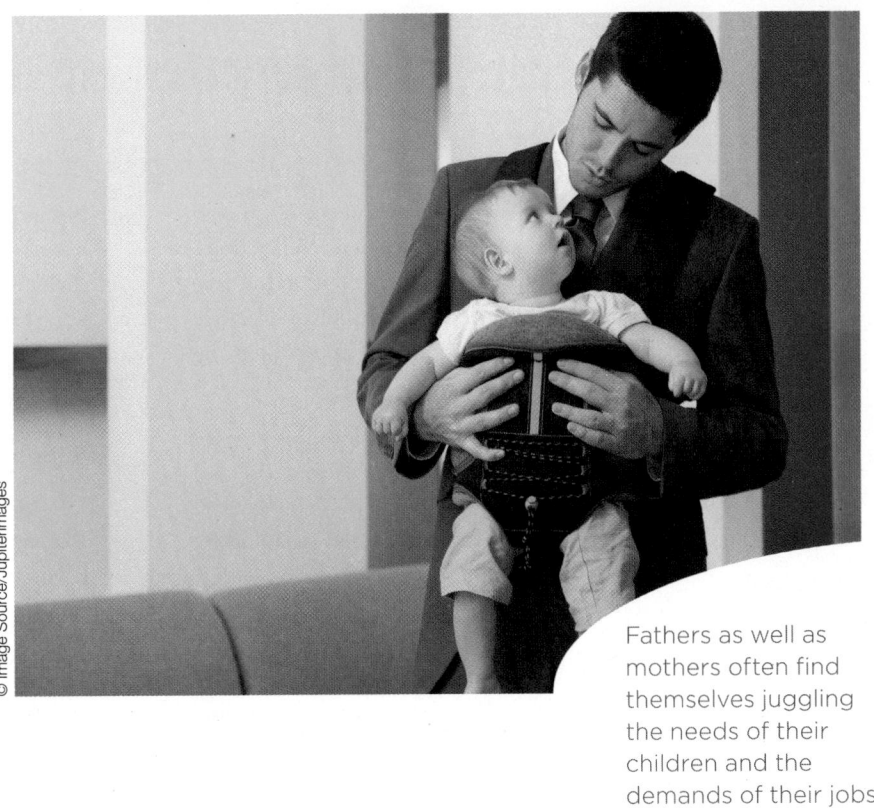

© Image Source/Jupiterimages

Fathers as well as mothers often find themselves juggling the needs of their children and the demands of their jobs.

# Creating Better Relationships

We are born social. From our first days of life, we reach out to others, struggle to express ourselves, strive to forge connections. The fabric of our lives becomes richer as family and friends weave through it the threads of their experiences. No solitary pleasure can match the gifts that we gain by reaching out and connecting with others.

As with other significant endeavors, good relationships require work—through hard times, despite conflicts, over months and years and decades. As you strive to improve the ties that bind you to others, keep in mind the characteristics of a good relationship. Check the ones that are most important to you.

____ **Trust**. Partners are able to confide in each other openly, knowing their confidences will be respected.

____ **Togetherness**. In a healthy relationship, two people create a sense of both intimacy and autonomy. They enjoy each other's company but also pursue solitary interests.

____ **Expressiveness**. Partners in healthy relationships say what they feel, need, and desire.

____ **Staying power**. People in committed relationships keep their bond strong through tough times by proving that they will be there for each other.

____ **Security**. Because a good relationship is strong enough to absorb conflict and anger, partners know they can express their feelings honestly. They also are willing to risk vulnerability for the sake of becoming closer.

____ **Laughter**. Humor keeps things in perspective—always crucial in any sort of ongoing relationship or enterprise.

____ **Support**. Partners in good relationships continually offer each other encouragement, comfort, and acceptance.

____ **Physical affection**. Sexual desire may fluctuate or diminish over the years, but partners in loving, long-term relationships usually retain some physical connection.

____ **Personal growth**. In the best relationships, partners are committed to bringing out the best in each other and have the other's best interests at heart.

____ **Respect**. Caring partners are aware of each other's boundaries, need for personal space, and vulnerabilities. They do not take each other or their relationship for granted.

## How Strong Are the Communication and Affection in Your Relationship?

Effective, caring communication and loving affection markedly enhance a couple's relationship. The following self-test may help you to assess the degree of good communication, love, and respect in your intimate relationship. If you agree or mostly agree with a statement, answer yes. If you disagree or mostly disagree, answer no. You may wish to have your partner respond to this assessment as well. If so, mark your answers on a separate sheet.

1. My partner seeks out my opinion.                    Yes    No

2. My partner cares about my feelings.                 Yes    No

3. I don't feel ignored very often.                    Yes    No

4. We touch each other a lot.                          Yes    No

5. We listen to each other.                            Yes    No

6. We respect each other's ideas.                      Yes    No

7. We are affectionate toward one another.             Yes    No

8. I feel my partner takes good care of me.            Yes    No

9. What I say counts.                                  Yes    No

10. I am important in our decisions.                   Yes    No

11. There's lots of love in our relationship.          Yes    No

12. We are genuinely interested in one another.        Yes    No

13. I love spending time with my partner.              Yes    No

14. We are very good friends.                           Yes    No

15. Even during rough times, we can be empathetic.     Yes    No

16. My partner is considerate of my viewpoint.　　Yes　No
17. My partner finds me physically attractive.　　Yes　No
18. My partner expresses warmth toward me.　　Yes　No
19. I feel included in my partner's life.　　Yes　No
20. My partner admires me.　　Yes　No

*Scoring:*

A preponderance of yes answers indicates that you enjoy a strong relationship characterized by good communication and loving affection. If you answered yes to fewer than seven items, it is likely that you are not feeling loved and respected and that the communication in your relationship is decidedly lacking.

*Source: John Gottman,* Why Marriages Succeed or Fail. *New York: Simon & Schuster, 1994.*

# *Making Change Happen*

## Listen Up

The essence of good listening is to seek to understand another person before you seek to be understood. In the process you not only will get an earful but also will learn more than you might imagine. If you would like to take a relationship to another level, see what happens when you listen up. And if you're shy or feel self-conscious in social settings, expect an added return on your investment. Knowing how to listen can help you—and the people around you—feel at ease. "Listen Up" in *Labs for IPC* shows you how to "be all ears." Here's a preview.

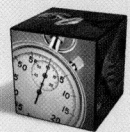

### Get Real

In this stage, you will replay three conversations you've had in the last 24 hours with three different people and answer 11 questions about them, including the following:

• What was the purpose of the conversation? Killing time? Flirting? Trying to get information you needed for a class or assignment?

• What questions did you ask, if any?

• What do you remember?

On the basis of your answers, rate your listening skills on a scale of 1 (you talkin' to me?) to 10 (competition for Oprah).

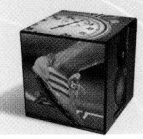

### Get Ready

In this stage, you will check your schedule and make time for listening opportunities.

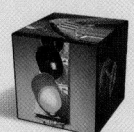

### Get Going

In this stage you will embark on a comprehensive program that includes four steps:

• **Enhance basic skills** by engaging in at least one conversation each day in which you focus on specifics such as making eye contact and reading body language.

• **Observe listening styles** in yourself and others as you converse in varied settings.

• **Master interviewing skills.** You will set up situations in which you might pretend you're a reporter doing a "person-on-the-street" interview or talk with an instructor about some class material that you're struggling to comprehend.

• **Apply listening skills.** You will seek out real-life encounters—for instance, with a friend seeking advice or with someone you don't like talking with and usually avoid.

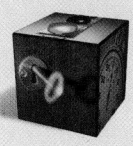

### Lock It In

To keep your listening muscles in shape, you will consciously practice intensive listening on a daily basis. You might ask a sales clerk how the day is going, and then listen—really listen—to the answer, or ask a classmate about . . .

# Making This Chapter Work for You

## Review Questions

1. Romantic love
   a. is associated with the depletion of the hormone oxytocin.
   b. is an emotional phenomenon between humans that has its roots in prehistoric times and occurs in almost all cultures.
   c. can only occur between people who share interests and goals.
   d. always results in a committed long-term relationship.

2. Which of the following is most likely a sign of a dysfunctional relationship?
   a. The partners have frequent disagreements about money.
   b. One partner makes all the decisions for the couple and the other partner.
   c. Each partner has a demanding career.
   d. One partner is much older than the other partner.

3. Smart suggestions for online dating include:
   a. Use your office or school computer so that contacts can't access your personal computer.
   b. Give out only your cell phone number, not your address.
   c. Plan a full-day outing so that you will have plenty of time to get to know each other.
   d. Plan to meet in a busy place, like the local coffeehouse.

4. In friendships and other intimate relationships, which of the following is *not* true?
   a. Friends can communicate feelings as well as facts.
   b. Listening is just as important as talking.
   c. Emotional investment is required but the rewards are great.
   d. There is no need to pay attention to nonverbal communication.

5. Which of these is an example of self-disclosure?
   a. Steve tells his friend Twana that he would really like to change jobs sometime in the next year.
   b. Mike and Nicole talk about which cars they prefer.
   c. Maria mentions to Carrie that she and her brother don't get along so he won't be at the picnic.
   d. Angela lets her boyfriend Paul know that she used to be bulimic.

6. Married people
   a. have sex less frequently than unmarried partners.
   b. are more likely to become alcoholics and drug users.
   c. typically have at least one extramarital affair during their marriage.
   d. live longer than single or divorced individuals.

7. Which of the following scenarios demonstrates what might be considered gender differences in verbal and nonverbal communication styles?
   a. While Alyssa and Peter are discussing their vacation plans, Alyssa is gazing at the television and Peter is looking at Alyssa.
   b. Good friends Eva and Julia see each other for the first time after Christmas break and greet each other with a nod and a quick "Hi."
   c. New bank manager Alejandro tells the staff that they should consider him "the team coach and the keeper of the playbook."
   d. During an argument, Tony complains to Nicki, "I don't appreciate your crude jokes and constant swearing."

8. Which of the following statements is *false*?
   a. College education increases your chances of a happy marriage.
   b. African American couples are more likely to divorce than white couples.
   c. Children whose parents divorced are more likely to stay married.
   d. The divorce rate is lower now than it was in 1980.

9. Partners in successful marital relationships
   a. are generally from the same social and ethnic background.
   b. usually lived together before marrying.
   c. were usually very young at the time of their marriage.
   d. have premarital agreements.

10. The characteristics of a good relationship include which of the following?
    a. trust
    b. financial stability
    c. identical interests
    d. physical attractiveness

*Answers to these questions can be found on page 672.*

## Critical Thinking

1. While our society has become more tolerant, marriages between people of different religious and racial groups still face special pressures. What issues might arise if a Christian marries a Jew or Muslim? What about the issues facing partners of different races? How could these issues be resolved? What are your own feelings about mixed marriages? Would you date someone of a different religion or race? Why or why not?

2. What are your personal criteria for a successful relationship? Develop a brief list of factors you consider important, and support your choices with examples or experiences from your own life.

## Media Menu

Visit www.cengagebrain.com to access course materials and companion resources for this text that will:

- Help you evaluate your knowledge of the material.

- Allow you to prepare for exams with interactive quizzing.

- Use the CengageNOW product to develop a Personalized Learning Plan targeting resources that address areas you should study.

- Coach you through identifying target goals for behavioral change and creating and monitoring your personal change plan throughout the semester using the Behavior Change Planner available in the CengageNOW resource.

## Internet Connections

**www.goaskalice.columbia.edu**
Sponsored by the health education and wellness program of the Columbia University Health Service, this site features educators' answers to questions on a wide variety of topics, including those related to relationships and marriage and family.

**www.apahelpcenter.org/articles/topic.php?id=2**
The American Psychological Association provides a wealth of articles and information on sustaining healthy relationships.

**www.cyfc.umn.edu**
This site offers research, programs, publications, and information on all types of parenting, relationships, and family issues.

## Key Terms

The terms listed are used on the page indicated. Definitions of the terms are in the Glossary at the end of the book.

altruism   125

blended family   144

codependency   134

cohabitation   137

dysfunctional   132

enabling   135

family   144

intimacy   129

same-sex marriage   140

self-disclosure   123

social phobia   125

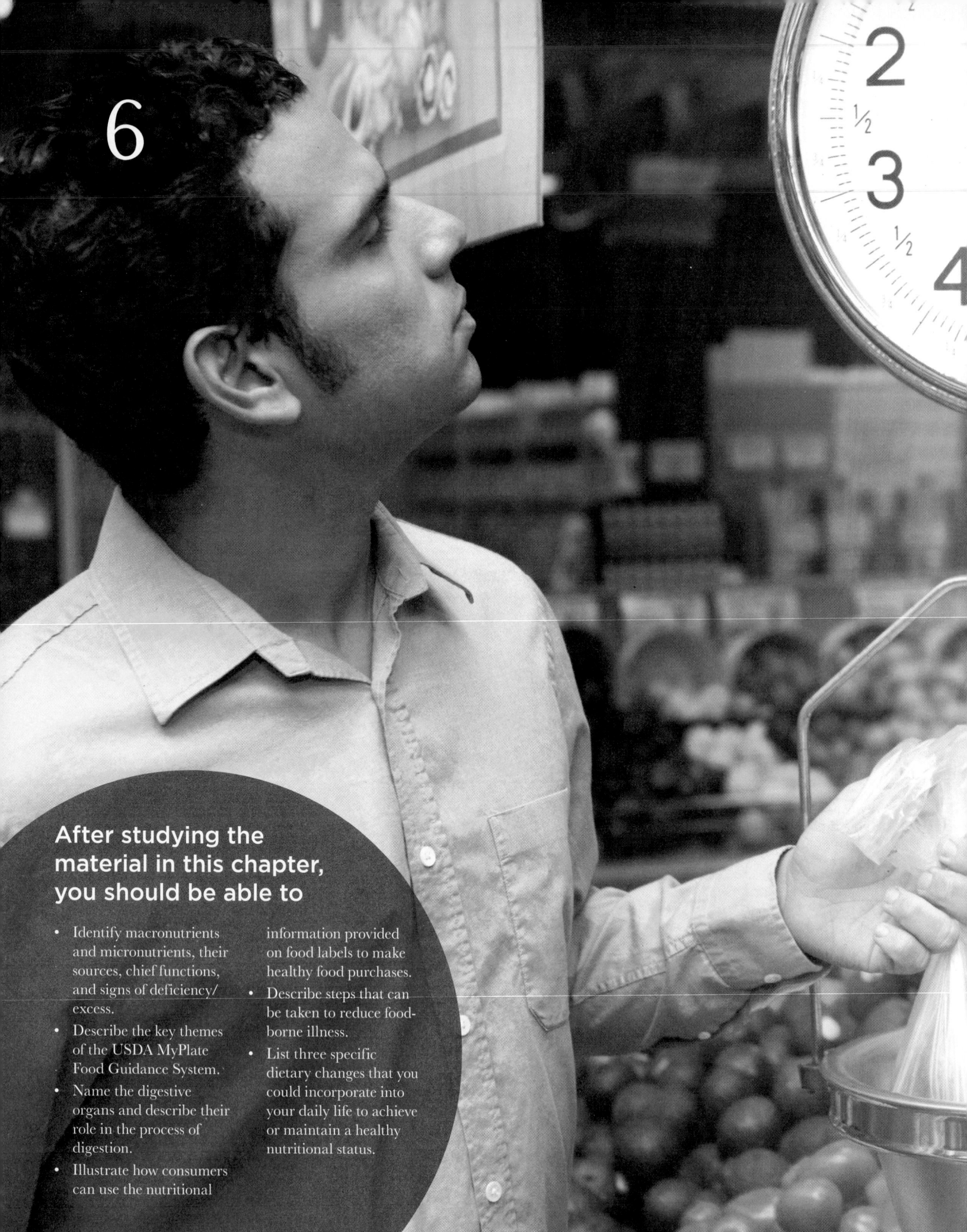

# 6

## After studying the material in this chapter, you should be able to

- Identify macronutrients and micronutrients, their sources, chief functions, and signs of deficiency/excess.
- Describe the key themes of the USDA MyPlate Food Guidance System.
- Name the digestive organs and describe their role in the process of digestion.
- Illustrate how consumers can use the nutritional information provided on food labels to make healthy food purchases.
- Describe steps that can be taken to reduce food-borne illness.
- List three specific dietary changes that you could incorporate into your daily life to achieve or maintain a healthy nutritional status.

The freshmen on the fifth floor of a university dormitory decided to test a dubious premise: that man—and woman—can live on pizza alone. For a month, they vowed to eat nothing but pizza in all its savory varieties—mushroom, pepperoni, sausage, anchovies, extra cheese, thin crust, double crust. "In less than a week," said one coed, "most of us cringed at the very sight of a cardboard delivery box." It wasn't just the boredom of having

# Personal Nutrition

the same meal that got to them. Some felt bloated. Others had stomachaches. A few complained of headaches and fatigue. One was convinced she had scurvy, a vitamin deficiency disease caused by a lack of fruit and vegetables. None of them managed to stick with pizza for an entire month.

As these students discovered, we are indeed what we eat—and it shows in everything from our stamina and strength to the sheen in our hair and the glow in our cheeks. Eating well helps us live and feel well.

As demonstrated by the science of **nutrition**, the field that explores the connections between our bodies and the foods we eat, our daily diet affects how long and how well we live. Sensible eating can provide energy for our daily tasks, can protect us from many chronic illnesses, and may even extend longevity. A high-quality diet also enhances day-to-day vitality, energy, and sense of well-being.

This chapter can help you make healthy food choices. It translates the latest scientific research and government dietary guidelines into specific advice designed both to promote health and to prevent chronic disease. By learning more about nutrients, food groups, eating patterns, nutrition labels, and safety practices, you can nourish your body with foods that not only taste good but also are good for you.

## What You Need To Know about Nutrients

Every day your body needs certain **essential nutrients** that it cannot manufacture for itself. They provide energy, build and repair body tissues, and regulate body functions. The six classes of essential nutrients, which are discussed in this section, are water, protein, carbohydrates, fats, vitamins, and minerals (Figure 6.1).

Water makes up about 60 percent of the body and is essential for health and survival. Besides water, we also need energy to live, and we

**nutrition** The science devoted to the study of dietary needs for food and the effects of food on organisms.

**essential nutrients** Nutrients that the body cannot manufacture for itself and must obtain from food.

Visit www.cengagebrain.com to access course materials for this text, including the Behavior Change Planner, interactive quizzes, tutorials, and more. See the preface on page xv for details.

© Jack Hollingsworth/Jupiterimages

## Figure 6.1 Six Categories of Nutrients

**1. CARBOHYDRATES** are substances in food that consist of a single sugar molecule, or of multiple sugar molecules in various forms. They provide the body with energy.

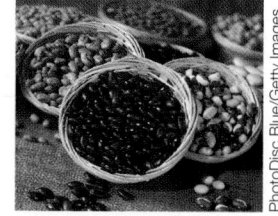

**Simple sugars** are the most basic type of carbohydrates. Examples include glucose (blood sugar), sucrose (table sugar), and lactose (milk sugar). **Starches** are complex carbohydrates consisting primarily of long, interlocking chains of glucose units. **Dietary fiber** consists of complex carbohydrates found principally in plant cell walls. Dietary fiber cannot be broken down by human digestive enzymes.

**2. PROTEINS** are substances in food that are composed of amino acids. Amino acids are specific chemical substances from which proteins are made. Of the 20 amino acids, 9 are "essential," or a required part of our diet.

**3. FATS** are substances in food that are soluble in fat, not water.

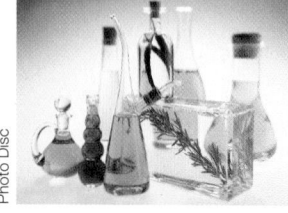

**Saturated fats** are found primarily in animal products, such as meat, butter, and cheese, and in palm and coconut oils. Diets high in saturated fat may elevate blood cholesterol levels. **Unsaturated fats** are found primarily in plant products, such as vegetable oil, nuts, and seeds, and in fish. Unsaturated fats tend to lower blood cholesterol levels. **Essential fatty acids** are two specific types of unsaturated fats that are required in the diet. **Trans fats** are a type of unsaturated fat present in hydrogenated oil, margarine, shortening, pastries, and some cooking oils that increase the risk of heart disease. **Cholesterol** is a fat-soluble, colorless liquid primarily found in animals. It can be manufactured by the liver.

**4. VITAMINS** are chemical substances found in food that perform specific functions in the body. Humans require 13 different vitamins in their diet.

**5. MINERALS** are chemical substances that make up the "ash" that remains when food is completely burned. Humans require 15 different minerals in their diet.

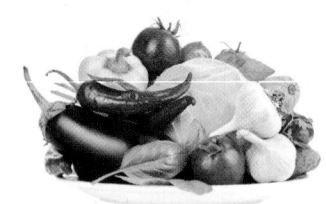

**6. WATER** is essential for life. Most adults need about 11–15 cups of water each day from food and fluids.

**macronutrients** Nutrients required by the human body in the greatest amounts, including water, carbohydrates, proteins, and fats.

**calorie** The amount of energy required to raise the temperature of 1 gram of water by 1 degree Celsius. In everyday usage related to the energy content of foods and the energy expended in activities, a calorie is actually the equivalent of a thousand such calories, or a kilocalorie.

**micronutrients** Vitamins and minerals needed by the body in very small amounts.

receive our energy from the carbohydrates, proteins, and fats in the foods we eat. The digestive system (Figure 6.2) breaks down food into these **macronutrients**. They are the nutrients required by the human body in the greatest amounts. The amount of energy that can be derived from the macronutrients is measured in **calories**. There are 9 calories in every gram of fat and 4 calories in every gram of protein or carbohydrate. The other two essential nutrients—the vitamins and minerals—are called **micronutrients** because our bodies need them in only very small amounts.

Your need for macronutrients depends on how much energy you expend. Because fats, carbohydrates, and protein can all serve as sources of energy, they can, to some extent, substitute for one another in providing calories. Adults, according to federal standards, should get 45 to 65 percent of calories from carbohydrates, 20 to 35 percent from fat, and 10 to 35 percent from protein. Children's fat intake should be slightly higher: 25 to 40 percent of their caloric intake.

To eat well without overeating, choose foods that are "nutrient-dense"—that is, foods that provide the most nutritional value. For example, both a cup of nonfat milk and an ounce and a half of cheddar cheese provide about 300 mg of calcium, but the milk offers the same amount of calcium for half the calories. Foods that are extremely low in nutrient density—such as potato chips, candy, and soft drinks—deliver only calories. Fruits and vegetables are nutrient-dense foods that provide many health benefits. (Take the Self Survey: How Healthful Is Your Diet? on pages 190–191 to evaluate how healthy your diet is.)

## Figure 6.2  The Digestive System

The organs of the digestive system break down food into nutrients that the body can use.

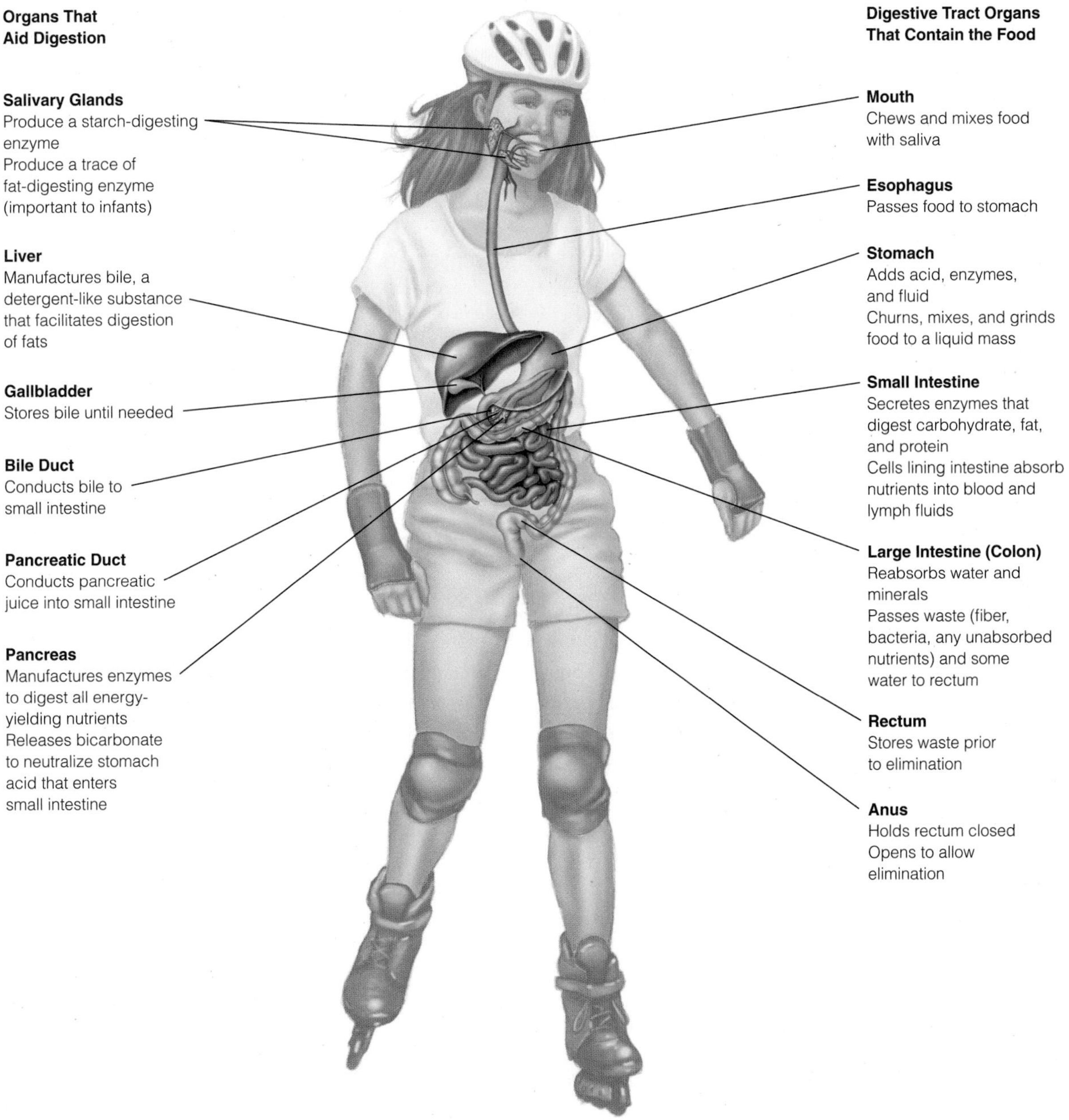

**Organs That Aid Digestion**

**Salivary Glands**
Produce a starch-digesting enzyme
Produce a trace of fat-digesting enzyme (important to infants)

**Liver**
Manufactures bile, a detergent-like substance that facilitates digestion of fats

**Gallbladder**
Stores bile until needed

**Bile Duct**
Conducts bile to small intestine

**Pancreatic Duct**
Conducts pancreatic juice into small intestine

**Pancreas**
Manufactures enzymes to digest all energy-yielding nutrients
Releases bicarbonate to neutralize stomach acid that enters small intestine

**Digestive Tract Organs That Contain the Food**

**Mouth**
Chews and mixes food with saliva

**Esophagus**
Passes food to stomach

**Stomach**
Adds acid, enzymes, and fluid
Churns, mixes, and grinds food to a liquid mass

**Small Intestine**
Secretes enzymes that digest carbohydrate, fat, and protein
Cells lining intestine absorb nutrients into blood and lymph fluids

**Large Intestine (Colon)**
Reabsorbs water and minerals
Passes waste (fiber, bacteria, any unabsorbed nutrients) and some water to rectum

**Rectum**
Stores waste prior to elimination

**Anus**
Holds rectum closed
Opens to allow elimination

## Calories

Calories are the measure of the amount of energy that can be derived from food. How many calories you need depends on your gender, age, body-frame size, weight, percentage of body fat, and your **basal metabolic rate (BMR)**—the number of calories needed to sustain your body at rest. Your activity level also affects your calorie requirements. Regardless of whether you consume fat, protein, or carbohydrates, if you take in more calories than required to maintain your size and don't work them off in some sort of physical activity, your body will convert the excess to fat (see Chapter 7). On average, daily calorie needs are:

- Most women, some older adults, children ages 2 to 6:  1,600
- Average adult:  2,000
- Most men, active women, teenage girls, older children:  2,200
- Active men, teenage boys:  2,800

(See Table 6.1.)

**basal metabolic rate (BMR)**  The number of calories required to sustain the body at rest.

Estimated amounts of calories needed to maintain calorie balance for various gender and age groups at three different levels of physical activity. The estimates are rounded to the nearest 200 calories. An individual's calorie needs may be higher or lower than these average estimates.

| Gender | Age (years) | Physical Activity Level | | |
|--------|-------------|-----------|-------------------|--------|
| | | Sedentary | Moderately Active | Active |
| **Female** | 19–30 | 1,800–2,000 | 2,000–2,200 | 2,400 |
| | 31–50 | 1,800 | 2,000 | 2,200 |
| | 51+ | 1,600 | 1,800 | 2,000–2,200 |
| **Male** | 19–30 | 2,400–2,600 | 2,600–2,800 | 3,000 |
| | 31–50 | 2,200–2,400 | 2,400–2,600 | 2,800–3,000 |
| | 51+ | 2,000–2,200 | 2,200–2,400 | 2,400–2,800 |

## Water

Water, which makes up 85 percent of blood, 70 percent of muscles, and about 75 percent of the brain, performs many essential functions: It carries nutrients, maintains temperature, lubricates joints, helps with digestion, rids the body of waste through urine, and contributes to the production of sweat, which evaporates from the skin to cool the body. Research has correlated high fluid intake with a lower risk of kidney stones, colon cancer, and bladder cancer. (See Chapter 19 for a discussion of bottled water.)

You lose about 64 to 80 ounces of water a day—the equivalent of eight to ten 8-ounce glasses—through perspiration, urination, bowel movements, and normal exhalation. You lose water more rapidly if you exercise, live in a dry climate or at a high altitude, drink a lot of caffeine or alcohol (which increases urination), skip a meal, or become ill. To ensure adequate water intake, nutritionists advise drinking enough so that your urine is not dark in color. Healthy individuals can get adequate hydration from beverages other than plain water, including juice.

## Protein

Every living cell in the body contains protein. Critical for growth and repair, **proteins** form the basic framework for our muscles, bones, blood, hair, and fingernails.

**proteins** Organic compounds composed of amino acids; one of the essential nutrients.

**amino acids** Organic compounds containing nitrogen, carbon, hydro—gen, and oxygen; the essential building blocks of proteins.

**complete proteins** Proteins that contain all the amino acids needed by the body for growth and maintenance.

**incomplete proteins** Proteins that lack one or more of the amino acids essential for protein synthesis.

**complementary proteins** Incomplete proteins that, when combined, provide all the amino acids essential for protein synthesis.

Twenty different **amino acids** join together to make all types of protein. Nine of these amino acids cannot be made by our bodies. These are known as *essential* amino acids that we must get from our diets. Dietary protein sources are categorized according to how many of the essential amino acids they provide:

- A *complete* or high-quality **protein** source provides all the essential amino acids. Animal-based foods such as meat, poultry, fish, milk, eggs, and cheese are considered complete protein sources.
- An *incomplete* **protein** source is low in one or more of the essential amino acids.
- *Complementary* proteins are two or more incomplete protein sources that together provide adequate amounts of all the essential amino acids. Two good examples are rice and dry beans, which together can provide adequate amounts of all the essential amino acids the body needs.

You need to eat protein every day, because your body doesn't store it the way it stores fats or carbohydrates. The average person needs 50 to 65 grams of protein daily. This is the amount in four ounces of meat plus a cup of cottage cheese.

Protein is found in the following foods:

- meats, poultry, and fish
- legumes (dry beans and peas)
- tofu
- eggs
- nuts and seeds
- milk and milk products
- grains, some vegetables, and some fruits (only small amounts relative to other sources)

Most people eat more protein than they need without harmful effects. However, protein contributes to calorie intake, so if you eat too much, your overall calorie intake could be greater than your calorie needs, and you can gain weight. Animal proteins also are sources of saturated fat, which has been linked to elevated low-density lipoprotein (LDL) cholesterol, a risk factor for cardiovascular disease.

Because some vegetarians avoid eating all (or most) animal foods, they must rely on plant-based sources of protein to meet their protein

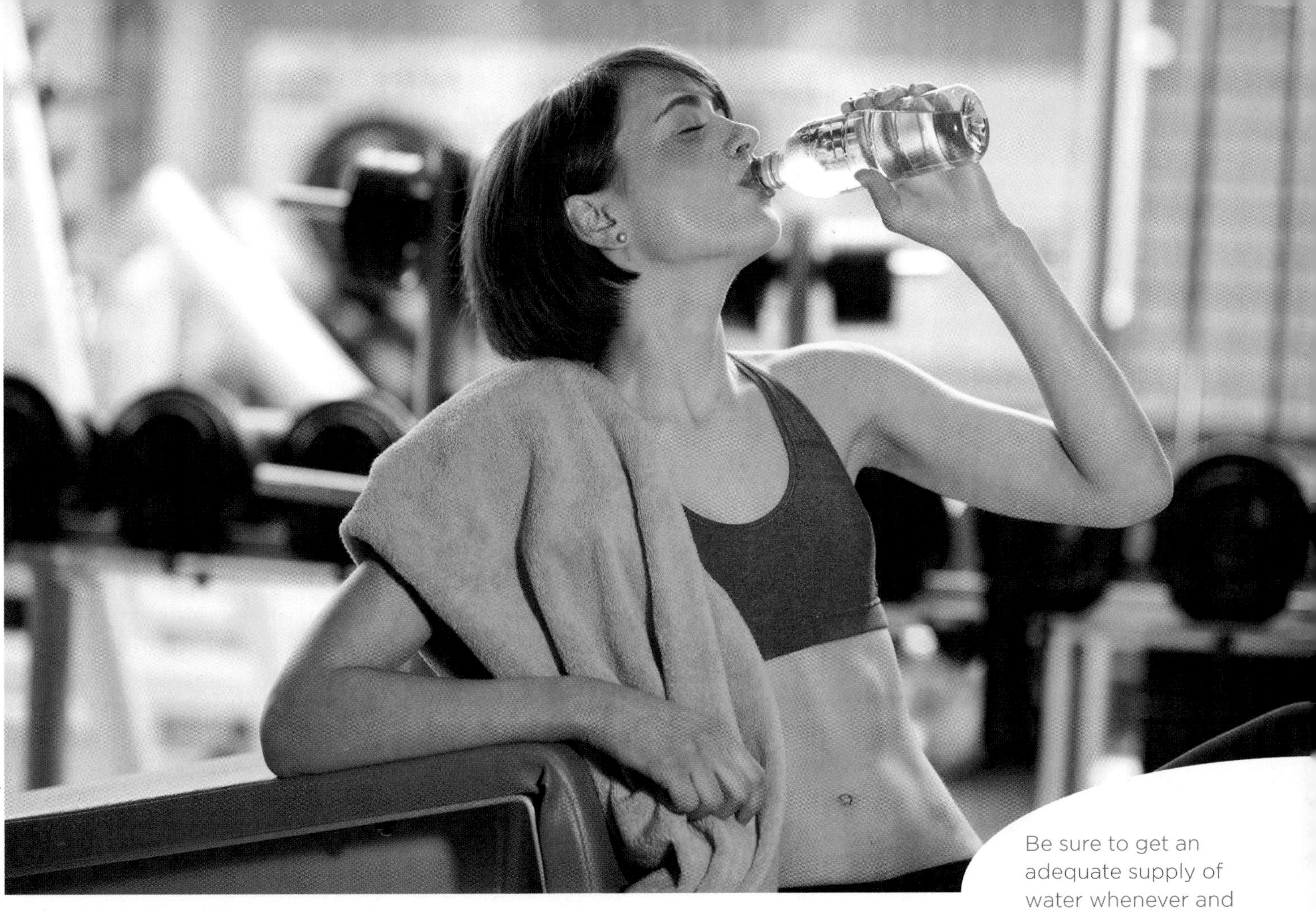

Be sure to get an adequate supply of water whenever and wherever you exercise.

needs. With some planning, a vegetarian diet can easily meet the recommended protein needs (see page 174).

## Carbohydrates

**Carbohydrates** are organic compounds that provide our brains and bodies with *glucose*, their basic fuel. The major sources of carbohydrates are plants—including grains, vegetables, fruits, and beans—and milk. There are two types: *simple carbohydrates* (sugars) and *complex carbohydrates* (starches and fiber). All provide 4 calories per gram. Both adults and children should consume at least 130 grams of carbohydrates each day, the minimum needed to produce enough glucose for the brain to function.

*Forms of Carbohydrates* **Simple carbohydrates** include *natural sugars*, such as the lactose in milk and the fructose in fruit, and *added sugars* that are found in candy, soft drinks, fruit drinks, pastries, and other sweets. Those whose diets are higher in added sugars typically have lower intakes of other essential nutrients.

On average Americans consume more than 20 teaspoons of sweet calories a day. Some come from the teaspoons of sucrose (simple sugar) you add to coffee or tea. But many come from high-fructose corn syrup, a common sweetener and preservative made by changing the sugar glucose in cornstarch to fructose. Because it extends the shelf life of processed foods and is cheaper than sugar, high-fructose corn syrup has become a popular ingredient in many sodas, fruit-flavored drinks, and other processed foods.

High-fructose corn syrup isn't intrinsically less healthy than other sweeteners. However, it makes beverages very sweet, which may increase consumption and contribute to obesity and other health problems.

**Complex carbohydrates** include grains, cereals, vegetables, beans, and nuts. Americans get most of their complex carbohydrates from refined grains, which have been stripped of fiber and many nutrients, in breads and desserts.

Far more nutritious are whole grains, which are made up of all components of the grain: the *bran* (or fiber-rich outer layer), the *endosperm* (middle

**carbohydrates** Organic compounds, such as starches, sugars, and glycogen, that are composed of carbon, hydrogen, and oxygen, and are sources of bodily energy.

**simple carbohydrates** Sugars; like all carbohydrates, they provide the body with glucose.

**complex carbohydrates** Starches, including cereals, fruits, and vegetables.

layer), and the *germ* (the nutrient-packed inner layer). Whole grains have proven effective in lowering the risk of diabetes and heart disease. Yet only 8 percent of American adults consume three or more servings of whole grains; 42 percent eat no whole grains on a given day. One excellent source: popcorn. Popcorn eaters have higher intakes of fiber and other nutrients.

*Low-Carb Foods* The popularity of diets that restrict carbohydrate intake, discussed in Chapter 7, prompted an explosion in products touted as "low-carb." You can get low-carb versions of everything from beer to bread. However, the Food and Drug Administration (FDA), which regulates health claims on food labels in the United States, hasn't defined what "low-carb" means. Words like "low-carb," "carb-wise," or "carb-free" are marketing terms created by manufacturers to sell their products.

Although many people may buy low-carb foods because they believe that they're healthier, that isn't necessarily the case. A low-carb nutrition bar, for instance, may be high in saturated fat and calories. Some low-carb food products cause digestive symptoms because food companies often replace the carbohydrates in a cookie or cracker with substances such as the sweetener sorbitol, which can cause diarrhea or stomach cramps.

Dieters often buy low-carb products in order to lose weight. According to proponents of low-carb diets, if carbohydrates raise blood sugar and insulin levels and cause weight gain, a decrease in carbs should result in lower blood sugar and insulin levels—and weight loss. With limited carbohydrates in the diet, the body would break down fat to provide needed energy.

Some people do lose weight when they switch to low-carb foods, but the reasons are probably that they consume fewer calories, lose water weight, and have decreased appetite because of a buildup of ketones (a by-product of fat metabolism) in the blood. As discussed in Chapter 7, a low-carb diet can lead to fairly rapid weight loss but is no easier to maintain over the long run than any other diet.

*Fiber* **Dietary fiber** is the nondigestible form of complex carbohydrates occurring naturally in plant foods, such as leaves, stems, skins, seeds, and hulls. **Functional fiber** consists of isolated, nondigestible carbohydrates that may be added to foods and that provide beneficial effects in humans. Total fiber is the sum of both.

The various forms of fiber enhance health in different ways: They slow the emptying of the stomach, which creates a feeling of fullness and aids weight control. They interfere with absorption of dietary fat and cholesterol, which lowers the risk of heart disease and stroke in both middle-aged and elderly individuals. In addition, fiber helps prevent constipation, diverticulosis (a painful inflammation of the bowel), and diabetes. The link between fiber and colon cancer is complex. Some studies have indicated that increased fiber intake reduces risk; others found no such correlation.

Fiber may also contribute to a longer lifespan. In a recent study of almost 400,000 people ages 50 to 71, those who ate a diet rich in whole grains, fruits, and vegetables (up to 29 grams of fiber per day for men and 26 grams for women) were significantly less likely to die of cardiovascular disease, infectious illnesses, and respiratory disorders over a nine-year period. A high-fiber diet also was associated with fewer cancer deaths in men, but not in women.[1]

The Institute of Medicine has set recommendations for daily intake levels of total fiber (dietary plus functional fiber): 38 grams of total fiber for men and 25 grams for women. For men and women over 50 years of age, who consume less food, the recommendations are, respectively, 30 and 21 grams. The American Dietetic Association recommends 25 to 35 grams of dietary fiber a day, much more than the amount Americans typically consume.

Good fiber sources include wheat and corn bran (the outer layer); leafy greens; the skins of fruits and root vegetables; oats, beans, and barley; and the pulp, skin, and seeds of many vegetables and fruits, such as apples and strawberries (see Table 6.2). Because sudden increases in fiber can cause symptoms like bloating and gas, experts recommend gradually adding more fiber to your diet with an additional serving or two of vegetables, fruit, or whole-wheat bread.

*Glycemic Index and Glycemic Load*
The glycemic index is a ranking of carbohydrates, gram for gram, based on their immediate effect on blood glucose (sugar) levels.

**dietary fiber** The nondigestible form of carbohydrates found in plant foods, such as leaves, stems, skins, seeds, and hulls.

**functional fiber** Isolated, nondigestible carbohydrates with beneficial effects in humans.

Table 6.2 **High-Fiber Foods**

### Grains

**Whole-grain products provide about 1 to 2 grams (or more) of fiber per serving:**

- 1 slice whole-wheat, pumpernickel, rye bread
- 1 oz ready-to-eat cereal (100% bran cereals contain 10 grams or more)
- ½ cup cooked barley, bulgur, grits, oatmeal, brown rice, quinoa

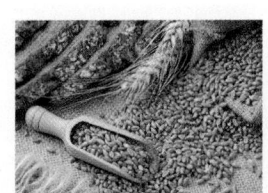

### Vegetables

**Most vegetables contain about 2 to 3 grams of fiber per serving:**

- 1 cup raw bean sprouts
- ½ cup cooked broccoli, brussels sprouts, cabbage, carrots, cauliflower, collards, corn, eggplant, green beans, green peas, kale, mushrooms, okra, parsnips, potatoes, pumpkin, spinach, sweet potatoes, swiss chard, winter squash
- ½ cup chopped raw carrots, peppers

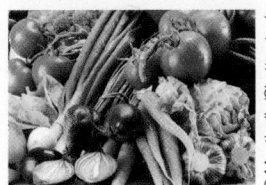

### Fruits

**Fresh, frozen, and dried fruits have about 2 grams of fiber per serving:**

- 1 medium apple, banana, kiwi, nectarine, orange, pear
- ½ cup applesauce, blackberries, blueberries, raspberries, strawberries

**Fruit juices contain very little fiber.**

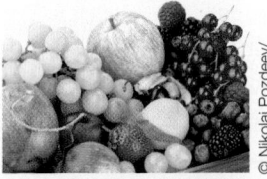

### Legumes

**Many legumes provide about 6 to 8 grams of fiber per serving:**

- ½ cup cooked baked beans, black beans, black-eyed peas, kidney beans, navy beans, pinto beans

**Some legumes provide about 5 grams of fiber per serving:**

- ½ cup cooked garbanzo beans, great northern beans, lentils, lima beans, split peas

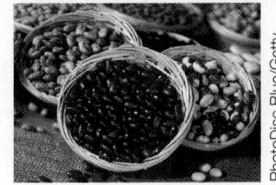

Carbohydrates that break down quickly during digestion and trigger a fast, high glucose response have the highest glycemic index rating. Those that break down slowly, releasing glucose gradually into the bloodstream, have low glycemic index ratings. Potatoes, which raise blood sugar higher and faster than apples, for instance, earn a higher glycemic index rating than apples. Glycemic index does not account for the amount of food you typically eat in a serving.

Glycemic load is a measure of how much a typical serving size of a particular food raises blood glucose. For example, the glycemic index of table sugar is high, but you use so little to sweeten your coffee or tea that its glycemic load is low.

## Fats

Fats carry the fat-soluble vitamins A, D, E, and K; aid in their absorption in the intestine; protect organs from injury; regulate body temperature; and play an important role in growth and development. They provide 9 calories per gram—more than twice the amount in carbohydrates or proteins.

Both high- and low-fat diets can be unhealthy. When people eat very low levels of fat and very high levels of carbohydrates, their levels of high-density lipoprotein, the so-called *good cholesterol*, decline. On the other hand, high-fat diets can lead to obesity and its related health dangers, discussed in Chapter 7.

*Forms of Fat* **Saturated fats** and **unsaturated fats** are distinguished by the type of fatty acids in their chemical structures. Unsaturated fats can be divided into monounsaturated or polyunsaturated, again depending on their chemical structure. All dietary fats are a mix of saturated and unsaturated fats but are predominantly one or the other. Unsaturated fats, like oils, are likely to be liquid at room temperature and saturated fats, like butter, are likely to be solid. In general, vegetable and fish oils are unsaturated, and animal fats are saturated. Table 6.3 lists the major sources of healthful monounsaturated and polyunsaturated fats.

**saturated fats** A chemical term indicating that a fat molecule contains as many hydrogen atoms as its carbon skeleton can hold. These fats are normally solid at room temperature.

**unsaturated fats** A chemical term indicating that a fat molecule contains fewer hydrogen atoms than its carbon skeleton can hold. These fats are normally liquid at room temperature.

## Table 6.3 **Major Sources of Various Fatty Acids**

### Healthful Fatty Acids

| Monounsaturated | Polyunsaturated | Omega-3 Polyunsaturated |
|---|---|---|
| Avocado | Margarine (nonhydrogenated) | Fatty fish (herring, mackerel, salmon, tuna) |
| Oils (canola, olive, peanut, sesame) | Oils (corn, cottonseed, safflower, soybean) | Flaxseed |
| Nuts (almonds, cashews, filberts, hazelnuts, macadamia nuts, peanuts, pecans, pistachios) | Nuts (pine nuts, walnuts) | Nuts (walnuts) |
| Olives | Mayonnaise | |
| Peanut butter | Salad dressing | |
| Seeds (sesame) | Seeds (pumpkin, sunflower) | |

### Unhealthful Fatty Acids

| Saturated | Trans | |
|---|---|---|
| Bacon | Fried foods (hydrogenated shortening) | |
| Butter | Margarine (hydrogenated or partially hydrogenated) | |
| Chocolate | Nondairy creamers | |
| Coconut | Many fast foods | |
| Cream cheese | Shortening | |
| Cream, half-and-half | Commercial baked goods (including doughnuts, cakes, cookies) | |
| Lard | Many snack foods (including microwave popcorn, chips, crackers) | |
| Meat | | |
| Milk and milk products (whole) | | |
| Oils (coconut, palm, palm kernel) | | |
| Shortening | | |
| Sour cream | | |

**trans fat** Fat formed when liquid vegetable oils are processed to make table spreads or cooking fats; also found in dairy and beef products; considered to be especially dangerous dietary fats.

Olive, soybean, canola, cottonseed, corn, and other vegetable oils are unsaturated fats. Olive oil is considered a good fat and one of the best vegetable oils for salads and cooking. Used for thousands of years, this staple of the Mediterranean diet (discussed later in this chapter) has been correlated with a lower incidence of heart disease, including strokes and heart attacks.

Omega-3 and omega-6 are polyunsaturated fatty acids with slightly different chemical compositions. Regular consumption of omega-3 fatty acids, found in fatty fish such as salmon and sardines, flaxseed, and walnuts, helps to prevent blood clots, protect against irregular heartbeats, and lower blood pressure, especially among people with high blood pressure or atherosclerosis.[2] Omega-6 fatty acids are found in vegetable oils, nuts, seeds, meat, poultry, and eggs. The recommended ratio for consumption of omega-6 and omega-3 fatty acids is 6 to 1.

Some fish, such as mackerel, shark, tilefish, tuna, and swordfish, contain potentially harmful levels of mercury. To balance the benefits and risks of eating fish, the American Heart Association recommends two servings of fish a week, although even a single fish meal a month may be beneficial. Nutritionists do not advise fish oil supplements as a source of omega-3 fatty acids because high intake may increase bleeding time, interfere with wound healing, and suppress immune function.

Saturated fats can increase the risk of heart disease and should be avoided as much as possible. In response to consumer and health professionals' demand for less saturated fat in the food supply, many manufacturers switched to partially hydrogenated oils.

The process of hydrogenation creates unsaturated fatty acids called **trans fat**. They are found in some margarine products and most foods made with partially hydrogenated oils, such as baked goods and fried foods. Even though trans fats are unsaturated, they have an even more harmful effect on cholesterol than saturated fats because they increase harmful LDL and, in large amounts, decrease helpful HDL. Epidemiological studies have suggested a possible link between cardiovascular disease risk and high intakes of trans fats, and researchers have concluded that they are, gram for gram, twice as damaging as saturated fats.[3] There is no safe level for trans fats, which occur naturally in meats as well as in foods prepared with partially hydrogenated vegetable oils.

Some food manufacturers have reduced or eliminated trans fats in snacks and other products. Cities and communities across the country have banned trans fats in restaurants. Some campuses also have stopped using trans fats in their dining halls and food outlets.

To cut down on both saturated and trans fats, choose oils such as soybean, canola, corn, olive, safflower, and sunflower, which are naturally free of trans fats and lower in saturated fats—see Table 6.3. Look for reduced-fat, low-fat, fat-free, and trans-fat-free versions of baked goods, snacks, and other processed foods. Some choices—such as butter versus margarine—are more difficult to make (see Figure 6.3).

Figure 6.3  **Butter or Margarine?**

Most of the fat in butter is saturated fat. Most of the fat in margarine is unsaturated, but the trans fats are twice as damaging as saturated fat. If the list of ingredients includes partially hydrogenated oils, you know the food contains trans fat. The closer "partially hydrogenated oil" is to the beginning of the ingredients list, the more trans fat the product contains. There are a handful of margarine alternatives that do not contain trans fats.

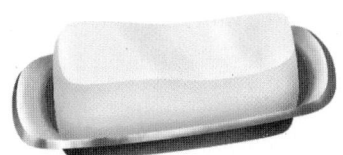

Butter

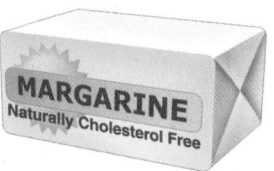

Margarine (stick)

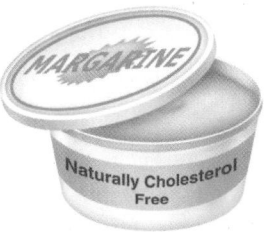

Margarine (tub)

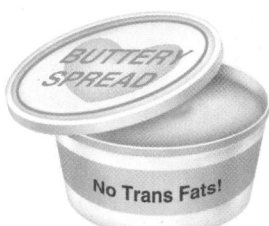

Buttery spread

**Nutrition Facts**

Serving Size 1 Tbsp (14g)
Servings per container about 32

| Amount per serving | |
|---|---|
| **Calories** 100 Calories from Fat 100 | |
| | %Daily Value* |
| **Total Fat** 11g | 17% |
| Saturated Fat 7g | 37% |
| Trans Fat 0g | |
| **Cholesterol** 30mg | 10% |
| **Sodium** 95mg | 4% |
| **Total Carbohydrate** 0g | 0% |
| **Protein** 0g | |
| Vitamin A 8% | |

Not a significant source of dietary fiber, sugars, vitamin C, calcium, and iron.

*Percent Daily Values are based on a 2,000 calorie diet.

**INGREDIENTS:** Cream, salt.

**Nutrition Facts**

Serving Size 1 Tbsp (14g)
Servings per container about 32

| Amount per serving | |
|---|---|
| **Calories** 100 Calories from Fat 100 | |
| | %Daily Value* |
| **Total Fat** 11g | 17% |
| Saturated Fat 2g | 11% |
| Trans Fat 2.5g | |
| Polyunsaturated Fat 3.5g | |
| Monounsaturated Fat 2.5g | |
| **Cholesterol** 0mg | 0% |
| **Sodium** 105mg | 4% |
| **Total Carbohydrate** 0g | 0% |
| **Protein** 0g | |
| Vitamin A 10% | |

Not a significant source of dietary fiber, sugars, vitamin C, calcium, and iron.

*Percent Daily Values are based on a 2,000 calorie diet.

**INGREDIENTS:** Liquid soybean oil, partially hydrogenated soybean oil, water, buttermilk, salt, soy lecithin, sodium benzoate (as a preservative), vegetable mono and diglycerides, artificial flavor, vitamin A palmitate, colored with beta carotene (provitamin A).

**Nutrition Facts**

Serving size 1 Tbsp (14g)
Servings per container about 32

| Amount per serving | |
|---|---|
| **Calories** 100 Calories from Fat 100 | |
| | %Daily Value* |
| **Total Fat** 11g | 17% |
| Saturated Fat 2.5g | 13% |
| Trans Fat 2g | |
| Polyunsaturated Fat 4g | |
| Monounsaturated Fat 2.5g | |
| **Cholesterol** 0mg | 0% |
| **Sodium** 80mg | 3% |
| **Total Carbohydrate** 0g | 0% |
| **Protein** 0g | |
| Vitamin A 10% | |

Not a significant source of dietary fiber, sugars, vitamin C, calcium, and iron.

*Percent Daily Values are based on a 2,000 calorie diet.

**INGREDIENTS:** Liquid soybean oil, partially hydrogenated soybean oil, buttermilk, water, butter (cream, salt), salt, soy lecithin, vegetable mono and diglycerides, sodium benzoate added as a preservative, artificial flavor, vitamin A palmitate, colored with beta carotene.

**Nutrition Facts**

Serving size 1 Tbsp (14g)
Servings per container about 24

| Amount per serving | |
|---|---|
| **Calories** 100 Calories from Fat 100 | |
| | %Daily Value* |
| **Total Fat** 11g | 17% |
| Saturated Fat 3.5g | 18% |
| Trans Fat 0g | |
| Polyunsaturated Fat 3.5g | |
| Monounsaturated Fat 3.5g | |
| **Cholesterol** 0mg | 0% |
| **Sodium** 120mg | 5% |
| **Total Carbohydrate** 0g | 0% |
| **Protein** 0g | |
| Vitamin A 0% | |

Not a significant source of dietary fiber, sugars, vitamin C, calcium, and iron.

*Percent Daily Values are based on a 2,000 calorie diet.

**INGREDIENTS:** Expeller pressed natural oil blend (soybean palm fruit, canola and olive), filtered water, pure salt, natural flavor, soy protein, soy lecithin, lactic acid (non-dairy, derived from sugar beets), and beta-carotene color (from natural source).

## Vitamins and Minerals

**Vitamins**, which help put proteins, fats, and carbohydrates to use, are essential to regulating growth, maintaining tissue, and releasing energy from foods. Together with the enzymes in the body, they help produce the right chemical reactions at the right times. They're also involved in the manufacture of blood cells, hormones, and other compounds.

The body produces some vitamins, such as vitamin D, which is manufactured in the skin after exposure to sunlight. Other vitamins must be ingested.

Vitamins A, D, E, and K are fat-soluble; they are absorbed through the intestinal membranes and stored in the body.

The B vitamins and vitamin C are water-soluble; they are absorbed directly into the blood and then used up or washed out of the body in urine and sweat. They must be replaced daily. Table 6.4 on pages 167–168 summarizes key information about the vitamins.

*Vitamin D* This vitamin is essential for bone health, cognitive function, pain control, and many other processes within the body. It comes in two forms: vitamin D, which comes from plants (that have been exposed to sunlight) and foods fortified with vitamin D, such as milk, cheese, bread, and juice; and vitamin D3, which is formed in the skin after exposure to the sun's ultraviolet rays and ingested from animal sources, including some fish.

Sunshine stimulates the production of vitamin D in the body, and many people can get a sufficient amount by spending five to ten minutes outside without sunscreen. (More unprotected time can cause sunburn and skin cancer.) During the winter months, Americans living north of an imaginary line stretching from San Francisco to St. Louis to Richmond, Virginia, may not be able to get an adequate amount of ultraviolet light simply by being outdoors.

Vitamin D, which we can also get from fortified milk, eggs, salmon, tuna, and sardines, aids in the absorption of calcium and helps to form and maintain strong bones. Other benefits include:

- **Lower risk of heart disease**. Calcium deposits that stiffen the arteries are more likely to develop in people with low levels of vitamin D. In one study, men low in vitamin D were twice as likely to develop heart disease.

- **Decreased blood pressure**. Vitamin D lowers the kidneys' production of rennin, a hormone that boosts blood pressure. Several studies suggest that getting more of the vitamin can help control blood pressure.

- **Protection against infection**. Adequate amounts of vitamin D can help the body fight off the flu, tuberculosis, and infections of the upper respiratory tract.

Too little vitamin D can contribute to heart disease, falls and broken bones, breast cancer, prostate cancer, depression, and memory loss. Low vitamin D levels also have been linked with Parkinson's disease, stroke risk, and exacerbation of multiple sclerosis.

Vitamin D may play a role in regulating weight and muscle strength. In one study of college-age young women (average age 19), those with too little vitamin D were heavier, weighing about 16 pounds more than those with adequate vitamin D intake.[4]

In recent years health officials have warned that most Americans might be deficient in calcium and vitamin D. However, an authoritative report by the Institute of Medicine (IOM) has determined that these claims were exaggerated. For the first time, the IOM has established a recommended dietary allowance (RDA) for both nutrients: 600 IU for vitamin D—a threefold increase for some age groups over previous suggested levels—and 1000 mg for calcium[5] (discussed on page 156).

Although extra vitamin D has been linked with prevention of cancer, heart disease, and diabetes, the report concluded that the scientific evidence is too weak to support its use for this purpose. Very large quantities, or megadoses, of vitamin D are not effective and could be harmful. The report also cautioned against spending more time in the sun to promote synthesis of vitamin D in the skin through ultraviolet rays.[6]

Many physicians remain convinced that the evidence for vitamin D's benefits, particularly to protect against cardiovascular disease, cancer, and premature death, will continue to accumulate.[7] Until the findings are conclusive, ask your doctor to test your vitamin D level. If it is low,

**vitamins** Organic substances that are needed in very small amounts by the body and carry out a variety of functions in metabolism and nutrition.

discuss the relative benefits and risks of taking a supplement.

*Antioxidants* **Antioxidants** prevent the harmful effects caused by oxidation within the body. They include vitamins C, E, and beta-carotene (a form of vitamin A), as well as compounds like carotenoids and flavonoids. All share a common enemy: renegade oxygen cells called free radicals released by normal metabolism as well as by pollution, smoking, radiation, and stress.

Diets high in antioxidant-rich fruits and vegetables have been linked with lower rates of esophageal, lung, colon, and stomach cancer. Nevertheless, scientific studies have not proved conclusively that any specific antioxidant, particularly in supplement form, can prevent cancer.

*Minerals* Carbon, oxygen, hydrogen, and nitrogen make up 96 percent of our body weight. The other 4 percent consists of **minerals** that help build bones and teeth, aid in muscle function, and help our nervous systems transmit messages. Every day we need about a tenth of a gram (100 milligrams) or more of the major minerals: sodium, potassium chloride, calcium, phosphorus, magnesium, and sulfur. We also need about a hundredth of a gram (10 milligrams) or less of each of the trace minerals: iron (although young women need more, particularly if they are physically active), zinc, selenium, molybdenum, iodine, copper, manganese, fluoride, and chromium. (See Table 6.5 on pages 162–163 for key information on minerals.)

*Calcium* Calcium, the most abundant mineral in the body, builds strong bone tissue throughout life and plays a vital role in blood clotting and muscle and nerve functioning. Pregnant or nursing women need more calcium to meet the additional needs of their babies' bodies. Calcium may also help control high blood pressure, prevent colon cancer in adults, and promote weight loss. Adequate calcium and vitamin D in—take during childhood, adolescence, and young adulthood is crucial to prevent osteoporosis, the bone-weakening disease that strikes one of every four women over the age of 60.

Most individuals can get adequate amounts of calcium from their diet, according to an Institute of Medicine report on this mineral and vitamin

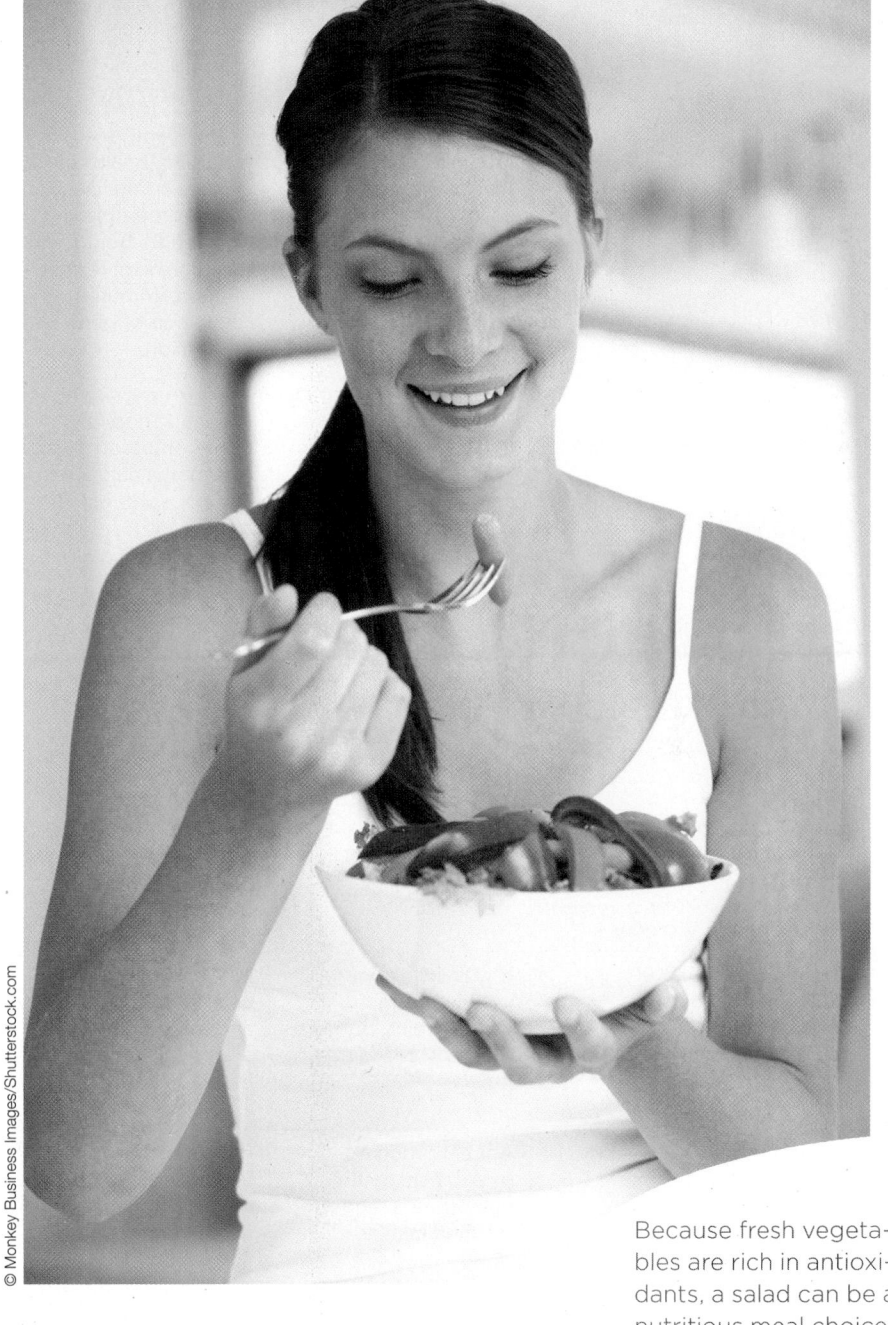

Because fresh vegetables are rich in antioxidants, a salad can be a nutritious meal choice.

D.[8] However, girls between ages 9 and 18 may fall short of getting the recommended 1300 mg for their age group. For women ages 19 to 50 and men ages 19 to 70, the recommended daily intake is 1000 mg. The recommended allowance for women older than 50 and men over 70 is 1200 mg. Amounts greater than 2000 mg can cause constipation and kidney stones and put individuals at risk for calcification within their blood vessels and other serious health threats.

**antioxidants** Substances that prevent the damaging effects of oxidation in cells.

**minerals** Naturally occurring inorganic substances, small amounts of some being essential in metabolism and nutrition.

## Table 6.4 **Key Information about Vitamins**

### Fat-Soluble Vitamins

| Vitamin/Recommended Intake per Day | Significant Sources | Chief Functions | Signs of Severe, Prolonged Deficiency | Signs of Extreme Excess |
|---|---|---|---|---|
| **Vitamin A**<br>Males 19–50: 900 μg RAE<br>Females 19–50: 700 μg RAE | Fortified milk, cheese, cream, butter, fortified margarine, eggs, liver, spinach and other dark leafy greens, broccoli, deep orange fruits (apricots, cantaloupes), and vegetables (carrots, sweet potatoes, pumpkins) | Antioxidant; needed for vision, health of cornea, epithelial cells, mucous membranes, skin health, bone and tooth growth, reproduction, immunity, regulation of gene expression | Cracks in teeth, tendency toward tooth decay, night blindness, keratinization, corneal degeneration | Overstimulated cell division, skin rashes, hair loss, hemorrhage, bone abnormalities, birth defects, fractures, liver failure, death |
| **Vitamin D**<br>Adults 19–50: 5 μg<br>51–70 years: 10 μg<br>>70 years: 15 μg | Exposure to sunlight; fortified milk or margarine, eggs, liver, sardines | Mineralization of bones and teeth (promotes calcium and phosphorus absorption) | Abnormal growth, misshapen bones (bowing of legs), soft bones, joint pain, malformed teeth, muscle spasms | Raised blood calcium, excessive thirst, headaches, irritability, weakness, nausea, kidney stones, deposits in arteries |
| **Vitamin E**<br>Males 19–50: 15 mg<br>Females 19–50: 15 mg | Polyunsaturated plant oils (margarine, salad dressings, shortenings), green and leafy vegetables, wheat germ, whole-grain products, nuts, seeds | Antioxidant; needed for stabilization of cell membranes, regulation of oxidation reactions | Red blood cell breakage, anemia, muscle degeneration, difficulty walking, leg cramps, nerve damage | Augments the effects of anticlotting medication; general discomfort; blurred vision |
| **Vitamin K**<br>Males 19–50: 120 μg<br>Females 19–50: 90 μg | Green leafy vegetables, cabbage-type vegetables, soybeans, vegetable oils | Synthesis of blood-clotting proteins and proteins important in bone mineralization | Hemorrhage, abnormal bone formation | Interference with anticlotting medication |

### Water-Soluble Vitamins

| Vitamin/Recommended Intake per Day | Significant Sources | Chief Functions | Signs of Severe, Prolonged Deficiency | Signs of Extreme Excess |
|---|---|---|---|---|
| **Vitamin B$_6$**<br>Males 19–50: 1.3 mg<br>Females 19–50: 1.3 mg | Meats, fish, poultry, liver, legumes, fruits, whole grains, potatoes, soy products | Part of a coenzyme used in amino acid and fatty acid metabolism, helps make red blood cells | Anemia, depression, abnormal brain wave pattern, convulsions, skin rashes | Impaired memory, depression, irritability, headaches, numbness, damage to nerves, difficulty walking, loss of reflexes |
| **Vitamin B$_{12}$**<br>Males 19–50: 2.4 μg<br>Females 19–50: 2.4 μg | Animal products (meat, fish, poultry, milk, cheese, eggs), fortified cereals | Part of a coenzyme used in new cell synthesis, helps maintain nerve cells | Anemia, nervous system degeneration progressing to paralysis, fatigue, memory loss, disorientation | None reported |
| **Vitamin C**<br>Males 19–50: 90 mg<br>Females 19–50: 75 mg<br>Smokers: +35 mg | Citrus fruits, cabbage-type vegetables, dark green vegetables, cantaloupe, strawberries, peppers, lettuce, tomatoes, potatoes, papayas, mangoes | Antioxidant, collagen synthesis (strengthens blood vessel walls, forms scar tissue, matrix for bone growth), amino acid metabolism, strengthens resistance to infection, aids iron absorption, restores vitamin E to active form | Anemia, pinpoint hemorrhages, frequent infections, bleeding gums, loosened teeth, bone fragility, joint pain, blotchy bruises, failure of wounds to heal | Nausea, abdominal cramps, diarrhea, headache, fatigue, rashes, interference with drug therapies and medical tests |
| **Thiamin**<br>Males 19–50: 1.2 mg<br>Females 19–50: 1.1 mg | Pork, ham, bacon, liver, whole grains, legumes, nuts; occurs in all nutritious foods in moderate amounts | Part of a coenzyme used in energy metabolism, supports normal appetite and nervous system function | Beriberi, edema, enlarged heart, nervous/muscular system degeneration, difficulty walking, loss of reflexes, mental confusion | None reported |

## Table 6.4 **Key Information about Vitamins (continued)**

| Vitamin/Recommended Intake per Day | Significant Sources | Chief Functions | Signs of Severe, Prolonged Deficiency | Signs of Extreme Excess |
|---|---|---|---|---|
| **Riboflavin**<br>Males 19–50: 1.3 mg<br>Females 19–50: 1.1 mg | Milk, yogurt, cottage cheese, meat, leafy green vegetables, whole-grain or enriched breads and cereals | Part of a coenzyme used in energy metabolism, supports normal vision and skin health | Cracks at corner of mouth, magenta tongue, hypersensitivity to light, reddening of cornea, skin rash, sore throat | None reported |
| **Niacin**<br>Males 19–50: 16 mg NE<br>Females 19–50: 14 mg NE | Meat, poultry, fish, whole-grain and enriched breads and cereals, nuts, and all protein-containing foods | Part of a coenzyme used in energy metabolism | Diarrhea, black smooth tongue, irritability, loss of appetite, weakness, dizziness, mental confusion, flaky skin rash on areas exposed to sun | Nausea, vomiting, painful flush and rash, sweating, liver damage, blurred vision, impaired glucose tolerance |
| **Folate**<br>Males 19–50: 400 $\mu$g<br>Females 19–50: 400 $\mu$g | Leafy green vegetables, legumes, seeds, liver, enriched breads, cereal, pasta, and grains | Part of a coenzyme needed for new cell synthesis | Anemia, heartburn, frequent infections, smooth red tongue, depression, mental confusion | Masks vitamin $B_{12}$ deficiency |
| **Pantothenic acid**<br>Males 19–50: 5 mg<br>Females 19–50: 5 mg | Widespread in foods | Part of a coenzyme used in energy metabolism | Vomiting, intestinal distress, insomnia, fatigue, increased sensitivity to insulin | None reported |
| **Biotin**<br>Males 19–50: 30 $\mu$g<br>Females 19–50: 30 $\mu$g | Widespread in foods | Used in energy metabolism, fat synthesis, amino acid metabolism, and glycogen synthesis | Abnormal heart action, loss of appetite, nausea, depression, muscle pain, drying of facial skin | None reported |

Source: Adapted from Sizer, Frances, and Ellie Whitney, *Nutrition: Concepts and Controversies*, 10th ed. (Belmont, CA: Wadsworth, 2006).

## Table 6.5 **Key Information about Minerals**

| Mineral | Significant Sources | Chief Functions | Signs of Severe, Prolonged Deficiency | Signs of Extreme Excess |
|---|---|---|---|---|
| **Sodium** | Salt, soy sauce, processed foods | Needed to maintain fluid balance and acid-base balance in body cells; critical to nerve impulse transmission | Mental apathy, poor appetite, muscle cramps | High blood pressure, edema |
| **Potassium** | All whole foods: meats, milk, fruits, vegetables, grains, legumes | Needed to maintain fluid balance and acid-base balance in body cells; needed for muscle and nerve activity | Muscle weakness, mental confusion, paralysis | Muscle weakness, irregular heartbeat, heart attacks, vomiting |
| **Chloride** | Salt, soy sauce, processed foods | Aids in digestion; needed to maintain fluid balance and acid-base balance in body cells | Does not occur under normal circumstances | Vomiting |
| **Calcium** | Milk and milk products, oysters, small fish (with bones), tofu, greens, legumes | Component of bones and teeth, needed for muscle and nerve activity, blood clotting | Stunted growth and weak bones in children, adult bone loss (osteoporosis) | Constipation; calcium deposits in kidneys, liver; decreased absorption of other minerals |

Table 6.5  **Key Information about Minerals (*continued*)**

| Mineral | Significant Sources | Chief Functions | Signs of Severe, Prolonged Deficiency | Signs of Extreme Excess |
|---|---|---|---|---|
| **Phosphorus** | All animal tissues, milk and milk products, legumes | Component of bones and teeth, energy metabolism, needed to maintain cell membranes | Muscle weakness, impaired growth, bone pain | Calcification of soft tissue, particularly the kidneys |
| **Magnesium** | Nuts, legumes, whole grains, dark green vegetables, seafoods, chocolate, cocoa | Component of bones and teeth, nerve activity, energy and protein formation, immune function | Stunted growth in children, weakness, muscle spasms, personality changes, hallucinations | From nonfood sources: diarrhea, dehydration, pH imbalance |
| **Sulfate** | All protein-containing foods | Component of certain amino acids; stabilizes protein shape | None known; protein deficiency would occur first | None reported |
| **Trace Minerals** | | | | |
| **Iron** | Red meats, fish, poultry, shellfish, eggs, legumes, dried fruits | Aids in transport of oxygen, component of myoglobin, energy metabolism | Anemia, weakness, fatigue, pale appearance, reduced attention span, developmental delays in children | Vomiting, abdominal pain, blue coloration of skin, shock, organ damage |
| **Zinc** | Protein-containing foods: fish, shellfish, poultry, grains, vegetables | Protein reproduction, component of insulin, activates many enzymes, transport of vitamin A | Growth failure, delayed sexual maturation, slow wound healing | Loss of appetite, impaired immunity, reduced copper and iron absorption, fatigue, metallic taste in mouth |
| **Selenium** | Meats and seafood, eggs, grains | Acts as an antioxidant in conjunction with vitamin E, regulates thyroid hormone | Anemia, heart failure | Hair and fingernail loss, weakness, skin rash, garlic or metallic breath |
| **Molybdenum** | Dried beans, grains, dark green vegetables, liver, milk and milk products | Aids in oxygen transfer from one molecule to another | Unknown | None reported |
| **Iodine** | Iodized salt, seaweed, seafood, bread | Component of thyroid hormones that helps regulate energy production and growth | Goiter, cretinism in newborns (mental retardation, hearing loss, growth failure) | Pimples, goiter, decreased thyroid function |
| **Copper** | Organ meats, whole grains, nuts and seeds, seafood, drinking water | Helps to form hemoglobin and collagen, component of enzymes involved in the body's utilization of iron and oxygen | Anemia, nerve and bone abnormalities in children, growth retardation | From nonfood sources: vomiting, diarrhea, liver disease |
| **Manganese** | Whole grains, coffee, tea, dried beans, nuts | Formation of body fat and bone | Rare | Infertility in men, disruptions in the nervous system, muscle spasms |
| **Fluoride** | Fluoridated water, foods, and beverages; tea; shrimp; crab | Component of bones and teeth (enamel), confers decay resistance on teeth | Tooth decay and other dental diseases | Fluorosis, brittle bones, mottled teeth, vomiting, diarrhea, chest pain |
| **Chromium** | Whole grains, liver, meat, beer, wine | Glucose utilization | Poor blood glucose control, weight loss | None reported |

Source: Adapted from Brown, Judith, *Nutrition Now*, 6th ed. (Belmont, CA: Wadsworth, Cengage Learning, 2011); Sizer, Frances, and Ellie Whitney, *Nutrition: Concepts and Controversies*, 12th ed. (Belmont, CA: Wadsworth, Cengage Learning, 2011).

Table 6.6 **Color-Coding Your Vegetables and Fruits**

| Color | Phytochemical Antioxidant | Vegetable and Fruit Sources |
|---|---|---|
| **Red** | Lycopene (*lie-co-peen*) | Tomatoes, red raspberries, watermelon, strawberries, red peppers |
| **Yellow-green** | Lutein zeaxanthin (*lou-te-in, ze-ah-zan-thun*) | Leafy greens, avocado, honey dew melon, kiwi fruit |
| **Red-purple** | Anthocyanins (*antho-sigh-ah-nin*) | Grapes, berries, wine, red apples, plums, prunes |
| **Orange** | Beta-carotene | Carrots, mangos, papayas, apricots, pumpkins, yams |
| **Orange-yellow** | Flavonoids (*fla-von-oids*) | Oranges, tangerines, lemons, plums, peaches, cantaloupe |
| **Green** | Glucosinolates (*glu-co-sin-oh-lates*) | Broccoli, brussels sprouts, kale, cabbage |
| **White-green** | Allyl sulfides (*al-lill sulf-ides*) | Onions, leeks, garlic |

Calcium is a special concern for African Americans who, as a group, have a higher risk for high blood pressure and obesity than the rest of the population but, on average, consume less than one serving of dairy foods a day. In fact, more than 80 percent of African Americans fail to get their daily recommended amount of calcium.

 National health organizations are promoting greater calcium consumption among college students, particularly women, to increase bone density and safeguard against osteoporosis. In both men and women, bone mass peaks between the ages of 25 and 35. Over the next 10 to 15 years, bone mass remains fairly stable. At about age 40, bone loss equivalent to 0.3 to 0.5 percent per year begins in both men and women. Women may experience greater bone loss, at a rate of 3 to 5 percent, at the time of menopause. This decline continues for approximately five to seven years and is the primary factor leading to postmenopausal osteoporosis.

The higher an individual's peak bone mass, the longer it takes for age- and menopause-related bone loss to increase the risk of fractures. Osteoporosis is less common in groups with higher peak bone mass—men versus women, blacks versus whites.

*Sodium*  Sodium helps maintain proper fluid balance, regulates blood pressure, transmits muscle impulses, and relaxes muscles. For those who are sodium-sensitive—as many as 30 percent of the population—too much sodium contributes to high blood pressure. African Americans, who have higher rates of high blood pressure and diseases related to hypertension, such as stroke and

kidney failure, tend to be more sensitive to salt. (See the discussion of sodium on pages 167–168.)

The average daily intake of sodium in the United States exceeds 4 grams (4000 mg). The National Heart, Lung, and Blood Institute recommends less than 2.4 grams (2400 mg) of sodium a day, the equivalent of about one tablespoon of table salt a day. For someone with high blood pressure, a daily intake of less than 1500 mg of sodium is better for lowering blood pressure. However, because individuals vary greatly in how they respond to sodium, some experts are dubious of the need for and potential benefits of uniform restrictions on dietary salt.[9]

*Phytochemicals*  **Phytochemicals**, compounds that exist naturally in plants, serve many functions, including helping a plant protect itself from bacteria and disease. Some phytochemicals such as solanine, an insect-repelling chemical found in the leaves and stalks of potato plants, are natural toxins, but many are beneficial to humans.

Phytochemicals give tomatoes their red color and hot peppers their "fire." In the body, they act as antioxidants, mimic hormones, and reduce the risk of various illnesses, including cancer and heart disease (see Table 6.6). Broccoli may contain as many as 10,000 different phytochemicals, each capable of influencing some action or organ in the body. Tomatoes provide lycopene, a powerful antioxidant that seems to offer protection against cancers of the esophagus, lungs, prostate, and stomach. Soybeans, a rich source of an array of phytochemicals, appear to slow the growth of breast and prostate cancer.

**phytochemicals** Chemicals such as indoles, coumarins, and capsaicin, which exist naturally in plants and have disease-fighting properties.

Americans get adequate amounts of most nutrients. However, the Advisory Committee for Dietary Guidelines reported that intakes of several nutrients are low enough to be of concern.

- For adults: vitamins A, C, and E, calcium, magnesium, potassium, and fiber.

- For children: vitamin E, calcium, magnesium, potassium, and fiber.

Are you getting enough of these nutrients?

Among the groups at highest risk of nutritional deficiencies are:

- Teenage girls.

- Women of child-bearing age (iron and folic acid).

- Persons over age 50 (vitamin $B_{12}$).

- The elderly, persons with dark skin, and those who do not get adequate exposure to sunshine (vitamin D).[10]

## Dietary Supplements

About two out of five Americans take a vitamin or mineral supplement regularly. Should you be among them? Or are you getting enough of the vitamins and minerals you need from your food? Despite intensive marketing of a host of supplements, large-scale studies have cast doubts on the benefits of many, especially antioxidants.

Multivitamin supplements, long believed to be beneficial, did not prevent cancer or heart disease in a recent eight-year study of more than 160,000 postmenopausal women. After controlling for age, physical activity, family history of cancer, and many other factors, supplements had no effect on the risk of breast cancer, colorectal cancer, endometrial cancer, lung cancer, ovarian cancer, heart attack, stroke, blood clots, or mortality. Individuals who are less well nourished than the study participants may benefit from supplements, but there is no convincing scientific evidence to justify routine use of dietary supplements by the general population. The bottom-line recommendation: Buying more fruits and vegetables might be a better choice than spending money on multivitamins.

In another study, supplements of vitamins C and E and beta-carotene had no impact on the cancer risk of middle-aged women, but vitamin C supplements may protect against gallstones.

Selenium and vitamin E also failed to protect men from prostate cancer.

Yet certain supplements may have an impact on the risk for certain conditions. Women over age 40 who took folic acid, vitamin $B_6$, and vitamin $B_{12}$ were less likely than a control group to develop a severe visual disorder called age-related macular degeneration.

High doses of vitamins carry potential risks. Certain antioxidants can interfere with the efficacy of cholesterol-lowering medications. High doses of vitamin E may increase the chances of earlier death. In cancer patients, those taking large doses had an increased risk of a new cancer.

In particular, the fat-soluble vitamins, primarily A and D, can build up in our bodies and cause serious complications, such as damage to the kidneys, liver, or bones. Large doses of water-soluble vitamins, including the B vitamins, may also be harmful. Excessive intake of vitamin $B_6$ (pyridoxine), often used to relieve premenstrual bloating, can cause neurological damage, such as numbness in the mouth and tingling in the hands. (An excessive amount in this case is 250 to 300 times the recommended dose.) High doses of vitamin C can produce stomachaches and diarrhea. Niacin, often taken in high doses to lower cholesterol, can cause jaundice, liver damage, and irregular heartbeats as well as severe, uncomfortable flushing of the skin.

If you do feel a need for vitamins, be sure not to exceed the recommended doses listed in Tables 6.4 and 6.5.

## Dietary Guidelines for Americans

Every five years the federal government reviews and updates its recommendations for healthy eating. Its most recent report, *Dietary Guidelines for Americans, 2010* (published in 2011), notes that poor diet and physical inactivity are contributing to an epidemic of overweight and obesity in men, women, and children in the United States, as well as to increased rates of illness and premature death. Diet-related chronic diseases include cardiovascular disease, hypertension, diabetes, cancer, and osteoporosis.

The key recommendations of the most recent *Dietary Guidelines* encompass two overarching concepts:

- **The key to achieving and sustaining a healthy weight is to maintain calorie balance**. People with healthy weights consume only enough calories from foods and beverages to meet their needs and expend excess calories through physical activity. (Weight control is discussed in depth in Chapter 7.)

- **Americans should focus on consuming nutrient-dense foods and beverages**. Rather than getting calories from solid fats, added sugars, and refined grains, we should limit such foods and increase our intake of foods that pack more nutritional power, such as vegetables, fruits, whole grains, non-fat or low-fat milk and milk products, seafood, lean meats and poultry, eggs, beans and peas, and nuts and seeds.[11]

## Balancing Calories to Manage Weight

**Calorie balance** refers to the relationship between calories consumed from foods and beverages and calories expended in normal body functions and through physical activity. You cannot control the calories your body burns to maintain temperature and other basic processes. However, you can control what you eat and drink and how many calories you use in physical activity. (See Health in the Headlines: Nutrition and Health.)

You must expend as much energy (calories) as you take in to stay at the same weight. Among the best ways to balance this energy equation are limiting portion sizes (discussed later in this chapter), substituting nutrient-dense foods (such as raw vegetables or low-fat soups) for nutrient-poor foods (such as candy and cake), and limiting added sugars, solid fats, and alcoholic beverages.

As discussed in Chapter 8, regular physical activity helps maintain a healthy weight and reduces risk for several chronic diseases. While 30 minutes of moderate physical activity (such

as walking at a pace of three or four miles an hour) on most days provides important benefits, exercising more often and more intensely yields additional health dividends. Many adults need up to 60 minutes of moderate to vigorous physical activity—the equivalent of 150 to 200 calories, depending on body size—daily to prevent unhealthy weight gain. Men and women who have lost weight may need 60 to 90 minutes to keep off excess pounds. Children and teenagers require at least 60 minutes of moderate physical activity every day.

## Foods and Food Components to Reduce

The *Dietary Guidelines* do not identify any single food as "bad" or "bad for you" but emphasize that excessive amounts of certain foods and food components—sodium, solid fats (major sources of saturated and trans-fatty acids), added sugars, refined grains, cholesterol, and alcohol—may increase the risks to your health. Because they add excess and often "empty" calories to a daily diet, they contribute to overweight and obesity. But even in normal-weight individuals, these foods can increase the risk of some of the most common chronic diseases in the United States.[12]

*Sodium* Virtually all Americans consume more sodium (primarily in the form of salt) than they need. The average intake for Americans over age 2 is about 3400 mg per day—much higher than the 1500 mg that the Institute of Medicine has set as the "adequate intake" for individuals ages 9 to 50 and its "tolerable upper limit" of 2300 mg for adolescents over age 14 and all adults.[13]

On average, the higher the sodium intake, the higher an individual's blood pressure. Conversely, reducing sodium can lower blood pressure. The *Dietary Guidelines* recommend that all Americans consume no more than 2300 mg per day. African Americans; individuals with hypertension, diabetes, or chronic kidney disease; and those older than age 51 should cut back to 1500 mg a day. However, because so many foods contain hidden sodium, only an estimated 15 percent of Americans currently meet this recommendation.

Salt added at the table and in cooking provides only a small proportion of the sodium

### Health in the Headlines

## Nutrition and Health

As a college student, you are faced with many choices about what you put in your body—from what to eat for breakfast to how much water you drink. It seems like every day there is a new study out about what we should and should not eat and drink. In fact, medical science is constantly expanding its understanding of nutrition and its impact on health. With this in mind, visit Global Health Watch to scan the latest articles on nutrition and health (Health & Wellness → Healthy Weight → Nutrition). How do you approach healthy and nutritious eating? Are there tools you use to help you eat a well-balanced diet? Use your online journal to answer these questions and record your thoughts.

**calorie balance** The relationship between calories consumed from foods and beverages and calories expended in normal body functions and through physical activity. If the calories consumed equals calories expended, you have calorie balance.

Americans consume. Most comes from salt added during food processing (see Figure 6.4). Here is what you can do to lower your sodium intake:

- **Look for labels that say "low sodium."** They contain 140 mg or less of sodium per serving.

- **Learn to use spices and herbs** rather than salt to enhance the flavor of food.

- **Go easy on condiments** such as soy sauce, pickles, olives, ketchup, and mustard, which can add a lot of salt to your food.

- **Always check the amount of sodium in processed foods,** such as frozen dinners, packaged mixes, cereals, salad dressings, and sauces. The amount in different types and brands can vary widely.

**Fats** The *Dietary Guidelines* call for reducing the number of calories from solid fats, which are abundant in the diets of Americans and contribute significantly to excess calorie intake. Solid fats make up an average of 19 percent of the total calories in the average daily diet, but contribute few essential nutrients and no dietary fiber. Reducing solid fats, most commonly consumed in grain-based desserts, pizza, regular cheese, processed meat products, and fried potatoes, can reduce intake of extra calories, saturated fats, trans-fatty acids, and cholesterol.

**Saturated Fats** According to the Institute of Medicine, the total fat intake of adults over age 19 should not exceed 20 to 35 percent of their daily calories. However, the types of fatty acid consumed are more important in influencing the risk of cardiovascular disease than is the total amount of fat in the diet.

Figure 6.4 **Less Food, Soda, and Salt**

**More of This, Less of That** Americans do not eat enough nutritious foods and eat too many fats, sugars, and refined grains, the government says. Here is how the average American diet compares to recommended levels.

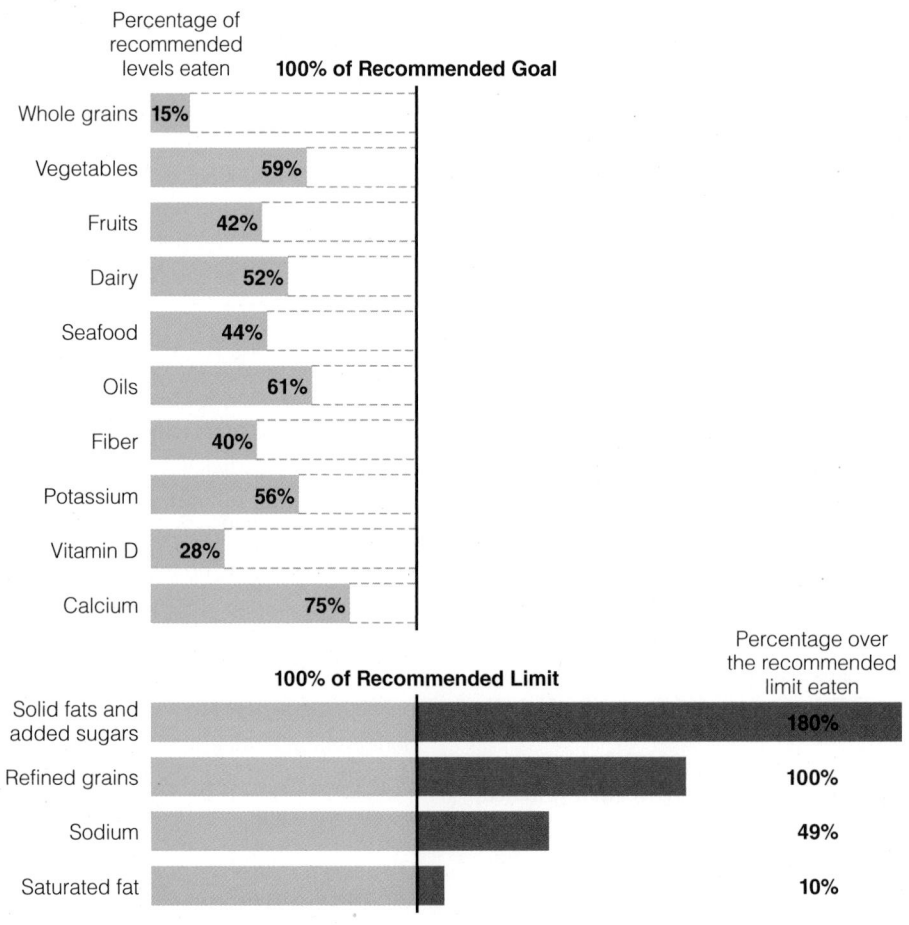

As discussed earlier in this chapter, animal fats tend to have a higher proportion of saturated fatty acids (the major exception is seafood), and plant foods tend to have a higher proportion of monounsaturated or polyunsaturated fatty acids or both.

The body makes adequate amounts of saturated fatty acids, and people have no dietary need for more. The *Dietary Guidelines* recommend consuming less than 10 percent of calories from saturated fatty acids and replacing them with monounsaturated or polyunsaturated fatty acids or both. Lowering saturated fats even more—to 7 percent of total calories—can further reduce the risk of cardiovascular disease.

To reduce your saturated fat intake:

- **Cut back on the major sources of saturated fats** in your diet: regular (full-fat) cheese, pizza, grain-based desserts (cakes, cookies, pies, sweet rolls, pastries, doughnuts, etc.), dairy-based desserts (ice cream, frozen yogurt, milkshakes, pudding, etc.), sausages, franks, bacon, and ribs.

- **Switch to nonfat or low-fat milk and dairy products.**

- When preparing or ordering fish, **choose grilled, baked, broiled, or poached fish,** not fried. Fried fish at fast food restaurants is often low in omega-3 fatty acids and high in trans and saturated fats.

- **Trim all visible fat from meat.**

- **Use oils that are rich in monounsaturated fatty acids,** such as canola, olive, and safflower oils, or polyunsaturated fatty acids, such as soybean, corn, and cottonseed oils.

**Trans-Fatty Acids**   These substances, found naturally in some foods and formed during food processing, are not essential in the diet. An increased intake of trans-fatty acids has been linked with higher levels of LDL (low-density lipoprotein) and heart-harming cholesterol and greater danger of cardiovascular disease. Check nutrition labels, and avoid products high in trans-fatty acids.

**Cholesterol**   The body makes more cholesterol than it uses, and people do not need additional amounts. Men are more likely than women to consume more than the recommended level of no more than 300 mg per day. The main sources of cholesterol, which is found only in animal foods, include eggs, chicken, beef, and all types of burgers.

*Added Sugars*   The majority of sugars that Americans consume are added to foods during processing, during preparation, or at the table. These "added sugars" contribute an average of 16 percent of the total calories in American diets. They include high fructose corn syrup, white sugar, brown sugar, corn syrup and solids, raw sugar, malt sugar, maple and pancake syrup, fructose sweetener, liquid fructose, honey, molasses, anhydrous dextrose, and crystal dextrose. As a percentage of calories from total added sugars, the major sources of added sugars are soda, energy drinks, and sports drinks; grain-based desserts; sugar-sweetened fruit drinks; dairy-based desserts; and candy.

The *Dietary Guidelines* recommend reducing consumption of products with added sugars to lower your daily calorie intake. For most people, no more than 5 to 15 percent of their daily calories should come from solid fats and added sugars.

*Refined Grains*   The refining of whole grains involves a process that removes vitamins, minerals, and fiber. Although most refined grains are enriched with iron, thiamin, riboflavin, niacin, and folic acid before being used as food ingredients, not all of the vitamins and minerals and none of the dietary fiber are routinely added back. Many refined grain products, such as cookies and cake, also are high in solid fats and added sugars.

On average Americans consume the equivalent of 6.3 ounces of refined grains per day. The recommended amount is no more than 3 ounce-equivalents. The *Dietary Guidelines* urge replacing refined grains with whole grains so that at least half of all the grains you consume are whole.

*Alcohol*   As discussed in Chapter 13, about half of Americans regularly drink alcohol. Depending on the amount consumed, age, and other factors, alcohol can have harmful or beneficial effects. However, there is no nutritional need for alcohol. The *Dietary Guidelines* note that no one should begin drinking or drink more frequently on the basis of potential health benefits because moderate alcohol consumption, though associated with a lower risk of cardiovascular disease, also is linked with an increased risk of breast cancer, violence, drowning, and injuries from falls and motor vehicle crashes.

## Foods and Nutrients to Increase

Even though many Americans have been consuming more calories, they are not getting enough of certain foods, including vegetables, fruits, whole grains, dairy products, and oils, and several nutrients, including potassium, dietary fiber, calcium, and vitamin D.

***Vegetables and Fruits***   The *Dietary Guidelines* recommend eating more vegetables and fruits for three reasons: They provide many nutrients that are underconsumed by many Americans. They lower the risk of many chronic illnesses and of cardiovascular disease (including heart attack and stroke) and may protect against certain types of cancer. And, when prepared without added fats or sugars, most are relatively low in calories.

Americans between the ages of 19 and 30 consume more than half of their fruit intake

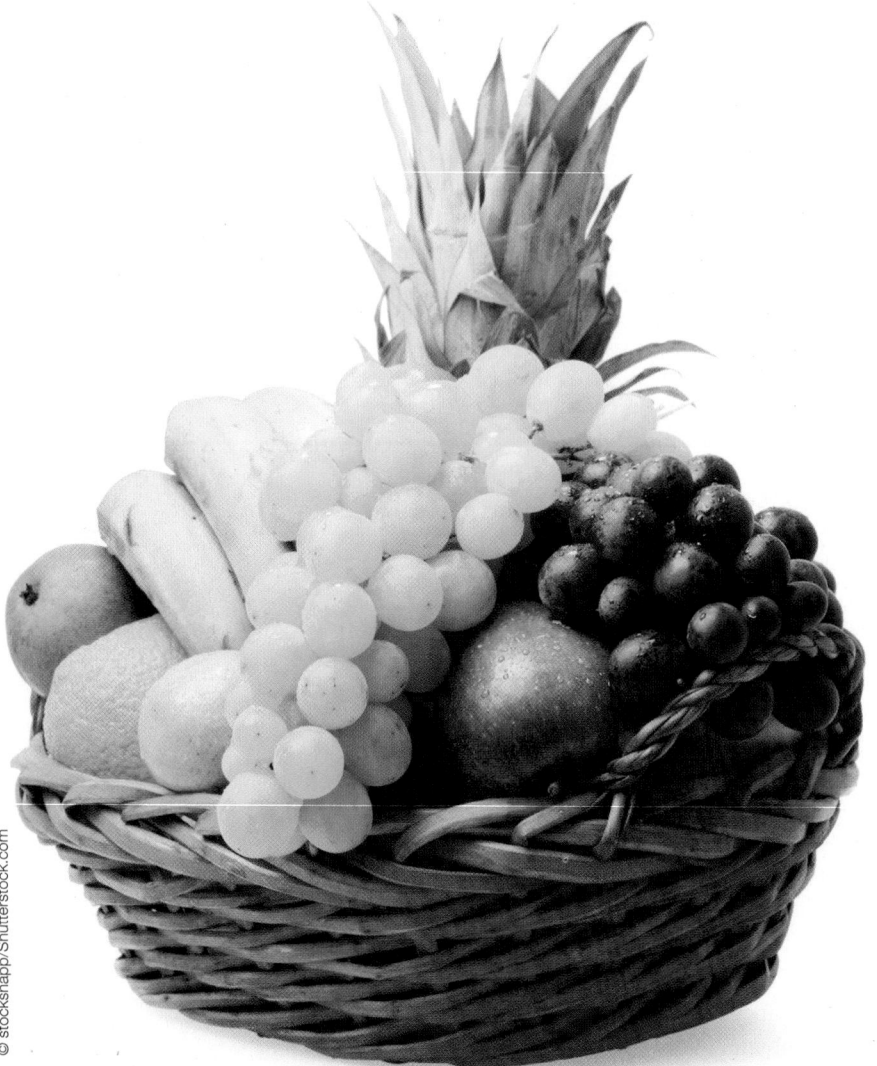

as juice. Juice labeled "100 percent" juice (not sweetened products with minimal juice content) can be part of a healthful diet, but it lacks fiber and can contribute extra calories. The *Dietary Guidelines* recommend whole fruits, including fresh, canned (in juice rather than syrup), frozen, and dried forms.

Fewer than a third of American adults eat the recommended amounts of fruits and vegetables. College-age young adults between ages 18 and 24 eat the fewest vegetables. Nearly four-fifths of this group don't put vegetables on their plates—or scrape them to the side if they do.

Greater consumption of fruits and vegetables (5 to 13 servings or 2½ to 6½ cups per day, depending on how many calories you burn) may reduce the risk of stroke, certain cancers, and type 2 diabetes (vegetables more so than fruit) as well as helping reach and maintain a healthy weight. There is an inverse relationship between fruit and vegetable consumption and the risk factors for cardiorespiratory disease. Plant-based foods also reduce the risk of rectal cancer in both men and women. To increase the fruits and vegetables in your diet, fill half of your plate with them. (See How Do You Compare? Are You Eating Your Veggies?)

Among the ways to increase your fruit and vegetable intake:

- **Toss fruit into a green salad** for extra flavor, variety, color, and crunch.
- **Start the day with a daily double**: a glass of juice and a banana or other fruit on cereal.
- **Buy pre-cut vegetables** for snacking or dipping (instead of chips).
- **Make or order sandwiches** with extra tomatoes or other vegetable toppings.

***Whole Grains***   Less than 5 percent of Americans consume the minimum recommended amount of whole grains—about 3 ounce-equivalents a day—which can reduce the risk of diabetes and cardiovascular disease. Half of the grains you consume every day should be whole grains. To get more grains in your diet:

- **Check labels of rolls and bread**, and choose those with at least 2 to 3 grams of fiber per slice.

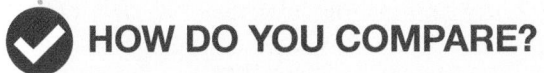
# ARE YOU EATING YOUR VEGGIES?

**College students who report:**

| | | | |
|---|---|---|---|
| Eating no servings of fruits and vegetables a day | **5.6 percent** | Eating three to four servings | **30 percent** |
| | | Eating five or more servings | **6 percent** |
| Eating one to two servings | **58.4 percent** | | |

## HOW DO YOU COMPARE?

For a three-day period (including one weekend day), keep track of your veggie intake. Put a star by those you like most. If you aren't getting at least five servings a day, add at least one of your favorites every day. Record your observations in your online journal.

Source: American College Health Association, *American College Health Association-National College Health Assessment II: Reference Group Executive Summary Spring 2010* (Linthicum, MD: American College Health Association, 2010).

---

- **Add brown rice or barley** to soups.
- **Choose whole-grain**, ready-to-eat cereals.
- **Have a whole-grain cereal for breakfast.** According to a recent study, people who eat breakfast cereal generally eat less total fat, saturated fat, and sugar than those who do not and have better intakes of protein and important micronutrients, such as iron, vitamins, and calcium, throughout the day.[14]

*Milk and Milk Products*  Dairy products provide many nutrients, including calcium, vitamin D, and potassium, and may improve bone health, lower blood pressure, and reduce the risk of cardiovascular disease and type 2 diabetes. The *Dietary Guidelines* recommend three cups a day or the equivalent for adults—ideally from no-fat or low-fat dairy products. Soy beverages fortified with calcium and vitamins A and D are considered part of the dairy product food group.

*Protein Foods*  These include seafood (both fish and shellfish), meat, poultry, eggs, beans and peas, soy products, and nuts. In addition to protein, these foods provide B vitamins, vitamin E, iron, zinc, and magnesium. Meat, poultry, and eggs are the most commonly consumed protein foods. The *Dietary Guidelines* recommend a balanced variety of protein sources to get more nutrients and health benefits. Certain nuts—peanuts,

walnuts, almonds, and pistachios—reduce risk factors for cardiovascular disease but, because they are high in calories, should be eaten only in small amounts.

The 2010 *Dietary Guidelines* include a new quantitative recommendation for seafood: 8 or more ounces a week or about 20 percent of total protein intake. Currently Americans consume about 3.5 ounces of seafood every week. Because it is rich in omega-3 fatty acids, seafood has been linked with fewer cardiac deaths among individuals with or without cardiovascular disease. These benefits outweigh the risks associated with methyl mercury, a heavy metal found in varying levels in different types of seafood. The types of seafood that are generally lower in mercury include salmon, anchovies, herring, sardines, Pacific oysters, trout, and Atlantic and Pacific mackerel (not king mackerel, which is high in mercury).

*Oils*  As discussed previously, fats with a high percentage of monounsaturated and polyunsaturated fatty acids are usually liquid at room temperature and so are referred to as oils. The *Dietary Guidelines* recommend replacing some solid fats with oils in order to lower cholesterol and promote heart health. However, because oils are high in calories, you should use them in small amounts. Some easy ways to replace solid with liquid fats are to use vegetable oils instead of butter for cooking and to use a soft margarine rather than stick margarine or butter. (See Figure 6.4.)

***Nutrients of Concern*** The *Dietary Guidelines* also recommend that Americans get adequate levels of several key nutrients, including potassium (discussed on page 163), dietary fiber (page 156), vitamin D (page 160), vitamin B$_{12}$, calcium (page 166), iron (page 161), and folate (page 163).

## Building Healthy Eating Patterns

There is no one "right" way to eat. As the *Dietary Guidelines* note, a healthy eating pattern is not a rigid prescription but an array of options that can accommodate cultural, ethnic, traditional, and personal preferences as well as food costs and availability.

Although healthy eating patterns vary around the world, most share common elements: They are abundant in vegetables and fruits. Many emphasize whole grains. They include moderate amounts and a variety of foods high in protein (seafood, beans and peas, nuts, seeds, soy products, meat, poultry, and eggs). They include only limited amounts of food high in added sugars and may include more oils than solid fats. Most are low in full-fat dairy products, although some include substantial amounts of low-fat milk and milk products. Compared to typical American diets, these patterns tend to have a high unsaturated to saturated fat ratio and a high dietary fiber and potassium content. Some are also relatively low in sodium compared to current American intake.

Among the research-based healthy eating patterns are the United States Department of Agriculture (USDA) Food Patterns, the Dietary Approaches to Stop Hypertension (DASH) Plan, and the Mediterranean Diet.

## MyPlate

In 2011 the USDA introduced a new food pattern icon: MyPlate. Rather than providing specific directives, it serves as a visual reminder for healthy eating. (See Figure 6.5.) The general messages it conveys reflect the key themes of the most recent Dietary Guidelines:

## Creating a Healthy Eating Pattern

- **Limit calorie intake to the amount needed** to attain or maintain a healthy weight.

- **Consume foods from all food groups** in nutrient-dense forms and in recommended amounts.

- **Reduce intake of solid fats.**

- **Replace solid fats with oils.**

- **Reduce intake of added sugars.**

- **Reduce intake of refined grains** and replace some refined grains with whole grains.

- **Reduce intake of sodium.**

- If consumed, **limit alcohol intake to moderate levels.**

- **Increase intake of vegetables and fruits.**

- **Increase intake of whole grains.**

- **Increase intake of milk and milk products** and replace whole milk and full-fat milk products with fat-free or low-fat choices to reduce solid fat intake.

- **Increase seafood intake** by replacing some meat or poultry with seafood.

Balancing Calories

- Enjoy your food, but eat less.
- Avoid oversized portions.

Foods to Increase

- Make half your plate fruits and vegetables.
- Make at least half your grains whole grains.
- Switch to fat-free or low-fat (1%) milk.

Foods to Reduce

- Compare sodium in foods like soup, bread, and frozen meals, and choose those with lower numbers.
- Drink water instead of sugary drinks.

***MyPlate vs. the MyPyramid System***
The MyPyramid Food Guidance System, developed in 2005, presented several key themes:

- **Variety.** Eating foods from all food groups and subgroups.

Figure 6.5 **The MyPlate System**

The most recent food pattern from the USDA reminds Americans to balance calories, increase foods such as fruits and vegetables, and drink fat-free or low-fat milk.

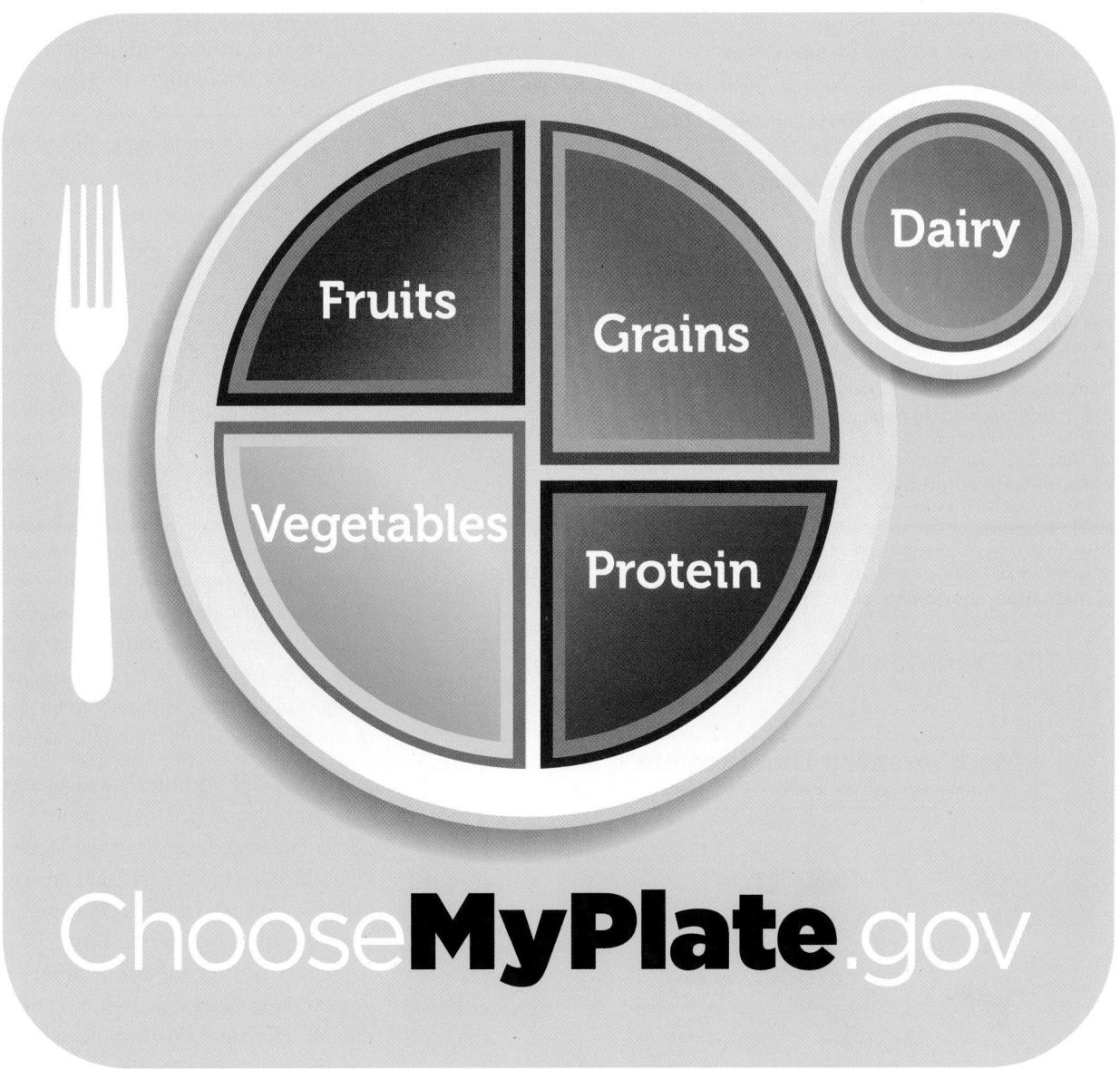

ChooseMyPlate.gov

- **Proportionality.** Eating more of some foods (fruits, vegetables, whole grains, fat-free or low-fat milk products) and less of others (foods high in saturated or trans fats, added sugars, cholesterol, salt, and alcohol).

- **Moderation.** Choosing forms of foods that limit intake of saturated or trans fats, added sugars, cholesterol, salt, and alcohol.

- **Activity.** Being physically active every day.

Critics of the MyPyramid System charged that it did not go far enough in urging Americans to cut back on harmful fats and simple carbohydrates and also lumped together various protein sources (red meat, poultry, fish, and beans) as equally healthy. MyPlate is designed to address these and other issues.

*The USDA Food Patterns* These approaches identify daily amounts of foods to eat from five major food groups and subgroups: vegetables, fruits and juices, grains, milk and milk products, and protein foods. (See Table 6.7). They also include an allowance for oils and limits on the maximum number of calories that should be consumed from solid fats and added sugars. Amounts and limits are given at different calorie levels, ranging from 1,000 to 3,200. All the USDA Food Patterns emphasize selection of

## Table 6.7 The DASH Eating Plan

USDA/DASH recommendations for a 2,000-calorie daily diet include:

- Fruit Group—2–2.5 cups (4–5 servings) of fresh, frozen, canned, or dried fruit, with only limited juice
  - Vegetable Group—2–2.5 cups (4–5 servings):
  - Dark greens, such as broccoli and leafy greens—three cups per week
  - Orange vegetables, such as carrots and sweet potatoes—two cups per week
  - Legumes, such as pinto or kidney beans, split peas, or lentils—three cups per week
  - Starchy vegetables—three cups per week
  - Other vegetables—6.5 cups per week
- Grain Group—6–8 ounce-equivalents of cereal, bread, crackers, rice, or pasta, with at least 50% whole grain
- Meat and Beans Group—5.5–6 ounce-equivalents of baked, broiled, or grilled lean meat, poultry, or fish, eggs, nuts, seeds, beans, peas, or tofu
- Milk Group—2–3 cups low-fat/fat-free milk, yogurt, or cheese, or lactose-free, calcium-fortified products
- Oils—2–6 teaspoons
- Discretionary—267 calories; for example, solid fats (saturated fat such as butter, margarine, shortening, or lard) or added sugar

## Figure 6.6 The Traditional Healthy Mediterranean Diet Pyramid

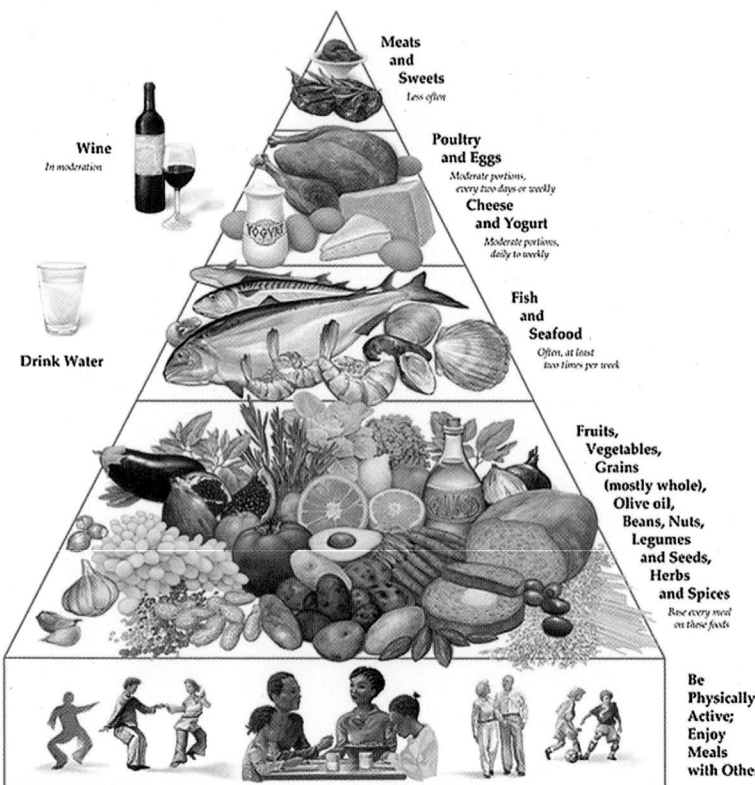

**Mediterranean Diet Pyramid**
*A contemporary approach to delicious, healthy eating*

Meats and Sweets
*Less often*

Wine
*In moderation*

Poultry and Eggs
*Moderate portions, every two days or weekly*

Cheese and Yogurt
*Moderate portions, daily to weekly*

Drink Water

Fish and Seafood
*Often, at least two times per week*

Fruits, Vegetables, Grains (mostly whole), Olive oil, Beans, Nuts, Legumes and Seeds, Herbs and Spices
*Base every meal on these foods*

Be Physically Active; Enjoy Meals with Others

Illustration by George Middleton

© 2009 Oldways Preservation and Exchange Trust    www.oldwayspt.org

a variety of foods in nutrient-dense forms—that is, with little or no solid fats and added sugars—from each food group.

The USDA Food Patterns include a vegan pattern, which consists of only plant foods and substitutes calcium-fortified beverages and foods for dairy products, and a lacto-ovo-vegetarian pattern, which includes milk, milk products, and eggs.

**The DASH Eating Plan**   DASH emphasizes vegetables, fruits, and low-fat milk and milk products; includes whole grains, poultry, seafood, and nuts; and is lower in sodium, red and processed meats, sweets, and sugar-containing beverages than typical intakes in the United States. In research studies, DASH approaches have proven to lower blood pressure, improve blood lipids, and reduce the risk of cardiovascular disease.

**The Mediterranean Diet**   Because many cultures and agricultural patterns exist in the countries that border the Mediterranean Sea, the "Mediterranean diet" is not one set way of eating but an eating pattern that emphasizes vegetables, fruits and nuts, olive oil, and grains (often whole grains), with only small amounts of meats and full-fat milk and milk products.

Scientists have identified antioxidants in red wine and olive oil that may account for the beneficial effects on the heart of the Mediterranean diet, which features lots of fruits and vegetables, legumes, nuts, and grains (see Figure 6.6). The Mediterranean diet also has beneficial effects on the lungs, reducing the risk of asthma and progressive lung disease as well as cardiovascular disease. The more closely individuals adhere to the diet, the greater the benefits to their hearts' health.

**Vegetarian Diets**   Not all vegetarians avoid all meats. Some, who call themselves *lacto-ovo-pesco-vegetarians*, eat dairy products, eggs, and fish but not red meat. **Lacto-vegetarians** eat dairy products as well as grains, fruits, and vegetables; **ovo-lacto-vegetarians** also eat eggs. Pure vegetarians, called **vegans**, eat only plant foods; often they take vitamin $B_{12}$ supplements because that vitamin is normally found only in animal products. If they select their food with care, vegetarians can get sufficient amounts of protein, vitamin $B_{12}$, iron, and calcium without supplements.

The key to getting sufficient protein from a vegetarian diet is understanding the concept of complementary proteins. Recall that meat, poultry, fish, eggs, and dairy products are complete proteins that provide the nine essential amino acids—substances that the human body cannot produce itself. Incomplete proteins, such as legumes or nuts, may have relatively low levels of one or two essential amino acids but fairly high levels of others. By combining complementary protein sources, vegetarians can make sure their bodies make the most of the nonanimal proteins they eat. Many cultures rely heavily on complementary foods for protein. In Middle Eastern cooking, sesame seeds and chickpeas are a popular combination; in Latin American dishes, beans and rice, or beans and tortillas; in Chinese cuisine, soy and rice.

According to the *Dietary Guidelines*, vegetarians can best meet their nutrient needs by paying special attention to protein, iron, vitamin $B_{12}$, calcium, and vitamin D. Instead of a 6-ounce serving of meat, they can substitute one egg, 1.5 ounces of nuts, or two-thirds cup of legumes. Those who avoid milk because of its lactose content may obtain all the nutrients of milk by using lactose-reduced milk or eating other calcium-rich foods, such as broccoli, calcium-fortified orange juice, and fortified soy milk.

Vegetarian diets have proven health benefits. Studies show that vegetarians' cholesterol levels are low, and vegetarians are seldom overweight. As a result, they're less apt to be candidates for heart disease than those who consume large quantities of meat. Vegetarians also have lower incidences of breast, colon, and prostate cancer; high blood pressure; and osteoporosis.

# The Way We Eat

Your ethnic background and family makeup influenced the way you ate as a child. In college, you probably will find yourself eating in different—and not necessarily better—ways. Because the United States is so diverse, you also will have the opportunity to sample the cuisines of many cultures. However, in this country and others, many do not have enough to eat.

## His Plate, Her Plate: Gender and Nutrition

Men and women do not need to eat different foods, but their nutritional needs are different. Because most men are bigger and taller than most women, they consume more calories. On average, a moderately active 125-pound woman needs 2,000 calories a day; a 175-pound man with a similar exercise pattern needs 2,800 calories. Eating more means it's easier for men to get the nutrients they need, even though many don't make the wisest food choices.

Women, particularly those who restrict their caloric intake or are chronically dieting, are more likely to develop specific deficiencies. Calcium is one example. Many teenage girls and young women under age 30 do not consume the recommended 800 to 1200 milligrams of calcium daily and may be at increased risk of bone-weakening osteoporosis.

Many women also get too little iron. Even in adolescence, girls are more prone to iron deficiency than boys; some suffer memory and learning impairments as a result. In adult women, menstrual blood loss and poor eating habits can lead to low iron stores, which puts them at risk for anemia. According to U.S. Department of Agriculture research, most women consume only 60 percent of the recommended 18 milligrams of iron per day. (The recommendation for men is 8 milligrams.) Regular blood tests can monitor a woman's iron status.

Both genders should increase their fruit and vegetable intake to ensure that they are getting adequate amounts of vitamins and fiber in their daily diet.

Here are some gender-specific strategies for better nutrition:

- **Men should cut back on fat and meat** in their diets, two things they eat too much.

- **Women should increase their iron intake** by eating meat (iron from animal sources is absorbed better than that from vegetable sources) or a combination of meat and vegetable iron sources together (for example, a meat and bean burrito). Those with iron deficiencies should consult a physician. Because large doses of iron can be toxic, iron supplements should be taken only with medical supervision.

**lacto-vegetarians** People who eat dairy products as well as fruits and vegetables (but not meat, poultry, or fish).

**ovo-lacto-vegetarians** People who eat eggs, dairy products, and fruits and vegetables (but not meat, poultry, or fish).

**vegans** People who eat only plant foods.

## How to Plan Vegetarian Meals

- **Choose a variety of foods,** including whole grains, vegetables, fruits, legumes, nuts, seeds, and, if desired, dairy products and eggs.

- **Choose whole, unrefined foods often** and minimize intake of highly sweetened, fatty, and highly refined foods.

- **Choose a variety of fruits and vegetables.**

- **If animal foods such as dairy products and eggs are used, choose lower-fat versions of these foods.** Cheeses and other high-fat dairy foods and eggs should be limited in the diet because of their saturated fat content and because their frequent use displaces plant foods in some vegetarian diets.

- **Vegans should include a regular source of vitamin B$_{12}$** in their diets along with a source of vitamin D if sun exposure is limited.

- **Do not restrict dietary fat in children younger than two years.** For older children, include some foods higher in unsaturated fats (for example, nuts, seeds, nut and seed butters, avocado, and vegetable oils) to help meet nutrient and energy needs.

Source: The American and Canadian Dietetic Associations

- **Women should consume more calcium-rich foods**, including low-fat and nonfat dairy products, leafy greens, and tofu. Women who cannot get adequate amounts of calcium from their daily diet should take calcium supplements. This is not advised for all men because of a possible connection between calcium and prostate cancer.

- **Women who could become pregnant should take a multivitamin** with 400 micrograms of **folic acid**, which helps prevent neural tube defects such as spina bifida. Folic acid is also useful to men because it may cut the risk of heart disease, stroke, and colon cancer.

**folic acid** A form of folate used in vitamin supplements and fortified foods.

# Campus Cuisine: How College Students Eat

 Often on their own for the first time, college students typically change their usual eating patterns. In one survey, 59 percent of freshmen said their diet had changed since they began college. When they are making meal choices, the top two influences on students are price and convenience, with nutrition coming in third. However, eating right doesn't have to cost more. (See Health on a Budget.)

According to various national samples, many students do not consume adequate amounts of fruits and vegetables and consume too many fried and fast foods. In one study that followed students through their freshman and sophomore years, more than half remained in the precontemplation stage for adopting healthier eating behaviors throughout this time. Only 30 percent of the students consumed at least five fruits and vegetables daily; more than half reported eating high-fat fried or fast foods at least three times during the previous week.

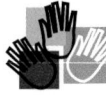 The proportion of 18- to 24-year-olds who eat the recommended amounts of fruits and vegetables is generally lower than in the population as a whole. College men eat fewer fruits and vegetables than women do; Caucasian and Asian students eat more than African American undergraduates. Both African American and Hispanic students consume less than multiracial or other racial/ethnic groups.

Student fruit-and-veggie eaters differ in other ways. According to an analysis of data from the ACHA-NCHA survey, they are more likely to exercise, use sunscreen, wear seatbelts and helmets, get more sleep, examine their breasts or testicles, report better health—and get better grades. They also are less likely to smoke, drink (and drink and drive), and feel hopeless. Researchers have found an association between higher fruit and vegetable consumption and lower BMI.

Time pressures often affect students' food choices. More than half say they tend to eat on the run, and they consume more soft drinks, fast food, total fat, and saturated fat. A significant number of undergraduates—35 percent of men and 42 percent of women—feel they don't have time to sit down and share a meal with friends or family. Yet students who take time for a social meal make better food choices, including eating more fruits and vegetables.[15]

Some colleges are doing their part to improve student nutrition. Many post nutritional information in dining halls; some have expanded their offerings to include more salads, fewer fried foods, and more ethnic dishes. On some campuses, students are taking the lead in demanding more healthful, fresher, and more varied dishes in their dining halls. (See Health in Action: Make Small Healthy Changes.)

## Fast Food: Nutrition on the Run

On any given day, about 25 percent of adults in the United States go to a fast-food restaurant. The typical American consumes three hamburgers and four orders of french fries every week. Many fast foods are high in calories, sugar, salt, and fat and low in beneficial nutrients (see Consumer Alert on page 178). A Burger King Whopper with cheese contains 760 calories and 47 grams of fat, 16 grams from saturated fat. A McDonald's Sausage McMuffin with egg has 450 calories and 27 grams of fat, 10 grams from saturated fat. Many fast-food chains have switched from beef tallow or lard to unsaturated vegetable oils for frying, but the total fat content of the foods remains the same.

 When provided with nutrition information on fast-food choices, college women chose meals significantly lower in calories than women who did not get such information. However, information on calories and nutrition had no effect on men's choices.[16]

## You Are What You Drink

About 20 percent of the calories consumed by Americans over age 2 come from sweetened beverages, predominantly soft drinks and fruit drinks. The consumption of sweetened beverages has surged in recent decades. Calories from these drinks, which some call "liquid candy," account for half the rise in caloric intake by Americans since the 1970s.

Water—tap or bottled, sparkling or still, chilled or room temperature—is the medical experts' beverage of choice. But don't think that "fortified" or "enriched" water is better. There is no evidence that nutrients added to water confer any health benefits. Consumers who assume they're getting vitamins in their drinks may think they don't need to eat healthful foods and could end up shortchanging themselves of vital nutrients.

*Soft Drinks*  According to a national survey, two-thirds of adults drink sugar-sweetened beverages, averaging 28 ounces per drink and almost 300 calories daily (15 percent of recommended total calories). Young adults, particularly those with lower incomes and education, consume the most soda.

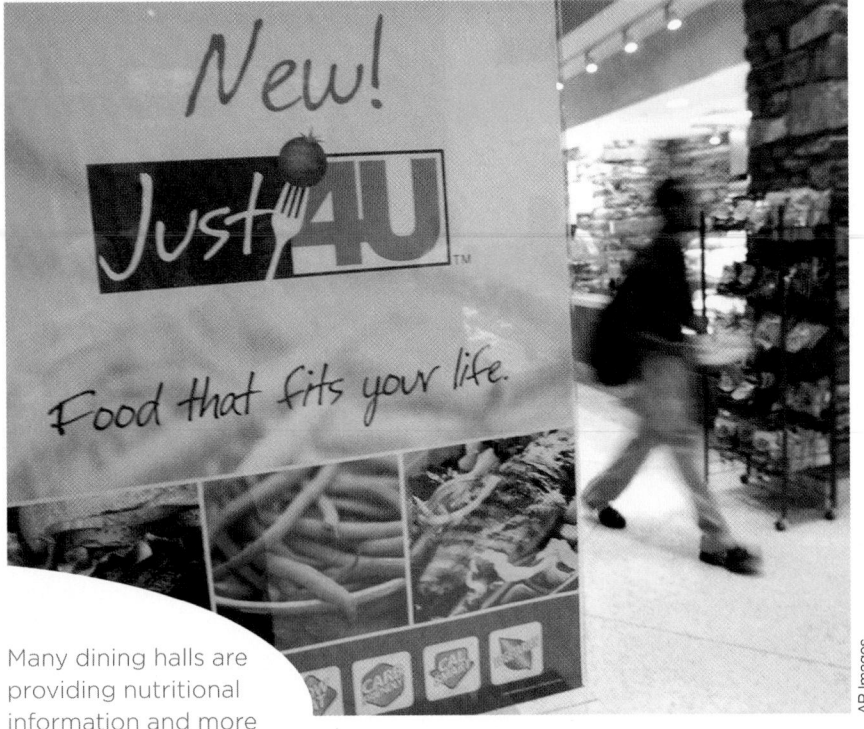

Many dining halls are providing nutritional information and more healthful food options for students.

## ⓘ CONSUMER ALERT

### More Healthful Fast-Food Choices

#### Facts to Know

Fast-food restaurants may be the cheapest option, but unfortunately, they are not usually the most healthful one.

- Eating just one fast-food meal can pack enough calories, sodium, and fat for an entire day.
- Just two or more high-fat fast-food meals a week have been linked to increased risk of diabetes.
- Seemingly healthful choices, such as a "Mac Snack Wrap," can be low in calories (330) but extremely high in fat (19 grams).

#### Steps to Take

- **Drink water instead of soda.** One 32-ounce Big Gulp with regular cola packs about 425 calories.
- **Eat your food naked.** Avoid calorie- and fat-packed spreads, cheese, sour cream, and so on. If you sample the salad bar, steer clear of mayonnaise, bacon bits, oily vegetable salads, and rich dressings.
- **Choose small portions.** Since an average fast-food meal can run as high as 1,000 calories or more, don't supersize anything. A single serving often provides enough for two meals. Take half home or divide with a friend.
- **Hold the salt.** Fast-food restaurant food tends to be very high in sodium, so don't add any more.

See the table on the following page for some specific choices.

These beverages can add five pounds every year. Cutting 300 liquid calories from your daily intake by cutting out sweetened beverages would translate into a 2.5-pound loss every month. In a recent review of 88 studies, researchers linked soft drinks with increased calorie intake, higher body weight, lower consumption of calcium and other nutrients, and greater risk of other medical problems, such as diabetes. Women who consume two or more cans of soda daily are almost twice as likely as other women to show early evidence of kidney disease. No one knows if the culprit is the amount of sugar they consume or the type. Some samples of the high-fructose syrup used to make and preserve soda have contained mercury, which is toxic to the kidneys.

Researchers also have found a strong association between soft drink consumption and greater risk of heart disease. A single daily soft drink, either diet or regular, also increases the likelihood of metabolic syndrome. Sweetened iced tea and many carbonated beverages can damage tooth enamel, especially when not consumed with food. Drinking regular and diet cola has been linked with the thinning of hip bones in women.

People who consume a lot of soft drinks generally take in more calories than others—and not just from the beverages. Instead of satisfying a sweet tooth, soft drinks seem to do the opposite. Although researchers cannot explain exactly why, soft drinks may increase hunger or decrease feelings of satiety or fullness. Even diet drinks made with artificial sweeteners may "condition" people to eat more sweets.

College students say they consume sugar-sweetened beverages—including soft drinks, energy drinks, and fruit-based drinks—on social occasions, sometimes mixed with alcohol. Some think of these drinks as part of the enjoyment

## A Fast-Food Nutrition Survival Guide

| Less Healthful Choices | More Healthful Choices |
|---|---|
| **Burger Chains** | |
| Double-patty hamburger with cheese, mayo, special sauce, and bacon | Regular, single-patty hamburger without mayo or cheese |
| Fried chicken sandwich | Grilled chicken sandwich |
| Fried fish sandwich | Veggie burger |
| Salad with toppings such as bacon, cheese, and ranch dressing | Garden salad with grilled chicken and low-fat dressing |
| Breakfast burrito with steak | Egg on a muffin |
| French fries | Baked potato or a side salad |
| Milkshake | Yogurt parfait |
| Chicken "nuggets" or tenders | Grilled chicken strips |
| Adding cheese, extra mayo, and special sauces | Limiting cheese, mayo, and special sauces |
| **Fried Chicken Chains** | |
| Fried chicken, original or extra-crispy | Skinless chicken breast without breading |
| Teriyaki wings or popcorn chicken | Honey BBQ chicken sandwich |
| Caesar salad | Garden salad |
| Chicken and biscuit "bowl" | Mashed potatoes |
| Adding extra gravy and sauces | Limiting gravy and sauces |
| **Taco Chains** | |
| Crispy shell chicken taco | Grilled chicken soft taco |
| Refried beans | Black beans |
| Steak chalupa | Shrimp ensalada |
| Crunch wraps or gordita-type burritos | Grilled "fresco"-style steak burrito |
| Nachos with refried beans | Veggie and bean burrito |
| Adding sour cream or cheese | Limiting sour cream or cheese |
| **Sub, Sandwich, and Deli Choices** | |
| Foot-long sub | Six-inch sub |
| High-fat meat such as ham, tuna salad, bacon, meatballs, or steak | Lean meat (roast beef, chicken breast, lean ham) or veggies |
| The "normal" amount of higher-fat (cheddar, American) cheese | One or two slices of lower-fat cheese (Swiss or mozzarella) |
| Adding mayo and special sauces | Low-fat dressing or mustard instead of mayo |
| An "as is" sub with all the toppings | Extra veggie toppings |
| White bread or "wraps," which are often higher in fat than normal bread | Choosing whole-grain bread or taking the top slice off your sub and eating it open-faced |
| **Asian Food Choices** | |
| Fried egg rolls, spare ribs, tempura | Egg drop, miso, wonton, or hot and sour soup |
| Battered or deep-fried dishes (sweet and sour pork, General Tso's chicken) | Stir-fried, steamed, roasted, or broiled entrées (shrimp chow mein, chop suey) |
| Deep-fried tofu | Steamed or baked tofu |
| Coconut milk, sweet and sour sauce, regular soy sauce | Sauces such as ponzu, rice-wine vinegar, wasabi, ginger, and low-sodium soy sauce |
| Fried rice | Steamed brown rice |
| Salads with fried or crispy noodles | Edamame, cucumber salad, stir-fried veggies |
| **Italian and Pizza Restaurant Choices** | |
| Thick-crust pizza with extra cheese and meat toppings | Thin-crust pizza with half the cheese and extra veggies |
| Garlic bread | Plain rolls or breadsticks |
| Antipasto with meat | Antipasto with vegetables |
| Pasta with cream or butter-based sauce | Pasta with tomato sauce and veggies |
| Entrée with side of pasta | Entrée with side of veggies |
| Fried ("frito") dishes | Grilled ("griglia") dishes |

of going to a movie or hanging out with friends; others drink more caffeinated beverages at exam times. Even when aware of negative health consequences, most do not feel these consequences pertain to them.

*Energy Drinks*   Coffee and tea, which both contain caffeine, are the classic "pick-me-up" beverages. As discussed in Chapter 12, regular coffee consumption may reduce the risk of several serious illnesses—including type 2 diabetes, colon cancer, and Parkinson's disease—and may protect against age-related memory and thinking defects. However, in adolescents and young adults, caffeine has been linked to elevated blood pressure and impaired sleep.

 The practice of mixing energy drinks with alcohol (discussed in Chapter 12) is especially dangerous. The FDA has identified caffeine as an unsafe food additive to alcoholic beverages and banned sale of pre-mixed alcoholic energy drinks. However, many college students add alcohol to energy drinks and assume that the caffeine counteracts the adverse effects of alcohol. In fact, caffeine may reduce sleepiness, but it leads to a state some call "wide-awake drunkenness," in which drinkers cannot fully assess their true level of impairment and are more likely to engage in risky behaviors, such as driving while intoxicated.[17]

Consumption of energy drinks such as Red Bull and Rockstar has more than doubled in the last three years, particularly among young people. The main ingredient in these drinks, including diet brands, is caffeine, sometimes in doses that can cause physical and psychological complications, including disrupted sleep, exaggerated stress response, heart palpitations, and increased risk of high blood pressure.

Red Bull, for instance, contains nearly 80 mg of caffeine per can, about the same amount of caffeine as a cup of brewed coffee and twice the caffeine of a cup of tea. Other energy drinks contain several times this amount—see Table 6.8.

The drink formulations vary widely, and manufacturers make many different claims about their effects. Some brands contain fruit juices, teas, and dietary supplements such as ginseng and glucuronolactone. One can of Red Bull contains 1000 mg of taurine, a substance that plays an important role in muscle contraction (especially in the heart) and the nervous system.

Some energy drinks contain guarana, a South American herbal caffeine source that could pose additional risks. We know very little about the effects of such combinations of ingredients, which may work synergistically with caffeine to boost its stimulant power.

Millions of college students consume energy drinks for the jolt provided or because they believe the drinks enhance sports performance or sexual function. Yet health experts warn that these sugar- and caffeine-laden drinks pose serious health risks, including dehydration, accidents, and alcohol poisoning.

## Ethnic Cuisines

Whatever your cultural heritage, you have probably sampled Chinese, Mexican, Indian, Italian, and Japanese foods. If you belong to any of these ethnic groups, you may eat these cuisines regularly. Each type of ethnic cooking has its own nutritional benefits and potential drawbacks.

The cuisine served in Mexico features rice, corn, and beans, which are low in fat and high in nutrients. However, the dishes Americans think of as Mexican are far less healthful. Burritos, especially when topped with cheese and sour cream, are very high in fat. Although guacamole has a high fat content, it contains mostly monounsaturated fatty acids, a better form of fat.

African American cuisine traces some of its roots to food preferences from west Africa (for example, peanuts, okra, and black-eyed peas), as well as to traditional American foods, such as fish, game, greens, and sweet potatoes. It uses many nutritious vegetables, such as collard greens and sweet potatoes, as well as legumes. However, some dishes include high-fat food products such as peanuts and pecans or involve frying, sometimes in saturated fat.

The mainland Chinese diet, which is plant-based, high in carbohydrates, and low in fats and animal protein, is considered one of the most healthful in the world. However, Chinese restaurants in the United States serve more meat and sauces than are generally eaten in China. According to laboratory tests of typical take-out dishes from Chinese restaurants, many have more fats and cholesterol than hamburger or egg dishes from fast-food outlets.

**Table 6.8 Energy Drinks: Caffeine in Cans and Cups**

| Type of Drink | Amount of Caffeine |
|---|---|
| Regular cola (12-oz can) | 40 mg |
| Red Bull (8.3-oz can) | 75 mg |
| Coffee (standard 8-oz cup) | 95 mg |
| Monster (16-oz container) | 140 mg |
| Rockstar (16-oz container) | 240 mg |

Table 6.9 **Ethnic Food Choices**

| | Grains | Vegetables | Fruits | Meats and Legumes | Milk |
|---|---|---|---|---|---|
| **Asian** <br> © Becky Luigart-Stayner/Corbis | Rice, noodles, millet | Amaranth, baby corn, bamboo shoots, chayote, bok choy, mung bean sprouts, sugar peas, straw mushrooms, water chestnuts, kelp | Carambola, guava, kumquat, lychee, persimmon, melons, mandarin orange | Soybeans and soy products such as soy milk and tofu, squid, duck eggs, pork, poultry, fish and other seafood, peanuts, cashews | Usually excluded |
| **Mediterranean** <br> PhotoDisc/Getty Images | Pita pocket bread, pastas, rice, couscous, polenta, bulgur, focaccia, Italian bread | Eggplant, tomatoes, peppers, cucumbers, grape leaves | Olives, grapes, figs | Fish and other seafood, gyros, lamb, chicken, beef, pork, sausage, lentils, fava beans | Ricotta, provolone, parmesan, feta, mozzarella, and goat cheeses; yogurt |
| **Mexican** <br> PhotoDisc/Getty Images | Tortillas (corn or flour), taco shells, rice | Chayote, corn, jicama, tomato salsa, cactus, cassava, tomatoes, yams, chilies | Guava, mango, papaya, avocado, plantain, bananas, oranges | Refried beans, fish, chicken, chorizo, beef, eggs | Cheese, custard |

Traditional French cuisine, which includes rich, high-fat sauces and dishes, has never been considered healthful. Yet, nutritionists have been stumped to explain the so-called French paradox. Despite a diet high in saturated fats, the French have had one of the lowest rates of coronary artery disease in the world. The French diet increasingly resembles the American diet, but French portions tend to be one-third to one-half the size of American portions.

Many Indian dishes highlight healthful ingredients such as vegetables and legumes (beans and peas). However, many also use *ghee* (a form of butter) or coconut oil; both are rich in harmful saturated fats. The best advice in an Indian restaurant is to ask how each dish is prepared. Good choices include *daal* or *dal* (lentils), *karbi* or *karni* (chickpea soup), and *chapati* (tortilla-like bread).

The traditional Japanese diet is very low in fat, which may account for the low incidence of heart disease in Japan. Dietary staples include soybean products, fish, vegetables, noodles, and rice. A variety of fruits and vegetables are also included in many dishes. However, Japanese cuisine is high in salted, smoked, and pickled foods. Watch out for deep-fried dishes such as tempura and salty soups and sauces.

Table 6.9 summarizes some of the ethnic food choices by food group.

# Taking Charge of What You Eat

You can't control what you don't know. Because of the Nutrition Labeling and Education Act, food manufacturers must provide information about fat, calories, and ingredients in large type on packaged food labels, and they must show how a food item fits into a daily diet of 2,000 calories. The law also restricts nutritional claims for terms such as *healthy, low-fat,* and *high-fiber.*

A growing number of cities and states are mandating calorie-posting by fast-food restaurants. Some national health reform proposals would require restaurant chains to post the number of calories, grams of saturated fat, and milligrams of sodium next to menu items, although menu labeling has not proven to affect dietary choices.[18] Often the problem is not a lack of information, health officials note, but a lack of self-control.[19] You can find detailed nutritional information for restaurants of all price levels at www.healthydiningfinder.com.

In evaluating food labels and product claims, keep in mind that while individual foods vary in their nutritional value, what matters is your total diet. If you eat too much of any one food—regardless of what its label states—you may not be getting the variety and balance of nutrients that you need.

## Portions and Servings

Consumers often are confused by what a *serving* actually is, especially since many American restaurants have supersized the amount of food they put on their customers' plates. The average bagel has doubled in size in the last 10 to 15 years. A standard fast-food serving of french fries is larger in the United States than in the United Kingdom.

A food-label *serving* is a specific amount of food that contains the quantity of nutrients described on the Nutrition Facts label. A *portion* is the amount of a specific food that an individual eats at one time. Portions can be bigger or smaller than the servings on food labels. According to nutritionists, "marketplace portions"—the actual amounts served to customers—are two to eight times larger than the standard serving sizes defined by the USDA. In fast-food chains, today's portions are two to five times larger than the original sizes. As studies have shown, people presented with larger portions eat 30 to 50 percent more than they otherwise would.

If you are trying to balance your diet or control your weight, it's important to keep track of the size of your portions so that you do not exceed recommended servings. For instance, a 3-ounce serving of meat is about the size of a pack of playing cards—see Figure 6.7. If you eat a larger amount, count it as more than one serving. (See "Mind over Platter" in Making Change Happen and in *Labs for IPC* for more on developing greater awareness of what and how you eat.)

## How to Read Nutrition Labels

The Nutrition Facts label on food products presents a wealth of information—if you know what to look for (Figure 6.8). The label focuses on those nutrients most clearly associated with disease risk and health: total fat, saturated fat, cholesterol, sodium, total carbohydrate, dietary fiber, sugar, and protein.

- **Calories.** Calories are the measure of the amount of energy that can be derived from food. Scientists define a calorie as the amount of energy required to raise the temperature of 1 gram of water by 1 degree Celsius. In the laboratory, the caloric content of food is measured in 1,000-calorie units called kilocalories. The calorie referred to in everyday usage is actually the equivalent of the laboratory kilocalorie.

  The Nutrition Facts label lists two numbers for calories: calories per serving and calories from fat per serving. This allows consumers to calculate how many calories they'll consume and to determine the percentage of fat in an item.

Figure 6.7 **Portion Sizes**
Quick and easy estimates of portion sizes

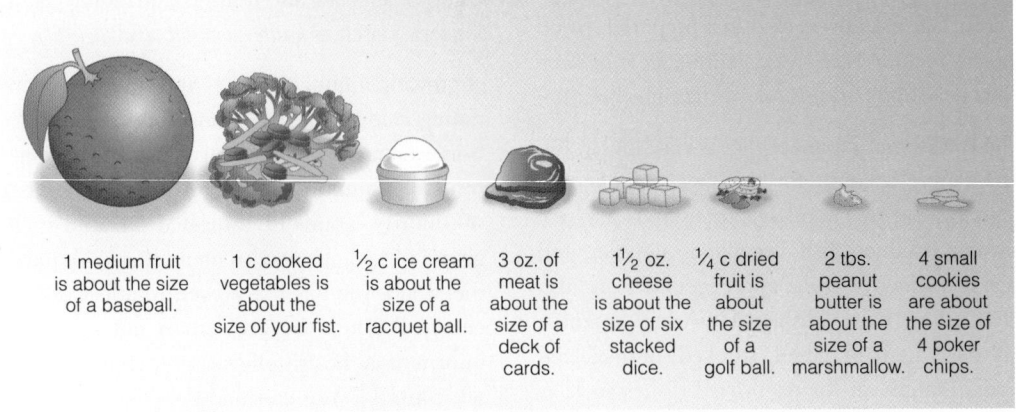

1 medium fruit is about the size of a baseball.

1 c cooked vegetables is about the size of your fist.

½ c ice cream is about the size of a racquet ball.

3 oz. of meat is about the size of a deck of cards.

1½ oz. cheese is about the size of six stacked dice.

¼ c dried fruit is about the size of a golf ball.

2 tbs. peanut butter is about the size of a marshmallow.

4 small cookies are about the size of 4 poker chips.

- **Serving size.** Rather than the tiny portions manufacturers sometimes used in the past to keep down the number of calories per serving, the new labels reflect more realistic portions. Serving sizes, which have been defined for approximately 150 food categories, must be the same for similar products (for example, different brands of potato chips) and for similar products (for example, snack foods such as pretzels, potato chips, and popcorn). This makes it easier to compare the nutritional content of foods.

- **Daily Values (DVs).** DVs refer to the total amount of a nutrient that the average adult should aim to get or not exceed on a daily basis. The DVs for cholesterol, sodium, vitamins, and minerals are the same for all adults. The DVs for total fat, saturated fat, carbohydrate, fiber, and protein are based on a 2,000-calorie daily diet—the amount of food ingested by many American men and active women. and trans fat numbers deserve special attention because of their link to several diseases.

- **Percent Daily Values (%DVs).** The goal for a full day's diet is to select foods that together add up to 100 percent of the DVs. The %DVs show how a particular food's nutrient content fits into a 2,000-calorie diet. Individuals who consume (or should consume) fewer than 2,000 total calories a day have to lower their DVs for total fat, saturated fat, and carbohydrates. For example, if their caloric intake is 10 percent less than 2,000 calories, they would lower the DV by 10 percent. Similarly, those who consume more than 2,000 calories should adjust the DVs upward.

- **Calories per gram.** The bottom of the food label lists the number of calories per gram for fat, carbohydrates, and protein.

People zero in on different figures on the food label—for example, calories if they're watching their weight, specific ingredients if they have food allergies.

- **Calories from fat.** Get into the habit of calculating the percentage of fat calories in a food before buying or eating it.

Watch out for statements such as "97 percent fat-free." All this means is that the product is 3 percent fat by weight, which has nothing to do

Figure 6.8 **Understanding Nutrition Labels**
Food labels can be misleading. Here are two examples of labels claiming "lean" ground beef. Only the 7% fat beef is actually lean; "20% fat" ground beef is far from lean, actually providing 21 grams of fat and 70% of total calories from fat per serving.

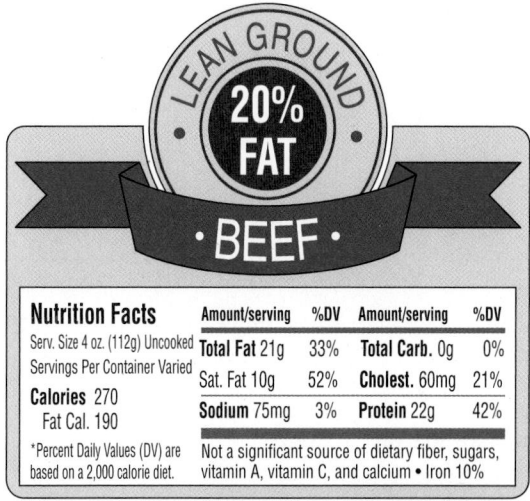

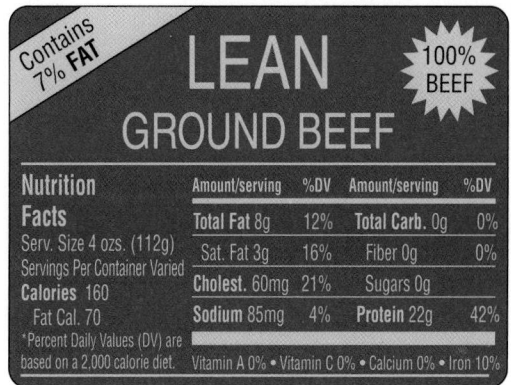

with the percentage of fat calories per serving. A product that's 97 percent fat-free may have as much as 30 percent of its calories from fat. See Table 6.10 for a list of the fat content of common food sources of fat including candy.

You can also figure out the percentage of fat with some simple calculations: Suppose that a slice of cherry pie provides 350 calories and 15 grams of fat. To calculate the percentage of fat calories, multiply 15 grams by 9 (the number of calories in each gram of fat), divide the result by 350 calories, and then multiply this result by 100:

15 grams fat ×
9 calories/gram = 135 calories from fat
135 calories/350 = 0.39
0.39 × 100 = 39% of total calories
from fat

Table 6.10 **The Fat Content of Some Foods**

| Food | Amount | Grams | Percentage of Total Calories from Fat |
|---|---|---|---|
| **Fat and oils** | | | |
| Butter | 1 tsp | 4.0 | 100% |
| Margarine | 1 tsp | 4.0 | 100 |
| Oil | 1 tsp | 4.7 | 100 |
| Mayonnaise | 1 tbs | 11.0 | 99 |
| Heavy cream | 1 tbs | 5.5 | 93 |
| Salad dressing | 1 tbs | 6.0 | 83 |
| **Meats and fish** | | | |
| Hot dog | 1 (2 oz) | 17.0 | 83 |
| Bologna | 1 oz | 8.0 | 80 |
| Sausage | 4 links | 18.0 | 77 |
| Bacon | 3 pieces | 9.0 | 74 |
| Salami | 2 oz | 11.0 | 68 |
| Hamburger, regular (20% fat) | 3 oz | 16.5 | 62 |
| Chicken, fried with skin | 3 oz | 14.0 | 53 |
| Steak (rib eye) | 3 oz | 9.9 | 47 |
| Veggie pita | 1 | 17.0 | 38 |
| Chicken, baked without skin | 3 oz | 4.0 | 25 |
| Flounder, baked | 3 oz | 1.0 | 13 |
| Shrimp, boiled | 3 oz | 1.0 | 10 |
| **Milk and milk products** | | | |
| Cheddar cheese | 1 oz | 9.5 | 74 |
| American cheese | 1 oz | 6.0 | 66 |
| Milk, whole | 1 cup | 8.5 | 49 |
| Cottage cheese, regular | 1/2 cup | 5.1 | 39 |
| Milk, 2% | 1 cup | 5.0 | 32 |
| Milk, 1% | 1 cup | 2.7 | 24 |
| Cottage cheese, 1% fat | 1/2 cup | 1.2 | 13 |
| Milk, skim | 1 cup | 0.4 | 4 |
| Yogurt, frozen | 3/4 cup | 0.0–6.6 | 0–3 |
| **Other** | | | |
| Olives | 4 medium | 1.5 | 90 |
| Avocado | 1/2 | 15.0 | 84 |
| Almonds | 1 oz | 15.0 | 80 |
| Sunflower seeds | 1/4 cup | 17.0 | 77 |
| Peanuts | 1/4 cup | 17.5 | 75 |
| Cashews | 1 oz | 13.2 | 73 |
| Egg | 1 | 6.0 | 61 |
| Potato chips | 1 oz (13 chips) | 11.0 | 61 |
| French fries | 20 fries | 20.0 | 49 |
| Taco chips | 1 oz (10 chips) | 6.2 | 41 |
| **Candy** | | | |
| Peanut butter cups, 2 regular | 1.6 oz | 15.0 | 54 |
| Milk chocolate | 1.6 oz | 14.0 | 53 |
| Almond Joy | 1.8 oz | 14.0 | 50 |
| Kit Kat | 1.5 oz | 12.0 | 47 |
| M & M's, peanut | 1.7 oz | 13.0 | 47 |

Source: Brown, Judith, *Nutrition Now*, 6th ed. (Belmont, CA: Wadsworth, Cengage Learning, 2011).

- **Total fat.** Since the average person munches on 15 to 20 food items a day, it's easy to overload on fat. Saturated fat and trans fat numbers deserve special attention because of their link to several diseases.

- **Cholesterol.** Cholesterol is made by animals and contained in products of animal origin only. Many high-fat products, such as potato chips, contain 0 percent cholesterol because they're made from plants and are cooked in vegetable fats. However, if the vegetable fats are hydrogenated, the resulting trans fat is more harmful to the heart than cholesterol.

- **Sugars.** There is no Daily Value for sugars because health experts have yet to agree on a daily limit. The figure on the label includes naturally present sugars, such as lactose in milk and fructose in fruit, as well as those added to the food, such as table sugar, corn syrup, or dextrose.

- **Fiber.** A "high-fiber" food has 5 or more grams of fiber per serving. A "good" source of fiber provides at least 2.5 grams. "More" or "added" fiber means at least 2.5 grams more per serving than similar foods—10 percent more of the DV for fiber.

- **Calcium.** "High" equals 200 mg or more per serving. "Good" means at least 100 mg, while "more" indicates that the food contains at least 100 mg more calcium—10 percent more of the DV—than the item usually would have.

- **Sodium.** Most of us routinely get more sodium than we need. Read labels carefully to avoid excess sodium, which can be a health threat.

- **Vitamins.** A Daily Value of 10 percent of any vitamin makes a food a "good" source; 20 percent qualifies it as "high" in a certain vitamin.

## What Is Organic?

Foods certified as **organic** by the USDA must meet strict criteria, including:

- Processing or preservation only with substances approved by the USDA for organic foods.

- Processing without genetic modification or ionizing radiation.

- No use of most synthetic chemicals, such as pesticides, herbicides, or fertilizers.
- Fertilization without sewage sludge.
- Food-producing animals grown without medication such as antibiotics or hormones, provided with living conditions similar to their natural habitat, and fed organic feed.

 The primary consumers of organic food are women ages 30 to 45 who have children at home and who are environmentally conscious. College students who are informed about organic products are more likely to choose them. In a recent study, more than half of undergraduates said they would support and purchase organic products on campus.

Are organic foods better for you? There has been limited research as to whether organic foods are nutritionally superior to conventional foods. Some studies have shown higher levels of specific nutrients, such as flavonoids, in organic produce, but no one knows if this translates into specific health benefits. However, you can avoid exposure to pesticides and other chemicals by opting for organic foods.

## Functional Foods

As the American Dietetic Association has noted, all foods are functional at some physiological level. However, the term *functional* generally applies to a food specifically created to have health-promoting benefits. The International Food Information Council defines functional foods as those "that provide health benefits beyond basic nutrition."

Some manufacturers are adding biologically active components such as beta-carotene to food products and promoting them as functional foods. However, the amounts added are often too low to have any effect, and many such foods are high-sugared drinks and snack foods. More research is needed to evaluate their claims of health benefits.

## Choosing Healthful Snacks

Snacking has become more widespread on campuses, as in other places. College students snack primarily "to satisfy hunger"; the second most common reason is "no time for meals." Other reasons for munching between meals: "for energy," "to be sociable," and "to relieve stress." One-third snack at 9:00 p.m. or later.

In response to consumer demands for smart snack choices, food manufacturers are offering "better-for-you" options that are lower in salt and sugar or free of trans fat and artificial colors. Some new snack items promoted as healthful options, such as sugar-free chocolate or organic potato chips, offer little nutritional value. Meat-based snacks, increasingly popular among young men, also can be high in fat and sodium. Read labels carefully, and be sure to check total calories and fat.

A best-for-you option is fruit such as bananas, apples, or berries—rich in vitamins, low in calories, and packed with fiber. Other nutritious snacks include nuts, trail mix, granola bars, yogurt, sunflower seeds, soy nuts, and dried fruit (such as cranberries). If you enjoy fruit juice, buy 100 percent fruit juice without added sugar. Limit yourself to one serving of these calorie-rich beverages a day.

If you rely on snacks to keep you energized throughout the day, take time to plan in advance so you have choices other than the nearest vending machine. Try to prepare snacks from different food groups: low- or no-fat milk and a few graham crackers, for instance, or celery sticks with peanut butter and raisins. Save part of one meal—half of your breakfast bagel or lunch sandwich—to eat a few hours later. If you're trying to add fiber to your diet, eat high-fiber snacks, such as prunes, popcorn, or sunflower seeds.

# Food Safety

Foodborne infections cause an estimated 76 million illnesses, 325,000 hospitalizations, and 5,000 deaths in the United States every year. Three organisms—*Salmonella*, *Listeria*, and *Toxoplasma*—are responsible for more than 75 percent of these deaths. Although most foodborne infections cause mild illness, severe infections and serious complications—including death—do occur.

Scares about tainted food have led to massive recalls of such popular foods as peanut butter, jalapenos, lettuce, spinach, and tomatoes. As a

**organic** Term designating food produced with, or production based on the use of, fertilizers originating from plants or animals, without the use of pesticides or chemically formulated fertilizers.

result, consumer advocates, as well as manufacturers and trade associations, are calling for stricter regulations.

What can you do to protect yourself? Pay attention when you hear that a food or product is under suspicion. Make note of the brands, the production dates, and the manufacturer(s) involved. Check the labels of the foods in your pantry and refrigerator, and throw out any that may be contaminated.

## Fight BAC!

To improve food safety awareness and practices, government and private agencies have developed the Fight BAC! campaign, which identifies four key culprits in foodborne illness:

- **Improper cooling**
- **Improper hand washing**
- **Inadequate cooking**
- **Failure to avoid cross-contamination**

## Avoiding *E. coli* Infection

Eating unwashed produce, such as spinach or lettuce, or undercooked beef, especially hamburger, can increase your risk of infection with *Escherichia coli* (*E. coli*) bacteria. These bacteria, which live in the intestinal tract of healthy people and animals, are usually harmless. However, infection with the strain *E. coli* O157:H7 produces symptoms that can range from mild to life-threatening. This strain has made its way into hamburger in fast-food chains and into packaged spinach. *E. coli* can cause severe bloody diarrhea, kidney failure, and even death. Symptoms usually develop within two to ten days and can include severe stomach cramps, vomiting, mild fever, and bloody diarrhea. Most people recover within seven to ten days. Others—especially older adults, children under the age of 5, and those with weakened immune systems—may develop complications that lead to kidney failure.

Proper handling and cooking of food can practically eliminate infection from meat. Especially if grilled, meat is likely to brown before it's completely cooked, so a meat thermometer should be used to ensure that meat is heated to at least 160°F at its thickest point. If a thermometer is

*Your Strategies for Prevention*

## How to Protect Yourself from Food Poisoning

- **Always wash your hands with liquid or clean bar soap before handling food.** Rub your hands vigorously together for 10 to 15 seconds; the soap combined with the scrubbing action dislodges and removes germs.

- **When preparing fresh fruits and vegetables, discard outer leaves, wash under running water, and when possible, scrub with a clean brush or hands.** Do not wash meat or poultry.

- **To avoid the spread of bacteria to other foods, utensils, or surfaces, do not allow liquids to touch or drip onto other items.** Wipe up all spills immediately.

- **Clean out your refrigerator regularly.** Throw out any leftovers stored for three or four days.

- **To kill bacteria and viruses, sterilize wet kitchen sponges by putting them in a microwave for two minutes.** Make sure they are completely wet to guard against the risk of fire.

not available, ground meat should be cooked until no pink shows in the center.

## Food Poisoning

*Salmonella* is a bacterium that contaminates many foods, particularly undercooked chicken, eggs, and sometimes processed meat. Eating contaminated food can result in salmonella poisoning, which causes diarrhea and vomiting. The Centers for Disease Control and Prevention (CDC) estimates 40,000 reported cases of salmonella poisoning a year; the actual number of cases could be anywhere from 400,000 to 4 million. The FDA has warned consumers about the dangers of unpasteurized orange juice because of the risk of salmonella contamination.

Another bacterium, *Campylobacter jejuni*, may cause even more stomach infections than salmonella. Found in water, milk, and some foods, campylobacter poisoning causes severe diarrhea and has been implicated in the growth of stomach ulcers.

Bacteria can also cause illness by producing toxins in food. *Staphylococcus aureus* is the most common culprit. When cooked foods are cross-contaminated with the bacteria from raw foods and not stored properly, staph infections can result, causing nausea and abdominal pain anywhere from 30 minutes to eight hours after ingestion.

An uncommon but sometimes fatal form of food poisoning is botulism, caused by the *Clostridium botulinum* organism. Improper home-canning procedures are the most common cause of this potentially fatal problem.

Even many healthful foods can pose dangers. The FDA has urged consumers to avoid eating raw sprouts because of the risk of getting sick. Sprouts, particularly alfalfa and clover, can be contaminated by *Salmonella* or *E. coli* bacteria. The FDA advises people to either cook sprouts before eating them or request that they be left off sandwiches and other food ordered in restaurants. Home-grown sprouts can also present a risk if they come from contaminated seeds.

There have been several outbreaks of listeriosis, caused by the bacterium *Listeria*, commonly found in deli meats, hot dogs, soft cheeses, raw meat, and unpasteurized milk. Although rare, listeriosis can be life-threatening. At greatest risk are pregnant women, infants, and those with weakened immune systems. You can reduce your risk by cooking meats and leftovers thoroughly and by washing everything that may come into contact with raw meat.

## Pesticides

Plants and animals naturally produce compounds that act as pesticides to aid in their survival. The vast majority of the pesticides we consume are therefore natural, not added by farmers or food processors. *Commercial pesticides* save billions of dollars of valuable crops from pests, but they also may endanger human health and life. Fearful of potential risks in pesticides, many consumers are purchasing organic foods.

## Food Allergies

Food allergies, which affect about 5 percent of young children and 4 percent of teens and adults, are much less common than many assume. As many as 50 to 90 percent of presumed food allergies are not allergic reactions.[20]

The National Institute of Allergy and Infectious Diseases has released the first comprehensive guidelines for diagnosing and treating a food allergy, which is defined as "an adverse health effect arising from a specific immune response that occurs reproducibly on exposure to a given food."[21]

Physicians disagree as to which foods are the most common triggers of food allergies. Cow's milk, eggs, seafood, wheat, soybeans, nuts, seeds, and chocolate have all been identified as culprits. The symptoms they provoke vary. One person might sneeze if exposed to an irritating food; another might vomit or develop diarrhea; others might suffer headaches, dizziness, hives, or a rapid heartbeat. Symptoms may not develop for up to 72 hours, making it hard to pinpoint which food was responsible.

If you suspect that you have a food allergy, see a physician with specialized training in allergy diagnosis. Medical opinion about the merits of many treatments for food allergies is divided. Once you've identified the culprit, the wisest and sometimes simplest course is to avoid it.

## Nutritional Quackery

The American Dietetic Association describes nutritional quackery as a growing problem for unsuspecting consumers. Because so much nutritional nonsense is garbed in scientific-sounding terms, it can be hard to recognize bad advice when you get it. One basic rule: If the promises of a nutritional claim sound too good to be true, they probably are (see Figure 6.9).

If you seek the advice of a nutrition consultant, carefully check his or her credentials and professional associations. Because licensing isn't required in all states, almost anyone can use the label "nutritionist," regardless of qualifications. Be wary of diplomas from obscure schools and organizations that allow anyone who pays dues to join. (One physician obtained a membership

Figure 6.9 **Spot the Hype!**

## Facts to Know

Nutritional supplements sold in health stores or through health and body-building magazines may contain ingredients that have not been tested and proven safe.

- Be wary of anyone who recommends megadoses of vitamins or nutritional supplements, which can be dangerous. High doses of vitamin A, which some people take to clear up acne, can be toxic.

- A quick way to spot a bad nutrition self-help book is to look in the index for a diet to prevent or treat rheumatoid arthritis (none exists). If you find one, don't buy the book.

## Steps to Take

- Before you try any new nutritional approach, check with your doctor or a registered dietitian or call the American Dietetic Association's consumer hotline, (800) 366-1655.

- Don't believe ads or advisers basing their nutritional recommendations on hair analysis, which is not accurate in detecting nutritional deficiencies.

- Question personal testimonies about the powers of some magical pill or powder, and be wary of "scientific articles" in journals that aren't reviewed by health professionals.

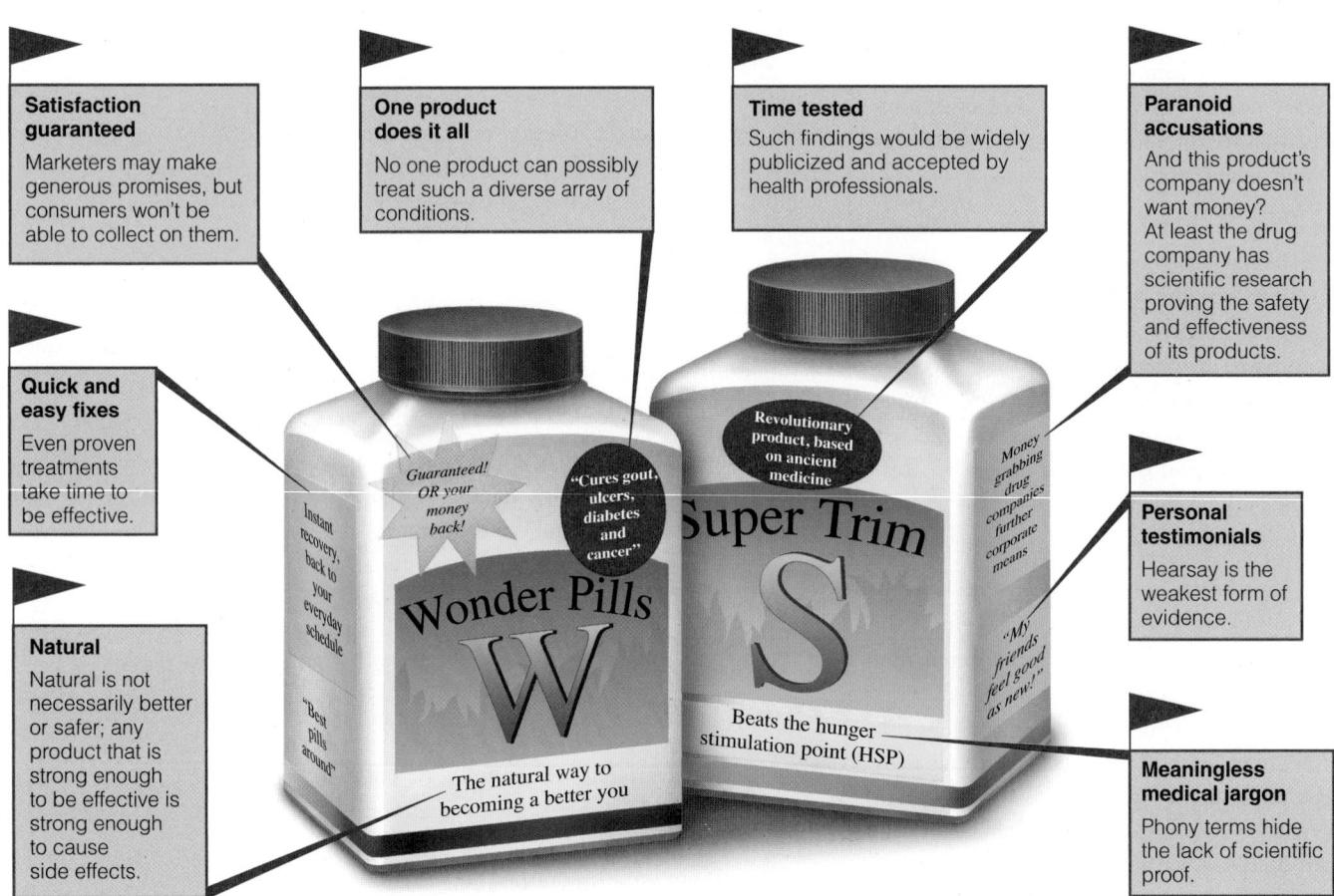

**Satisfaction guaranteed**
Marketers may make generous promises, but consumers won't be able to collect on them.

**One product does it all**
No one product can possibly treat such a diverse array of conditions.

**Time tested**
Such findings would be widely publicized and accepted by health professionals.

**Paranoid accusations**
And this product's company doesn't want money? At least the drug company has scientific research proving the safety and effectiveness of its products.

**Quick and easy fixes**
Even proven treatments take time to be effective.

**Natural**
Natural is not necessarily better or safer; any product that is strong enough to be effective is strong enough to cause side effects.

**Personal testimonials**
Hearsay is the weakest form of evidence.

**Meaningless medical jargon**
Phony terms hide the lack of scientific proof.

for his dog!) A registered dietitian (R.D.), who has a bachelor's degree and specialized training (including an internship) and who passed a certification examination, is usually a member of the American Dietetic Association (ADA), which sets the standard for quality in diets. A nutrition expert with an M.D. or Ph.D. generally belongs to the ADA, the American Institute of Nutrition, or the American Society of Clinical Nutrition; all have stringent membership requirements.

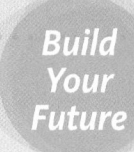

# Making Healthful Food Choices

As nutritional knowledge expands and evolves, it's easy to be confused by changing advice on which foods to avoid and which to eat. But even though research may challenge or change thinking on a specific food, some basic principles always apply. Which of the following do you practice most days of the week?

_____ **Eat breakfast.** Easy-to-prepare breakfasts include cold cereal with fruit and low-fat milk, whole-wheat toast with peanut butter, yogurt with fruit, or whole-grain waffles.

_____ **Don't eat too much of one thing.** Your body needs protein, carbohydrates, fat, and many different vitamins and minerals, such as vitamins C and A, iron, and calcium, from a variety of foods.

_____ **Eat more grains, fruits, and vegetables.** These foods give you carbohydrates for energy, plus vitamins, minerals, and fiber. Try breads such as whole-wheat, bagels, and pita. Spaghetti and oatmeal are also in the grain group.

_____ **Don't ban any food.** Fit in a higher-fat food, like pepperoni pizza, at dinner by choosing lower-fat foods at other meals. And don't forget about moderation. If two pieces of pizza fill you up, don't eat a third.

_____ **Make every calorie count.** Load up on nutrients, not on big portions. Choosing foods that are nutrient dense will help protect against disease and keep you healthy.

_____ **Eat five servings of fruits and vegetables per day.** For breakfast, have 100% fruit juice or add raisins, berries, or sliced fruit to cereal, pancakes, or waffles. For lunch, have vegetable soup or salad with your meal or pile vegetables on your sandwich. For dinner, choose vegetables that are green, orange (such as carrots or squash), and red (such as tomatoes or bell peppers).

_____ **Include three servings of whole-grain foods every day.** To identify whole-grain products, check the ingredient list. The first ingredient should be a whole-grain, such as "whole-grain oats," "whole-grain wheat," or "whole wheat."

_____ **Consume a calcium-rich food at each meal.** Good options include low-fat and nonfat milk, cheese, or yogurt; tofu; broccoli; dried beans; spinach; and fortified soy milk.

_____ **Eat less meat.** Rather than making meat the heart of a meal, think of it as a flavoring ingredient.

_____ **Avoid high-fat fast foods.** Hot dogs, fried foods, packaged snack foods, and pastries are most likely to be laden with fat.

_____ **Check the numbers.** When buying prepared foods, choose items that contain no more than 3 grams of fat per 100 calories.

_____ **Think small.** A dinner-size serving of meat should be about the size of a deck of cards; half a cup is the size of a woman's fist; a pancake is the diameter of a CD.

_____ **Read labels carefully.** Remember that "cholesterol-free" doesn't necessarily mean fat-free. Avoid products that contain saturated coconut oil, palm oil, lard, or hydrogenated fats.

_____ **Switch to low-fat and nonfat dairy products.** Rather than buying whole-fat dairy products, choose skim milk, fat-free sour cream, and low- or nonfat yogurt.

_____ **The brighter the better.** When selecting fruits and vegetables, choose the most intense color. A bright orange carrot has more beta-carotene than a pale one. Dark green lettuce leaves have more vitamins than lighter ones. Orange sweet potatoes pack more vitamin A than yellow ones.

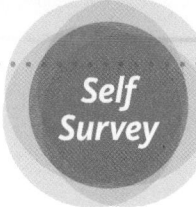

# How Healthful Is Your Diet?

*STEP 1*

Keep a food diary for a week, writing down everything you eat and drink for meals and snacks. Include the approximate amount eaten (for example, 1/2 cup, 1 large, 12-oz can, and so on).

|  | Mon | Tues | Wed | Thurs | Fri | Sat | Sun |
|---|---|---|---|---|---|---|---|
| Grains |  |  |  |  |  |  |  |
| Vegetables |  |  |  |  |  |  |  |
| Fruits |  |  |  |  |  |  |  |
| Milk, yogurt, cheese |  |  |  |  |  |  |  |
| Meat, poultry, dry beans, eggs, nuts |  |  |  |  |  |  |  |
| Fats, oil, sweets |  |  |  |  |  |  |  |

*STEP 2: Are You Getting Enough Vegetables, Fruits, and Grains?*

| How often do you eat: | Seldom/ Never | 1–2 times a week | 3–5 times a week | Almost daily |
|---|---|---|---|---|
| At least three servings of vegetables a day? |  |  |  |  |
| Starchy vegetables like potatoes, corn, or peas? |  |  |  |  |
| Foods made with dry beans, lentils, or peas? |  |  |  |  |
| Dark green or deep yellow vegetables (broccoli, spinach, collards, carrots, sweet potatoes, squash)? |  |  |  |  |
| At least two servings of fruit a day? |  |  |  |  |
| Citrus fruits and 100% fruit juices (oranges, grapefruit, tangerines)? |  |  |  |  |
| Whole fruit with skin or seeds (berries, apples, pears)? |  |  |  |  |
| At least six servings of breads, cereals, pasta, or rice a day? |  |  |  |  |

The best answer for each is "almost daily." Use your food diary to see which foods you should be eating more often.

## STEP 3: Are You Getting Too Much Fat?

| How often do you eat: | Seldom/ Never | 1–2 times a week | 3–5 times a week | Almost daily |
|---|---|---|---|---|
| Fried, deep-fat fried, or breaded food? | | | | |
| Fatty meats, such as sausages, luncheon meat, fatty steaks or roasts? | | | | |
| Whole milk, high-fat cheeses, ice cream? | | | | |
| Pies, pastries, rich cakes? | | | | |
| Rich cream sauces and gravies? | | | | |
| Oily salad dressings or mayonnaise? | | | | |
| Butter or margarine on vegetables, rolls, bread, or toast? | | | | |

Ideally, you should be eating these foods no more than one or two times a week. If your food diary indicates that you're eating them more frequently, your fat intake may well be too high.

## STEP 4: Are You Getting Too Much Sodium?

| How often do you eat: | Seldom/ Never | 1–2 times a week | 3–5 times a week | Almost daily |
|---|---|---|---|---|
| Cured or processed meats, such as ham, sausage, frankfurters, or luncheon meats? | | | | |
| Canned vegetables or frozen vegetables with sauce? | | | | |
| Frozen TV dinners, entrées, or canned or dehydrated soups? | | | | |
| Salted nuts, popcorn, pretzels, corn chips, or potato chips? | | | | |
| Seasoning mixes or sauces containing salt? | | | | |
| Processed cheese? | | | | |
| Salt added to table foods before you taste them? | | | | |

Ideally, you should be eating these high-sodium items no more than one or two times a week. If your food diary indicates that you're eating them more frequently, your sodium intake may well be too high.

# Making Change Happen

## Mind over Platter

If you want to transform your three daily meals from mundane chores to life-enhancing experiences, you have to learn to eat with your mind as well as your mouth. When you bring your mind to the table, you are practicing basic principles of personal change: You are making conscious choices. You are doing what's best for you. You are taking control of your care and feeding. And you are adding another dimension of pleasure to your life.

Whatever your eating circumstances, you always have choices. Maybe you eat in the dining hall every day. Maybe you commute home for meals with your family. Maybe you're rushing to and from a job and wolfing down the fastest food you can find. Even when you feel you can't completely control what you eat, you can control how you eat. By working through "Mind over Platter" in *Labs for IPC*, you can learn to bring to your meals a sense of awareness and appreciation that can transform even an ordinary doughnut into something worth savoring. Here's a preview.

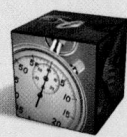

### Get Real

Among other activities in this stage, you will monitor what you put in your mouth for three days (including one weekend day) and record what you eat as well as when, where, and how (standing by a vending machine, sitting at the kitchen table with your husband, lying on your bed and watching a game, etc.). Include coffee, soda, the nibbles you took from your friend's dessert. You will analyze your food diary by answering several questions, including:

- If we are what we eat, what does you food log say about you?

- Are you a junk food junkie? A nonstop grazer? A breakfast skipper? A speed eater? A nocturnal nosher?

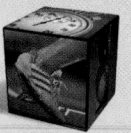

### Get Ready

In this preparatory stage, you will plan and purchase specific foods and find time and a place to eat them. If your idea of a meal is inhaling some ramen noodles at your desk or munching on a pita on the way to class, you will need to make meals more of a time priority . . .

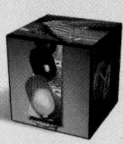

### Get Going

The action stage of this lab includes activities on building bite awareness, mastering the mindful bite, and taste testing, as well as the exercises we call "The Mindful Doughnut" and "The Mindful Meal." However, our favorite is "Mindful Indulgence." Rather than banishing a particular food from your plate, you limit the amount you eat to four bites, which can deliver the maximum taste sensation.

If you're a chocoholic, for instance, mindful eating can take you to a new level of appreciation. Here's how:

- **Go for quality.** Buy a piece or two of handmade or gourmet chocolate rather than the biggest chocolate bar the supermarket sells.

- **Set aside time to savor the chocolate.** Enjoy the anticipation . . . Don't multitask or even watch television while you're eating it.

- **Don't chew the chocolate.** Put a piece in your mouth, and let it melt. Make each piece last at least 90 seconds . . .

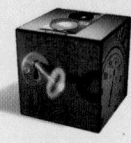

### Lock It In

In this stage, you will learn how to maintain mindfulness by exercises such as trying one new taste every week. The reason: When people try a new food, they generally "sample" the food by taking a very small piece and chewing it slowly but shallowly. This natural taste testing engages all the senses because . . .

# Making This Chapter Work for You

## Review Questions

1. An example of an unhealthy saturated fat would be
   **a.** olive oil.
   **b.** canola oil.
   **c.** corn oil.
   **d.** coconut oil.

2. The *Dietary Guidelines 2010* for Americans include:
   **a.** Maintain intake of added sugars.
   **b.** Decrease consumption of olive oil.
   **c.** Control calorie intake to manage body weight.
   **d.** Eat dessert no more than three days a week.

3. Common causes of foodborne infections include which of the following?
   **a.** the influenza virus
   **b.** *Salmonella* and *E. coli* bacteria
   **c.** avian flu virus
   **d.** pesticides

4. The classes of essential nutrients include which of the following?
   **a.** amino acids, antioxidants, fiber, and cholesterol
   **b.** proteins, calcium, calories, and folic acid
   **c.** carbohydrates, minerals, fat, and water
   **d.** iron, whole grains, fruits, and vegetables

5. Some vegetarians may
   **a.** include fish in their diets.
   **b.** avoid vitamin B₁₂ supplements if they eat only plant foods.
   **c.** eat only legumes or nuts because these provide complete proteins.
   **d.** have high cholesterol levels because of the saturated fats in fruits and vegetables.

6. Which nutrient has the greatest number of calories?
   **a.** protein
   **b.** carbohydrate
   **c.** vitamins
   **d.** fats

7. Because Sam plays poker, it's been easy for him to remember that a recommended serving of 3 ounces of meat means a piece of meat about the size of
   **a.** one deck of cards.
   **b.** eight poker chips.
   **c.** two decks of cards.
   **d.** a roll of quarters.

8. It is recommended that no greater than 30% of a healthy diet come from
   **a.** fats.
   **b.** sugars.
   **c.** starches.
   **d.** protein.

9. Food labels on packaged foods include all of the following *except*
   **a.** total weight of the package.
   **b.** total amount of nutrients contained in the food.
   **c.** the percent of nutrient Daily Values provided in the food.
   **d.** serving size.

10. Antioxidants
    **a.** are nutrients important in the production of hemoglobin.
    **b.** are substances added to foods to make them more flavorful or physically appealing.
    **c.** are suspected triggers of food allergies.
    **d.** are substances that prevent the harmful effects of free radicals.

*Answers to these questions can be found on page 672.*

## Critical Thinking

1. Which alternative or ethnic diet do you think has the best tasting food? Which is the most healthy? Why?

2. Is it possible to meet nutritional requirements on a limited budget? Have you ever been in this situation? What would you recommend to someone who wanted to eat healthfully on $30 a week?

3. Consider the number of times a week you eat fast food. How much money would you have saved if you had eaten home-prepared meals? Which fast foods could you have selected that would have provided more nutritional value?

## Media Menu

Visit www.cengagebrain.com to access course materials and companion resources for this text that will:

- Help you evaluate your knowledge of the material.

- Allow you to prepare for exams with interactive quizzing.

- Use the CengageNOW product to develop a Personalized Learning Plan targeting resources that address areas you should study.

- Coach you through identifying target goals for behavioral change and creating and monitoring your personal change plan throughout the semester using the Behavior Change Planner available in the CengageNOW resource.

## Internet Connections

### www.nal.usda.gov/fnic
This comprehensive governmental website features reports and scientific studies on a variety of nutrition information, including the USDA *Dietary Guidelines 2010*, MyPlate, dietary supplements, dietary assessment, food composition searchable databases, educational brochures, historical food guides, and a topics "A–Z" section.

### www.choosemyplate.gov
This interactive site features the MyPlate Plan, which provides suggestions for applying the most recent *Dietary Guidelines*.

## Key Terms

The terms listed are used on the page indicated. Definitions of the terms are in the Glossary at the end of the book.

amino acids   154

antioxidants   161

basal metabolic rate (BMR)   153

calorie   152

calorie balance   165

carbohydrates   155

complementary proteins   154

complete proteins   154

complex carbohydrates   155

dietary fiber   156

essential nutrients   151

folic acid   175

functional fiber   156

incomplete proteins   154

lacto-vegetarians   175

macronutrients   152

micronutrients   152

minerals   161

nutrition   151

organic   185

ovo-lacto-vegetarians   175

phytochemicals   165

proteins   154

saturated fats   157

simple carbohydrates   155

trans fat   158

unsaturated fats   157

vegans   174

vitamins   160

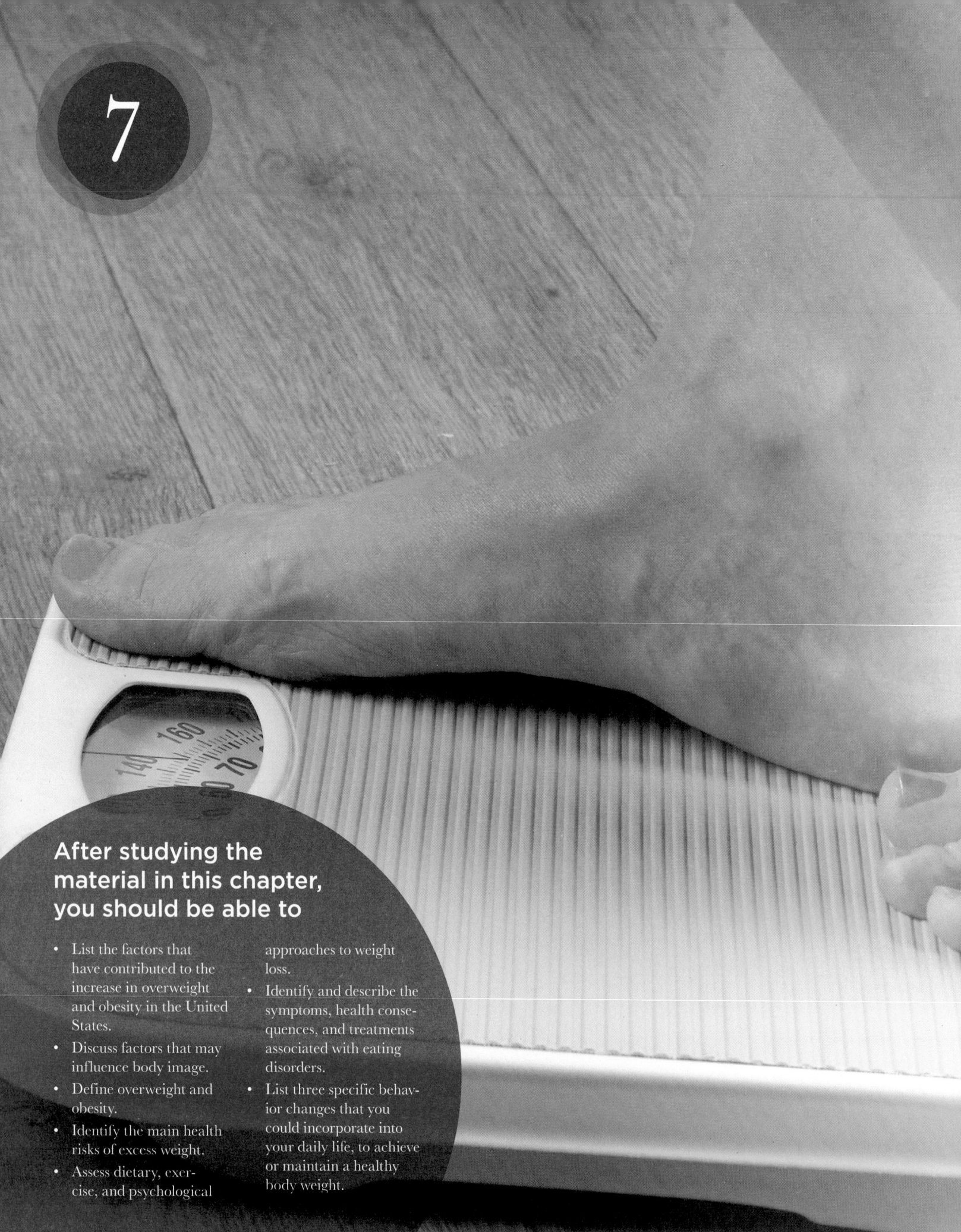

# 7

## After studying the material in this chapter, you should be able to

- List the factors that have contributed to the increase in overweight and obesity in the United States.
- Discuss factors that may influence body image.
- Define overweight and obesity.
- Identify the main health risks of excess weight.
- Assess dietary, exercise, and psychological

approaches to weight loss.
- Identify and describe the symptoms, health consequences, and treatments associated with eating disorders.
- List three specific behavior changes that you could incorporate into your daily life, to achieve or maintain a healthy body weight.

Lina's mother called it "baby fat." "You'll outgrow it soon enough," she said. Yet Lina's cheeks grew chubbier and her waist wider every year. "Wait for your growth spurt," her mother reassured her. But Lina remained one of the shortest girls in her class—and, she was convinced, the roundest.

# Managing Your Weight

Lina went on her first diet in high school. For three days she ate nothing but carrot sticks, cottage cheese, and apples. Then she scarfed down two double cheeseburgers with fries and a chocolate shake. Her other attempts at dieting didn't last much longer. By graduation Lina was grateful to hide under the flowing black robe as she walked on stage to get her diploma.

When Lina heard about the "freshman 15," the extra pounds many students acquire during their first year at college, she groaned at the prospect of putting on more weight. In her Personal Health class, Lina set one primary goal: not to gain another pound. Rather than going on—and inevitably falling off—one diet after another, she developed a weight management plan that included healthful food choices and regular exercise. Armed with the information and tools provided in this chapter, Lina, for the first time in her life, took charge of her weight.

You can do the same.

This chapter explains how we grew so big, tells what obesity is and why excess pounds are dangerous, describes current approaches to weight loss, discusses diets that work (and some that don't), offers practical guidelines for exercise and behavioral approaches to losing weight, and examines unhealthy eating patterns and eating disorders. If you're already at a healthy weight, this chapter can ensure that you remain so in the future. If, like two-thirds of Americans, you are overweight, you will find help in these pages. Remember: You *can* choose to lose.

© Voronin76/Shutterstock.com

## The Global Epidemic

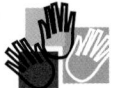

An estimated 1.1 billion people around the world—seven in ten of the Dutch and Spanish, two in three Americans and Canadians, and one in two Britons, Germans, and Italians—are overweight or obese. Overall one in ten adults worldwide is obese.[1] In Europe, excess weight ranks as the most common childhood disorder. Since 1980, obesity rates have tripled in parts of Eastern Europe, the Middle East, China, and the Pacific Islands. More than 20 percent of Chinese children between the ages of 7 and 17 living in large cities are overweight. One in five Chinese adults is overweight or obese. In South Africa some 60 percent of women are overweight or obese.[2]

The World Health Organization, in its first global diet, exercise, and health program to combat obesity, recommends that governments promote public knowledge about diet, exercise, and health; offer information that makes

Visit www.cengagebrain.com to access course materials for this text, including the Behavior Change Planner, interactive quizzes, tutorials, and more. See the preface on page xv for details.

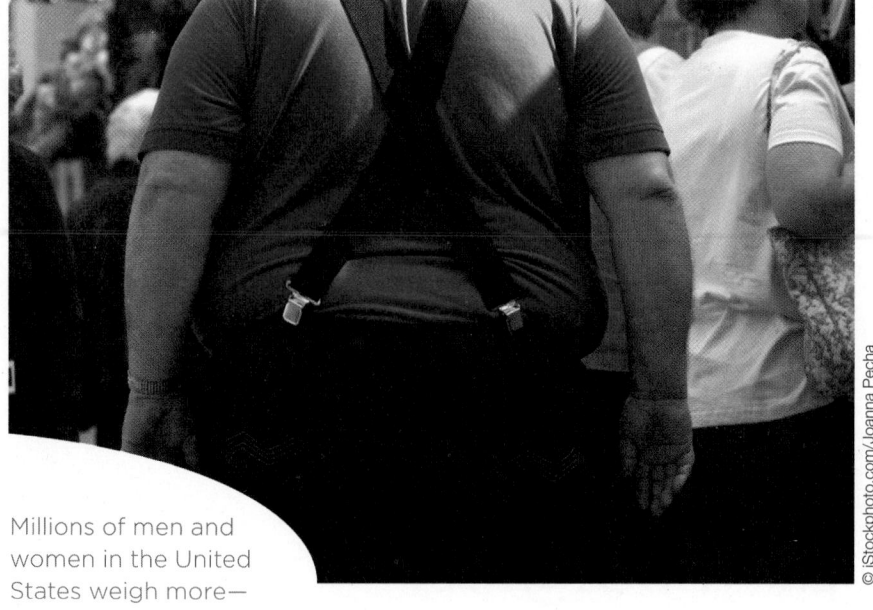

Millions of men and women in the United States weigh more—often two times more—than their recommended ideal weight.

Hawaiians who follow a more traditional diet and lifestyle also have lower rates of obesity and cardiovascular disease.

## Supersized Nation

Over the last 30 years the proportion of Americans considered to be overweight (with a body mass index, or BMI, of 25 or higher) or obese (with a BMI of 30 or higher) has steadily increased. (Body mass index is discussed in Chapter 8.)

Five percent of the U.S. population is morbidly obese, a number far higher than previously thought.[4] In the most recent National Health and Nutrition Examination Survey (NHANES), 68 percent of adults in the United States were overweight; 34 percent of these individuals were obese. More men (72 percent) than women (64 percent) were overweight or obese. Obesity rates among young adults ages 20 to 39 have tripled in the last three decades, rising to 28 percent of men and 34 percent of women.

By some estimates, Americans are collectively more than 5 billion pounds overweight. Some 200 million men and women weigh more—often much more—than their recommended target weights. If this trend were to continue, almost half of American adults would be considered obese by the year 2020. However, there are indications that obesity rates may have reached a plateau, at least for women and most children.[5]

healthy choices easier for consumers to make; and require accurate, comprehensible food labels.[3] Although ultimately each individual decides what and how much to eat, policy makers agree that governments also must act to reverse the obesity epidemic.

Exposure to a Western lifestyle seems to bring out susceptibility to excess weight. Obesity is much more common among the Pima Indians of Arizona compared to Pimas living in Mexico, who have maintained a more traditional lifestyle, with more physical activity and a diet lower in fat and richer in complex carbohydrates. Native

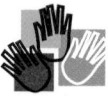 Obesity rates have risen among Americans of all ages and incomes, although there are some gender and racial differences. Among black and Hispanic men, obesity tended to rise along with income. Among women, higher income correlates with lower weight. Women with college degrees also are less likely to be obese than those with less education.[6] About 33 percent of white Americans are obese, compared with 44 percent of African Americans and 39 percent of Mexican Americans. In some Native American communities, up to 70 percent of all adults are dangerously overweight. Differences in metabolic rates may be one factor. (See Table 7.1.)

Children have become part of this epidemic. According to the NHANES data, almost 17 percent of children and adolescents have BMIs

Table 7.1 **Prevalence of Obesity and Overweight**

| | (Percentage of Adults over Age 20) | | | | |
|---|---|---|---|---|---|
| | All | White | Black | Hispanic | Mexican American |
| **Obese (BMI ≥ 30)** | | | | | |
| All | 34 | 33 | 44 | 38 | 39 |
| Men 20–39 | 28 | 26 | 35 | 32 | 34 |
| Women 20–39 | 34 | 31 | 47 | 38 | 40 |
| **Overweight (BMI ≥ 25)** | | | | | |
| All | 68 | 67 | 74 | 77 | 78 |
| Men 20–39 | 64 | 63 | 62 | 74 | 75 |
| Women 20–39 | 60 | 55 | 78 | 69 | 70 |

Source: K. Flegal, et al. "Prevalence and Trends in Obesity among U.S. Adults, 1999–2008." *Journal of the American Medical Association,* Vol. 303, No. 3, January 20, 2010.

that categorize them as overweight or obese. This percentage seems to have reached a plateau, except for the heaviest boys, who are getting even heavier over time.[7] Young adults from immigrant families are at particular risk of becoming overweight or obese by age 25. The reasons may be that they replace outdoor activities with more sedentary ones, such as video games and Internet use; eat more fast food; and consume fewer fruits and vegetables. At highest risk are black and Hispanic youth.[8]

Early obesity strongly predicts later cardiovascular disease, and excess weight may explain the drastic increase in type 2 diabetes, a major risk factor for cardiovascular disease (discussed in Chapter 15). Among obese children, over 70 percent have at least one additional risk factor for cardiovascular disease; almost 40 percent have two or more. Being overweight in late adolescence is as hazardous as heavy smoking in increasing the risk of dying over a 38-year period.[9] Obese children are twice as likely to die before age 55 than normal-weight youngsters; those with elevated blood sugar levels face an even greater risk of premature death.

## How Did We Get So Fat?

A variety of factors, ranging from behavior to environment to genetics, played a role in the increase in overweight and obesity. They include:

- **More calories.** Bombarded by nonstop commercials for taste treats, tempted by foods in every form to munch and crunch, in the last 30 years the average man has added 168 calories and the average woman 335 calories to their daily diets.

- **Bigger portions.** As Table 7.2 shows, the size of many popular restaurant and packaged foods has increased two to five times during the past 20 years. Some foods, like chocolate bars, have grown more than ten times since they were first introduced. Popular 64-ounce sodas can pack a whopping 800 calories. According to studies of appetite and satiety, people presented with larger portions eat up to 30 percent more than they otherwise would.

- **Fast food.** Young adults who eat frequently at fast-food restaurants gain more weight

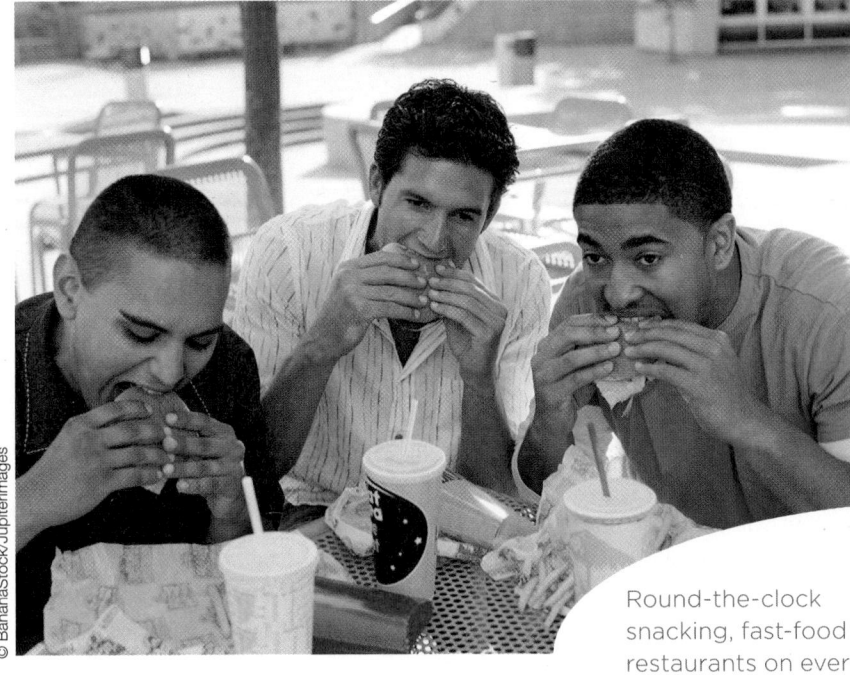

Round-the-clock snacking, fast-food restaurants on every corner, and hours in front of the TV have all contributed to the increase in overweight and obesity.

and develop metabolic abnormalities that increase their risk of diabetes in early middle age. (See discussion of fast food in Chapter 6.)

- **Physical inactivity.** As Americans eat more, they exercise less. Experts estimate that most adults expend 200 to 300 fewer calories than people did 25 years ago. The most dramatic drop in physical activity often occurs during the college years.

Table 7.2 **Supersized Portions**

| Food/Beverage | Original Size (year introduced) | Today (largest available) |
|---|---|---|
| Soda (Coca-Cola) | 6.5 oz (1916) | 34 oz |
| French fries (Burger King) | 2.6 oz (1954) | 6.9 oz |
| Hamburger (McDonald's; beef only) | 1.6 oz (1965) | 8 oz |
| Nestlé Crunch | 1.6 oz (1938) | 5 oz |
| Budweiser (bottle) | 7 oz (1976) | 40 oz |

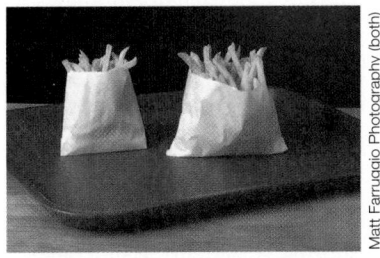
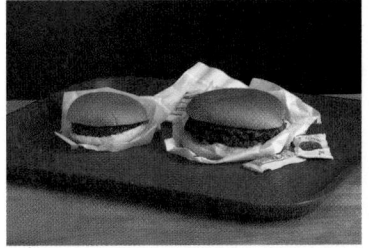

Source: "Are Growing Portion Sizes Leading to Expanding Waistlines?" American Dietetic Association, www.eatright.org.

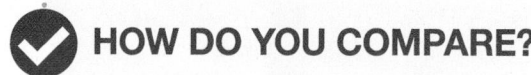

## HOW DO YOU COMPARE?

# THE WEIGHT OF STUDENT BODIES

| BMI | Male | Percent (%) Female | Total |
|---|---|---|---|
| <18.5 Underweight | 3.2 | 5.8 | 4.9 |
| 18.5–24.9 Healthy Weight | 56.2 | 64.6 | 61.6 |
| 25–29.9 Overweight | 28.3 | 18.3 | 21.9 |
| 30–39.9 Obesity | 10.9 | 9.3 | 9.9 |
| ≥40 Morbid Obesity | 1.3 | 1.9 | 1.7 |

## HOW DO YOU COMPARE?

Using the chart on page 258 in Chapter 8, determine your BMI. Which of the above categories do you fit in? Have you ever been overweight or obese? Are you now? Do you want to lose weight? Why or why not? Record your feelings on your weight today and in the past in your online journal.

Source: American College Health Association. *American College Health Association-National College Health Assessment II: Reference Group Executive Summary Spring 2010*. Linthicum, MD: American College Health Association, 2010.

**Passive entertainment.** Television is a culprit in an estimated 30 percent of new cases of obesity. TV viewing may increase weight in several ways: It takes up time that otherwise might be spent in physical activities. It increases food intake since people tend to eat more while watching TV.[10] And compared with sewing, reading, driving, or other relatively sedentary pursuits, watching television lowers metabolic rate so viewers burn fewer calories. The combination of watching television (at least two and one-half hours a day) and eating fast food more than twice a week can triple the risk of obesity.

**Genetics.** Scientists have identified a specific gene, found in one-sixth of people of European descent, that increases the risk of obesity by 30 percent or more. It also may be that various genes contribute a small increase in risk or that rare abnormalities in many genes create a predisposition to weight gain and obesity. Individuals with a family history of alcoholism—women more so than men—are more likely to become obese, perhaps because junk foods stimulate the same parts of the brain as alcohol.[11]

**Prenatal factors.** A woman's weight before conception and weight gain during pregnancy influence her child's weight. A substantial number of children are prone to gaining weight because their mothers developed gestational diabetes during their pregnancies. Children born to obese women are more than twice as likely to be overweight by age four.

**Childhood development.** Today's children don't necessarily eat more food than in the past, but they eat more high-fat, high-calorie foods and they exercise much, much less. These habits have more impact on their weight than does genetics.[12] On days when they eat fast food, youngsters consume an average of 187 more calories per day. Fewer than half of grade schoolers participate in daily physical education classes. Many spend five hours or more a day in front of a computer or television screen.

**Emotional influences.** Obese people are neither more nor less psychologically troubled than others. Psychological problems, such as irritability, depression, and anxiety, are more likely to be the result of obesity than the cause. As discussed later in this chapter, emotions do play a role in weight problems. Just as some people reach for a drink or a drug when they're upset, others cope by overeating, bingeing, or purging.

**Social networks.** Friends may have a significant effect on a person's risk of obesity.

A 32-year detailed analysis of a large social network of 12,067 people found that when one close friend became obese, the others' chances of doing the same increased by 171 percent. Young adults who are overweight or obese tend to befriend and date people who also have weight problems, according to a recent study. Researchers are not sure if overweight people seek out other overweight people or whether normal-weight individuals become heavier as a result of their relationships with people who are above-normal weight.[13] The scientists' suggestion: If you need to lose weight, join with your social contacts who also are heavy and work on shedding pounds together. (See Chapter 5, "Social Health," for further discussion.)

- **Marriage and children.** Women often blame weight gain in early adulthood on having a baby, but that is not the only influence on weight. In a study that followed young women between ages 18 and 23 for ten years, most of the women put on extra pounds but the women who remained childless and single gained least. Those who got married or moved in with a partner gained significantly more weight; those who had a child gained still more (although only with a first baby).[14]

## Living in an "Obesogenic" Environment

Is obesity an individual or a societal problem? Some experts argue that modern America has become an "obesogenic" environment that contributes to obesity by promoting overconsumption of calories and discouraging physical activity.[15] Although each of us chooses what and how much we eat and how physically active we are, environmental factors affect our choices.

Whatever your age, wherever you live, the less money you make, the more likely you are to be overweight. One in four adults below the poverty level is obese, compared with one in six in households earning $67,000 or more. Minorities are at even greater risk. One in three poor African Americans is obese.

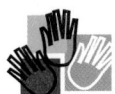 Location is important because where you live influences the availability of healthful food choices and the quality of your diet. In studies of diverse neighborhoods in Baltimore, Maryland, researchers found a much lower availability of healthful foods in predominantly black, low-income areas, compared with more affluent white ones.[16] Lower-income and minority neighborhoods generally have greater access to fast-food restaurants and high-calorie foods.[17] Obesity rates are consistently higher in neighborhoods with more small grocery stores and fast-food restaurants and fewer supermarkets.

However, suburban sprawl also directly contributes to obesity, according to research. People who live in neighborhoods where they must drive to get anywhere are significantly more likely to be obese than those who can easily walk to their destinations.

# Body Image

Throughout most of history, bigger was better. The great beauties of centuries past, as painted by such artistic masters as Rubens and Renoir, were soft and fleshy, with rounded bellies and dimpled thighs. Culture often shapes views of beauty and health.

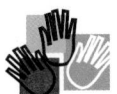 Many developing countries still regard a full figure, rather than a thin one, as the ideal. Fattening huts, in which brides-to-be eat extra food to plump up before marriage, still exist in some African cultures. Among certain Native American tribes of the Southwest, if a girl is thin at puberty, a fat woman places her foot on the girl's back so she will magically gain weight and become more attractive.

Influenced by the media, many Americans are paying more attention to their body images than ever before, but body image fluctuates throughout life. Women of all ages tend to be less satisfied with their bodies than are men. The "perfect body" ideal popularized by television, magazines, and movies can undermine a positive body image and cause girls and women to go to extreme measures to control their weight. The more time that women spend reading fashion magazines, the more "antifat" their attitudes are and the greater dissatisfaction with their bodies. Boys' body images also are influenced by media images depicting superstrong, highly muscular males.

Being overweight for a long period of time has a cumulative negative impact on body image. In a study of 266 college women, those who described themselves as "always overweight" ranked much lower in current body self-esteem than those with more recent weight problems.

 College students of different ethnic and racial backgrounds, including Asians, express as much—and sometimes more—concern about their body shape and weight as whites. In a study of university students, African American and Caucasian men were similar in their ideals for body size and in their perceptions of their own shapes. Both African American and white women perceive themselves as smaller than they actually were and desire an even smaller body size. However, African American women are more accepting of larger size.

## Male and Female Body Image

Although women generally report a more negative body image, many men are dissatisfied with their bodies but for different reasons. Often they want either to lose or gain weight or to add muscle and bulk. Women compare their appearance to that of celebrities and models as well as peers more frequently than men and worry more that others will think negatively about their looks.[18] Yet appearance matters just as much to men, who are as likely as women to engage in efforts to improve their bodies.

Women have long been bombarded by idealized images in the media of female bodies that bear little resemblance to the way most women look. Increasingly, more advertisements and men's magazines are featuring idealized male bodies. Sleek, strong, and sculpted, they do not resemble the bodies most men inhabit. The gap between reality and ideal is getting bigger for both genders. (See Chapter 8 for a discussion of "bigorexia" or muscle dysmorphia.)

College women are more likely to overestimate their weight, while men tend to underestimate their actual weight. The greater the discrepancy between a woman's current view of her body shape and the ideal she considers most attractive to men, the more likely she is to worry about how others will view her and to doubt her ability to make a desirable impression. Such "social physique anxiety" occurs often in women who feel they do not measure up to what they or others consider most desirable in terms of weight or appearance. Women with high BMIs and greater body-related anxiety may exercise to become thinner or more attractive. Those reporting the greatest distress because of body image are at highest risk of disordered eating or actual eating disorders (discussed later in this chapter).

Health educators are tackling the thorny issue of body image in various ways, including discussions of the media's role in influencing how people perceive their bodies. "Health educators should demand that airbrushed, touched up, and computer-enhanced images be replaced with those of real, beautiful women complete with freckles, stretch marks, scars, and, on occasion, cellulite," argues Catherine Rasberry of

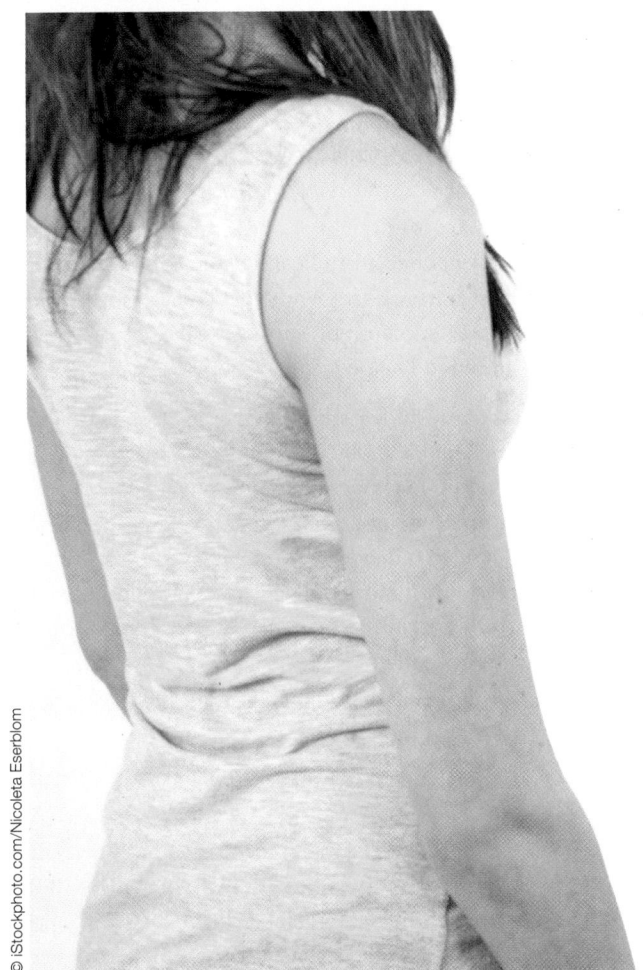

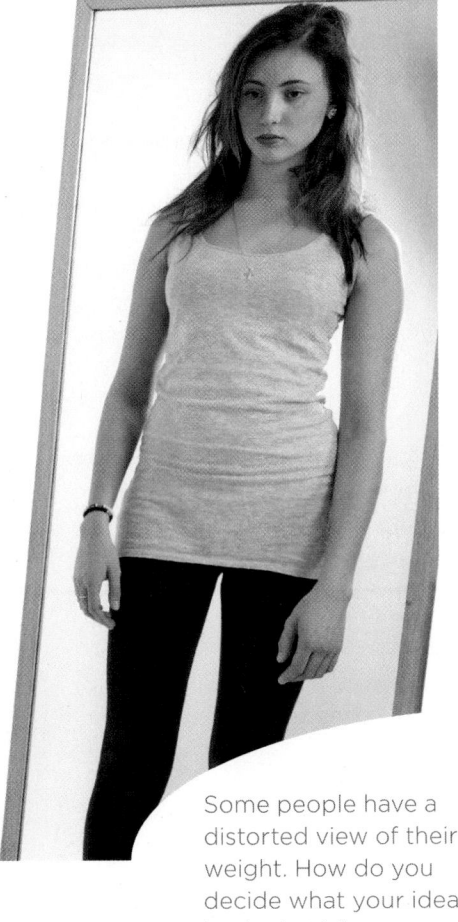

Some people have a distorted view of their weight. How do you decide what your ideal body size is?

Texas A&M University. Do you think more realistic media images would affect how you feel about your body?

## Understanding Weight Problems

Weight problems don't develop overnight. Fat accumulates meal by meal, day by day, pound by pound. Ultimately, all weight problems are the result of a prolonged energy imbalance—of consuming too many calories and burning too few in daily activities.

How many calories you need depends on your gender, age, body-frame size, weight, percentage of body fat, and your *basal metabolic rate* (BMR)—the number of calories needed to sustain your body at rest. Your activity level also affects your calorie requirements. Regardless of whether you consume fat, protein, or carbohydrates, if you take in more calories than required to maintain your size and don't work them off in some sort of physical activity, your body will convert the excess to fat.

The average American consumes about 1 million calories a year. Given that number, what difference does an extra 100-calorie soda or 300-calorie brownie make? A lot, because the extra calories that you don't burn every day accumulate, adding an average of two to four pounds to your weight every year.

### What Is a Healthy Weight?

Rather than relying on a range of ideal weights for various heights, as they did in the past, medical experts use various methods to assess body composition and weight. The best indicators of weight-related health risks are body mass index

# Hold the Line!

You can leave college a whole lot smarter but no heavier than when you entered—without spending extra money. Here are some suggestions:

- **Plan meals.** Most campus cafeterias post the week's menus in advance. Plan which items you will eat before you see or smell high-fat dishes.

- **Don't linger.** If you use the cafeteria as a social gathering place, you may end up eating with two or three different groups of people. Set a time limit to eat—then leave.

- **Develop alternative behavior.** People who eat when they are stressed or bored need substitute activities ready when they need them. Make a list of things you can do—shower, phone a friend, take a hike—when stress strikes.

- **Eat at "home."** If the dormitory has a small kitchen, cook some healthful dishes and invite friends to join you.

- **Take advantage of physical activity programs.** Many college students become less active during their years in college. Aim to maintain or increase the amount of exercise you did in high school. Join a biking club, take a salsa class, learn yoga, try tennis or racquetball.

## Weight and the College Student

Obesity rates have increased most rapidly among young adults. An estimated 43 percent of 18- to 24-year-olds are overweight or obese. One in five college students has an unhealthy weight as well as at least one risk factor for metabolic disorder, an important cause of cardiovascular disease (discussed in Chapter 15).

As many students discover, it's easy to gain weight on campuses, which are typically crammed with vending machines, fast-food counters, and cafeterias serving up hearty meals. As discussed in Chapter 6, students who eat on the run often opt for fast food and consume more fatty foods and soft drinks, which increase their risk of obesity and other health problems. However, it is possible to hold the line on calories—and costs. (See Health on a Budget.)

Only about 5 percent of students gain the legendary "freshman 15." According to an overview of recent research, from 62 to 76 percent of freshmen gain an average of 2.8 to 3.8 pounds. Percent body fat, absolute body fat, and BMI also tend to increase in the first semester at school. However, a certain percentage of incoming students—27 to 34 percent in different studies—lose weight their first year. The students who gain the most weight tend to be less physically active and sleep more than their peers.

Researchers have found gender differences in first-year weight gain. In men, increased alcohol consumption and peer pressure to drink account for extra pounds. In women, the strongest correlation of weight gain was with an increased workload, which may lead to more stress-related eating, greater snacking, or less exercise.

Sexual orientation also correlates with the weight of college women. In a recent study of female undergraduates between the ages of 18 and 25, lesbian and bisexual women were almost twice as likely to be overweight or obese as heterosexual women. The reason may be that these women have more available partners and less motivation to exercise. Studies have shown that lesbians report a lower drive for thinness and generally have a higher ideal weight than heterosexual women.[19]

(BMI); waist circumference (WC); and waist-to-hip ratio (WHR). (All are discussed in depth in Chapter 8.)

If you have a BMI higher than 25, you are **overweight** and at greater risk of health problems. If your BMI is between 30 and 34.9, you have class 1 **obesity**. If it is between 35 and 39.9, you have class 2 obesity. Both indicate increased risk of dying of weight-related problems. A BMI over 40 signifies class 3 or severe obesity and poses the greatest threat to health and longevity.

If you're a young adult, even mild to moderate overweight poses a threat to your health because it puts you at risk for gaining even more weight—and for facing greater health risks. Obesity has been implicated as a culprit in rising rates of disability among younger Americans as well as a factor in chronic health problems. If you are older than a traditional-age student, the risks to your health are more immediate.

**overweight** A condition of having a BMI between 25.0 and 29.9.

**obesity** The excessive accumulation of fat in the body; class 1 obesity is defined by a BMI between 30.0 and 34.9; class 2 obesity by a BMI between 35.0 and 39.9; class 3, or severe obesity, is a BMI of 40 or higher.

Although students do put on the most weight in their first term of college, many continue to gain weight as sophomores. Among the suspected culprits in college weight gain are alcohol, socializing that involves eating, high-fat foods in dorm cafeterias, and less physical activity.

## If You're Too Thin: How to Gain Weight

Being underweight is not an uncommon problem, particularly among adolescent and young adult men as well as among those who diet excessively or suffer from an eating disorder (discussed later in this chapter). If you lose weight suddenly and don't know the reason, talk to a doctor. Rapid weight loss can be an early symptom of a health problem.

If you're trying to put on pounds, you need to do the opposite of dieters: Consume more calories than you burn. But as with losing weight, you should try to gain weight in healthy ways. Here are some suggestions:

- **Eat more of a variety of foods** rather than more high-fat, high-calorie foods. Get no more than 30 percent of your daily calories from fat. A higher percentage poses a threat to your heart and your health.

- **If your appetite is small, eat more frequently.** Try for five or six smaller meals rather than a big lunch and dinner.

- **Choose some calorie-rich foods,** such as dried fruits rather than fresh ones. Add nuts and cheese to salads and main dishes.

- **Drink juice** rather than regular or diet soda.

- **Try adding a commercial liquid meal** replacement as a snack.

- **Exercise regularly** to build up both appetite and muscle.

## Health Dangers of Excess Weight

The federal government has recognized obesity as a serious, potentially fatal disease. This designation cleared the way for insurance coverage for obesity treatments, rather than just for the medical problems it can cause.

The effects of obesity on health are the equivalent of 20 years of aging. They include increased risk of cardiovascular disease, diabetes, and cancer, as well as rheumatoid arthritis, sleep apnea, gout, and liver disease (Figure 7.1). Being overweight or obese at age 25 increases your likelihood of difficulties in walking, balance, and rising from a chair. Obesity, according to recent analysis, robs people of about 2.5 healthy, pain-free years.[20] Total medical costs, both direct and indirect, amount to more than $117 billion a year.

Obesity kills. Researchers attribute 112,000 to 280,000 deaths every year to excess weight. Your weight in early adulthood and middle age can have an impact on how long and how well you live. Life expectancy at age 20 is five years less for someone who is obese. Obesity may be responsible for one-fifth to one-third of the life expectancy gap between the United States and other developed countries.[21]

***The Impact on the Body*** The incidence of diabetes, gallstones, hypertension, heart disease, and colon cancer increases with the degree of overweight in both sexes. Those with BMIs of 35 or more are approximately 20 times more likely to develop diabetes. Overweight men and women are at least three times more likely to suffer knee injuries that require surgery to repair.

Health risks may vary in different races, ethnic groups, and at-risk populations. Even relatively small amounts of excess fat—as little as five pounds—can add to the dangers in those already at risk for hypertension and diabetes. Obesity also causes alterations in various measures of immune function and increases the risk of kidney stones and disease. It may also affect the brain and contribute to cognitive problems and dementia.

Overweight young adults have a 70 percent chance of becoming overweight or obese adults. They are two to three times more likely to have high total cholesterol levels and more than 43 times more likely to have cardiovascular disease risk factors such as elevated blood pressure. They also have a higher prevalence of type 2 diabetes.

Excess pounds affect people around the clock. Overweight and obese individuals sleep less than those with normal weights. The lost sleep

## The Impact of Obesity

The obesity epidemic is affecting many aspects of our society, from health care costs to food labeling to longevity. Get a sense of the impact of obesity in the United States by researching the topic on Global Health Watch. Access the latest research on the "Healthy Weight" portal (Health and Wellness → Healthy Weight → Obesity). Look at the articles in the Latest News feed. What are the latest developments in this area? Does obesity affect you personally? Use the articles and your personal experience with obesity to write a journal entry.

Figure 7.1 **Health Dangers of Excess Weight**

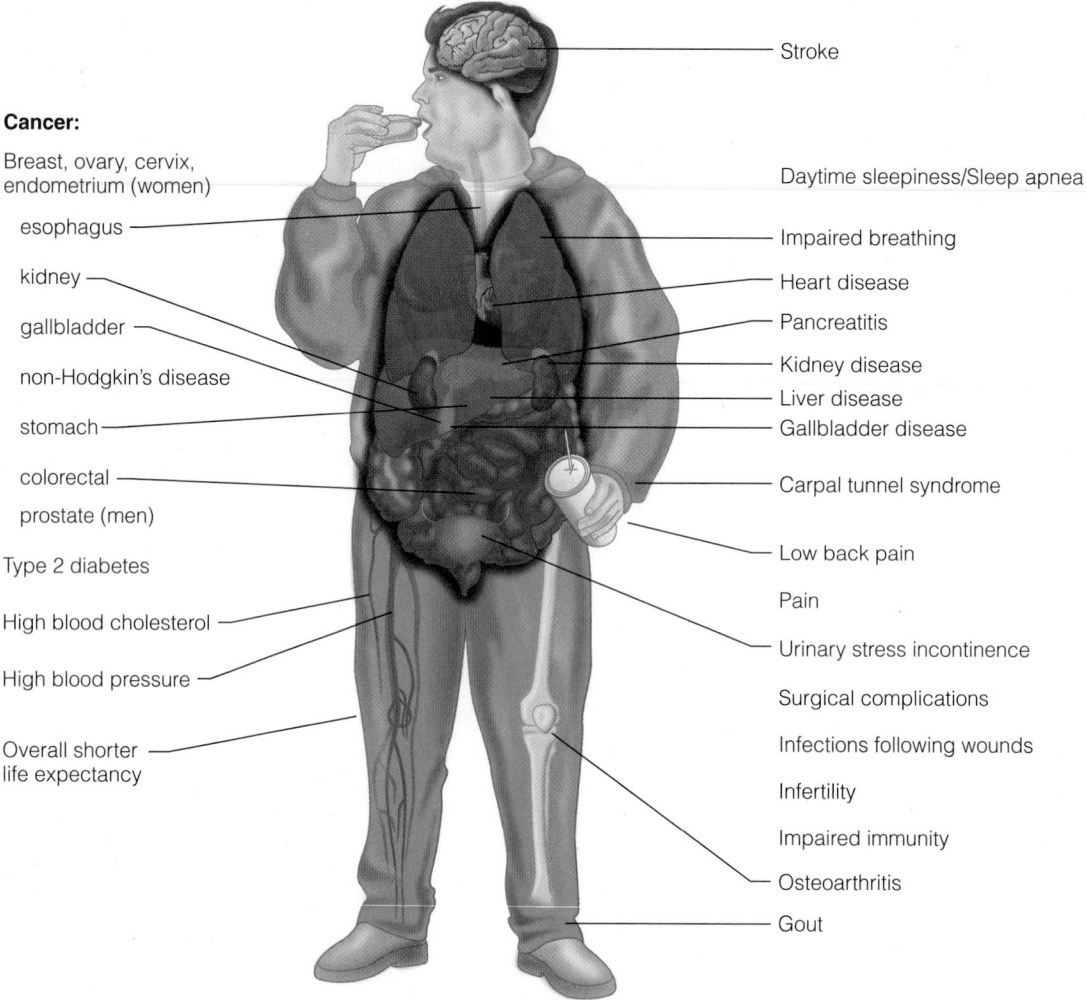

**Cancer:**

Breast, ovary, cervix, endometrium (women)

esophagus

kidney

gallbladder

non-Hodgkin's disease

stomach

colorectal

prostate (men)

Type 2 diabetes

High blood cholesterol

High blood pressure

Overall shorter life expectancy

Stroke

Daytime sleepiness/Sleep apnea

Impaired breathing

Heart disease

Pancreatitis

Kidney disease

Liver disease

Gallbladder disease

Carpal tunnel syndrome

Low back pain

Pain

Urinary stress incontinence

Surgical complications

Infections following wounds

Infertility

Impaired immunity

Osteoarthritis

Gout

could add to the risk of medical problems. (See Chapter 2 for a discussion of sleep.) The lost sleep could add to the risk of medical problems.

Major diseases linked to obesity include:

- **Type 2 diabetes.** More than 80 percent of people with type 2 diabetes are overweight. Although the reasons are not known, being overweight may make cells less efficient at using sugar from the blood. This then puts stress on the cells that produce insulin (a hormone that carries sugar from the blood to cells) and makes them gradually fail. You can lower your risk for developing type 2 diabetes by losing weight and increasing the amount of physical activity you do. If you have type 2 diabetes, losing weight and becoming more physically active can help you control your blood sugar levels and may allow you to reduce the amount of diabetes medication you take.

- **Heart disease and stroke.** People who are overweight are more likely to suffer from high blood pressure, high levels of triglycerides (blood fats) and harmful LDL cholesterol, and low levels of beneficial HDL cholesterol. In addition, people with more body fat have higher blood levels of substances that cause inflammation, which may raise heart disease risk. Losing 5 to 15 percent of your weight can lower your chances for developing heart disease or having a stroke. Obese men face a much greater risk of dying from a heart attack, regardless of whether they have other risk factors.[22]

People who both smoke and are obese are at especially high risk of cardiovascular disease.

Although some smokers have felt that they couldn't lose weight until they stopped smoking, researchers have found that weight loss among smokers is possible and beneficial, leading to a reduction in other risk factors, such as lower blood pressure and lower cholesterol.

- **Cancer.** Obesity contributes to more than 100,000 cases of cancer—among them cancers of the endometrium, esophagus, pancreas, gallbladder, kidney, breast, and colon—in the United States every year. Excess weight may account for 14 percent of all cancer deaths in men and 20 percent of those in women. Losing weight, researchers estimate, could prevent as many as one of every six cancer deaths.

Body size and higher BMI are linked with increased risk of breast cancer in premenopausal women and in postmenopausal women not using hormone replacement therapy. Women who are overweight or obese tend to have more aggressive cancers and lower survival rates.[23]

*The Emotional Toll* In our calorie-conscious and thinness-obsessed society, obesity also affects quality of life, including sense of vitality and physical pain. Many see it as a psychological burden, a sign of failure, laziness, or inadequate willpower. Overweight men and women often blame themselves for becoming heavy and feel guilty and depressed as a result. In fact, the psychological problems once considered the cause of obesity may be its consequence.

Obesity also has social consequences. Heavy women are less likely to marry, earn less, and have lower rates of college graduation. In a recent study, obese individuals who felt discriminated against because of their weight developed more physical problems over time than those who did not.[24]

# A Practical Guide to Weight Loss

More than half of college women and about a third of college men intend to lose weight. Readiness to change is the key to successful weight loss. However, individuals vary in their readiness to change their diets, increase their physical activity, and seek professional counseling. Take the Self Survey at the end of this chapter to determine your readiness to lose weight.

## Why We Overeat

The answer lies not just in the belly but in the brain. Both **hunger**, the physiological drive to consume food, and **appetite**, the psychological desire to eat, influence and control our desire for food. Scientists have discovered appetite receptors within the brain that specifically respond to hunger messages carried by hormones produced in the digestive tract (Figure 7.2).

Although usually a direct result of hunger, appetite is easily led into temptation. In one famous experiment, psychologists bought high-calorie goodies—peanut butter, marshmallows, chocolate-chip cookies, and salami—for their test rats. The animals ate so much on this "supermarket diet" that they gained more weight than any laboratory rats ever had before. The snack-food diet that fattened up these rats was particularly high in fats. Biologists speculate that creamy, buttery, or greasy foods may cause internal changes that increase appetite and, consequently, weight.

**hunger** The physiological drive to consume food.

**appetite** A desire for food, stimulated by anticipated hunger, physiological changes within the brain and body, the availability of food, and other environmental and psychological factors.

Figure 7.2 **Hormones Help Regulate Our Appetites**

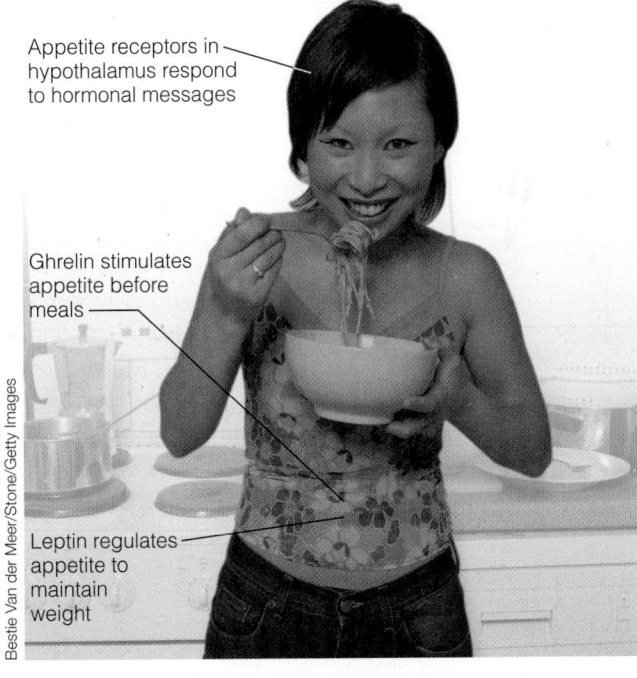

Appetite receptors in hypothalamus respond to hormonal messages

Ghrelin stimulates appetite before meals

Leptin regulates appetite to maintain weight

Bestie Van der Meer/Stone/Getty Images

A hormone called leptin, produced by fat cells, sends signals that regulate appetite to the brain. When leptin levels are normal, people eat just enough to maintain weight. When leptin is low, the brain responds as if fat stores had been depleted and slows down metabolism. This may be one reason why it is so difficult to lose weight by dieting alone. However, vigorous exercise can lower the hormone ghrelin, which is a natural appetite stimulant. When given shots of ghrelin, people become very hungry and eat 30 percent more than they normally would. Ghrelin typically rises before meals and falls afterward. Dieters tend to have high levels of ghrelin, as if their bodies were trying to stimulate appetite so they regain lost fat.

We usually stop eating when we feel satisfied; this is called **satiety**, a feeling of fullness and relief from hunger. The neurotransmitter serotonin has been shown to produce feelings of satiety. In addition, several peptides, released from the digestive tract as we ingest food, may signal the brain to stop or restrict eating. However, it takes 20 minutes for the brain to register fullness.

Many people eat without regard for their bodies' signals. This "non-hunger" or "emotional" eating is almost always overeating, since it's eating for reasons other than sustenance. The psychological aspect of overeating is discussed later in the chapter.

## Weight Loss Diets

The diet debates over low-fat versus low-carbohydrate versus high-protein have raged for years. Which is best? Several studies over recent years found little difference in the ultimate results. It doesn't matter whether you count carbohydrates, protein, or fat—as long as you eat less.

Although people lose weight on any diet that helps them eat less, most dieters only lose about 5 percent of their initial weight and gain some of that back. However, even a modest weight loss can lower cardiovascular risk factors, such as blood pressure, total cholesterol, and elevated blood glucose.[25]

Although a variety of dietary approaches will result in weight loss and reduce cardiac risk factors, individuals who have been identified as insulin-resistant may lose more weight, at least in the short term, from a high-protein, low-carbohydrate rather than a low-fat diet.[26] Medical researchers do not fully understand why this is so. It could be that increased protein promotes weight loss by inducing satiety and increasing energy expenditure.[27] It is still not clear whether high-protein, low-carbohydrate diets are safe for very long periods.[28]

In a large-scale European study that compared more than a thousand overweight individuals on different diets, the greatest long-term success—in terms of sticking with the diet and maintaining weight loss—came with a modest increase in protein and a modest reduction in carbohydrates and the glycemic index (discussed in Chapter 6).[29]

Following is a brief overview of some of the current approaches to dieting.

### High-Carbohydrate, Low-Fat (Ornish)

The basic principle of Dr. Dean Ornish's approach is that by strictly limiting fat (whether animal or vegetable) by eating high-fiber, low-fat foods, you eat fewer calories without eating less food.

**Promise**

- Weight loss plus significant health benefits, including lower blood pressure and cholesterol.

**Pitfalls**

- Many people find low-fat diets so unsatisfying that they cannot stay on them.

- The diet limits the healthy fats in fish, nuts, and olive oil.

- With so little fat, some people may not get adequate essential fatty acids.

### Low-Carbohydrate, High-Protein (Atkins)

The late Dr. Robert Atkins theorized that eating too many carbohydrates could create a metabolic imbalance that leads to overweight or obesity. Restricting carbohydrates corrects these imbalances so people can lose weight without having to eat fewer calories.

**Promise**

- Quick, short-term weight loss without hunger.

**satiety** A feeling of fullness after eating.

**Pitfalls**

- Severe restriction of carbohydrates can induce ketosis, which is caused by an incomplete breakdown of fats that can lead to nausea, fatigue, and light-headedness and can worsen kidney disease and other medical problems.

- The plan is so rigid, restrictive, and complicated that many find it hard to follow.

- There is no sound scientific basis for the diet's health claims.

### Carbohydrate-Modified (South Beach)

This diet encourages eating "good carbohydrates," such as vegetables, whole-wheat pasta, and brown rice, in order to feel full and resist cravings for "bad carbs," such as potatoes and white rice.

**Promise**

- Enhanced health due to emphasis on nutritious foods such as fish, lean meats, vegetables, and unsaturated oils and restriction on fatty meats, cheeses, and sweets.

**Pitfalls**

- The complete exclusion of starchy carbohydrates and all fruits during the first two weeks is difficult for many people.

### Low-Calorie (Weight Watchers)

Nothing is forbidden on this diet. Instead, a point system assigns a value to portions of all sorts of foods, and dieters track the number of points taken in every day.

**Promise**

- Steady weight loss with portion control and moderation.

**Pitfalls**

- Hunger makes the diet hard to maintain.
- Low-carb diets may impair memory and cognition.
- A high-fat diet may increase the long-term risk of heart disease and some cancers.

### Low-Carbohydrate (Zone)

The premise of this approach is that eating the correct proportions of carbohydrates, fat, and protein leads to hormonal balance, weight loss, greater vitality, and less risk of disease.

**Promise**

- Quick weight loss because of low calorie intake.

**Pitfalls**

- Hunger makes the diet hard to maintain.

## How to Design a Diet

There is no one perfect diet that will work for everyone who needs to lose weight. "Experiment with various methods for weight control," suggests Dr. Walter Willett of the Harvard School of Public Health. "Patients should focus on finding ways to eat that they can maintain indefinitely rather than seeking diets that promote rapid weight loss." In other words, design an eating plan that you can stick with for the rest of your life.

Whether you decide to focus on carbohydrates, fat, or calories, the following strategies can help you get to and maintain a healthy weight:

- **Avoid "bad" fats,** including trans-fatty acids and partially hydrogenated fats.

- **Consume "good" fats, such as omega-3 fatty acids,** every day.

- **Eat fewer "bad" carbohydrates,** such as sugar and white flour.

- **Eat more "good" carbs,** including fruits, vegetables, legumes, and unrefined grains like whole-wheat flour and brown rice.

- **Opt for quality over quantity.** Eating a smaller amount of something delicious and nutritious can be far more satisfying than larger portions of junk foods.

- **Exercise more.** The key to balancing the equation between calories consumed and calories used is physical activity.

- **Eliminate sweetened soft drinks** and drink water instead.

## Avoiding Diet Traps

Whatever your eating style, there are only two effective strategies for losing weight: eating less and exercising more. Unfortunately, most people search for easier alternatives that almost invariably turn into dietary dead ends or unexpected dangers (see Consumer Alert). Common traps to avoid are very-low-calorie diets, diet pills, diet foods, and the yo-yo syndrome. Among young people the most successful weight loss strategies include drinking less soda, eating less junk food, drinking more water, increasing physical activity, weighing themselves regularly, adding more protein to their diets, and watching less television.

*Over-the-Counter Diet Pills* An estimated 15 percent of adults—21 percent of women and 10 percent of men—have used weight loss supplements. Women between ages 18 and 34 are the highest users. In the 1920s, some women swallowed patented weight loss capsules that turned out to be tapeworm eggs. In the 1960s and 1970s, addictive amphetamines were common diet aids. In the 1990s, appetite suppressants known as fen-phen became popular but were taken off the market after being linked to heart valve problems.

In the last decade dieters tried ephedra products for weight loss, but a major study reported more than 16,000 adverse events associated with the use of ephedra-containing dietary supplements, including heart palpitations, tremors, and insomnia. The study also found little evidence that ephedra is effective in boosting physical activities and weight loss. The Food and Drug Administration has prohibited the sale of dietary supplements containing ephedra, because they present an unreasonable risk of illness or injury.

The weight loss prescription drug Orlistat is available as an over-the-counter weight loss pill called Alli. The drug, which blocks about a quarter of the fat consumed, works best with a low-fat diet. If dieters eat a meal made up of more than 15 fat grams, they can suffer nasty side effects, including flatulence, an urgent need to defecate, oily stools, and diarrhea.

*Diet Foods* According to the Calorie Control Council, 90 percent of Americans choose some foods labeled "light." But even though these foods keep growing in popularity, Americans' weight keeps rising. There are several reasons: Many people think choosing a food that's lower in calories, fat-free, or light gives them a license to eat as much as they want. What they don't realize is that many foods that are low in fat are still high in sugar and calories. Refined carbohydrates, rapidly absorbed into the bloodstream, raise blood glucose levels. As those levels fall, appetite increases.

Diet products, including diet sodas and low-fat foods, are a very big business. Many people rely

on meal replacements, usually shakes or snack bars, to lose or keep off weight. If used appropriately—as actual replacements rather than supplements to regular meals and snacks—they can be a useful strategy for weight loss. Yet people who use these products often gain weight because they think that they can afford to add high-calorie treats to their diets.

What about the artificial sweeteners and fake fats that appear in many diet products? Nutritionists caution to use them in moderation and not to substitute them for basic foods, such as grains, fruits, and vegetables. Foods made with fat substitutes may have fewer grams of fat, but they don't necessarily have significantly fewer calories. Many people who consume reduced-fat, fat-free, or sugar-free sodas, cookies, chips, and other snacks often cut back on more nutritious foods, such as fruits and vegetables. They also tend to eat more of the low- or no-fat foods so that their daily calorie intake either stays the same or actually increases.

*The Yo-Yo Syndrome* On-and-off-again dieting, especially by means of very-low-calorie diets (under 800 calories a day), can be self-defeating and dangerous. Some studies have shown that weight cycling may make it more difficult to lose weight or keep it off (Figure 7.3). Repeated cycles of rapid weight loss followed by weight gain may even change food preferences. Chronic crash dieters often come to prefer foods that combine sugar and fat, such as cake frosting.

To avoid the yo-yo syndrome and overcome its negative effects: Exercise. Researchers at the University of Pennsylvania found that when overweight women who also exercised went off a very-low-calorie diet, their metabolism did not stay slow but bounced back to the appropriate level for their new, lower body weight. The reason may be exercise's ability to preserve muscle tissue. The more muscle tissue you have, the higher your metabolic rate.

If you've been losing (and regaining) the same five or ten pounds for years, try the following suggestions for long-term success:

- **Set a danger zone.** Once you've reached your desired weight, don't let your weight climb more than three or four pounds higher. Take into account normal fluctuations, but watch out for an upward trend. Once you hit your upper weight limit, take action immediately rather than waiting until you gain ten pounds.
- **Be patient.** Think of weight loss as a road trip. If you're going across town, you expect to get there in 20 minutes. If your destination is 400 miles away, you know it'll take

## Figure 7.3 **Weight Cycling Effect of Repeated Dieting**
Each round of dieting is typically followed by a rebound leading to a greater weight gain.

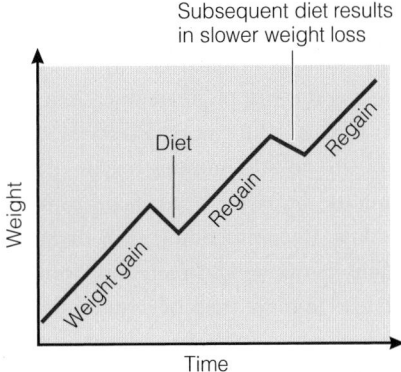

longer. Give yourself the time you need to lose weight safely and steadily.

- **Try, try again.** Dieters don't usually keep weight off on their first attempt. The people who eventually succeed don't give up. Through trial and error, they find a plan that works for them.

However, in the long run, dieting usually doesn't keep off excess pounds. Regardless of the diets they follow, people lose only about 5 percent of their initial weight after one year. Even in programs that provide intensive counseling by doctors, nurses, or dietitians, participants regain about half the weight they lost within three years. Five years after a successful diet, they typically have put on all the weight they lost. What can keep off extra pounds for good? A minimum of 200–300 minutes of exercise a week.

## Physical Activity

Unplanned daily activity, such as fidgeting or pacing, can make a difference in preventing weight gain. Scientists use the acronym **NEAT**—for **nonexercise activity thermogenesis**—to describe such "nonvolitional" movement, which may be an effective way of burning calories. In research on self-confessed couch potatoes, the thinner ones sat an average of two hours less and moved and stood more often than the heavier individuals. However, NEAT levels seem at least partially genetically predetermined.

**NEAT (nonexercise activity thermogenesis)** Nonvolitional movement that can be an effective way of burning calories.

Although physical activity and exercise can prevent weight gain and improve health, usually they do not lead to significant weight loss. However, when combined with diet, exercise ensures that you lose fat rather than muscle, helps keep off excess pounds, and promotes greater fitness. Moderate exercise, such as 30 to 60 minutes of daily physical activity, has proved effective in reducing the risk of heart disease and other health threats. But more exercise—a minimum of 200 to 300 minutes weekly of moderately intense activity—is necessary to maintain weight loss. Recommending such higher levels of activity to overweight men and women does indeed lead to more exercise—and more lasting weight loss.

Exercise has other benefits: It increases energy expenditure, builds up muscle tissue, burns off fat stores, and stimulates the immune system. Exercise also may reprogram metabolism so that more calories are burned during and after a workout.

An exercise program designed for both health benefits and weight loss should include both aerobic activity and resistance training. (See Chapter 8.) People who start and stick with an exercise program during or after a weight loss program are consistently more successful in keeping off most of the pounds they've shed.

***Can a Person Be Fat and Fit?*** Most people assume that fitness comes in only one size: small. That's not necessarily so. There is considerable controversy over how to define a healthy weight. But individuals of every size can improve their physical fitness.

Physical fitness can buffer some, but not all, of the ill effects of obesity. Individuals who are both overweight and sedentary face the greatest risk of disease and premature death. Those who are obese but physically active can be healthier, in many ways, than sedentary individuals whose weight is considered healthy. But working out cannot overcome all the dangers of weighing too much. In a recent study that followed participants for 30 years, overweight and obese men were at higher risk of suffering a heart attack or stroke and of dying from such a cardiovascular event than normal-weight men. "There appears to be no such thing as metabolically healthy obesity," the authors concluded.[30]

# The Psychology of Losing Weight

Diets change what you eat. Exercise changes body composition, stamina, and strength. But changing your food-related thoughts and behaviors can be the key to lasting weight loss. If you think that you can shed pounds, if you think that you can control what you put in your mouth, if you think that there is a form of exercise that you could enjoy, then you are on your way to reaching your weight loss goals. (See "Health in Action: Thinking Thinner.")

## Get a Grip on Emotional Eating

Occasionally all of us seek comfort at the tip of a spoon. However, many people use food as a way of coping with anger, frustration, stress, boredom, or fatigue. Whatever its motivation, emotional eating always involves eating for reasons other than physiological hunger. If you're not sure whether you do this, ask yourself the following questions:

- Do you eat when you're not hungry?
- Do you eat or continue eating even if the food doesn't taste good?
- Do you eat when you can't think of anything else to do?
- Do you eat when you're emotionally vulnerable—tired, frustrated, or worried?
- Do you eat after an argument or stressful situation to calm down?
- Do you eat as one of your favorite ways of enjoying yourself?
- Do you eat to reward yourself?
- Do you keep eating even after you're full?

If you answer yes to more than three of these, you're eating in response to what you feel, not what you need. Diets may work for you, but the extra weight will inevitably creep back unless you confront your hidden motives for overeating. Since neither emotions nor food ever go away, you have to learn to deal with both for as long as you live.

To get a grip on your emotional eating, try this three-step plan:

**Step 1: Know Your Triggers**  Whatever its specific motivation, emotional eating always involves eating for reasons other than physiological hunger. The key to getting it under control is awareness.

Did any of these possibilities hit home? If so, train yourself to take a step back and ask yourself a series of questions before you take a bite: Are you hungry? If not, what are you feeling? Stressed, tired, bored, anxious, sad, happy? Once you identify your true feeling, push deeper and ask why you feel this way. Try writing down your answers in a notebook. This is an even more effective way to help make sure that every bite you take is a conscious one.

**Step 2: Put Your Body, Not Your Emotions, in Charge of What You Eat**  To keep mind and body on an even keel, avoid getting so hungry and feeling so deprived that you become desperate and panicky. If you're facing an emotionally intense period—exam week or a visit from an ornery relative—plan your meals and snacks in advance and try, as much as you can, to stick with your program.

**Step 3: Focus on Your Feelings**  Let yourself feel how you're feeling without eating. Breathe deeply for a minute or two. Focus on the places in your body that feel tense. Rate the intensity of the emotion on a scale from ten (life or death) to one (truly trivial). Ask yourself: What's the worst-case scenario of feeling this way? Is food going to make it better in any way? Will it make it worse?

# Maintaining Weight Loss

Surveys of people who lost significant amounts of weight and kept it off for several years show that most did so on their own—without medication, meal substitutes, or membership in an organized weight loss group. When a National Institutes of Health panel reviewed 48 separate weight loss trials, they found that participants lost about 8 percent of their body weight on average and kept it off. "Weight loss

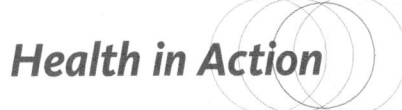

## Health in Action

### Thinking Thinner

Do you ease onto your scale, hoping for a certain number to appear—maybe what you weighed when you graduated from high school? If so, you may be setting yourself up for disappointment. Rather than focus on just one number, consider other ways to think about weight:

| | |
|---|---|
| "If-only weight" | A weight you would choose if you could weigh whatever you wanted—just like the height or eye color you'd have chosen if you could |
| "Happy weight" | A weight that is not the one you'd choose as your ideal but that you'd be happy with |
| "Acceptable weight" | A weight that would not make you particularly happy but that you could be satisfied with |
| "Disappointed weight" | A weight that would not be acceptable |
| "Never-again weight" | The all-time high you never want to hit again. |

In your online journal, jot down your if-only weight, happy weight, acceptable weight, disappointed weight, and never-again weight. Then write down your actual weight, as of today. How many pounds is your real weight from your acceptable weight?

Assuming you can lose a pound a week, how many weeks would it take to get to that weight? How do you envision yourself feeling and behaving once you reach your acceptable weight? Do you have any plans once you reach your acceptable weight, such as buying clothes or taking a weekend trip? How will your life be different?

You can find the complete "Thinking Thinner" lab in *Labs for Invitation to Personal Change.*

maintainers" are more active, have fewer TVs in their homes, and don't keep high-fat foods in their pantries.

Rather than focusing on why dieters fail, the creators of the National Weight Control Registry study the habits and lifestyles of those who've maintained a weight loss of at least 30 pounds for at least a year. The nearly 6,000 people in the registry have maintained their weight loss for almost six years.

No one diet or commercial weight loss program helped all these formerly overweight individuals. Many, through years of trial and error, eventually came up with a permanent exercise and eating program that worked for them. Despite the immense variety, their customized approaches share certain characteristics:

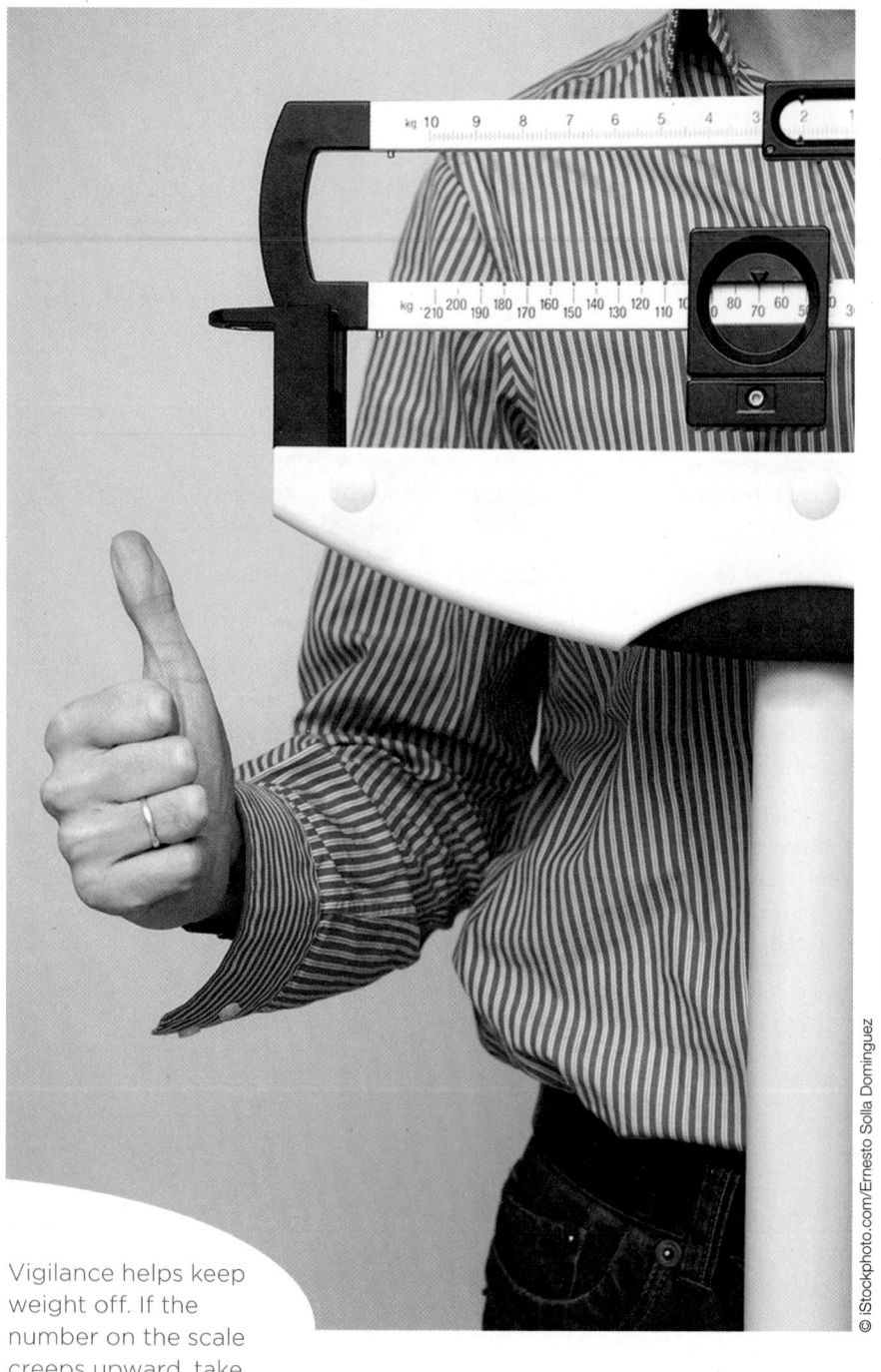

Vigilance helps keep weight off. If the number on the scale creeps upward, take action immediately.

On average, they burn about 2,545 calories per week through physical activity.

- **Monitoring.** About 44 percent of registry members count calories, and almost all keep track of their food intake in some way, written or not.

- **Vigilance.** Rather than avoiding the scale or telling themselves their jeans shrank in the wash, successful losers keep tabs on their weight and size. About a third check the scale every week. If the scale notches upward or their waistbands start to pinch, they take action.

- **Breakfast.** Although about eight in ten successful dieters in the registry always eat breakfast, recent research has challenged the impact of a morning meal on total calories consumed during the day. In one study, both normal-weight and obese individuals who ate a high-calorie breakfast consumed more calories throughout the day.[31] The key to weight loss success may be monitoring calorie intake at every meal of the day.

# Treating Severe Obesity

The biggest Americans are getting bigger. The prevalence of severe or "morbid" obesity is increasing faster than obesity itself. The number of extremely obese adults—those at least 100 pounds overweight with BMIs over 40—has quadrupled in the last two decades from 1 in 200 to about 1 in every 50 men and women. The number with BMIs greater than 50 has jumped from 1 in 2,000 in the 1980s to 1 in 400.

Extreme obesity poses extreme danger to health and survival and undermines quality of life. White women report more impairment than men or African American women, even when they have lower BMIs. Severe obesity also has a profound effect on every aspect of an adolescent's life.

## Drug Therapy

Obesity medications are recommended only for patients with BMIs equal to or greater than 30 or those with a BMI equal to or greater than 27 with risk factors (like high blood pressure) that

- **Personal responsibility for change.** Weight loss winners develop an internal locus of control. Rather than blaming others for their weight problem or relying on a doctor or trainer to fix it, they believe that the keys to a healthy weight lie within themselves.

- **Exercise.** Registry members report an hour of moderate physical activity almost every day. Their favorite exercise? Three in four say walking, followed by cycling, weight lifting, aerobics, running, and stair climbing.

increase their risk of disease. Researchers are experimenting with other medications, such as rimonabant and the epilepsy drug zonisamide, to enhance weight loss. Currently, only two weight loss drugs are FDA approved.

Xenical (orlistat) (also available in a lower dose as the over-the-counter drug Alli) blocks fat absorption by the gut but also inhibits absorption of water and vitamins in some patients and may cause cramping and diarrhea. It produces a weight loss of 2 to 3 percent of initial weight beyond the weight lost by dieting over the course of a year.

Meridia (sibutramine) is in the same chemical class as amphetamines and works by suppressing appetite. It also may increase blood pressure, heart rate, or both. Other side effects include headache, insomnia, dry mouth, and constipation. Patients taking these drugs generally lose less than 10 percent of their body weight, and many regain weight after they stop treatment.

## Obesity Surgery

Obesity, or bariatric, surgery is becoming the most popular weight loss approach for the estimated 15 million men and women who qualify as "morbidly obese" (100 or more pounds overweight) because of their increased health risks. This year as many as 200,000 Americans will undergo obesity surgery—four times the number who did so in 2000. Eight in ten are women. A growing number are teenagers, although adolescents make up less than 1 percent of patients having such procedures. According to the Agency for Healthcare Research and Quality, three in four bariatric patients lose 50 to 75 percent of their excess weight within two years and keep it off.

As recent research has shown, bariatric surgery eliminates or improves diabetes, high cholesterol, hypertension, and sleep apnea, and reduces patients' odds of dying by nearly half. Weight loss surgery also may "remodel" the heart so it returns to more normal functioning.[32] However, these operations—particularly in the hands of poorly trained or inexperienced surgeons—pose serious risks, including potentially fatal leaks, infection, bleeding, hernias, and pneumonia. According to federal estimates, four in ten patients suffer complications within six months. The mortality rate averages about

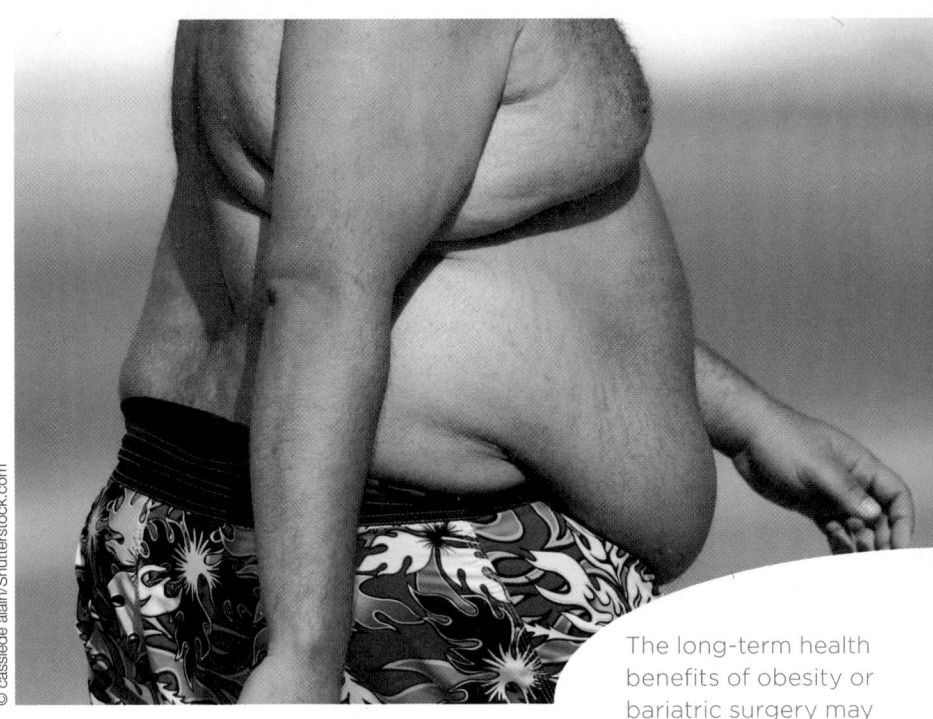

© cassiede alain/Shutterstock.com

The long-term health benefits of obesity or bariatric surgery may outweigh the risks for individuals who are "morbidly obese" (100 or more pounds overweight).

two deaths in 1,000 operations. Even with excellent medical results, extreme weight loss creates drapes of excess skin that sag over the belly, buttocks, thighs, breasts, or upper arms.

Long-term dangers—both physical and psychological—are unknown, particularly for adolescents. Following gastric bypass surgery, obese teenagers lose weight and no longer suffer from diabetes, according to recent research. The benefits extend beyond the physical, with many reporting better psychological health and social ease.

The two most common types of procedures are:

- **Gastric bypass.** Surgeons create an egg-sized pouch with staples and reroute food around part of the upper intestine to block absorption of calories and nutrients. About 75 percent of bypass patients lose 50 to 75 percent of their excess weight within two years. For the "super obese," a more extensive procedure that bypasses most of the small intestine can lead to a loss of 80 percent of excess weight. However, the latter procedure carries the highest risks of complications, including serious vitamin and mineral deficiencies. Too little thiamine, for instance, can lead to a serious neurological condition called Wernicke encephalopathy.

- **Banding.** In this newer, less risky procedure, surgeons slip an inflatable silicon band around the stomach; it can be tightened or loosened at a doctor's office without the need for further surgery. Patients lose about 40 to 55 percent of excess weight but may be more likely to regain lost pounds. The band also may slip or erode.

The individuals most likely to benefit from obesity surgery generally:

- Have a body mass index over 40.

- Have a BMI over 35 and a serious obesity-related problem, such as type 2 diabetes or severe sleep apnea (when breathing stops for brief periods during sleep).

- Have made repeated unsuccessful attempts to lose weight.

- Do not have any significant or untreated psychological problems.

- Are well-informed about the risks of the surgery.

- Recognize the need for lifestyle changes and daily vitamin and mineral supplements.

# Unhealthy Eating Behavior

Unhealthy eating behavior takes many forms, ranging from not eating enough to eating too much too quickly. Its roots are complex. In addition to media and external pressures, family history can play a role. Researchers have linked specific genes to some cases of anorexia nervosa and binge eating, but most believe that a variety of factors, including stress and culture, combine to cause disordered eating.

Sooner or later many people don't eat the way they should. They may skip meals, thereby increasing the likelihood that they'll end up with more body fat, a higher weight, and a higher blood cholesterol level. They may live on diet foods, but consume so much of them that they gain weight anyway. Some even engage in more extreme eating behavior: Dissatisfied with almost all aspects of their appearance, they continuously go on and off diets, eat compulsively, or binge on high-fat treats. Such behaviors can be warning signs of potentially serious eating disorders that should not be ignored.

## Unhealthy Eating in College Students

 College students—particularly women, including varsity athletes—are at risk for unhealthy eating behaviors. Researchers estimate that only about a third of college women maintain healthy eating patterns.[33] Some college women have full-blown eating disorders; others develop "partial syndromes" and experience symptoms that are not severe or numerous enough for a diagnosis of anorexia nervosa or bulimia nervosa. Distress over body image increases the risk of all forms of disordered eating in college women.

 In a survey at a large, public, rural university in the mid-Atlantic states, 17 percent of the women were struggling with disordered eating. Younger women (ages 18 to 21) were more likely than older students to have an eating disorder. In this study, eating disorders did not discriminate, equally affecting women of different races (white, Asian, African American, Native American, and Hispanic), religions, athletic involvement, and living arrangements (on or off campus; with roommates, boyfriends, or family). Although the students viewed eating disorders as both mental and physical problems and felt that individual therapy would be most helpful, all said that they would first turn to a friend for help. Women in sororities are at slightly increased risk of an eating disorder compared with those in dormitories. Loneliness also has emerged as a risk factor for eating disorders in college women.

## Extreme Dieting

Extreme dieters go beyond cutting back on calories or increasing physical activity. They become preoccupied with what they eat and weigh. Although their weight never falls below 85 percent of normal, their weight loss is severe enough to cause uncomfortable physical consequences, such as weakness and sensitivity to cold. Technically, these dieters do not have anorexia nervosa (discussed later in this chapter), but they are at increased risk for it.

Extreme dieters may think they know a great deal about nutrition, yet many of their beliefs about food and weight are misconceptions or myths. For instance, they may eat only protein because they believe complex carbohydrates, including fruits and whole-grain breads, are fattening.

Sometimes nutritional education alone can help change these eating patterns. However, many avid dieters who deny that they have a problem with food may need counseling (which they usually agree to only at their family's insistence) to correct dangerous eating behavior and prevent further complications.

## Compulsive Overeating

People who eat compulsively cannot stop putting food in their mouths. They eat fast and they eat a lot. They eat even when they're full. They may eat around the clock rather than at set mealtimes, often in private because of embarrassment over how much they consume.

Some mental health professionals describe compulsive eating as a food addiction that is much more likely to develop in women. According to Overeaters Anonymous (OA), an international 12-step program, many women who eat compulsively view food as a source of comfort against feelings of inner emptiness, low self-esteem, and fear of abandonment.

The following behaviors may signal a potential problem with compulsive overeating:

- **Turning to food** when depressed or lonely, when feeling rejected, or as a reward.
- **A history of failed diets** and anxiety when dieting.
- **Thinking about food** throughout the day.
- **Eating quickly** and without pleasure.
- **Continuing to eat** even when no longer hungry.
- **Frequently talking about food** or refusing to talk about food.
- **Fear of not being able to stop** eating after starting.

Recovery from compulsive eating can be challenging because people with this problem cannot give up entirely the substance they abuse. Like everyone else, they must eat. However, they can learn new eating habits and ways of dealing with underlying emotional problems. An OA survey found that most of its members joined to lose weight but later felt the most important effect was their improved emotional, mental, and physical health. As one woman put it, "I came for vanity but stayed for sanity."

## Binge Eating

**Binge eating**—the rapid consumption of an abnormally large amount of food in a relatively short time—often occurs in compulsive eaters. The 25 million Americans with a binge-eating disorder typically eat a larger than ordinary amount of food during a relatively brief period, feel a lack of control over eating, and binge at least twice a week for at least a six-month period. During most of these episodes, binge eaters experience at least three of the following:

- **Eating much more rapidly** than usual.
- **Eating until they feel uncomfortably full.**
- **Eating large amounts of food** when not feeling physically hungry.
- **Eating large amounts of food** throughout the day with no planned mealtimes.
- **Eating alone** because they are embarrassed by how much they eat and by their eating habits.

Binge eaters may spend up to several hours eating, and consume 2,000 or more calories worth of food in a single binge—more than many people eat in a day. After such binges, they usually do not do anything to control weight, but simply get fatter. As their weight climbs, they become depressed, anxious, or troubled by other psychological symptoms to a much greater extent than others of comparable weight.

Binge eating is probably the most common eating disorder. An estimated 8 to 19 percent of obese patients in weight loss programs are binge eaters.

If you occasionally go on eating binges, use the behavioral technique called *habit reversal*, and replace your bingeing with a competing behavior. For example, every time you're tempted to binge, immediately do something— text-message a friend, play solitaire, check your e-mail—that keeps food out of your mouth.

**binge eating** The rapid consumption of an abnormally large amount of food in a relatively short time.

If you binge twice a week or more for at least a six-month period, you may have binge-eating disorder, which can require professional help. Short-term talk treatment, such as cognitive-behavioral therapy, either individually or in a group setting, has proven most effective for binge eating.[34]

# Eating Disorders

According to the American Psychiatric Association, patients with **eating disorders** display a broad range of symptoms that occur along a continuum between those of anorexia nervosa and those of bulimia nervosa.

As many as 10 percent of teenage girls develop symptoms of or full-blown eating disorders. Among the factors that increase the risk are preoccupation with a thin body; social pressure; and childhood traits such as perfectionism and excessive cautiousness, which can reflect an obsessive-compulsive personality. Teenage girls who diet and have four specific risk factors—a high BMI, menarche (first menstruation) before sixth grade, extreme concern with weight or shape, and teasing by peers—are most likely to have an eating disorder.

The best known eating disorders are anorexia nervosa, which affects fewer than 1 percent of adolescent women, and bulimia nervosa, which strikes 2 to 3 percent. The American Psychiatric Association has developed practice guidelines for the treatment of patients with eating disorders, which include medical, psychological, and behavioral approaches. One of the most scientifically supported is cognitive-behavioral therapy.

## Who Develops Eating Disorders?

Eating disorders affect an estimated 5 to 10 million women and 1 million men. Despite evidence that 5 to 10 percent of those with eating disorders are male, many college students believe mainly young white women develop eating disorders.

More people—and more types of people—are developing full-blown or "partial syndrome" eating disorders, including more young children, boys and men, people of color, and individuals

with lower socioeconomic backgrounds. Among young people, those at highest risk are athletes (including gymnasts and wrestlers), performers, dancers, and models.[35]

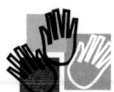  In the few studies of eating disorders in minority college students that have been completed, African American female undergraduates had a slightly lower prevalence of eating disorders than did whites. Asian Americans reported fewer symptoms of eating disorders but more body dissatisfaction, concerns about shape, and more intense efforts to lose weight.

In a survey of health-care professionals at the country's largest colleges and universities, 69 percent have professionals on staff who specialize in diagnosing and treating eating disorders. Of all the hurdles to helping students with eating disorders, 39 percent said denial is the biggest, while 24 percent felt it was unwillingness to seek treatment, and 20 percent blamed pressure from peers and the media to stay thin.

Eating disorders affect every aspect of college students' lives, including dating. Both men and women tend to avoid dating individuals with eating disorders, but men are far less accepting of obesity than women.

Male and female athletes are vulnerable to eating disorders, because of the pressure either to maintain ideal body weight or to achieve a weight that might enhance their performance. Many female athletes, particularly those participating in sports or activities that emphasize leanness (such as gymnastics, distance running, diving, figure skating, and classical ballet) have subclinical eating disorders that could undermine their nutritional status and energy levels. Male wrestlers, cyclists, triathletes, and Nordic skiers are also developing unhealthy eating behaviors. However, there is often little awareness or recognition of their disordered eating. On the other hand, a recent study found that many female athletes rely on exercise rather than vomiting or diet pills to control their weight.[36] Websites and smart phone "apps" that count calories and monitor every morsel eaten may push some vulnerable teens and young adults over the edge of self-motivating into an eating disorder.

**eating disorders** Bizarre, often dangerous patterns of food consumption, including anorexia nervosa and bulimia nervosa.

## Do You Have an Eating Disorder?

Physicians have developed a simple screening test for eating disorders, consisting of the following questions:

- Do you make yourself sick because you feel uncomfortably full?

- Do you worry you have lost control over how much you eat?

- Have you recently lost more than 14 pounds in a three-month period?

- Do you believe yourself to be fat when others say you are too thin?

- Would you say that food dominates your life?

Score one point for every "yes." A score of two or more is a likely indication of anorexia nervosa or bulimia nervosa.

Source: Karl Miller, "Treatment Guideline for Eating Disorders," *American Family Physician*, Vol. 62, No. 1, July 1, 2000.

---

If someone you know has an eating disorder, let your friend know you're concerned and that you care. Don't criticize or make fun of his or her eating habits. Encourage your friend to talk about other problems and feelings, and suggest that he or she talk to the school counselor or someone at the mental health center, the family doctor, or another trusted person. Offer to go along if you think that will make a difference.

## Anorexia Nervosa

Although *anorexia* means "loss of appetite," most individuals with **anorexia nervosa** are, in fact, hungry all the time. For them, food is an enemy—a threat to their sense of self, identity, and autonomy. In the distorted mirror of their mind's eye, they see themselves as fat or flabby even at a normal or below-normal body weight. Some simply feel fat; others think that they are thin in some places and too fat in others, such as the abdomen, buttocks, or thighs.

The characteristics of anorexia nervosa include:

- A refusal to maintain normal body weight (weight loss leading to body weight of less than 85 percent of that expected for age and height).

- An intense fear of gaining weight or becoming fat, even though underweight.

- A distorted body image so that the person feels fat even when emaciated.

- In women, the absence of at least three menstrual cycles.

The incidence of anorexia nervosa has increased in the last three decades in most developed countries. The peak ages for its onset are 14½ to 18 years. According to the American Psychiatric Association's Work Group on Eating Disorders, cases are increasing among males, minorities, women of all ages, and possibly preteens. About 1 percent of American women develop anorexia.

In the *restricting type* of anorexia, individuals lose weight by avoiding any fatty foods and by dieting, fasting, and exercising. Some start smoking as a way of controlling their weight. Some college women may numb their pain by drinking alcohol, a problem the media have dubbed "drunkorexia."[37] In the *binge-eating/purging* type, they engage in binge eating, purging (through self-induced vomiting, laxatives, diuretics, or enemas), or both. Obsessed with an intense fear of fatness, they may weigh themselves several times a day, measure various parts of their body, check mirrors to see if they look fat, and try on different items of clothing to see if they feel tight.

*What Causes Anorexia Nervosa?* Many complex factors interact and contribute to this disorder, including biological, psychological, and social ones. Anorexia is more common among close relatives, particularly sisters, than it is in the general population. The relatives of anorexics also have a higher than expected frequency of depressive disorders.

Anorexia is associated with changes within the brain, including abnormalities in the stress hormone cortisol and the neurotransmitters dopamine, serotonin, and norepinephrine—all of which influence appetite and satiety. Brain chemistry returns to normal after treatment and recovery.

Anorexia also may be a response to a personal loss or a sign of a driven, perfectionist personality. Often young anorexics have above-average grades and an unwarranted fear of failure. Girls who develop anorexia often have little insight into or awareness of their feelings, needs, and wants.

**anorexia nervosa** A psychological disorder in which refusal to eat and/or an extreme loss of appetite leads to malnutrition, severe weight loss, and possibly death.

In one study that followed 21 college women with eating disorders for six years, 11 got better during their post-college years, while 10 continued to struggle with disordered eating. The major difference between the two groups revolved around issues of autonomy and relation. Those who could better negotiate the tension between being independent and relating to others had higher self-esteem, a more positive self-concept, and a healthier relationship with food.

About one-third of those with anorexia initially were mildly overweight and cut back on food just to lose a few pounds. Others had normal weights but began to diet to look more attractive or, in the case of male and female athletes and dancers, to gain a performance advantage. Sometimes illness, stress, or surgery triggers weight loss. Often the initial response to their weight loss—from parents, coaches, or friends—is positive. However, starvation seems to take on a life of its own, and anorexics cannot return to a healthy eating pattern. In time, they may place so much value on thinness that they cannot recognize the dangers to their health.

*Health Dangers and Treatment* The medical consequences of anorexia nervosa are serious (Figure 7.4). Menstrual periods stop in women; testosterone levels decline in men. Adolescents with this disorder do not undergo normal sexual maturation, such as breast development, and may not reach their anticipated height. Even individuals who look and feel reasonably healthy may have subtle or hidden abnormalities, including heart irregularities and arrhythmias that can increase their risk of sudden death. Women who do not menstruate for six months or more may develop osteoporosis and suffer irreversible weakening and thinning of their bones as a result.

Even when they realize that they are jeopardizing their health, people with anorexia tend to fear that treatment will make them worse—that is, fatter. They need repeated reassurance that they will not become overweight and that they can and will find healthier ways of coping with life.

According to current practice guidelines, treatment of anorexia nervosa includes medical therapy (such as "refeeding" to overcome malnutrition) and behavioral, cognitive, psychodynamic, and family therapy. Antidepressant medication sometimes can help, particularly when there is a personal or family history of depression. Most people who get help do return to normal weight, but it can take a long time for their eating behaviors to become normal and for them to deal with troubling body image issues. Nutritional therapy is critical for a return to regular menstrual periods and an improvement in bone density.

## Bulimia Nervosa

Individuals with **bulimia nervosa** go on repeated eating binges and rapidly consume large amounts of food, usually sweets, stopping only because of severe abdominal pain or sleep, or because they are interrupted. Those with *purging bulimia* induce vomiting or take large doses of laxatives to relieve guilt and control their weight. In *nonpurging bulimia*, individuals use other means, such as fasting or excessive exercise, to compensate for binges.

The characteristics of bulimia nervosa include:

- Repeated binge eating.
- A feeling of lack of control over eating behavior.

**bulimia nervosa** Episodic binge eating, often followed by forced vomiting or laxative abuse, and accompanied by a persistent preoccupation with body shape and weight.

Figure 7.4  **Medical Complications of Weight Loss from Anorexia Nervosa**

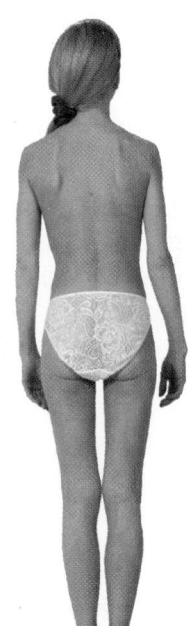

Loss of fat and muscle mass, including heart muscle

Increased sensitivity to cold

Irregular heartbeats

Bloating, constipation, abdominal pain

Amenorrhea (absence of menstruation)

Growth of fine, babylike hair over body

Abnormal taste sensations

Osteoporosis

Depression

Sudden death

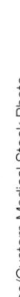
B.Bodine/Custom Medical Stock Photo

- Regular reliance on self-induced vomiting, laxatives, or diuretics.
- Strict dieting or fasting, or vigorous exercise, to prevent weight gain.
- A minimum average of two bingeing episodes a week for at least three months.
- A preoccupation with body shape and weight.

An estimated 1 to 3 percent of adolescent and young American women develop bulimia. Some experiment with bingeing and purging for a few months and then stop when they change their social or living situation. Others develop longer-term bulimia. Among males, this disorder is about one-tenth as common. The average age for developing bulimia is 18.

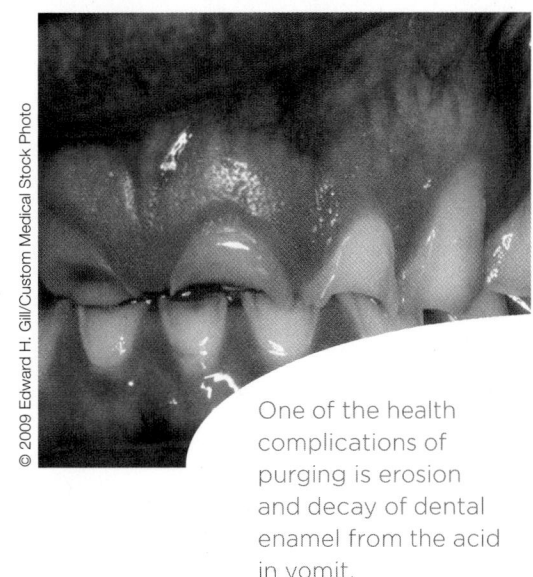

One of the health complications of purging is erosion and decay of dental enamel from the acid in vomit.

*What Causes Bulimia Nervosa?* Bulimia usually begins after a rigid diet that lasted from several weeks to a year or more. Strict dieting may affect brain chemistry in such a way as to disrupt the normal mechanisms for appetite and satiety. Semi-starvation eventually sets off a binge; bingeing leads to purging. Once dieters realize that vomiting reduces the anxiety triggered by gorging, they no longer fear overeating. When this happens, bingeing may become more frequent and severe until, in time, it becomes an all-purpose way of coping with stress. However, the driving force in this disorder may not be the overeating but the vomiting or laxative use. If individuals felt they couldn't get rid of food, they might not overeat.

Obesity in adolescence may increase the likelihood of bulimia in adulthood. Extremely obese individuals may lose weight by vomiting and not want to stop because they fear regaining it. Sometimes bulimia develops after recovery from anorexia. Purging becomes an alternative way of staying thin. People with bulimia may spend thousands of dollars—a third of their food budget—on foods for binge episodes and for laxatives and diet pills.[38]

As with anorexia, bulimia is associated with changes in brain chemistry, particularly low levels of the peptide cholescystokinin, which produces feelings of satiety. The cycle of bingeing and purging seems to wreak havoc on the biological controls that keep weight at a certain level. Neuroimaging scans show differences in areas of the brain responsible for regulating behavior in individuals with bulimia.[39]

Family conflicts, life stresses such as going away to school, and struggles with the transition to independent adulthood also may play a role. Bulimia also may be a symptom of depression. About 20 to 30 percent of those with this problem are chronically depressed; others have a history of depressive episodes. Bulimic individuals also are more likely to experience other problems, including anxiety disorders, substance abuse, and impulse disorders, such as shoplifting (kleptomania) and cutting themselves. A significant percentage of bulimics—from a quarter to a half, by some estimates—may have been victims of incest, sexual molestation, or rape, but this correlation is controversial.

*Health Dangers and Treatment* Bulimia may continue for many years, with binges alternating with periods of normal eating. Physiological consequences are cumulative. Often dentists are the first to detect bulimia because they notice damage to teeth and gums, including erosion of the enamel from the stomach acids in vomit. Repeated vomiting can lead to other complications as it robs the body of essential nutrients and fluids, causes dehydration and electrolyte imbalances, and impairs the ability of the heart and other muscles to function. Bulimia can trigger cardiac arrhythmias and, occasionally, sudden death.

Cognitive-behavioral therapy has proved more effective than other approaches in improving bulimia symptoms.[40]

# Taking Control of Your Weight

No diet—high-protein, low-fat, or high-carbohydrate—can produce permanent weight loss. Successful weight management, the American Dietetic Association has concluded, "requires a lifelong commitment to healthful lifestyle behaviors emphasizing sustainable and enjoyable eating practices and daily physical activity." Studies have shown that successful dieters are highly motivated, monitor their food intake, increase their activity, set realistic goals, and receive social support from others. Another key to long-term success is tailoring any weight loss program to an individual's gender, lifestyle, and cultural, racial, and ethnic values.

Are you following these practical guidelines?

- **Be realistic.** Trying to shrink to an impossibly low weight dooms you to defeat. Start off slowly and make steady progress. If your weight creeps up five pounds, go back to the basics of your program. Take into account normal fluctuations, but watch out for an upward trend. If you let your weight continue to creep up, it may not stop until you have a serious weight problem—again.

- **Recognize that there are no quick fixes.** Ultimately, quick-loss diets are very damaging physically and psychologically because when you stop dieting and put the pounds back on, you feel like a failure.

- **Note your progress.** Make a graph, with your initial weight as the base, to indicate your progress. View plateaus or occasional gains as temporary setbacks rather than disasters.

- **Adopt the 90 percent rule.** If you practice good eating habits 90 percent of the time, a few indiscretions won't make a difference. In effect, you should allow for occasional cheating, so that you don't have to feel guilty about it.

- **Look for joy and meaning beyond your food life.** Make your personal goals and your relationships your priorities, and treat food as the fuel that allows you to bring your best to both.

- **Try again and again.** Remember, dieters usually don't keep weight off on their first attempt. The people who eventually succeed try various methods until they find the plan that works for them.

# Are You Ready to Lose Weight?

As discussed in Chapter 1, people change the way they behave stage by stage and step by step. The same is true for changing behaviors related to weight. If you need to lose excess pounds, knowing your stage of readiness for change is a crucial first step. Here is a guide to identifying where you are right now.

If you are still in the *precontemplation* stage, you don't think of yourself as having a weight problem, even though others may. If you can't fit into some of your clothes, you blame the dry cleaners. Or you look around and think, "I'm no bigger than anyone else in this class." Unconsciously, you may feel helpless to do anything about your weight. So you deny or dismiss its importance.

In the *contemplation* stage, you would prefer not to have to change, but you can't avoid reality. Your coach or doctor may comment on your weight. You wince at the vacation photos of you in a swimsuit. You look in the mirror, try to

suck in your stomach, and say, "I've got to do something about my weight."

In the *preparation* stage, you're gearing up by taking small but necessary steps. You may buy athletic shoes or check out several diet books from the library. Maybe you experiment with some minor changes, such as having fruit instead of cookies for an afternoon snack. Internally, you are getting accustomed to the idea of change.

In the *action* stage of change, you are deliberately working to lose weight. You no longer snack all evening long. You stick to a specific diet and track calories, carbs, or points. You hop on a treadmill or stationary bike for 30 minutes a day. Your resolve is strong, and you know you're on your way to a thinner, healthier you.

In the *maintenance* stage, you strengthen, enhance, and extend the changes you've made. Whether or not you have lost all the weight you want, you've made significant progress. As you continue to watch what you eat and to be physically active, you lock-in healthy new habits.

Where are you right now? Read each of the following statements and decide which best applies to you.

| | |
|---|---|
| 1. I never think about my weight. | Precontemplation Stage |
| 2. I'm trying to zip up a pair of jeans and wondering when was the last time they fit. | Contemplation Stage |
| 3. I'm downloading a food diary to keep track of what I eat. | Preparation Stage |
| 4. I have been following a diet for three weeks and have started working out. | Action Stage |
| 5. I have been sticking to a diet and engaging in regular physical activity for at least six months. | Maintenance Stage |

For a guide to strategies most likely to help you at your particular stage of readiness to change, see "Making Change Happen: A Stage-by-Stage Approach to Weight Loss."

## *Making Change Happen*

## A Stage-by-Stage Approach to Weight Loss

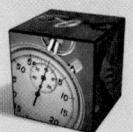

### Get Real
- **Start paying attention** to what, when, where, and why you eat. Take note of the times you eat or continue eating even though you're not hungry.

- **List what you see** as the cons of physical activity. For example, do you fear it will take up too much time? Write down three activities you could do if you woke up half an hour earlier.

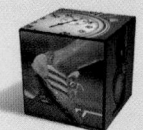

### Get Ready
- **Start drinking more water.** Get used to the idea of ending every meal with water to wash away the taste of what you've eaten and signal that you've stopped putting food in your mouth.

- **Find an image of a slimmer body** you'd like to have—from a magazine advertisement, for example—and post it where you can see it often.

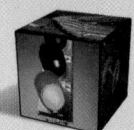

### Get Going
- **Record everything you put in your mouth.** List calories and carbs next to each entry. Also describe how you feel as you eat.

- **Find new comfort foods.** Good options include air-popped popcorn, chocolate fruit sundaes (fresh fruit with a spoonful of rich syrup), hot chocolate (with skim milk), and fudgsicles (creamy but low in calories).

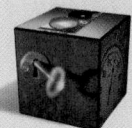

### Lock It In
- **Avoid boredom.** Think through ways to vary your exercise routine. Take different routes on your walks. Invite different friends to join you. Alternate working with free weights with resistance machines at the gym.

- **Try new athletic and sports skills.** Try snowshoeing, kayaking, rock climbing, dancing. Don't expect instant expertise. It usually takes four to six weeks to feel competent and get in the swing of a new activity.

# Making This Chapter Work for You

## Review Questions

1. If you have gone online to check out weight reduction support groups in your area, which stage of readiness for weight behavior change are you in?
   a. precontemplation stage
   b. contemplation stage
   c. preparation stage
   d. action stage

2. Successful weight management strategies include which of the following?
   a. Learn to distinguish between actual and emotional hunger.
   b. Ask friends for recommendations for methods that helped them to lose weight quickly.
   c. Practice good eating habits 50 percent of the time so that you can balance your cravings with healthy food.
   d. Look at celebrity photos and pick one for a model.

3. Jacob is an average-build, 26-year-old college student who is much thinner than his friends. What should he focus on to gain more weight?
   a. Consume more calories than he burns on an average day.
   b. Eat a large lunch and dinner each day.
   c. Eat foods that will provide at least 50 percent of caloric intake from fats.
   d. Bench press more weights to build up muscle mass.

4. Individuals with anorexia nervosa
   a. believe they are overweight even if they are extremely thin.
   b. typically feel full all the time, which limits their food intake.
   c. usually look overweight, even though their body mass index is normal.
   d. have a reduced risk for heart-related abnormalities.

5. What is basal metabolic rate?
   a. Another way to define body mass index.
   b. The number of calories needed to maintain the body after physical activity.
   c. Another term for breathing rate.
   d. The number of calories needed to sustain the body at rest.

6. People gain weight when
   a. their basal metabolic rate increases.
   b. they consume more calories than they use up in daily activity.
   c. they eat fast food more than two times a week.
   d. they watch two hours of television a day.

7. Bulimia nervosa
   a. is characterized by excessive sleeping followed by periods of insomnia.
   b. is found primarily in older women who are concerned with the aging process.
   c. is associated with the use of laxatives or excessive exercise to control weight.
   d. does not have serious health consequences.

8. Which of the following statements is *incorrect*?
   a. I can lose weight successfully on a low-carbohydrate diet.
   b. I can lose weight successfully on a low-fat diet.
   c. I can lose weight successfully on a low-calorie diet.
   d. I can lose weight successfully by working out once a week.

9. Which of the following statements is true?
   a. Ephedra supplements are a safe and effective way to increase metabolism.
   b. An individual eating low-calorie or fat-free foods can increase the serving sizes.
   c. Low-carbohydrate diets have been shown safe over the short term but long-term studies have not been completed.
   d. Yo-yo dieting works best for long-term weight loss.

10. Satiety occurs when
    a. one's caloric needs have been met.
    b. one feels full.
    c. one has had dessert.
    d. one has no appetite.

*Answers to these questions can be found on page 672.*

## Critical Thinking

1. Do you think you have a weight problem? If so, what makes you think so? Is your perception based on your actual BMI measurement or on how you believe you look? If you found out that your BMI was within the ideal range, would that change your opinion about your body? Why or why not?

2. Suppose a good friend appears to have symptoms of an eating disorder. You have told him or her of your concerns, but your friend has denied having a problem and brushed off your fears. What can you do to help this individual? Should you contact his or her parent or spouse? Why or why not?

## Media Menu

Visit www.cengagebrain.com to access course materials and companion resources for this text that will:

- Help you evaluate your knowledge of the material.

- Allow you to prepare for exams with interactive quizzing.

- Use the CengageNOW product to develop a Personalized Learning Plan targeting resources that address areas you should study.

- Coach you through identifying target goals for behavioral change and creating and monitoring your personal change plan throughout the semester using the Behavior Change Planner available in the CengageNOW resource.

## Internet Connections

**www.obesity.org**
The American Obesity Association is the leading organization for advocacy and education on the nation's obesity epidemic. This comprehensive website features statistics on overweight and obesity in the United States, research articles, consumer protection links, prevention topics, library resources, fact sheets on a variety of weight management topics, and more.

**http://win.niddk.nih.gov**
This government-sponsored website features a variety of publications in English and Spanish on nutrition, physical activity, and weight control for the general public and for health-care professionals. In addition, there are links for research, a newsletter, statistical data, and a bibliographic collection of journal articles on various aspects of weight management and obesity.

**www.something-fishy.org**
This very comprehensive and popular site features the latest news on eating disorders, as well as links regarding signs to watch for, "Recovery: Reach Out," treatment finders, doctors and patients, cultural issues, and a support chat.

## Key Terms

The terms listed are used on the page indicated. Definitions of the terms are in the Glossary at the end of the book.

| | | |
|---|---|---|
| anorexia nervosa   219 | eating disorders   218 | obesity   204 |
| appetite   207 | hunger   207 | overweight   204 |
| binge eating   217 | NEAT (nonexercise activity thermogenesis)   211 | satiety   206 |
| bulimia nervosa   220 | | |

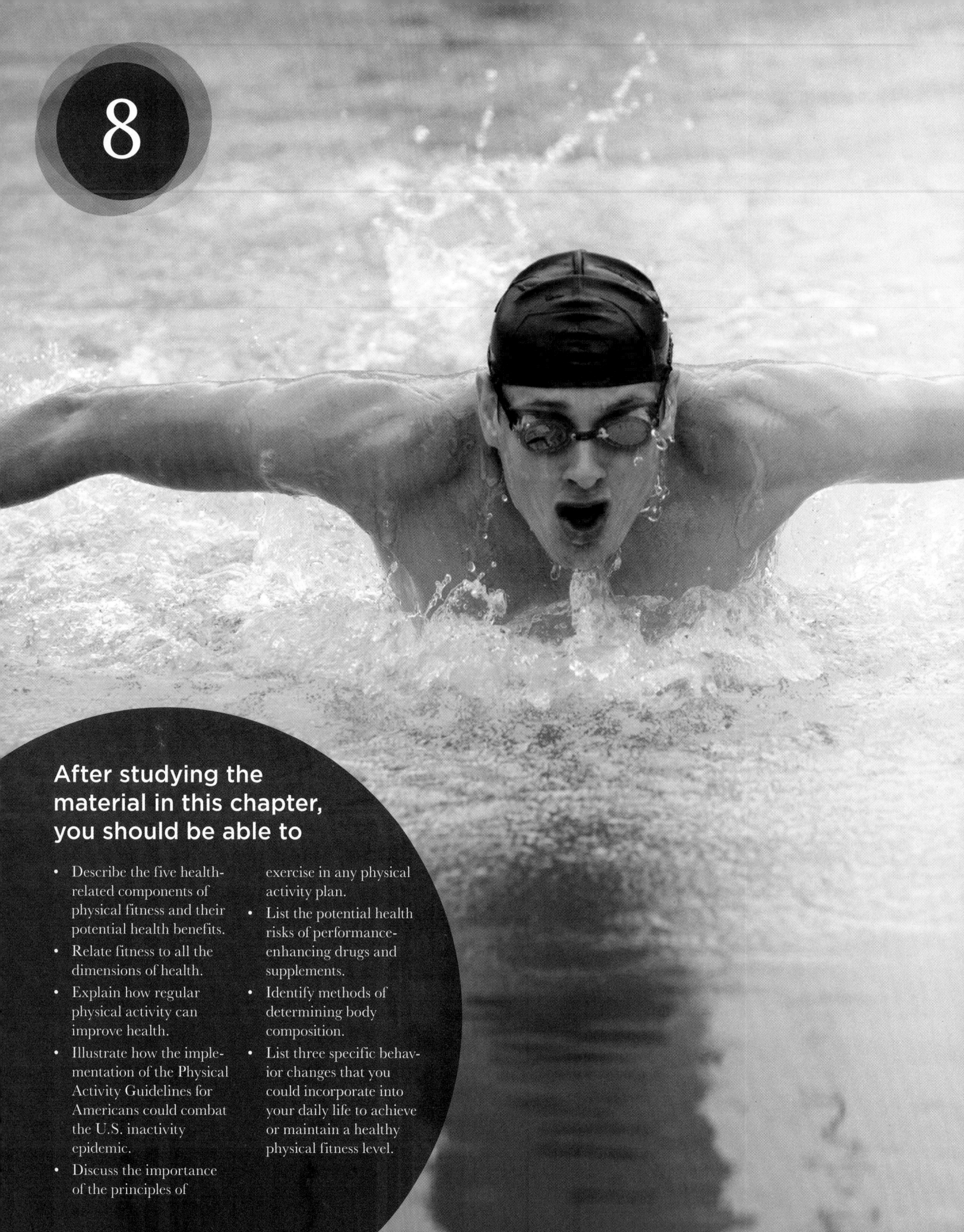

# 8

## After studying the material in this chapter, you should be able to

- Describe the five health-related components of physical fitness and their potential health benefits.

- Relate fitness to all the dimensions of health.

- Explain how regular physical activity can improve health.

- Illustrate how the implementation of the Physical Activity Guidelines for Americans could combat the U.S. inactivity epidemic.

- Discuss the importance of the principles of

- exercise in any physical activity plan.

- List the potential health risks of performance-enhancing drugs and supplements.

- Identify methods of determining body composition.

- List three specific behavior changes that you could incorporate into your daily life to achieve or maintain a healthy physical fitness level.

As a boy, Derek never thought about doing anything special to stay physically fit. He loved sports so much that he spent every free moment on a softball field or basketball court. He could sprint faster, jump higher, and hit a ball harder than any of his friends. In high school Derek's life revolved around practices and games. He was a varsity athlete and a regional all-star.

# The Joy of Fitness

Early in his first year in college, an injury sidelined Derek. Frustrated that he had to sit out the season, he gave up his rigorous training routine. As he became immersed in academics and other activities, Derek stopped going to the gym or working out on his own. Yet he continued to think of himself as an athlete in excellent physical condition. When Derek went home for spring break, he joined his younger brothers on a neighborhood basketball court. While he wasn't surprised that his long shots were off, Derek was amazed by how quickly he got winded. In 15 minutes, he was panting for breath. "Getting old," one of his brothers joked. "Getting soft," the other teased.

Often the college years represent a turning point in physical fitness. Like Derek, many students, busy with classes and other commitments, devote less time to physical activity. However, the choices you make and the habits you develop now can affect how long and how well you'll live. As you'll see in this chapter, exercise yields immediate rewards: It boosts energy, improves mood, soothes stress, improves sleep, and makes you look and feel better. In the long term, physical activity slows many of the

changes associated with chronological aging such as loss of calcium and bone density, lowers the risk of serious chronic illnesses, and extends the lifespan.

This chapter can help you reap these rewards. It presents the latest activity recommendations, documents the benefits of exercise, describes types of exercise, and provides guidelines for getting into shape and exercising safely.

## What Is Physical Fitness?

The simplest, most practical definition of **physical fitness** is the ability to respond to routine physical demands, with enough reserve energy to cope with a sudden challenge. You can consider yourself fit if you meet your daily energy needs; can handle unexpected extra demands; and are protecting yourself against potential health problems, such as heart disease. Fitness is important both for health and for athletic performance.

**physical fitness** The ability to respond to routine physical demands, with enough reserve energy to cope with a sudden challenge.

Visit www.cengagebrain.com to access course materials for this text, including the Behavior Change Planner, interactive quizzes, tutorials, and more. See the preface on page xv for details.

## Health-Related Fitness

The five health-related components of physical fitness include aerobic or cardiorespiratory endurance, muscular strength, muscular endurance, flexibility, and body composition (the ratio of fat and lean body tissue).

**Cardiorespiratory fitness** refers to the ability of the heart to pump blood through the body efficiently. It is achieved through aerobic exercise—any activity, such as brisk walking or swimming, in which sufficient or excess oxygen is continually supplied to the body. In other words, aerobic exercise involves working out strenuously without pushing to the point of breathlessness.

**Muscular strength** refers to the force within muscles; it is measured by the absolute maximum weight that you can lift, push, or press in one effort. Strong muscles help keep the skeleton in proper alignment, improve posture, prevent back and leg aches, help in everyday lifting, and enhance athletic performance. Muscle mass increases along with strength, which makes for a healthier body composition and a higher metabolic rate.

**Muscular endurance** is the ability to perform repeated muscular effort; it is measured by counting how many times you can lift, push, or press a given weight. Important for posture, muscular endurance helps in everyday work as well as in athletics and sports.

**Flexibility** is the range of motion around specific joints—for example, the stretching you do to touch your toes or twist your torso. Flexibility depends on many factors: your age, gender, and posture; how muscular you are; and how much body fat you have. As children develop, their flexibility increases until adolescence. Then a gradual loss of joint mobility begins and continues throughout adult life. Both muscles and connective tissue, such as tendons and ligaments, shorten and become tighter if not consistently used through their full range of motion.

**Body composition** refers to the relative amounts of fat and lean tissue (bone, muscle, organs, water) in the body. As discussed later in this chapter, a high proportion of body fat has serious health implications, including increased incidence of heart disease, high blood pressure, diabetes, stroke, gallbladder problems, back and joint problems, and some forms of cancer.

Physical conditioning (or training) refers to the gradual building up of the body to enhance cardiorespiratory, or aerobic, fitness; muscular strength; muscular endurance; flexibility; and a healthy body composition.

**Functional fitness**, which is gaining greater emphasis among professional trainers, refers to the performance of activities of daily living. Exercises that mimic job tasks or everyday movements can improve an individual's balance, coordination, strength, and endurance.

## Athletic, or Performance-Related, Fitness

You may jog five miles, work out with weights, and start each day with a stretching routine. This doesn't qualify you for the soccer team. Most sports, such as softball, tennis, and basketball, require additional skills, including:

- **Agility,** the ability to change direction rapidly.
- **Balance,** or equilibrium, the ability to maintain a certain body position.
- **Coordination,** the ability to integrate the movement of body parts to produce smooth, fluid movements.
- **Power,** the product of force and speed.
- **Reaction time,** the time required to respond to a stimulus.
- **Speed,** or velocity, the ability to move rapidly.

While many amateur and professional athletes are in superb overall condition, you do not need athletic skills to keep your body operating at maximum capacity throughout life.

## Fitness and the Dimensions of Health

The concept of fitness is evolving. Rather than focusing only on miles run or weight lifted, instructors, coaches, and consumers are pursuing a broader vision of total fitness that encompasses every dimension of health:

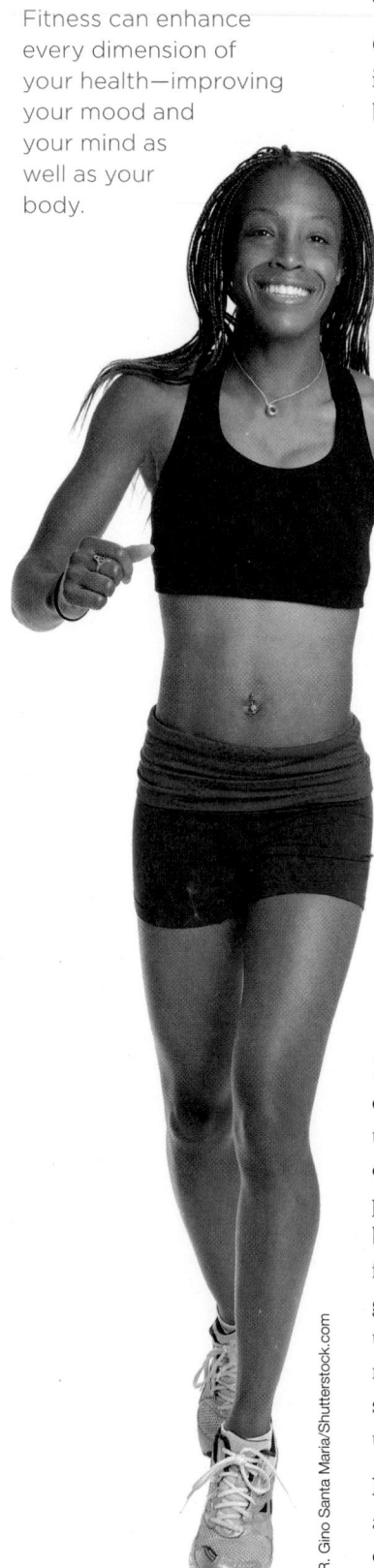

Fitness can enhance every dimension of your health—improving your mood and your mind as well as your body.

© R. Gino Santa Maria/Shutterstock.com

Section II  Healthy Lifestyles

- **Physical.** As described later in this chapter, becoming fit reduces your risk of major diseases, increases energy and stamina, and may prolong your life.
- **Emotional.** Fitness lowers tension and anxiety, lifts depression, relieves stress, improves mood, and promotes a positive self-image.
- **Social.** Physical activities provide opportunities to meet new people and to work out with friends or family.
- **Intellectual.** Fit individuals report greater alertness, better concentration, more creativity, and improved personal health habits.
- **Occupational.** Fit employees miss fewer days of work, are more productive, and incur fewer medical costs.
- **Spiritual.** Fitness fosters appreciation for the relationship between body and mind and may lead to greater realization of your potential.
- **Environmental.** Fit individuals often become more aware of their need for healthy air and food and develop a deeper appreciation of the physical world.

## Gender, Race, and Fitness

Men and women of all racial backgrounds benefit equally from fitness. However, there are some physiological differences between men and women, many of which are related to size. On average, men are 10 to 15 percent bigger than women, with roughly twice the percentage of muscle mass and half the percentage of body fat. They have more sweat glands and a greater maximum oxygen uptake. A man's bigger heart pumps more blood with each beat. His larger lungs take in 10 to 20 percent more oxygen (Figure 8.1). His longer legs cover more distance with each stride. If a man jogs along at 50 percent of his capacity, a woman has to push to 73 percent of hers to keep up.

Women have a higher percentage of body fat than men, and more is distributed around the hips and thighs; men carry more body fat around the waist and stomach.

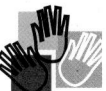 College-age men average 15 percent body fat; college-age women, 23 percent. On average, women have 11 percent more body fat and 8 percent less muscle mass than men.

Figure 8.1 **Physiological Differences between Men and Women**

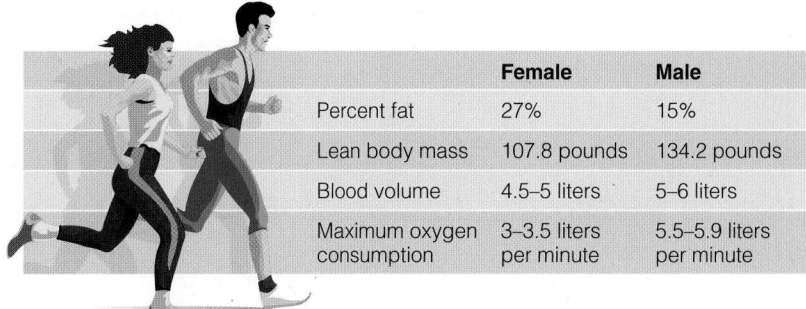

| | Female | Male |
|---|---|---|
| Percent fat | 27% | 15% |
| Lean body mass | 107.8 pounds | 134.2 pounds |
| Blood volume | 4.5–5 liters | 5–6 liters |
| Maximum oxygen consumption | 3–3.5 liters per minute | 5.5–5.9 liters per minute |

 Women are generally less active than men. Fewer than 12 percent of white women, 25 percent of African American women, and 27 percent of Hispanic women are active enough to improve their fitness levels. Among women who do exercise, most choose aerobic activities, and relatively few do any strength training. Yet women may benefit more from strength training than men because they typically have more body fat and face greater risk of osteoporosis.

The average woman has a smaller heart and blood volume than a man. Because women have a lower concentration of red blood cells, their bodies are less effective at transporting oxygen to their working muscles during exercise.

Even though training produces the same relative increases for both genders, a woman's maximum oxygen intake remains about 25 to 30 percent lower than that of an equally well-conditioned man. In elite athletes, the gender difference is smaller. Because the angle of the upper leg bone (femur) to the pelvis is greater in a woman, she is less efficient at running. Intense exercise provokes a rise in the stress hormone cortisol in men, but not women.

In some endurance events, such as ultramarathon running and long-distance swimming, female anatomy and physiology may have some aerobic advantages. The longer a race—on land, water, or ice—the better women perform.

In absolute terms, men are 30 percent stronger, but gender differences in absolute strength do not apply to all muscle groups. Women have about 40 to 60 percent of the upper-body strength of men but 70 to 75 percent of the lower-body strength.

**cardiorespiratory fitness** The ability of the heart and blood vessels to circulate blood through the body efficiently.

**muscular strength** Physical power; the maximum weight one can lift, push, or press in one effort.

**muscular endurance** The ability to withstand the stress of continued physical exertion.

**flexibility** The range of motion allowed by one's joints; determined by the length of muscles, tendons, and ligaments attached to the joints.

**body composition** The relative amounts of fat and lean tissue (bone, muscle, organs, water) in the body.

**functional fitness** The ability to perform real-life activities, such as lifting a heavy suitcase.

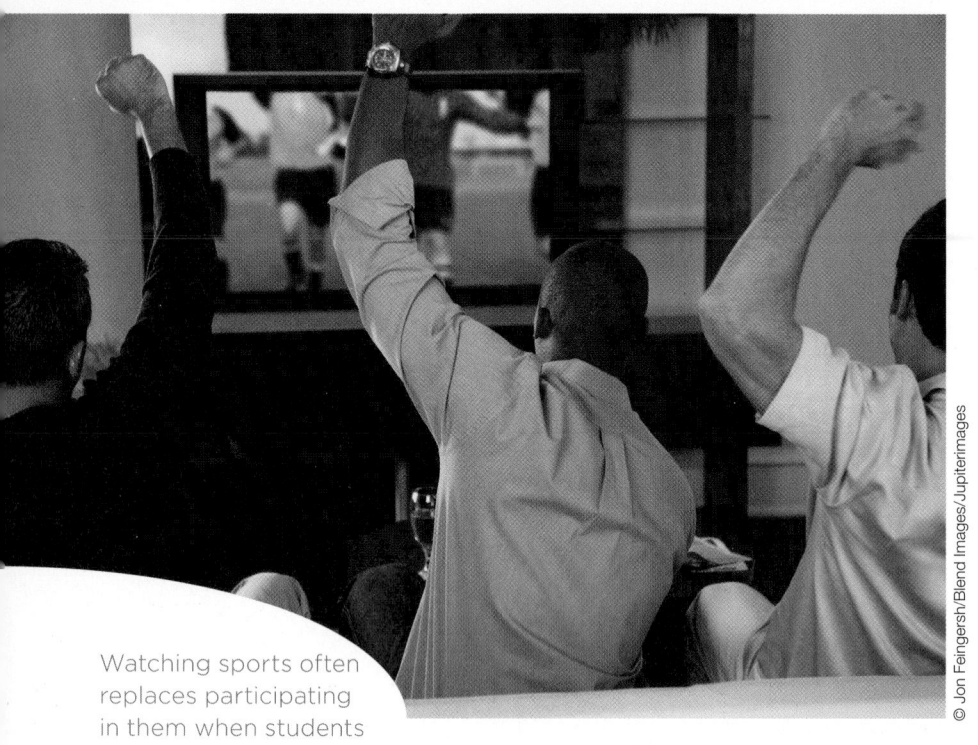

Watching sports often replaces participating in them when students enter college. Many students exercise less with each succeeding year.

 Exercise capacity, an indicator of how much your body can do and how much oxygen it needs to do it, is the most accurate predictor of a person's potential lifespan. This holds true for both men and women, for healthy individuals and those with cardiovascular disease, and, as the largest study ever of exercise capacity and mortality recently showed, for African Americans and whites. African Americans, whose mortality rates from all causes are as much as 60 percent higher than those of whites, benefit just as much from increased fitness as other racial groups. Yet in one recent sampling, only 22 percent of African Americans reported getting the recommended levels of exercise.[1]

# The Inactivity Epidemic

In the most recent National Health Interview Survey, 59 percent of adults said they engaged in no vigorous physical activity (one that causes heavy sweating and large increases in breathing and heart rate).[2] More than a third of U.S. adults don't engage in any leisure-time physical activity. According to another national survey, about a third of adolescents and 14 percent of adults between ages 20 and 49 fall into the category of "low fitness" because they engage in little or no physical activity.

People who don't exercise are significantly more likely to develop diabetes, hypertension, and metabolic syndrome (discussed in Chapter 15) than those with higher fitness levels. Many factors affect physical activity levels, including geographic location, gender, education, and income. According to the CDC, city dwellers are more active than country folks, westerners more active than those in other regions. Americans who live in parts of Appalachia and the South are the least physically active.[3] Men, people with higher education levels, and high-income earners work out more often.

Where you live as a student has an impact on your weight, eating, and exercise patterns. In a study of Texas undergraduate women, those who lived on campus were significantly more physically active than those who lived off campus. As measured by pedometers, they walked an average of 90,000 steps per week, compared to 42,000 steps for off-campus students. The reasons may be the greater distance from classrooms to dormitories than to bus stops or parking lots and higher levels of participation in intramural sports.

Regardless of where they live, Americans spend most of their leisure time watching television: on average, more than 30 hours a week. Yet the more time spent in "recreational sitting" in front of a television or screen, the greater the risk of obesity, chronic diseases, and premature death.[4] Compared with other sedentary activities, such as reading, writing, or driving, watching TV lowers metabolic rate, so people burn fewer calories. Every hour spent watching television may increase your risk of dying prematurely from any cause by 11 percent, from cardiorespiratory disease by 18 percent, and from cancer by 9 percent, according to recent research. Compared with those who watched less than two hours per day, individuals who watched more than four hours had an 80 percent greater risk of premature death from heart-related causes.[5]

## SWEATING IT OUT ON CAMPUS

College students reported the following behaviors within the past seven days:

**Do moderate-intensity cardio or aerobic exercise for at least 30 minutes:**

| | Percentage (%) | | |
| --- | --- | --- | --- |
| | Male | Female | Total |
| 0 days | 21.6 | 22.8 | 22.5 |
| 1–4 days | 57.0 | 59.2 | 58.3 |
| 5–7 days | 21.4 | 17.9 | 19.2 |

**Do vigorous-intensity cardio or aerobic exercise for at least 20 minutes:**

| | Percentage (%) | | |
| --- | --- | --- | --- |
| | Male | Female | Total |
| 0 days | 31.8 | 40.9 | 37.6 |
| 1–2 days | 32.6 | 30.3 | 31.1 |
| 3–7 days | 35.7 | 28.8 | 31.3 |

### HOW DO YOU COMPARE?

Did you engage in moderate-intensity aerobic exercise for at least 30 minutes in the last seven days? Or did you exercise vigorously for at least 20 minutes? How often do you exercise? Are you in better shape now than you were a year ago? Would you like to improve your fitness? Record your feelings on your fitness today and in the past in your online journal.

Source: American College Health Association. *American College Health Association-National College Health Assessment II: Reference Group Executive Summary, Spring 2010.* Linthicum, MD: American College Health Association, 2010.

## The Toll of Sedentary Living

Physical inactivity, along with smoking, high body mass index, and low levels of income and education, may accelerate the aging process. A recent study found a significant difference in one biological indicator of human aging—the length of the telomeres (segments of DNA at the end of chromosomes) of white blood cells—between active and inactive twins. The most active individuals, regardless of age and sex, had telomeres the same length as sedentary individuals up to ten years younger. This means that sedentary individuals may be biologically ten years older.

Sedentary living claims some 250,000 lives, accounting for 10 percent of all deaths in America every year, and contributes to four of the six leading causes of death: heart disease, cancer, stroke, and diabetes. Inactivity doubles the risk of cardiorespiratory diseases, diabetes, and obesity and increases the risk of colon cancer, high blood pressure, osteoporosis, depression, and anxiety. As a risk factor for heart disease, physical inactivity ranks as high as elevated cholesterol, high blood pressure, or cigarette smoking.

# Working Out on Campus: Student Bodies in Motion

 By various estimates, only 15 to 30 percent of college students meet the recommended amount of physical activity for health benefits.

College men are generally more active than women; full-time students and those without jobs exercise more than part-time or employed students. Undergraduates living on campus are more active than those living off campus; students living in fraternity or sorority housing engage in more exercise than those living in a house or an apartment. Single students report more days of vigorous workouts than married, divorced, or separated ones. Only 16 percent of students who are parents get the recommended levels of physical activity, compared with about half of those without children. How do you compare?

While two in three high school seniors engaged in regular vigorous physical activity (defined in one study as at least 20 minutes of an activity, such as basketball, soccer, running, swimming

### Health Benefits of Physical Activity—A Review of the Strength of the Scientific Evidence

**Strong Evidence**

Lower risk of:
- Early death
- Heart disease
- Stroke
- Type 2 diabetes
- High blood pressure
- Adverse blood lipid profile
- Metabolic syndrome
- Colon and breast cancers

Prevention of weight gain
Weight loss when combined with diet
Improved cardiorespiratory and muscular fitness
Prevention of falls
Reduced depression
Better cognitive function (older adults)

**Moderate to Strong Evidence**

Better functional health (older adults)
Reduced abdominal obesity

**Moderate Evidence**

Weight maintenance after weight loss
Lower risk of hip fracture
Increased bone density
Improved sleep quality
Lower risk of lung and endometrial cancers

Source:
http://www.health.gov/paguidelines/factSheetProf.aspx

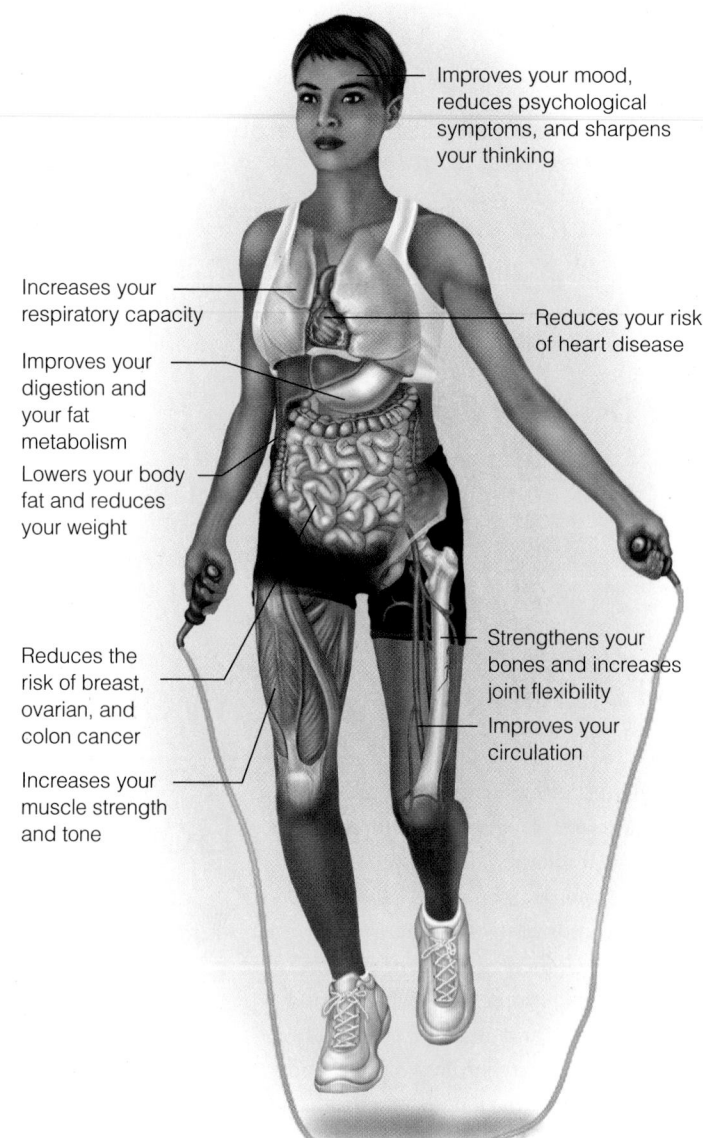

Improves your mood, reduces psychological symptoms, and sharpens your thinking

Increases your respiratory capacity

Reduces your risk of heart disease

Improves your digestion and your fat metabolism

Lowers your body fat and reduces your weight

Reduces the risk of breast, ovarian, and colon cancer

Increases your muscle strength and tone

Strengthens your bones and increases joint flexibility

Improves your circulation

laps, or bicycling, that made them sweat), fewer than half of college students report the same level of exercise. Once active in high school, one-third of students become insufficiently active in the first three weeks at college.

 Asian males were more active than whites, while Asian females were less active. Hispanic men and women were more active than their white peers.

As students progress from their first to fourth year of studies, they exercise less. The most drastic drop in physical activity occurs in the freshman year. In a recent study, physical fitness declined, and levels of total cholesterol, harmful LDL (low-density lipoprotein) cholesterol, and fasting glucose (blood sugar) levels increased over undergraduates' first 14-week school term. (See Chapter 15 for a complete discussion of these risk factors for heart disease.)

In research on influences on students' health behaviors, peer pressure to exercise, having an exercise partner, a flexible class schedule, access to fitness facilities, and a sense of being stressed all increase physical activity. Female students report exercising more at college, particularly when their workload is heavy and their stress levels rise. Peers have a greater impact on men than on women.

College courses that require regular exercise in order to earn academic credit have proven effective in motivating students and in teaching them specific skills, such as how to monitor their heart rates.[6]

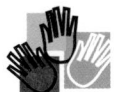 In a study of college students in the United States, Costa Rica, India, and South Korea, vigorous physical activity correlated with perceived overweight and fruit and vegetable consumption everywhere. However, physical activity was not consistently linked with gender or TV/video watching cross culturally.

# Physical Activity and Health

## Why Exercise?

If exercise could be packed into a pill, it would be the single most widely prescribed and beneficial medicine in the nation. Why? Because nothing can do more to help your body function at its best—a fact that not all students know. In a survey, eight in ten undergraduates realized that physical activity can prevent heart disease and prevent and treat obesity. However, fewer than half knew that it maintains bone density and can help prevent diabetes.

As Figure 8.2 illustrates, exercise provides head-to-toe benefits. With regular activity, your heart muscles become stronger and pump blood more efficiently. Your heart rate and resting pulse slow down. Your blood pressure may drop slightly from its normal level.

Exercise thickens the bones and can slow the loss of calcium that normally occurs with age. Physical activity increases flexibility in the joints and improves digestion and elimination. It speeds up metabolism and builds lean body mass, so the body burns more calories and body fat decreases. It heightens sensitivity to insulin (a great benefit for diabetics) and may lower the risk of developing diabetes. In addition, exercise enhances clot-dissolving substances in the

blood, helping to prevent strokes, heart attacks, and pulmonary embolisms (clots in the lungs), and it helps lower the risk of certain cancers.

Numerous studies have documented the benefits of physical activity in preventing or delaying many age-related conditions, including osteoarthritis, falls, hip fractures, cardiovascular disease, respiratory diseases, cancer, diabetes mellitus, osteoporosis, obesity, and decreased functional ability.[7] In a recent study, women who regularly participated in physical activity during middle age were more likely to be in better health at age 70 than those with lower fitness levels.[8] But it's never too late to get in shape. Women who started an exercise program at age 65 or older developed higher bone density and greatly reduced their risk of falls.[9]

Regular exercise can actually extend your lifespan and sharpen your memory and mind by combating the ongoing damage done to cells, tissue, and organs that underlie many chronic conditions. It also lowers blood pressure, reduces bad cholesterol, and cuts the incidence of type 2 diabetes. Exercise lengthens telomeres, the strands of DNA at the tips of chromosomes. When telomeres get too short, cells no longer can divide and become inactive—a process associated with aging, cancer, and higher risk of death. In a recent study of professional athletes (some in their twenties, some middle-aged) and healthy nonsmokers in the same age groups, the athletes had significantly less erosion in telomeres.

If you start exercising now and keep working out, you're less likely to put on pounds and inches as you age. In a recent study that followed men and women (initially between ages 18 and 30) for 20 years, those who put in at least 150 minutes of moderate to vigorous physical activity a week—running, fast walking, basketball, exercise classes, or housework—remained leaner than their less active peers. Men gained an average of 5.7 fewer pounds and 1.2 fewer inches around the gut. Women put on 13.4 fewer pounds and 1.5 fewer inches around their waists.[10]

*Healthier Heart and Lungs* Regular physical activity makes blood less likely to clot and cause a stroke or heart attack. Sedentary people are about twice as likely to die of a heart attack as people who are physically active.

Although rigorous exercise somewhat increases the risk of sudden cardiac death for men, regular physical activity lowers the overall danger, especially in women. (See Chapter 15 for a discussion of heart disease.)

Exercise also lowers levels of the indicators of increased risk of heart disease, such as high cholesterol. Exercise itself, even without weight loss, may reduce dangerous blood fats in obese individuals. It also lowers the risk of developing the prediabetic condition called metabolic syndrome, which if untreated can lead to type 2 diabetes and increase the risk of heart disease.

In women exercise lowers the risk of a fatal heart attack by slowing a rapid heart rate. The faster the resting heart rate (beats per minute), the greater the risk of dying from a heart attack in both sexes, although the risk is higher in women.[11]

In addition to its effects on the heart, exercise makes the lungs more efficient. The lungs take in more oxygen, and their vital capacity (the maximum amount of air volume the lungs can take in and expel) increases, providing more energy for you to use.

Even in young men, physical fitness is associated with improvements in blood pressure and the makeup of blood fats, including cholesterol and triglycerides. Exercise, along with a healthy weight, keeps blood fats at healthy levels over time. Prolonged, sustained endurance training prevents the stiffening of the heart muscle once thought to be an inevitable consequence of aging. Cardiorespiratory fitness declines more rapidly after age 45, but exercising regularly, maintaining a healthy weight, and not smoking can help maintain cardiorespiratory health throughout life.

**Protection Against Cancer** Physical activity lowers the likelihood of getting some forms of cancer and, according to preliminary research, may lessen the risk of recurrence or a second cancer. According to the American Institute for Cancer Research, physical activity may lower the risk of colon cancer by 40 to 50 percent, the risk of breast, endometrial, and lung cancers by 30 to 40 percent, and the risk of prostate cancer by 10 to 30 percent. Along with a healthful diet and limited alcohol intake, regular exercise could prevent about 340,000 cancer cases a year.[12]

The combination of excess weight and physical inactivity may account for a quarter to a third of all breast cancer cases. Regular, lifelong exercise may lower a woman's breast cancer risk by 20 percent, possibly by reducing weight and body mass and preventing metabolic syndrome and chronic inflammation (discussed in Chapter 15). It is not clear whether exercise can prevent a recurrence in women who have had breast cancer, but it does improve their overall survival rates. Women who exercised regularly in the year before a diagnosis of breast cancer have higher survival rates than sedentary women. Exercise also lowers the risk of recurrence in colon cancer, perhaps by lowering levels of substances such as insulin and insulin-like growth factor that drive the growth of cancer cells. Men who regularly get moderate exercise may have a lower risk of developing prostate cancer; those who do get the disease are less likely to have aggressive, fast-growing tumors.

**Greater Immunity** Exercise may enhance immune function by reducing stress hormones like cortisol that can dampen resistance to disease, and by increasing the circulation of natural killer cells that fight off viruses and bacteria. Exercise also improves the body's response to the influenza vaccine so it is more effective at keeping the virus at bay.

In a recent study, people who walked briskly for 45 minutes five days a week over 12 to 15 weeks had fewer and less severe upper respiratory infections, such as colds and flu, and reduced their number of sick days by 25 to 50 percent compared to a sedentary control group.[13]

**Brighter Mood and Less Stress** Exercise makes people feel good from the inside out. Exercise boosts mood, elevates self-esteem, increases energy, reduces anxiety, improves concentration and alertness, and may help ward off dementia. During long workouts, some people experience what is called "runner's high," which may be the result of increased levels of mood-elevating brain chemicals called **endorphins**.

A highly effective stress reducer, exercise reduces muscle tension and cortisol secretion. According to a recent study, psychological improvements occur even after a 20-minute bout of exercise, regardless of how intensely you exercise. Physical activity also may boost memory and other

**endorphins** Mood-elevating, pain-killing chemicals produced by the brain.

cognitive abilities in certain individuals. Brisk walks three times a week boost seniors' scores on memory tests and increase the size of the hippocampus, a portion of the brain involved with memory formation.[14]

### Better Mental Health and Functioning

Exercise is an effective—but underused—treatment for mild to moderate depression and may help in treating other mental disorders. Regular, moderate exercise—such as walking, running, or lifting weights—three times a week has proved helpful for depression and anxiety disorders, including panic attacks. Exercise is as effective as medication in improving mood and also helps prevent relapse.

Lifelong fitness may protect the brain as we age. According to numerous long-term studies, physically fit adults perform better on cognitive tests than their less fit peers. Improving cardio-respiratory fitness reduces the harmful effects of aging on brain structures as well as on memory and other functions.

Exercise appears to help prevent and improve mild cognitive impairment. People who were moderately active at midlife or later were less likely to suffer cognitive declines, while those with mild cognitive impairment improved after six months of high-intensity aerobic exercise. Exercise may protect the aging brain by means of increased blood flow, improved development and survival of neurons, and decreased risk of heart and blood vessel diseases.[15]

Among older women, those who did an hour or two of strength training every week showed improved cognition a year later, scoring higher on tests of memory and thinking than those who did toning and balance exercises.[16] In another study, moderate to high physical activity lowered seniors' risk of cognitive impairment over a two-year period.[17]

### Better Bones

By 2020, one in two Americans over age 50 may suffer from **osteoporosis**—a condition in which bones lose their mineral density and become susceptible to injury. Most are unaware that their bone health is in jeopardy. Four times as many men and almost three times as many women actually have osteoporosis than those that realize they do. (See Chapter 20 for more on osteoporosis and aging.)

You may think that weak, brittle bones are a problem only for the elderly. However, 2 percent of college-age women have osteoporosis; another 15 percent have already sustained significant losses in bone density and are at high risk of osteoporosis.

Exercise during adolescence and young adulthood may prevent bone weakening and fractures in old age. Women who did not participate in high school sports are seven times more likely to have low bone density than those who did. The college women at greatest risk often are extremely skinny and maintain their low weights and slim looks by dieting and by avoiding exercise so as not to increase their muscle mass. Some eliminate dairy products, an important source of calcium, from their diets. Depo-Provera, a method of birth control that consists of hormone injections every three months, also is associated with low bone density, especially with long-term use. (See Chapter 10 on contraception.)

What are the best exercises to boost bone density? According to a study of college women, high-impact aerobics, such as step exercising, "may offer the quickest route to building bone in young women." Resistance exercises such as squats, leg presses, and calf presses strengthened leg muscles but had no effect on bone density. The American College of Sports Medicine recommends moderate- to high-intensity weight-bearing activities to maintain bone mass in adults.

### Lower Weight

For individuals on a diet, exercise provides extra benefits: Dieters who work out lose more fat than lean muscle tissue, which improves their body composition. Exercise also may help to control weight by suppressing appetite. Aerobic activity, such as a vigorous 60-minute workout on a treadmill, affects the release of two key appetite hormones. Resistance training, such as 90 minutes of weightlifting, affects only one of these hormones.

In a recent study, dieters who exercised as well as cut calories lost about the same amount of weight over a six-month period. But those who worked out had better health outcomes, including lower blood pressure and cholesterol.[18]

### Sexuality

By improving physical endurance, muscle tone, blood flow, and body composition, exercise improves sexual functioning.

**osteoporosis** A condition in which the bones become increasingly soft and porous, making them susceptible to injury.

Simply burning 200 extra calories a day can significantly lower the risk of erectile dysfunction in sedentary men. Exercise also may increase sexual drive, activity, and sexual satisfaction in people of all ages.

 ***Benefits for Students*** Unlike middle-aged and older individuals, traditional-age college students cite improved fitness as the number one advantage that exercise offers, followed by improved appearance and muscle tone. Undergraduates who recognize the benefits of exercise are more likely to be physically active than those who focus on barriers to working out.

Their brains may also benefit. According to a very large recent study of more than 1.2 million men, strong cardiorespiratory fitness in young adulthood was associated with higher intelligence, better grades, and greater success in life. The reasons may be improved blood flow to the brain, diminished anxiety, enhanced mood, and less fatigue.

### A More Active and Fulfilling Old Age
Exercise slows the changes that are associated with advancing age: loss of lean muscle tissue, increase in body fat, and decrease in work capacity. In addition to lowering the risk of heart disease and stroke, exercise helps older men and women retain the strength and mobility needed to live independently. In a study of overweight, post-menopausal women, exercise improved both physical and mental well-being—and the more the women exercised, the greater the improvements in their quality of life. Even in old age, exercise boosts strength and stamina, lessens time in wheelchairs, and improves outlook and sense of control.

***Longer Life*** People who are physically active for approximately seven hours a week have a 40 percent lower risk of dying early than those who are active for less than 30 minutes a week.[19] Those who exercise regularly enjoy 3.7 years of additional life expectancy when compared with sedentary individuals. Formerly sedentary people, even the elderly, who begin to exercise live longer, on average, than those who remain inactive.

## Exercise Risks

Beyond doubt exercise is good for you. But despite its many benefits, exercise can pose risks—and not just for those over age 40. Even young college athletes who seem in perfect health have collapsed and died while playing sports such as football, running, and basketball.[20]

The most common cause is hypertrophic cardiomyopathy (HCM), a genetic disease that results in thickening or enlargement of the heart that affects up to 1 in 500 people. HCM accounts for 40 percent of all deaths on athletic fields in the United States.[21] An average of 66 athletes younger than age 40 die each year from cardiac arrest in the United States.[22] HCM can be detected and treated. Medical experts urge screening for all young athletes, beginning in elementary school. However, screening results in a high number of false positives and has not proven to reduce young athlete deaths.[23]

Other college athletes may also be at cardiovascular risk. In a recent study of an ethnically diverse sample of university players, one in four had a BMI in the overweight range (discussed later in this chapter). One in five had elevated blood pressure and was considered "prehypertensive" (discussed in Chapter 15), and one in four had lower-than-recommended levels of beneficial HDL cholesterol. Those with the largest waist circumferences were at greater risk.

## Physical Activity Guidelines for Americans

The most recent U.S. Department of Health and Human Services *Physical Activity Guidelines for Americans*, based on the most significant research findings on the health benefits of physical activity, recognize that some activity is better than none. However, the *Guidelines* emphasize that more activity—consisting of both aerobic (endurance) and muscle-strengthening (resistance) physical activity—is more beneficial. People of every age—children, adolescents, adults, seniors—and those in every racial and ethnic

## How to Meet the ACSM Guidelines

- **Work in short bouts.** Ten-minute intervals of exercise can be just as effective as exercising for 30 minutes straight.

- **Mix it up.** Combine moderate- and vigorous-intensity exercises to meet the guidelines. For instance, you can walk briskly two days a week and jog at a faster pace on other days.

- **Set aside exercise times.** Schedule exercise in advance so you can plan your day around it.

- **Find exercise buddies.** Recruit roommates, friends, family, coworkers. You'll have more fun on your way to getting fit.

group, along with those with disabilities, can benefit from physical activity.[24]

Here are the government's key recommendations:

- **All adults should avoid inactivity.** Some physical activity is better than none, and adults who participate in any amount of physical activity gain some health benefits.

- For substantial health benefits, **adults should do at least 150 minutes (2 hours and 30 minutes) a week** of moderate-intensity, or 75 minutes (1 hour and 15 minutes) a week of vigorous-intensity aerobic physical activity, or an equivalent combination of moderate- and vigorous-intensity aerobic activity. Aerobic activity should be performed in episodes of at least 10 minutes, and, preferably, it should be spread throughout the week.

- For additional and more extensive health benefits, **adults should increase their aerobic physical activity to 300 minutes** (5 hours) a week of moderate-intensity, or 150 minutes a week of vigorous-intensity aerobic physical activity, or an equivalent combination of moderate- and vigorous-intensity activity. Additional health benefits

are gained by engaging in physical activity beyond this amount.

- Adults should also do muscle-strengthening activities that are moderate or high intensity and involve all major muscle groups **on two or more days a week,** as these activities provide additional health benefits.

The American College of Sports Medicine (ACSM) and the American Heart Association (AHA) have released similar guidelines that call for:

Moderately intense cardiorespiratory exercise 30 minutes a day, 5 days a week

*or*

Vigorously intense cardiorespiratory exercise 20 minutes a day, 3 days a week

*and*

8 to 10 strength-training exercises, with 8 to 12 repetitions of each exercise, twice a week.

According to the ACSM, moderate-intensity physical activity means working hard enough to raise your heart rate and break a sweat, yet still being able to carry on a conversation. The 30-minute recommendation is for the average healthy adult to maintain health and reduce the risk for chronic disease.

If you need to lose weight or want to keep off pounds you lost, you will need to exercise more. According to the ACSM's statement on "appropriate physical activity intervention strategies for weight loss and prevention of weight regain," long-term weight loss requires 250 or more minutes (2 hours and 30 minutes) of moderately intense physical activity per week. Less exercise can prevent a gain greater than 3 percent of current weight but provides what the ACSM describes as "only modest" weight loss. In addition to aerobic workouts, the ACSM recommends resistance training to increase lean tissue and decrease fat.

The timing of exercise may make a difference in weight loss. In a recent study, volunteers who exercised in the morning before eating breakfast but ate the same amount of calories as late-day exercisers were less likely to gain weight, burned fat more efficiently, and metabolized foods more efficiently.[25]

## Health in Action

### *Excise Exercise Excuses*

In your online journal, write down as many reasons as you can think of not to exercise. Then come up with quick excuse busters. Here are some ideas:

**I can't afford a gym.**
- Who needs a gym? You can get all the exercise you need on your own.
- Check out campus or community facilities.
- Walk or jog outdoors.
- Invest in inexpensive hand weights.

**The school gym is always crowded.**
- Always? Have you tried Sunday mornings, Friday evening at 7:00, Tuesdays at 3:00 p.m.? Ask the staff what the quietest hours are.
- If there are lines for the weight machines, use hand weights. If the treadmills are occupied, go to the outdoor track.
- Sign up for small-group training or classes to guarantee yourself a spot.

**It's finals week.**
- Break up study sessions with mini-workouts.
- Burn off tension with a jog.
- Unwind after studying with stretches, yoga, or pilates.

**I go to my dorm and just don't feel like leaving.**
- Arrange to meet friends at the gym. If you know they're waiting, you'll go out even if it's rainy and cold.
- Sign up for a gym class during the day so that you don't have to make an extra trip.
- Recruit an exercise buddy so that the two of you can motivate each other to get moving.

See the complete "Excise Exercise Excuses" in *Labs for Invitation to Personal Change.*

## Table 8.1 **Exercise Options**

Vigorous activities take more effort than moderate ones. Here are just a few moderate and vigorous aerobic physical activities. Do these for 10 minutes or more at a time.

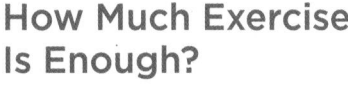

| Moderate Activities (I can talk while I do them, but I can't sing.) | Vigorous Activities (I can only say a few words without stopping to catch my breath.) |
|---|---|
| • Ballroom and line dancing | • Aerobic dance |
| • Biking on level ground or with few hills | • Biking faster than 10 miles per hour |
| • Canoeing | • Fast dancing |
| • General gardening (raking, trimming shrubs) | • Heavy gardening (digging, hoeing) |
| • Sports where you catch and throw | • Hiking uphill (baseball, softball, volleyball) |
| • Tennis (doubles) | • Jumping rope |
| • Using your manual wheelchair | • Martial arts (such as karate) |
| • Using hand cyclers—also called ergometers | • Race walking, jogging, or running |
| • Walking briskly | • Sports with a lot of running (basketball, hockey, soccer) |
| • Water aerobics | • Swimming fast or swimming laps |
| | • Tennis (singles) |

Image copyright Sean Nel, 2010 Used under license from Shutterstock.com

## How Much Exercise Is Enough?

In developing federal physical activity guidelines, experts considered dozens of studies and concluded that the "amount of physical activity necessary to produce health benefits cannot yet be identified with a high degree of precision." However, they did determine the minimum amount of exercise required for a significant lowering of the risk of premature dying: 500 MET minutes of exercise a week.

A single **MET**, or **metabolic equivalent of task**, is the amount of energy a person uses at rest. Two METs represent twice the energy burned at rest; four METs, four times the energy used at rest; and so on. Walking at three miles per hour is a 3.3-MET activity, while running at six miles per hour is a ten-MET activity. Moderate exercise is defined by the Department of Health and Human Services as activities of between three and six METs, equivalent

to about 45 to 64 percent of your maximum heart rate (discussed on page 241)—or, in simpler terms, activities during which you can carry on a conversation but cannot sing out loud. (See Table 8.1.)

The weekly minimum of 500 MET minutes of exercise does not mean 500 minutes of exercise. Instead, 150 minutes a week (two and a half hours) of a moderate, three- to five-MET activity, such as walking, works out to be about 500 MET minutes. Half as much time (an hour and 15 minutes per week) spent on a six-plus-MET activity like easy jogging produces similar health effects. As a rule of thumb, one minute of vigorous-intensity activity is as beneficial as two minutes of moderate-intensity activity.

Are more METS better? To a certain extent, the answer is yes. Activity of 500 MET minutes a week substantially reduces the risk of premature death, but a significant reduction in breast cancer risk requires more METs. Exercise in the range of 500 to 1,000 MET minutes a week, experts generally agree, delivers substantial benefits.

# The Principles of Exercise

Your body is literally what you make of it. Superbly designed for multiple uses, it adjusts to meet physical demands. If you need to sprint for a bus, your heart will speed up and pump more blood. Beyond such immediate, short-term adaptations, physical training can produce long-term changes in heart rate, oxygen consumption, and muscle strength and endurance. Although there are limits on the maximum levels of physical fitness and performance that any individual can achieve, regular exercise can produce improvements in everyone's baseline wellness and fitness.

The following principles of exercise are fundamental to any physical activity plan.

## Overload Principle

The **overload principle** requires a person exercising to provide a greater stress or demand on the body than it's usually accustomed to

**MET (metabolic equivalent of task)** The amount of energy a person uses at rest.

**overload principle** Providing a greater stress or demand on the body than it is normally accustomed to handling.

handling. For any muscle, including the heart, to get stronger, it must work against a greater-than-normal resistance or challenge. To continue to improve, you need further increases in the demands—but not too much too quickly. **Progressive overloading**—gradually increasing physical challenges—provides the benefits of exercise without the risk of injuries (Figure 8.3).

Overloading is specific to each body part and to each component of fitness. Leg exercises develop only the lower limbs; arm exercises, only the upper limbs. This is why you need a comprehensive fitness plan that includes a variety of exercises to develop different parts of the body. If you play a particular sport, you also need training to develop sports-specific skills, such as a strong, efficient stroke in swimming.

## FITT

Although low-intensity activity can enhance basic health, you need to work harder—that is, at a greater intensity—to improve fitness. Whatever exercise you do, there is a level, or threshold, at which fitness begins to improve; a target zone, where you can achieve maximum benefits; and an upper limit, at which potential risks outweigh any further benefits. The acronym **FITT** sums up the four dimensions of progressive overload: *frequency* (how often you exercise), *intensity* (how hard), *time* (how long), and *type* (specific activity).

*Frequency*   To attain and maintain physical fitness, you need to exercise regularly, but the recommended frequency varies with different types of exercise and with an individual's fitness goals. Health officials urge Americans to engage in moderate-intensity aerobic activity most days and in resistance and flexibility training two or three days a week.

*Intensity*   Exercise intensity varies with the type of exercise and with personal goals. To improve cardiorespiratory fitness, you need at a minimum to increase your heart rate to a target zone (the level that produces benefits). To develop muscular strength and endurance, you need to increase the amount of weight you lift or the resistance you work against and/or the number of repetitions. For enhanced flexibility, you need to stretch muscles beyond their normal length.

Figure 8.3   **The Overload Principle**
By increasing frequency, intensity, or duration, you will improve your level of fitness. Once your body adapts to (becomes comfortable with) the demands, you can again apply the overload principle to achieve a higher level of fitness.

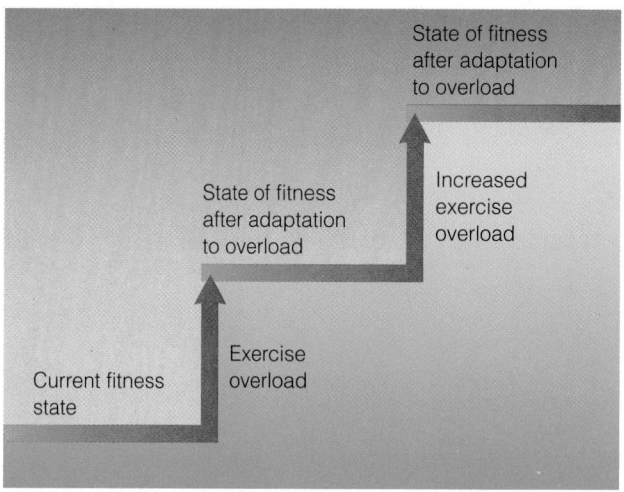

*Time (Duration)*   The amount of time, or duration, of your workouts is also important, particularly for cardiorespiratory exercise. The American College of Sports Medicine recommends 30 to 45 minutes of aerobic exercise, preceded by 5 to 10 minutes of warm-up and followed by 5 to 10 minutes of stretching. However, experts have found similar health benefits from a single 30-minute session of moderate exercise as from several shorter sessions throughout the day. Duration and intensity are interlinked. If you're exercising at high intensity (biking or running at a brisk pace, for instance), you don't need to exercise as long as when you're working at lower intensity (walking or swimming at a moderate pace). For muscular strength and endurance and for flexibility, duration is defined by the number of sets or repetitions rather than total time.

*Type (Specificity)*   The **specificity principle** refers to the body's adaptation to a particular type of activity or amount of stress placed upon it. Jogging, for instance, trains the heart and lungs to work more efficiently and strengthens certain leg muscles. However, it does not build upper body strength or enhance flexibility.

## Reversibility Principle

The **reversibility principle** is the opposite of the overload principle. Just as the body adapts to greater physical demands, it also adjusts to

**progressive overloading** Gradually increasing physical challenges once the body adapts to the stress placed upon it to produce maximum benefits.

**FITT** A formula that describes the frequency, intensity, type, and length of time for physical activity.

**specificity principle** Each part of the body adapts to a particular type and amount of stress placed upon it.

**reversibility principle** The physical benefits of exercise are lost through disuse or inactivity.

# Improving Cardiorespiratory Fitness

Cardiorespiratory endurance refers to the ability of the heart, lungs, and circulatory system to deliver oxygen to muscles working rhythmically over an extended period of time. Unlike muscular endurance (discussed later in this chapter), which is specific to individual muscles, cardiorespiratory endurance involves the entire body. **Aerobic exercise**, which improves cardiorespiratory endurance, can take many forms, but all involve working strenuously without pushing to the point of breathlessness. A person who builds up good aerobic capacity can maintain long periods of physical activity without great fatigue.

In **anaerobic exercise**, the amount of oxygen taken in by the body cannot meet the demands of the activity. This quickly creates an oxygen deficit that must be made up later. Anaerobic activities are high in intensity but short in duration, usually lasting only about ten seconds to two minutes. An example is sprinting the quarter-mile, which leaves even the best-trained athletes gasping for air. In *nonaerobic exercise*, such as bowling, softball, or doubles tennis, there is frequent rest between activities. Because the body can take in all the oxygen it needs, the heart and lungs don't get much of a workout.

## Monitoring Intensity

To use your pulse, or heart rate, as a guide, feel your pulse in the carotid artery in your neck. Slightly tilt your head back and to one side. Use your middle finger or forefinger, or both, to feel for your pulse. (Do not use your thumb; it has a beat of its own.) To determine your heart rate, count the number of pulses you feel for 10 seconds and multiply that number by six, or count for 30 seconds and multiply that number by two. Learn to recognize the pulsing of your heart when you're sitting or lying down. This is your **resting heart rate**.

Start taking your pulse during, or immediately after, exercise, when it's much more pronounced than when you're at rest. Three minutes after heavy exercise, take your pulse again. The

Group sports provide a fun alternative way to exercise, but an occasional game is no substitute for regular physical activity.

**aerobic exercise** Physical activity in which sufficient or excess oxygen is continually supplied to the body.

**anaerobic exercise** Physical activity in which the body develops an oxygen deficit.

**resting heart rate** The number of heartbeats per minute during inactivity.

lower levels. If you stop exercising, you can lose as much as 50 percent of your fitness improvements within two months. If you have to curtail your usual exercise routine because of a busy schedule, you can best maintain your fitness by keeping the intensity constant and reducing frequency or duration. The principle of reversibility is aptly summed up by the phrase, "Use it or lose it."

© Ariel Skelley/Blend Images/Jupiterimages

closer that reading is to your resting heart rate, the better your condition. If it takes a long time for your pulse to recover and return to its resting level, your body's ability to handle physical stress is poor. As you continue working out, however, your pulse will return to normal much more quickly.

*Target Heart Rate*  You don't want to push yourself to your maximum heart rate. The ACSM recommends working at 55 to 65 percent of that maximum to get cardiorespiratory benefits from your training. This range is called your **target heart rate**. If you don't exercise intensely enough to raise your heart rate at least this high, your heart and lungs won't reap the most benefit from the workout. If you push too hard, and exercise at or near your absolute maximum heart rate, you run the risk of placing too great a burden on your heart.

In order to find the best "zone" for your goals and activity, you must first know how to calculate your maximum heart rate. The following formula offers a rough baseline:

$$220 - \text{Age} = \text{maximum heart rate (MHR)}$$

The ACSM recommends that for endurance training and general aerobic conditioning, you calculate 50 to 65 percent of your maximum heart rate if you're a beginner; 60 to 75 percent for intermediate level exercisers; and 70 to 85 percent for established aerobic exercisers. For example, if you're a 45-year-old beginner with no known health issues, your maximum heart rate is approximately 175 beats a minute. Fifty to 65 percent of that maximum is 87 to 113 beats per minute.

For weight loss, use interval training to burn the most calories. Short bursts of high-intensity exercise (80 to 85 percent of your maximum heart rate) followed by lower-intensity recovery periods (50 to 65 percent of your maximum heart rate) burn more calories than exercising at a consistent level of exertion for the same amount of time.

Your heart rate can also help you keep tabs on your progress: measure your heart rate 15 to 60 minutes after exercising and compare these numbers over time as you get in better shape. The numbers decrease as your heart becomes stronger.[26]

## Figure 8.4  Revised Scale for Rating of Perceived Exertion (RPE)

You can learn to rate your exertion based on this scale.

Source: Original scale from G. Borg, "Psychophysical Bases of Perceived Exertion," *Medicine and Science in Sports and Exercise*, Vol. 14, No. 5, 2003, pp. 377–381.

| Rating of Perceived Exertion (RPE) | |
| --- | --- |
| 0 | Nothing at all |
| 0.5 | Extremely weak (just noticeable) |
| 1 | Very weak |
| 2 | Weak (light) |
| 3 | Moderate |
| 4 | Somewhat strong |
| 5 | Strong (heavy) |
| 6 | — |
| 7 | Very strong |
| 8 | — |
| 9 | — |
| 10 | Extremely strong (almost maximum) |

4 and 5: Correlate to target heart rate

*Rating of Perceived Exertion (RPE)*
Another option besides heart rate for monitoring your exercise intensity is the **Rating of Perceived Exertion (RPE)**, a self-assessment scale that rates symptoms of breathlessness and fatigue. You can use the RPE scale to describe your sensation of effort when exercising and gauge how hard you are working. The ACSM revised the original RPE scale to a range of 0 to 10 (Figure 8.4). Most exercisers should aim for a perceived exertion of "somewhat strong" or "strong," the equivalent of 4 or 5 on the RPE scale.

RPE is considered fairly reliable, but about 10 percent of the population tends to over- or underestimate their exertion. Your health or physical education instructor can help you learn to match what your body is feeling to the RPE scale. By paying attention to how you feel at different exercise intensities, you can learn to challenge yourself without risking your safety.

You can also experiment with alternative ways for determining exercise intensity. One of the easiest follows.

**target heart rate** Sixty to 85 percent of the maximum heart rate; the heart rate at which one derives maximum cardiovascular benefit from aerobic exercise.

**Rating of Perceived Exertion (RPE)** A self-assessment scale that rates symptoms of breathlessness and fatigue.

*"Talk Test"* During "aerobic" exercise you should be able to carry on a somewhat stilted conversation if you are indeed "with oxygen"—which is what the word "aerobic" means.

If you are gasping for air and unable to talk, you are most likely working at or beyond the anaerobic "without oxygen" threshold—a very, very, very hard intensity level at or beyond the high end of the aerobic zone.

If you can sing the entire "Star Spangled Banner," you are probably not exerting much effort. If you can sing "Row Row Row Your Boat," but have to take a breath after every other word, you are probably working pretty hard—and just where you should be.

## Designing an Aerobic Workout

Whatever activity you choose, your aerobic workout should consist of several stages: a warm-up, an aerobic activity, and a cool-down.

*Warm-Up* Just as you don't get in your car and immediately gun your engine to 60 miles per hour, you shouldn't do the same with your body. You need to prepare your cardiorespiratory system for a workout, speed up the blood flow to your lungs, and increase the temperature and elasticity of your muscles and connective tissue to avoid injury.

After reviewing more than 350 scientific studies, the ACSM concluded that preparing for sports or exercise should involve a variety of activities and not be limited to stretching alone. Researchers found little to no relationship between stretching and injuries or postexercise pain. A better option is a combination of warm-up, strength training, and balance exercises.

*Aerobic Activity* The two key components of this part of your workout are intensity and duration. As described in the previous section, you can use your target heart rate range to make sure you are working at the proper intensity. The current recommendation is to keep moving for 30 to 60 minutes, either in one session or several briefer sessions, each lasting at least 10 minutes.

*Cool Down* After you've pushed your heart rate up to its target level and kept it there for a while, the worst thing you can do is slam on the brakes. If you come to a sudden stop, you put your heart at risk. When you stand or sit immediately after vigorous exercise, blood can pool in your legs. You need to keep moving at a slower pace to ensure an adequate supply of blood to your heart. Ideally, you should walk for 5 to 10 minutes at a comfortable pace before you end your workout session.

## Your Long-Term Fitness Plan

One of the most common mistakes people make is to push too hard too fast. Often they end up injured or discouraged and quit entirely. If you are just starting an aerobic program, think of it as a series of phases: beginning, progression, and maintenance:

- **Beginning (4–6 weeks).** Start slow and low (in intensity). If you're walking, monitor your heart rate and aim for 55 percent of your maximum heart rate. Another good rule of thumb to make sure you're moving at the right pace: If you can sing as you walk, you're going too slow; if you can't talk, you're going too fast.
- **Progression (16–20 weeks).** Gradually increase the duration and/or intensity of your workouts. For instance, you might add 5 minutes every two weeks to your walking time. You also can gradually pick up your pace, using your target heart rate as your guide. Keep a log of your workouts so you can chart your progress until you reach your goal.
- **Maintenance (lifelong).** Once you've reached the stage of exercising for an hour every day, you may want to develop a repertoire of aerobic activities you enjoy. Combine or alternate activities to avoid monotony and keep up your enthusiasm (cross-training).

## Aerobic Options

You have lots of choices for aerobic exercise, so experiment. Focus on one for a few weeks; alternate different activities on different days; try something new every month.

*Stepping Out: Walk the Walk* More men and women are taking to their feet. Some are casualties of high-intensity sports and can no longer withstand the wear and tear of rigorous workouts. Others want to shape up, slim down, or ward off heart disease and other health problems. The good news for all is that walking is good exercise.[27] Walking may reduce the risk factors for cardiorespiratory disease, such as insulin resistance, as much as vigorous activity does.

*Why Walk?* One major study of women, the Nurses Health Study, found that women who walk briskly three hours a week are as well protected from heart disease as women who spend an hour and a half a week in more vigorous activities, such as aerobics or running. Women engaged in either form of exercise had a rate of heart attacks 30 to 40 percent lower than that of sedentary women.

Walking also protects men's hearts, whether they're healthy or have had heart problems. Men who regularly engage in light exercise, including walking, have a significantly lower risk of death than their sedentary counterparts.

Walking has proved to be one of the safest and most effective ways of preventing bone and joint disorders in obese individuals. In a study that followed healthy men and women between the ages of 18 and 30 for 15 years, the regular walkers gained less weight over time and were more likely to lose weight and keep pounds off.

*America on the Move* How many steps do you walk every day? The typical adult averages about 5,310 steps; a child from 11,000 to 13,000. According to the American College of Sports Medicine, college students who used a pedometer to count their daily steps took an average of 7,700 steps per day. This falls short of the 10,000 steps recommended as part of the national "America on the Move" program.

How far is 10,000 steps? The average person's stride length is approximately 2.5 feet. That means it takes just over 2,000 steps to walk one mile, and 10,000 steps is close to five miles. Wearing a pedometer is an easy way to track your steps each day. Start by wearing the pedometer every day for one week. Put it on when you get up in the morning and wear it until bedtime. Record your daily steps in a log or diary. By the end of the week, you can calculate your average daily steps. To increase your steps, add 500 daily steps every week until you reach 10,000. The more steps you take, the lower your risk of health problems such as diabetes.[28]

Why 10,000 steps? According to researchers' estimates, you take about 5,000 steps just to accomplish your daily tasks. Adding about 2,000 steps brings you to a level that can improve your health and wellness. Another 3,000 steps can help you lose excess pounds and prevent weight gain. People who walk at least 10,000 steps a day are more likely to have healthy weights. In addition, 10,000 steps generally translates into 30 minutes of activity, the minimum recommended by the U.S. Surgeon General.

Regular use of pedometers has proven effective in helping overweight individuals increase their steps per day. However, pedometers alone do not measure exercise intensity. In order to meet the current physical activity guidelines, researchers have determined that individuals should walk a minimum of 3,000 steps in 30 minutes or three bouts of 1,000 steps in ten minutes on five days of the week.

Treadmills are a good alternative to outdoor walks—and not just in bad weather. They keep you moving at a certain pace, they're easier on the knees, and they allow you to exercise in a climate-controlled, pollution-free environment—a definite plus for many city dwellers. Holding onto the handrails while walking on a treadmill reduces both heart rate and oxygen consumption, so you burn fewer calories. Experts advise slowing the pace if necessary so you can let go of the handrails while working out.

*Jogging and Running* The difference between jogging and running is speed. You should be able to carry on a conversation with someone on a long jog or run; if you're too breathless to talk, you're pushing too hard.

If your goal is to enhance aerobic fitness, long, slow, distance running is best. If you want to improve your speed, try *interval training*—repeated hard runs over a certain distance, with intervals of relaxed jogging in between. Depending on what suits you and what your training goals are, you can vary the distance, duration, and number of fast runs, as well as the time and activity between them.

If you have been sedentary, it's best to launch a walking program before attempting to jog or run. Start by walking for 15 to 20 minutes three times a week at a comfortable pace. Continue at this same level until you no longer feel sore or unduly fatigued the day after exercising. Then

## The Right Way to Walk and Run

Here are some guidelines for putting your best foot forward, whether you are walking or running:

- **Take time to warm up.**

- **Maintain good posture.** Keep your back straight, your head up, and your eyes looking straight ahead. Hold your arms slightly away from your body—your elbows should be bent slightly so that your forearms are almost parallel to the ground.

- **Use the heel-to-toe method.** The heel of your leading foot should touch the ground before the ball or toes of that foot do. Push off the ball of your foot, and bend your knee as you raise your heel. You should be able to feel the action in your calf muscles.

- **Pump your arms back and forth.** This burns more calories and gives you an upper-body workout as well.

- **Do not walk or run on the balls of your feet.** This produces soreness in the calves because the muscles must contract for a longer time. Avoid running on hard surfaces and making sudden stops and turns.

- **End your walk or run with a cool-down period.** Let your pace become more leisurely for the last five minutes.

increase your walking time to 20 to 25 minutes, speeding up your pace as well.

When you can handle a brisk 25-minute walk, alternate fast walking with slow jogging. Begin each session walking, and gradually increase the amount of time you spend jogging. If you feel breathless while jogging, slow down and walk. Continue to alternate in this manner until you can jog for ten minutes without stopping. If you gradually increase your jogging time by one or two minutes with each workout, you'll slowly build up to 20 or 25 minutes per session. For optimal fitness, you should jog at least three times a week.

**Other Aerobic Activities** Because variety is the spice of an active life, many people prefer different forms of aerobic exercise. All can provide many health benefits. Among the popular options:

- **Swimming.** For aerobic conditioning, you have to swim laps using the freestyle, butterfly, breaststroke, or backstroke. (The sidestroke is too easy.) You must also be a good enough swimmer to keep churning through the water for at least 20 minutes. Your heart will beat more slowly in water than on land, so your heart rate while swimming is not an accurate guide to exercise intensity. Try to keep up a steady pace that's fast enough to make you feel pleasantly tired, but not completely exhausted, by the time you get out of the pool.

- **Cycling.** Bicycling, indoors and out, can be an excellent cardiovascular conditioner, as well as an effective way to control weight—provided you aren't just along for the ride. If you coast down too many hills, you'll have to ride longer up hills or on level ground to get a good workout. An 18-speed bike can make pedaling too easy unless you choose gears carefully. To gain aerobic benefits, mountain bikers have to work hard enough to raise their heart rates to their target zone and keep up that intensity for at least 20 minutes.

- **Spinning™.** Spinning is a cardiovascular workout for the whole body that utilizes a special stationary bicycle. Led by an instructor, a group of bikers listens to music, and participants modify their individual bike's resistance and their own pace according to the rhythm. An average spinning class lasts 45 minutes.

- **Cardio kick-boxing.** Also referred to as kick-boxing or boxing aerobics, this hybrid of boxing, martial arts, and aerobics offers an intense total-body workout. An hour of kick-boxing burns an average of 500 to 800 calories, compared to 300 to 400 calories in a typical step aerobics class.

- **Rowing.** Whether on water or a rowing machine, rowing provides excellent aerobic exercise as well as working the upper and lower body and toning the shoulders, back, arms, and legs. Correct rowing techniques are important to avoid back injury.

- **Skipping rope.** Essentially a form of stationary jogging with some extra arm action thrown in, skipping rope is excellent as both a heart conditioner and a way of losing weight. Always warm up before starting and cool down afterward.

- **Aerobic dancing.** This activity combines music with kicking, bending, and jumping. A typical class (you can also dance at home to a video or TV program) consists of stretching exercises and sit-ups, followed by aerobic dances and cool-down exercises. "Soft," or low-impact, aerobic dancing doesn't put as much strain on the joints as "hard," or high-impact, routines.

- **Step training, or bench aerobics.** "Stepping" combines step, or bench, climbing with music and choreographed movements. Basic equipment consists of a bench 4 to 12 inches high. The fitter you are, the higher the bench—but the higher the bench, the greater the risk of knee injury.

- **Stair climbing.** You could run up the stairs in an office building or dormitory, but most people use stair-climbing machines available in home models and at gyms and health clubs.

- **Inline skating.** Inline skating can increase aerobic endurance and muscular strength and is less stressful on joints and bones than running or high-impact aerobics. Skaters can adjust the intensity of their workout by varying the terrain.

- **Tennis.** As with other sports, tennis can be an aerobic activity—depending on the number of players and their skill level. In general, a singles match requires more continuous exertion than playing doubles.

# Building Muscular Fitness

Although aerobic workouts condition your insides (heart, blood vessels, and lungs), they don't exercise many of the muscles that shape your outsides and provide power when you need it. Strength workouts are important because they enable muscles to work more efficiently and reliably. Conditioned muscles function

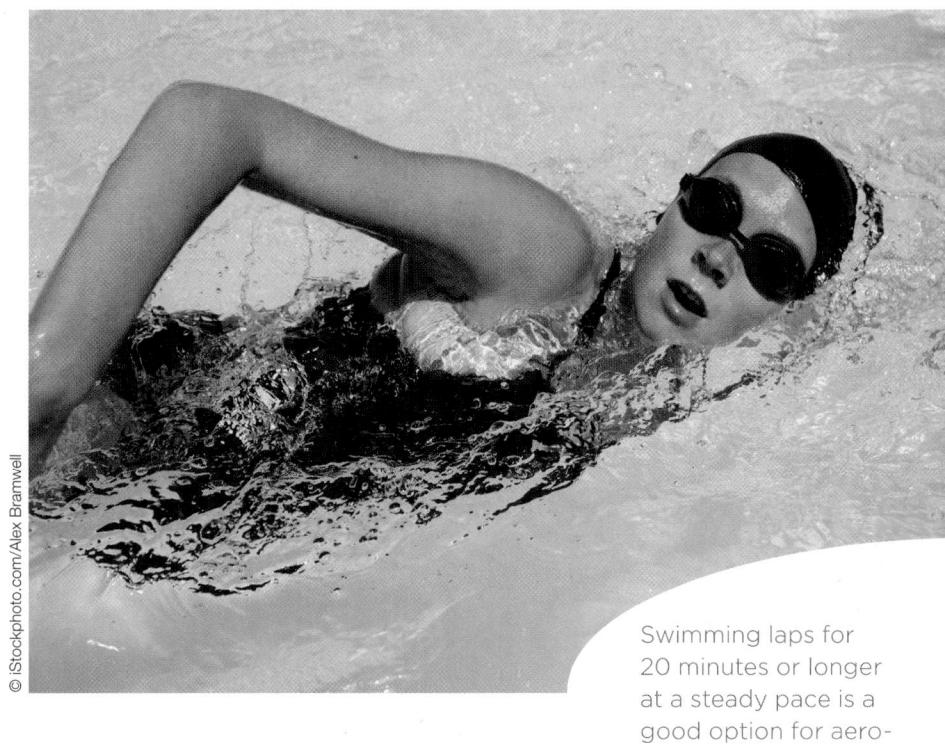

© iStockphoto.com/Alex Bramwell

Swimming laps for 20 minutes or longer at a steady pace is a good option for aerobic exercise.

more smoothly and contract somewhat more vigorously and with less effort. With exercise, muscle tissue becomes firmer and can withstand much more strain—the result of toughening the sheath protecting the muscle and developing more connective tissue within it (Figure 8.5).

The two dimensions of muscular fitness are strength and endurance. Muscular strength is the maximal force that a muscle or group of muscles can generate for one movement. Muscular endurance is the capacity to sustain repeated muscle actions. Both are important. You need strength to hoist a shovelful of snow—and endurance so you can keep shoveling the entire driveway.

The latest research on fat-burning shows that the best way to reduce your body fat is to add muscle-strengthening exercise to your workouts. Muscle tissue is your very best calorie-burning tissue, and the more you have, the more calories you burn, even when you are resting. You don't have to become a serious body-builder. Using handheld weights (also called *free weights*) two or three times a week is enough. Just be sure you learn how to use them properly, because you can tear or strain muscles if you don't practice the proper weight-lifting techniques. As more people have begun to lift weights, injuries have soared.

## Figure 8.5 Benefits of Strength Training on the Body

Strength training increases blood circulation to body tissues and develops muscles.

**Strength workouts increase circulation**

The heart's right half pumps oxygen-poor blood to capillary beds in lungs. There, $O_2$ diffuses into blood and $CO_2$ diffuses out. The oxygenated blood flows into the heart's left half where it is then pumped to capillary beds throughout the body.

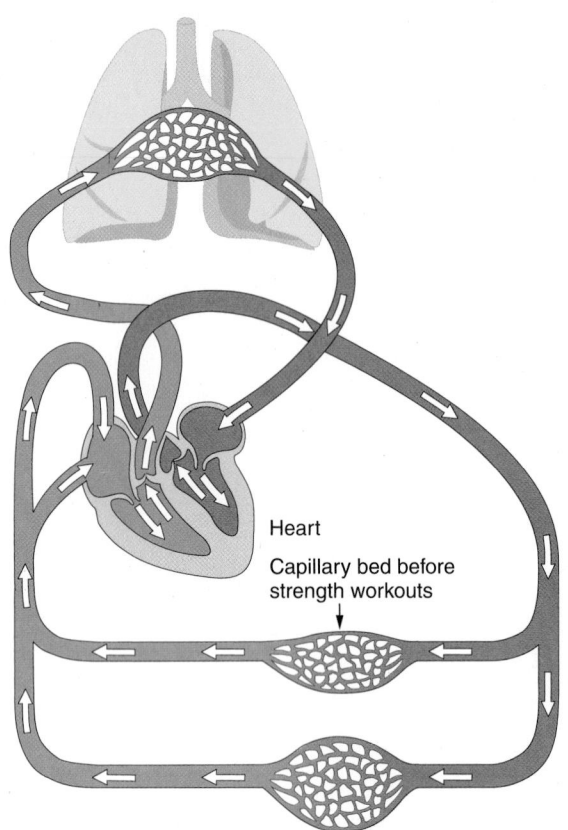

Heart

Capillary bed before strength workouts

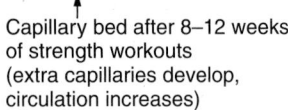

Capillary bed after 8–12 weeks of strength workouts (extra capillaries develop, circulation increases)

**Strength workouts build muscles**

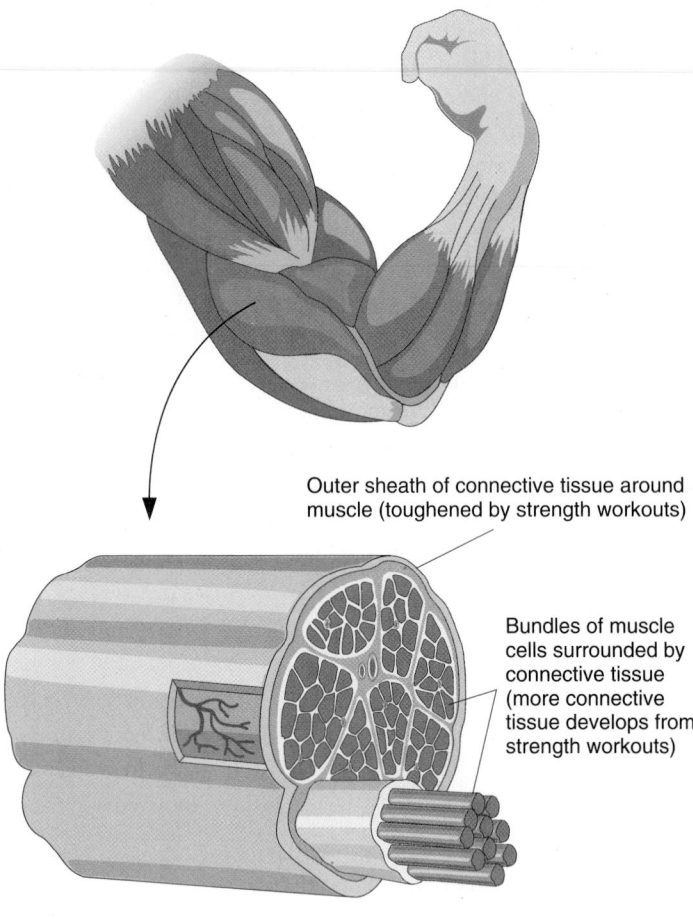

Outer sheath of connective tissue around muscle (toughened by strength workouts)

Bundles of muscle cells surrounded by connective tissue (more connective tissue develops from strength workouts)

**overloading** Method of physical training involving increasing the number of repetitions or the amount of resistance gradually to work the muscle to temporary fatigue.

A balanced workout regimen of muscle building and aerobic exercise does more for you than just burn fat. It gives you more endurance by promoting better distribution of oxygen to your tissues and increasing the blood flow to your heart.

Strength training has particular benefits for women: As numerous studies have documented, it makes their muscles stronger, their bodies leaner, and their bones more resistant to falls. In young women, it boosts self-esteem, body image, and emotional well-being. In middle-aged and older women, it enhances self-concept, boosts psychological health, and prevents weight gain. According to a recent study, both female and male seniors with greater muscle strength are less likely to suffer mild cognitive impairment and Alzheimer's disease. Regular resistance training can slow age-related loss of lean body mass and prevent sarcopenia, the deterioration of the muscles that can lead to disability and loss of independence in the elderly.[29]

## Muscles at Work

Your muscles never stay the same. If you don't use them, they atrophy, weaken, or break down. If you use them rigorously and regularly, they grow stronger. The only way to develop muscles is by demanding more of them than you usually do. This is called **overloading**. (Remember the overload principle?) As you train, you have to gradually increase the number of repetitions or the amount of resistance and work the muscle to temporary fatigue. That's why it's important not to quit when your muscles start to tire. Progressive overload—steadily increasing the stress placed on the body—builds stronger muscles.

You need to exercise differently for strength than for endurance. *To develop strength*, do a few repetitions with heavy loads. As you increase the weight your muscles must move, you increase your strength. *To increase endurance*, do many more repetitions with lighter loads. If your muscles are weak and you need to gain strength in your upper body, you may have to work for weeks to do a half-dozen regular push-ups. Then you can start building endurance by doing as many push-ups as you can before collapsing in exhaustion.

Muscles can do only two things: contract or relax. As they do so, skeletal muscles either pull on bones or stop pulling on bones. All exercise involves muscles pulling on bones across a joint. The movement that takes place depends on the structure of the joint and the position of the muscle attachments involved.

In an **isometric** contraction, the muscle applies force while maintaining an equal length. The muscle contracts and tries to shorten but cannot overcome the resistance. An example is pushing against an immovable object, like a wall, or tightening an abdominal muscle while sitting. The muscle contracts, but there is no movement. Push or pull against the immovable object, with each muscle contraction held for five to eight seconds; repeat five to ten times daily.

An **isotonic** contraction involves movement, but the muscle tension remains the same. In an isotonic exercise, the muscle moves a moderate load several times, as in weight lifting or calisthenics. The best isotonic exercise for producing muscular strength involves high resistance and a low number of repetitions. On the other hand, you can develop the greatest flexibility, coordination, and endurance with isotonic exercises that incorporate lower resistance and frequent repetitions.

True **isokinetic** contraction is a constant speed contraction. Isokinetic exercises require special machines that provide resistance to overload muscles throughout the entire range of motion.

## Designing a Muscle Workout

A workout with weights should exercise your body's primary muscle groups: the *deltoids* (shoulders), *pectorals* (chest), *triceps* and *biceps* (back and front of upper arms), *quadriceps* and *hamstrings* (front and back of thighs), *gluteus maximus* (buttocks), *trapezius* and *rhomboids* (back), and *abdomen* (Figure 8.6). Various machines and free-weight routines focus on each muscle group, but the principle is always the same: Muscles contract as you raise and lower a weight, and you repeat the lift-and-lower routine until the muscle group is tired.

A weight-training program is made up of **reps** (the single performance, or **repetition**, of an exercise, such as lifting 50 pounds one time) and **sets** (a *set* number of repetitions of the same movement, such as a set of 20 push-ups). You should allow your breath to return to normal before moving on to each new set. Pushing yourself to the limit builds strength. Although the ideal number of sets in a resistance-training program remains controversial, recent evidence suggests that multiple sets lead to additional benefits in short- and long-term training in young and middle-aged adults.

Maintaining proper breathing during weight training is crucial. To breathe correctly, inhale when muscles are relaxed and exhale when you push or lift. Don't ever hold your breath, because oxygen flow helps prevent muscle fatigue and injury.

No one type of equipment—free weight or machine—has a clear advantage in terms of building fat-free body mass, enhancing strength and endurance, or improving a sport-specific skill. Each type offers benefits but also has drawbacks.

Free weights offer great versatility for strength training. With dumbbells, for example, you can perform a variety of exercises to work specific muscle groups, such as the chest and shoulders. Machines, in contrast, are much more limited; most allow only one exercise.

Strength-training machines have several advantages. They ensure correct movement for a lift, which helps protect against injury and prevent cheating when fatigue sets in. They isolate specific muscles, which is good for rehabilitating

**isometric** Of the same length; exercise in which muscles increase their tension without shortening in length, such as when pushing an immovable object.

**isotonic** Having the same tension or tone; exercise requiring the repetition of an action that creates tension, such as weight lifting or calisthenics.

**isokinetic** Having the same force; exercise with specialized equipment that provides resistance equal to the force applied by the user throughout the entire range of motion.

**rep (or repetition)** In weight training, a single performance of a movement or exercise.

**set** In weight training, the number of repetitions of the same movement or exercise.

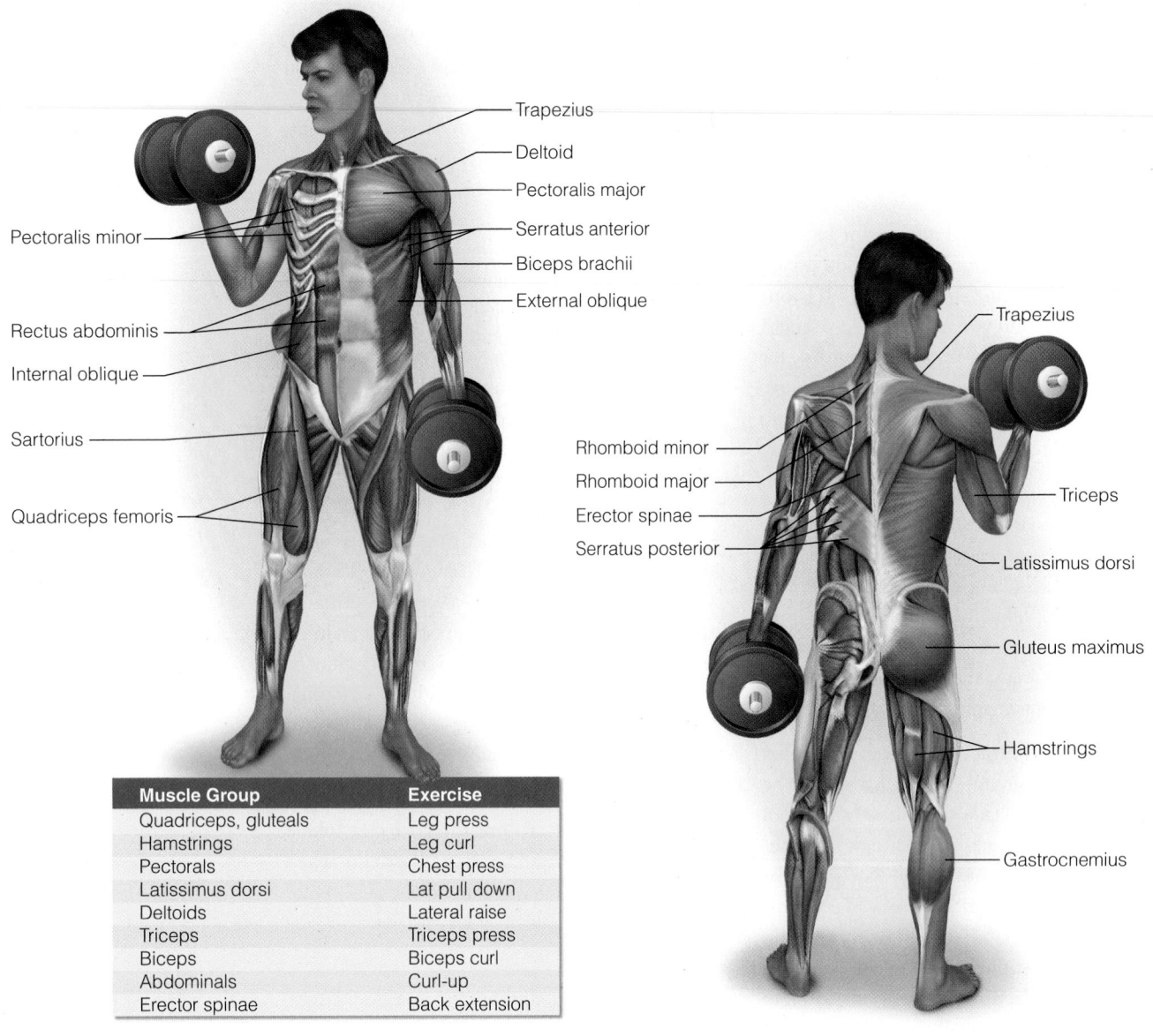

| Muscle Group | Exercise |
|---|---|
| Quadriceps, gluteals | Leg press |
| Hamstrings | Leg curl |
| Pectorals | Chest press |
| Latissimus dorsi | Lat pull down |
| Deltoids | Lateral raise |
| Triceps | Triceps press |
| Biceps | Biceps curl |
| Abdominals | Curl-up |
| Erector spinae | Back extension |

an injury or strengthening a specific body part. Because they offer high-tech options like varying resistance during the lifting motion, they can tax muscles in ways that a traditional barbell cannot.

Resistance training with whole-body vibration (WBV) has become popular among professional and amateur athletes and in fitness centers and clubs as either a substitute for or supplement to conventional weight work. Despite claims that WBV increases muscle strength and power, a recent study found that 12 weeks of such exercise did not provide any meaningful changes in muscle performance or lean body mass in healthy young men and women.[30]

## Recovery

The American College of Sports Medicine recommends a minimum of eight to ten exercises involving the major muscle groups two to three days a week. Remember that your muscles need sufficient time to recover from a weight-training session. Never work a sore muscle, because soreness may indicate that too-heavy weights have caused tiny tears in the fibers. Allow no

## How to Work with Free Weights

If you plan to work with free weights, here are some guidelines for using them safely and effectively:

- **Don't train alone—for safety's sake.** Work with a partner so you can serve as spotters for each other and help motivate each other as well.

- **Always warm up before weight training; also be sure to stretch after training.**

- **Breathe!** Holding your breath during exertion can produce a dangerous rise in blood pressure.

- **Begin with relatively light weights** (50 percent of the maximum you can lift), and increase the load slowly until you find the weight that will cause muscle failure at anywhere from 8 to 12 repetitions. (Muscle failure is the point during a workout at which you can no longer perform or complete a repetition through the entire range of motion.)

- **In the beginning, don't work at maximum intensity.** Increase your level of exertion gradually over two to six weeks to allow your body to adapt to new stress without soreness.

- **Always train your entire body, starting with the larger muscle groups.** Don't focus only on specific areas, although you may want to concentrate on your weakest muscles.

- **Always use proper form.** Unnecessary twisting, lurching, lunging, or arching can cause serious injury. Remember, quality matters more than quantity. One properly performed set of lifts can produce a greater increase in strength and muscle mass than many sets of improperly performed lifts.

- **Work through the full range of motion.** Be careful not to hyperextend or overextend.

less than 48 hours, but no more than 96 hours, between training sessions, so your body can recover from the workout and you avoid overtraining. Workouts on consecutive days do more harm than good because the body can't recover that quickly. Strength training twice a week at greater intensity and for a longer duration can be as effective as working out three times a week. However, your muscles will begin to atrophy if you let more than three or four days pass without exercising them.

## Core Strength Conditioning

"Core strength," a popular trend in exercise and fitness, refers to the ability of the muscles to support your spine and keep your body stable and balanced. When you have good core stability, the muscles in your pelvis, lower back, hips, and abdomen work in harmony. This improves your posture, breathing, appearance, and performance in sports, while reducing your risk of muscle strain. When your core is weak, you become more susceptible to lower back pain and injury.

The major muscles of your core include the transverse abdominis, the deepest of the abdominal muscles; the external and internal obliques on the side and front of the abdomen around your waist; and the rectus abdominis, a long muscle that extends along the front of the abdomen. Strengthening all of your core muscles provides stability, improves balance, and protects you from injury.

## Muscle Dysmorphia

Also referred to as "bigorexia" or "reverse anorexia," muscle dysmorphia is a condition that primarily affects male bodybuilders. Convinced that they are too small or insufficiently muscular, they spend hours working out at the gym, invest large sums in exercise equipment, take various supplements including potentially harmful drugs, and obsess about their appearance.

Some researchers believe muscle dysmorphia is a form of body dysmorphic disorder; others view it as an eating disorder. Its primary characteristics are:

- Frequently giving up important social, occupational, or recreational activities because of a compulsive need to maintain a workout and diet regimen.

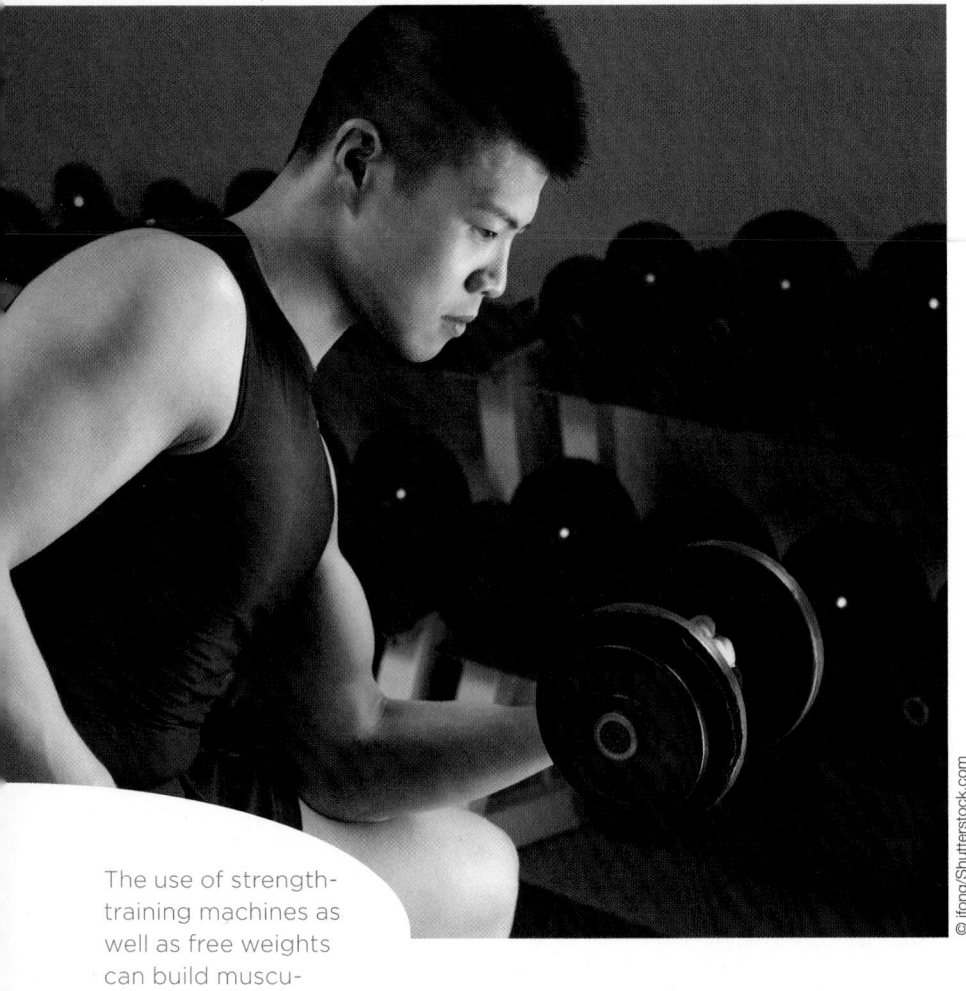

The use of strength-training machines as well as free weights can build muscular strength and endurance.

© ifong/Shutterstock.com

- Avoiding situations that involve bodily exposure (such as swimming) or enduring them only with great distress.
- Preoccupation with body size or musculature that causes significant distress or interferes with work, socializing, or other important aspects of daily life.
- Continued exercise, diet, or use of performance-enhancing substances despite knowledge of their potential for physical or psychological harm.

# Drugs Used to Boost Athletic Performance

In recent years, revelations that many athletes have used performance-enhancing drugs have shaken the sports profession. Some sports stars have served time in prison. Others have had to end their careers and see their reputations forever tarnished. Fiercely competitive and driven by the pursuit of fame and fortune, some professional athletes continue to use steroids and other agents despite the threat of cancer, liver disease, blood diseases, severe arthritis, or sexual dysfunction. The number of college athletes using or at least checking into performance-enhancing drugs is believed to be growing. Some feel the stakes are high enough to outweigh the risks: being even a little faster and stronger and finding that extra edge can be worth millions. (See Consumer Alert, p. 251.)

Public attitudes about sports doping vary. Some blame team owners, who want to sell tickets and bring in revenues at any cost. Others criticize the athletes for letting down fans and acting as bad role models for children. In a study of college students' attitudes, more women than men felt that sports doping was unacceptable, but not at statistically significant levels.[31]

Despite the hype, in a review of more than 7,500 scientific investigations all but two found that performance-enhancing drugs do not provide strength benefits. The drugs have been shown to increase lean body mass, heart rate, and metabolic rate but these do not translate into improved performance.

Here's what we know—and don't know—about the most widely used performance boosters.

- **Anabolic steroids** are synthetic derivatives of the male hormone testosterone that promote the growth of skeletal muscle and increase lean body mass. Taking them to improve athletic performance is illegal.

  Anabolic steroids have been reported to increase lean muscle mass, strength, and ability to train longer and harder, but they pose serious health hazards, including liver tumors, jaundice (yellowish pigmentation of skin, tissues, and body fluids), fluid retention, high blood pressure, decreased immune function, and severe acne. Men may experience shrinking of the testicles, reduced sperm count, infertility, baldness, and development of breasts. Women may experience growth of facial hair, acne, changes in or cessation of the menstrual cycle, enlargement of the clitoris, and deepened voice. In women, these changes are irreversible. In men, side effects may be reversible once abuse stops. In adolescents, steroids may bring about a premature halt in skeletal maturation.

Anabolic steroid abuse may lead to aggression and other psychiatric side effects. Many users report feeling good about themselves while on anabolic steroids, but researchers report that anabolic steroid abuse can cause wild mood swings including maniclike symptoms leading to "'roid rage," or violent, even homicidal, episodes. Researchers have reported that users may suffer from paranoid jealousy, extreme irritability, delusions, and impaired judgment stemming from feelings of invincibility. Stopping the drugs abruptly can lead to depression.

- **Androstenedione ("andro").** This testosterone precursor is normally produced by the adrenal glands and gonads. Manufacturers claim that androstenedione improves testosterone concentration, increases muscular strength and mass, helps reduce body fat, enhances mood, and improves sexual performance. Studies have shown that supplemental androstenedione doesn't increase testosterone and muscles don't get stronger with andro use. Andro has been classified as a controlled substance, making its use illegal.

- **Creatine.** This amino acid is made by the body and stored predominantly in skeletal muscle. Creatine serves as a reservoir to replenish adenosine triphosphate (ATP), a substance involved in energy production. Some studies show creatine may increase strength and endurance. Other effects on the body remain unknown.

The Food and Drug Administration has warned consumers to consult a physician before taking creatine supplements. Creatine may cause dehydration and heat-related illnesses, reduced blood volume, and electrolyte imbalances. Some athletes drink quantities of water hoping to avoid such effects. However, many coaches forbid or discourage creatine use because its long-term effects remain unknown.

- **GBL (gamma butyrolactone).** This unapproved drug is being studied as a treatment for narcolepsy, a disabling sleep disorder. Nevertheless, it is marketed on the Internet

## ⚠ CONSUMER ALERT

### Watch Out for "Pump Fiction"

Shape up in seven days! Burn calories without breaking a sweat! A brand-new body in minutes a day!

Too good to be true? Absolutely. Advertisers promise no-sweat, no-effort ways to fitness with pills, potions, flab-melting belts, and thigh-slimming paddles. These claims amount to nothing more than what the American Council on Exercise calls "pump fiction." The benefits of fitness are real and well documented, but the only way to reap them is through regular exercise.

#### Facts to Know

- **Be wary** of any program or product that promises "easy" or "effortless" results. Athletes in peak condition might use them without breaking a sweat. Chances are that you, like most people, won't.

- **Watch out for "spot" reducers.** You can't lose a "spare tire" or firm flabby thighs by targeting only that area of your body. You need to lose weight and tone your entire body.

- **Don't believe testimonials** or celebrity endorsements. Slim, trim, smiling celebrities are paid well for their enthusiasm.

#### Steps to Take

- **Read the fine print.** Often it states that the results are based not just on the device but on dieting and exercise as well.

- **Be skeptical** of dramatic "before and after" photos. With today's technology, you never know if photos were doctored or if the results lasted.

- **Check the details** on warranties, guarantees, and return policies. The ads may promise a "30-day money-back guarantee" but fail to mention hefty shipping costs.

and in some professional gyms as a muscle-builder and performance-enhancer.

The Food and Drug Administration has warned consumers to avoid any products containing GBL, noting that they have been associated with at least one death and several incidents in which users became comatose or unconscious.

- **Ergogenic aids.** These are substances used to enhance energy and provide athletes with a competitive advantage. These include everyday substances. *Caffeine*, for instance, may boost alertness in some people but cause jitteriness in others. *Baking soda* (sodium bicarbonate) is believed to delay fatigue by neutralizing lactic acid in the muscles, but its potential drawbacks include explosive diarrhea, abdominal cramps, bloating, and nausea.

  *Glycerol* is a natural element derived from fats. Some sports-drink manufacturers are testing formulations that include glycerol, which they claim can lower heart rate and stave off exhaustion in marathon events. Glycerol-induced hyperhydration (holding too much water in the blood) can have a negative impact on performance, however, and may be hazardous to health.

- **Human growth hormone.** According to an analysis of all existing research, human growth hormone increases lean body mass but does not affect exercise capacity or aerobic endurance. Previous studies found no beneficial effect on aging in healthy older people. Congress is considering legislation to make human growth hormone a controlled substance.

# Becoming More Flexible

Flexibility is the characteristic of body tissues that determines the **range of motion** achievable without injury at a joint or group of joints. There are two types of flexibility: static and dynamic. **Static flexibility**—the type most people think of as flexibility—refers to the ability to assume and maintain an extended position at one end point in a joint's range of motion. **Dynamic flexibility**, by comparison, involves movement. It is the ability to move a joint quickly and fluidly through its entire range of motion with little resistance. The static flexibility in the hip joint determines whether you can do a split; dynamic flexibility is what would enable you to perform a split leap.

Static flexibility depends on many factors, including the structure of a joint and the tightness of the muscles, tendons, and ligaments attached to it. Dynamic flexibility is influenced by static flexibility but also depends on additional factors, such as strength, coordination, and resistance to movement.

Genetics, age, gender, and body composition all influence how flexible you are. Girls and women tend to be more flexible than boys and men to a certain extent because of hormonal and anatomical differences. The way females and males use their muscles and the activities they engage in can also have an effect. Over time, the natural elasticity of muscles, tendons, and joints decreases in both genders, resulting in stiffness.

## The Benefits of Flexibility

Just as cardiorespiratory fitness benefits the heart and lungs and muscular fitness builds endurance and strength, a stretching program produces unique benefits, including enhancement of the ability of the respiratory, circulatory, and neuromuscular systems to cope with the stress and demands of our high-pressure world (Figure 8.7). Among the other benefits of flexibility are:

- **Prevention of injuries.** Flexibility training stretches muscles and increases the elasticity of joints. Strong, flexible muscles resist stress better than weak or inflexible ones. Adding flexibility to a training program for sports such as soccer, football, or tennis can reduce the rate of injuries by as much as 75 percent. However, stretching before a run neither prevents nor causes injury, according to a study of several thousand athletes who ran ten or more miles a week. Half performed a three- to five-minute stretching routine immediately before running; the others did not. There was no difference in the number or severity of injuries they suffered.[32]

- **Relief of muscle strain.** Muscles tighten as a result of stress or prolonged sitting. If you study or work in one position for several hours, you'll often feel stiffness in your back or neck. Stretching helps relieve this tension and enables you to work more effectively.

**range of motion** The fullest extent of possible movement in a particular joint.

**static flexibility** The ability to assume and maintain an extended position at one end point in a joint's range of motion.

**dynamic flexibility** The ability to move a joint quickly and fluidly through its entire range of motion with little resistance.

Figure 8.7 **Basic Stretching Program**
Just doing a few minutes of stretching to your major muscle groups can reap many benefits. Here is a simple yet comprehensive program.

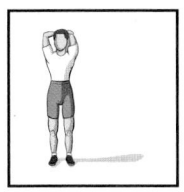

**Triceps Stretch**
1. Starting position: This exercise may be done while standing or seated. Reach both arms overhead, bend the right elbow, and grasp it with the left hand. The right hand should be pointing straight down the back.
2. Pull the elbow up and slightly back and hold for at least 20 seconds.
3. Repeat on the other side.

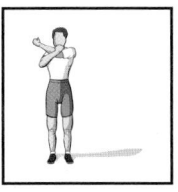

**Deltoid Stretch—Rear**
1. Starting position: Sit or stand with good posture. Cross the right arm across the front of the body at neck level. Grasp the elbow with the left hand while keeping the shoulders down and relaxed.
2. Press the elbow toward the neck and hold for at least 20 seconds.
3. Repeat on the other side.

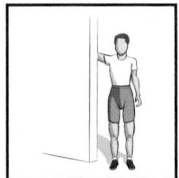

**Chest Stretch**
1. Starting position: Stand beneath a doorway. Bend the left arm and place the forearm against the wall with the elbow at shoulder height.
2. Rotate the body away from the arm and hold for at least 20 seconds.
3. Repeat on the other side.

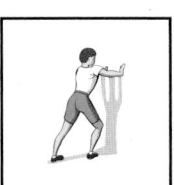

**Calf Stretch—Wall**
1. Starting position: Stand approximately two feet away from a wall and place hands on wall at about shoulder height. Place one foot at the base of the wall with the heel on the floor and toes against the wall.
2. Slowly straighten the knees and press the chest toward the wall to feel a stretch in the back of the lower leg.
3. Hold for at least 20 seconds and repeat on the other side.

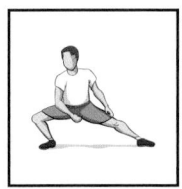

**Inner Thigh**
1. Starting position: Stand with feet three or more feet apart and toes turning outward. Bend one knee and lunge to one side, being careful not to allow the knee to extend beyond the toes.
2. Keeping weight on bent leg, lift the toes of the extended leg to increase the stretch in the inner thigh. Keep torso upright and head lifted.
3. Hold for at least 20 seconds.

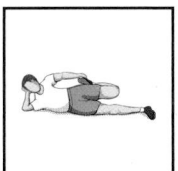

**Quadriceps Stretch—Lying**
1. Starting position: Lie on your side with your legs extended and your lower arm or hand supporting your head. Bend the top knee and grasp the top of the foot with your hand. Knees should be in alignment.
2. Press the top hip forward to feel a stretch along the front of the thigh.
3. Hold for at least 20 seconds and repeat on the other side.

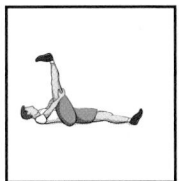

**Hamstring Stretch—Lying**
1. Starting position: Lie on your back with your legs extended. Lift one leg up and grasp behind the thigh or knee with both hands as you bring the knee to the chest.
2. Press the heel up toward the ceiling as you straighten the leg.
3. Hold for at least 20 seconds and repeat on the other side.

• **Relaxation.** Flexibility exercises are great stress-busters that reduce mental strain, slow the rate of breathing, and reduce blood pressure.

• **Relief of soreness after exercise.** Many people develop delayed-onset muscle soreness (DOMS) one or two days after they work out. This may be the result of damage to the muscle fibers and supporting connective tissue.

- **Improved posture.** Bad posture can create tight, stressed muscles. If you slump in your chair, for instance, the muscles in the front of your chest may tighten, causing those in the upper spine to overstretch and become loose.

## Stretching

When you stretch a muscle, you are primarily stretching the connective tissue. The stretch must be intense enough to increase the length of the connective tissue without tearing it.

**Static stretching** involves a gradual stretch held for a short time (10 to 30 seconds). A shorter stretch provides little benefit; a longer stretch does not provide additional benefits. Since a slow stretch provokes less of a reaction from the stretch receptors, the muscles can safely stretch farther than usual. Fitness experts most often recommend static stretching because it is both safe and effective. An example of such a stretch is letting your hands slowly slide down the front of your legs (keeping your knees in a soft, unlocked position) until you reach your toes and holding this final position for several seconds before slowly straightening up. You should feel a pull, but not pain, during this stretch.

In **passive stretching**, your own body, a partner, gravity, or a weight serves as an external force or resistance to help your joints move through their range of motion. You can achieve a more intense stretch and a greater range of motion with passive stretching. There is a greater risk of injury, however, because the muscles themselves are not controlling the stretch.

**Active stretching** involves stretching a muscle by contracting the opposing muscle (the muscle on the opposite side of the limb). This method allows the muscle to be stretched farther with a low risk of injury.

**Ballistic stretching** is characterized by rapid bouncing movements, such as a series of up-and-down bobs as you try again and again to touch your toes with your hands. These bounces can stretch the muscle fibers too far, causing the muscle to contract rather than stretch. They also can tear ligaments and weaken or rupture tendons, the strong fibrous cords that connect muscles to bones. The heightened activity to

**static stretching** A gradual stretch held for a short time of 10 to 30 seconds.

**passive stretching** A stretching technique in which an external force or resistance (your body, a partner, gravity, or a weight) helps the joints move through their range of motion.

**active stretching** A technique that involves stretching a muscle by contracting the opposing muscle.

**ballistic stretching** Rapid bouncing movements.

## How to Avoid Stretching Injuries

Before you begin, increase your body temperature by slowly marching or running in place. Sweat signals that you're ready to start stretching.

- **Don't force body parts beyond their normal range of motion.** Stretch to the point of tension, back off, and hold for ten seconds to a minute.

- **Do a minimum of four repetitions of each stretch, with equal repetitions on each side.**

- **Don't hold your breath.** Continue breathing slowly and rhythmically throughout your stretching routine.

- **Don't attempt to stretch a weak or injured muscle.**

- **Start small.** Work the muscles of the smaller joints in the arms and legs first and then work the larger joints like the shoulders and hips.

- **Stretch individual muscles before you stretch a group of muscles**, for instance, the ankle, knee, and hip before a stretch that works all three.

- **Don't make any quick, jerky movements while stretching.** Stretches should be gentle and smooth.

- **Certain positions can be harmful to the knees and lower back.** In particular, avoid stretches that require deep knee bends or full squats, because they can harm your knees and lower back.

stretch receptors caused by the rapid stretches can continue for some time, possibly causing injuries during any physical activities that follow. Because of its potential dangers, fitness experts generally recommend against ballistic stretching.

*Stretching and Warming Up*   Warming up means getting the heart beating, breaking a sweat, and readying the body for more vigorous activity. Stretching is a specific activity intended to elongate the muscles and keep joints limber, not simply a prelude to a game of tennis or a three-mile run. According to a review of recent studies, the value of stretching varies with different activities. While it does not prevent injuries from jogging, cycling, or swimming, stretching may be beneficial in sports, like soccer and football, that involve bouncing and jumping.

For aerobic activities, one of the best times to stretch is after an aerobic workout. Your muscles will be warm, more flexible, and less prone to injury. In addition, stretching after aerobic activity can help a fatigued muscle return to its normal resting length and possibly helps reduce delayed-onset muscle soreness.

## Stretching and Athletic Performance

Conventional wisdom holds that stretching improves athletic performance, but a review of the research finds that this isn't necessarily so. In some cases, active stretching can impede rather than improve performance in terms of muscle force and jumping height. Passive stretching prior to a sprint—a common practice—also has proved to reduce runners' speed. On the other hand, regular stretching can improve athletic performance in a variety of sports.

# Mind-Body Approaches

Yoga, Pilates, and t'ai chi—increasingly popular on campuses and throughout the country, can help reduce stress, enhance health and wellness, and improve physical fitness, including balance.

## Yoga

One of the most ancient of mind-body practices, *yoga* comes from the Sanskrit word meaning "union." Traditionally associated with religion, yoga consists of various breathing and stretching exercises that unite all aspects of a person.

Once considered an exotic pursuit, yoga has gained acceptance as part of a comprehensive stress management and fitness program. Scientific studies have demonstrated its benefits, which include:

- **Improved flexibility**, which may offer protection from back pain and injuries.

- **Protection of joints** because yoga postures take joints through their full range of motion, providing a fresh supply of nutrients to joint cartilage.
- **Stronger, denser bones** from yoga's weight-bearing postures.
- **Enhanced circulation**, which also boosts the supply of oxygen throughout the body.
- **Lower blood pressure**.
- **Lower levels of stress hormones**, which (as discussed in Chapter 4) can affect the immune system, interfere with memory, and increase the risk of depression and osteoporosis.
- **Lower blood sugar** in people with diabetes, which reduces the risk of complications.
- **Reduced pain** in people with back problems, arthritis, carpal tunnel syndrome, fibromyalgia, and other chronic problems.
- **Improved lung function** in people with asthma.

The best way to get started is to find a class that appeals to you and learn a few yoga moves and breathing techniques. Once you have mastered these, you can easily integrate yoga into your total fitness program.

The ACSM cautions that yoga should help, not hurt. To prevent injuries to your knees, back, neck, shoulders, wrists, or ankles, avoid forcing your body into difficult postures. Proper technique is essential to safety.

## Pilates

Used by dancers for deep-body conditioning and injury rehabilitation, Pilates (pronounced Pilahteez) was developed more than seven decades ago by German immigrant Joseph Pilates. Increasingly used to complement aerobics and weight training, Pilates exercises improve flexibility and joint mobility and strengthen the core by developing pelvic stability and abdominal control.

Pilates-trained instructors offer "mat" or "floor" classes that stress the stabilization and strengthening of the back and abdominal muscles. Fitness centers also may offer training on Pilates equipment, primarily a device called the Reformer, a wooden contraption with various cables, pulleys, springs, and sliding boards

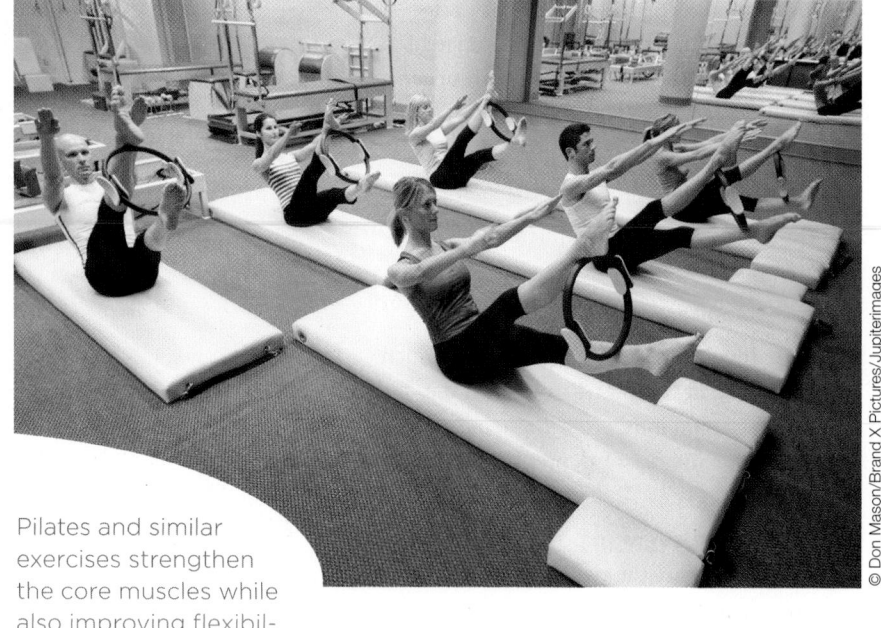

© Don Mason/Brand X Pictures/Jupiterimages

Pilates and similar exercises strengthen the core muscles while also improving flexibility and joint mobility.

attached that is used for a series of progressive, range-of-motion exercises. Instructors typically work one on one or with small groups of two or three participants and tailor exercise sessions to individual flexibility and strength limitations. Unlike exercise techniques that emphasize numerous repetitions in a single direction, Pilates exercises involve very few, but extremely precise, repetitions in several planes of motion.

According to research from the ACSM, Pilates enhances flexibility and muscular endurance, particularly for intermediate and advanced practitioners, but its potential to increase cardiorespiratory fitness and reduce body weight is limited. The intensity of a Pilates workout increases from basic to intermediate to advanced levels, as does the number of calories burned. For intermediate practitioners, a 30-minute session burns 180 calories, with each additional quarter-hour burning another 90 calories. A single weekly session enhances flexibility but has little impact on body composition.

## T'ai Chi

This ancient Chinese practice, designed to exercise body, mind, and spirit, gently works muscles, focuses concentration, and improves the flow of "qi" (often spelled "chi"), the vital life energy that sustains health. Popular with all ages, from children to seniors, t'ai chi is easy to learn and perform. Because of its focus on breathing and

flowing gestures, t'ai chi is sometimes described as "meditation in motion."

Classes are available on campuses, in fitness centers, community centers, and some martial arts schools. According to recent research, t'ai chi enhances college students' self-assessed mental and physical well-being. Physicians may recommend t'ai chi for those with musculoskeletal disorders like arthritis to improve flexibility and build muscle strength gently and gradually. The ACSM reports that t'ai chi has proved effective in reducing falls in the elderly and those with balance disorders. (See Health in the Headlines.)

# Keeping Your Back Healthy

The average person has an 80 percent chance of experiencing low-back pain in the course of a lifetime. Back pain strikes slightly more women than men and is most common between the ages of 20 and 55. You are at greater risk if you smoke or if you're overstressed, overweight, or out of shape. Back pain, which accounts for 40 percent of sickness absences, causes more lost workdays and costs the country more than any other malady.

In most cases the most effective treatment for low back pain, which usually is caused by degeneration of the lumbar spinal disks, is a combination of physical therapy and anti-inflammatory medication. According to a review of research on this common problem, 90 percent of patients with low back pain recover within three months, most within six weeks. One of the most effective ways to prevent or recover from back problems is to strengthen the core muscles.

Once bedrest was the primary treatment for back pain, but now doctors urge patients to avoid it. Even two to seven days of bedrest may provide little, if any, benefit. Acetaminophen (Tylenol) is the first-line therapy for pain relief. If it is not effective, doctors recommend nonsteroidal anti-inflammatory drugs, such as ibuprofen (Motrin or Advil). Muscle relaxants seem to be effective for a spasm in the lower back. The sooner that back patients return to normal activity, the less pain medication they require

## How to Protect Your Back

- **When standing, shift your weight from one foot to the other.** If possible, place one foot on a stool, step, or railing four to six inches off the ground. Hold in your stomach, tilt your pelvis toward your back, and tuck in your buttocks to provide crucial support for the lower back.

- **Because sitting places more stress on the lower back than standing, try to get up from your seat at least once an hour to stretch or walk around.** Whenever possible, sit in a straight chair with a firm back. Avoid slouching in overstuffed chairs or dangling your legs in midair. When driving, keep the seat forward so that your knees are raised to hip level; your right leg should not be fully extended. A small pillow or towel can help support your lower back.

- **Sleep on a flat, firm mattress.** The best sleep position is on your side, with one or both knees bent at right angles to your torso. The pillow should keep your head in line with your body so that your neck isn't bent forward or to the side.

- **When lifting, bend at the knees, not from the waist.** Get close to the load. Tighten your stomach muscles, but don't hold your breath. Let your leg muscles do the work.

and the less long-term disability they suffer. Fewer than 1 percent of patients with chronic low-back pain benefit from surgery.

# Body Composition

Body composition, the fifth component of fitness, can tell you a lot about risk for cardiorespiratory disease and diabetes.

A combination of regular exercise and good nutrition is the best way to maintain a healthy body composition. Aerobic exercise helps by burning calories and increasing metabolic rate (the rate at which the body uses calories) for several hours after a workout. Strength training increases the proportion of lean body tissue by building muscle mass, which also increases the metabolic rate.

Experts debate which measure of body composition—body mass index (BMI), waist circumference, or waist-to-hip ratio—is the best indicator of central or visceral obesity, which increases the risk of heart disease, metabolic syndrome, diabetes, and other illnesses.

## Body Mass Index (BMI)

**Body mass index (BMI)**, a ratio between weight and height, is a mathematical formula that correlates with body fat. You can determine your BMI from Figure 8.8. A healthy BMI ranges from 18.5 to 24.9.

A BMI of 25 or greater defines **overweight** and marks the point at which excess weight increases the risk of disease. If your BMI is between 25 (23.4 for Asians) and 29.9, your weight is undermining the quality of your life. You suffer more aches and pains. You find it harder to perform everyday tasks. You run a greater risk of serious health problems.

A BMI of 30 or greater defines **obesity** and marks the point at which excess weight increases the risk of death. If your BMI is between 30 and 34.9 (class 1 obesity), you face all the preceding dangers plus one more: dying. The risk of premature death increases even more if your BMI is between 35 and 39.9 (class 2 obesity). A BMI of 40 or higher indicates class 3 or severe obesity.

Doctors use BMI to determine whether a person is at risk for weight-related diseases like diabetes. However, using BMI as an assessment tool has limitations. Muscular individuals, including athletes and body builders, may be miscategorized as overweight or obese because they have greater lean muscle mass. BMI also does not reliably reflect body fat, an independent predictor of health risk, and is not useful for growing children, women who are pregnant or nursing, or the elderly. In addition, BMI, which was developed in Western nations,

## Getting Fit

As you learned in this chapter, there are many components to fitness. Using Global Health Watch, investigate the latest news on a fitness topic of particular interest to you. From the Fitness menu, you can investigate Aerobic and Endurance Training, Cardiovascular Exercise, Endurance Testing, Steroids, Strength Training, or Stretching—simply mouse over Fitness and select the topic that interests you. Scan the Latest News feed. Are there any new developments in this area? Are you taking steps to make fitness a priority in your life? Use your online journal to record your answers to these questions.

**body mass index (BMI)** A mathematical formula that correlates with body fat; the ratio of weight to height squared.

**overweight** A condition of having a BMI between 25.0 and 29.9.

**obesity** The excessive accumulation of fat in the body; class 1 obesity is defined by a BMI between 30 and 34.9; class 2 obesity is defined by a BMI between 35 and 39.9; class 3, or severe obesity, is a BMI of 40 or higher.

Figure 8.8 **BMI Values Used to Assess Weight for Adults**

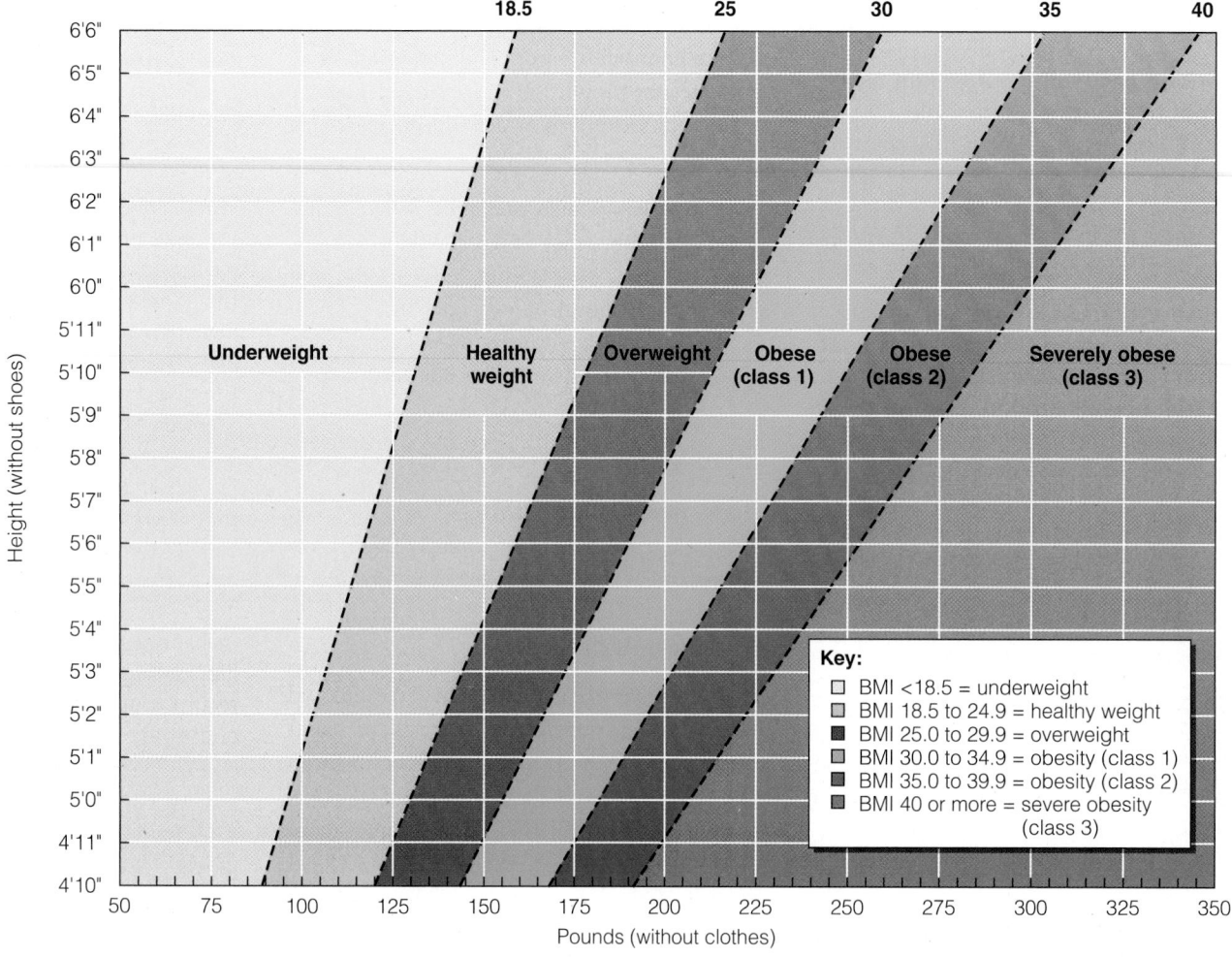

may not accurately indicate the risk of obesity-related diseases in Asian men and women.

Scientists have developed a still-experimental way of assessing body composition called the Body Adiposity Index (BAI), which relies on height and hip measurements and may be a better predictor of health outcomes in certain age, gender, and ethnic groups. However, to date, it has been tested only on African American and Mexican American volunteers.[33]

## Waist Circumference

Even if your scale shows that you haven't gained a lot of weight, your waist may widen—particularly if you've been under stress. Because of the physiological impact of stress hormones, fat accumulates around your midsection in times of tension and turmoil.

A widening waist or "apple" shape is a warning signal. In women, a wider waist correlates with high levels of harmful blood fats, such as LDL cholesterol and triglycerides. In both sexes, abdominal fat, unlike fat in the thighs or hips, increases the risk of high blood pressure, type 2 diabetes, high cholesterol, and metabolic syndrome (a perilous combination of overweight, high blood pressure, and high levels of cholesterol and blood sugar, discussed in Chapter 15.

To measure your waist circumference, place a tape measure around your bare abdomen just above your hip bone. Be sure that the tape is snug but does not compress your skin. Relax, exhale, and measure.

When is a waist too wide? Various studies have produced different results, but the general guideline is that a waist measuring more than 35 inches in a woman or more than 40 inches in a man signals greater health risks. These waist circumferences indicate "central" obesity, which is characterized by fat deposited deep within the central abdominal area of the body. Such "visceral" fat is more dangerous than "subcutaneous" fat just below the skin because it moves more readily into the bloodstream and directly raises levels of harmful cholesterol. Individuals with a large belly at midlife also are at increased risk of dementia later in life.[34]

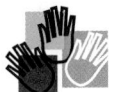 Body composition varies with race and ethnicity. Asians, for instance, may be more likely and African Americans less likely to accumulate visceral fat than Caucasians.

## Waist-to-Hip Ratio (WHR)

Another way of determining your health risk is your **waist-to-hip ratio** (**WHR**). In addition to measuring your waist, measure your hips at the widest part. Divide your waist measurement by your hip measurement. For women, a ratio of 0.80 or less is considered safe; for men, the recommended ratio is 0.90 or less. For both men and women, a 1.0 or higher is considered "at risk" or in the danger zone for undesirable health consequences, such as heart disease and other ailments associated with being overweight.

Men of all ages are more prone to develop the "apple" shape characteristic of central obesity; women in their reproductive years are more likely to accumulate fat around the hips and thighs and acquire a pear shape (Figure 8.9).

## Measuring Body Fat

Knowing your specific body composition can provide useful information about body fat and health. Ideal body fat percentages for men range from 7 to 25 percent and for women from 16 to 35 percent. Methods of assessing body composition range from skin calipers to more high-tech methods.

*Skinfold Measurement* *Skinfold measurement* is determined using a caliper to measure the amount of skinfold. The usual sites include the chest, abdomen, and thigh for men, and the tricep, hip, and thigh for women. Various equations determine body fat percentage, including

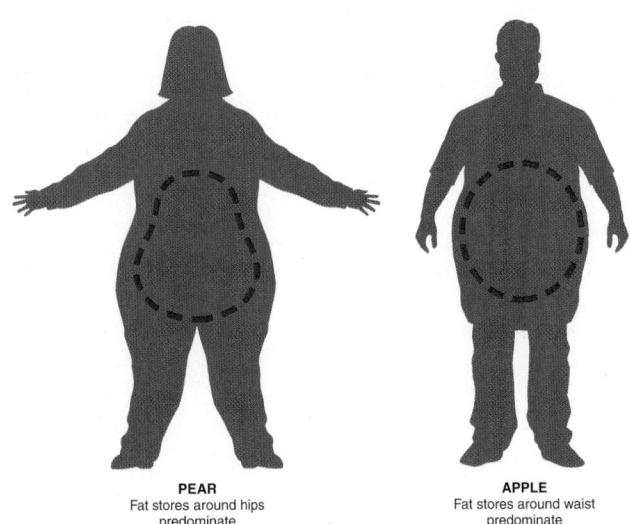

Figure 8.9 **Pear-Shaped versus Apple-Shaped Bodies**

**PEAR**
Fat stores around hips predominate

**APPLE**
Fat stores around waist predominate

calculations that take into account age, gender, race, and other factors. This relatively simple and low-cost method requires considerable technical skill for an accurate reading.

*Home Body Fat Analyzers* Handheld devices and stand-on monitors sold online and in specialty stores promise to make measuring your body fat percentage as easy as finding your weight. None has been extensively tested.

## Laboratory Methods

- **Bioelectrical Impedance Analysis (BIA).** This noninvasive method is based on the principle that electrical current applied to the body meets greater resistance with different types of tissue. Lean tissue, which contains large amounts of water and electrolytes, is a good electrical conductor; fat, which does not, is a poor conductor. In theory, the easier the electrical conduction, the greater an individual's lean body mass.

- **Hydrostatic (underwater) weighing.** According to the Archimedes Principle, a body immersed in a fluid is buoyed by a force equal to the weight of the displaced fluid. Since muscle has a higher density than water and fat has a lower density, fat people tend to displace less water than lean people.

- **Dual-energy X-ray absorptiometry (DXA).** X-rays are used to quantify the skeletal and soft tissue components of body

**waist-to-hip-ratio (WHR)**
The proportion of one's waist circumference to one's hip circumference.

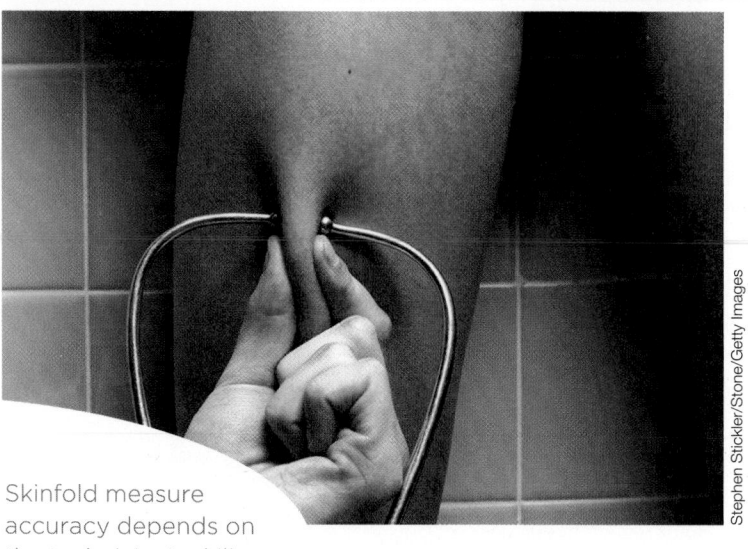

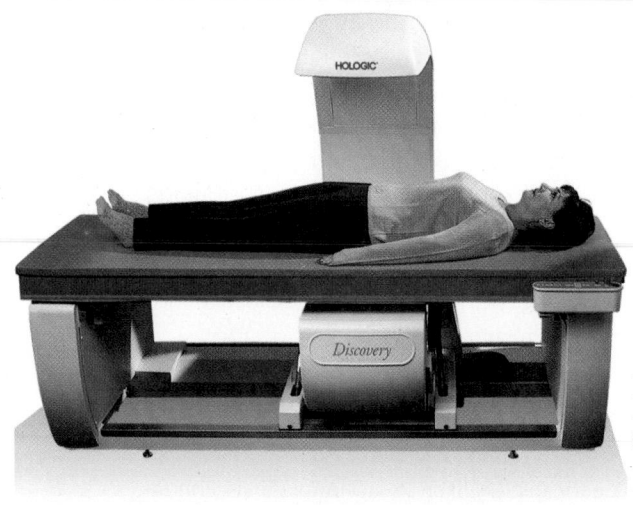

Stephen Stickler/Stone/Getty Images

Courtesy of Hologic, Inc.

Skinfold measure accuracy depends on the technician's skill; laboratory methods such as DXA don't have that subjective component.

mass. The test requires just 10 to 20 minutes, and radiation dosage is low (800 to 2,000 times lower than a typical chest X-ray). Some researchers believe that DXA will supplant hydrostatic testing as the standard for body composition assessment.

- **The Bod Pod®.** This large, egg-shaped fiberglass chamber uses an approach based on air displacement plethysmography—that is, the calculation of the relationship between pressure and volume—to derive body volume.

# Evaluating Fitness Products and Programs

As fitness has become a major industry in the United States, consumers have been bombarded with pitches for products that promise to do everything from whittle a waistline to build up biceps. As always, you have to ask questions and do your own research—whether you're buying basic exercise aids or joining a health club. Beware of any promise that sounds too good to be true. And keep in mind that nothing matters more than your own commitment.

Individuals who are overweight or obese, even when they believe in the benefits of exercise, often don't work out because they're self-

conscious about sweating pounds off in a health club or public gym.[35] If you feel self-conscious about joining a spinning class or swimming laps at the university pool, start with short walks or working with hand weights.

## Exercise Equipment

Always try out equipment before buying it. If you decide to purchase a stationary bicycle, for instance, read all the product information. Ask someone in your physical education department or at a local gym for recommendations. Try out a bicycle at the gym. Any equipment you purchase should be safe and durable, but not necessarily expensive (see Health on a Budget, p. 263).

## Athletic Shoes

Footwear has come a long way from the days of canvas sneakers. With so many new materials and high-tech options, choosing the right shoe for working out can be confusing. The best shoes aren't necessarily the most expensive but the ones that fit you best. (See Figure 8.10.) Here are some basic guidelines:

- **Choose the right shoe for your sport.** If you're a walker or runner, you want maximum overall shock absorption for the foot, with extra cushioning in the heel and under the ball of the foot (the metatarsal area) to prevent pain, burning, and tenderness. If you also participate in other types of exercise, consider "cross-trainers," shoes that are flexible enough in the front for running but

Figure 8.10 **What to Look for When You Buy Running Shoes**

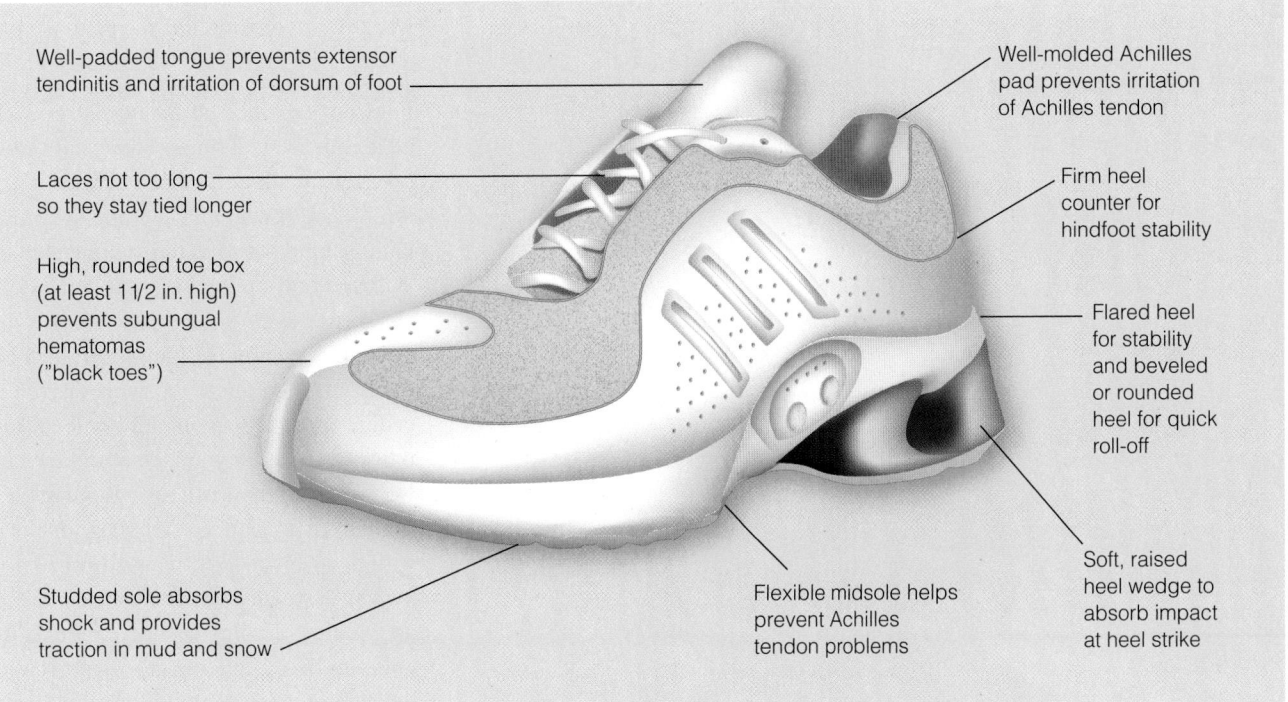

Well-padded tongue prevents extensor tendinitis and irritation of dorsum of foot

Laces not too long so they stay tied longer

High, rounded toe box (at least 1 1/2 in. high) prevents subungual hematomas ("black toes")

Studded sole absorbs shock and provides traction in mud and snow

Well-molded Achilles pad prevents irritation of Achilles tendon

Firm heel counter for hindfoot stability

Flared heel for stability and beveled or rounded heel for quick roll-off

Soft, raised heel wedge to absorb impact at heel strike

Flexible midsole helps prevent Achilles tendon problems

provide the side-to-side, or lateral, control you need for aerobics or tennis.

- **Check out the shoe.** A "slip-lasted" shoe, made by sewing together the upper like a moccasin and gluing it to the sole, is lightweight and flexible. A "board-lasted" shoe has a leather, nylon mesh, or canvas upper sewn to a cardboardlike material, which provides more support and control. A "combination-lasted" shoe offers the advantages of both and works well for a variety of foot types.

- **Shop late.** Try on shoes at the end of the day or after a workout, when your foot size is at its maximum (sometimes half a shoe size larger than in the morning).

- **Give your toes room.** Allow a half-inch, or the width of your index finger, between the end of your longest toe and the tip of the shoe. Try on both shoes. If one foot is larger than the other, buy the larger size.

- **Check the width.** A shoe should be as wide as possible across the forefoot without allowing the heel to slip. Lace up the shoe completely and walk or jog a few steps to make sure the shoes are comfortable.

- **Replace shoes when they lose their cushioning.** After about 300 to 500 miles of running or 300 hours of aerobic activity, your shoes are no longer absorbing the pounding and jarring of your sport. Don't put yourself at increased risk of knee and ankle injuries.

## Alternatives to Conventional Running Shoes

In recent years a trend to run barefoot or in so-called minimalist shoes has taken off. Advocates argue that running shoes encourage people to strike the ground hard with their heels, which may weaken muscles in the feet. Barefoot runners, they contend, take shorter strides and land more softly on the middle or front of their soles, which some believe reduces injuries and strengthens foot muscles. In cold or very hot weather or on rough surfaces, some runners opt for lightweight shoes with thin soles that simulate the barefoot experience. However, without socks, they can promote foot odor and fungal infections. There is no scientific evidence that either conventional or low-tech shoes provide a health benefit.[36]

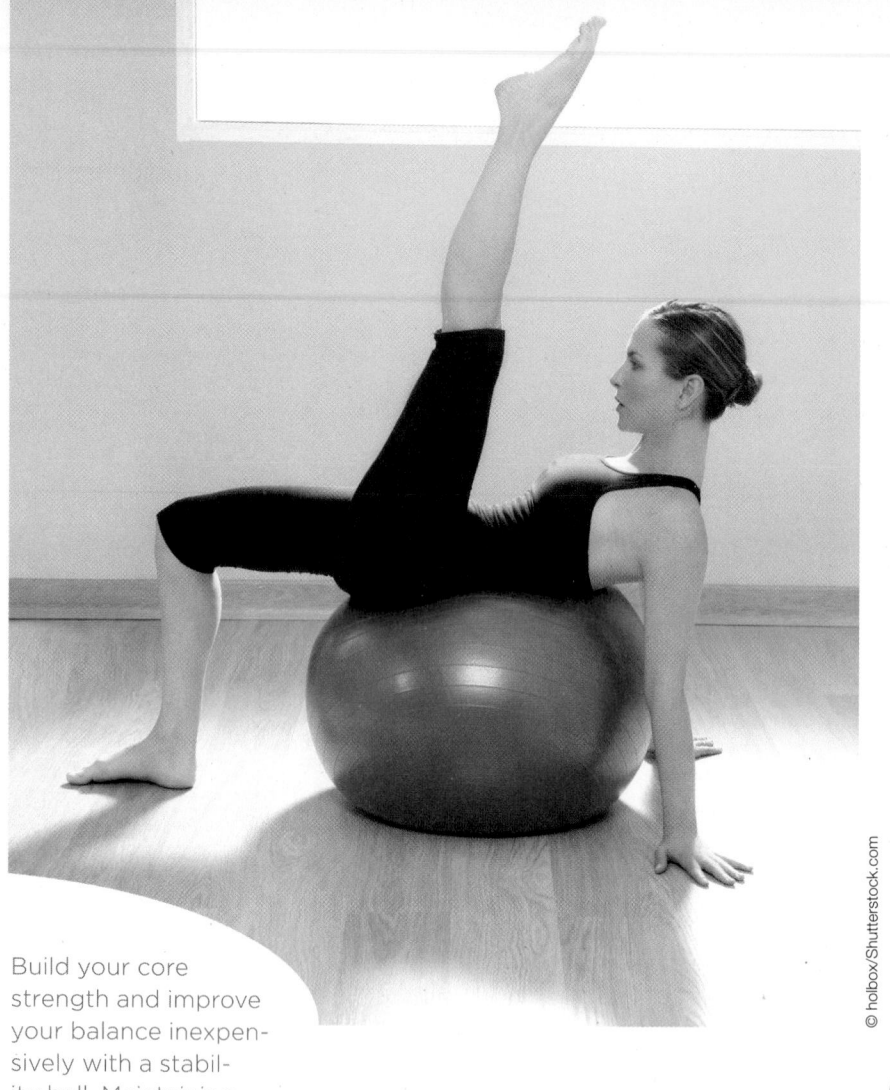

Build your core strength and improve your balance inexpensively with a stability ball. Maintaining appropriate air pressure is important—the exercise will become more difficult as pressure increases.

a running track, aerobics classes, a swimming pool, strength-training equipment, and, if it's what you're looking for, racquetball courts and a large gym for basketball and volleyball.

Find out whether all facilities are available to all members at all times. Some clubs reserve the pool for families only or kids' lessons at certain times. Ask if you can try out the club before joining. Find out what the membership includes. Will you end up paying extra for lockers, towels, classes, and the like? Are student discounts offered? Beware of long-term memberships; many clubs go out of business or change ownership often. Do the members seem to be significantly older or younger, or in much better or worse shape, than you are? Remember: You're more likely to work out regularly in a place, and with people, you like. In a study of undergraduates in university physical activity classes (such as spinning, aerobic water exercise, kickboxing, and aerobics), students reported greater effort, enjoyment, and commitment to future exercise and lower tension and anxiety about their physiques when they perceived the atmosphere in the class as caring and positive.[37]

## Fitness Centers

Begin by checking out the recreational facilities on your own campus. Is there a gym, running track, pool, basketball court, athletic fields? Are they crowded at certain times? Are they convenient? Are classes in spinning or Pilates available?

If you decide to join a private gym or health club, find out exactly what facilities and programs it offers. The club should be located close to home, campus, or work and should be open at convenient hours. Think about your schedule and when you'll have time to work out. Visit the club at the times you're most likely to use it.

A club should have facilities for a complete workout, including both aerobic and muscle workouts: exercycles, rowing machines, treadmills, stair-climbing machines, stationary bicycles,

# Sports Nutrition

In general, active people need the same basic nutrients as others and should follow the recommendations in Chapter 6. However, athletes in competitive sports—amateur as well as professional—may have increased energy requirements.

 Contrary to a common misconception, athletes generally do not need more protein; the exception may be those engaged in intense strength training. Like most Americans, athletes typically consume more than the Recommended Daily Allowance for protein and do not need increased protein. A high-protein diet can be high in fat and low in the nutrients supplied by fruits, vegetables, and grains and can put a strain on the liver and kidneys. However, in a recent study of undergraduates, college men and women who engaged in vigorous exercise ate more fruits and vegetables than their less active classmates.

Although complex carbohydrates are essential in an athlete's diet, fat also plays a role. Including the right types of fat in the daily diet can actually improve athletic performance—not just by providing calories, but by replenishing intramuscular fat stores (fat stored within the muscle and used to fuel extended exercise).

Not just *what* you eat but *when* you eat can affect your exercise performance. If you eat immediately prior to a workout, you may feel sluggish or develop nausea, cramping, or diarrhea. If you don't eat, you may feel weak, faint, or tired.

Time your meals so that you exercise three to four hours after a large meal and one to two hours after a small one. Most people can eat a snack right before exercise. After a workout, eat a meal containing both protein and carbohydrates within two hours to help your muscles recover and to replace fuel stores.

## Water

Water, which we need more than any other nutrient, is even more important during exercise and exertion. Thirst, the body's way of telling you to replace lost fluids, is not a good way for athletes to monitor their fluid needs. Rather than waiting until you're already somewhat dehydrated, you should be fully hydrated when you begin your activity or exercise and, depending on the duration and intensity of your workout, continue to replace fluids both during and afterward.

The American College of Sports Medicine (ACSM) recommends fluid intake before, during, and after exercise to regulate body temperature and replace body fluids lost through sweating. The failure to replace fluids during exercise can lead to dehydration, which can cause muscle fatigue, loss of coordination, heat exhaustion, and an elevation of body-core temperature to dangerously high levels. To avoid this danger, the ACSM advises:

- **Consume a nutritionally balanced diet and drink adequate fluids** in the 24 hours before an exercise event.
- **Drink about 17 ounces of fluid** about two hours before.
- **During exercise, start drinking early** and at regular intervals to replace all the

water lost through sweating (i.e., body weight loss).
- **Drink fluids with carbohydrates and/or electrolytes** for exercise lasting more than an hour. For shorter periods, there is little evidence of differences between drinking a carbohydrate–electrolyte drink and plain water.

Too much water during prolonged bouts of exercise, such as a marathon, can lead to *hyponatremia*, or water intoxication. This condition occurs when the body's sodium level falls below normal as a result of salt loss from sweat and dilution of sodium in the bloodstream by overdrinking. Symptoms of hyponatremia include nausea, vomiting, weakness, and in severe cases, seizures, coma, and death.

# Low-Cost Fitness Aids

Not all fitness equipment comes with a big price tag. Here are some affordable ways to expand and enhance a home workout:

- **Dumbbells.** You can purchase light weights to carry when walking and jogging to build and firm arm muscles. Training with heavier weights increases muscle strength and endurance, improves balance and body composition, and may reverse some bone loss. An adjustable dumbbell set allows you to add more weight as you build strength.

- **Stability balls.** A large inflatable rubber ball can be a fun, effective way of building core strength, improving posture, and increasing balance. When performing standard exercises like crunches and abdominal curls, the ball provides an additional challenge: maintaining a stable trunk throughout each exercise. You also can sit on the ball while working with hand weights to build core strength and balance. Introductory videos and DVDs are available for rental or purchase.

- **Resistance tubing.** Developed by physical therapists for rehabilitation after injuries, elastic bands and tubing come in different strengths, based on the thickness of the plastic. If you're a beginner, start with a thin band, particularly for the upper body. The lightweight, inexpensive, and easy-to-carry bands aren't particularly risky, but you should check for holes or worn spots, choose a smooth surface, maintain good posture, and perform the exercises in a slow, controlled manner.

## Sports Drinks

More than 20 "power" beverages compete for the $1 billion market of drinks for active people. As noted earlier, water best meets the fluid needs of most athletes, but you have other choices. According to a recent study, nonfat milk is more effective than even a soy protein beverage or sports drink such as Gatorade at burning fat and building lean muscle mass. Young men who consistently drank fat-free milk after resistance training gained 40 percent more muscle mass than those who consumed soy drinks, and 60 percent more than those consuming carbohydrate-based sport drinks.

What you are actually consuming in a sports drink is a mixture of simple sugars, sodium, and other electrolytes. Sugars help maintain hydration and blood glucose and may be especially beneficial for strenuous endurance workouts that last longer than 45 minutes or during prolonged competitive games that demand repeated intermittent activity.

Most sports drinks contain about 7 percent carbohydrate (about half the sugar of ordinary soft drinks). Less than 6 percent may not enhance performance; more than 8 percent could cause abdominal cramping, nausea, and diarrhea.

Sodium and other electrolytes in sports drinks help replace those lost during physical activity. However, most exercisers do not have to replace minerals lost in sweat immediately. A meal eaten within several hours does so soon enough.

If you exercise to lose weight, sports drinks may be counterproductive since you take in 50 to 100 calories with every 8-ounce drink. Water, on the other hand, replenishes lost fluids without adding empty calories. (See Chapter 6 for a discussion of sodas and energy drinks.)

## Dietary Supplements

Athletes and active individuals of all ages take dietary supplements, sometimes to ensure that they're getting the nutrients they need and sometimes to enhance their performance. Vitamin and mineral supplements, as discussed in Chapter 6, are safe when taken at recommended doses. Excess amounts can contribute to serious health problems. Vitamin supplements marketed for athletes are poorly regulated, and some may be adulterated with banned substances, such as ephedrine. Always look for the USP (United States Pharmacopeia) certification on the label when buying vitamins.

Athletes involved in heavy training may need more of several vitamins, such as thiamin, riboflavin, and $B_6$, which are involved in energy production. The best source, nutritionists advise, is vitamin-rich foods, such as fruits and vegetables.

Mineral deficiencies, such as too little iron in female athletes, can impair athletic performance. Women who exercise rigorously should undergo regular blood testing and, if needed, take iron supplements. In general, calcium, magnesium, iron, zinc, and copper supplements do not enhance sport performance in well-nourished athletes. Chromium, boron, and vanadium have been studied as possible performance boosters, but researchers have not reported any beneficial effects on body composition or muscular strength and endurance.

## Energy Bars

Sold as snacks, meal substitutes, or performance enhancers, energy bars come in different forms. High-carbohydrate bars derive more than 70 percent of their calories from carbohydrates (such as corn syrup, grape and pear juice concentrate, oat bran, and brown rice) and are low in protein and fat. Another type gets 40 percent of its energy from carbohydrate, 30 percent from protein, and 30 percent from fat.

Little scientific research has studied the actual benefits of the various types of energy bars, including their effects on blood glucose levels and athletic performance. According to one nutritional analysis, high-carbohydrate energy bars are similar to candy bars in their impact on glucose—even though sugars composed 31 percent of the high-carbohydrate energy bar and 86 percent of the candy bar. In fact, the high-carbohydrate energy bar caused a more rapid peak in blood glucose followed by a sharper decline than did the candy bar. This effect may be desirable for athletes involved in short-duration events who want a quick increase in blood glucose.

Energy bars with a lower carbohydrate level produce a more moderate, sustained increase in blood glucose level, possibly because the protein and fat in a 40–30–30 bar diminish blood glucose response. These bars would be a better choice for athletes involved in endurance events. As an alternative, try fiber-rich whole foods, like nuts and fruit, that provide a steady release of energy.

# Safe and Healthy Workouts

Whenever you work out, you don't want to risk becoming sore or injured. Starting slowly when you begin any new fitness activity is the smartest strategy. Keep a simple diary to record the time and duration of each workout. Get accustomed to an activity first and then begin to work harder or longer. In this way, you strengthen your musculoskeletal system so you're less likely to be injured, you lower the cardiorespiratory risk, and you build the exercise habit into your schedule.

To prevent exercise-related problems before they happen, use common sense and take appropriate precautions, including the following:

- **Get proper instruction** and, if necessary, advanced training from knowledgeable instructors.
- **Make sure you have good equipment** and keep it in good condition. Know how to check and do at least basic maintenance on the equipment yourself. Always check your equipment prior to each use (especially if you're renting it).
- **Always warm up before and cool down** after a workout.
- Rather than being sedentary all week and then training hard on weekends, try to stay active throughout the week **and not overdo on weekends**.
- **Use reasonable protective measures,** including wearing a helmet when cycling or skating.
- For some sports, such as boating, **always go with a buddy**.

- **Take each outing seriously**—even if you've dived into this river a hundred times before, even if you know this mountain like you know your own backyard. Avoid the unknown under adverse conditions (for example, hiking unfamiliar terrain during poor weather or kayaking a new river when water levels are unusually high or low) or when accompanied by a beginner whose skills may not be as strong as yours.
- **Never combine alcohol or drugs with any workout or sport**.

## Temperature

Prevention is the wisest approach to heat and cold problems. And knowing what can go wrong is part of that preventive approach.

*Heat Cramps*   These muscle cramps are caused by profuse sweating and the consequent loss of electrolytes (salts). They occur most often during exercise in hot weather. Salty snacks and sports beverages like Gatorade can help, but be aware that sports drinks can be very high in calories. Salt tablets usually aren't necessary except in cases of extreme sweating.

*Heat Syndromes*   More serious temperature-related conditions include heat exhaustion and heat stroke. These are most likely to occur when both temperature and humidity are high, because sweat does not evaporate as quickly, preventing the body from releasing heat quickly. Other conditions that limit the body's ability to regulate temperature are old age, fever, obesity, dehydration, heart disease, poor circulation, sunburn, and drug and alcohol use. Some medicines that increase the risk include allergy medicines (antihistamines), some cough and cold medicines, blood pressure and heart medicines, diet pills, laxatives, and psychiatric medications.

**Heat Exhaustion**   Heat exhaustion is a mild form of heat-related illness that can be caused by exercise or hot weather. The signs of heat exhaustion are heavy sweating, paleness, muscle cramps, tiredness, weakness, dizziness, headache, nausea or vomiting, and/or fainting. Your pulse rate or heart rate may be fast and weak, and your breathing fast and shallow.

If you think you may have heat exhaustion, get out of the heat quickly. Rest in a cool, shady place and drink plenty of water or other fluids. Do *not* drink alcohol, which can make heat exhaustion worse. If you do not feel better within 30 minutes, see your doctor. If left untreated, heat exhaustion may lead to a heat stroke.

**Heat Stroke**   A heat stroke can occur when the body temperature rises to 106 degrees Fahrenheit or higher within 10 to 15 minutes. A heat stroke is a medical emergency that can be fatal. The warning signs are extremely high temperature; red, hot, and dry skin; rapid, strong pulse; throbbing headache; dizziness; nausea; confusion or unconsciousness.

If you think someone might have heat stroke, you should take him or her to a cool, shady place quickly, and call a doctor. Remove unnecessary clothing and bathe or spray the victim with cool water. People with heat stroke may seem confused. They may have seizures or go into a coma.

### Protecting Yourself from the Cold

The tips of the toes, fingers, ears, nose, and chin and the cheeks are most vulnerable to exposure to high wind speeds and low temperatures, which can result in *frostnip*.

Because frostnip is painless, you may not even be aware that it is occurring. Watch for a sudden blanching or lightening of your skin. The best early treatment is warming the area by firm, steady pressure with a warm hand; blowing on it with hot breath; holding it against your body; or immersing it in warm (not hot) water. As the skin thaws, it becomes red and starts to tingle. Be careful to protect it from further damage. Don't rub the skin vigorously or with snow, as you could damage the tissue.

More severe is *frostbite*. There are two types of frostbite: *superficial* and *deep*. Superficial frostbite, the freezing of the skin and tissues just below the skin, is characterized by a waxy look and firmness of the skin, although the tissue below is soft. Initial treatment should be to slowly rewarm the area. As the area thaws, it will be numb and bluish or purple, and blisters may form. Cover the area with a dry, sterile dressing, and protect the skin from further exposure to cold. See a doctor for further treatment. Deep frostbite, the freezing of skin, muscle, and even bone, requires medical treatment. It usually involves the tissues of the hands and feet, which appear pale and feel frozen. Keep the victim dry and as warm as

## How to Cope with Climate

### Heeding Heat

- **Increase your fluid intake** during hot temperatures by two to four glasses of cool fluids each hour. Cold beverages can cause stomach cramps; alcoholic beverages can cause you to lose more fluid.

- **Cool off with a cool shower or sponge bath.**

- **Move into an air-conditioned environment.**

- **Wear lightweight clothing.**

- **Check weather conditions.** The National Weather Service has produced a Heat Index chart that can be accessed online at www.crh.noaa.gov/pub/heat.php.

### Handling Cold

- **Dress appropriately.** Choose several layers of loose clothing made of wool, cotton, down, or synthetic down. Make sure your head, feet, and hands are well protected. A pair of cotton socks inside a pair of wool socks will keep your feet warm.

- **Don't go out in the cold after drinking.** Alcohol can make you more susceptible to cold and can impair your judgment and sense of time.

- When snowshoeing or cross-country skiing, **always let a responsible person know where you're heading and when you expect to be back.** Stick to marked trails.

- **Carry a small emergency kit** that includes waterproof matches, a compass, a map, high-energy food, and water.

- **Don't eat snow.** It could lower your body temperature.

possible on the way to a medical facility. Cover the frostbitten area with a dry, sterile dressing.

The center of the body may gradually cool at temperatures above, as well as below, freezing—usually in wet, windy weather. When body temperature falls below 95 degrees Fahrenheit, the body is incapable of rewarming itself because of the breakdown of the internal system that regulates its temperature. This state is known as **hypothermia**. The first sign of hypothermia is severe shivering. Then the victim becomes uncoordinated, drowsy, listless, and confused and is unable to speak properly. Symptoms become more severe as body temperature continues to drop, and coma or death can result.

Hypothermia requires emergency medical treatment. Try to prevent any further heat loss. Move the victim to a warm place, cover him or her with blankets, remove wet clothing, and replace it with dry garments. If the victim is conscious, administer warm liquids, not alcohol.

Protect yourself in cold weather (or cold indoor gyms) by covering as much of your body as possible, but don't overdress. Wear one layer less than you would if you were outside but not exercising. Don't use warm-up clothes made of waterproof material, because they tend to trap heat and keep perspiration from evaporating. Make sure your clothes are loose enough to allow movement and exercise of the hands, feet, and other body parts, thereby maintaining proper circulation. Choose dark colors that absorb heat. And because 40 percent or more of your body heat is lost through your head and neck, wear a hat, turtleneck, or scarf. Make sure you cover your hands and feet as well; mittens provide more warmth and protection than gloves.

Warm up and cool down. Cold weather constricts muscles, so you need to allow enough time for proper stretching to warm up muscles before you exercise.[38]

## Exercise Injuries

According to the American Physical Therapy Association, the most common exercise-related injury sites are the knees, feet, back, and shoulders, followed by the ankles and hips. **Acute injuries**—sprains, bruises, and pulled muscles—are the result of sudden trauma, such as a fall or collision. **Overuse injuries**, on the other hand, are the result of overdoing a repetitive activity, such as running. When one particular joint is overstressed—such as a tennis player's elbow or a swimmer's shoulder—tendonitis, an inflammation at the point where the tendon meets the bone, can develop. Other overuse

## Figure 8.11  PRICE: How to Cope with an Exercise Injury

- **P**rotect the area with an elastic wrap, a sling, splint, cane, crutches, or an air cast.
- **R**est to promote tissue healing. Avoid activities that cause pain, swelling, or discomfort.
- **I**ce the area immediately, even if you're seeking medical help (don't put the ice pack directly on the skin). Repeat every two or three hours while you're awake for the first 48 to 72 hours. Cold reduces pain, swelling, and inflammation in injured muscles, joints, and connecting tissues and may slow bleeding if a tear has occurred.
- **C**ompress the area with an elastic bandage until the swelling stops. Begin wrapping at the end farthest from your heart. Loosen the wrap if the pain increases, the area becomes numb, or swelling is occurring below the wrapped area.
- **E**levate the area above your heart, especially at night. Gravity helps reduce swelling by draining excess fluid.
- After 48 hours, if the swelling is gone, you may apply warmth or gentle heat, which improves the blood flow and speeds healing.

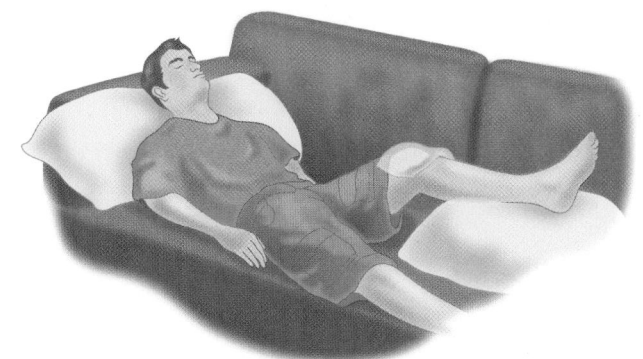

injuries include muscle strains and aches and stress fractures, which are hairline breaks in a bone, usually in the leg or foot.

Men and women may be vulnerable to different types of injuries. Studies of male and female college basketball and soccer players have shown that gender differences in the neuromuscular control of the knee places female athletes at higher risk for knee injuries. Balance training may reduce the risk.

Sooner or later most active people suffer an injury. Although most are minor, they all require attention. Ignoring a problem or trying to push through the pain can lead to more serious complications.

***PRICE*** If you develop aches and pains beyond what you might expect from an activity, stop. Never push to the point of fatigue. If you do, you could end up with sprained or torn muscles. Figure 8.11 gives the PRICE prescription for coping with an exercise injury.

**hypothermia** An abnormally low body temperature; if not treated appropriately, coma or death could result.

**acute injuries** Physical injuries, such as sprains, bruises, and pulled muscles, which result from sudden traumas, such as falls or collisions.

**overuse injuries** Physical injuries to joints or muscles, such as strains, fractures, and tendonitis, which result from overdoing a repetitive activity.

**overtrain** Working muscles too intensely or too frequently, resulting in persistent muscle soreness, injuries, unintended weight loss, nervousness, and an inability to relax.

*Overtraining*   About half of all people who start an exercise program drop out within six months. One common reason is that they **overtrain**, pushing themselves to work too intensely too frequently. Signs of overdoing it include persistent muscle soreness, frequent injuries, unintended weight loss, nervousness, and an inability to relax.

If you develop any of the symptoms of overtraining, reduce or stop your workout sessions temporarily. Make gradual increases in the intensity of your workouts. Allow 24 to 48 hours for recovery between workouts. Make sure you get adequate rest.

*Exercise Addiction*   Excessive exercise can become a form of addiction, and "exercise dependence" is not uncommon among young men and women. Although most physically active college students work out at healthy levels, some exercise to an extent that could signal dependence.

# Shaping Up

This chapter has given you the basic information you need to launch a fitness program. However, you're more likely to succeed if you create a plan and follow it. Check off these basic steps to help you determine where you are now and how to get to where you want to be.

____ **Motivate yourself.** See this chapter's Making Change Happen and "Excise Exercise Excuses" in *Labs for IPC*.

____ **Set fitness goals.** Do you have an overall conditioning goal, such as losing weight? Or do you have a training goal, such as preparing for a 5K race or trying out for the volleyball team? Break down your goal into smaller "step" goals that lead you toward it. For more about exercise options, read "Your Health Plan for Physical Fitness: Keep It Simple" in Your *Personal Wellness Guide*.

____ **Think through your personal preferences.** What are your physical strengths and weaknesses? Do you have good upper body strength but easily get winded? Do you have a stiff back? Do your allergies flare up when you exercise outdoors? By paying attention to your needs, likes, and dislikes, you can choose activities you enjoy—and are more likely to continue.

____ **Schedule exercise into your daily routine.** If you can, block out a half-hour for working out at the beginning of the day, between classes, or in the evening. Write it into your schedule as if it were a class or doctor's appointment. If you can't find 30 minutes, look for two 15-minute or three 10-minute slots that you can use for "mini-workouts." Once you've worked out a schedule, write it down. A written plan encourages you to stay on track.

____ **Assemble your gear.** Make sure you put your athletic shoes in your car or in the locker at the gym. Lay out the clothes you'll need to shoot hoops or play racquetball.

____ **Start slowly.** If you are just beginning regular activity or exercise, begin at a low level. If you have an injury, disability, or chronic health problem, be sure you get medical clearance from a physician.

____ **Progress gradually.** If you have not been physically active, begin by incorporating a few minutes of physical activity into each day, building up to 30 minutes or more of moderate-intensity activities. If you have been active but not as often or as intensely as recommended, become more consistent. Continue to increase the frequency, intensity, and duration of your workouts.

____ **Take stock.** After a few months of leading a more active life, take stock. Think of how much more energy you have at the end of the day. Ask yourself if you're feeling any less stressed, despite the push and pull of daily pressures. Focus on the unanticipated rewards of exercise. Savor the exhilaration of an autumn morning's walk; the thrill of feeling newly toughened muscles bend to your will; or the satisfaction of a long, smooth stretch after a stressful day. Enjoy the pure pleasure of living in the body you deserve.

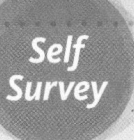

*Self Survey*

# Are You Ready to Become More Active?

*Physical Activity Stages of Change Questionnaire*

For each of the following questions, please circle Yes or No. Please be sure to read the questions carefully.

Physical activity or exercise includes activities such as walking briskly, jogging, bicycling, swimming, or any other activity in which the exertion is at least as intense as these activities.

1. I am currently physically active.    NO    YES

2. I intend to become more physically active in the next 6 months.    NO    YES

For activity to be regular, it must add up to a total of 30 minutes or more per day and be done at least 5 days per week. For example, you could take one 30-minute walk or take three 10-minute walks for a daily total of 30 minutes.

3. I currently engage in regular physical activity.    NO    YES

4. I have been regularly physically active for the past 6 months.    NO    YES

| Scoring Algorithm | Question | | | |
|---|---|---|---|---|
| | 1 | 2 | 3 | 4 |
| Precontemplation | No | No | | |
| Contemplation | No | Yes | | |
| Preparation | Yes | | No | |
| Action | Yes | | Yes | No |
| Maintenance | Yes | | Yes | Yes |

*Sources: From B. H. Marcus & L. H. Forsyth, 2003, Motivating People to be Physically Active, page 21. © 2003 by Bess H. Marcus and Leigh Ann H. Forsyth. Reprinted with permission from Human Kinetics (Champaign, IL).*

# Making Change Happen

## A Stage-by-Stage Shape-Up Plan

### Physical Activity Stages of Change Questionnaire

Once you know your stage of motivational readiness, you can employ the cognitive and behavioral strategies most likely to work for you now. As you progress through the stages of change, you can shift to other approaches. Here are some suggestions:

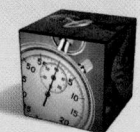

### Get Real

- List what you see as the cons of physical activity. For example, do you fear it would take time you need for your studies? Think of small changes that don't require time—for instance, standing rather than sitting when talking on the phone, doing stretches while watching television, or taking a quick walk down the hall or up the stairs while waiting for a friend or a class.

- Identify barriers to physical activity, such as lack of money. Take advantage of your student status, and check out facilities, such as the swimming pool at the athletic center, or opportunities, such as an intramural soccer team, available to you free (or almost).

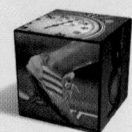

### Get Ready

- Determine the types of activity you can realistically fit into your daily schedule. You might join friends for softball every Saturday, or sign up for an evening body-sculpting class.

- Visualize success. Focus on the person you want to become: How would you look? What would you do differently? Find an image—from a magazine advertisement, for example—and post it where you can see it often.

- Plan your rewards. Use a technique called shaping, which reinforces progress on the way to a goal. For instance, initially you might reward yourself once you engage in physical activity for 15 minutes a day. After a week, you get the reward only after 20 minutes a day. Over time you increase the number of days you are physically active as well as the number of minutes of activity per day.

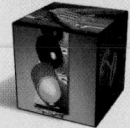

### Get Going

- Identify specific barriers that limit your activity. If your daily jogs are rained or snowed out, develop a list of indoor alternatives, such as walking stairs or working out to an exercise video.

- Set specific daily and weekly goals. Your daily goal might begin with 10 or 15 minutes of activity. Your weekly goal might be to try a new activity, such as spinning or a dance class.

- Divide physical activity over the course of the day with a 10- or 15-minute walk in the morning, another at lunch, and a third at the end of the day.

- Document your progress. You could use a monthly calendar to keep track of the number of days you've exercised as well as the length of each workout. Or you can keep a more detailed record, noting the types of exercise you do every day, the intensity you work at, the duration of each workout, and so forth.

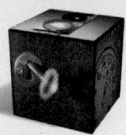

### Lock It In

- Reach out for support. Find a friend, family member, or classmate who is willing or able to provide support for being active. Or join an organized martial arts class or an informal team.

- Identify risk factors that might lead to relapse. If vacations or holiday breaks disrupt your routine, make a plan for alternative ways to remain active before you leave campus.

- Stress-proof your fitness program. In crunch times, you may feel you don't have time to spare for exercise. Multiple 10-minute walks during the day may be particularly useful both to keep up your fitness and to relieve stress buildup.

# Making This Chapter Work for You

## Review Questions

1. The benefits of regular physical activity include
   a. decreased bone mass.
   b. lowered risk of shin splints.
   c. enhanced immune response.
   d. altered sleep patterns.

2. Which of the following precautions could help to prevent a serious sports injury from occurring?
   a. Wear swimming goggles when doing laps to decrease the irritating effects of chlorine.
   b. Wear knee pads when cycling to prevent knee gashes if you fall off your bicycle.
   c. To eliminate persistent muscle soreness, increase the frequency and/or time period of your workout.
   d. Wear a helmet, wrist guards, and knee pads when inline skating to help prevent fractures and head injuries.

3. Michael started a walking program two weeks ago. Which of these workouts would you recommend to him for aerobic exercise?
   a. 5 minutes of brisk walking, 30 minutes of flexibility exercises, 5 minutes of brisk walking
   b. 5 minutes of stretching, 15 minutes of slow walking, 5 minutes of brisk walking, 15 minutes of slow walking
   c. 10 minutes of slow walking, 35 minutes of brisk walking, 5 minutes of slow walking
   d. 10 minutes of stretching, 45 minutes of brisk walking

4. Which of the following statements is true?
   a. Inactivity does not affect health until middle age.
   b. Total fitness includes emotional and social dimensions of health besides the physical.
   c. Men and women have the same physiological capacities.
   d. Total fitness is one dimension of physical fitness.

5. A regular flexibility program provides which of the following benefits?
   a. stronger heart and lungs
   b. relief of muscle strain and soreness

   c. increased strength and endurance
   d. increased bone mass and leaner muscles

6. To motivate yourself to stick to an exercise program:
   a. Watch professional athletic competitions.
   b. Set a long-term goal, then break it down into short-term goals that can be achieved in a few months.
   c. Keep a detailed record of all the times that you avoided working out.
   d. Join an expensive health club so that you feel pressured to get your money's worth.

7. For any muscle to get stronger, it must work against a greater-than-normal resistance. This is called the
   a. reversibility principle.
   b. overload principle.
   c. FITT principle.
   d. principle of compound interest.

8. Jessica takes a step aerobics class three times a week. Which component of physical fitness does her exercise routine emphasize?
   a. muscular strength and endurance
   b. flexibility
   c. cardiorespiratory fitness
   d. body composition

9. If you are a healthy weight,
   a. you are always hungry.
   b. your BMI is between 18.5 and 24.9.
   c. your waist measurement is 25 to 28 inches.
   d. your waist-to-hip ratio is greater than 1.0.

10. Which nutrient is the most important during exercise and exertion?
    a. water
    b. carbohydrates
    c. fat
    d. protein

*Answers to these questions can be found on page 672.*

## Critical Thinking

1. Allison knows that exercise is good for her health, but she figures she can keep her weight down by dieting and worry about her heart and health when she gets older. "I look good. I feel okay. Why should I bother exercising?" she asks. What would you reply?

2. Your younger brother Andre is hoping to get a starting position on his high school football team. Practices began in July. You are aware that a couple of other players have suffered heat-related incidents, but according to Andre, these players just weren't tough enough. What can you do to help your brother protect his health?

3. Research is mixed on whether stretching can decrease delayed-onset muscle soreness. Do you think a placebo effect can occur in studies on exercise and training as it does in research on medications? Why or why not?

## Media Menu

Visit www.cengagebrain.com to access course materials and companion resources for this text that will:

- Help you evaluate your knowledge of the material.

- Allow you to prepare for exams with interactive quizzing.

- Use the CengageNOW product to develop a Personalized Learning Plan targeting resources that address areas you should study.

- Coach you through identifying target goals for behavioral change and creating and monitoring your personal change plan throughout the semester using the Behavior Change Planner available in the CengageNOW resource.

## Internet Connections

**www.acefitness.org**
This website features information for the general public as well as for certified fitness trainers. The comprehensive site includes health and fitness news headlines, Fit Facts information sheets, a question and answer site, whole-body exercise workouts, daily fitness tips, discussion boards, newsletters, and information on ACE certification.

**www.aahperd.org**
This organization provides legislative advocacy for healthy lifestyles through high-quality programs in health and physical education. The website features consumer news, career links, listing of graduate programs, research, and a link for the *International Electronic Journal of Health Education*.

**www.shapeup.org/fitness/index.php**
At this site, you can perform a battery of physical fitness assessments, including activity level, strength, flexibility, and an aerobic fitness test. You get started by entering your weight, height, age, and gender and then take a quick screen test to assess your physical readiness for physical activity. Your final results in each area will be based on your personal data.

## Key Terms

The terms listed are used on the page indicated. Definitions of the terms are in the Glossary at the end of the book.

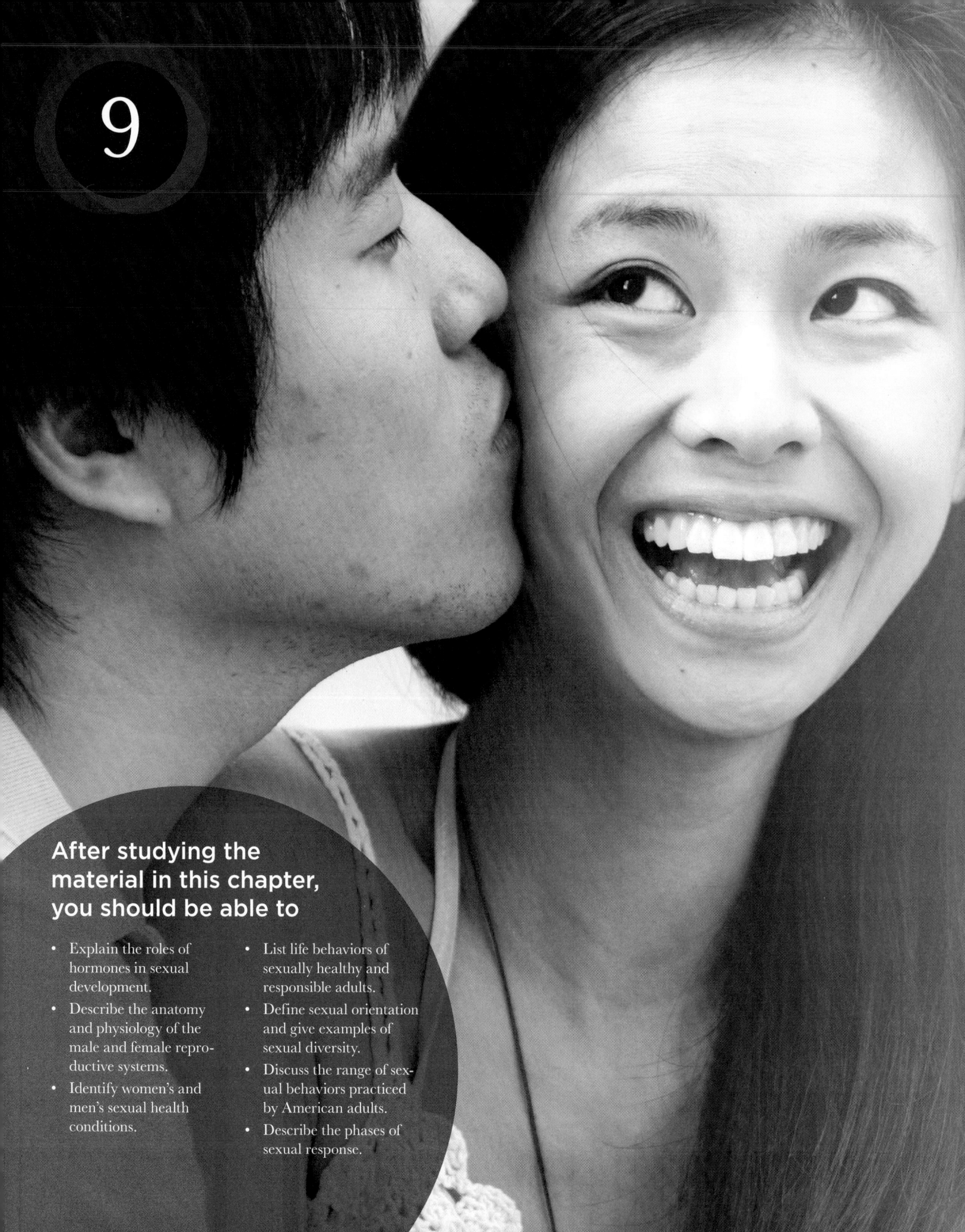

# 9

## After studying the material in this chapter, you should be able to

- Explain the roles of hormones in sexual development.
- Describe the anatomy and physiology of the male and female reproductive systems.
- Identify women's and men's sexual health conditions.

- List life behaviors of sexually healthy and responsible adults.
- Define sexual orientation and give examples of sexual diversity.
- Discuss the range of sexual behaviors practiced by American adults.
- Describe the phases of sexual response.

Charles, several years older than the typical college freshman, usually doesn't think much about the age difference—until the conversation turns to sex. He understands his younger classmates' seemingly endless fascination with sex, but his perspective is different. As a teenager, he had plunged recklessly into dangerous territory of every type. Sex—casual and sometimes unprotected—was one of them. "Looking back," Charles muses, "I feel lucky that I didn't end up a statistic." But he still regrets the irresponsible ways he acted.

# Personal Sexuality

At 28 Charles is a veteran of military service, a married man, and an expectant father. His enjoyment of sex hasn't faded—in many ways, it's deepened and become more gratifying. He now realizes that there is no such thing as casual sex, that sexual choices have consequences and effects on one's own life and on other people. These are the lessons he hopes someday to pass on to his own children.

As Charles learned with time and experience, you are ultimately responsible for your sexual health and behavior. You make decisions that affect how you express your sexuality, how you respond sexually, and how you give and get sexual pleasure. Yet most sexual activity involves another person. Therefore, your decisions about sex—more so than those you make about nutrition, drugs, or exercise—have important effects on other people. Recognizing this fact is the key to responsible sexuality.

Sexual responsibility means learning about your body, your partner's body, your sexual development and preferences, and the health risks associated with sexual activity. This chapter is an introduction to your sexual self and an exploration of sexual issues in today's world. It provides the information and insight you can use in making decisions and choosing behaviors that are responsible for all concerned.

## Human Sexuality

Human **sexuality**—the quality of being sexual—is as rich, varied, and complex as life itself. Along with our **sex**, or biological maleness or femaleness, it is an integral part of who we are, how we see ourselves, and how we relate to others. Of all of our involvements with others, sexual **intimacy**, or physical closeness, can

**sexuality** The behaviors, instincts, and attitudes associated with being sexual.

**sex** Maleness or femaleness, resulting from genetic, structural, and functional factors.

**intimacy** A state of closeness between two people, characterized by the desire and ability to share one's innermost thoughts and feelings with each other either verbally or nonverbally.

Visit www.cengagebrain.com to access course materials for this text, including the Behavior Change Planner, interactive quizzes, tutorials, and more. See the preface on page xv for details.

© iStockphoto.com/zhang bo

be the most rewarding. But while sexual expression and experience can provide intense joy, they also can involve great emotional turmoil.

# Sexuality and the Dimensions of Health

Our sexuality both affects and is affected by the various dimensions of health. Responsible sexuality and high-level **sexual health** contribute to the fullest possible functioning of body, mind, spirit, and social relationships. In turn, other aspects of health enhance our sexuality. Here are some examples:

- **Physical.** As described in Chapter 11, safer sex practices reduce the risk of sexually transmitted infections that can threaten sexual health, physical health, and even survival. When our bodies are healthy and well, we feel better about how we look and move—which enhances both self-esteem and healthy sexuality.

- **Emotional.** By acknowledging and respecting the intimacy of a sexual relationship, responsible sexuality builds trust and commitment. When our emotional health is high, we can better understand and cope with the complex feelings related to being sexual.

- **Social.** From dating to mating, we express and fulfill our sexual identities in the context of families, friends, and society as a whole. Having strong friendships, intimate relationships, and caring partnerships enables us to explore our sexuality in safe and healthy ways.

- **Intellectual.** Our most fulfilling relationships involve a meeting of minds as well as bodies. High-level intellectual health enables us to acquire and understand sexual information, analyze it critically, and make healthy sexual decisions.

- **Spiritual.** At its deepest, most fulfilling level, sexuality uplifts the soul by allowing us to connect to something greater than ourselves. Individuals who have developed their spirituality bring to their most intimate relationships an awareness and appreciation that lifts them beyond the physical.

- **Environmental.** Responsible sexuality makes people more aware of the impact of their decisions on others. Protecting yourself from sexual threats and creating a supportive environment in which to study and work are crucial to high-level health and to healthy sexuality.

# Becoming Male or Female

Physiological maleness or femaleness, or biological sex, is indicated by the sex chromosomes, hormonal balance, and genital anatomy. **Gender** refers to the psychological and sociological, as well as the physical, aspects of being male or female. You are born with a certain *sexual identity* based on your sexual anatomy and appearance; you, your parents, and society mold your gender identity.

## Are You an X or a Y?

Biologically, few absolute differences separate the sexes: Males alone can make sperm and contribute the chromosome that causes embryos to develop as males; females alone are born with sex cells (eggs, or ova), menstruate, give birth, and breast-feed babies. But the process of becoming male or female is a long and complex one.

In the beginning, all human embryos have undifferentiated sex organs. Only after several weeks do the sex organs differentiate, becoming either male or female *gonads* (testes or ovaries), the structures that produce the future reproductive cells of an individual. This initial differentiation process depends on genetic instructions in the form of the sex chromosomes, referred to as X and Y. If a Y (or male) chromosome is present in the embryo, about seven weeks after conception, it signals the sex organs to develop into testes. If a Y chromosome isn't present, an embryo begins developing ovaries in the eighth week. From this point on, the sex hormones produced by the gonads, not the chromosomes, play the crucial role in making a male or female.

**sexual health** The integration of the physical, emotional, intellectual, social, and spiritual aspects of sexual being in ways that are positively enriching and that enhance personality, communication, and love.

**gender** Maleness or femaleness, as determined by a combination of anatomical and physiological factors, psychological factors, and learned behaviors.

Figure 9.1 **Puberty**
The body's endocrine system produces hormones that trigger body changes, including growth spurts, in boys and girls.

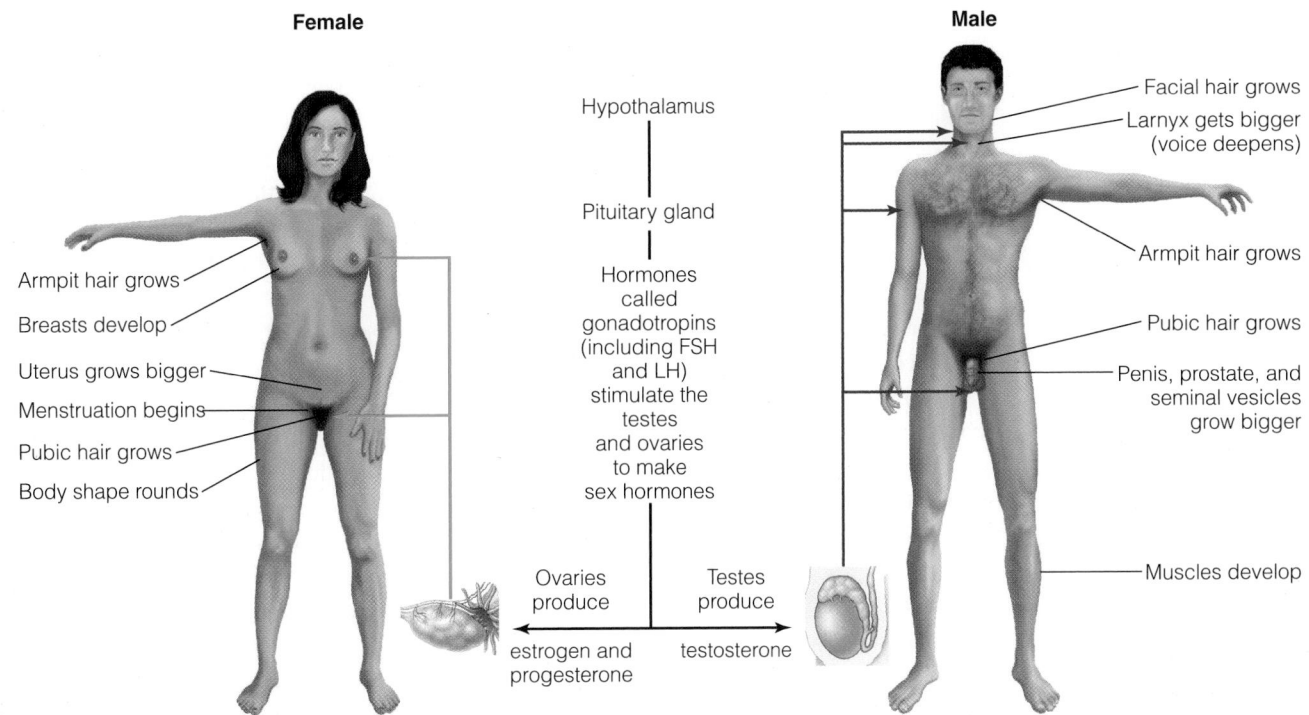

**Female**

Armpit hair grows

Breasts develop

Uterus grows bigger

Menstruation begins

Pubic hair grows

Body shape rounds

Hypothalamus

Pituitary gland

Hormones called gonadotropins (including FSH and LH) stimulate the testes and ovaries to make sex hormones

Ovaries produce

Testes produce

estrogen and progesterone

testosterone

**Male**

Facial hair grows

Larnyx gets bigger (voice deepens)

Armpit hair grows

Pubic hair grows

Penis, prostate, and seminal vesicles grow bigger

Muscles develop

## How Hormones Work

In Greek, *hormone* means "set into motion"—and that's exactly what our **hormones** do. These chemical messengers, produced by various organs in the body, including the sex organs, and carried to target structures by the bloodstream, arouse cells and organs to specific activities and influence the way we look, feel, develop, and behave.

The group of organs that produce hormones is referred to as the **endocrine system**. Except for the sex organs, males and females have identical endocrine systems. Directing the endocrine system is the hypothalamus, a pea-sized section of the brain. The pituitary gland, directly beneath the hypothalamus, turns the various glands on and off in response to messages from it.

The ovaries produce the sex hormones most crucial to women, **estrogen** and **progesterone**. The primary sex hormone in men is **testosterone**, which is produced by the testes and the adrenal glands. However, both men and women have small amounts of the hormones of the opposite sex. Estrogen, in fact, is crucial to male fertility and gives sperm what researchers describe as their "reproductive punch."

The sex hormones begin their work early in an embryo's development. As soon as the testes are formed, they start releasing testosterone, which stimulates the development of other structures, such as the penis. The absence of testosterone in an embryo causes female genitals to form. (If the testes of a genetic male don't produce testosterone, the fetus will develop female genitals. Similarly, if a genetic female is exposed to excessive testosterone, the fetus will have ovaries but will also develop male genitals.)

As puberty begins, the pituitary gland initiates the changes that transform boys into men and girls into women (Figure 9.1). When a boy is about 14 years old and a girl about 12, their brains stimulate the hypothalamus to secrete a hormone called gonadotropin-releasing hormone (GnRH). This substance causes the pituitary gland to release hormones called **gonadotropins**. These, in turn, stimulate the gonads to make sex hormones.

The gonadotropins are *follicle-stimulating hormone (FSH)* and *luteinizing hormone (LH)*. In girls, these hormones travel to the ovary and stimulate the production of estrogen. As estrogen increases, a girl's **secondary sex characteristics** develop. Her breasts become fuller, her external genitals

**hormone** Substance released in the blood that regulates specific bodily functions.

**endocrine system** The group of ductless glands that produce hormones and secrete them directly into the blood for transport to target organs.

**estrogen** The female sex hormone that stimulates female secondary sex characteristics.

**progesterone** The female sex hormone that stimulates the uterus, preparing it for the arrival of a fertilized egg.

**testosterone** The male sex hormone that stimulates male secondary sex characteristics.

**gonadotropins** Gonad-stimulating hormones produced by the pituitary gland.

**secondary sex characteristics** Physical changes associated with maleness or femaleness, induced by the sex hormones.

enlarge, and fat is deposited on her hips and buttocks. Estrogen keeps her hair thick and skin smooth. She begins menstruating because she has begun ovulating, the process that prepares her body to conceive and carry a baby.

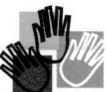 This process seems to be beginning earlier than in the past. "By eight, 15 percent of white girls and 48 percent of African American girls show signs of sexual development," says Marcia Herman-Giddens, Ph.D., of the University of North Carolina at Chapel Hill, who analyzed 17,077 growth charts from pediatricians around the country. In her study, the mean ages for breast development were 8.87 years for African American girls and 9.96 years for white girls. African American girls reach **menarche**—the term for first menstruation—at a mean age of 12.16 years; white girls, at 12.88 years. By comparison, a hundred years ago girls didn't reach menarche until the relatively ripe age of fifteen.

Improved nutrition and good health seem to be the primary factors. Girls today are bigger, taller, better fed, and more sedentary and have a higher percentage of body fat (one of the triggers of sexual maturation). They also grow up amid a host of environmental influences that may further speed development.

Cultural influences affect a girl's response to menarche. In a cross-cultural study of college students, the most common emotions expressed by American women at menarche were embarrassment, pride, and anxiety. Malaysian women cited fear, embarrassment, and worry. Lithuanian women described themselves as happy or scared, while Sudanese women cited fear, anxiety, embarrassment, and anger. On the positive side, the Lithuanian women reported feeling more valuable and believing they had entered the world of women. American girls worried about whether they could still play sports but felt superior to friends who had not reached menarche and became eager to learn about sex. Malaysians described feeling wise, respected, and mature. In several countries women felt more beautiful because they could now have children.

In boys, the gonadotropins stimulate the testes to produce testosterone, which triggers the development of male secondary sex characteristics. Their voices deepen, hair grows on their faces and bodies, their penises become thicker and longer, and their muscles become stronger.

The sex hormones released during puberty change the growth pattern of childhood, so that a boy or girl may now spurt up four to six inches in a single year. The skeleton matures very rapidly until, at the end of puberty (usually around age 18), the growth centers at the ends of the bones close off. Estrogen causes girls' bones to stop growing at an earlier age than boys' bones.

## Sexual and Gender Identity

It's a boy! It's a girl! These statements confer an instant identity on a newborn. However, in recent years, researchers have challenged such either/or distinctions as male or female, masculine or feminine, heterosexual or homosexual. Although most people have the biological characteristics of a male or a female, some possess some degree of both male and female reproductive structures. They are referred to as intersexual.

The continuum for gender identity ranges from extreme stereotypical masculine notions to extreme stereotypical feminine behaviors. Different cultures vary in defining what is masculine or feminine. Individuals who consider themselves androgynous choose not to conform to sexual stereotypes. **Androgyny** includes those who are "positively androgynous," combining positive attributes linked with both sexes—for example, feminine compassion and masculine independence—and individuals who are "negatively androgynous" and might show less desirable characteristics of each gender, such as feminine dependency and masculine assertiveness. (Transgenderism is discussed on page 293.)

# Women's Sexual Health

Only recently has medical research devoted major scientific investigations to issues in women's health. Until about a decade ago, the National Institutes of Health routinely excluded women from experimental studies because of

**menarche** The onset of menstruation at puberty.

**androgyny** The expression of both masculine and feminine traits.

**mons pubis** The rounded, fleshy area over the junction of the female pubic bones.

**labia majora** The fleshy outer folds that border the female genital area.

**labia minora** The fleshy inner folds that border the female genital area.

**clitoris** A small erectile structure on the female, corresponding to the penis on the male.

**urethral opening** The outer opening of the thin tube that carries urine from the bladder.

concerns about menstrual cycles and pregnancy. In clinical settings, women are more likely to have their symptoms dismissed as psychological and not to be referred to a specialist than are men with identical complaints. Some physicians are suggesting the creation of a new medical specialty (distinct from obstetrics and gynecology) that would be devoted to women's health.

## Female Sexual Anatomy

As illustrated in Figure 9.2a, the **mons pubis** is the rounded, fleshy area over the junction of the pubic bones. The folds of skin that form the outer lips of a woman's genital area are called the **labia majora**. They cover soft flaps of skin (inner lips) called the **labia minora**. The inner lips join at the top to form a hood over the **clitoris**, a small elongated erectile organ, and the most sensitive spot in the entire female genital area. Below the clitoris is the **urethral opening**, the outer opening of the thin tube that carries urine from the bladder. Below that is a larger opening, the mouth of the **vagina**, the canal that leads to the primary internal organs of reproduction. The **perineum** is the area between the vagina and the anus (the opening to the rectum and large intestine).

At the back of the vagina is the **cervix**, the opening to the womb, or **uterus** (see Figure 9.2b). The uterine walls are lined by a layer of tissue called the **endometrium**. The **ovaries**, about the size and shape of almonds, are located on either side of the uterus and contain egg cells called **ova** (singular, **ovum**). Extending outward and back from the upper uterus are the **fallopian tubes**, the canals that transport ova from the ovaries to the uterus. When an egg is released from an ovary, the fingerlike ends of the adjacent fallopian tube "catch" the egg and direct it into the tube.

Discharge and changes in odor normally occur in a healthy vagina. They typically fluctuate through the menstrual cycle, depending on hormone level. In the past, many women practiced douching, the introduction of a liquid into the vagina, to cleanse the vagina. However, particularly if done frequently, douching may increase the risk of pelvic inflammatory disease (discussed in Chapter 11) and ectopic or out-of-uterus pregnancy. Despite the potential dangers,

Figure 9.2 **The Female Sex Organs and Reproductive Structures**

**(a) External structure**

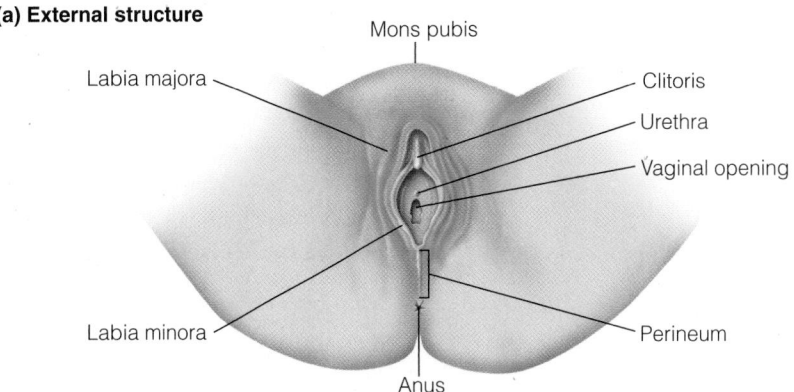

**(b) Internal structure**

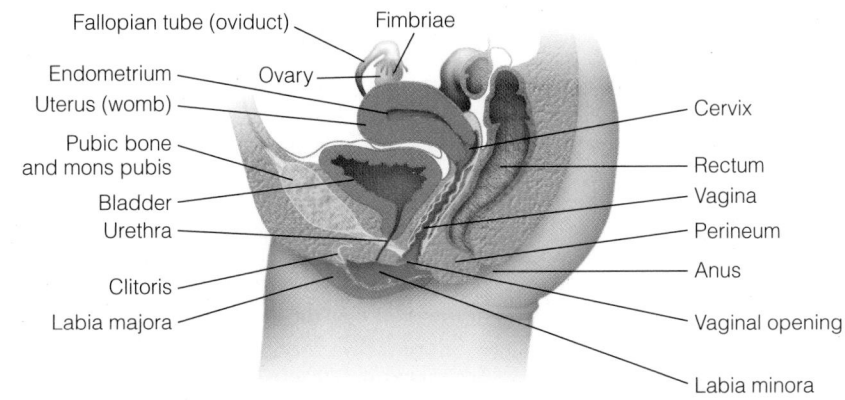

according to data from a southern university, four in ten female students had douched in the past; half currently douche.

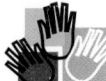 African American women were encouraged to douche by their mothers; white women were more influenced by television advertisements. When advised to stop douching by a doctor or nurse, most students do so.

## The Menstrual Cycle

Scientists have discovered that the menstrual cycle actually begins in the brain with the production of gonadotropin-releasing hormone (GnRH). Each month a surge of GnRH sets into motion the sequence of steps that lead to ovulation, the potential for conception, and if conception doesn't occur, menstruation. The hypothalamus monitors hormone levels in the blood and sends messages to the pituitary gland

**vagina** The canal leading from the exterior opening in the female genital area to the uterus.

**perineum** The area between the anus and vagina in the female and between the anus and scrotum in the male.

**cervix** The narrow, lower end of the uterus that opens into the vagina.

**uterus** The female organ that houses the developing fetus until birth.

**endometrium** The mucous membrane lining the uterus.

**ovary** The female sex organ that produces egg cells, estrogen, and progesterone.

**ovum** (plural, ova) The female gamete (egg cell).

**fallopian tubes** The pair of channels that transport ova from the ovaries to the uterus; the usual site of fertilization.

to release follicle-stimulating hormone (FSH) and luteinizing hormone (LH).

As shown in Figure 9.3, in the ovaries, these hormones stimulate the growth of a few of the immature eggs, or ova, stored in follicles in every woman's body. Usually, only one ovum matures completely during each monthly cycle. As it does, it increases its production of the female sex hormone estrogen, which in turn triggers the release of a larger surge of LH.

At midcycle, the increased LH hormone levels trigger **ovulation**, the release of the egg cell, or ovum, from the follicle. Estrogen levels drop, and the remaining cells of the follicle then enlarge, change character, and form the **corpus luteum**, or yellow body. In the second half of the menstrual cycle, the corpus luteum secretes estrogen and larger amounts of progesterone. The endometrium (uterine lining) is stimulated by progesterone to thicken and become more engorged with blood in preparation for nourishing an implanted, fertilized ovum.

If the ovum is not fertilized, the corpus luteum disintegrates. As the level of progesterone drops, **menstruation** occurs; the uterine lining is shed during the course of a menstrual period. If the egg is fertilized and pregnancy occurs, the cells that eventually develop into the placenta secrete *human chorionic gonadotropin (HCG)*, a messenger hormone that signals the pituitary not to start a new cycle. The corpus luteum then steps up its production of progesterone.

Many women experience physical or psychological changes, or both, during their monthly cycles. Usually the changes are minor, but more serious problems can occur. One recently recognized culprit is work stress. Women who are overcommitted or in jobs in which they put in a great deal of effort are more likely to report painful periods, possibly because of the effect of stress on the hormones that regulate menstruation.[1]

*Premenstrual Syndrome* Women with **premenstrual syndrome (PMS)** experience bodily discomfort and emotional distress for up to two weeks, from ovulation until the onset of menstruation. Up to 75 percent of menstruating women report one or more premenstrual symptoms; 3 to 9 percent experience disabling, incapacitating symptoms.

Once dismissed as a psychological problem, PMS has been recognized as a very real physiological disorder that may be caused by a hormonal deficiency; abnormal levels of thyroid hormone; an imbalance of estrogen and progesterone; or social and environmental factors, particularly stress. Recent studies indicate that PMS may originate in the brain. Changes in brain receptors during the ovarian cycle may be responsible.

Women with a high dietary intake of the B vitamins thiamine and riboflavin have a significantly lower risk of PMS. It is not known if vitamin B supplements also might be effective.[2]

The most common symptoms of PMS are mood changes, anxiety, irritability, difficulty concentrating, forgetfulness, impaired judgment, tearfulness, digestive symptoms (diarrhea, bloating, constipation), hot flashes, palpitations, dizziness, headache, fatigue, changes in appetite, cravings (usually for sweets or salt), water retention, breast tenderness, and insomnia. For a diagnosis to be made, women—using a self-rating symptom scale or calendar—must report troubling premenstrual symptoms in the period before menstruation in at least two successive menstrual cycles.

*Treatments* Treatments for PMS depend on specific symptoms. Diuretics (drugs that speed up fluid elimination) can relieve water retention and bloating. Relaxation techniques have led to a 60 percent reduction in anxiety symptoms. Sleep deprivation, or the use of bright light to adjust a woman's circadian or daily rhythm, also has proven beneficial. Behavioral approaches, such as exercise or charting cycles, help by letting women know when they're vulnerable.

Low doses of medications known as *selective serotonin-reuptake inhibitors (SSRIs)* (discussed in Chapter 3), such as fluoxetine (marketed as Prozac and Sarafem and in generic forms) provide relief for symptoms such as tension, depression, irritability, and mood swings, even when taken only during the premenstrual phase rather than daily throughout the month. SSRIs are not effective in all women with PMS, and other factors, including a genetic susceptibility, may play a role. YAZ, a low-dose combination birth control pill made up of the hormones drospirenone and ethinyl estradiol, is the only oral contraceptive

**ovulation** The release of a mature ovum from an ovary approximately 14 days prior to the onset of menstruation.

**corpus luteum** A yellowish mass of tissue that is formed, immediately after ovulation, from the remaining cells of the follicle; it secretes estrogen and progesterone for the remainder of the menstrual cycle.

**menstruation** Discharge of blood from the vagina as a result of the shedding of the uterine lining at the end of the menstrual cycle.

**premenstrual syndrome (PMS)** A disorder that causes physical discomfort and psychological distress prior to a woman's menstrual period.

## Figure 9.3 Menstrual Cycle

(a) In response to the hypothalamus, the pituitary gland releases the gonadotropins FSH and LH. Levels of FSH and LH stimulate the cycle (and in turn are affected by production of estrogen and progesterone).

(b) FSH does what its name says—it stimulates follicle development in the ovary. The follicle matures and ruptures, releasing an ovum (egg) into the fallopian tube.

(c) The follicle produces estrogen, and the corpus luteum produces estrogen and progesterone. The high level of estrogen at the middle of the cycle produces a surge of LH, which triggers ovulation.

(d) Estrogen and progesterone stimulate the endometrium, which becomes thicker and prepares to receive an implanted, fertilized egg. If a fertilized egg is deposited in the uterus, pregnancy begins. If the egg is not fertilized, progesterone production decreases, and the endometrium is shed (menstruation). At this point, both estrogen and progesterone levels have dropped, so the pituitary responds by producing FSH, and the cycle begins again.

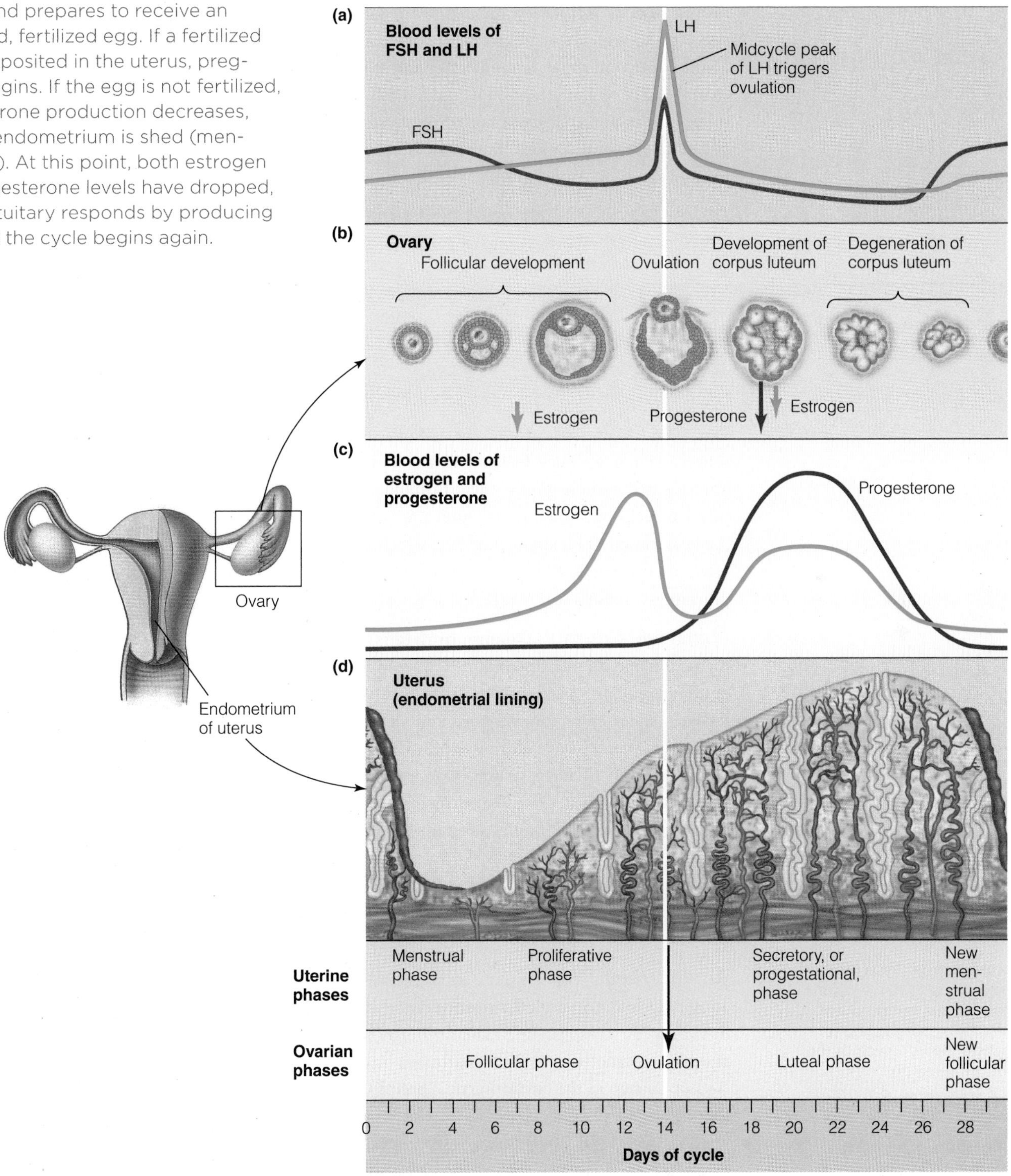

(a) **Blood levels of FSH and LH**
LH
Midcycle peak of LH triggers ovulation
FSH

(b) **Ovary**
Follicular development — Ovulation — Development of corpus luteum — Degeneration of corpus luteum
↓ Estrogen — Progesterone ↓ Estrogen

(c) **Blood levels of estrogen and progesterone**
Estrogen
Progesterone

(d) **Uterus (endometrial lining)**

Ovary
Endometrium of uterus

| Uterine phases | Menstrual phase | Proliferative phase | | Secretory, or progestational, phase | New menstrual phase |
|---|---|---|---|---|---|
| Ovarian phases | | Follicular phase | Ovulation | Luteal phase | New follicular phase |

Days of cycle: 0 2 4 6 8 10 12 14 16 18 20 22 24 26 28

approved by the FDA to treat emotional and physical premenstrual symptoms. (See Chapter 10 on birth control.)

A diet rich in calcium and vitamin D reduces the risk of PMS; supplements of the two decrease the severity of symptoms.[3] Cognitive-behavioral therapy, described in Chapter 3, may be the most effective psychological approach; simply educating women about PMS has not proven useful.[4] Other treatments with some reported success include exercise; less caffeine, alcohol, salt, and sugar; acupuncture; and stress management techniques such as meditation or relaxation training. Chinese herbal medicine is popular in several nations, but there is insufficient evidence to support its use.

*Premenstrual Dysphoric Disorder* **Premenstrual dysphoric disorder** (**PMDD**), which is not related to PMS, occurs in an estimated 3 to 5 percent of all menstruating women. It is characterized by regular symptoms of depression (depressed mood, anxiety, mood swings, diminished interest or pleasure) during the last week of the menstrual cycle. Women with PMDD cannot function as usual at work, school, or home. They feel better a few days after menstruation begins. Certain birth control pills can help by stopping ovulation and stabilizing hormone fluctuations.[5] SSRIs, which are often used to treat PMS, also are effective in relieving symptoms of PMDD.

*Menstrual Cramps* **Dysmenorrhea** is the medical name for the discomforts—abdominal cramps and pain, back and leg pain, diarrhea, tension, water retention, fatigue, and depression—that can occur during menstruation. About half of all menstruating women suffer from dysmenorrhea. The cause seems to be an overproduction of bodily substances called prostaglandins, which typically rise during menstruation. Medications that inhibit prostaglandins can reduce menstrual pain, and exercise can also relieve cramps.

*Amenorrhea* Women may stop menstruating—a condition called **amenorrhea**—for a variety of reasons, including a hormonal disorder, drastic weight loss, strenuous exercise, or change in the environment. "Boarding-school amenorrhea" is common among young women who leave home for school. Distance running and strenuous exercise also can lead to

**premenstrual dysphoric disorder (PMDD)** A disorder that causes symptoms of psychological depression during the last week of the menstrual cycle.

**dysmenorrhea** Painful menstruation.

**amenorrhea** The absence or suppression of menstruation.

amenorrhea. The reason may be a drop in body fat from the normal range of 18 to 22 percent to a range of 9 to 12 percent. To be considered amenorrheic, a woman's menstrual cycle is typically absent for three or more consecutive months. Prolonged amenorrhea can have serious health consequences, including a loss of bone density that may lead to stress fractures or osteoporosis.

Scientists have developed chemical mimics, or analogues, of GnRH—usually administered by nasal spray—that trigger ovulation in women who don't ovulate or menstruate normally.

*Toxic Shock Syndrome* This rare, potentially deadly bacterial infection primarily strikes menstruating women under the age of 30 who use tampons. Both *Staphylococcus aureus* and group

Figure 9.4  **Male Sex Organs and Reproductive Structures**

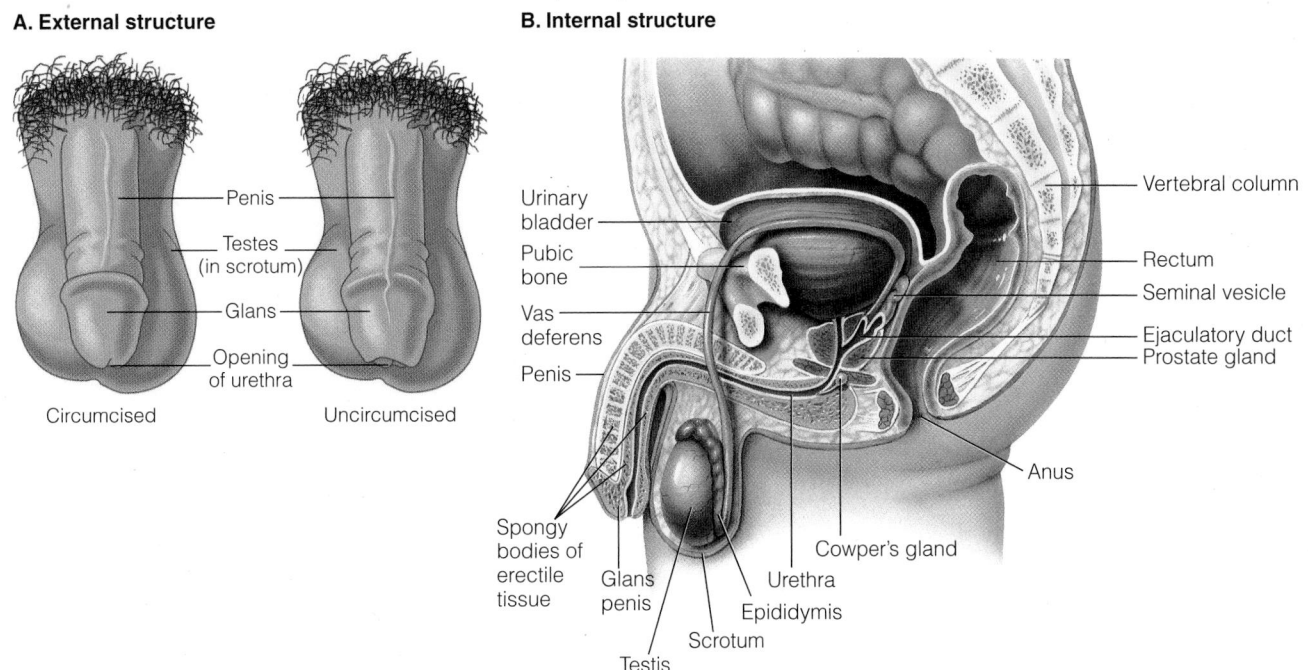

**A. External structure**

- Penis
- Testes (in scrotum)
- Glans
- Opening of urethra

Circumcised    Uncircumcised

**B. Internal structure**

- Urinary bladder
- Pubic bone
- Vas deferens
- Penis
- Spongy bodies of erectile tissue
- Glans penis
- Testis
- Scrotum
- Epididymis
- Urethra
- Cowper's gland
- Anus
- Vertebral column
- Rectum
- Seminal vesicle
- Ejaculatory duct
- Prostate gland

A *Streptococcus pyogenes* can produce **toxic shock syndrome** (**TSS**). Symptoms include a high fever; a rash that leads to peeling of the skin on the fingers, toes, palms, and soles; dizziness; dangerously low blood pressure; and abnormalities in several organ systems (the digestive tract and the kidneys) and in the muscles and blood. Treatment usually consists of antibiotics and intense supportive care; intravenous administration of immunoglobulins that attack the toxins produced by these bacteria also may be beneficial.

# Men's Sexual Health

Because the male reproductive system is simpler in many ways than the female, it's often ignored—especially by healthy young men. However, men should make regular self-exams (including checking the penis and testes, as described in Chapter 15) part of their routine.

## Male Sexual Anatomy

The visible parts of the male sexual anatomy are the **penis** and the **scrotum**, the pouch that contains the **testes** (Figure 9.4). The testes manufacture testosterone, the hormone that stimulates the development of a male's secondary sex characteristics, and **sperm**, the male reproductive cells. Immature sperm are stored in the **epididymis**, a collection of coiled tubes adjacent to each testis.

The penis contains three hollow cylinders loosely covered with skin. The two major cylinders, the corpora cavernosa, extend side by side through the length of the penis. The third cylinder, the corpus spongiosum, surrounds the urethra, the channel for both seminal fluid and urine; see Figure 9.4.

When hanging down loosely, the average penis is about 3¾ inches long. During erection, its internal cylinders fill with so much blood that they become rigid, and the penis stretches to an average length of 6¼ inches. About 90 percent of all men have erect penises measuring between 5 and 7 inches in length. There is no relation, however, between penis size and female sexual satisfaction: A woman's vagina naturally adjusts during intercourse to the size of her partner's penis.

Inside the body are several structures involved in the production of seminal fluid, or **semen**, the liquid in which sperm cells are carried out of

**toxic shock syndrome (TSS)** A disease characterized by fever, vomiting, diarrhea, and often shock, caused by a bacterium that releases toxic waste products into the bloodstream.

**penis** The male organ of sex and urination.

**scrotum** The external sac or pouch that holds the testes.

**testes** (singular, testis) The male sex organs that produce sperm and testosterone.

**sperm** The male gamete produced by the testes and transported outside the body through ejaculation.

**epididymis** That portion of the male duct system in which sperm mature.

**semen** The viscous whitish fluid that is the complete male ejaculate; a combination of sperm and secretions from the prostate gland, seminal vesicles, and other glands.

## Sexual Health

There are many aspects of sexuality. To investigate the latest news on sexual health, log in to Global Health Watch and ender the phrase "sexual health" in the search box. Scan the search results and find a recent article related to any aspect of sexual health. In your online journal, write a brief summary of the article and use it to start a personal reflection about your sexual health.

**vas deferens** Two tubes that carry sperm from the epididymis into the urethra.

**urethra** The canal through which urine from the bladder leaves the body; in the male, also serves as the channel for seminal fluid.

**seminal vesicles** Glands in the male reproductive system that produce the major portion of the fluid of semen.

**ejaculatory duct** The canal connecting the seminal vesicles and vas deferens.

**prostate gland** A structure surrounding the male urethra that produces a secretion that helps liquefy the semen from the testes.

**Cowper's glands** Two small glands that discharge into the male urethra; also called bulbourethral glands.

**circumcision** The surgical removal of the foreskin of the penis.

the body during ejaculation. The **vas deferens** are two tubes that carry sperm from the epididymis into the **urethra**. The **seminal vesicles**, which make some of the seminal fluid, join with the vas deferens to form the **ejaculatory ducts**. The **prostate gland** produces some of the seminal fluid, which it secretes into the urethra during ejaculation. The **Cowper's glands** are two pea-sized structures on either side of the urethra (just below where it emerges from the prostate gland) and connected to it via tiny ducts. When a man is sexually aroused, the Cowper's glands often secrete a fluid that appears as a droplet at the tip of the penis. This fluid is not semen, although it occasionally contains sperm.

## Circumcision

In its natural state, the tip of the penis is covered by a fold of skin called the *foreskin*. About 60 percent of baby boys in the United States undergo **circumcision**, the surgical removal of the foreskin.

An estimated 1.2 million newborn males are circumcised in the United States annually for reasons that vary from religious traditions to preventive health measures. Circumcision rates are highest in the Midwest and Northeast and lowest in the West. They are significantly higher in states that provide Medicaid coverage for routine circumcision.[6] Until the last half century, scientific evidence to support or repudiate routine circumcision was limited.

According to recent research, circumcision significantly reduces the risk of infection with human immunodeficiency virus (HIV), herpes simplex virus type 2, and human papillomavirus (HPV).[7] Female partners of circumcised men are less likely to develop bacterial vaginosis and *Trichomonas vaginalis* infection. (Sexually transmitted infections are discussed in Chapter 11.)

Additional health benefits of circumcision include:

- Lower risk of cancer of the penis, a rare type.
- Less risk of urinary tract infections during the first year of life. An uncircumcised baby boy has a 1 in 100 chance of getting a urinary tract infection, compared with a 1 in 1,000 chance for a circumcised baby boy.

- Prevention of foreskin infections and retraction.
- Easier genital hygiene.

Complications may include bleeding, infection, improper healing, or cutting the foreskin too long or too short. Analgesic creams or anesthetic shots are typically used to minimize discomfort. There is little consensus on what impact the presence or absence of a foreskin has on sexual functioning or satisfaction.

# Responsible Sexuality

The World Health Organization defines sexual health as "the integration of the physical, emotional, intellectual, and social aspects of sexual being in ways that are positively enriching, and that enhance personality, communication, and love. . . . Every person has a right to receive sexual information and to consider sexual relationships for pleasure as well as for procreation."

Sexuality education is a lifelong process. Your own knowledge about sex may not be as extensive as you might assume. Most people grow up with a lot of myths and misconceptions about sex. (See this chapter's Self Survey: "How Much Do You Know about Sex?"). Rather than relying on what peers say or what you've always thought was true, find out the facts. This textbook is a good place to start. The student health center and the library can provide additional materials on sexual identity, orientation, behavior, and health, as well as on options for reducing your risk of acquiring sexually transmitted infections (discussed in Chapter 11) or becoming pregnant.

## Creating a Sexually Healthy Relationship

A sexually healthy relationship, as defined by the Sexuality Information and Education Council of the United States (SIECUS), is based on shared values and has five characteristics: It is

- Consensual.
- Nonexploitative.

- Honest.
- Mutually pleasurable.
- Protected against unintended pregnancy and sexually transmitted infections.

All individuals also have sexual rights, which include the right to the information, education, skills, support, and services they need to make responsible decisions about their sexuality consistent with their own values, as well as the right to express their sexual orientation without violence or discrimination.

Communication is vital in a sexually healthy relationship, even though these discussions can be awkward. Yet if you have a need or a problem that relates to your partner, it is your responsibility to bring it up. (See Health on a Budget, p. 288.)

## Making Sexual Decisions

Sexual decision making should always take place within the context of an individual's values and perceptions of right and wrong behavior. Making responsible sexual decisions means considering all the possible consequences—including emotional consequences—of sexual behavior for both yourself and your partner.

Even after they have entered into a relationship, many young people are not clear on whether they will have sex only with one another. According to a recent study of heterosexual married and unmarried couples between ages 18 and 25, in 40 percent of the cases, one partner said the couple had agreed to be monogamous while the other said there was no such understanding. Even among couples who had agreed to have sex exclusively with each other, nearly 30 percent broke this commitment, with at least one partner having sex outside the relationship. Married couples were no more likely than unmarried ones to have an explicit monogamy agreement.[8]

Prior to any sexual activity that involves a risk of sexually transmitted infection or pregnancy, both partners should talk about their prior sexual histories (including number of partners and exposure to STIs) and other high-risk behavior, such as the use of injection drugs. They should also discuss the issue of birth control and which methods might be best for them to use. If you know someone well enough to consider having

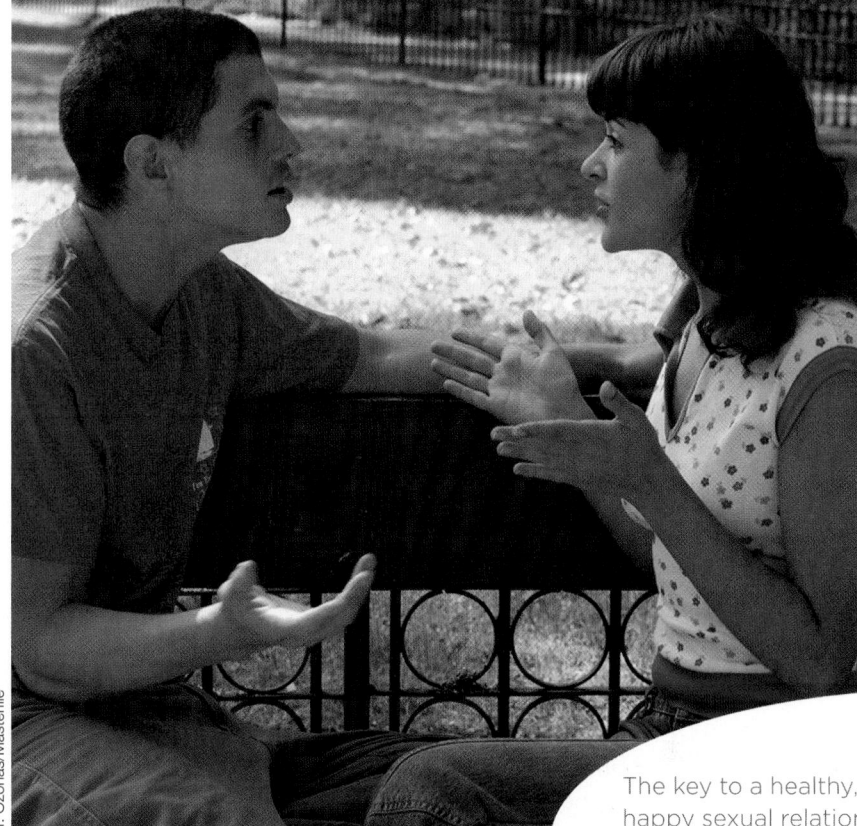

© T. Ozonas/Masterfile

The key to a healthy, happy sexual relationship is open, honest communication—even when you and your partner have different points of view.

sex with that person, you should be able to talk about such sensitive subjects. If a potential partner is unwilling to talk or hedges on crucial questions, you shouldn't be engaging in sex.

Here are some questions to consider as you think and talk about the significance of becoming sexually intimate with a partner:

- **What role do we want relationships and sex to have in our life at this time?**

- **What are my values and my potential partner's values as they pertain to sexual relationships?** Does each of us believe that intercourse should be reserved for a permanent partnership or committed relationship?

- **Will a decision to engage in sex enhance my positive feelings about myself or my partner?** Does either of us have questions about sexual orientation or the kinds of people we are attracted to?

- **Do I and my partner both want to have sex?** Is my partner pressuring me in any way? Am I pressuring my partner? Am

# Health in Action

## Developing Sexual Responsibility

The Sexuality Information and Education Council of the United States (SIECUS) has worked with nongovernmental organizations around the world to develop a consensus about the life behaviors of a sexually healthy and responsible adult. These include:

- Appreciating one's own body.
- Seeking information about reproduction as needed.
- Affirming that sexual development may or may not include reproduction or genital sexual experience.
- Interacting with both genders in respectful and appropriate ways.
- Affirming one's own sexual orientation and respecting the sexual orientation of others.
- Expressing love and intimacy in appropriate ways.
- Developing and maintaining meaningful relationships.
- Avoiding exploitative or manipulative relationships.
- Making informed choices about family options and lifestyles.
- Enjoying and expressing one's sexuality throughout life.
- Expressing one's sexuality in ways congruent with one's values.
- Discriminating between life-enhancing sexual behaviors and those that are harmful to oneself and/or others.

From the preceding list, choose three characteristics that you would like to improve in your intimate relationships. Why did you choose these three? Do they have special significance for you? How will you go about strengthening them? Do you have other goals for responsible sexuality? Record your reflections in your online journal.

I making this decision for myself or for my partner?

**Have my partner and I discussed our sexual histories and risk factors?** Have I spoken honestly about any STIs I've had in the past? Am I sure that neither my partner nor I have a sexually transmitted infection?

**Have we taken precautions against unwanted pregnancy and STIs?**

## Saying No to Sex

Whether couples are on a first date or have been married for years, each partner always has the right not to have sex. Unfortunately, "no" sometimes seems to mean different things to men and women.

The following strategies can help you assert yourself when saying no to sex:

- **First of all, recognize** your own values and feelings. If you believe that sex is something to be shared only by people who've already become close in other ways, be true to that belief.

- **Be direct.** Look the person in the eyes, keep your head up, and speak clearly and firmly.

- **Just say no.** Make it clear you're rejecting the offer, not the person. You don't owe anyone an explanation for what you want, but if you want to expand on your reasons, you might say, "I enjoy your company, and I'd like to do something together, but no," or "Thank you. I appreciate your interest, but no."

- **If you're still at a loss for words,** try these responses: "I like you a lot, but I'm not ready to have sex." "You're a great person, but sex isn't something I do to prove I like someone." "I'd like to wait until I'm married to have sex."

- **If you're feeling pressured,** let your date know that you're uncomfortable. Be simple and direct. Watch out for emotional blackmail. If your date says, "If you really like me, you'd want to make love," point out that if he or she really likes you, he or she wouldn't try to force you to do something you don't want to do.

- **If you're a woman, monitor your sexual signals.** Men impute more sexual meaning to gestures (such as casual touching) that women perceive as friendly and innocent.

- **Communicate your feelings** to your date sooner rather than later. It's far easier to say, "I don't want to go to your apartment" than to fight off unwelcome advances once you're there.

- **Remember that if saying no to sex** puts an end to a relationship, it wasn't much of a relationship in the first place.

# Sexual Behavior

From birth to death, we are sexual beings. Our sexual identities, needs, likes, and dislikes emerge in adolescence and become clearer as we enter adulthood, but we continue to change and evolve throughout our lives. In men, sexual interest is most intense at age 18; in women, it reaches a peak in the 30s. Although age brings changes in sexual responsiveness, we never outgrow our sexuality.

## Adolescent Sexuality

Early in adolescence, sexual curiosity explodes, and sexual exploration—both alone and with a partner—takes on new meaning and intensity. Sexual education programs can make a difference by helping young people become sexually responsible, enabling them to form satisfying relationships, helping them assess their own attitudes toward sex, and giving them information on sexuality. Good programs can clarify values and enhance communication.

It's not unusual for teenage boys to experience frequent erections during the day and night, including **nocturnal emissions**, or wet dreams, during which ejaculation occurs. **Masturbation** (discussed later in this chapter) is the primary form of sexual expression for many teenagers, especially boys. Self-stimulation helps teens learn about their bodies and their sexual potential and serves as an outlet for sexual tension. By the end of adolescence, the majority of teens have masturbated to orgasm.

Other common sexual activities during adolescence include kissing and petting—erotic physical contact that may include holding, touching, manual stimulation of the genitals, and oral sex. As many as 25 percent of teens experience some same-sex attractions. Although many experiment with heterosexual and homosexual sexual experiences, adolescent sexual behavior does not always foretell sexual orientation. Young people, who often feel confused about their sexual identity, may engage in sexual activity with members of the same or the other sex as a way of testing how they really feel.

## Teen Sexual Activity

More than half of adolescents (58 percent) in the United States have never had sexual intercourse. According to the CDC's most recent report on teen sexual activity, the percentage of virgins among teens ages 15 to 19 has grown steadily in recent decades.[9] The reasons teens give for not having sex include the following:

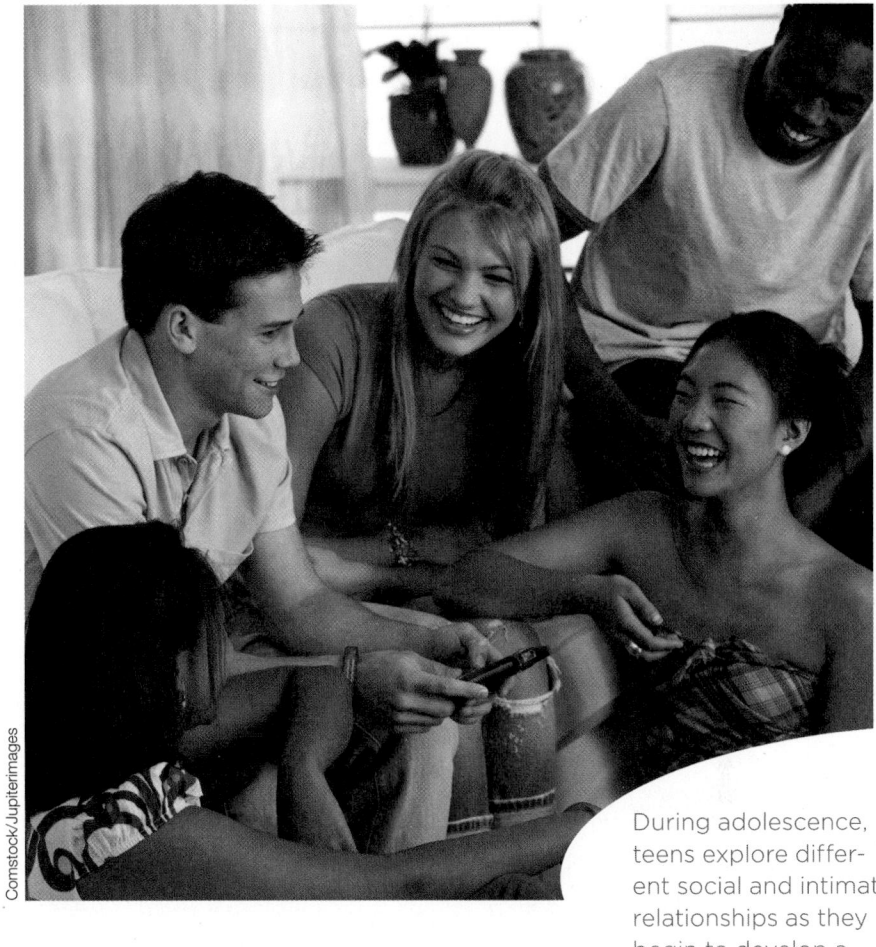

During adolescence, teens explore different social and intimate relationships as they begin to develop a sexual identity.

- against religion or morals
- don't want to get pregnant/get a girl pregnant
- don't want to get a sexually transmitted infection
- haven't found the right person yet
- in a relationship but waiting for the right time.[10]

Among sexually active teens, their most common first partner was someone with whom they were going steady. Boys were more likely than girls to report that their first sexual experience was with someone they had just met. Seven percent of the young women reported that their first sexual experience was not voluntary, particularly when their partner was older.

Teenagers were more likely to become sexually active if their mothers had their first births as teenagers, and if they did not live with both parents at age 14. The younger that teens were at first intercourse, the greater the number of total partners that they reported. Girls who lost

**nocturnal emissions** Ejaculations while dreaming; wet dreams.

**masturbation** Manual (or nonmanual) self-stimulation of the genitals, often resulting in orgasm.

# The Secret to a Good Sexual Relationship

The secret to a healthy, happy sexual relationship isn't a hot car or sexy outfit. It's the ability to communicate openly, honestly, and respectfully with your partner. Here are some specific suggestions:

- **Choose an appropriate time and place for an intimate discussion.** In a new relationship, talking in a public place, such as a park bench or a quiet table at a coffee house, can seem safer. If you're in an established relationship, choose a time when you can give each other complete attention and a setting in which you can both relax.

- **Ask open-ended questions that encourage a dialogue—** for instance, "How do you feel about . . . ?" or "What are your thoughts about . . . ?"

- **Listen actively rather than passively when your partner speaks.** Show that you're paying attention by nodding, smiling, and leaning forward. Paraphrase what he or she says to show you understand it fully.

(See "Listen Up" in *Labs for IPC*.)

- **Use "I" statements, such as "I really enjoy making love, but I'm so tired right now that I won't be a responsive partner.** Why don't we get the kids to bed early tomorrow so we can enjoy ourselves a little earlier?"

- **If you would like to try something different, say so.** Practice saying the words first if they embarrass you. If your partner feels uncomfortable, don't force the issue, but do try talking it through.

- **If you want to request changes or tackle a touchy topic, start with positive statements.** Let your partner know how much you enjoy having sex, and then express your desire to enjoy lovemaking more often or in different ways.

- **Encourage small changes.** If you want your partner to be less inhibited, start slowly, perhaps by suggesting sex in a different room or place.

their virginity before age 15 were significantly more likely to have multiple unintended pregnancies.[11] Among never-married, sexually experienced teens, 79 percent used birth control at first intercourse—68 percent relied on condoms and 15 percent on the pill. (See Chapter 10 for more on birth control and teens.)

Among teens who had sex at least once, the vast majority had not had sex in the previous year (62 percent) or three months (72 percent). An even higher percentage—76 percent of girls and 79 percent of boys—had not had intercourse in the month before the interview. In the previous year, 25 percent of sexually active teenage girls and 22 percent of boys had sex with only one partner. A small percentage—3 percent of the girls and 4 percent of the boys—had sex with four or more partners.[12]

## Sex on Campus

 Sexual behavior on campus has changed dramatically in the last 25 years. Surveys conducted in the United States and in Canada since 1980 reveal a steady increase in the number of students who have had intercourse and an increase in safer sex practices among sexually active students. Today's undergraduates are more likely to question potential partners about their past, use condoms with a new partner, and maintain fairly long-term monogamous relationships.

College students see sexual activity as normal behavior for their peer group. College students tend to overestimate how much sex their peers are having. According to the American College Health Association National College Health Assessment, about a third of undergraduates reported having no sexual partners within the last 12 months. Among sexually active students, the mean number of partners was two.[13] (See How Do You Compare? The Sex Lives of College Students.)

College students who binge drink or participate in drinking games, which often involve physical skills (such as bouncing a coin into a glass) or word play, increase their odds of sexually risky behavior. Both men and women report being taken advantage of sexually, including someone having sex with them when they were too drunk to give consent, after such games.

Annual spring breaks provide what researchers describe as "ideal conditions for the potentially lethal interaction between alcohol, drugs, and sexual risk-taking." Students typically engage in binge drinking, illicit drug use, and unsafe sexual practices. The likelihood of casual sex depends on several factors, including peer influences, prior experiences with casual sex, alcohol consumption prior to sex, and impulsivity.

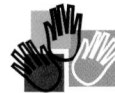 As with other aspects of health, cultural, religious, and personal values affect students' sexual behaviors.

# THE SEX LIVES OF COLLEGE STUDENTS

Students reporting having:

### Oral sex within the past 30 days:

| | Percent (%) | | |
|---|---|---|---|
| | Male | Female | Total |
| No, have never done this sexual activity | 26.5 | 27.6 | 27.2 |
| No, have done this sexual activity but not in the last 30 days | 28.7 | 27.2 | 27.7 |
| Yes | 44.8 | 45.2 | 45.1 |

### Vaginal sex within the past 30 days:

| | Percent (%) | | |
|---|---|---|---|
| | Male | Female | Total |
| No, have never done this sexual activity | 31.8 | 29.1 | 30.1 |
| No, have done this sexual activity but not in the last 30 days | 22.8 | 18.6 | 20.1 |
| Yes | 45.4 | 52.3 | 49.8 |

### Anal sex within the past 30 days:

| | Percent (%) | | |
|---|---|---|---|
| | Male | Female | Total |
| No, have never done this sexual activity | 73.0 | 77.9 | 76.0 |
| No, have done this sexual activity but not in the last 30 days | 20.6 | 18.2 | 19.1 |
| Yes | 6.4 | 3.9 | 4.9 |

### College students reporting having the following number of sexual partners (oral sex, vaginal or anal intercourse) within the last 12 months:

| | Percent (%) | | |
|---|---|---|---|
| | Male | Female | Total |
| None | 30.3 | 28.5 | 29.2 |
| 1 | 40.8 | 47.0 | 44.7 |
| 2 | 10.5 | 11.0 | 10.8 |
| 3 | 6.6 | 5.8 | 6.1 |
| 4 or more | 11.7 | 7.7 | 9.2 |

## HOW DO YOU COMPARE?

Most college students assume that their classmates are more sexually active than they are. As the preceding data indicate, a significant percentage have never had sexual intercourse. Those who are sexually active report a median of two partners. Do these statistics change your perception of sexual activity on campus? Do they have any influence on your own intimate relationships? Record your thoughts in your online journal.

Source: American College Health Association. *American College Health Association-National College Health Assessment II: Reference Group Executive Summary, Spring 2010*. Linthicum, MD: American College Health Association, 2010.

Researchers raised concern about young Latina women, who have the highest teen birth rate in the United States (twice the national rate) and are at greater risk of sexually transmitted infections. Although Latinas represent about 10 percent of women over age 21, they account for 20 percent of female AIDS cases. Among college students and other populations, Latinas are more likely to engage in unprotected intercourse than women from other ethnic groups.

Acculturation—the process of adaptation that occurs when immigrants enter a new country— also affects sexual behavior. As Latina immigrants become more acculturated in the United States, some aspects of their sexual behavior become more Americanized; for instance, they become more likely to engage in nonmarital sexual activity and to have multiple partners. In a study of Cuban American college women, older, less religious, and U.S.-born Latinas were more likely to be sexually active and to engage in risky sexual behavior than other Latinas.

## The Sex Life of American Adults

The scientific study of Americans' sexual behavior began in 1938, when Alfred Kinsey, Ph.D.,

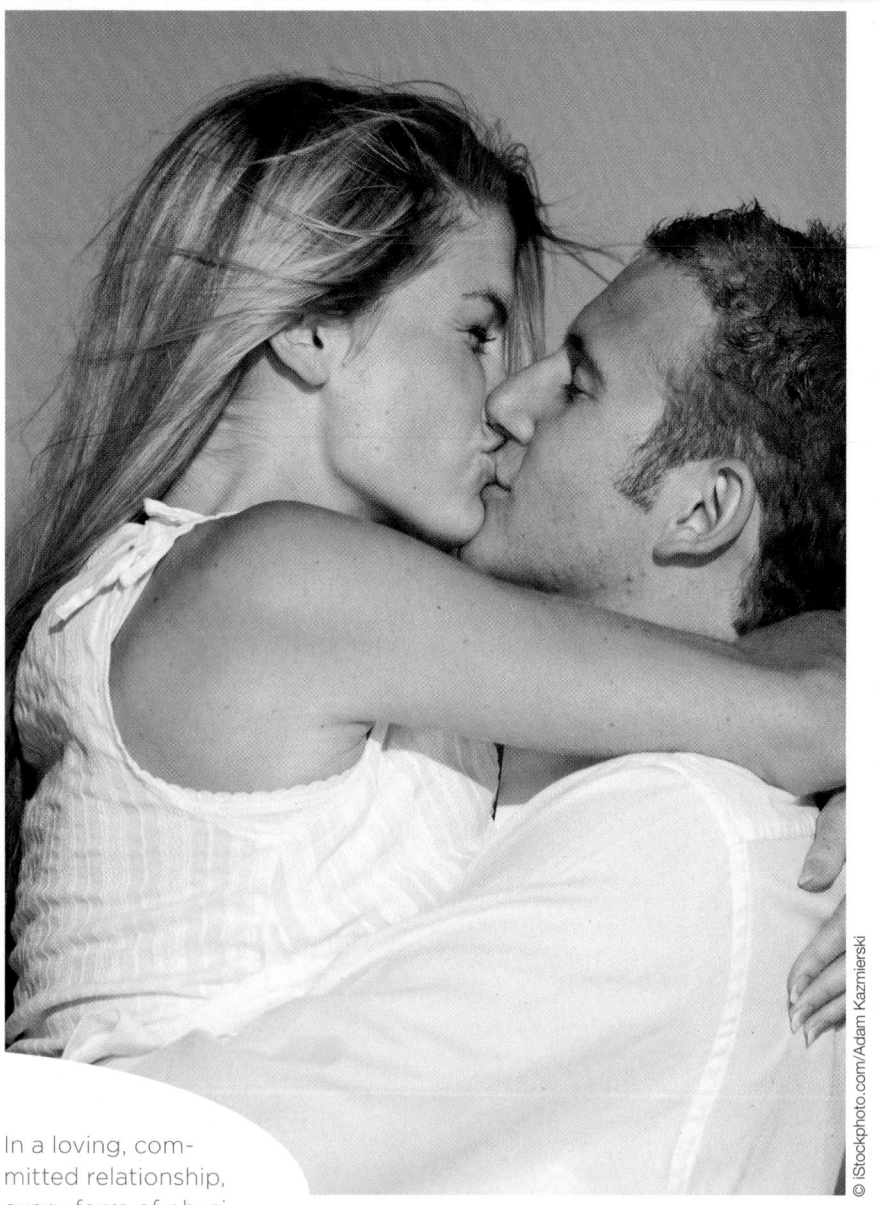

In a loving, committed relationship, every form of physical contact can serve as an intimate form of expressing deep emotion.

individuals across the United States. A larger survey, conducted by researchers at the University of Chicago, was based on face-to-face interviews with 3,432 Americans, ages 18 to 59. It became the basis for two books published in 1994: *Sex in America,* aimed at a lay audience, and *The Social Organization of Sexuality,* a more scholarly work. Since then, the researchers' General Social Survey (GSS) database on sexual activity has grown to nearly 10,000 respondents.

College students tend to believe that they engage in fewer risky sex behaviors than their peers—yet only about a third report using condoms regularly. Generally they are more likely to do so with a partner they have not known long or well, such as a hookup or one-night stand. Undergraduates who believe they "know" their partners often see safe practices as unnecessary—even though there is no way of "knowing" whether a potential partner has a sexually transmitted infection.[14]

The average American adult reports having sex about once a week. However, 1 in 5 Americans has been celibate for at least a year, and 1 in 20 engages in sex at least every other day. Men report more sexual frequency than women—not because men are more boastful about their prowess, the researchers contend, but because the sample of women includes many widows and older women without partners. Among married people, the frequency reports of husbands and wives (not in the same couples) are within one episode per year—58.6 for married men and 57.9 for married women. If other differences between men and women are statistically controlled (such as sexual preference, age, and educational attainment), married women actually report a slightly higher frequency than men.

 Sexual frequency peaks among those with some college education, then decreases among four-year college graduates, and declines even further among those with professional degrees. Americans who have attended graduate school are the least sexually active educational group in the population. These respondents may be more honest than others in reporting sexual activity, or they may be more precise in their definition of what counts as sex.

a professor of biology at the University of Indiana, and his colleagues asked 5,300 white men and 5,940 white women about their sexual practices. In his landmark studies—*Sexual Behavior in the Human Male,* published in 1948, and *Sexual Behavior in the Human Female,* published in 1953—Kinsey reported that 73 percent of men and 20 percent of women had premarital intercourse by age 20, and 37 percent of men and 17 percent of women had some homosexual experience in their lifetime.

The Janus Report on Sexual Behavior, published in 1993, was based on a survey of 2,765

Does sex make people happier or healthier? Researchers have concluded that the more sex a person has, the more likely he or she is to report having a happy life and a happy marriage. This connection is stronger among women than among men. A second and more important predictor of sexual frequency is the feeling that one's life is exciting rather than routine or dull. "Being excited by life is most strongly associated with being happier," the researchers noted. "It seems that increased sexual activity is one of the many benefits of having a positive attitude."

## Why People Have Sex

The reasons people engage in sex long seemed so obvious that scientists didn't bother to investigate them. They assumed that heterosexuals had sex primarily to reproduce, experience sexual pleasure, and relieve sexual tension.

In the most extensive study of why humans have sex, researchers identified 237 motivations. The study sample included 1,549 undergraduates ranging in age from 16 to 42. The reasons people gave fell into nine categories:

- Pure attraction to the other person in general.
- Experiencing physical pleasure.
- Expressing love.
- Feeling desired by the other.
- Escalating the depth of a relationship.
- Curiosity or seeking new adventures.
- Marking a special occasion for celebration.
- Mere opportunity.
- Sex "just happening" due to seemingly uncontrollable circumstances.

The responses of men and women were generally similar. However, men were significantly more likely to report having sex for reasons of opportunity and experience—for instance, because a person "was available" or wanting "to increase the number of partners I experienced." Women were more likely to endorse certain emotional motivations, such as, "I wanted to express my love for the person," or "I realized I was in love." Men also endorsed more reasons related to pure physical pleasure, such as wanting to have sex because it felt good or because they were "horny."

# Sexual Diversity

Human beings are diverse in all ways—including sexual preferences and practices. Physiological, psychological, and social factors determine whether we are attracted to members of the same sex or the other sex. This attraction is our **sexual orientation**. Sigmund Freud argued that we all start off **bisexual**, or attracted to both sexes. But by the time we reach adulthood, most males prefer female sexual partners, and most females prefer male partners. **Heterosexual** is the term used for individuals whose primary orientation is toward members of the other sex. In virtually all cultures, some men and women are **homosexuals**, preferring partners of their own sex.

In our society, we tend to view heterosexuality and homosexuality as very different. In reality, these orientations are opposite ends of a spectrum. Sex researcher Alfred Kinsey devised a seven-point continuum representing sexual orientation in American society. At one end of the continuum are those exclusively attracted to members of the other sex; at the opposite end are people exclusively attracted to members of the same sex. In between are varying degrees of homosexual, bisexual, and heterosexual orientation.

According to Kinsey's original data, 4 percent of men and 2 percent of women are exclusively homosexual. More recent studies have found lower numbers. For instance, in the University of Chicago's national survey, 2.8 percent of men and 1.4 percent of women defined themselves as homosexual. However, when asked if they'd had sex with a person of the same gender since age 18, about 5 percent of men and 4 percent of women said yes. When asked if they found members of the same gender sexually attractive, 6 percent of men and 5.5 percent of women said yes.

Most lesbian and bisexual women report that their first sexual experience occurred with a man (at the median age of 18) and that sex with a woman followed a few years later (at median age 21).

## Heterosexuality

Heterosexuality, the most common sexual orientation, refers to sexual or romantic attraction

**sexual orientation** The direction of an individual's sexual interest, either to members of the opposite sex or to members of the same sex.

**bisexual** Sexually oriented toward both sexes.

**heterosexual** Primary sexual orientation toward members of the other sex.

**homosexual** Primary sexual orientation toward members of the same sex.

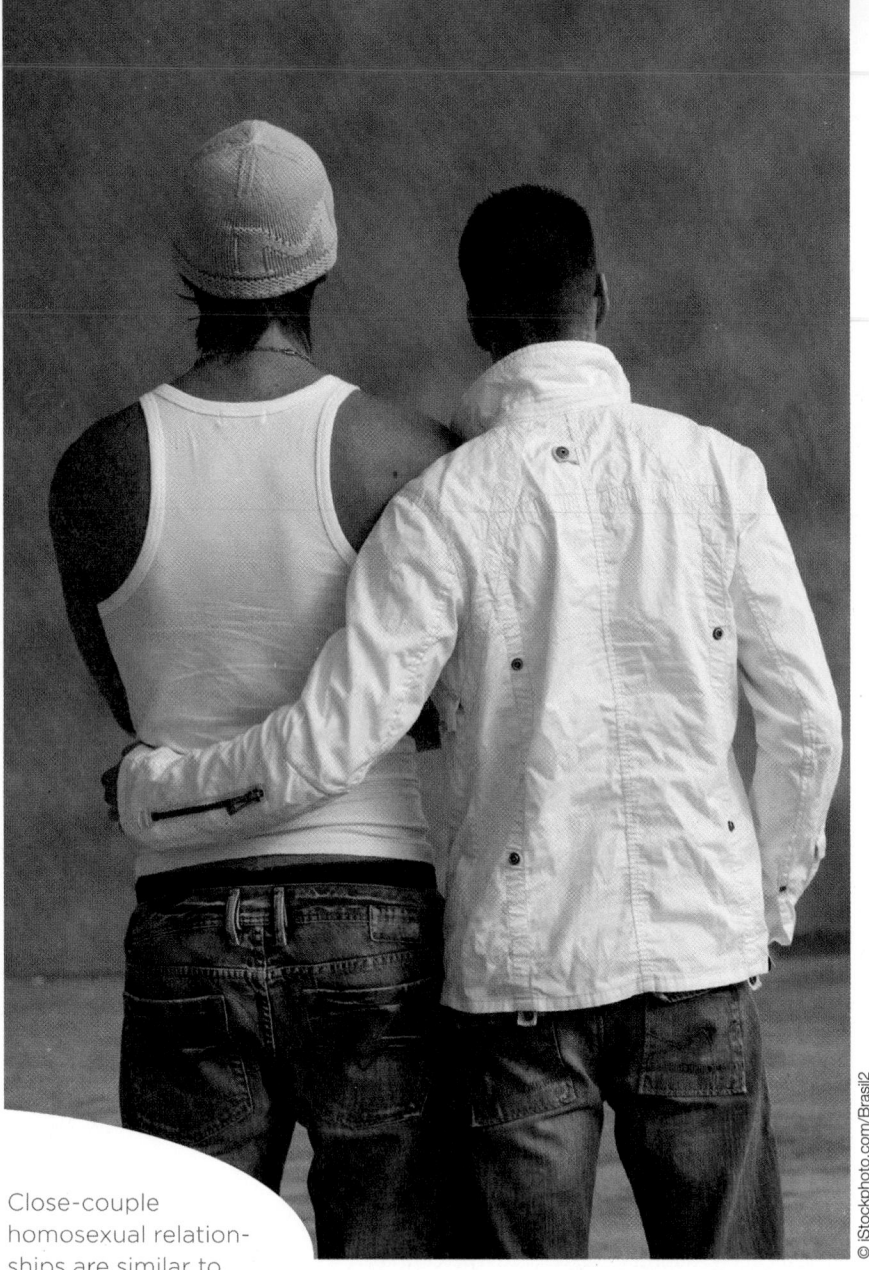

Close-couple homosexual relationships are similar to stable heterosexual relationships.

considered part of normal sexual experimentation. Among the Sambia Highlanders in Papua New Guinea, for instance, boys perform oral sex on one another as part of the rites of passage into manhood.

Some people identify themselves as bisexual even if they don't behave bisexually. Some are *serial bisexuals*—that is, they are sexually involved with same-sex partners for a while and then with partners of the other sex, or vice versa. An estimated 7 to 9 million men, about twice the number thought to be exclusively homosexual, could be described as bisexual during some extended period of their lives. The largest group are married, rarely have sexual relations with women other than their wives, and have secret sexual involvements with men.

Fear of HIV infection has sparked great concern about bisexuality, particularly among heterosexual women who worry about becoming involved with a bisexual man. About 20 to 30 percent of women with AIDS were infected by bisexual partners, and health officials fear that bisexual men who hide their homosexual affairs could transmit HIV to many more women.

## Homosexuality

Homosexuality—social, emotional, and sexual attraction to members of the same sex—exists in almost all cultures. Men and women homosexuals are commonly referred to as *gays;* women homosexuals are also called *lesbians.*

Homosexuality threatens and upsets many people, perhaps because homosexuals are viewed as different, or perhaps because no one understands why some people are heterosexual and others homosexual. *Homophobia* has led to an increase in *gay bashing* (attacking homosexuals) in many communities, including college campuses. Some blame the emergence of AIDS as a societal danger. However, researchers have found that fear of AIDS has not created new hostility but has simply given bigots an excuse to act out their hatred.

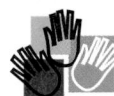 Different ethnic groups respond to homosexuality in different ways. To a greater extent than white homosexuals, gays and lesbians from ethnic groups tend to stay in the closet longer rather than risk

between opposite sexes. The adjective *heterosexual* describes intimate relationships and/or sexual relations between a man and a woman. The term *straight* is used predominantly for self-identified heterosexuals of either sex. In his landmark research in the 1940s, Alfred Kinsey reported that while many men and women were exclusively heterosexual, a significant number (37 percent of men and 13 percent of women) had at least one adult sexual experience with a member of the same sex.

## Bisexuality

Bisexuality—sexual attraction to both males and females—can develop at any point in one's life. In some cultures, bisexual activity is

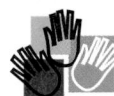© iStockphoto.com/Brasil2

alienation from their families and communities. Often they feel forced to choose between their gay and their ethnic identities.

In general, the African American community has stronger negative views of homosexuals than whites, possibly because of the influence of strong fundamentalist Christian beliefs. Stigma may contribute to a phenomenon called "the Down Low" or DL, which refers to African American men who publicly present themselves as heterosexuals while secretly having sex with other men. This practice, which is neither new nor limited to African American men, can increase the risk of HIV infection in unsuspecting female partners. Hispanic culture, with its emphasis on machismo, also has a very negative view of male homosexuality. Asian cultures, which tend to view an individual as a representative of his or her family, tend to view open declarations of sexual orientation as shaming the family and challenging their reputation and future.

*Roots of Homosexuality* Most mental health experts agree that nobody knows what causes a person's sexual orientation. Research has discredited theories tracing homosexuality to troubled childhoods or abnormal psychological development. Sexual orientation probably emerges from a complex interaction that includes biological and environmental factors.

 *Homosexuality on Campus* In a study of almost 700 heterosexual students at six small liberal arts colleges, attitudes toward homosexuals and homosexuality varied, depending on students' membership in fraternities or sororities, sex-role attitudes, religion and religiosity, and contact with and knowledge of gays, lesbians, and bisexuals. The students most likely to be accepting were those who were women, had less traditional sex-role attitudes, were less religious, attended colleges that did not have Greek social clubs, and had gay, lesbian, and/or bisexual friends.

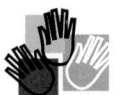 In a study of heterosexual African American college students, women expressed positive attitudes toward homosexuality, whereas men's attitudes were slightly negative. A survey of colleges and universities found great variation in the resources available to gay, lesbian, and bisexual students.

Most have a student organization; about a third provide a paid staff member to deal with the students' needs and issues, provide a support identification program, or offer at least one course on gay, lesbian, and bisexual issues.

## Transgenderism and Transsexuality

The term **transgender** is used as an umbrella term to describe people who have gender identities, expressions, or behaviors not traditionally associated with their birth sex. Male-to-female transgenders have been assigned a male gender at birth, but identify their gender as female. Female-to-male people were assigned a female gender at birth, but identify their gender as male.

Transgender individuals may be happy with the biological sex in which they are born but enjoy dressing up and behaving like the other sex. Most do so for psychological and social pleasure rather than sexual gratification.

Transsexuals feel trapped in the body of the wrong gender—a condition called *gender dysphoria*. In general, more men than women have this experience. Transsexualism is now viewed as a disorder that can be treated with sexual reassignment surgery. However, this intervention, which requires long psychological counseling, hormonal treatments, and complicated operations, remains controversial. Some studies report healthy postoperative functioning, while others note that many male and female transsexuals do not escape their psychological misery.[15]

Transgender individuals face varied health risks, including unprotected sex, sexually transmitted diseases, and HIV infection. Violence, including rape, sexual abuse, physical abuse, and suicide, is a major public health issue.

# Sexual Activity

Part of learning about your own sexuality is having a clear understanding of human sexual behaviors. Understanding frees us from fear and anxiety so that we can accept ourselves and others as the natural sexual beings we all are.

**transgender** Having a gender identity opposite one's biological sex.

## Celibacy

A celibate person does not engage in sexual activity. Complete **celibacy** means that the person doesn't masturbate (stimulate himself or herself sexually) or engage in sexual activity with a partner. In partial celibacy, the person masturbates but doesn't have sexual contact with others. Many people decide to be celibate at certain times of their lives. Some don't have sex because of concerns about pregnancy or STIs; others haven't found a partner for a permanent, monogamous relationship. Many simply have other priorities, such as finishing school or starting a career, and realize that sex outside of a committed relationship is a threat to their physical and psychological well-being.

## Abstinence

The CDC defines **abstinence** as "refraining from sexual activities which involve vaginal, anal, and oral intercourse." The definition of abstinence remains a subject of debate and controversy, with some emphasizing positive choices and others avoidance of specific behaviors. In reality, abstinence means different things to different people, cultures, and religious groups.

Increasing numbers of adolescents and young adults are choosing to remain virgins and abstain from sexual intercourse until they enter a permanent, committed, monogamous relationship. About 2.5 million teens have taken pledges to abstain from sex.

Many people who were sexually active in the past also are choosing abstinence because the risk of medical complications associated with STIs increases with the number of sexual partners a person has. Practicing abstinence is the safest, healthiest option for many. However, there is confusion about what it means to abstain, and individuals who think they are abstaining may still be engaging in behaviors that put them at risk for HIV and STIs. (See Chapter 10 for more on abstinence as a form of birth control.)

Why abstain? Among the reasons students give are:

- Remaining a virgin until you meet someone you love and see as a life partner.
- Being true to your religious and moral values.
- Getting to know a partner better.
- If you're heterosexual, to avoid pregnancy.
- To be sure you're safe from sexually transmitted infections.

Abstinence education programs, which received federal support and became widespread in American schools, have had little, if any, impact on teen sexual behavior.

## Fantasy

The mind is the most powerful sex organ in the body, and erotic mental images can be sexually stimulating. Sexual fantasies can accompany sexual activity or be pleasurable in themselves.

Fantasies generally enhance sexual arousal, reduce anxiety, and boost sexual desire. They're also a way to anticipate and rehearse new sexual experiences, as well as to bolster a person's self-image and feelings of desirability. Part of what makes fantasies exciting is that they provide an opportunity for expressing forbidden desires, such as sex with a different partner or with a past lover.

Men and women have different types of sexy thoughts, with men's fantasies containing more explicit genital images and culminating in sexual acts more quickly than women's. In women's fantasies, emotional feelings play a greater role, and there is more kissing and caressing rather than genital contact. For many women, fantasy helps in reaching orgasm during intercourse; a loss of fantasy often is a sign of low sexual desire.

Fantasies lived out via the Internet are becoming more common but may also be harmful to psychological health. (See Consumer Alert.)

## Masturbation

Not everybody masturbates, but most people do. Kinsey estimated that 7 out of 10 women and 19 out of 20 men masturbate (and admit they do). Their reason is simple: It feels good. Masturbation produces the same physical responses as sexual activity with a partner and can be an enjoyable form of sexual release.

Masturbation has been described as immature; unsocial; tiring; frustrating; and a cause of hairy

**celibacy** Abstention from sexual activity; can be partial or complete, permanent or temporary.

**abstinence** Voluntary refrainment from sexual intercourse.

## Sex in Cyberspace

Sex is the number one word searched for online. About 15 percent of Americans logging onto the Internet visit sexually oriented sites. Most people who check out sex sites on the Internet do not suffer any negative impact, but be aware of some potential risks.

### Facts to Know

- Men are the largest consumers of sexually explicit material and outnumber women by a ratio of six to one. However, while men look for visual erotica, women are more likely to visit chat rooms, which offer more interactions.

- While most individuals use their home computers when surfing the Internet for sex-related sites, one in ten has used a school computer. Some universities have strict policies barring such practices and may take punitive actions against students or employees who violate the rules.

### Steps to Take

- **Limit time online.** Individuals who spend 11 hours or more a week online in sexual pursuits show signs of psychological distress and admit that their behavior interferes with some areas of their lives.

- **Be skeptical.** Most Internet surfers admit that they occasionally "pretend" about their age on the Internet. Most keep secret how much time they spend on sexual pursuits in cyberspace.

- **Monitor yourself for signs of compulsivity.** A small but significant number of users are at risk of a serious problem as a result of their heavy Internet use.

- **Don't do anything "virtually" that you wouldn't do in real life.** For instance, "sexting" a photo of yourself nude or partially nude to your boyfriend or girlfriend might seem funny and flirty at the time. But would you flash your body on the quad or at a mall? Remember that nothing remains totally private once it makes its way into cyberspace.

palms, warts, blemishes, and blindness. None of these myths is true. Sex educators recommend masturbation to adolescents as a means of releasing tension and becoming familiar with their sexual organs.

 In a recent survey of college students, nearly all learned about masturbation through the media or from peers, rather than from parents or teachers. Most of the women reported struggling with feelings of stigma and taboo and enjoying this pleasurable act. Most of the men saw masturbation as part of healthy sexual development.[16]

Throughout adulthood, masturbation often is the primary sexual activity of individuals not involved in a sexual relationship and can be particularly useful when illness, absence, divorce, or death deprives a person of a partner. In the University of Chicago survey, about 25 percent of men and 9 percent of women said they masturbate at least once a week.

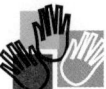 White men and women have a higher incidence of masturbation than African American men and women. Latina women have the lowest rate of masturbation, compared with Latino men, white men and women, and African American men and women. Individuals with a higher level of education are more likely to masturbate than those with less schooling, and people living with sexual partners masturbate more than those who live alone.

## Nonpenetrative Sexual Activity (Outercourse)

Various pleasurable behaviors can lead to orgasm with little risk of pregnancy or sexually transmitted infection. The options for "outercourse" include kissing, hugging, and touching but do not involve genital-to-genital, mouth-to-genital, or insertive anal sexual contact.

A kiss is a universal sign of affection. A kiss can be just a kiss—a quick press of the lips—or it can lead to much more. Usually kissing is the first sexual activity that couples engage in, and even after years of sexual experimentation and sharing, it remains an enduring pleasure for partners.

Touching is a silent form of communication between friends and lovers. Although a touch

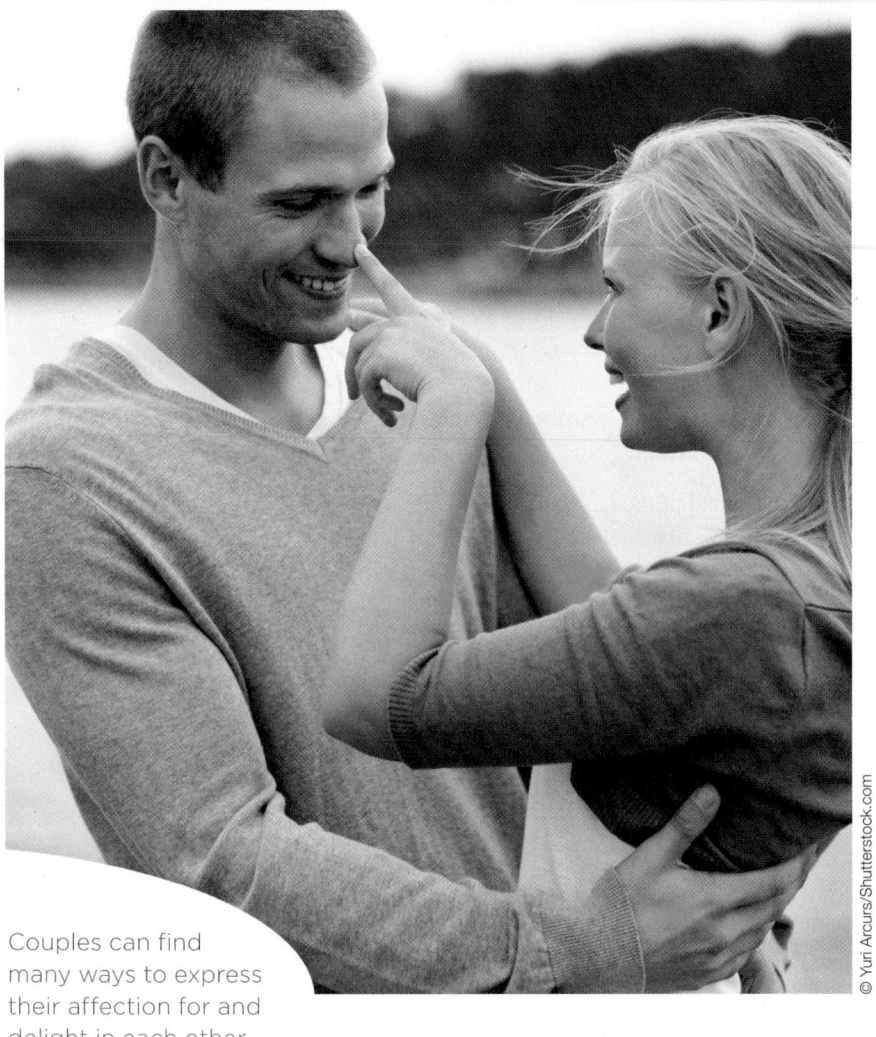

Couples can find many ways to express their affection for and delight in each other.

the woman, his penis entering her vagina from the rear); lying with the man on top of the woman in a rear-entry position; and kneeling or standing (again, in either a face-to-face or rear-entry position). Many couples move into several different positions for intercourse during a single episode of lovemaking; others may have a personal favorite or may choose different positions at different times.

Sexual activity, including intercourse, is possible throughout a woman's menstrual cycle. However, some women prefer to avoid sex while menstruating because of uncomfortable physical symptoms, such as cramps, or concern about bleeding or messiness. Others use a diaphragm or cervical cap (see Chapter 10) to hold back menstrual flow. Since different cultures have different views on intercourse during a woman's period, partners should discuss their own feelings and try to respect each other's views. If they choose not to have intercourse, there are other gratifying forms of sexual activity.

Vaginal intercourse, like other forms of sexual activity involving an exchange of body fluids, carries a risk of sexually transmitted infections, including HIV infection. In many other parts of the world, in fact, heterosexual intercourse is the most common means of HIV transmission (see Chapter 11).

## Oral Sex

The formal terms for oral sex are **cunnilingus**, which refers to oral stimulation of the woman's genitals, and **fellatio**, oral stimulation of the man's genitals. For many couples, oral sex is a regular part of their lovemaking. For others, it's an occasional experiment. Oral sex with a partner carrying a sexually transmitted infection, such as herpes or HIV infection, can lead to infection, so a condom should be used (with cunnilingus, a condom cut in half to lay flat can be used). According to the CDC, 90 percent of men and 88 percent of women ages 25 to 44 report having had oral sex with a partner of the opposite sex.

## Anal Stimulation and Intercourse

Because the anus has many nerve endings, it can produce intense erotic responses. Stimulation of

to any part of the body can be thrilling, some areas, such as the breasts and genitals, are especially sensitive. Stimulating these **erogenous** regions can lead to orgasm in both men and women. Though such forms of stimulation often accompany intercourse, more couples are gaining an appreciation of these activities as primary sources of sexual fulfillment—and as safer alternatives to intercourse.

### Intercourse

Vaginal **intercourse**, or coitus, refers to the penetration of the vagina by the penis (Figure 9.5). This is the preferred form of sexual intimacy for most heterosexual couples, who may use a wide variety of positions. The most familiar position for intercourse in our society is the so-called missionary position, with the man on top, facing the woman. An alternative is the woman on top, either lying down or sitting upright. Other positions include lying side by side (either face-to-face or with the man behind

**erogenous** Sexually sensitive.

**intercourse** Sexual stimulation by means of entry of the penis into the vagina; coitus.

**cunnilingus** Sexual stimulation of a woman's genitals by means of oral manipulation.

**fellatio** Sexual stimulation of a man's genitals by means of oral manipulation.

the anus by the fingers or mouth can be a source of sexual arousal; anal intercourse involves penile penetration of the anus. An estimated 25 percent of adults have experienced anal intercourse at least once. However, anal sex involves important health risks, such as damage to sensitive rectal tissues and the transmission of various intestinal infections, hepatitis, and STIs, including HIV.

## Cultural Variations

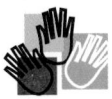 While the biological mechanisms underlying human sexual arousal and response are essentially universal, the particular sexual stimuli or behaviors that people find arousing are greatly influenced by cultural conditioning. For example, in Western societies, where the emphasis during sexual activity tends to be heavily weighted toward achieving orgasm, genitally focused activities are frequently defined as optimally arousing. In contrast, devotees to Eastern Tantric traditions (where spirituality is interwoven with sexuality) often achieve optimal pleasure by emphasizing the sensual and spiritual aspects of shared intimacy rather than orgasmic release.

Kissing on the mouth, a universal source of sexual arousal in Western society, may be rare or absent in many other parts of the world. Certain North American Eskimo people and inhabitants of the Trobriand Islands would rather rub noses than lips, and among the Thonga of South Africa, kissing is viewed as odious behavior. The Hindu people of India are also disinclined to kiss because they believe such contact symbolically contaminates the act of sexual intercourse. One survey of 190 societies found that mouth kissing was acknowledged in only 21 societies and practiced as a prelude or accompaniment to coitus in only 13.

Oral sex (both cunnilingus and fellatio) is a common source of sexual arousal among island societies of the South Pacific, in industrialized nations of Asia, and in much of the Western world. In contrast, in Africa (with the exception of northern regions), such practices are likely to be viewed as unnatural or disgusting behavior.

Foreplay in general, whether it be oral sex, sensual touching, or passionate kissing, is subject to wide cultural variation. In some societies, most notably those with Eastern traditions,

**A Cross-Sectional View of Sexual Intercourse**
Sperm are formed in each of the testes and stored in the epididymis. When a man ejaculates, sperm carried in semen travel up the vas deferens. (The prostate gland and seminal vesicles contribute components of the semen.) The semen is expelled from the penis through the urethra and deposited in the vagina, near the cervix. During sexual excitement and orgasm in a woman, the upper end of the vagina enlarges and the uterus elevates. After orgasm, these organs return to their normal states, and the cervix descends into the pool of semen.

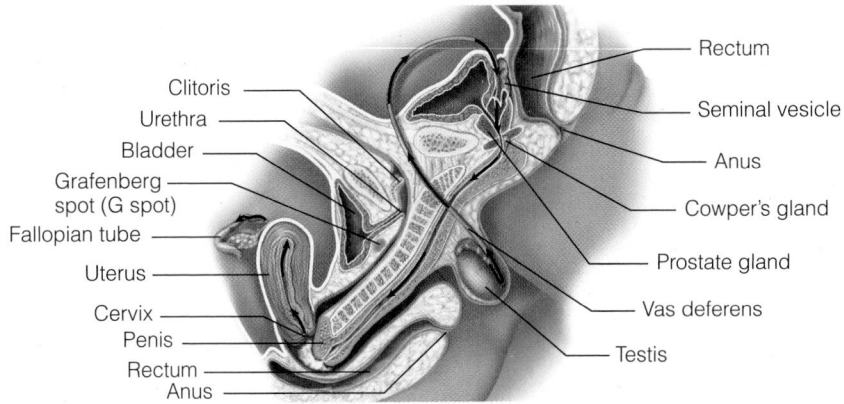

couples may strive to prolong intense states of sexual arousal for several hours. While varied patterns of foreplay are common in Western cultures, these activities often are of short duration as lovers move rapidly toward the "main event" of coitus. In still other societies, foreplay is either sharply curtailed or absent altogether. For example, the Lepcha farmers of the southeastern Himalayas limit foreplay to men briefly caressing their partners' breasts, and among the Irish inhabitants of Inis Beag, precoital sexual activity is reported to be limited to mouth kissing and rough fondling of the woman's lower body by her partner.

# Sexual Response

Sexuality involves every part of you: mind and body, muscles and skin, glands and genitals. The pioneers in finding out exactly how human beings respond to sex were William Masters and Virginia Johnson, who first studied more than 800 individuals in their laboratory in the 1950s. They discovered that sexual response is a well-ordered sequence of events, so predictable it could be divided into four phases: excitement, plateau, orgasm, and resolution (Figure 9.6). In real life, individuals don't necessarily follow this well-ordered pattern. But the responses for

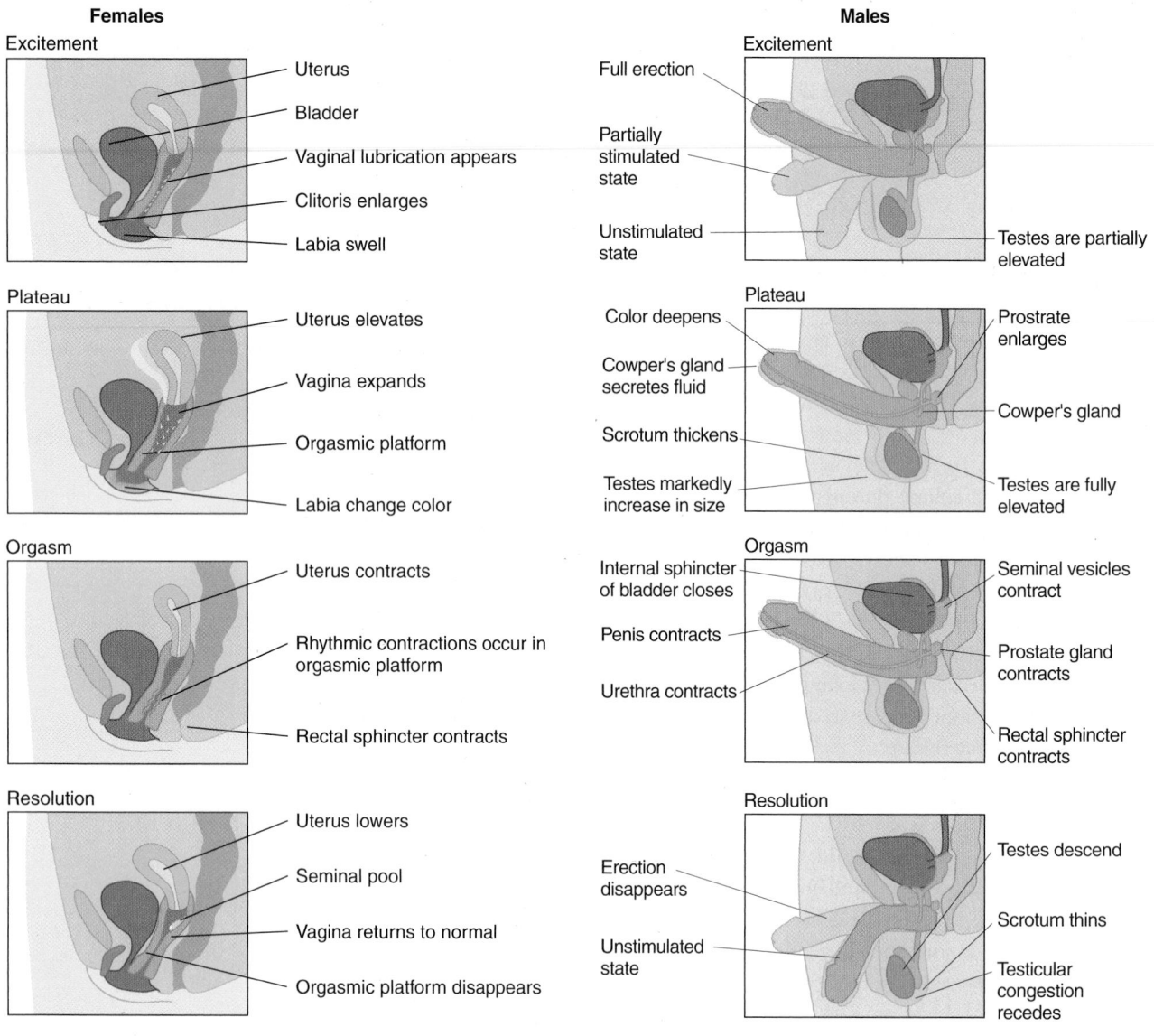

**Females**

Excitement
- Uterus
- Bladder
- Vaginal lubrication appears
- Clitoris enlarges
- Labia swell

Plateau
- Uterus elevates
- Vagina expands
- Orgasmic platform
- Labia change color

Orgasm
- Uterus contracts
- Rhythmic contractions occur in orgasmic platform
- Rectal sphincter contracts

Resolution
- Uterus lowers
- Seminal pool
- Vagina returns to normal
- Orgasmic platform disappears

**Males**

Excitement
- Full erection
- Partially stimulated state
- Unstimulated state
- Testes are partially elevated

Plateau
- Color deepens
- Cowper's gland secretes fluid
- Scrotum thickens
- Testes markedly increase in size
- Prostrate enlarges
- Cowper's gland
- Testes are fully elevated

Orgasm
- Internal sphincter of bladder closes
- Penis contracts
- Urethra contracts
- Seminal vesicles contract
- Prostate gland contracts
- Rectal sphincter contracts

Resolution
- Erection disappears
- Unstimulated state
- Testes descend
- Scrotum thins
- Testicular congestion recedes

both sexes are remarkably similar. And sexual response always follows the same sequence, whatever the means of stimulation.

## Excitement

Stimulation is the first step: a touch, a look, a fantasy. In men, sexual stimuli set off a rush of blood to the genitals, filling the blood vessels in the penis. Because these vessels are wrapped in a thick sheath of tissue, the penis becomes erect. The testes lift.

Women respond to stimulation with vaginal lubrication within 10 to 20 seconds of exposure to sexual stimuli. The clitoris becomes larger, as

do the vaginal lips (the labia), the nipples, and later the breasts. The vagina lengthens, and its inner two-thirds increase in size. The uterus lifts, further increasing the free space in the vagina.

## Plateau

During this stage, the changes begun in the excitement stage continue and intensify. The penis further increases in both length and diameter. The outer one-third of the vagina swells. During intercourse, the vaginal muscles grasp the penis to increase stimulation for both partners. The upper two-thirds of the vagina become wider as the uterus moves up; eventually its diameter is $2\frac{1}{2}$ to 3 inches.

## Orgasm

Men and women have remarkably similar **orgasm** experiences. Both men and women typically have 3 to 12 pelvic muscle contractions approximately four-fifths of a second apart and lasting up to 60 seconds. Both undergo contractions and spasms of other muscles, as well as increases in breathing and pulse rates, and blood pressure. Both can sometimes have orgasms simply from kisses, stimulation of the breasts or other parts of the body, or fantasy alone.

The process of **ejaculation** (the discharge of semen by a male) requires two separate events. First, the vas deferens, the seminal vesicles, the prostate, and the upper portion of the urethra contract. The man perceives these subtle contractions deep in his pelvis just before the point of no return—which therapists refer to as the point of "ejaculatory inevitability." Then, seconds later, muscle contractions force semen out of the penis via the urethra.

Female orgasms follow several patterns. Some women experience a series of mini-orgasms—a response sometimes described as "skimming." Another pattern consists of rapid excitement and plateau stages, followed by a prolonged orgasm. This is the most frequent response to stimulation by a vibrator.

Female orgasms are primarily triggered by stimulating the clitoris. When stimulation reaches an adequate level, the vagina responds by contracting. Although it sometimes seems that vaginal stimulation alone can set off an orgasm, the clitoris is usually involved—at least indirectly during full penile penetration.

Some researchers have identified what they call the *Grafenberg* (or G) *spot* (or area) just behind the front wall of the vagina, between the cervix and the back of the pubic bone (see Figure 9.5). When this region is stimulated, women report various sensations, including slight discomfort, a brief feeling that they need to urinate, and increasing pleasure. Continued stimulation may result in an orgasm of great intensity, accompanied by ejaculation of fluid from the urethra. However, other researchers have failed to confirm the existence and importance of the G spot, and sex therapists disagree about its significance for a woman's sexual satisfaction.

Is sexual satisfaction different for lesbians and heterosexual women? Not according to a recent study of married heterosexual women and lesbian/bisexual women in committed same-sex relationships. The same factors—the quality of the relationship, sexual functioning, social support, symptoms of depression—affected all the women's sexual satisfaction more than a partner's gender.[17]

## Resolution

The sexual organs of men and women return to their normal, nonexcited state during this final phase of sexual response. Heightened skin color quickly fades after orgasm, and the heart rate, blood pressure, and breathing rate soon return to normal. The clitoris also resumes its normal position and appearance very shortly thereafter, whereas the penis may remain somewhat erect for up to 30 minutes.

After orgasm, men typically enter a **refractory period**, during which they are incapable of another orgasm. The duration of this period varies from minutes to days, depending on age and the frequency of previous sexual activity. If either partner doesn't have an orgasm after becoming highly aroused, resolution may be much slower and may be accompanied by a sense of discomfort.

## Other Models of Sexual Response

Since Masters and Johnson's pioneering work, other researchers have challenged and expanded their theories. Some argue that their model neglects the importance of desire in sexual response and that the plateau stage is virtually indistinguishable from excitement. Others note that arousal may come before desire, particularly for women who may not have spontaneous feelings of sexual desire.

As many experts have concluded, physiology alone can never explain the complexity of human sexual response. Desire, arousal, pleasure, and satisfaction are highly subjective. Positive feelings like trust and happiness enhance them. Negative emotions like anger and anxiety can undermine them. For women, sexual satisfaction cannot be defined, as it typically is for men, by whether or not they achieved orgasm.

**orgasm** A series of contractions of the pelvic muscles occurring at the peak of sexual arousal.

**ejaculation** The expulsion of semen from the penis.

**refractory period** The period of time following orgasm during which the male cannot experience another orgasm.

# Sexual Concerns

Many sexual concerns stem from myths and misinformation. There is no truth, for instance, behind these misconceptions: men are always capable of erection, sex always involves intercourse, partners should experience simultaneous orgasms, or people who truly love each other always have satisfying sex lives.

Cultural and childhood influences can affect our attitudes toward sex. Even though America's traditionally puritanical values have eased, our society continues to convey mixed messages about sex. Some children, repeatedly warned of the evils of sex, never accept the sexual dimensions of their identity. Others—especially young boys—may be exposed to macho attitudes toward sex and feel a need to prove their virility. Young girls may feel confused by media messages that encourage them to look and act provocatively and a double standard that blames them for leading boys on. In addition, virtually everyone has individual worries. A woman may feel self-conscious about the shape of her breasts; a man may worry about the size of his penis; both partners may fear not pleasing the other.

The concept of sexual normalcy differs greatly in different times, cultures, or racial and ethnic groups. In certain times and places, only sex between a husband and wife has been deemed normal. In other circumstances, "normal" has been applied to any sexual behavior—alone or with others—that does not harm others or produce great anxiety and guilt. The following are some of the most common contemporary sexual concerns.

## Safer Sex

Having sex is never completely safe; the only 100 percent risk-free sexual choice is abstinence. By choosing not to be sexually active with a partner, you can safeguard your physical health, your fertility, and your future.

For men and women who are sexually active, a mutually faithful sexual relationship with just one healthy partner is the safest option. For those not in such relationships, safer-sex practices are essential for reducing risks. See Chapter 11 and "The Seduction of Safer Sex" in *Labs for IPC* for a complete discussion of safer sex.

## Difficulties and Sexual Dysfunctions

SIECUS defines **sexual dysfunction** as the inability to react emotionally and/or physically to sexual stimulation in a way expected of the average healthy person or according to one's own standards. Sexual dysfunctions, which have a wide range of psychological and physiological origins, can affect different stages in the sexual response cycle. They are not all-or-nothing problems but vary considerably in how severe they are and how frequently they occur. In as many as one-third of people with sexual problems, the partner also has a sexual dysfunction.

Most men and women at one time or another experience some sort of sexual difficulty, but they tend to develop different types. The most common male sexual problems are early ejaculation, reported by 26 percent of men in a recent survey; erectile difficulties, reported by 23 percent; and lack of sexual interest, reported by 18 percent. The most common female problems are lack of sexual interest (reported by 33 percent), lubrication difficulties (reported by 22 percent), inability to reach orgasm (21 percent), and lack of sexual pleasure (20 percent).

Although sexual problems are common, fewer than 25 percent of men and women sought help from a health professional.[18] Why don't more people seek help? Many are hesitant about bringing up the subject. Others are not informed about available treatments. Some are fatalistic and feel that nothing can help.[19] Men are more likely to seek and receive treatment for sexual problems. Nevertheless, they find them very difficult to talk about and may delay or avoid seeking help.

***Erectile Dysfunction (ED)*** An NIH consensus conference has defined **erectile dysfunction (ED)**, also referred to as *impotence*, as the consistent inability to maintain a penile erection sufficient for adequate sexual relations. Virtually all men are occasionally unable to achieve or maintain an erection because of fatigue, stress, alcohol, or drug use, but the incidence

**sexual dysfunction** The inability to react emotionally and/or physically to sexual stimulation in a way expected of the average healthy person or according to one's own standards.

**erectile dysfunction (ED)** The consistent inability to maintain a penile erection sufficient for adequate sexual relations.

of erectile disorders increases with age. Recent research has overturned many common misconceptions about ED. Rather than a chronic condition that worsens with age, ED can be a temporary symptom that improves on its own much more commonly than was thought.[20]

Erectile dysfunction affects an estimated 18 million men—about 18 percent of those over age 20—in the United States. Only 5 percent of men between ages 20 and 40 report ED, which becomes more prevalent with age and illness. Almost 90 percent of men with ED have at least one risk factor for cardiovascular disease, including hypertension or diabetes.

Psychological factors, such as anxiety about performance, may cause erectile dysfunction. But in as many as 80 percent of cases, the problem has physical origins. Diabetes and reactions to drugs—including an estimated 200 prescription medications—are the most frequent organic causes. Even cigarettes can create erection problems for men sensitive to nicotine.

**Preventing Erectile Dysfunction** "The way a man lives can affect the way he loves." This was the conclusion of the Harvard's Health Professionals Follow-up Study, which found that healthy habits directly affect a man's risk of ED. Here are their key findings:

- **Smoking.** Men who smoke are twice as likely to develop ED than nonsmokers.

- **Exercise.** Men who exercise for 30 minutes a day are less likely to develop erectile dysfunction than sedentary men.

- **Obesity.** Overweight men are more likely to have ED, even after age, diabetes, exercise, and other risk factors are taken into account. For example, a man with a 42-inch waist is 50 percent more likely to be impotent than a man with a 32-inch waist.

- **Alcohol.** The effects of alcohol are complex: A man who averages one to two drinks a day is less likely to have erectile dysfunction than a nondrinker, but a man who drinks more will increase his risk of sexual dysfunction.

- **Cycling.** Sitting on a bicycle for a long time puts pressure on the perineum, the area between the genitals and anus. This pressure can harm nerves and temporarily block

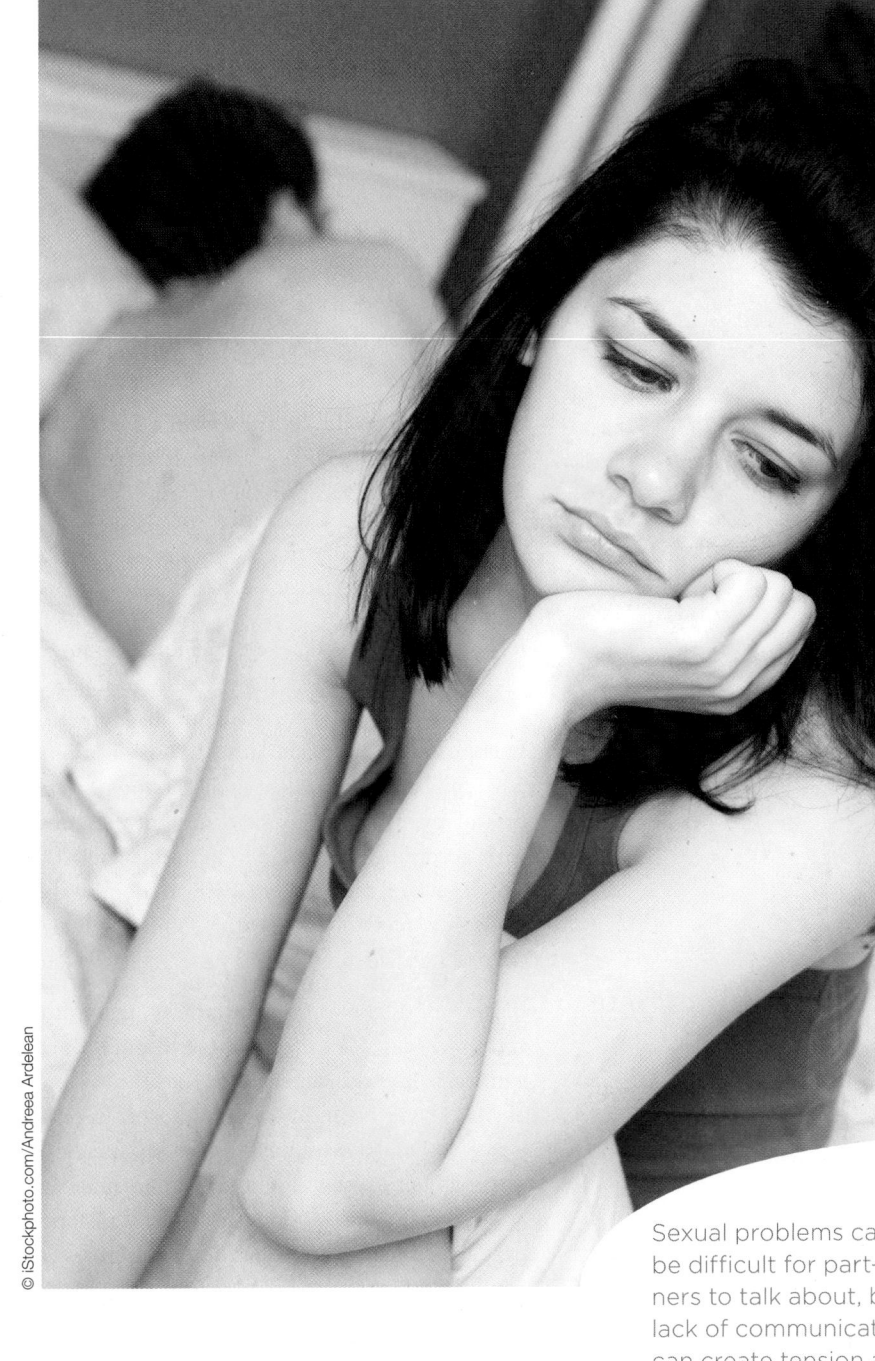

© iStockphoto.com/Andreea Ardelean

Sexual problems can be difficult for partners to talk about, but lack of communication can create tension and increase anxiety.

blood flow, causing tingling or numbness in the penis and eventually leading to ED. To prevent this problem:

- Wear padded biking shorts.
- Raise the handlebars so you sit relatively upright, which shifts pressure from the perineum to the buttocks.
- Use a wide, well-padded or gel-filled seat rather than a narrow one. Position the seat so you don't have to extend your legs fully

at the bottom of your pedal stroke. Don't tilt the seat upward.

- Shift position and take regular breaks during long rides.
- If you feel tingling or numbness in the penis, stop riding for a week or two.

Lifestyle therapy has promise for erectile dysfunction, but men have to make changes early enough to prevent irreversible changes in the arteries and nerves required for normal sexual function.

**Treating Erectile Dysfunction**   Men with erectile dysfunction can get help. If medication for a chronic medical problem is the culprit, a change in treatment may work. Treating underlying diseases, such as diabetes, may also help restore erectile function.

 Millions of men, including about 1 percent of male undergraduates, have used the "erection pills": Viagra, Levitra, and Cialis.[21] The three ED medications have similar success rates. In all, about 70 percent of men respond to the drugs but the rates vary according to what is responsible for ED. About half of men with diabetes respond well, while 90 percent of those without an underlying disease benefit.

Because of their effects on the arteries, men with cardiovascular disease should try ED pills only with their doctors' supervision, and some cannot use them under any circumstances. Recent research has shown that erectile dysfunction drugs do not cause vision loss or abnormalities as once was thought.[22] Some side effects include headache, facial flushing, nasal congestion, indigestion, and diarrhea.

Men can purchase ED drugs on the Internet, but they are taking a risk in using them without a legitimate medical evaluation. Other men turn to herbal remedies. The FDA warns that "all-natural" supplements may actually contain prescription-strength levels of Viagra that could be life-threatening for men with heart disease.

Erection drugs are not aphrodisiacs, but they can improve the erectile response to erotic stimulation. They correct impotence but do not enhance sexual performance. However, successful treatment correlates with greater emotional well-being. Wives of men treated for ED also report high levels of satisfaction with their sexual lives.

*Orgasm Problems in Men*   About 20 percent of men complain of **premature ejaculation**, which is defined as ejaculating within 30 to 90 seconds of inserting the penis into the vagina, or after 10 to 15 thrusts. Another definition is that a premature ejaculator cannot control or delay his ejaculation long enough to satisfy a responsive partner at least half the time. By this definition, a man may be premature with some women but not with others.

To delay orgasm, men may try to think of baseball or other sports, but this just makes sex boring. Others may masturbate before intercourse, hoping to take advantage of the refractory period, during which they cannot ejaculate again. Others may bite their lips or dig their nails into their palms—although usually this just results in premature ejaculators with bloody lips and scarred palms. Topical anesthetics used to prevent climax dull pleasurable sensations for the woman as well as for the man.

Researchers are studying several medications, including clomipramine, SSRIs, and Viagra, in the treatment of premature ejaculation. The combination of medication and psychological and behavioral counseling seems most effective.

Men can learn to control their ejaculation by concentrating on their sexual responses, rather than by trying to distract themselves or ignore their reactions. Some men find that they have greater control by lying on their backs with their partner on top, by relaxing during intercourse, and by communicating with their partner about when to stop or slow down movements.

Other techniques for delaying ejaculation include *stop-start*, in which a man learns to sense the feelings that precede ejaculation and stop his movements before the point of ejaculatory inevitability, allowing his arousal to subside slightly before restarting sexual activity. In the *squeeze technique*, a man's partner applies strong pressure with the thumb on the frenum (the thin strip of skin that connects the glans to the shaft on the underside of the penis) and the second and third fingers on the top side of the penis, one above and one below the corona (rim of penile glans), until the man loses the urge to ejaculate.

**premature ejaculation** A sexual difficulty in which a man ejaculates so rapidly that his partner's satisfaction is impaired.

***Female Sexual Dysfunction*** The American Foundation for Urological Disease classifies female sexual dysfunction into four categories: sexual desire disorders, arousal disorders, orgasmic disorders, and sexual pain disorders. How common are these problems? That's hard to estimate. Some sex therapists have speculated that as many as 43 percent of American women may have some form of sexual dysfunction.

Many health professionals remain dubious about the "medicalization" of various patterns of female sexual response. Scientists at the Kinsey Institute for Research in Sex, Gender, and Reproduction, for instance, caution that a pill, whatever its nature, may not be the solution to many women's sexual concerns. Among the medications that have been tried for female sexual dysfunction are tibolone, a steroid used to treat osteoporosis in Europe that has been linked to improved sexual functioning in postmenopausal women, and phosphodiesterase inhibitors, which help erectile dysfunction in men but have been less effective in women.[23] In women, psychology often is as important as or even more important than physiology, and effective therapy must address psychological problems in a sexual relationship as well as social constraints and inhibitions.

Some forms of female sexual dysfunction do respond to various therapies. These include **dyspareunia**, or pain during intercourse, and **vaginismus**, an extreme form of painful intercourse in which involuntary contractions of the muscles of the outer third of the vagina are so intense that they totally or partially close the vaginal opening. This problem often derives from a fear of being penetrated. Relaxation techniques, such as Kegel exercises (alternately tightening and relaxing the muscles of the pelvic floor), or the use of fingers or dilators to gradually open the vagina, can make penetration easier.

The female orgasm has long been a controversial sexual topic. According to recent estimates, about 90 percent of sexually active women have experienced orgasm, but only a much smaller percentage achieve orgasm through intercourse alone. Even fewer reach orgasm if intercourse isn't accompanied by direct stimulation of the clitoris. Is intercourse without orgasm a sexual problem? The best answer is that it is a problem if a woman wants to experience orgasm during intercourse but doesn't.

Many counseling programs urge women who have never had orgasms to masturbate. They are then encouraged to share with their partners what they've learned, communicating with words or gestures what is most pleasing to them. Some women want more than a single orgasm during intercourse. Partners can help by varying positions and experimenting with sexual techniques. However, in sexual response, more is not necessarily better, and the couple should keep in mind that no one else is counting.

## Sex Therapy

Modern sex therapy, pioneered by Masters and Johnson in the 1960s, views sex as a natural, healthy behavior that enhances a couple's relationship. Their approach emphasizes education, communication, reduction of performance anxiety, and sexual exercises that enhance sexual intimacy.

Today most sex therapists, working either alone or with a partner, have modified Masters and Johnson's approach. Most see couples once a week for eight to ten weeks; the focus of therapy is on correcting dysfunctional behavior, not exploring underlying psychodynamics.

Contrary to common misconceptions, sex therapy does not involve conducting sexual activity in front of therapists. The therapist may review psychological and physiological aspects of sexual functioning and evaluate the couple's sexual attitudes and ability to communicate. The core of the program is the couple's "homework"—a series of exercises, carried out in private, that enhances their sensory awareness and improves nonverbal communication. These techniques have proved effective for couples regardless of their age or general health.

You and your partner should consider consulting a sex therapist if any of the following is true for you:

- Sex is painful or physically uncomfortable.
- You're having sex less and less frequently.
- You have a general fear of, or revulsion toward, sex.

**dyspareunia** A sexual difficulty in which a woman experiences pain during sexual intercourse.

**vaginismus** A sexual difficulty in which a woman experiences painful spasms of the vagina during sexual intercourse.

- Your sexual pleasure is declining.
- Your sexual desire is diminishing.
- Your sexual problems are increasing in frequency or persisting for longer periods.

## Drugs and Sex

Many recreational drugs, such as alcohol and marijuana, are believed to enhance sexual performance. However, none of the popular drugs touted as *aphrodisiacs*—including amphetamines, barbiturates, cantharides ("Spanish fly"), cocaine, LSD and other psychedelics, marijuana, amyl nitrite ("poppers"), and L-dopa (a medication used to treat Parkinson's disease)—is truly a sexual stimulant. In fact, these drugs often interfere with normal sexual response. Researchers are studying one drug that may truly enhance sexual performance: yohimbine hydrochloride, which is derived from the sap of the tropical yohimbe tree that grows in West Africa.

Because many psychiatric problems can lower sexual desire and affect sexual functioning, medications appropriate to the specific disorders can help. In addition, psychiatric drugs may be used as part of therapy. Drugs such as certain antidepressants may be used to prolong sexual response in conditions such as premature ejaculation.

Medications can also cause sexual difficulty. In men, drugs that are used to treat high blood pressure, anxiety, allergies, depression, muscle spasms, obesity, ulcers, irritable colon, and prostate cancer can cause impotence, breast enlargement, testicular swelling, priapism (persistent erection), loss of sexual desire, inability to ejaculate, and reduced sperm count. In women, they can diminish sexual desire, inhibit or delay orgasm, and cause breast swelling or secretions.

# Atypical Behavior

Although sexual desire and response are universal, some individuals develop sexual appetites or engage in activities that are not typical sexual behaviors.

## Sexual Addiction

Some men and women can get relief from their feelings of restlessness and worthlessness only through sex (either masturbation or with a partner). Once the sexual high ends, however, they're overwhelmed by the same negative feelings and driven, once more, to have sex.

Some therapists describe this problem as sexual addiction; others, as sexual compulsion. Professionals continue to debate exactly what this controversial condition is, how to diagnose it, and how to overcome it. However, most agree that for some people, sex is more than a normal pleasure: It is an overwhelming need that must be met, even at the cost of their careers and marriages.

Sex addicts can be heterosexual or homosexual, male or female. Their behaviors include masturbation, phone sex, reading or viewing pornography, attending strip shows, having affairs, engaging in anonymous sex with strangers or prostitutes, exhibitionism, voyeurism, child molestation, incest, and rape. Many were physically and emotionally abused as children or have family members who abuse drugs or alcohol. They typically feel a loss of control and a compulsion for sexual activity, and they continue their unhealthy (and sometimes illegal) sexual behavior despite the dangers, including the risk of contracting STIs.

With help, sex addicts can deal with the shame that both triggers and follows sexual activity. Professional therapy may begin with a month of complete sexual abstinence, to break the cycle of compulsive sexual behavior. Several organizations, such as Sexaholics Anonymous and Sexual Addicts Anonymous, offer support from people who share the same problem.

*Sexual Deviations*  Sexual deviations listed by the American Psychiatric Association include the following:

- **Fetishism**. Obtaining sexual pleasure from an inanimate object or an asexual part of the body, such as the foot.
- **Transvestitism.** Becoming sexually aroused by wearing the clothing of the opposite sex.
- **Exhibitionism.** Exposing one's genitals to an unwilling observer.

- **Voyeurism.** Obtaining sexual gratification by observing people undressing or involved in sexual activity.
- **Sadism.** Becoming sexually aroused by inflicting physical or psychological pain.
- **Masochism.** Obtaining sexual gratification by suffering physical or psychological pain.

Another, increasingly common sexual variation, hypoxyphilia, involves attempts to enhance the pleasure of orgasm by reducing oxygen intake. Individuals who do so by tying a noose around the neck have accidentally killed themselves.

Psychiatrists distinguish between passive sexual deviancy, which doesn't involve actual contact with another, and aggressive deviancy. Most voyeurs and obscene phone callers don't seek physical contact with the objects of their sexual desire. These behaviors are performed predominantly, but not exclusively, by males.

## The Business of Sex

Sex, without affection and individuality, becomes a product to be packaged, marketed, traded, bought, and sold. Two of the billion-dollar industries that treat sex as a commodity are prostitution and pornography.

Prostitution, described as the world's oldest profession, is a nationwide industry grossing more than $1 billion annually. In every state except Nevada (and in all but a few counties there), prostitution is illegal. Besides the threat of jail and fines, prostitutes and their clients face another danger: sexually transmitted infections, including HIV infection and hepatitis B.

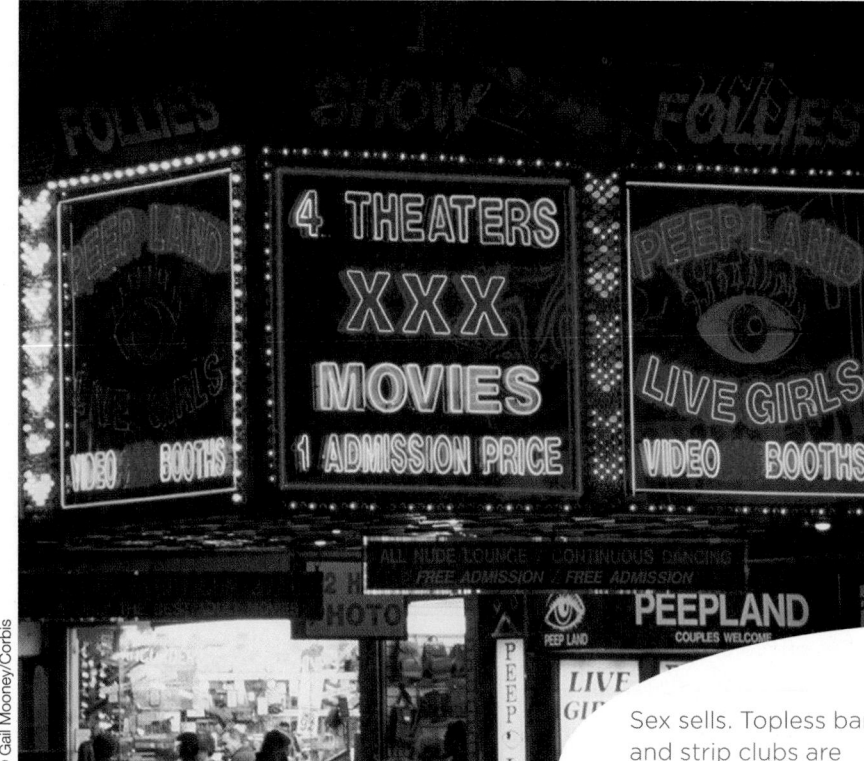

© Gail Mooney/Corbis

Sex sells. Topless bars and strip clubs are among the businesses that cater to those who enjoy sexual stimulation outside a loving relationship.

Pornography is a multimedia industry—books, magazines, movies, the Internet, phone lines, and computer games are available to those who find sexually explicit material entertaining or exciting. Most laws against pornography are based on the assumption that such materials can set off uncontrollable, dangerous sexual urges, ranging from promiscuity to sexual violence. Research indicates that exposure to scenes of rape or other forms of sexual violence against women, or to scenes of degradation of women, does lead to tolerance of these hostile and brutal acts.

# Being Sexually Responsible

We remain sexual beings throughout life. At different ages and stages, sexuality can take on different meanings. As you forge relationships and explore your sexuality, you may encounter difficult situations and unfamiliar feelings. But sex is never just about hormones and body parts. People describe the brain as the sexiest of our organs. Using your brain to make responsible sexual decisions leads to both a smarter and a more fulfilling sex life.

Which of the following characterize your behavior or the way you would want to behave in an intimate relationship?

_____ **Communicate openly.** If you or your partner cannot talk openly and honestly about your sexual histories and contraception, you should avoid having sex. For the sake of protecting your sexual health, you have to be willing to ask—and answer—questions that may seem embarrassing.

_____ **Share responsibility in a sexual relationship.** Both partners should be involved in protecting themselves and each other from STIs and, if heterosexual, unwanted pregnancy.

_____ **Respect sexual privacy.** Revealing sexual activities violates the trust between two partners. Bragging about a sexual conquest demeans everyone involved.

_____ **Never sexually harass others.** Pinches, pats, sexual comments or jokes, and suggestive gestures are offensive and disrespectful.

_____ **Be considerate.** A public display of sexual affection can be extremely embarrassing to others. Roommates, in particular, should be sensitive and discreet in their sexual behavior.

_____ **Be prepared.** If there's any possibility that you may be engaging in sex, be sure you have the means to protect yourself against unwanted pregnancy and sexually transmitted infections.

_____ **In sexual situations, always think ahead.** For the sake of safety, think about potential dangers—parking in an isolated area, going into a bedroom with someone you hardly know, and the like—and options to protect yourself.

_____ **Be aware of your own and your partner's alcohol and drug intake.** The use of such substances impairs judgment and reduces the ability to say no. While under their influence, you may engage in sexual behavior you'll later regret.

_____ **Be sure sexual activity is consensual.** Coercion can take many forms: physical, emotional, and verbal. All cause psychological damage and undermine trust and respect. At any point in a relationship, whether the couple is dating or married, either individual has the right to say no.

Source: Adapted from Robert Hatcher, et al., *Sexual Etiquette 101 and More* (Atlanta, GA: Emory University School of Medicine, 2002).

---

**Self Survey**

# How Much Do You Know about Sex?

*Mark each of the following statements True or False:*

1. Men and women have completely different sex hormones.

2. Premenstrual syndrome (PMS) is primarily a psychological problem.

3. Circumcision diminishes a man's sexual pleasure.

4. Sexual orientation may have a biological basis.

5. Masturbation is a sign of emotional immaturity.

6. Only homosexual men engage in anal intercourse.

7. Despite their awareness of AIDS, many college students do not practice safe sex.

8. After age 60, lovemaking is mainly a fond memory, not a regular pleasure of daily living.

9. Doctors advise against having intercourse during a woman's menstrual period.

10. Only men ejaculate.

11. It is possible to be infected with HIV during a single sexual encounter.

12. Impotence is always a sign of emotional or sexual problems in a relationship.

*Answers:*

1. False. Men and women have the same hormones, but in different amounts.

2. False. PMS has been recognized as a physiological disorder that may be caused by a hormonal deficiency, abnormal levels of thyroid hormone, or social and environmental factors, such as stress.

3. False. Sex therapists have not been able to document differences in sensitivity to stimulation between circumcised and uncircumcised men.

4. True. Researchers documented structural differences in the brains of homosexual men and women.

5. False. Throughout a person's life, masturbation can be a form of sexual release and pleasure.

6. False. As many as one in every four married couples under age 35 have reported that they occasionally engage in anal intercourse.

7. True. In one recent study, more than a third of college students had engaged in vaginal or anal intercourse at least once in the previous year without using effective protection from conception or sexually transmitted infections (STIs).

8. False. More than a third of American married men and women older than 60 make love at least once a week, as do 10 percent of those older than 70.

9. False. There's no medical reason to avoid intercourse during a woman's menstrual period.

10. False. Some researchers say that stimulation of the Grafenberg spot in a woman's vagina may lead to a release of fluid from her urethra during orgasm.

11. True. Although the risk increases with repeated sexual contact with an infected partner, an individual can contract HIV during a single sexual encounter.

12. False. Many erection difficulties have physical causes.

# Making Change Happen

## Creating True Intimacy

Intimacy doesn't happen at first sight—or in a day or a week or a string of weeks. Intimacy needs time and nurturing. It is a process of self-revelation, of exposing rather than hiding, or expressing rather than suppressing, or wanting someone to know us as fully as possible, and of wanting to know that someone as fully as possible. Although intimacy isn't the same as sex, it often includes a sexual relationship.

Like every other worthwhile endeavor in life, quality relationships require attention and effort—but of the most delightful and rewarding type. "What's Your Intimacy Quotient?" in *Labs for IPC* assesses and strengthens the skills you need to enrich your life with warm, close, supportive intimate relationships. Here's a preview.

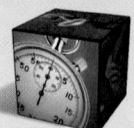

### Get Real

To create and maintain intimate relationships, you need to assess nine essential skills, including the following three:

- **Receptivity.** If you are text-messaging or checking e-mail while talking to your partner, friend, or child, the message you're sending them is, "Don't bother me. I've got something better to do" . . .

  Do you spend some time every day simply sitting and reconnecting with your partner? Do you spend some time every day simply sitting and reconnecting with you?

- **Expressing yourself.** Don't expect your partner to read your mind. Avoid the "If-you-loved-me-you'd-know" trap. Avoid fuzzy expressions like "sort of" and "kind of maybe."

  Do you spend time every day communicating your thoughts, needs, and wishes to yourself and your partner?

- **Trust.** In an intimate relationship, trust creates a safe harbor where you can be who you are without being attacked, rejected, or abandoned—and without attacking, rejecting, or abandoning.

  Do you honor the trust between you every day by following a basic rule: no secrets, no lies, no deceptions, no excuses, no illusions?

On a scale of 0 (clueless) to 10 (masterful), how did you rate yourself?

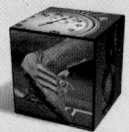

### Get Ready

For the sake of your future, you and your partner need to coordinate your schedules and, if necessary, make appointments for quality time together. You also have to ask whether you spend more time on intimacy substitutes like blogging, gaming, gambling, shopping, or working out than you do enjoying your relationship.

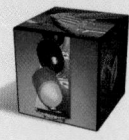

### Get Going

This section consists of seven exercises, each with daily, weekly, and monthly components and designed to create more intimacy in your most personal relationship. Here are three examples:

- **Receptivity.**

  Every day: Clear the decks for some real one-on-one time. But beware . . .

  Every week: Make a date to go out for a meal, walk together, or curl up on the couch and just talk . . .

- **Expressing yourself.**

  Every day: Let your partner in on things you know would be of interest . . .

  Every week: Share your perspective on the issues that came up during your week . . .

  Every month: If you journal, review the themes that have been on your mind. Are you rethinking your major? Concerned about expenses?

- **Trust.**

  Every day: Honor your partner's trust by not discussing private matters with friends.

  Every week or so: Confide in your partner to demonstrate your trust.

  Every month or so: Let your partner know how much you value the trust you have in each other. Be consistently trustworthy.

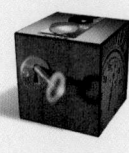

### Lock It In

In this stage you set a goal for which intimacy skills to focus on in the coming week. Continue working to deepen and enrich your relationships throughout your life.

# Making This Chapter Work for You

## Review Questions

1. Which of the following behaviors is most likely to be a characteristic of sexually healthy and responsible adults?
   a. engages in frequent sexual encounters with many partners
   b. avoids the use of condoms in order to heighten sexual enjoyment for both partners
   c. uses alcohol sparingly and only to help loosen the inhibitions of a resistant partner
   d. engages in sex that is unquestionably consensual

2. Which statement about sexual activity is *not* true?
   a. College students consider sexual activity normal for their peer group.
   b. The frequency of sexual activity is highest among those with some college education.
   c. Men and women have sex for generally similar reasons.
   d. Masters and Johnson discovered five stages in human sexual response.

3. Which of the following statements about erectile dysfunction (ED) is *false*?
   a. ED is usually caused by physical factors.
   b. A popular treatment for ED is Viagra.
   c. ED is usually caused by psychological factors.
   d. Men who are heavy smokers are at risk for developing ED.

4. The hormones that influence the early development of sexual organs
   a. are released by the ovaries in the female and the testes in the male.
   b. begin to work soon after conception during the embryo's development.
   c. begin to work during puberty, when they stimulate the development of secondary male and female sex characteristics.
   d. determine one's biological sex.

5. Women may experience which of the following problems during intercourse?
   a. vaginismus
   b. excitement
   c. vaginal expansion
   d. amenorrhea

6. Which of the following statements is true about sexual orientation?
   a. Most individuals who identify themselves as bisexual are really homosexual.
   b. Homosexuality is caused by a poor family environment.
   c. Homosexual behavior is found only in affluent and well-educated cultures.
   d. The African American, Hispanic, and Asian cultures tend to be less accepting of homosexuality than the white community.

7. Which of the following statements about the menstrual cycle is true?
   a. The pituitary gland releases estrogen and progesterone.
   b. Ovulation occurs at the end of the menstrual cycle.
   c. Premenstrual syndrome is a physiological disorder that usually results in amenorrhea.
   d. The endometrium becomes thicker during the cycle and is shed during menstruation.

8. According to the Centers for Disease Control, abstinence is defined as
   a. refraining from all sexual behaviors that result in arousal.
   b. refraining from all sexual activities that involve vaginal, anal, and oral intercourse.
   c. having sexual intercourse with only one partner exclusively.
   d. refraining from drinking alcohol before sexual activity.

9. Atypical sexual behaviors include which of the following?
   a. masochism
   b. sexual desire
   c. masturbation
   d. celibacy

10. Which statement about male anatomy is *incorrect*?
    a. The testes manufacture testosterone and sperm.
    b. Sperm cells are carried in the liquid semen.
    c. Cowper's glands secrete semen.
    d. Circumcision is the surgical removal of the foreskin of the penis.

*Answers to these questions can be found on page 672.*

## Critical Thinking

1. Amara signed an abstinence pledge through her church group before leaving for college. She feels strongly that sex should be saved for marriage. Early in her sophomore year, Amara fell deeply in love with Raul, and she now wonders if she will be able to maintain her commitment to abstinence. Raul respects her choice, but expresses frustration that they can't fully express their feelings. What would you advise Amara to do? What would you say to Raul?

2. Sex education is always a controversial topic. In SIECUS national surveys, nine in ten parents believe it is important to have sex education as part of the curriculum. Other parents feel that boys and girls should learn about sex and sexual values in the home. Did you have "sex ed" in junior high or high school? What do you think about such classes—and why?

3. Do you think it is okay to read or look at pornographic books, magazines, websites, and videos? Why or why not?

## Media Menu

Visit www.cengagebrain.com to access course materials and companion resources for this text that will:

- Help you evaluate your knowledge of the material.

- Allow you to prepare for exams with interactive quizzing.

- Use the CengageNOW product to develop a Personalized Learning Plan targeting resources that address areas you should study.

- Coach you through identifying target goals for behavioral change and creating and monitoring your personal change plan throughout the semester using the Behavior Change Planner available in the CengageNOW resource.

## Internet Connections

**www.siecus.org**
This website is sponsored by SIECUS, a national nonprofit organization that promotes comprehensive education about sexuality and advocates the right of all individuals of all sexual orientations to make responsible sexual choices. The site features a library of fact sheets and articles on a variety of sexuality topics and STIs designed for educators, adults, teens, parents, media, international audiences, and religious organizations.

**www.hrc.org**
The Human Rights Campaign is America's largest gay, lesbian, bisexual, and transgender civil rights organization.

Its website features up-to-date information on issues related to gay rights and suggests courses of action to change government policies.

**www.goaskalice.columbia.edu/**
Sponsored by the health education and wellness program of the Columbia University Health Service, this site features educators' answers to questions on a wide variety of topics of concern to young people, including those related to sexual orientation and healthy sexuality.

## Key Terms

The terms listed are used on the page indicated. Definitions of the terms are in the Glossary at the end of the book.

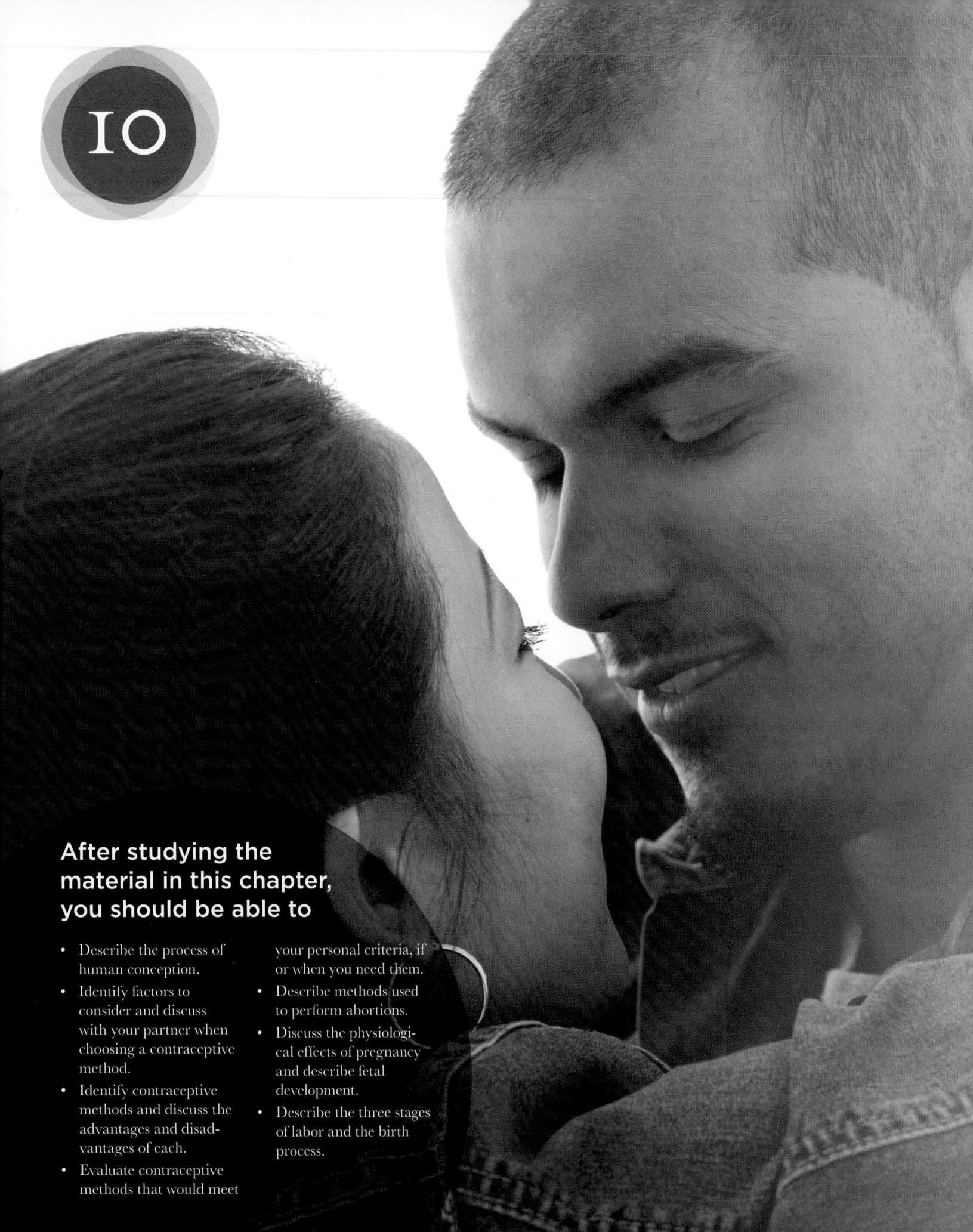

# IO

## After studying the material in this chapter, you should be able to

- Describe the process of human conception.
- Identify factors to consider and discuss with your partner when choosing a contraceptive method.
- Identify contraceptive methods and discuss the advantages and disadvantages of each.
- Evaluate contraceptive methods that would meet your personal criteria, if or when you need them.
- Describe methods used to perform abortions.
- Discuss the physiological effects of pregnancy and describe fetal development.
- Describe the three stages of labor and the birth process.

Justin and Sara, sophomores at the same community college, can't remember a time when abortion was illegal, when AIDS wasn't a deadly threat, and when safe sex wasn't a concern of every sexually active individual. Yet even though they were aware of the risks and the realities involved, neither used contraception during every single sexual encounter. Then one of Justin's partners had a pregnancy scare. He decided never again to engage in unprotected sex. Sara had a different reality check: At

# Reproductive Choices

her regular physical, she learned that she had contracted chlamydia, the most common sexually transmitted infection in the United States.

"When we started dating," Sara recalls, "both of us felt that something was special about our relationship." Despite their mutual attraction, they decided to take every step toward intimacy slowly. Both considered and talked about their personal priorities and concerns. Even though it was awkward, they also discussed their own sexual histories and underwent tests for STIs.

Looking toward a continuing committed relationship, they decided on not one but two forms of contraception: the birth control pill and a condom. In the future, they realized that they might switch to other forms of birth control or consider different options, including both marriage and parenthood.

As human beings, we have a unique power: the ability to choose to conceive or not to conceive. No other species on earth can separate sexual activity and pleasure from reproduction.

However, simply not wanting to get pregnant is never enough to prevent conception, nor is wanting to have a child always enough to get pregnant. Both desires require individual decisions and actions.

This chapter provides information on conception, birth control, abortion, infertility, adoption, and the processes by which a new human life develops and enters the world.

## Reproductive Responsibility

Anyone who engages in vaginal intercourse must be willing to accept the consequences of that activity—the possibility of pregnancy and responsibility for the child who might be conceived—or take action to avoid those consequences. Although many people are concerned about the risks associated with contraception,

Visit www.cengagebrain.com to access course materials for this text, including the Behavior Change Planner, interactive quizzes, tutorials, and more. See the preface on page xv for details.

using birth control is safer and healthier than not using it. According to the Population Reference Bureau, the use of contraceptives, including oral contraceptives, saves millions of lives each year.

An additional health benefit from contraception for women is a lower risk of ovarian cancer. Birth control pills and tubal ligation have the greatest protective effect, but recent research has found that any type of contraception, including barrier methods, intrauterine devices, and vasectomy, lowers a woman's risk.[1]

The typical American woman who wants two children spends about five years pregnant or trying to become pregnant and three decades— more than three-quarters of her reproductive life—trying to avoid pregnancy. About half of all pregnancies in the United States each year— more than 3 million—are unintended. By age 45, more than half of all American women will have experienced an unintended pregnancy, and about one-third will have had an abortion.

 Among all young women ages 20 to 24, 45 percent of pregnancies are unintended. Among African American women in this age group, the percentage rises to 55 percent. Racial differences in unintended pregnancy rates persist even when socioeconomic variables, such as income and education, are accounted for.

 In a study that compared college students and nonstudents of the same age, African American undergraduates were more likely to put themselves at risk of unwanted pregnancy by choosing less effective contraceptive methods than African Americans who weren't enrolled in college.[2]

There are racial differences in students' contraceptive choices. Compared with white undergraduates, black students report greater condom use for oral, anal, and vaginal sex. However, black students are less likely to use hormonal contraceptives and have higher rates of unprotected intercourse and unintended pregnancy.[3]

Women who reported having sex at age 15 or younger are at increased risk of multiple unintended pregnancies throughout their lives.[4] Girls are almost twice as likely to have a baby before age 20 if they did not use a contraceptive the first time they had sex or if their mothers had a baby when they were teenagers.[5]

# Conception

The equation for making a baby is quite simple: One sperm plus one egg equals one fertilized egg, which can develop into an infant. But the processes that affect or permit **conception** are quite complicated. The creation of sperm, or **spermatogenesis**, starts in the male at puberty, and the production of sperm is regulated by hormones. Sperm cells form in the seminiferous tubules of the testes and are passed into the epididymis, where they are stored until ejaculation; a single male ejaculation may contain 500 million sperm. Each sperm released into the vagina during intercourse moves on its own, propelling itself toward its target, an ovum.

To reach its goal, the sperm must move through the acidic secretions of the vagina, enter the uterus, travel up the fallopian tube containing the ovum, then fuse with the nucleus of the egg (**fertilization**). Just about every sperm produced by a man in his lifetime fails to accomplish its mission.

There are far fewer human egg cells than there are sperm cells. Each woman is born with her lifetime supply of ova, and between 300 and 500 eggs eventually mature and leave her ovaries during ovulation. As discussed in Chapter 9, every month, one or the other of the woman's ovaries releases an ovum to the nearby fallopian tube. It travels through the fallopian tube until it reaches the uterus, a journey that takes three to four days. An unfertilized egg lives for about 24 to 36 hours, disintegrates, and during menstruation is expelled along with the uterine lining.

Even if a sperm, which can survive in the female reproductive tract for two to five days, meets a ripe egg in a fallopian tube, its success is not ensured. A mature ovum releases the chemical allurin, which attracts the sperm. A sperm is able to penetrate the ovum's outer membrane because of a protein called fertilin. The egg then pulls the sperm inside toward its nucleus (Figure 10.1). The fertilized egg, called the **zygote**, travels down the fallopian tube, dividing to form a tiny clump of cells called a **blastocyst**. When it reaches the uterus, about a week after fertilization, it burrows into the endometrium, the lining of the uterus. This process is called **implantation**.

**conception** The merging of a sperm and an ovum.

**spermatogenesis** The process by which sperm cells are produced.

**fertilization** The fusion of sperm and egg nucleus.

**zygote** A fertilized egg.

**blastocyst** In embryonic development, a ball of cells with a surface layer and an inner cell mass.

**implantation** The embedding of the fertilized ovum in the uterine lining.

**contraception** The prevention of conception; birth control.

Conception can be prevented by **contraception**. Some contraceptive methods prevent ovulation or implantation, and others block the sperm from reaching the egg. Some methods are temporary; others permanently alter one's fertility.

# Birth Control Basics

Most sexually active women use some form of birth control. According to the Centers for Disease Control and Prevention, more than 98 percent of women between the ages of 15 and 44 who have ever had intercourse have used at least one contraceptive method. Most of the women not using any form of contraception are pregnant, trying to get pregnant, unable to conceive, or not having intercourse.

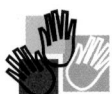 The use of contraception has declined in recent years, particularly among poor women. As a result, they are more likely to get pregnant unintentionally and to have abortions. An estimated 11 percent of sexually active women, including white, Hispanic, and African American women, who are not trying to get pregnant do not use birth control, up from 7 percent in 1994. Half of unintended pregnancies are carried to term. Annually, about 14,000 women who continue their pregnancies put the children up for adoption; 1.2 million women have abortions.[6]

If you are engaging in sexual activity that could lead to conception, you have to be realistic about your situation. This means assuming full responsibility for your reproductive ability, whether you're a man or a woman. The more you know about contraception, the more likely you are to use birth control. Contraceptives cost money; not using contraception can cost much more. (See Health on a Budget, p. 317.)

You also have to recognize the risks associated with various methods of contraception. If you're a woman, the risks are chiefly yours. Various methods of birth control have side effects, but pregnancy and childbirth account for much higher rates of medical complications and deaths than any contraceptive. Although most women never experience any serious

Figure 10.1 **Fertilization**

(a) The efforts of hundreds of sperm may allow one to penetrate the ovum's corona radiate, an outer layer of cells, and then the zona pellucida, a thick inner membrane. (b) The nuclei of the sperm and the egg cells merge, and the male and female chromosomes in the nuclei come together, forming a zygote. (c) The zygote divides into two cells, then four cells, and so on. (d) As fluid enters the ball, cells form a ball of cells called a blastocyst. (e) The blastocyst implants itself in the endometrium.

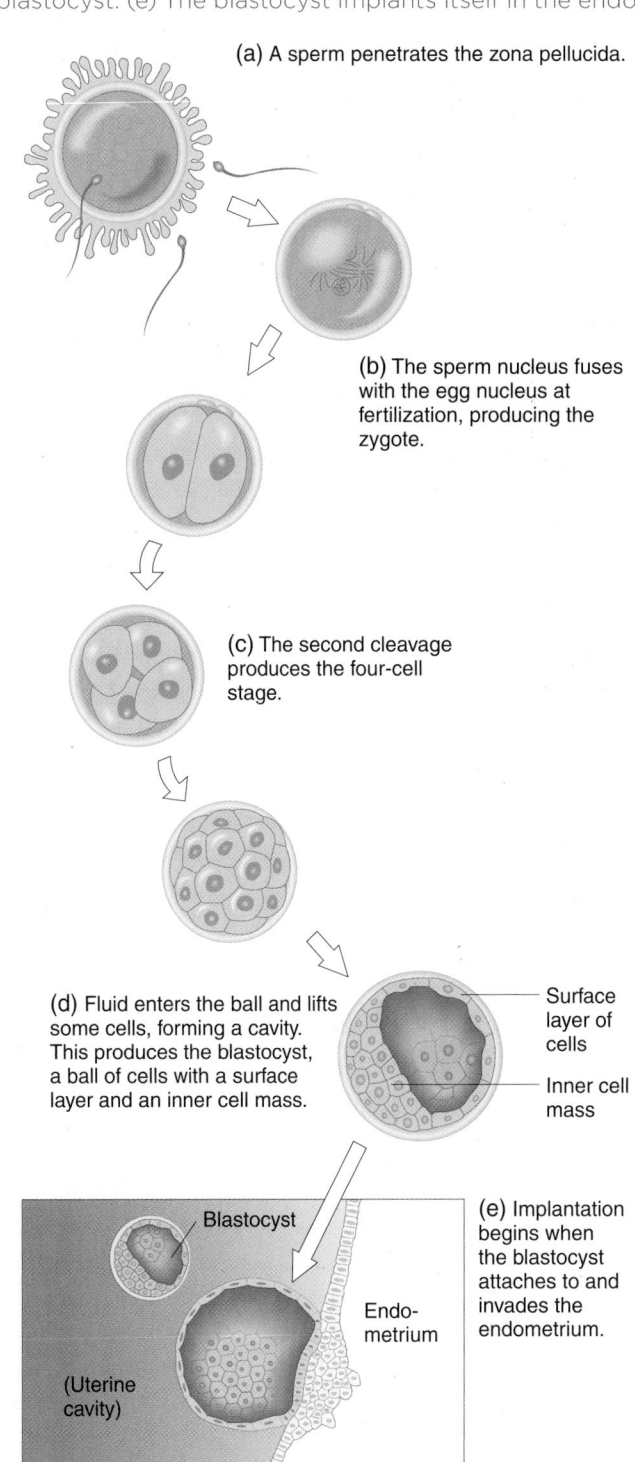

(a) A sperm penetrates the zona pellucida.

(b) The sperm nucleus fuses with the egg nucleus at fertilization, producing the zygote.

(c) The second cleavage produces the four-cell stage.

(d) Fluid enters the ball and lifts some cells, forming a cavity. This produces the blastocyst, a ball of cells with a surface layer and an inner cell mass.

Surface layer of cells

Inner cell mass

Blastocyst

(Uterine cavity)

Endo-metrium

(e) Implantation begins when the blastocyst attaches to and invades the endometrium.

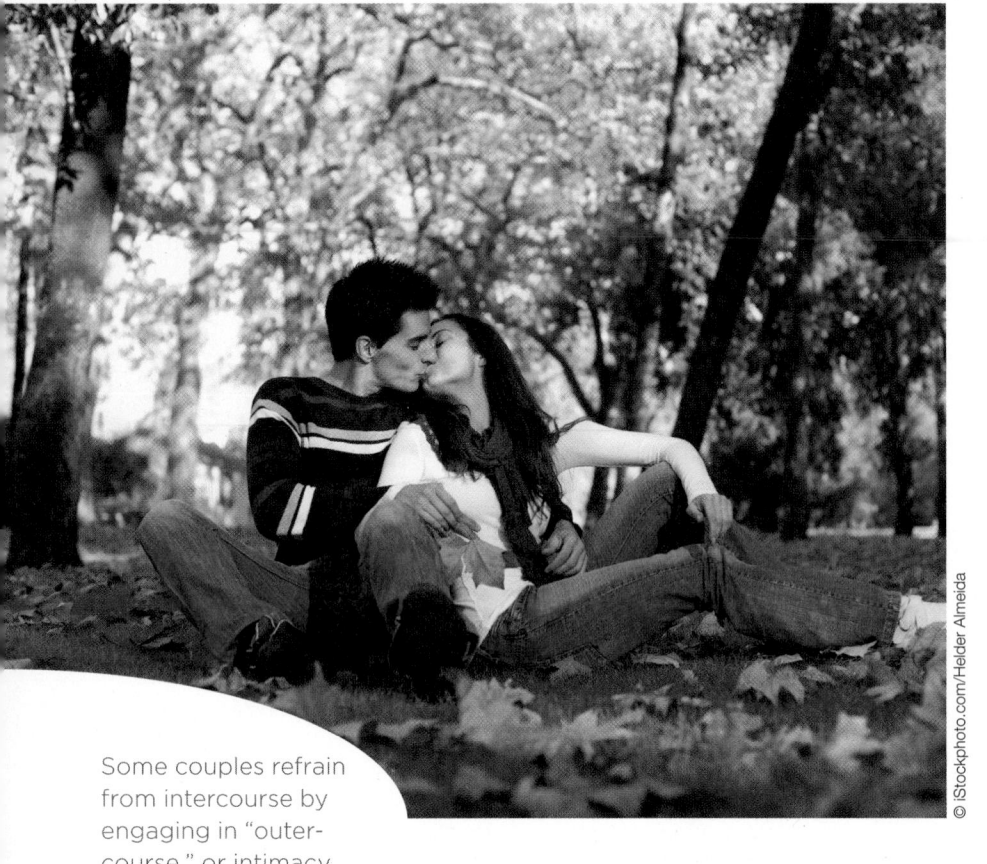

Some couples refrain from intercourse by engaging in "outercourse," or intimacy that includes kissing and hugging.

for various reasons, including waiting until they are ready for a sexual relationship or until they find the "right" partner, respecting religious or moral values, enjoying friendships without sexual involvement, recovering from a breakup, or preventing pregnancy and sexually transmitted infection.

Practicing abstinence is the only form of birth control that is 100 percent effective and risk-free. It is also an important, increasingly valued lifestyle choice. A growing number of individuals, including some who have been sexually active in the past, are choosing abstinence until they establish a relationship with a long-term partner.

Abstinence offers special health benefits for women. Those who abstain until their twenties and engage in sex with fewer partners during their lifetime are less likely to get sexually transmitted infections, to suffer infertility, or to develop cervical cancer. However, some people find it difficult to abstain for long periods of time. There also is a risk that people will abruptly end their abstinence without being prepared to protect themselves against pregnancy or infection.

Individuals who choose abstinence from vaginal intercourse often engage in activities sometimes called *outercourse*, such as kissing, hugging, sensual touching, and mutual masturbation. Outercourse is nearly 100 percent effective as a contraceptive measure, but pregnancy is possible if there is genital contact. If the man ejaculates near the vaginal opening, sperm can swim up into the vagina and fallopian tubes to fertilize an egg. Outercourse also may lower the risk of contracting sexually transmitted infections. It is an effective form of safe sex as long as no body fluids are exchanged.

Some couples routinely restrict themselves to outercourse; others temporarily choose such sexual activities when it is inadvisable for them to have vaginal intercourse—for example, after childbirth. Other benefits: Outercourse has no medical or hormonal side effects; it may prolong sex play and enhance orgasm; it can be used when no other birth control methods are available.

complications, it's important to be aware of the potential for long-term risks. Risks that are acceptable to others may not be acceptable to you. Table 10.1 on pages 319–320 presents your contraceptive choices.

# Abstinence and Nonpenetrative Sexual Activity

The contraceptive methods discussed in this chapter are designed to prevent pregnancy as a consequence of vaginal intercourse. Couples who choose abstinence make a very different decision—to abstain from vaginal intercourse and forms of nonpenetrative sexual activity that could result in conception (any in which ejaculation occurs near the vaginal opening).

For many individuals, abstinence represents a deliberate choice regarding their bodies, minds, spirits, and sexuality. People choose abstinence

# A Cross-Cultural Perspective

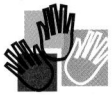 Culture, religion, gender roles, and folklore can affect birth control options and decisions. In countries that are predominantly Catholic, such as Ireland, Italy, and the Philippines, the Church promotes fertility awareness and the rhythm method and condemns other contraceptive methods. Because Jewish law teaches men not to "spill their seed," methods that can cause damage to sperm, such as vasectomy, condoms, or spermicides, are less acceptable in Israel than oral contraceptives are. In Japan, which has one of the lowest birth rates in the world, men are primarily responsible for birth control decisions. In Kenya, married couples view the use of a condom as an indicator of a husband's infidelity. In Scandinavian countries, where birth control is free and easily accessible, many women begin taking oral contraceptives before becoming sexually active.[7]

Worldwide, sterilization is used by more people than any other birth control method. The intra-uterine device (IUD) is the most commonly used reversible form of contraception. Among the countries with the highest usage rates are Turkey, China (where an IUD is often inserted immediately after a woman gives birth to her first child), Nigeria, England, Russia, and Korea. About 2 percent of women in the United States rely on IUDs for birth control.[8]

In developing countries, conception and contraception are life-and-death issues. One in three women give birth before age 20. Some 20 million women have unsafe abortions, which claim the lives of about 70,000 women between the ages of 15 and 19. Effective contraception could prevent about 90 percent of these deaths.[9]

The reasons why young women in developing countries do not use effective birth control are complex. In a recent analysis of studies in four African countries and Vietnam, the key factors were:

- Lack of education and information about sex and reproduction.
- Limited access to modern birth control methods.
- Limited understanding of how they work (for example, the belief that a woman only needs to take a birth control pill before or after sex).
- Fears that hormonal contraceptives would endanger future fertility.
- Association of condoms with disease and promiscuity.
- Partners' refusal to use condoms.

Even when premarital sex is widespread, many of these young women view birth control as appropriate only for married couples and feel ashamed to visit a family planning center. These women rely on traditional methods, such as

## Health on a Budget

# The Cost of Contraception

The only free forms of birth control are abstinence and the rhythm method. But even the most expensive methods cost less (much, much less) than having and caring for a child. If you're on a tight budget, you might want to consider the relative cost of a year's prescription of oral contraceptives compared to the annual cost of condoms or spermicidal foam or jelly.

Here are some cost estimates from the FDA that can help you make sense of the dollars-and-cents of contraception:

| | |
|---|---|
| Spermicide | Less than a dollar per time |
| Contraceptive sponge | $2.50 to $3 per sponge |
| Cervical cap | $65 or more for cap; $50 to $200 for fitting |
| Diaphragm | $30 to $50 plus fitting |
| Female condom | $2 to $4 each |
| Male condom | $.50 to $2 each |
| Progestin-only pill | $15 to $60 a month |
| Injection | $30 to $70 per shot plus exam |
| Combination pill | $15 to $60 per cycle |
| Contraceptive patch | $35 to $70 a month |
| NuvaRing | $25 to $35 a month |
| Seasonale | $90 to $100 for three-month supply |
| Copper-coated IUD | $150 to $300 |
| Mirena | $150 to $300 every five years |
| Female sterilization | $2,000 to $4,000 |
| Male sterilization | $300 to $1,000 |
| Emergency contraception | $8 to $25 for Plan B |

The cost of each method depends on where you purchase it. Contraceptives are generally less expensive at health care clinics than in pharmacies or private medical practices.

Source of cost estimates: Janell Carroll, *Sexuality Now*, 3rd ed. (Belmont, CA: Wadsworth-Cengage, 2010).

# Health in Action

## Choosing a Contraceptive

You may choose different types of birth control at different stages of your life, or switch contraceptives for various reasons. (See Self Survey: Which Contraceptive Method Is Best for You?) You and your partner should always consider and discuss these factors:

- **Effectiveness.** Keep in mind that your own conscientiousness will play an important role. If you forget to take your daily pill, or if you decide not to use a condom "just this once," you'll increase the odds of pregnancy by interfering with effective birth control.

- **Suitability.** If you don't have sex very often, a contraceptive with many risks and side effects, such as the pill, may be wrong for you. If you have many sexual partners and are at risk of contracting a sexually transmitted infection, a condom may provide protection against pregnancy and infection, especially if used with a diaphragm or cervical cap.

- **Side effects.** Some complications related to contraceptives are serious health threats. Be sure to ask questions and gather as much information as possible about what side effects to expect.

- **Safety.** The risks of certain contraceptives, such as the pill, may be too great to allow their use if, for example, you have high blood pressure. Be honest in describing your medical history to your physician.

- **Future fertility.** Some women don't return to regular menstrual cycles for six months to a year after discontinuing oral contraceptives. This possibility may or may not be important to you now, but you should try to look ahead.

- **Reduced risk of sexually transmitted infections.** Some forms of contraception, in particular barrier contraceptives and spermicides, help reduce the risk of transmission of some STIs. However, none provides complete protection.

What is your top priority for any form of birth control? Why? What is your top concern or source of hesitation? Record your reflections in your online journal.

herbs or withdrawal, and seek abortions if they become pregnant.[10]

Costs and insurance coverage also influence contraceptive choices (see Health on a Budget). Young women between ages 18 and 24 who lack insurance coverage are less likely to use prescription contraceptives, which are generally more effective, than women with private insurance.[11]

**failure rate** The number of pregnancies that occur per year for every 100 women using a particular method of birth control.

**coitus interruptus** The removal of the penis from the vagina before ejaculation.

# Choosing a Birth Control Method

When it comes to deciding which form of birth control to use, there's no one "right" decision. Good decisions are based on sound information. You should consult a physician or family-planning counselor if you have questions or want to know how certain methods might affect existing or familial medical conditions, such as high blood pressure or diabetes.

Table 10.1 presents your contraceptive choices. As the table indicates, contraception doesn't always work. When you evaluate any contraceptive, always consider its effectiveness (the likelihood that it will indeed prevent pregnancy). The **failure rate** refers to the number of pregnancies that occur per year for every 100 women using a particular method of birth control.

The reliability of contraceptives in actual, real-life use is much lower than that reported in national surveys or clinical trials. In general, failure rates are highest among cohabiting and other unmarried women, very poor families, African American and Hispanic women, adolescents, and women in their twenties. (See Figure 10.2.)

Some couples use withdrawal or **coitus interruptus** (removal of the penis from the vagina before ejaculation), to prevent pregnancy, even though this is not a reliable form of birth control. About half the men who have tried coitus interruptus find it unsatisfactory, either because they don't know when they're going to ejaculate or because they can't withdraw quickly enough. Also, the Cowper's glands, two pea-size structures located on each side of the urethra, often produce a fluid that appears as drops at the tip of the penis any time from arousal and erection to orgasm. This fluid can contain active sperm and, in infected men, human immunodeficiency virus (HIV).

Many unintentional pregnancies are the result of contraceptive failure, either from problems with the drug or device itself or from improper use. Partners can lower the risk of unwanted pregnancy by using backup methods—that is, more than one form of contraception simultaneously. Emergency or after-intercourse contraception (discussed later in this chapter) could prevent as many as 1.7 million unwanted pregnancies each year.

The bottom line is that it takes two people to conceive a baby, and two people should be involved in deciding not to conceive a baby. In the process, they can also enhance their skills in communication, critical thinking, and negotiating. (See Health in Action: Choosing a Contraceptive.)

Table 10.1 **Birth Control Guide**

| Methods | Number of Pregnancies Expected per 100 Women | MD Visit | How to Use It | Some Risks | Noncontraceptive Benefits |
|---|---|---|---|---|---|
| **Sterilization Surgery for Women** | 1 | yes | One-time procedure; nothing to do or remember | • Pain<br>• Bleeding<br>• Infection or other complications after surgery<br>• Ectopic (tubal) pregnancy | Reduces risk of ovarian cancer |
| **Surgical Sterilization Implant for Women** | 1 | yes | One-time procedure; nothing to do or remember | • Mild to moderate pain after insertion<br>• Ectopic (tubal) pregnancy | Reduces risk of ovarian cancer |
| **Sterilization Surgery for Men** | 1 | yes | One-time procedure; nothing to do or remember | • Pain<br>• Bleeding<br>• Infection | Possible reduction in risk for prostate cancer |
| **Implantable Rod** | 1 | yes | One-time procedure; nothing to do or remember | • Acne<br>• Hair loss<br>• Weight gain<br>• Headache<br>• Cysts of the ovaries<br>• Upset stomach<br>• Mood changes<br>• Dizziness<br>• Depression<br>• Sore breasts | Can use while breast-feeding; reduced menstrual flow and cramping |
| **IUD** | 1 | yes | One-time procedure; nothing to do or remember | • Cramps<br>• Lower interest in sexual activity<br>• Bleeding<br>• Pelvic inflammatory disease<br>• Changes in your periods<br>• Infertility<br>• Tear or hole in the uterus | Decreased menstrual flow and cramping; can use while breast-feeding; reduced risk of endometrial cancer |
| **Shot/Injection** | 1 | yes | Need a shot every 3 months | • Bone loss<br>• Bleeding between periods<br>• Weight gain<br>• Breast tenderness<br>• Headaches | |
| **Oral Contraceptives (Combined Pill) "The Pill"** | 5 | yes | Must swallow a pill every day | • Dizziness<br>• High blood pressure<br>• Nausea<br>• Blood clots<br>• Changes in your cycle (period)<br>• Heart attack<br>• Changes in your mood<br>• Strokes<br>• Weight gain | Decreases menstrual flow and cramping, PMS, acne, ovarian and endometrial cancers, and the development of ovarian cysts |
| **Oral Contraceptives (Progestin-only) "The Pill"** | 5 | yes | Must swallow a pill every day | • Irregular bleeding<br>• Weight gain<br>• Breast tenderness | May have similar non-contraceptive benefits as combined pills; reduction of uterine and ovarian cancers |

*(continued)*

Table 10.1 **Birth Control Guide** *(continued)*

| Methods | Number of Pregnancies Expected per 100 Women | MD Visit | How to Use It | Some Risks | Noncontraceptive Benefits |
|---|---|---|---|---|---|
| Oral Contraceptives Extended/Continued Use "The Pill" | 5 | yes | Must swallow a pill every day | • Risks are similar to other oral contraceptives<br>• Bleeding<br>• Spotting between periods | Four periods per year and fewer menstrual-related problems; may reduce uterine fibroids and endometriosis systems |
| Patch | 5 | yes | Must wear a patch every day | • Exposure to higher average levels of estrogen than most oral contraceptives | Decreases menstrual flow and cramping, PMS, acne, ovarian and endometrial cancers, and the development of ovarian cysts |
| Vaginal Contraceptive Ring | 5 | yes | Must leave the ring in every day for 3 weeks | • Vaginal discharge<br>• Swelling of the vagina<br>• Irritation<br>• Similar to oral contraceptives | Decreases menstrual flow and cramping, PMS, acne, ovarian and endometrial cancers, and the development of ovarian cysts |
| Male Condom | 11–16 | no | Must use every time you have sex; requires partner's cooperation | • Allergic reactions | Protects against STIs; delays premature ejaculation<br><br>Except for abstinence, latex condoms are the best protection against HIV/AIDS and other STIs |
| Diaphragm with Spermicide | 15 | yes | Must use every time you have sex | • Irritation<br>• Urinary tract infection<br>• Allergic reactions<br>• Toxic shock | |
| Sponge with Spermicide | 16–32 | no | Must use every time you have sex | • Irritation<br>• Allergic reactions<br>• Hard time removing<br>• Toxic shock | Possible STI protection |
| Cervical Cap with Spermicide | 17–23 | yes | Must use every time you have sex | • Irritation<br>• Allergic reactions<br>• Abnormal Pap test<br>• Toxic shock | |
| Female Condom | 20 | no | Must use every time you have sex | • Irritation<br>• Allergic reactions | Possible STI protection |
| Spermicide | 30 | no | Must use every time you have sex | • Irritation<br>• Allergic reactions<br>• Urinary tract infection | |

Emergency Contraception—If your primary method of birth control fails

| Methods | Number of Pregnancies Expected per 100 Women | MD Visit | How to Use It | Some Risks | Noncontraceptive Benefits |
|---|---|---|---|---|---|
| Emergency Contraceptives "The Morning-After Pill" | 15 | no, if over 18 | Must be used within 72 hours of unprotected sex<br>It should not be used as a regular form of birth control | • Nausea<br>• Vomiting<br>• Abdominal pain<br>• Fatigue<br>• Headache | |

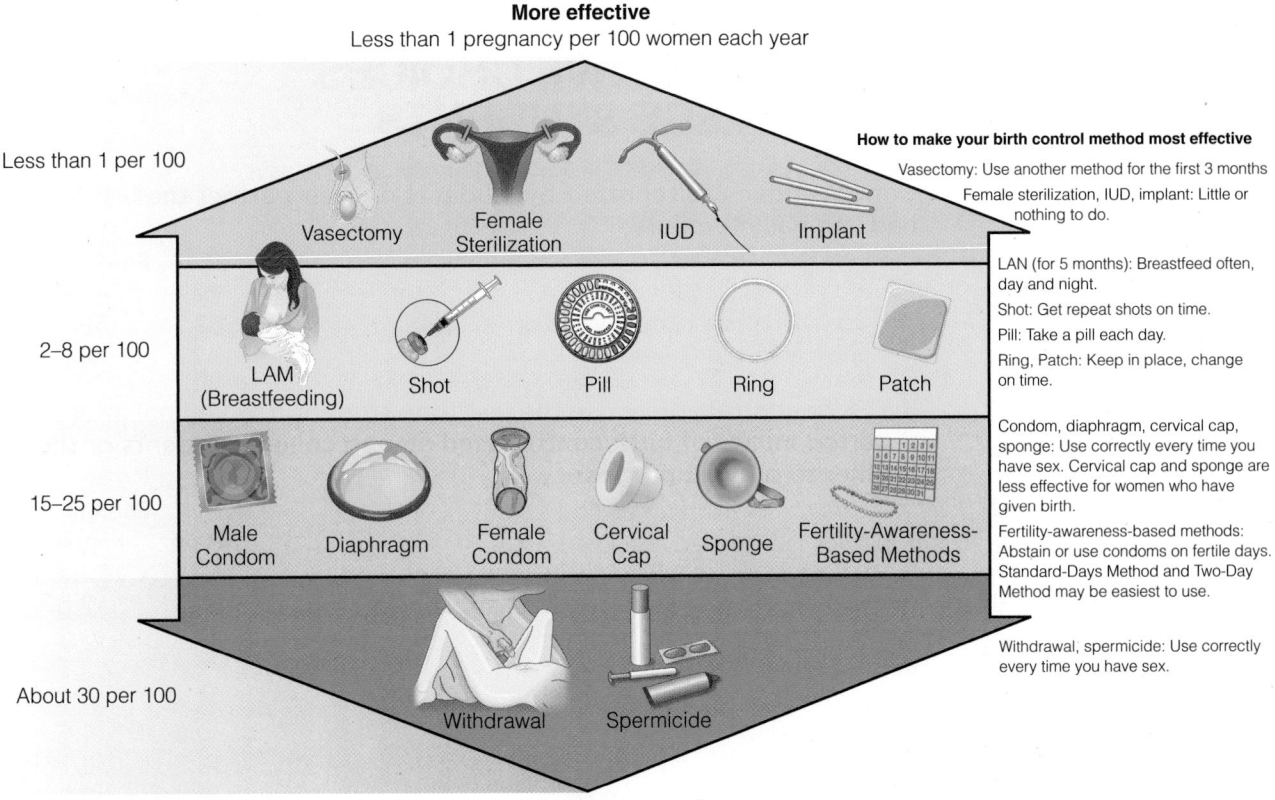

**More effective**
Less than 1 pregnancy per 100 women each year

Less than 1 per 100

Vasectomy
Female Sterilization
IUD
Implant

2–8 per 100

LAM (Breastfeeding)
Shot
Pill
Ring
Patch

15–25 per 100

Male Condom
Diaphragm
Female Condom
Cervical Cap
Sponge
Fertility-Awareness-Based Methods

About 30 per 100

Withdrawal
Spermicide

**Less effective**
About 30 pregnancies per 100 women each year

**How to make your birth control method most effective**

Vasectomy: Use another method for the first 3 months

Female sterilization, IUD, implant: Little or nothing to do.

LAN (for 5 months): Breastfeed often, day and night.

Shot: Get repeat shots on time.

Pill: Take a pill each day.

Ring, Patch: Keep in place, change on time.

Condom, diaphragm, cervical cap, sponge: Use correctly every time you have sex. Cervical cap and sponge are less effective for women who have given birth.

Fertility-awareness-based methods: Abstain or use condoms on fertile days. Standard-Days Method and Two-Day Method may be easiest to use.

Withdrawal, spermicide: Use correctly every time you have sex.

# Contraception on Campus

In the NCHA *American College Health Assessment*, 56.6 percent of students—52.7 percent of men and 59 percent of women—reported using contraception the last time they had vaginal intercourse. (See How Do You Compare? Contraceptive Choices of College Students.) Among students who had vaginal intercourse in the last 12 months, 16.4 percent reported that they or their partner had used emergency contraception (the morning-after pill), discussed later in this chapter, while 2.2 percent reported an unintentional pregnancy.[12]

Even students who know and understand the risks associated with unprotected sex often do not take steps to prevent pregnancy or sexually transmitted infections. One reason is that many believe that "a known partner is a safe partner" and that sex with someone they know as a friend

or have been dating for a while is safe. Students are more likely to use condoms with one-night stands or hookups than with someone they feel familiar with. Even when they acknowledge that this is not a wise strategy for others, most consider themselves "better than average" about sexual decision-making and trust their ability to judge a potential partner.[13]

# Barrier Contraceptives

As their name implies, **barrier contraceptives** block the meeting of egg and sperm by means of a physical barrier (condom, sponge, diaphragm, cervical cap, or FemCap) or a chemical one (vaginal spermicide in jellies, foams, creams, suppositories, or film).

**barrier contraceptives** Birth control devices that block the meeting of egg and sperm, either by physical barriers, such as condoms, diaphragms, or cervical caps, or by chemical barriers, such as spermicide, or both.

# CONTRACEPTIVE CHOICES OF COLLEGE STUDENTS

**Contraceptive use reported by students or their partner the last time they had vaginal intercourse:**

| | Percent (%) | | |
|---|---|---|---|
| | Male | Female | Total |
| Yes, used a method of contraception | 52.7 | 59.0 | 56.6 |
| Not applicable/Didn't use a method/Don't know | 47.3 | 41.0 | 43.4 |

**If YES to contraceptive use the last time student had vaginal intercourse, reported means of birth control used among college students or their partner to prevent pregnancy:**

| | Percent (%) | | |
|---|---|---|---|
| | Male | Female | Total |
| Birth control pills (monthly or extended cycle) | 61.4 | 60.9 | 60.9 |
| Birth control shots | 3.3 | 2.8 | 3.0 |
| Birth control implants | 1.5 | 0.9 | 1.1 |
| Birth control patch | 1.6 | 1.1 | 1.3 |
| Vaginal ring | 4.8 | 4.9 | 4.9 |
| Intrauterine device | 3.6 | 4.6 | 4.3 |
| Male condom | 66.3 | 58.7 | 61.2 |
| Female condom | 0.9 | 0.5 | 0.7 |
| Diaphragm or cervical cap | 0.7 | 0.3 | 0.5 |
| Contraceptive sponge | 0.5 | 0.3 | 0.4 |
| Spermicide (foam, jelly, cream) | 7.0 | 4.0 | 5.0 |
| Fertility awareness (calendar, mucus, basal body temperature) | 4.7 | 5.8 | 5.4 |
| Withdrawal | 24.8 | 27.2 | 26.3 |
| Sterilization (hysterectomy, tubes tied, vasectomy) | 2.2 | 3.1 | 2.8 |
| Other method | 2.6 | 2.2 | 2.3 |
| Male condom use plus another method | 48.3 | 43.9 | 45.2 |
| Any two or more methods (excluding male condoms) | 25.5 | 25.8 | 25.6 |

## HOW DO YOU COMPARE?

If you engage in heterosexual intercourse, do you always use a form of birth control? If not, why not? If so, which type? How did you choose it? Did you discuss contraception with your sexual partner? Did you find this difficult? Write down your reflections in your online journal.

American College Health Association, *American College Health Association-National College Health Assessment II: Reference Group Executive Summary Spring 2010* (Linthicum, MD: American College Health Association, 2010).

**condom** A latex sheath worn over the penis during sexual acts to prevent conception and/or the transmission of disease; the female condom lines the walls of the vagina.

## Nonprescription Barriers

The nonprescription barrier contraceptives include the male and female condom, the contraceptive sponge, and vaginal spermicides. Condoms provide some protection against HIV infection and other STIs; spermicides, sponges, and films do not.

*Male Condom* The male **condom** covers the erect penis and catches the ejaculate, thus preventing sperm from entering the woman's reproductive tract (Figure 10.3). Most are made of thin surgical latex or sheep membrane; a new type is made of polyurethane, which is thinner, stronger, more heat sensitive, and more

## Figure 10.3 **Male Condom**

Condoms effectively reduce the risk of pregnancy as well as STIs if used consistently and correctly.

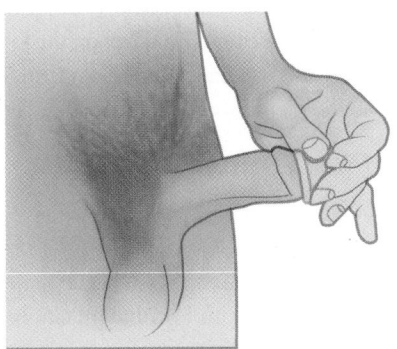

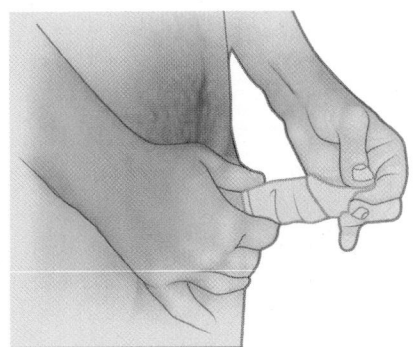

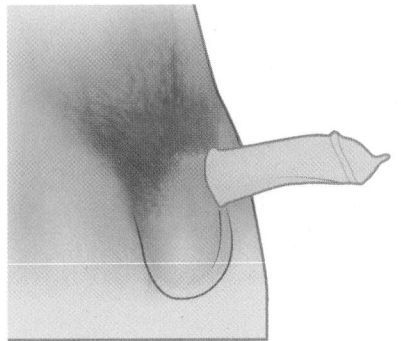

Pinch or twist the tip of the condom, leaving one-half inch at the tip to catch the semen.

Holding the tip, unroll the condom.

Unroll the condom until it reaches the pubic hairs.

comfortable than latex. In a study of 901 couples over six months, the polyurethane condom was not as effective as the latex condom for pregnancy prevention. Experts now advise against use of condoms with nonoxynol-9, which may increase rather than lower the risk of sexual infections (see discussion in Chapter 11).

Although the theoretical effectiveness rate for condoms is 97 percent, the actual rate is only 80 to 85 percent. The condom can be torn during the manufacturing process or during its use; testing by the manufacturer may not be as strenuous as it could or should be. Careless removal can also decrease the effectiveness of condoms. However, the major reason that condoms have such a low actual effectiveness rate is that couples don't use them each and every time they have sex. Users who have little experience with condoms—who are young, single, or childless, or who engage in risky behaviors—are more likely to have condoms break.

Most teenagers—79 percent—report using contraception at first intercourse, most often a condom. Condoms are the most widely used method of contraception among sexually experienced teenage girls; 95 percent report using them at least once.[14]

Condoms are second only to the pill in popularity among college-age adults. Half of sexually active students report using condoms the last time they had vaginal intercourse. College men give various reasons for not using a condom, including not having one available, a partner's objection, the belief that proposing its use could lead to problems between the couple, fear of irritation, and the belief that it doesn't feel natural.[15] Comfort is also an issue. Ill-fitting condoms lead to more problems with slippage and breakage as well as diminished sexual pleasure. Men also may be more likely to remove a condom that doesn't fit well.[16]

 College men also may try to avoid condom use because of concern about erectile dysfunction (ED), the inability to maintain a penile erection sufficient for sexual relations. In an anonymous survey of 234 sexually active males between the ages of 18 and 25 on three university campuses, 25 percent reported ED with condom use. These men were much more inconsistent in their use of condoms than other students. Six percent of all the students surveyed had taken ED medications, such as Viagra. Almost two-thirds mixed these medications with alcohol and drugs, such as ecstasy or methamphetamine.

*Female Condom* The female condom, made of polyurethane or nitrile (a form of rubber), consists of two rings and a polyurethane sheath, and is inserted into the vagina with a tamponlike applicator (Figure 10.4). Once in place, the device loosely lines the walls of the vagina. Internally, a thickened rubber ring keeps it anchored near the cervix. Externally, another rubber ring, two inches in diameter, rests on the labia and resists slippage.

Although not widely used in the West, female condoms have been distributed in 142 countries. Properly used, they are believed to be as good

## Figure 10.4 **Female Condom**

No spermicide is used with the female condom. Like the male condom, this method does not require a prescription.

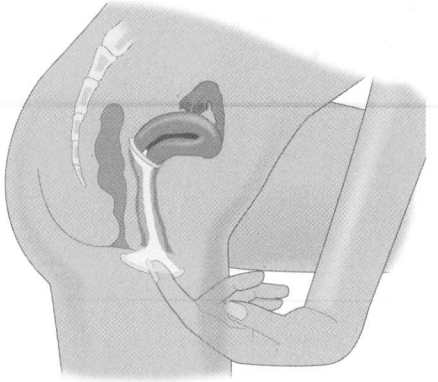
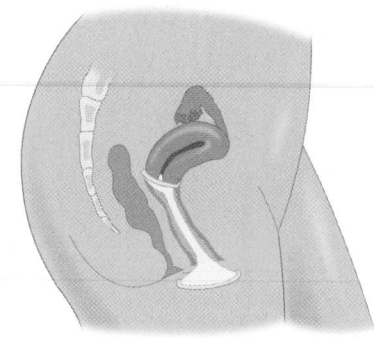

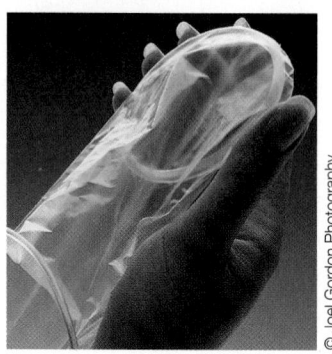

applicator from the wrapper and inserts the condom slowly by gently pushing the applicator toward the small of the back. When properly inserted, the outer ring should rest on the folds of skin around the vaginal opening, and the inner ring (the closed end) should fit against the cervix.

**Advantages**

- Effective when used correctly.
- Lowers a woman's risk of pelvic inflammatory disease (PID) and may protect against some urinary tract and genital infections.
- No side effects, unless the woman is allergic to latex.
- No prescription required.
- Inexpensive.
- The female condom gives women more control in reducing their risk of pregnancy and STIs and does not require a prescription or medical appointment.

**Disadvantages**

- Requires consistent and diligent use.
- Not 100 percent effective in preventing pregnancy or STIs.
- Risk of manufacturing defects, such as pin-size holes, and breaking or slipping off during intercourse.
- May inhibit sexual spontaneity.
- Users or partners may complain about odor, lubrication (too much or too little), feel, taste, difficulty opening the packages, and disposal.
- Some men dislike reduced penile sensitivity or cannot sustain an erection while putting on a condom.
- Some women complain that the female condom is difficult to use, squeaks, and looks odd.

as or better than the male condom for preventing infections, including HIV, because they are stronger and cover a slightly larger area. Female condoms may be more prone to slipping and other mechanical problems but are as effective as male condoms in blocking semen. The efficacy of female condoms does increase with a woman's experience in using them.

### How They Work

**Male Condom** Most physicians recommend prelubricated, spermicide-treated, American-made latex or polyurethane condoms, not membrane condoms ("natural" or "sheepskin"). Before using a condom, check the expiration date and make sure it's soft and pliable. If it's yellow or sticky, throw it out. Don't check for leaks by blowing up a condom before using it; you may weaken or tear it.

The condom should be put on at the beginning of sexual activity, before genital contact occurs. There should be a little space left at the top of the condom to catch the semen (see Figure 10.3). Any vaginal lubricant should be water-based. Petroleum-based creams or jellies (such as Vaseline, baby oil, massage oil, vegetable oils, or oil-based hand lotions) can deteriorate the latex. After ejaculation, the condom should be held firmly against the penis so that it doesn't slip off or leak during withdrawal. Couples engaging in anal intercourse should use a water-based lubricant as well as a condom, but should never assume the condom will provide 100 percent protection from HIV infection or other STIs.

**Female Condom** As illustrated in Figure 10.4, a woman removes the condom and

### Do Men and Women Use Condoms for Different Reasons?
The genders have very different motives both for engaging in sex and for using condoms. In focus groups, young women say they engage in sexual relations because of a desire for physical intimacy and a committed relationship. They generally report having sex only with men they care for and deeply trust and expect that these men would be honest and forthright about their sexual history. This trust plays a significant role in their decision whether to insist on condom use.

In contrast, few young men say relationships are an important dimension of their sexual involvements. Their primary motivation is a desire for physical and sexual satisfaction. Most say they are not interested in commitment and view emotional expectations as a complication of becoming sexually involved with a woman. Young men also admit to making judgments about types of girls. To them, young women they didn't care about were "sluts" with whom they used a condom for their own protection.

Which partner determines whether a couple uses a condom? The answer is often the women—if they choose to do so. Regardless of race or ethnicity, many young women are adamant in demanding that their partners use condoms—and many young men say they would not challenge such a demand out of fear of losing the opportunity for sex. Men often expect potential partners to want to use condoms and describe themselves as "suspicious" of women who do not.

Both sexes name two primary reasons for using condoms: preventing pregnancy and protecting against sexually transmitted infections. Young women see an unwanted pregnancy as an occurrence that would be disruptive and expensive and that could "ruin" their lives and their parents' lives. Young men see condom use as a way of protecting themselves against emotional entanglements and paternity issues. But young adults of both sexes tend to overestimate how consistently they use condoms.

*Contraceptive Sponge* The Today Sponge, which is made of soft polyurethane foam laced with spermicide, was sold as an over-the-counter contraceptive in the United States from 1983 to 1995, when it was withdrawn because of contamination problems at the manufacturing plant. It has returned to stores several times.

**How It Works** The contraceptive sponge acts as a barrier by blocking the entrance to the uterus and absorbing and deactivating sperm. Prior to inserting it in the vagina, moisten the sponge with water to activate the spermicide. Then fold it in half and insert deep into the vagina. Check to make sure it is covering the cervix. Intercourse can occur immediately or at any time during the next 24 hours. However, the sponge must remain in place for six hours after

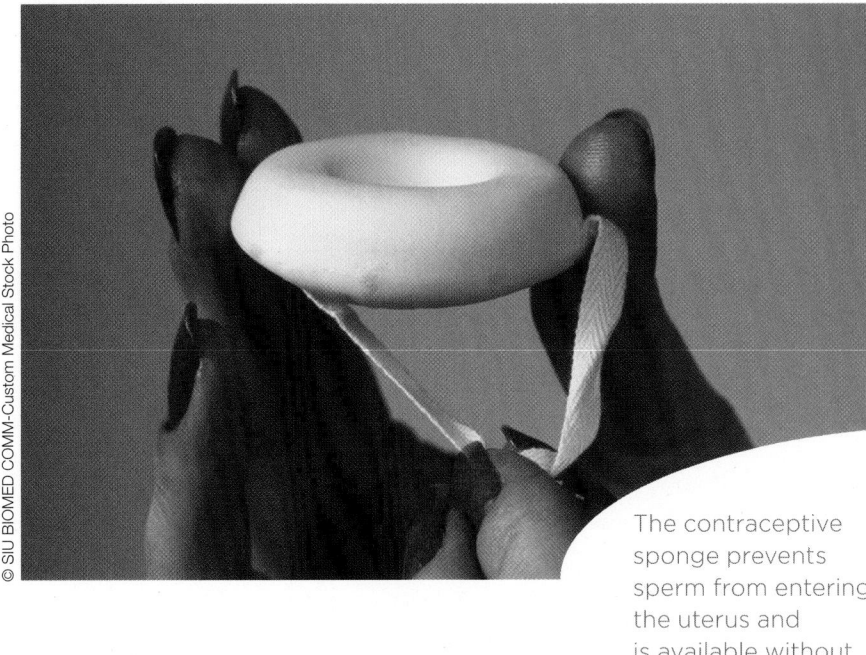

© SIU BIOMED COMM–Custom Medical Stock Photo

The contraceptive sponge prevents sperm from entering the uterus and is available without a prescription.

intercourse. To remove, gently pull the cloth loop or the tabs on the outside.

**Advantages**

- Easy to carry and use.
- Can be inserted up to 24 hours before intercourse.
- Effective immediately if used correctly.
- No effect on fertility.
- Generally cannot be felt by a woman or her partner.
- Can be used by women who are breast-feeding.

**Disadvantages**

- May be difficult to remove.
- May be less effective in women who have had children.
- No reliable protection against STIs.
- Requires advance planning to place the sponge.
- Side effects include vaginal irritation and allergic reactions.
- Should not be used during menstruation.
- Slightly increased risk of toxic shock syndrome (see Chapter 16).

*Vaginal Spermicides and Film* The various forms of **vaginal spermicide** include chemical foams, creams, jellies, vaginal suppositories, gels, and film. Some creams and jellies

**vaginal spermicide** A substance that kills or neutralizes sperm, inserted into the vagina in the form of a foam, cream, jelly, suppository, or film.

## Figure 10.5 **Vaginal Contraceptive Film**

The effectiveness of this thin film, laced with spermicide, is similar to other spermicides and greatest when used with a condom.

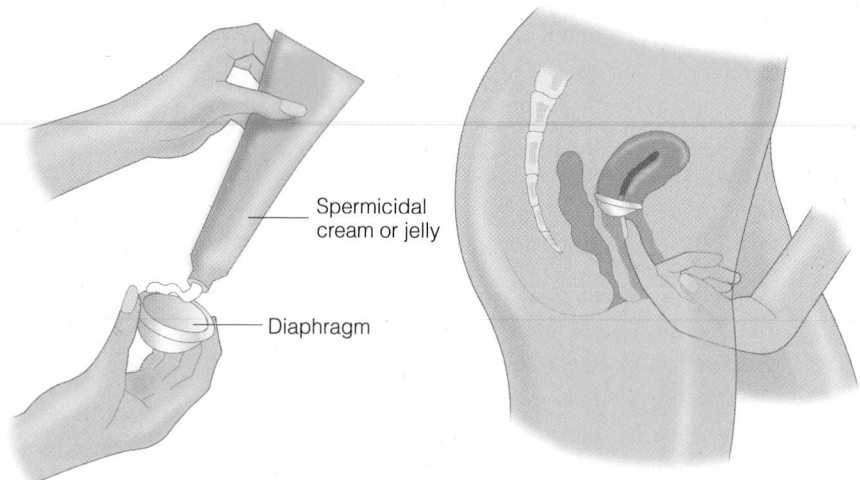

## Figure 10.6 **Diaphragm**

When used correctly and consistently with a spermicide, the diaphragm is effective in preventing pregnancy. It must be fitted by a health-care professional.

Spermicidal cream or jelly

Diaphragm

Squeeze spermicide into dome of diaphragm and around the rim.

Squeeze rim together; insert jelly-side up.

Check placement to make certain cervix is covered.

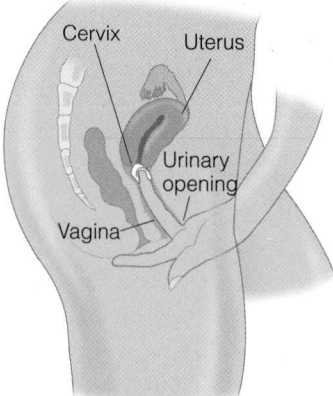

Cervix
Uterus
Urinary opening
Vagina

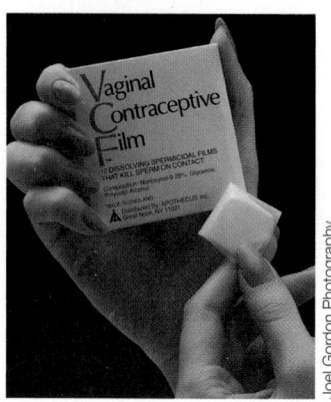

Joel Gordon Photography

**vaginal contraceptive film (VCF)** A small dissolvable sheet saturated with spermicide that can be inserted into the vagina and placed over the cervix.

are made for use with a diaphragm; others can be used alone. Several vaginal suppositories claim high effectiveness, but no American studies have confirmed these claims. In general, failure rates for vaginal suppositories are as high as 10 to 25 percent.

One widely used spermicide, nonoxynol-9, has proven to be less effective than once believed. It does not protect against many STIs, including chlamydia and gonorrhea. Nonoxynol-9 also may increase the risk of infection with human papillomavirus (HPV). The CDC has concluded that it is ineffective against HIV, and the World Health Organization describes it as only "moderately effective" for pregnancy prevention.

**Vaginal contraceptive film (VCF)**, a thin two-inch-square film laced with spermicide, is folded and inserted into the vagina, where it dissolves into a stay-in-place gel (see Figure 10.5). VCF, which can be used by people allergic to foams and jellies, is as effective as most spermicides and almost 100 percent effective when paired with a condom.

Although more effective methods of birth control now provide good alternatives to spermicides, they remain popular as a means of lowering the risk of STIs.

**How They Work** Spermicides consist of a chemical that kills sperm and potential pathogens and an inert base, such as jelly, cream, foam, or film, that holds the spermicide close to the cervix. The jelly, cream, or foam spermicide is inserted into the vagina with an applicator or finger. Vaginal suppositories take about 20 minutes to dissolve and cover the vaginal walls. Follow package directions precisely.

You must apply additional spermicide or insert another VCF film before each additional intercourse. After sex, women should shower rather than bathe to prevent the spermicide from being rinsed out of the vagina, and they should not douche for at least six hours.

### Advantages

- Easy to use.
- Effective if used with another form of contraception, such as condoms.
- Reduces the risk of some vaginal infections, PID, and STIs.
- No effect on fertility.

### Disadvantages

- Insertion interrupts sexual spontaneity.
- May cause irritation.
- Some people cannot use foams or jellies because of an allergic reaction.
- Some users complain that spermicides are messy or interfere with oral-genital contact.
- Spermicidal suppositories that do not dissolve completely can feel gritty.

# Prescription Barriers

The prescription barrier contraceptives are used by women: the diaphragm, cervical cap, and FemCap. They are placed in the vagina with a spermicide. They do not protect against HIV infection and most STIs.

*Diaphragm*   The **diaphragm** is a bowl-like rubber cup with a flexible rim that is inserted into the vagina to cover the cervix and prevent the passage of sperm into the uterus during sexual intercourse (Figure 10.6). When used with a spermicide, the diaphragm is both a physical and a chemical barrier to sperm. The effectiveness of the diaphragm in preventing pregnancy depends on strong motivation (to use it faithfully) and a precise understanding of its use. If diaphragms with spermicide are used consistently and carefully, they can be 95 to 98 percent effective. Without a spermicide, the diaphragm is not effective.

*Cervical Cap*   Like the diaphragm, the **cervical cap** combined with spermicide serves as both a chemical and physical barrier blocking the path of the sperm to the uterus. The rubber or plastic cap is smaller and thicker than a diaphragm. It resembles a large thimble that fits snugly around the cervix and may work better for some women. It is about as effective as a diaphragm (95 to 98 percent).

*FemCap*   The FemCap is a nonhormonal, latex-free barrier contraceptive that works with a spermicide (Figure 10.7). The FemCap, designed to conform to the anatomy of the cervix and vagina, comes in three sizes. The smallest usually best suits women who have never been pregnant; the medium size, for women who have been pregnant but have not had a vaginal delivery; the largest, for those who have delivered a full-term baby vaginally.

## How They Work

**Diaphragm**   Diaphragms are fitted and prescribed by a qualified health-care professional in diameter sizes ranging from two to four inches (50 to 105 millimeters). The diaphragm's main function is to serve as a container for a spermicidal (sperm-killing) foam or jelly, which is available at pharmacies without a prescription. A diaphragm should remain in the vagina for at least six hours after intercourse to ensure that all sperm are killed. If intercourse occurs again during this period, additional spermicide must be inserted with an applicator tube.

The key to proper use of the diaphragm is having it available. A sexually active woman should keep it in the most accessible place—her purse, bedroom, bathroom. Before every use, a diaphragm should be checked for tiny leaks (hold up to the light or place water in the dome). A health-care provider should check its fit and condition every year when the woman has her annual Pap smear. Oil-based lubricants will deteriorate the latex of the diaphragm and should not be used.

**Cervical Cap**   Like the diaphragm, the cervical cap is fitted by a qualified health-care professional. For use, the woman fills it one-third to two-thirds full with spermicide and inserts it by holding its edges together and sliding it into the vagina. The cup is then pressed onto the cervix. (Most women find it easiest to do so while squatting or in an upright sitting position.) The cap can be inserted up to six hours prior to intercourse and should not be removed for at least six hours afterward. It can be left in place up to 24 hours. Pulling on one side of the rim breaks the suction and allows easy removal. Oil-based lubricants should not be used with the cap because they can deteriorate the latex.

**FemCap**   A prescription is required to purchase FemCap, and the woman selects the appropriate size. Apply spermicide to the bowl of the FemCap (which goes over the cervix), to the outer brim, and to the groove that will face into the vagina. Insert the squeezed, flattened cap into the vagina with the bowl facing upward. The FemCap must be pushed all the way in to cover the cervix completely and left in place at least six hours after intercourse.

### Advantages

- Relatively inexpensive.
- Doesn't interrupt sexual activity; can be inserted hours ahead of time.
- Usually not felt by either partner.
- Can easily be carried in pocket or purse.
- No hormones or side effects.
- Cervical caps are an alternative for women who cannot use diaphragms or find them too messy.

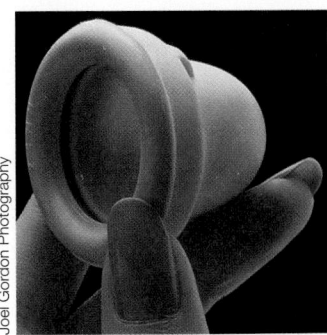

The cervical cap, preferred by some women, is about as effective as a diaphragm.

**diaphragm**  A bowl-like rubber cup with a flexible rim that is inserted into the vagina to cover the cervix and prevent the passage of sperm into the uterus during sexual intercourse; used with a spermicidal foam or jelly, it serves as both a chemical and a physical barrier to sperm.

**cervical cap**  A thimble-size rubber or plastic cap that is inserted into the vagina to fit over the cervix and prevent the passage of sperm into the uterus during sexual intercourse; used with a spermicidal foam or jelly, it serves as both a chemical and a physical barrier to sperm.

Figure 10.7 **FemCap**
The FemCap must be used with spermicide and correctly positioned to cover the cervix completely.

Source: Reproduced with permission from FemCap, Inc., and Alfred Shihata, MD

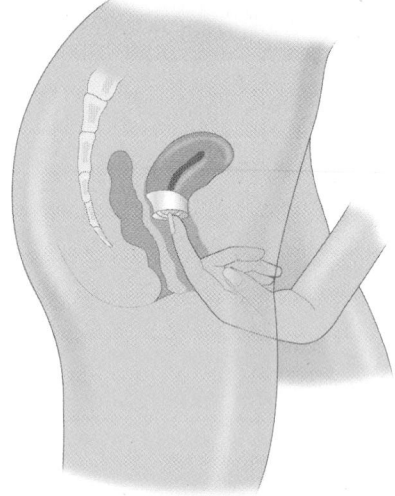

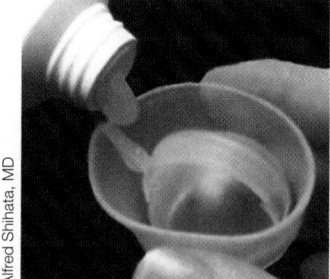

Courtesy of FemCap, Inc., and Alfred Shihata, MD

**oral contraceptives** Preparations of synthetic hormones that inhibit ovulation; also referred to as birth control pills or simply the pill.

### Disadvantages

- Less effective than hormonal contraceptives.
- Available by prescription only.
- Requires advance planning or interruption of sexual activity to position the device before intercourse.
- May slip out of place during intercourse.
- May be uncomfortable for some women and their partners.
- Spermicidal foams, creams, and jellies may be messy, cause irritation, and detract from oral–genital sex.
- Some diaphragm users report bladder discomfort, urethral irritation, or recurrent cystitis.
- Some cap users find it difficult to insert and remove and uncomfortable to wear.
- Slightly increased risk of toxic shock syndrome.

# Hormonal Contraceptives

In recent years, birth control methods made with synthetic hormones have become available in a variety of forms. Oral contraceptives have been available for decades, and the birth control pill is one of the most well-researched medications. Other options for hormonal birth control include a skin patch, a vaginal ring, a three-month injection, and a three-year implant. All are extremely effective when used consistently and conscientiously.

Hormonal contraceptives can provide benefits beyond birth control, including:

- Regular menstrual cycles.
- Reduction of menstrual pain and excess bleeding.
- Treatment of premenstrual syndrome.
- Prevention of menstrual migraines.
- Decreased risk of endometrial cancer, ovarian cancer, and colorectal cancer.
- Treatment of acne and excess facial hair.
- Improved bone mineral density.[17]

Hormonal contraceptives do not protect against HIV infection and other STIs, so condoms and spermicides should also be used to get protection against infections.

## Oral Contraceptives

The *pill*—the popular term for **oral contraceptives**—is the method of birth control preferred by unmarried women and by those under age 30, including college students. About one in five American women of childbearing age uses the pill. Women 18 to 24 years old are most likely to choose oral contraceptives. In use for 40 years, the pill is one of the most researched, tested, and carefully followed medications in medical history—and one of the most controversial.

Although many women incorrectly think that the risks of the pill are greater than those of pregnancy and childbirth, long-term studies show that oral contraceptive use does not increase mortality rates. In fact, women who took the birth control pill beginning in the late 1960s lived longer than those never on the pill, according to a British study that followed more than 46,000 women for nearly four decades. The pill cut women's risk of dying from colon cancer by 38 percent and from any other diseases by about 12 percent.[18] Combination oral contraceptives significantly reduce the risk of ovarian and endometrial cancer and produce no increase in diabetes, multiple sclerosis, rheumatoid arthritis, and liver disease. However, there is evidence of increased risk of breast cancer in women who have taken the pill within the last ten years for more than a year.

Common antibiotics, including many prescribed for dental procedures or skin conditions, may lower the effectiveness of oral contraceptives, particularly low-dose birth control pills. Always ask a dentist or doctor who prescribes an antibiotic about its potential effect on your oral contraceptive, and check with your gynecologist or primary physician about using an additional nonhormonal means of contraception (such as a condom) to ensure protection against an unwanted pregnancy. Other medicines and supplements that may make hormonal contraceptives less effective include St. John's wort, certain pills prescribed for yeast infections, certain HIV medications, and certain antiseizure medication.

Doctors have debated making birth control pills available over-the-counter without a prescription. Women given six or more packets of pills at a time are less likely to stop using the pill.[19] However, women with certain health conditions may put themselves at risk by taking the pill without medical supervision.[20]

*Combination Pills* These pills consist of two hormones, synthetic estrogen and progestin, which play important roles in controlling ovulation and the menstrual cycle. The doses in today's oral contraceptives are much lower—less than one-fourth the amount of estrogen and one-twentieth the progestin in the original pill. This means fewer side effects and lower risk of heart disease and stroke.[21] Stroke risk among women taking newer, low-dose formulations of oral contraceptive pills may be extremely low. However, these pills appear to be less effective than those approved decades ago, with twice the failure rate of previous products.[22] The reason seems to be lower doses of hormones that stop ovulation. Women on low-dose oral contraceptives should take their pills at the same time every day and follow their doctor's advice if they miss a dose.

**Monophasic pills** release a constant dose of estrogen and progestin throughout a woman's menstrual cycle. **Multiphasic pills** mimic normal hormonal fluctuations of the natural menstrual cycle by providing different levels of estrogen and progesterone at different times of the month. Multiphasic pills reduce total hormonal dose and side effects. Both monophasic and multiphasic pills block the release of hormones that would stimulate the process leading to ovulation. They also thicken and alter the cervical mucus, making it more hostile to sperm, and they make implantation of a fertilized egg in the uterine lining more difficult.

One combination pill, Yasmin, contains a unique progestin that works like a mild diuretic and prevents fluid retention. YAZ, a lower-dose 24-day version, can ease the emotional and physical symptoms of premenstrual dysphoric disorder (discussed in Chapter 9). Women who are taking potassium supplements, daily anti-inflammatory drugs, or heparin (a blood-thinner) should talk with their doctor because of potentially dangerous drug interactions. Other pills offer different benefits, such as clearer skin and reduced facial hair, and less spotting.

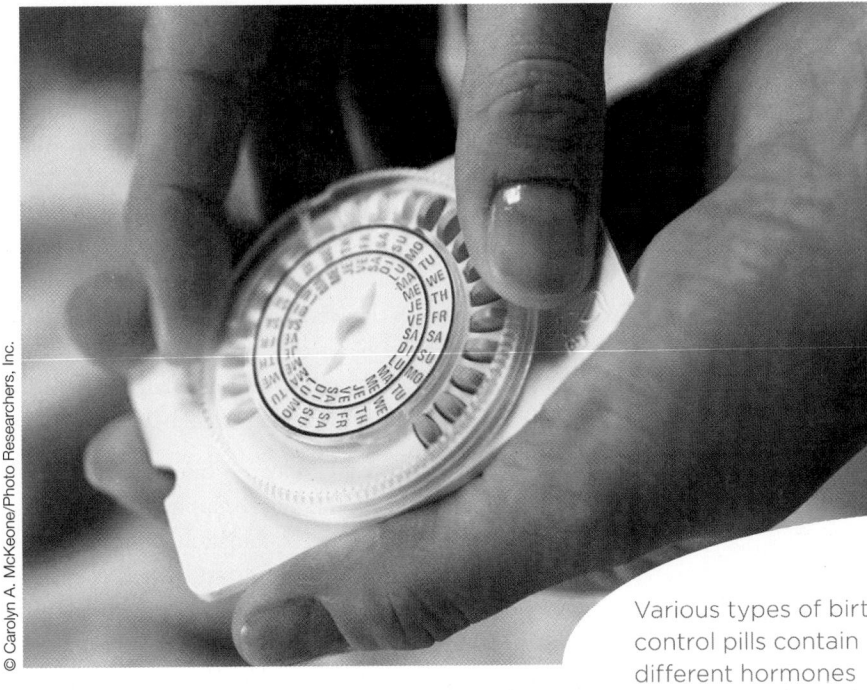

© Carolyn A. McKeone/Photo Researchers, Inc.

Various types of birth control pills contain different hormones and combinations of hormones.

*Progestin-Only Pills* Progestin-only **"mini-pills"** contain only a small amount of progestin and no estrogen. They work somewhat differently than combination pills. Women taking **progestin-only pills** probably ovulate, at least occasionally. In those cycles, the pills prevent pregnancy by thickening cervical mucus, making it hard for sperm to penetrate, and by interfering with implantation of a fertilized egg.[23]

The risk of heart disease and stroke is lower with progestin-only pills than with any combination pill. For this reason, they are a good choice for women over age 35 and others who cannot take estrogen-containing pills because of high blood pressure, diabetes, or clotting disorders.[24] Because they do not affect the quality or quantity of breast milk, progestin-only pills often are recommended for nursing mothers, and they are recommended for smokers. Because progestin can affect mood and worsen the symptoms of depression, progestin-only pills are not recommended for women with a history of depression. Antiseizure medications, such as Dilantin, which accelerate liver metabolism, may make the minipill less effective.

Users of progestin-only pills have to be conscientious about taking these pills, not just every day, but at the same time every day. If you take a progestin-only pill three or more hours later than usual, use a backup method of contraception,

**monophasic pill** An oral contraceptive that releases synthetic estrogen and progestin at constant levels throughout the menstrual cycle.

**multiphasic pill** An oral contraceptive that releases different levels of estrogen and progestin to mimic the hormonal fluctuations of the natural menstrual cycle.

**minipill, progestin-only pill** An oral contraceptive containing a small amount of progestin and no estrogen, which prevents contraception by making the mucus in the cervix so thick that sperm cannot enter the uterus.

such as a condom, for two days after you resume taking the pill.

*How They Work*  The pill usually comes in 28-day packets: 21 of the pills contain the hormones, and 7 are "blanks," included so that the woman can take a pill every day, even during her menstrual period. If a woman forgets to take one pill, she should take it as soon as she remembers. However, if she forgets during the first week of her cycle or misses more than one pill, she should rely on another form of birth control until her next menstrual period.

Even if you experience no discomfort or side effects while on the pill, see a physician at least once a year for an examination, which should include a blood pressure test, a pelvic exam, and a breast exam. Notify your doctor at once if you develop severe abdominal pain, chest pain, coughing, shortness of breath, pain or tenderness in the calf or thigh, severe headaches, dizziness, faintness, muscle weakness or numbness, speech disturbance, blurred vision, a sensation of flashing lights, a breast lump, severe depression, or yellowing of your skin.

Generally, when a woman stops taking the pill, her menstrual cycle resumes the next month, but it may be irregular for the next couple of months. However, 2 to 4 percent of pill users experience prolonged delays. Women who become pregnant during the first or second cycle after discontinuing use of the pill may be at greater risk of miscarriage; they also are more likely to conceive twins.

### Advantages

- Extremely effective when taken consistently.
- Convenient.
- Moderately priced.
- Does not interrupt sexual activity.
- Reversible within three months of stopping the pill.
- Reduces the risk of benign breast lumps, ovarian cysts, iron-deficiency anemia, pelvic inflammatory disease, endometrial and ovarian cancer.
- May relieve painful menstruation.

### Disadvantages

- In real life, rates of unintended pregnancies among pill users are much higher: as high as 2.8 percent in the first year of use and 5.7 percent after three years, according to a recent study.[25]
- Requires a prescription.
- Increases risk of cardiovascular problems, primarily for women over age 35 who smoke and those with high blood pressure or other health problems.
- Side effects vary with different brands but include spotting between periods, weight gain or loss, nausea and vomiting, breast tenderness, and decreased sex drive.
- Must be taken at the same time every day (especially critical with low-dose estrogen and progestin-only pills).
- No protection against STIs.
- Must use a secondary form of birth control for the initial seven days of use.

*Before Using Oral Contraceptives*  Before starting on the pill, you should undergo a thorough physical examination that includes the following tests:

- Routine blood pressure test.
- Pelvic exam, including a Pap smear.
- Breast exam.
- Blood test.
- Urine sample.

Let your doctor know about any personal or family incidence of high blood pressure or heart disease; diabetes; liver dysfunction; hepatitis; unusual menstrual history; severe depression; sickle-cell anemia; cancer of the breast, ovaries, or uterus; high cholesterol levels; or migraine headaches. (See Consumer Alert, p. 331.)

## Extended-Use Pills

For years physicians have prescribed prolonged use of birth control pills to lessen the number of menstrual cycles for women with asthma, migraines, rashes, or other conditions that flare up during their periods. Eliminating periods eliminates symptoms, and having fewer cycles also may lower a woman's long-term risk of ovarian cancer. However, some women are wary of long-term hormone use or consider a lack of menstrual cycles unnatural.

*Seasonale and Seasonique*  Seasonale and Seasonique are prescription forms of oral contraception that prevent pregnancy as

## The Risks of Contraceptives

For individuals with certain medical conditions, specific types of birth control can pose a health risk.

### Facts to Know

If you have one of the following conditions, you should talk with your doctor about which types of contraceptive may increase your health risks:

- High blood pressure.
- Episodes of depression.
- Seizure disorder.
- Ectopic pregnancy.
- Hepatitis.

### Steps to Take

- High blood pressure (180/110 mmHg or higher): Avoid birth control pills or injections containing estrogen, which may increase your risk of a heart attack or stroke.

- Episodes of depression: Avoid products that contain progestin, such as Depo-Provera, the contraceptive implant, and the minipill. In some women with depression, progestin may worsen depressive symptoms. Also, check with your doctor if you are taking an antidepressant medication; it may affect or be affected by oral contraceptives and you may require a different dose.

- Seizure disorder: Avoid low-dose birth control pills. Some antiseizure medications, such as Dilantin, accelerate liver metabolism of all substances, including oral contraceptives, and make them less effective.

- Ectopic pregnancy: Avoid IUDs. Although IUDs do not cause ectopic pregnancies, if your fallopian tubes have been scarred by a previous ectopic gestation, you're more likely to have another ectopic if you use an IUD.

- Hepatitis: Avoid birth control pills or injections containing estrogen, which is metabolized in the liver—an organ damaged by hepatitis.

effectively as other birth control pills but produce only four menstrual periods a year.

**How They Work** Unlike traditional birth control pills, women take "active" pills continuously for three months or 84 days. During this time, Seasonale prevents the uterine lining from thickening enough to produce a full menstrual period. Every three months, a woman takes one week of inactive pills to produce a "pill period," which may be lighter than a regular period. With Seasonique, women take a very low dose of estrogen for seven days to eliminate any symptoms of complete hormone withdrawal.

The chance of getting pregnant ranges from 5 percent with typical use to 1 percent with perfect use. For maximum effectiveness, each pill should be taken at the same time of day.

### Advantages

- Fewer periods.
- Tri-monthly periods are usually lighter, with less blood flow.

### Disadvantages

- Similar to those of other oral contraceptives in terms of health risks, costs, and side effects. Cigarette smoking increases these risks.
- No protection from STIs.
- More spotting and breakthrough bleeding than with a 28-day pill.
- Determining pregnancy is difficult without a monthly period.

*The "No-Period" Pill* Lybrel, described as a continuous contraceptive, works the same way as other combination hormonal birth control pills. However, women take the "365-day" pill every single day without interruption.

**How It Works** Like other oral contraceptives, Lybrel stops the body's monthly preparation for pregnancy by lowering the production of hormones that make pregnancy possible. However, it does not include the "week-off" of placebo pills that leads to vaginal bleeding. Most women resume menstruation within 90 days of stopping Lybrel.

Medical experts see no long-term risk in doing away with regular monthly periods, but the long-term safety of menstrual suppression is unknown.

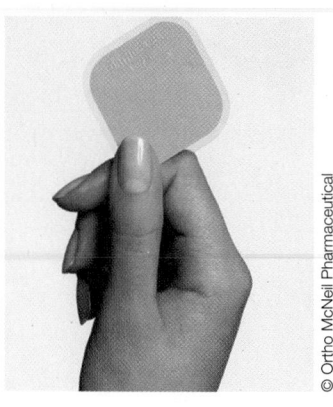

Contraceptive hormones can be delivered through the skin with the patch.

© Ortho McNeil Pharmaceutical

### Advantages

- No menstrual periods, cramps, or other symptoms.
- No need to stop taking pills or to switch to dummy pills for a week.
- Relief from menstruation-linked conditions such as endometriosis and menstrual migraine.

### Disadvantages

- Spotting, which generally tapers off over the first year of use.
- Health risks similar to those of other combination pills.
- Determining pregnancy is difficult without a monthly period.
- Some women feel that eliminating periods is unnatural.

## The Patch (Ortho Evra)

The Ortho Evra birth control patch, the first transdermal (through the skin) contraceptive, works like a combination pill but looks like a Band-Aid. Embedded in its adhesive layer are two hormones, a low-dose estrogen and a progestin. It prevents pregnancy by delivering continuous levels of estrogen and progestin through the skin directly into the bloodstream so women are exposed to higher overall levels of estrogen, which may increase their risk of blood clots. The patch is waterproof and stays on in the shower, swimming pool, or hot tub.

*How It Works* A woman applies the 1¾-inch square to her back, upper arm, lower abdomen, or buttocks and changes it every seven days for three weeks. During the patch-free week, she experiences menstrual bleeding. A user should check every day to make sure the patch is still in place. If you don't replace a detached patch within 24 hours, use a backup method of contraception until your next period.

### Advantages

- Good alternative for women who can't remember, don't like, or have problems swallowing daily pills.
- Highly effective when used correctly.
- Does not interrupt sexual activity.

- Fewer side effects, such as nausea, breakthrough bleeding, and mood swings, than pills.
- Fertility returns quickly after you stop using it.

### Disadvantages

- Must apply a new patch every week.
- Requires a prescription.
- No protection against STIs.
- Increases risk of blood clots, heart attack, and stroke, particularly for women who smoke or have certain health conditions. The risk of dying or suffering a survivable blood clot while using the patch is estimated to be about two times higher than while using birth control pills.[26]
- Less effective in women who weigh more than 198 pounds.
- Some women report breast tenderness, headaches, bleeding between periods, upper respiratory infections, or self-consciousness wearing the patch.
- Contact lens wearers may experience vision changes.
- Five percent of women report that at least one patch slipped off; 2 percent report skin irritation.
- Must use another form of birth control for the initial seven days of use.

## Vaginal Ring (NuvaRing)

The silver-dollar-size NuvaRing, a two-inch ring made of flexible, transparent plastic, slowly emits the same hormones as oral contraceptives through the vaginal tissues (Figure 10.8). Smaller than the smallest diaphragm, it contains less estrogen than any pill. As effective as the pill, it provides a steady dose of hormones and causes fewer side effects. In a campus-based study, women were equally satisfied with birth control pills and with the vaginal ring, but were more likely to forget to take pills.[27]

*How It Works* Unlike a diaphragm, the NuvaRing does not have to be exactly positioned within the vagina or used with a spermicide. The flexible, plastic two-inch ring compresses so a woman can easily insert it. Each ring stays in place for three weeks, then is removed for the fourth week of the menstrual cycle.

If a NuvaRing pops out (uncommon but possible), it should be washed, dried, and replaced within three hours. If a longer time passes, users should rely on a backup form of birth control until the ring has been reinserted for a week and the medications have risen to protective levels again.

### Advantages

- Under medical supervision, may be safer than birth control pills for women with mild hypertension or diabetes.
- Less likelihood of pill-related side effects, such as nausea, mood swings, spotting, and cramping.
- No need to remember a daily pill or weekly patch.
- Fertility returns quickly when ring is removed.

### Disadvantages

- Some women do not feel comfortable placing and removing something inside their vagina.
- Possible side effects include vaginal discharge, irritation, and infection.
- Cannot use oil-based vaginal medications for yeast infections while ring is in place.
- No protection against STIs.

## Contraceptive Injection

A progestin-only contraceptive is available in the form of a birth control "shot" or injection. Depo-Provera or its newer form, Depo-subQ Provera, must be given every 12 weeks. Contraceptive injections provide no protection against HIV and other STIs.

Because of the risk of significant bone mineral loss, the FDA has recommended that women not use Depo-Provera for longer than two years. Although mineral loss is common and greater in the first year of use, most individuals regain bone density after discontinuing its use.[28]

*How It Works* One injection of this synthetic version of the natural hormone progesterone provides three months of contraceptive protection. This long-acting hormonal contraceptive raises levels of progesterone, thereby simulating pregnancy. The pituitary gland doesn't produce FSH and LH, which normally cause egg ripening and release. The endometrial

lining of the uterus thins, preventing implantation of a fertilized egg.

### Advantages

- Because it contains only progestin, it is safe for women who cannot take combination birth control pills.
- No risk of user error.
- No worry about buying, storing, or using contraceptives.
- No need to think about contraception for three months at a time.
- Possible protection against endometrial and ovarian cancer.
- Can be used by women who are breast-feeding.

### Disadvantages

- Must visit a doctor or clinic every three months for injection.
- Menstrual cycles become irregular. After a year, 50 percent of women stop having periods.
- Potential side effects include decreased sex drive, depression, headaches, dizziness, frequent urination, allergic reactions, hair loss or increased hair growth.
- Increased weight gain, especially for obese women and teenage girls.
- No protection against STIs.
- According to a recent NIH study, appears to triple risk of acquiring chlamydia and gonorrhea compared with women not using a hormonal contraceptive. Scientists do not know the reason for this increased risk.
- Delayed return of fertility.
- Long-term use may significantly reduce bone density, particularly for women who smoke, don't get enough calcium, and have never been pregnant.[29]

## Contraceptive Implant (Implanon)

This thin, flexible, plastic implant—about the size of a matchstick—is inserted under the skin of the upper arm to provide birth control that is 99 percent effective for up to three years. Easier to insert and remove than earlier implants, Implanon has been used in other countries for years, and is now available in all 50 states in the U.S.

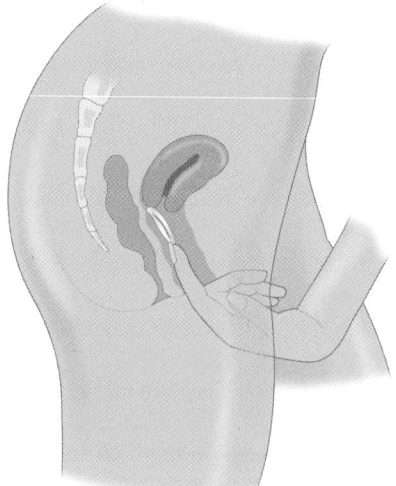

Figure 10.8 **NuvaRing**
The NuvaRing releases estrogen and progestin, preventing ovulation. The exact position of the NuvaRing in the vagina is not critical.

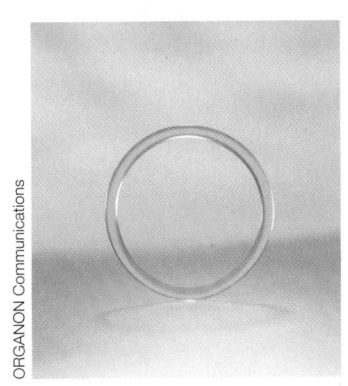

ORGANON Communications

Teenage mothers who used Implanon were less likely to become pregnant again.[30]

*How It Works*   Implanon works primarily by releasing progestin and suppressing ovulation. It also thickens cervical mucus, which inhibits sperm movement, inhibits the development and growth of the uterine lining, and limits secretion of progesterone during the second half of the menstrual cycle.

### Advantages

- Can be used while breast-feeding.
- Can be used by women who cannot take estrogen.
- Provides continuous long-lasting birth control without sterilization.
- No medicine to take every day.
- Does not interfere with sexual foreplay.
- Ability to become pregnant returns quickly once Implanon is removed.

### Disadvantages

- Irregular bleeding, especially in the first 6 to 12 months of use. After one year, one in three women stop having periods completely.
- Side effects, such as dizziness, acne, hair loss, headache, nausea, nervousness, pain at the insertion site.
- No protection against STIs.
- Change in appetite.
- Change in sex drive.
- Cysts on the ovaries.
- Depression.
- Discoloring or scarring of the skin over the implant.

If implanted during the first five days of a woman's period, Implanon protects against pregnancy immediately. Otherwise, a woman needs to use some form of backup birth control for the first week after getting the implant.

# Intrauterine Contraceptives

An **intrauterine device (IUD)** is a small piece of molded plastic, with a nylon string attached, that is inserted into the uterus through the cervix. It prevents pregnancy by interfering with implantation. Once widely used, IUDs became less popular after most brands were removed from the market because of serious complications such as pelvic infection and infertility. The ParaGuard IUD, which contains copper, protects against pregnancy for 12 years. As confirmed in a recent study, neither copper IUDs nor those releasing levonorgestrel increase a woman's risk of breast cancer.[31]

## Mirena (Hormonal IUD)

The Mirena intrauterine system consists of a T-shaped device inserted in the uterus by a physician. It releases a continuous low dose of progestin and provides five years of protection from pregnancy. Used in Europe, Asia, and Latin America for years, it is 99 percent effective.

Mirena is increasingly being used, not just for contraception, but as an alternative to hysterectomy for extremely heavy menstrual bleeding and as a treatment for problems such as iron-deficiency anemia.

*How It Works*   A physician must insert the Mirena in a woman's uterus. In a five-year clinical trial, about 5 in every 100 women reported that the Mirena had slipped out of the uterus. Users should check for the string that extends from the device through the vagina at least once a month.

### Advantages

- Highly effective at preventing pregnancy.
- No need to think about contraception for five years.
- Allows sexual spontaneity; neither partner can feel it.
- Starts working immediately.
- New mothers can breast-feed while using it.
- Periods become shorter and lighter or stop altogether.
- Low incidence of side effects.
- Can be removed at any time.

### Disadvantages

- Spotting or breakthrough bleeding in first three to six months.
- No protection against STIs.
- Potential side effects include acne, headaches, nausea, breast tenderness, mood changes.

**intrauterine device (IUD)** A device inserted into the uterus through the cervix to prevent pregnancy by interfering with implantation.

- Increased risk of benign ovarian cysts.
- May take up to a year for fertility to return after discontinuation.

# Fertility Awareness Methods

Awareness of a woman's cyclic fertility can help in both contraception and conception. The different methods of birth control based on a woman's menstrual cycle are sometimes referred to as *natural family planning* or *fertility awareness methods*. They include the calendar method, the basal-body-temperature method, and the cervical mucus method. New fertility monitors that use saliva to determine time of ovulation can improve the accuracy of these methods.

Women's menstrual cycles vary greatly. To use one of the fertility awareness methods, a woman must know and understand her cycle. She should track her cycle for at least eight months—marking day one (the day bleeding begins) on a calendar and counting the length of each cycle. Figure 10.9 shows the days in a 28-day cycle when abstinence or other contraceptive methods would be necessary.

*How It Works* The calendar method, often called the **rhythm method**, is based on counting the woman's safe days based on her individual menstrual cycle. The basal-body-temperature method determines the safe days based on the woman's *basal body temperature*, which rises after ovulation. The cervical mucus method, also called the *ovulation method*, is based on observation of changes in the consistency of the woman's vaginal mucus throughout her menstrual cycle. The period of maximum fertility occurs when the mucus is smooth and slippery.

### Advantages
- No expense.
- No side effects.
- No need for a prescription, medical visit, or fittings.
- Nothing to insert, swallow, or check.

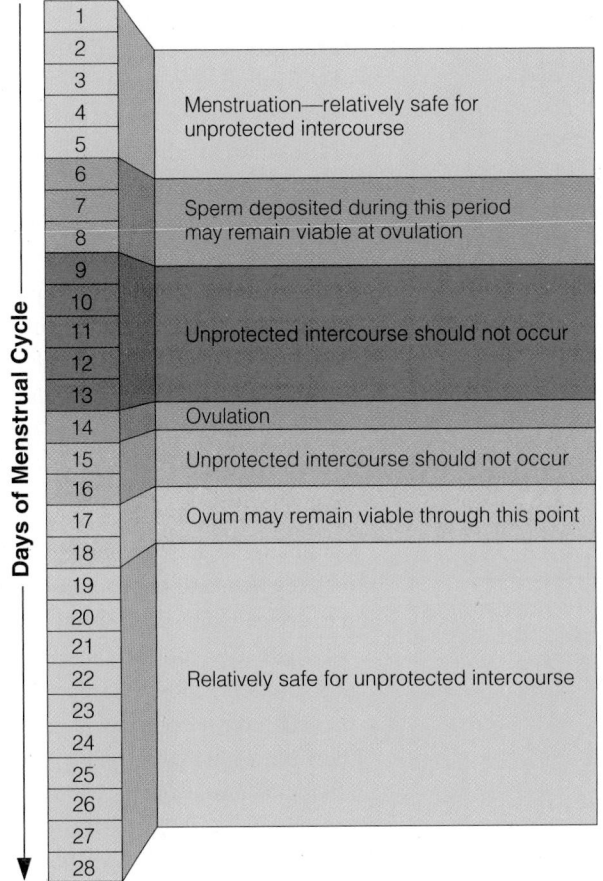

Figure 10.9 **Safe and Unsafe Days**
Events in the menstrual cycle determine the relatively safe days for avoiding pregnancy in unprotected intercourse.

*Days of Menstrual Cycle*

|  |  |
|-----|-------|
| 1–5 | Menstruation—relatively safe for unprotected intercourse |
| 6–8 | Sperm deposited during this period may remain viable at ovulation |
| 9–13 | Unprotected intercourse should not occur |
| 14 | Ovulation |
| 15–16 | Unprotected intercourse should not occur |
| 17 | Ovum may remain viable through this point |
| 18–28 | Relatively safe for unprotected intercourse |

- No effect on fertility.
- Complies with the teachings of the Roman Catholic Church.

### Disadvantages
- Less reliable than other forms of birth control.
- Couples must abstain from vaginal intercourse 8 to 11 days a month or use some form of contraception.
- Conscientious planning and scheduling are essential.
- May not work for women with irregular menstrual cycles.
- Some women find the mucus or temperature methods difficult to use.

**rhythm method** A birth control method in which sexual intercourse is avoided during those days of the menstrual cycle in which fertilization is most likely to occur.

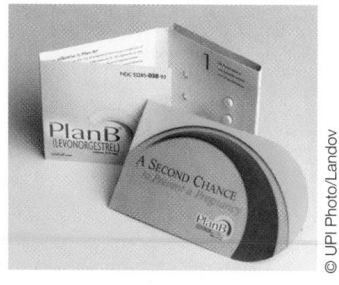

Emergency contraception can prevent unintended pregnancy after unprotected intercourse or when another form of contraception fails.

© UPI Photo/Landov

# Emergency Contraception

**Emergency contraception (EC)** is the use of a method of contraception to prevent unintended pregnancy after unprotected intercourse or the failure of another form of contraception, such as a condom breaking or slipping off. EC is available without prescription to women as young as 17. However, EC remains controversial because, unlike other contraceptives, it prevents pregnancy after fertilization has occurred. EC has proved extremely safe in almost all women, as confirmed by numerous health organizations, including the World Health Organization and the American College of Obstetricians and Gynecologists.

Combination estrogen-progestin pills, progestin-only pills, and the copper-bearing intrauterine device (IUD) have been used as methods of emergency contraception for decades. The progestin-only pills, referred to as Plan B, have proved more effective with fewer side effects than the combination pills.[32] Plan B morning-after pills are available without a prescription for anyone over age 17. Plan B, which should be taken within five days (120 hours) of unprotected sex, can reduce the risk of pregnancy up to 89 percent. An alternative agent, ulipristal acetate, also has proven effective if taken up to five days after unprotected intercourse.[33] The most common side effects are headache, nausea, and abdominal pain.[34] Men can and do purchase emergency contraception for their partners.[35]

Most women can safely use emergency contraception pills (ECPs), even if they cannot use birth control pills as their regular method of birth control. (Although ECPs use the same hormones as birth control pills, not all brands of birth control pills can be used for emergency contraception.) Some women may experience spotting or a full menstrual period a few days after taking ECPs, depending on where they were in their cycle when they began therapy. Most women have their next period at the expected time.

The easier availability of EC has not yet resulted in a decrease in unintended pregnancies because many women, particularly foreign-born Hispanic women, women with incomes below the poverty level, and women who did not complete high school, are unaware of this option. Providing an advance supply of emergency contraception to teens who have given birth may lower their odds of becoming pregnant again.[36]

Among sexually active college women, 11 percent report having used emergency contraception in the past year. According to a national survey of colleges and universities, slightly more than half of student health centers offer emergency contraception. The primary reasons for not dispensing EC are religious affiliation, insufficient staff, and lack of funding. None of the two-year colleges surveyed provide EC. More public institutions, rural schools, four-year institutions, and schools with enrollments smaller than 15,000 are offering EC than in the past.

Among college students who have heard of emergency contraception, few say they know "quite a bit" or "a lot" about it, know if it is available on campus, or are aware of where to obtain EC off-campus. In a recent survey of University of Michigan undergraduates, more than nine in ten knew of EC, yet only 10 percent of the female respondents said that their health-care providers had spoken to them about EC in a routine health visit. A majority—60 percent—felt EC should be available over-the-counter, and a third indicated they would purchase EC in advance "just in case."

***How It Works*** Emergency contraception pills stop pregnancy in the same way as other hormonal contraceptives: They delay or inhibit ovulation, inhibit fertilization, or block implantation of a fertilized egg, depending on a woman's phase of the menstrual cycle. They have no effect once a pregnancy has been established.

Combined ECPs may be moderately effective even if started between the third and fifth days (up to 120 hours) after unprotected sexual intercourse or contraceptive failure. At least one EC agent, levonorgestrel, can be used in a single dose (1.5 mg) rather than two doses of .75 mg 12 hours apart.

**emergency contraception (EC)** Types of oral contraceptive pills, usually taken within 72 hours after intercourse, that can prevent pregnancy.

The morning-after pill also may be safe for use as a regular birth control method and may appeal to women who do not have sex regularly and who could use it before or after sex. However, it is not as effective as regular birth control pills, patches, or rings, with an estimated 5 percent risk of unintentional pregnancy each year. The most common side effect is irregular bleeding.[37]

# Sterilization

The most popular method of birth control among married couples in the United States is **sterilization** (surgery to end a person's reproductive capability). Each year an estimated 1 million men and women in the United States undergo sterilization procedures. Fewer than 25 percent ever seek reversal.

## Male Sterilization

In men, the cutting of the vas deferens, the tube that carries sperm from one of the testes into the urethra for ejaculation, is called **vasectomy**. During the 15- or 20-minute office procedure, done under a local anesthetic, the doctor makes small incisions in the scrotum, lifts up each vas deferens, cuts it, and ties off the ends to block the flow of sperm (Figure 10.10). Sperm continue to form, but they are broken down and absorbed by the body.

The man usually experiences some local pain, swelling, and discoloration for about a week after the procedure. More serious complications, including the formation of a blood clot in the scrotum (which usually disappears without treatment), infection, and an inflammatory reaction, occur in a small percentage of cases.

Sometimes men want to reverse their vasectomies, usually because they want to have children with a new spouse. Although anyone who chooses to have a vasectomy should consider it permanent, surgical reversal (*vasovasostomy*) is sometimes successful. New microsurgical techniques have led to annual pregnancy rates for the wives of men having undergone vasovasostomies of about 50 percent, depending on such factors as the doctor's expertise and the time elapsed since the vasectomy.

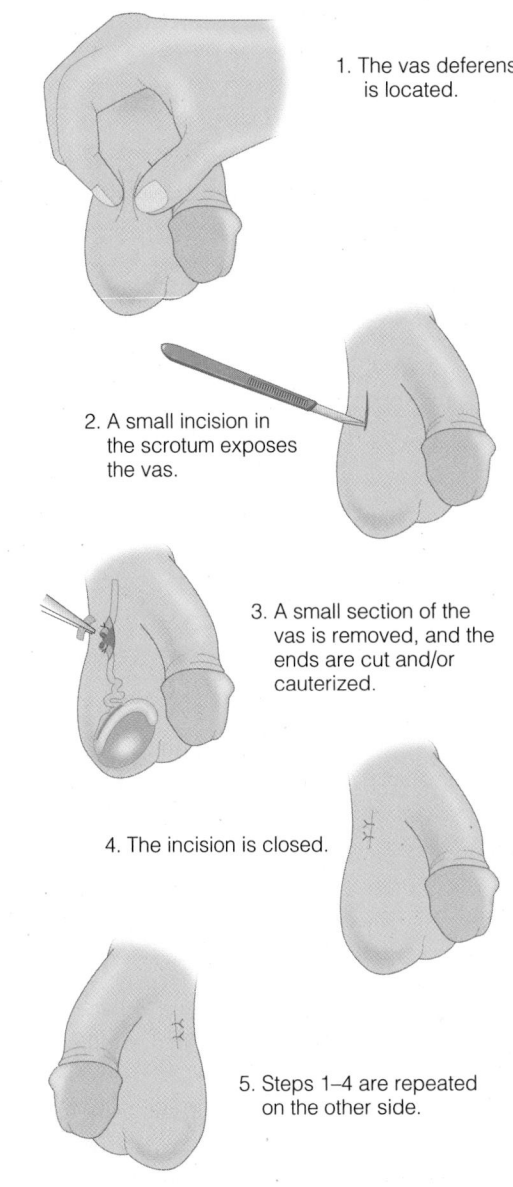

Figure 10.10 **Male Sterilization, or Vasectomy**

1. The vas deferens is located.

2. A small incision in the scrotum exposes the vas.

3. A small section of the vas is removed, and the ends are cut and/or cauterized.

4. The incision is closed.

5. Steps 1–4 are repeated on the other side.

## Female Sterilization

Eleven million U.S. women ages 15 to 44 rely on tubal sterilization for contraception. An estimated 750,000 tubal sterilization procedures are performed each year in the United States. The average age of sterilization is about 30. Female sterilization procedures modify the fallopian tubes, which each month normally carry an egg from the ovaries to the uterus. The two terms used to describe female sterilization are **tubal ligation** (the cutting or tying of the fallopian tubes) and **tubal occlusion** (the blocking

**sterilization** A surgical procedure to end a person's reproductive capability.

**vasectomy** A surgical sterilization procedure in which each vas deferens is cut and tied shut to stop the passage of sperm to the urethra for ejaculation.

**tubal ligation** The suturing or tying shut of the fallopian tubes to prevent pregnancy.

**tubal occlusion** The blocking of the fallopian tubes to prevent pregnancy.

## Figure 10.11 Female Sterilization, or Tubal Ligation

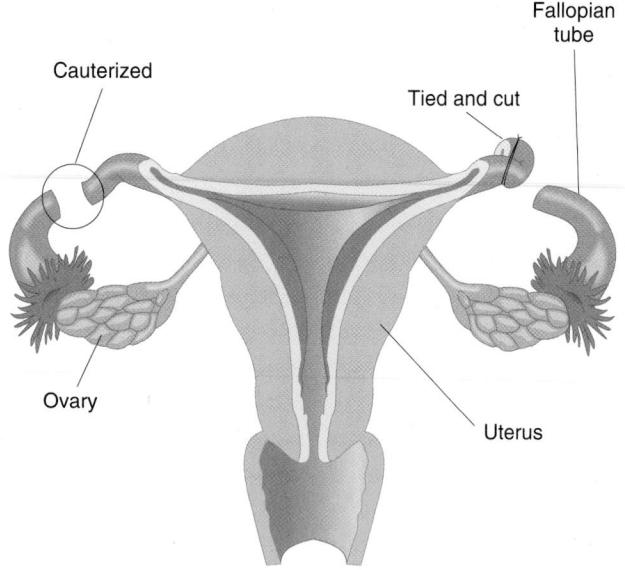

Cauterized

Fallopian tube

Tied and cut

Ovary

Uterus

**laparoscopy** A surgical sterilization procedure in which the fallopian tubes are observed with a laparoscope inserted through a small incision, and then cut or blocked.

of the tubes). The tubes may be cut or sealed with thread, a clamp, or a clip, or by electrical coagulation to prevent the passage of eggs from the ovaries (Figure 10.11). They also can be blocked with bands of silicone.

One of the common methods of tubal ligation or occlusion uses **laparoscopy**, commonly called *belly-button* or *band-aid surgery*. This procedure is done on an outpatient basis and takes 15 to 30 minutes. A lighted tube called a laparoscope is inserted through a half-inch incision made right below the navel, giving the doctor a view of the fallopian tubes. Using surgical instruments that may be inserted through the laparoscope or through other tiny incisions, the doctor then cuts or seals the tubes, most commonly by electrical coagulation.

The cumulative failure rate of tubal sterilization is about 1.85 percent during a ten-year period. Complications include problems with anesthesia, hemorrhage, organ damage, and mortality.

***Essure*** Essure involves placement of small, flexible microcoils into the fallopian tubes via the vagina by a physician. Unlike other methods, it does not require the risks of general anesthesia and surgery. The procedure itself does not require incisions and takes an average of about 35 minutes. Recovery occurs quickly. In clinical trials, about 90 percent of women returned to work within 24 hours. For the first three months after insertion, women should use

another form of contraception. An X-ray called a hysterosalpingogram must confirm that the inserts are correctly placed and the fallopian tubes are completely blocked.

Like traditional forms of tubal ligation, Essure cannot be reversed. It is recommended only for women who definitely do not want more children and especially for those with medical and health problems (such as diabetes, heart disease, or obesity) that make surgery and anesthesia more dangerous. There is a risk that the micro-inserts may not be placed correctly at the first attempt (this occurred in 14 percent of women in one study). Long-term data on the effectiveness of Essure are not yet available.

### Advantages

- Offers permanent protection against unwanted pregnancy.

- No effect on sex drive in men or women. Many couples report greater sexual activity and pleasure because they no longer have to worry about pregnancy or deal with contraceptives.

- Vasectomy and tubal ligation are performed as outpatient procedures, with a quick recovery time.

- Use of Essure requires no incision, so there's less discomfort and very rapid recovery. Essure may be an option for women with chronic health conditions, such as obesity, diabetes, or heart disease.

### Disadvantages

- All procedures should be considered permanent and used only if both partners are certain they want no more children.

- No protection against STIs.

- Must use another form of birth control for first three months.

- Many long-term risks remain unknown, but there is no evidence of any link between vasectomy and prostate cancer.

## Abortion

No woman in any country ever chooses to be in a situation where she has to consider abortion. But if faced with an unwanted pregnancy, many women consider *elective abortion* as an option.

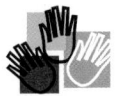 The U.S. abortion rate, which has declined in the last two decades, still remains higher than that of many Western countries, including Canada, Great Britain, the Netherlands, and Sweden. Although there is no one single or simple explanation for this difference, researchers focus on America's high rate of unintended pregnancies. In many nations with fewer unwanted pregnancies and lower abortion rates, contraceptives are generally easier and cheaper to obtain, and early sex education strongly emphasizes their importance.

After rising steadily through the 1970s, the number of legal abortions leveled off in the 1980s and has declined since. Although women of all backgrounds have abortions, abortion in the United States is most likely to occur among single women, racial or ethnic minorities, low-income women, and women who have had at least one child.

Claims that abortion increases the risk of breast cancer, based on retrospective studies that are less accurate because they rely on individuals' recall, have proved false. Research has found no correlation between the termination of a pregnancy, whether induced or spontaneous, and increased risk of breast cancer.

## Thinking Through the Options

A woman faced with an unwanted pregnancy—often alone, unwed, and desperate—can find it extremely difficult to decide what to do. The political debate over the right to life almost always is secondary to practical and emotional matters, such as the quality of her relationship with the baby's father, their capacity to provide for the child, the impact on any children she already has, and other important life issues.

Giving up her child for adoption is an option for women who do not feel abortion is right for them. Because the number of would-be adoptive parents greatly exceeds the number of available newborns, some women considering adoption may feel pressured by offers of money from couples eager to adopt. Others, particularly minority women, may feel cultural pressures to keep a child—regardless of their age, economic situation, or ability to care for an infant. Advocates of adoption reform are pressing for mandatory counseling for all pregnant women considering adoption (available now in agency-arranged, but not private, adoptions) and for extending the period of time during which a new mother can change her mind about giving up her child for adoption.

## Medical Abortion

The term **medical abortion** describes the use of drugs, also called *abortifacients*, to terminate a pregnancy. In 2000, the abortion pill mifepristone (*Mifeprex*), formerly known as RU-486, became available for use in the United States. Mifepristone, which is 97 percent effective in inducing abortion, blocks progesterone, the hormone that prepares the uterine lining for pregnancy. Two days after taking this compound, a woman takes a prostaglandin to increase uterine contractions. The uterine lining is expelled along with the fertilized egg (Figure 10.12).

Women have compared the discomfort of this experience to severe menstrual cramps. Common side effects include excessive bleeding, nausea, fatigue, abdominal pain, and dizziness. About 1 woman in 100 requires a blood transfusion. The FDA has warned doctors about rare but deadly bloodstream infections in women using mifepristone. The rate of infection is about 1 in 100,000 uses, comparable to infection risks with surgical abortions and childbirth.

Although condemned by right-to-life advocates, abortion medications may in time lower the public profile of pregnancy termination. They are not painless, cheap, or equally available to all, but they do offer women a chance to carry through on their personal choice in greater privacy and safety.

Medical abortion does not require anesthesia and can be performed very early in pregnancy. However, women experience more cramping and bleeding during medical abortion than during surgical abortion, and bleeding lasts for a longer period.

## Other Abortion Methods

About half of all abortions (54 percent) are performed within the first 8 weeks of pregnancy. Only about 1 percent of abortions occur after 20 weeks. Medically, first-trimester abortion is less risky than childbirth. However, the likelihood

**medical abortion** Method of ending a pregnancy within nine weeks of conception using hormonal medications that cause expulsion of the fertilized egg.

## Figure 10.12 **Medical Abortion**

Mifepristone works by blocking the action of progesterone, a hormone produced by the ovaries that is necessary for the implantation and development of a fertilized egg.

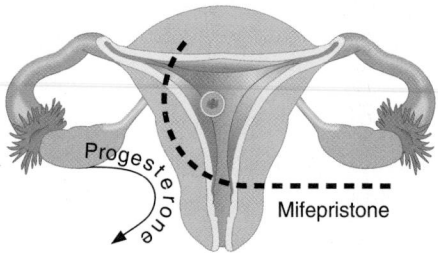

Step 1. Taken early in pregnancy, mifepristone blocks the action of progesterone and makes the body react as if it weren't pregnant.

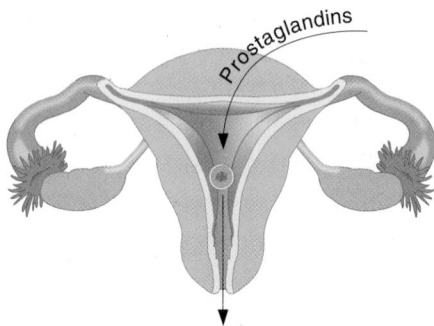

Step 2. Prostaglandins, taken two days later, cause the uterus to contract and the cervix to soften and dilate. As a result, the fertilized egg is expelled in 97 percent of cases.

**suction curettage** A procedure in which the contents of the uterus are removed by means of suction and scraping.

**dilation and evacuation (D and E)** A medical procedure in which the contents of the uterus are removed through the use of instruments.

(Figure 10.13). A *curette* (a spoon-shaped surgical instrument used for scraping) is used to check for complete removal of the contents of the uterus. With suction curettage, the risks of complication are low. Major complications, such as perforation of the uterus, occur in fewer than 1 in 100 cases.

For early second-trimester abortions, physicians generally use a technique called **dilation and evacuation (D and E)**, in which they open the cervix and use medical instruments to remove the fetus from the uterus. D and E procedures are performed under local or general anesthesia.

To induce abortion from week 16 to week 20, prostaglandins (natural substances found in most body tissues) are administered as vaginal suppositories or injected into the amniotic sac by inserting a needle through the abdominal wall. They induce uterine contractions, and the fetus and placenta are expelled within 24 hours. Injecting saline or urea solutions into the amniotic sac also can terminate the pregnancy by triggering contractions that expel the fetus and placenta. Sometimes vaginal suppositories or drugs that help the uterus contract are used. Complications from abortion techniques that induce labor include nausea, vomiting, diarrhea, tearing of the cervix, excessive bleeding, and possible shock and death.

## The Psychological Impact of Abortion

Abortion can have various psychological effects. As decades of research have shown, the primary emotion of women who have just had an abortion is relief. Although many women also express feelings of guilt or sadness, usually their anxiety levels drop to lower levels than immediately before the abortion. Women who experienced violence, including rape, or high anxiety levels prior to becoming pregnant have more anxiety symptoms following an abortion. A Scandinavian study recently found a higher prevalence of depression among young adult women who have had an abortion.

A woman's responses to abortion often change with passing days, weeks, months, or years. Anniversaries—of conception, of the date a woman found out she was pregnant, of the abortion, of the delivery date—can trigger memories and a

of complications increases when abortions are performed in the second trimester (the second three-month period) of pregnancy.

The majority of abortions performed in the United States today are surgical. **Suction curettage**, usually done from 7 to 13 weeks after the last menstrual period, involves the gradual dilation (opening) of the cervix, often by inserting into the cervix one or more sticks of *laminaria* (a sterilized seaweed that absorbs moisture and expands, thus gradually stretching the cervix). Some women feel pressure or cramping with the laminaria in place. Occasionally, the laminaria itself starts to bring on a miscarriage.

At the time of abortion, the laminaria is removed, and dilators are used to further enlarge the cervical opening, if needed. The physician inserts a suction tip into the cervix, and the uterine contents are drawn out via a vacuum system

sense of loss, but most women deal with these and move on with their lives.

The best predictor of psychological well-being after abortion is a woman's emotional well-being prior to pregnancy. At highest risk are women who have had a psychiatric illness, such as an anxiety disorder or clinical depression, prior to an abortion, and those whose abortions occurred among complicated circumstances (such as a rape, or coercion by parents or a partner). The vast majority of women manage to put the abortion into perspective as one of many life events.

## The Politics of Abortion

Abortion is one of the most controversial political, religious, and ethical issues of our time (see Health in the Headlines). The issues of when life begins, a woman's right to choose, and an unborn child's right to survival are among the most divisive Americans face. Abortions were legal in the United States until the 1860s. For decades after that, women who decided to terminate unwanted pregnancies did so by attempting to abort on their own or by obtaining illegal abortions—often performed by untrained individuals using unsanitary and unsafe procedures. In the late 1960s, some states changed their laws to make abortions legal. In 1973, the U.S. Supreme Court, following a 1970 ruling on the case of *Roe v. Wade* by the New York Supreme Court, said that an abortion in the first trimester of pregnancy was a decision between a woman and her physician and was protected by privacy laws. The Court further ruled that abortion during the second trimester could be performed on the basis of health risks and that abortion during the final trimester could be performed only for the sake of the mother's health.

The debate over abortion continues to stir passionate emotions, with pro-life supporters arguing that life begins at conception and that abortion is therefore immoral, and pro-choice advocates countering that an individual woman should have the right to make decisions about her body and health. The controversy over abortion has at times become violent: Physicians who perform abortions have been shot and killed; abortion clinics have been bombed,

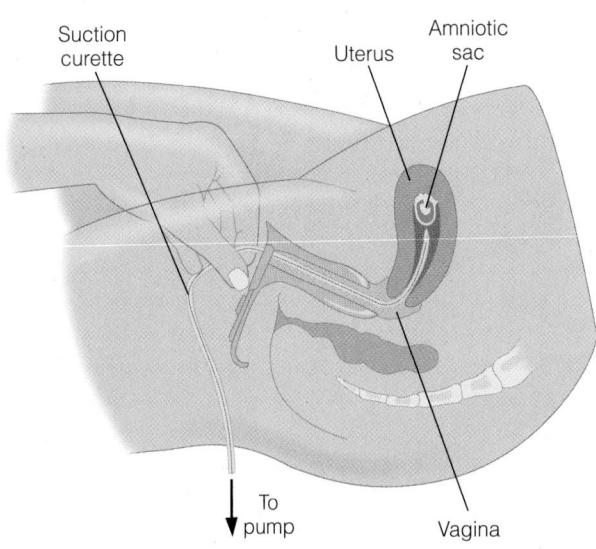

Figure 10.13 **Suction Curettage**
The contents of the uterus are extracted through the cervix with a vacuum apparatus.

wounding and killing patients and staff members. Although the majority of Americans continue to support abortion, many feel that it should be more restricted and difficult to obtain.

The Supreme Court has upheld a federal law banning "partial-birth" abortions, a late-term procedure involving the removal of a fetus from the uterus and the collapsing of its skull. Pro-life groups hailed this ruling as a step toward the overthrow of *Roe v. Wade*. More than 40 years after this landmark ruling, the controversy over abortion and the conflict between pro-lifers and pro-choicers remains intense.

## A Cross-Cultural Perspective

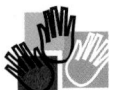 More than one in four pregnancies worldwide ends in abortion. Of the estimated 46 million global abortions, an estimated 20 million are illegal and lead to the death of about 70,000 women.

More than 50 countries now allow abortion up to at least the twelfth week of pregnancy. Some, such as Great Britain, permit it up to 24 weeks; others have no time limit. In recent years abortion has become more restrictive in terms of limits on timing, grounds, or methods in the United States, Russia, Hungary, and Poland.

**Health in the Headlines**

### Abortion

Abortion is one of the most controversial medical, political, religious, and ethical issues of our time. Access Global Health Watch, and search for the most recent articles on abortion. Choose one of the recent articles and use it as a starting point for a personal reflection on the topic. Record your thoughts in your online journal.

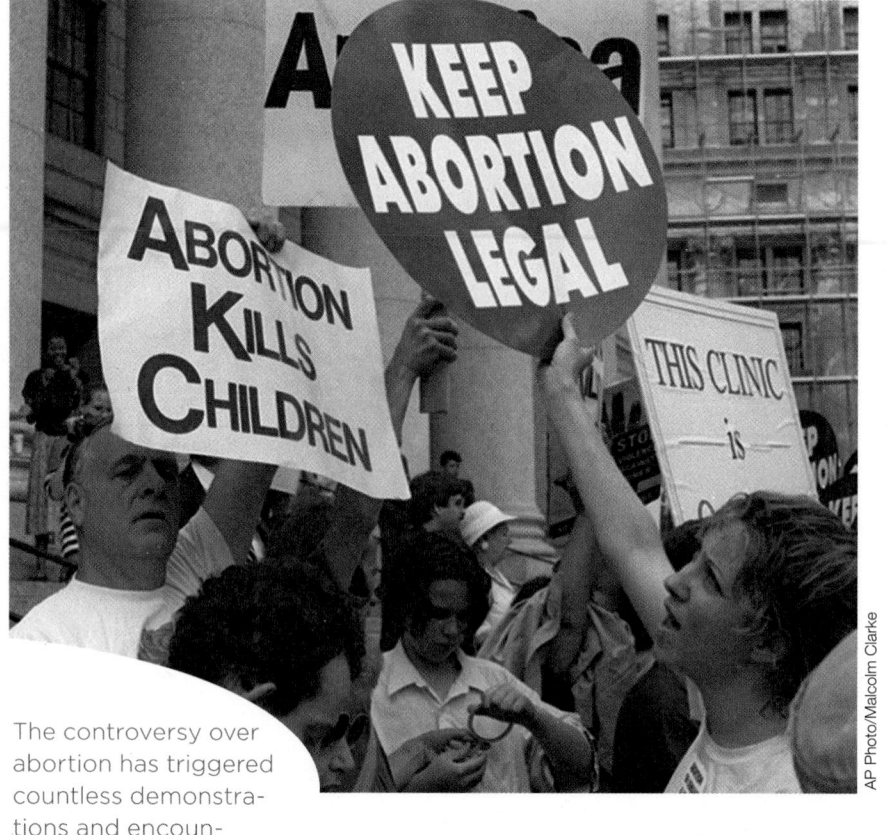

The controversy over abortion has triggered countless demonstrations and encounters between pro-choice and pro-life supporters.

AP Photo/Malcolm Clarke

Nicaragua and El Salvador have banned the practice outright. Romania has the world's highest abortion rate; three in four pregnancies are terminated. In the United States, Australia, Canada, Great Britain, and most of Western Europe, around 15 to 25 percent of pregnancies end in abortion.

## Childfree by Choice

More women and men are deliberately choosing to remain "childfree." According to the limited data available, single childfree women tend to be better educated, more cosmopolitan, less religious, and more professional than those in the general population. In general, childfree women are high achievers, often in demanding careers, who describe their work as exciting and satisfying. Childfree couples are predominantly urban, well-educated, and upper middle class, with egalitarian and long-running marriages.

Their reasons for not having children are diverse: a desire to maintain their freedom and have more time with their partners, career ambitions, concern about overpopulation and the fate of the earth. Some women cite the hostile work environment for mothers and the inadequacy of day care. Others say they're disillusioned with the have-it-all hopes of baby boomers and believe in a have-most-of-it philosophy.

## Pregnancy

Birth rates have risen to the highest ever recorded in the U.S. Births rose among all racial and age groups, including teenagers and unmarried women. Although the average age of mothers in the United States has risen, about 70 percent of babies are born to women in their twenties. Mothers are now averaging about two children each.

The number of never-married, college-educated career women who are becoming single parents has risen dramatically. They want children—with or without an ongoing relationship with a man—and may feel that, because of their age, they can't delay getting pregnant any longer.

### Preconception Care

The time *before* a child is conceived can be crucial in ensuring that an infant is born healthy, full-size, and full-term. Women who smoke, drink alcohol, take drugs, eat poorly, are too thin or too heavy, suffer from unrecognized infections or illnesses, or are exposed to toxins at work or home may start pregnancy with one or more strikes against them and their unborn babies. The best chance for lowering the infant mortality rate and preventing birth defects is before pregnancy. **Preconception care**—the enhancement of a woman's health and well-being prior to conception in order to ensure a healthy pregnancy and baby—includes risk assessment (evaluation of medical, genetic, and lifestyle risks), health promotion (such as teaching good nutrition), and interventions to reduce risk (such as treatment of infections and other diseases, and assistance in quitting smoking or drug use).

**preconception care** Health care to prepare for pregnancy.

## Home Pregnancy Tests

The sooner a woman realizes she is pregnant, the more she can do to take care of herself and her child. Home pregnancy tests detect the presence of human chorionic gonadotropin (hCG), which is secreted as the fertilized egg implants in the uterus. If the concentration of hCG is high enough, a woman will test positive for pregnancy. If the test is done too early, the result will be a false negative. A follow-up test a week later can usually confirm a pregnancy. Although home pregnancy tests are 85 to 95 percent accurate, medical laboratory tests provide definitive confirmation of a pregnancy.

## How a Woman's Body Changes during Pregnancy

The 40 weeks of pregnancy transform a woman's body. At the beginning of pregnancy, the woman's uterus becomes slightly larger, and the cervix becomes softer and bluish due to increased blood flow. Progesterone and estrogen trigger changes in the milk glands and ducts in the breasts, which increase in size and feel somewhat tender. The pressure of the growing uterus against the bladder causes a more frequent need to urinate. As the pregnancy progresses, the woman's skin stretches as her body shape changes, her center of gravity changes as her abdomen protrudes, and her internal organs shift as the baby grows (Figure 10.14). Pregnancy is typically divided into three-month periods called trimesters.

## How a Baby Grows

Silently and invisibly, over a nine-month period, a fertilized egg develops into a human being. When the zygote reaches the uterus, it's still smaller than the head of a pin. Once nestled into the spongy uterine lining, it becomes an **embryo**. The embryo takes on an elongated shape, rounded at one end. A sac called the **amnion** envelops it (see photo in Fig. 10.15). As water and other small molecules cross the amniotic membrane, the embryo floats freely in the absorbed fluid, cushioned from shocks and bumps. At nine weeks the embryo is called a **fetus**.

A special organ, the **placenta**, forms. Attached to the embryo by the umbilical cord, it supplies the growing baby with fluid and nutrients from the maternal bloodstream and carries waste back to the mother's body for disposal (Figure 10.15).

## Complications of Pregnancy

In about 10 to 15 percent of all pregnancies, there is increased risk of some problem, such as a baby's failure to grow normally. *Perinatology*, or maternal-fetal medicine, focuses on the special needs of high-risk mothers and their unborn babies. Perinatal centers, with state-of-the-art equipment and 24-hour staffs of specialists in this field, have been set up around the country.

**embryo** An organism in its early stage of development; in humans, the embryonic period lasts from the second to the eighth week of pregnancy.

**amnion** The innermost membrane of the sac enclosing the embryo or fetus.

**fetus** The human organism developing in the uterus from the ninth week until birth.

**placenta** An organ that develops after implantation and to which the embryo attaches, via the umbilical cord, for nourishment and waste removal.

## Figure 10.14   **Physiological Changes of Pregnancy**

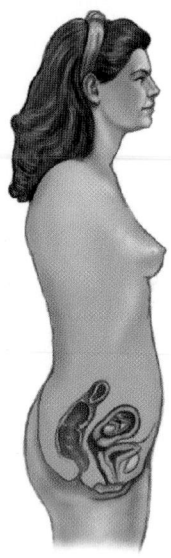

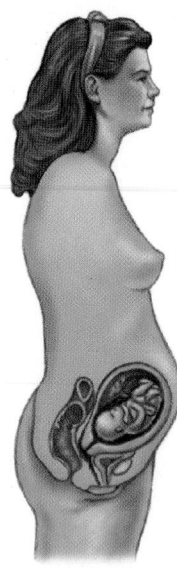

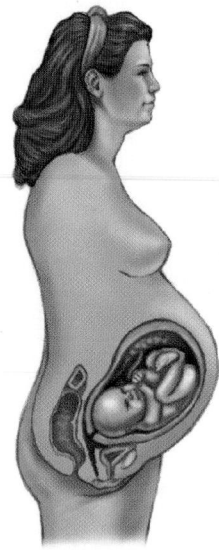

### First Trimester

Increased urination because of hormonal
  changes and the pressure of the enlarging
  uterus on the bladder.
Enlarged breasts as milk glands develop.
Darkening of the nipples and the area around them.
Nausea or vomiting, particularly in the morning,
  may occur.
Fatigue.
Increased vaginal secretions.
Pinching of the sciatic nerve, which runs from
  the buttocks down through the back of the legs,
  may occur as the pelvic bones widen and begin
  to separate.

### Second Trimester

Thickening of the waist as the
  uterus grows.
Weight gain.
Increase in total blood volume.
Slight increase in size and change
  in position of the heart.
Darkening of the pigment around
  the nipple and from the navel to the pubic region.
Darkening of the face.
Increased salivation and perspiration.
Secretion of colostrum from the breasts.

### Third Trimester

Increased urination because of
  pressure from the uterus.
Tightening of the uterine muscles
  (called Braxton-Hicks
  contractions).
Shortness of breath because of
  increased pressure by the uterus
  on the lungs and diaphragm.
Interrupted sleep because of the
  baby's movements or the need to urinate.
Descending ("dropping") of the baby's
  head into the pelvis about two to
  four weeks before birth.
Navel pushed out.

## Figure 10.15   **The Placenta**

The placenta supplies the growing embryo with fluid and nutrients from the maternal bloodstream and carries waste
back for disposal.

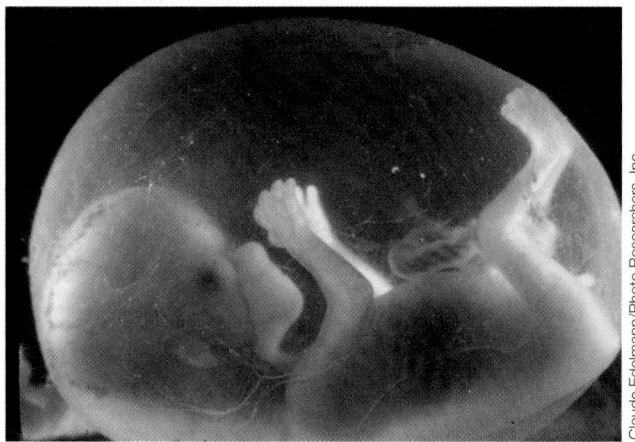

Claude Edelmann/Photo Researchers, Inc.

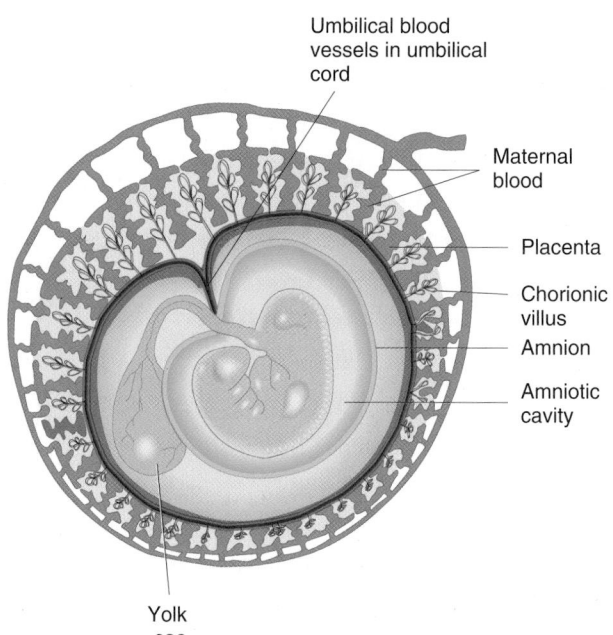

Umbilical blood
vessels in umbilical
cord

Maternal
blood

Placenta

Chorionic
villus

Amnion

Amniotic
cavity

Yolk
sac

Several of the most frequent potential complications of pregnancy are discussed next.

*Ectopic Pregnancy*  Any woman who is of childbearing age, has had intercourse, and feels abdominal pain with no reasonable cause may have an **ectopic pregnancy**. In this type of pregnancy, the fertilized egg remains in the fallopian tube instead of traveling to the uterus. Ectopic, or tubal, pregnancies have increased dramatically in recent years, now accounting for 2 percent of all reported pregnancies. STIs, particularly chlamydia infections (discussed in Chapter 11), have become a major cause of ectopic pregnancy. Other risk factors include previous pelvic surgery, particularly involving the fallopian tubes; pelvic inflammatory disease; infertility; and use of an IUD.

*Miscarriage*  About 10 to 20 percent of pregnancies end in **miscarriage**, or spontaneous abortion, before the twentieth week of gestation. Major genetic disorders may be responsible for 33 to 50 percent of pregnancy losses. The most common cause is an abnormal number of chromosomes. About 0.5 to 1 percent of women suffer three or more miscarriages, possibly because of genetic, anatomic, hormonal, infectious, or autoimmune factors. An estimated 70 to 90 percent of women who miscarry eventually become pregnant again.

*Infections*  The infectious disease most clearly linked to birth defects is **rubella** (German measles). All women should be vaccinated against this disease at least three months prior to conception, to protect themselves and any children they may bear. (See Chapter 16 for more on immunization.) The most common prenatal infection today is *cytomegalovirus*. This infection produces mild flu-like symptoms in adults but can cause brain damage, retardation, liver disease, cerebral palsy, hearing problems, and other malformations in unborn babies.

STIs, such as syphilis, gonorrhea, and genital herpes, can be particularly dangerous during pregnancy if not recognized and treated. If a woman has a herpes outbreak around the date her baby is due, her physician will deliver the baby by caesarean section to prevent infecting the baby. HIV infection endangers both a pregnant woman and her unborn baby, and all pregnant women and new mothers should be aware of the HIV epidemic, the risks to them

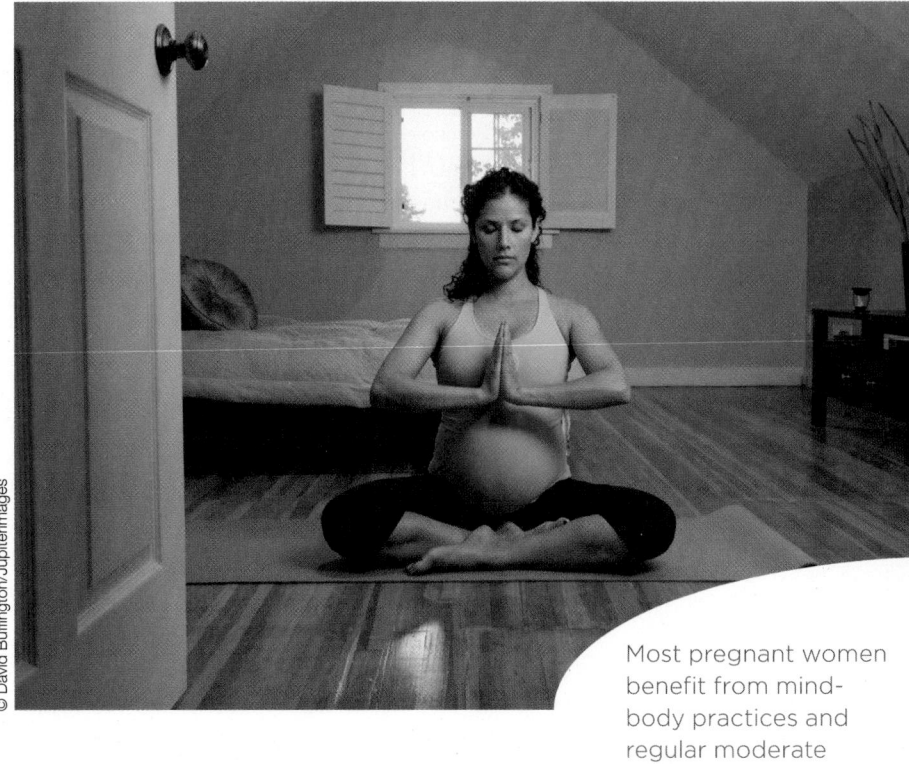

Most pregnant women benefit from mind-body practices and regular moderate exercise.

and their babies, and the availability of anonymous testing.

*Genetic Disorders*  In some sense, each of us is a carrier of a genetic problem. Every individual has an estimated four to six defective genes, but the chances of passing them on to a child are slim. Almost all are recessive, which means they are "masked" by a more influential dominant gene. The likelihood of a child inheriting the same faulty recessive gene from both parents is remote—unless the parents are so closely related that they have very similar genetic makeup.

The child of a parent with an abnormal dominant gene has a 50 percent likelihood of inheriting it. The most common of such defects are minor, such as the growth of an extra finger or toe. However, some single-gene defects can be fatal. Huntington's chorea, for example, is a degenerative disease that in the past was usually not diagnosed until midlife.

Genetic tests can identify "carriers" of abnormal recessive genes for diseases such as sickle-cell anemia (the most common genetic disorder among African Americans), beta-thalassemia (found in families of Mediterranean origin), and Tay-Sachs (found in Jews of Eastern European origin). Two carriers of the same abnormal

**ectopic pregnancy** A pregnancy in which the fertilized egg has implanted itself outside the uterine cavity, usually in the fallopian tube.

**miscarriage** A pregnancy that terminates before the twentieth week of gestation; also called spontaneous abortion.

**rubella** An infectious disease that may cause birth defects if contracted by a pregnant woman; also called German measles.

recessive genes can pass such problems on to their children.

The American College of Obstetricians and Gynecologists recommends a blood test for biochemical markers and ultrasound to screen for chromosomal abnormalities for all women in their first trimester. More invasive techniques, such as chorionic villus sampling (CVS) and second-trimester amniocentesis, can provide a precise diagnosis but carry a small risk for pregnancy loss.

*Premature Labor*   Approximately 10 percent of all babies are born too soon (before the thirty-seventh week of pregnancy). According to researchers, prematurity is the main underlying cause of stillbirth and infant deaths within the first few weeks after birth. Bed rest, close monitoring, and, if necessary, medications for at-risk women can buy more time in the womb for their babies. But women must recognize the warning signs of **premature labor**—dull, low backache; a feeling of tightness or pressure on the lower abdomen; and intestinal cramps, sometimes with diarrhea. Low–birth weight premature babies face the highest risks, but comprehensive, enriched programs can reduce developmental and health problems.

# Childbirth

A generation ago, delivering a baby was something a doctor did in a hospital. Today parents can choose from many birthing options, including a birth attendant, who can be a physician or a nurse-midwife, and a birthing center, hospital, or home birth.

## Preparing for Childbirth

The most widespread method of childbirth preparation is the **Lamaze method** (*psychoprophylaxis*). Fernand Lamaze, a French doctor, instructed women to respond to labor contractions with prelearned, controlled breathing techniques. As the intensity of each contraction increases, the laboring woman concentrates on increasing her breathing rate in a prescribed way. Her partner coaches her during each contraction and helps her cope with discomfort.

Women who attend prenatal classes are less likely to undergo caesarean deliveries and more likely to breast-feed. They also tend to have fewer complications and require fewer medications. However, painkillers or anesthesia are always an option if labor is longer or more painful than expected. The lower body can be numbed with an *epidural block*, which involves injecting an anesthetic into the membrane around the spinal cord, or a spinal block, in which the injection goes directly into the spinal canal. General anesthesia is usually used only for emergency caesarean births.

## Labor and Delivery

There are three stages of **labor**. The first starts with *effacement* (thinning) and *dilation* (opening up) of the cervix. Effacement is measured in percentages, and dilation in centimeters or finger-widths. Around this time, the amniotic sac of fluids usually breaks, a sign that the woman should call her doctor or midwife.

The first contractions of the early, or *latent*, phase of labor are usually not uncomfortable; they last 15 to 30 seconds, occur every 15 to 30 minutes, and gradually increase in intensity and frequency. The most difficult contractions come after the cervix is dilated to about 8 centimeters, as the woman feels greater pressure from the fetus. The first stage ends when the cervix is completely dilated to a diameter of 10 centimeters (or five finger-widths) and the baby is ready to come down the birth canal (Figure 10.16). For women having their first baby, this first stage of labor averages 12 to 13 hours. Women having another child often experience shorter first-stage labor.

When the cervix is completely dilated, the second stage of labor occurs, during which the baby moves into the vagina, or birth canal, and out of the mother's body. As this stage begins, women who have gone through childbirth preparation training often feel a sense of relief from the acute pain of the transition phase and at the prospect of giving birth.

This second stage can take up to an hour or more. Strong contractions may last 60 to 90 seconds and occur every two to three minutes. As the baby's head descends, the mother feels an urge to push. By bearing down, she helps the baby complete its passage to the outside.

**premature labor** Labor that occurs after the twentieth week but before the thirty-seventh week of pregnancy.

**Lamaze method** A method of childbirth preparation taught to expectant parents to help the woman cope with the discomfort of labor; combines breathing and psychological techniques.

**labor** The process leading up to birth: effacement and dilation of the cervix; the movement of the baby into and through the birth canal, accompanied by strong contractions; and contraction of the uterus and expulsion of the placenta after the birth.

Figure 10.16 **Birth**

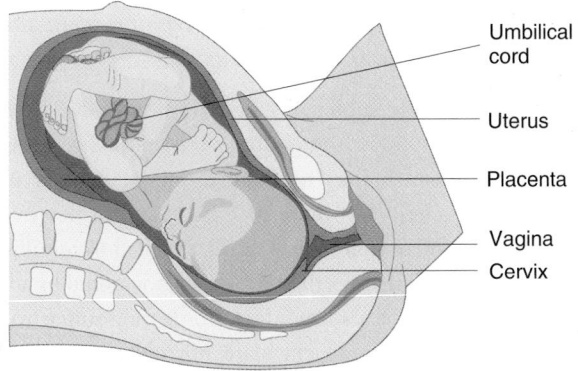

Umbilical cord

Uterus

Placenta

Vagina

Cervix

(a) The cervix is partially dilated, and the baby's head enters the birth canal.

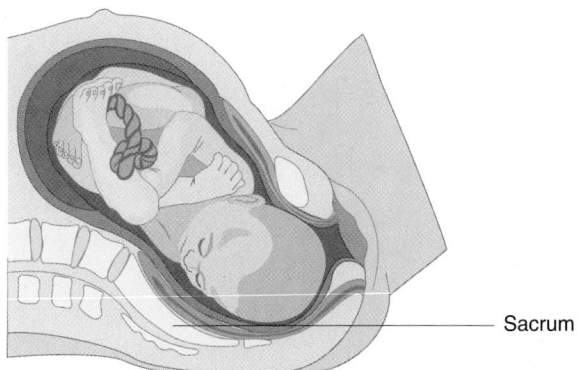

Sacrum

(b) The cervix is nearly completely dilated. The baby's head rotates so that it can move through the birth canal.

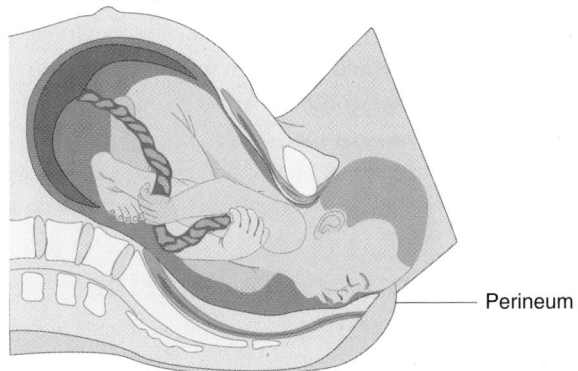

Perineum

(c) The baby's head extends as it reaches the vaginal opening, and the head and the rest of the body pass through the birth canal.

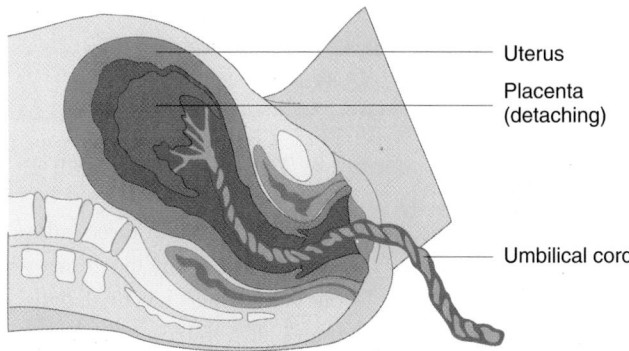

Uterus

Placenta (detaching)

Umbilical cord

(d) After the baby is born, the placenta detaches from the uterus and is expelled from the woman's body.

As the baby's head appears, or *crowns*, the doctor may perform an *episiotomy*—an incision from the lower end of the vagina toward the anus to enlarge the vaginal opening. The purpose of the episiotomy is to prevent the baby's head from causing an irregular tear in the vagina, but routine episiotomies have been criticized as unnecessary. Women may be able to avoid this procedure by trying different birthing positions or having an attendant massage the perineal tissue.

Usually the baby's head emerges first, then its shoulders, then its body. With each contraction, a new part is born. However, the baby can be in a more difficult position, facing up rather than down, or with the feet or buttocks first (a *breech birth*), and a caesarean birth may then be necessary.

In the third stage of labor, the uterus contracts firmly after the birth of the baby and, usually within five minutes, the placenta separates from the uterine wall. The woman may bear down to help expel the placenta, or the doctor may exert gentle external pressure. If an episiotomy has been performed, the doctor sews up the incision. To help the uterus contract and return to its normal size, it may be massaged manually, or the baby may be put to the mother's breast to stimulate contraction of the uterus.

## Caesarean Birth

In a **caesarean delivery** (also referred to as a *caesarean section*, or *C-section*), the doctor lifts the baby out of the woman's body through an incision made in the lower abdomen and uterus. The most common reason for caesarean birth is *failure to progress*, a vague term indicating that labor has gone on too long and may put the baby or mother at risk. Other reasons include the baby's position (if feet or buttocks are first) and signs that the fetus is in danger.

**caesarean delivery** The surgical procedure in which an infant is delivered through an incision made in the abdominal wall and uterus.

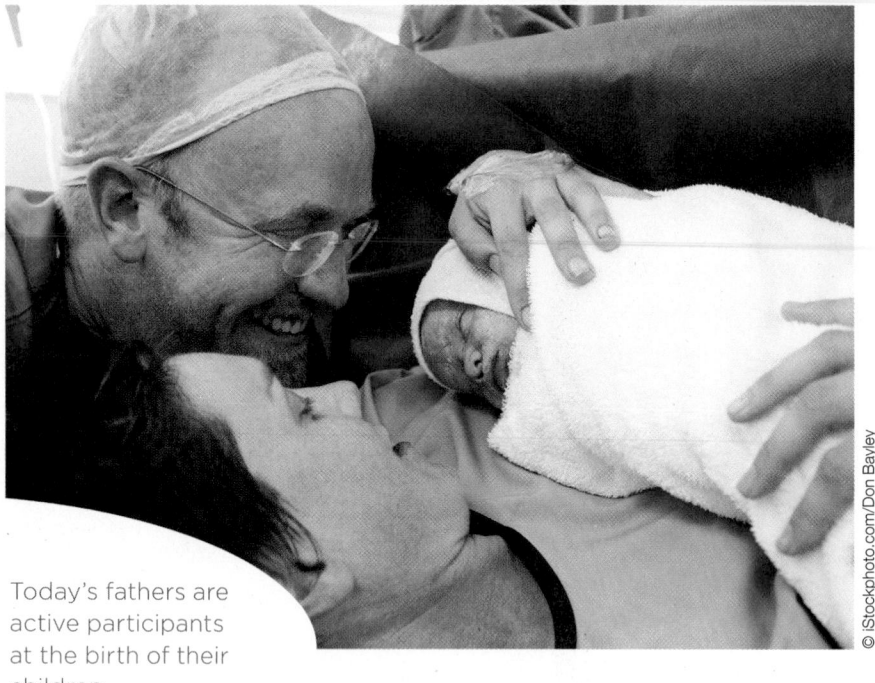

Today's fathers are active participants at the birth of their children.

©iStockphoto.com/Don Bayley

Thirty years ago, only 5 percent of babies born in America were delivered by caesarean birth. Now, nearly one in three babies is delivered by this method, many in women who had a previous C-section. A recent analysis of data on more than half a million caesarean births found that more than 95 percent are performed because of risk factors complicating labor or delivery.

# Infertility

The World Health Organization defines **infertility** as the failure to conceive after one year of unprotected intercourse. Infertility affects one in seven couples. Women between ages 35 and 44 are about twice as likely to have fertility problems as women ages 30 to 34.

Infertility is a problem of the couple, not of the individual man or woman. In 40 percent of cases, infertility is caused by female problems, in 40 percent by male problems, in 10 percent by a combination of male and female problems, and in 10 percent by unexplained causes. A thorough diagnostic workup can reveal a cause for infertility in 90 percent of cases.

In women, the most common causes of subfertility or infertility are age, abnormal menstrual patterns, suppression of ovulation, and blocked

**infertility** The inability to conceive a child.

**artificial insemination** The introduction of viable sperm into the vagina by artificial means for the purpose of inducing conception.

fallopian tubes. A woman's fertility peaks between ages 20 and 30 and then drops quickly: by 20 percent after 30, by 50 percent after 35, and by 95 percent after 40.

Male subfertility or infertility is usually linked to either the quantity or the quality of sperm, which may be inactive, misshapen, or insufficient (less than 20 million sperm per milliliter of semen in an ejaculation of 3 to 5 milliliters). Sometimes the problem is hormonal or a blockage of a sperm duct. Some men suffer from the inability to ejaculate normally, or from retrograde ejaculation, in which some of the semen travels in the wrong direction, back into the body of the male.

Infertility can have an enormous emotional impact. Many women long to experience pregnancy and childbirth and feel great loss if they cannot conceive. Women in their thirties and forties fear that their biological clock is running out of time. Men may be confused and surprised by the intensity of their partner's emotions.

## Options for Infertile Couples

The treatment of infertility has become a $2 billion a year enterprise in the United States. The odds of successful pregnancy range from 30 to 70 percent, depending on the specific cause of infertility. One result of successful infertility treatments has been a boom in multiple births, including quintuplets and sextuplets. Multiple births are associated with greater risk, both to the babies—including prematurity, low birth weight, neonatal death, and lifelong disability—and to the mothers, including caesarean section and hemorrhage.

*Artificial Insemination* **Artificial insemination**—the introduction of viable sperm into the vagina by artificial means—is used primarily by couples in which the husband is infertile. Some states do not recognize such children as legitimate; others do, but only if the woman's husband gives consent for the insemination.

*Assisted Reproductive Technology* An estimated 500,000 babies have been born in the United States through assisted reproductive technology (ART) since 1985. The most common ART procedure is *in vitro fertilization (IVF)*, which removes the ova from a woman's ovary and places the woman's egg and her mate's sperm in a laboratory dish for fertilization. If the fertilized egg cell shows signs of development, within several days it is returned to the woman's uterus, the egg cell implants itself in the lining of the uterus, and the pregnancy continues as normal.

One of the most common complications of ART is the birth of as many as eight babies. More than half of ART-conceived twins and more than 95 percent of ART triplets are born prematurely or have low birth weights. Born too soon or too small, they face greater risks of short- and long-term complications.

## Adoption

Men and women who cannot conceive children biologically can still become parents. **Adoption** matches would-be parents yearning for youngsters to love with infants or children who need loving. Couples interested in adoption can work with either public agencies or private counselors who contact obstetricians directly. Or they can contact organizations that arrange adoptions of children in need from other countries.

There are no reliable statistics on the annual number of adoptions in the United States, but

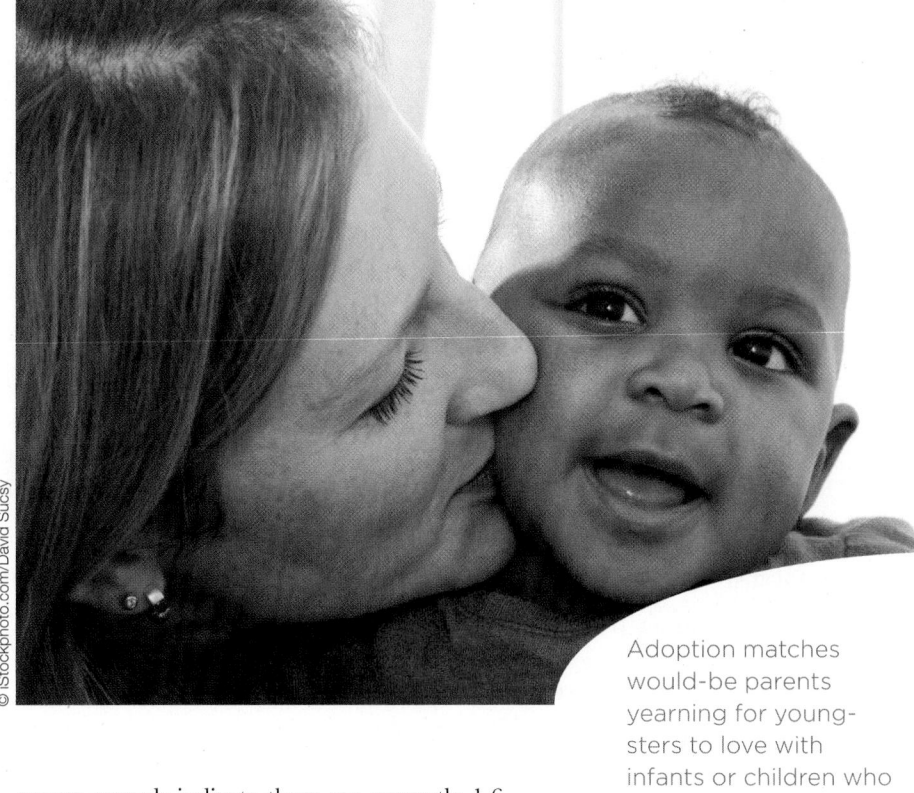

© iStockphoto.com/David Sucsy

census records indicate there are currently 1.6 million adopted children in the United States. Each year some 50,000 U.S. children become available for adoption—far fewer than the number of would-be parents looking for youngsters to adopt. An estimated 13 percent of adopted children are foreign-born.

Adoption matches would-be parents yearning for youngsters to love with infants or children who need loving homes.

**adoption** The legal process for becoming the parent to a child of other biological parents.

# Protecting Your Reproductive Health

The decisions you make about birth control can affect your reproductive health—and your partner's. Here are guidelines that can help prevent pregnancy and protect your reproductive well-being. Check those that you have used or think you will use in the future.

_____ **Abstinence.** The only 100 percent safe and effective way to avoid unwanted pregnancy is not to engage in heterosexual intercourse.

_____ **Limiting sexual activity to outercourse or oral sex.** You can engage in many sexual activities—kissing, hugging, touching, massage, oral–genital sex—without risking pregnancy.

_____ **Talking about birth control with any potential sex partner.** If you are considering sexual intimacy with a person, you should feel comfortable enough to talk about contraception.

_____ **Knowing what doesn't work—and not relying on it.** There are many misconceptions about ways to avoid getting pregnant, such as having sex in a standing position or during menstruation. Only the methods described in this chapter are reliable forms of birth control.

_____ **Talking with a health-care professional.** A great deal of information and advice is available—in writing, from family planning counselors, from physicians on the Internet. Check it out.

_____ **Choosing a contraceptive method that matches your personal habits and preferences.** If you can't remember to take a pill every day, oral contraceptives aren't for you. If you're constantly forgetting where you put things, a diaphragm might not be a good choice.

_____ **Considering long-term implications.** Since you may well wish to have children in the future, find out about the reversibility of various methods and possible effects on future fertility.

_____ **Resisting having sex without contraceptive protection "just this once."** It only takes once—even the very first time—to get pregnant. Be wary of drugs and alcohol. They can impair your judgment and make you less conscientious about using birth control—or using it properly.

_____ **Using backup methods.** If there's a possibility that a contraceptive method might not offer adequate protection (for instance, if it's been almost three months since your last injection of Depo-Provera), use an additional form of birth control.

_____ **Informing yourself about emergency contraception.** Just in case a condom breaks or a diaphragm slips, find out about the availability of forms of after-intercourse contraception.

# Which Contraceptive Method Is Best for You?

Answer Yes or No to each statement as it applies to you and, if appropriate, your partner.

1. You have high blood pressure or cardiovascular disease.
2. You smoke cigarettes.
3. You have a new sexual partner.
4. An unwanted pregnancy would be devastating to you.
5. You have a good memory.
6. You or your partner have multiple sexual partners.
7. You prefer a method with little or no bother.
8. You have heavy, crampy periods.
9. You need protection against STIs.
10. You are concerned about endometrial and ovarian cancer.
11. You are forgetful.
12. You need a method right away.
13. You're comfortable touching your own and your partner's genitals.

14. You have a cooperative partner.

15. You like a little extra vaginal lubrication.

16. You have sex at unpredictable times and places.

17. You are in a monogamous relationship and have at least one child.

*Scoring:*

Recommendations are based on Yes answers to the following numbered statements:

The combination pill: 4, 5, 6, 8, 10, 16

The progestin-only pill: 1, 2, 5, 7, 16

The patch: 4, 7, 8, 11, 16

The NuvaRing: 4, 7, 8, 11, 13, 16

Condoms: 1, 2, 3, 6, 9, 12, 13, 14

Depo-Provera: 1, 2, 4, 7, 11, 16

Diaphragm, cervical cap, or FemCap: 1, 2, 13, 14

Mirena IUD: 1, 2, 7, 8, 11, 13, 16, 17

Spermicides: 1, 2, 12, 13, 14, 15

Sponge: 1, 2, 12, 13

# Making Change Happen

## To Have or Have Not

Maybe you can't imagine not having a child. Maybe you feel that you're still a kid yourself but maybe someday you'll want a baby. Or maybe you're married and are seriously thinking about starting a family. Regardless of whether your answer to the question of wanting a child is yes, no, maybe, not yet, or it depends, "To Have or Have Not" in *Labs for IPC* can help you sort through your feelings so you can make a conscious, responsible decision. Here's a preview.

In this stage, you test your parental readiness by answering 17 questions including the following three:

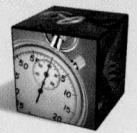

### Get Real
• How much experience have you had in caring for children in the past? As an older sibling, babysitter, camp counselor? What did you enjoy about it? What didn't you enjoy?

• What did you enjoy about being a child? What didn't you enjoy?

• What did you get from your parents that you would like to pass on to your children? What wouldn't you want to pass on?

You also complete several exercises, including this one:

Imagine that you or your partner (or a woman you slept with a few weeks ago) will take a pregnancy test tomorrow. Spend the next 24 hours thinking about how you might feel if it turns out positive and how you might feel if it's negative . . .

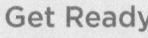

### Get Ready
In this stage you complete several preparatory exercises, including the following:

• Make a wish list. In your *IPC Journal*, write down everything you want for any child you bring into the world. This list might include:

• A loving home.

• Two committed parents.

• Financial security.

• An excellent education.

Put a check mark next to every one that you are confident you and your partner could give to a child at this point in your life. Write a second set of check marks for what you could give to this child if for some reason you become solely responsible for this child . . .

• **Budget for a baby.** Make a list of all the supplies, equipment, and furniture new parents have to get for their baby's first year. "Shop" for these items online, and calculate how much they would cost . . .

### Get Going
Over an eight-week period, you will engage in five exercises, such as:

• **"Shadowing" a new parent.** Ask a friend with a baby, or a friend of a friend, or a cousin or neighbor, if you can follow her or him during a typical day. Take notes of when the baby wakes, cries, frets, and sleeps. You get extra credit if you volunteer to change a diaper . . .

• **Having a virtual baby.** Based on your research, come up with a typical day in the life of a three-month-old baby. Name your baby boy or girl. Record when your baby wakes up. Calculate how much time you would need to drop the baby off at day care on your way to class . . . Throw in some unexpecteds, such as the baby fussing all afternoon so you don't have time to study . . .

### Lock It In
Keep talking—with your partner, your friends, parents you know. Also seek out and talk to people who have decided not to have children. Imagine that you have decided not to have children, and live with this decision for a week. Then imagine you've decided to have a child. Think of all the ways your life would change. How does that make you feel?

# Making This Chapter Work for You

## Review Questions

1. Which statement about prescription contraceptives is *not* true?
   a. Prescription contraceptives do not offer protection against STIs.
   b. Some prescription contraceptives contain estrogen and progestin, and some contain only progestin.
   c. The contraceptive ring must be changed every week.
   d. IUDs prevent pregnancy by preventing or interfering with implantation.

2. Which of the following statements is true about infertility?
   a. Infertility is most often caused by female problems.
   b. In men, infertility is usually caused by a combination of excess sperm production and an ejaculation problem.
   c. In vitro fertilization involves introducing sperm into the vagina with a long needle.
   d. In some cases of infertility, no cause can be demonstrated.

3. Conception occurs
   a. when a fertilized egg implants in the lining of the uterus.
   b. when sperm is blocked from reaching the egg.
   c. when a sperm fertilizes the egg.
   d. after the uterine lining is discharged during the menstrual cycle.

4. Which of the following statements is true about sterilization?
   a. In women, the most frequently performed sterilization technique is Essure.
   b. Many couples experience an increase in sexual encounters after sterilization.
   c. Vasectomies are easily reversed with surgery.
   d. Sterilization is recommended for single men and women who are unsure about whether they want children.

5. Factors to consider when choosing a contraceptive method include all of the following *except*
   a. cost.
   b. failure rate.
   c. effectiveness in preventing sexually transmitted infections.
   d. preferred sexual position.

6. During childbirth,
   a. breech birth can be prevented by practicing the Lamaze method.
   b. the cervix thins and dilates so that the baby can exit the uterus.
   c. the intensity of contractions decreases during the second stage of labor.
   d. the placenta is expelled immediately before the baby's head appears.

7. When used correctly, which is the most effective non-hormonal contraceptive method?
   a. male condom
   b. female condom
   c. spermicide
   d. diaphragm

8. Which statement about abortion is *false*?
   a. The abortion rate in the United States started declining in the 1990s.
   b. The U.S. abortion rate is higher than the rate in Canada and England.
   c. Most women are traumatized by an abortion.
   d. Mifepristone is 97 percent effective in inducing abortion.

9. Which of the following contraceptive choices offers the best protection against STIs?
   a. condom alone
   b. condom plus spermicide
   c. abstinence
   d. IUD plus spermicide

10. In the third trimester of pregnancy,
    a. the woman experiences shortness of breath as the enlarged uterus presses on the lungs and diaphragm.
    b. the embryo is now called a fetus.
    c. the woman should begin regular prenatal checkups.
    d. the woman should increase her activity level to ensure that she is fit for childbirth.

*Answers to these questions can be found on page 672.*

## Critical Thinking

1. After reading about the various methods of contraception, which do you think would be most effective for you? What factors enter into your decision (convenience, risks, effectiveness, etc.)?

2. If you are sexually active, how do you start the conversation about contraception with a potential partner? What do you say and do if your partner is not ready for sex? What would you do if you do not have condoms with you to prevent sexually transmitted infection and do not have another form of birth control, such as a diaphragm?

3. Suppose that you and your partner were told that your only chance of having a child is by using fertility drugs. After taking the drugs, you and your partner are informed that there are seven fetuses. Would you carry them all to term? What if you knew that the chances of them all surviving were very slim and that eliminating some of them would improve the odds for the others? What ethical issues do cases like this raise?

## Media Menu

Visit www.cengagebrain.com to access course materials and companion resources for this text that will:

- Help you evaluate your knowledge of the material.

- Allow you to prepare for exams with interactive quizzing.

- Use the CengageNOW product to develop a Personalized Learning Plan targeting resources that address areas you should study.

- Coach you through identifying target goals for behavioral change and creating and monitoring your personal change plan throughout the semester using the Behavior Change Planner available in the CengageNOW resource.

## Internet Connections

**www.guttmacher.org**
This site offers excellent resources on teen pregnancy rates and sexual health for teens and young adults, including discussions on contraceptives versus abstinence.

**www.arhp.org**
ARHP calls its website "the ultimate resource offering comprehensive information and education on all reproductive health topics to healthcare professionals, policymakers, the media, and the public."

**www.naral.org**
The website of this national organization provides information on the politics of the pro-choice movement.

**www.nrlc.org**
The website of this national organization provides information on the politics of the pro-life movement.

**www.plannedparenthood.org**
The website for the Planned Parenthood Federation of America offers a wealth of information on sexual and reproductive health, reproductive choices, methods of contraception, and reproductive policy.

## Key Terms

The terms listed are used on the page indicated. Definitions of the terms are in the Glossary at the end of the book.

**II**

"Use Condoms Like Your Life Depended On It."

© CALIFORNIA AIDS PREVENTION CA...

Use a condom. Get tested. 1-800-367-AIDS

1009

## After studying the material in this chapter, you should be able to

- Classify common STIs by transmission mode, symptoms, and treatments.
- Discuss STI risk factors, calculate your risk, and identify behaviors you can modify to reduce your risk.
- Recite the ABCs of safer sex, and explain some

- specific steps for safeguarding sexual health.
- Identify criteria for receiving the HPV vaccination.
- Discuss the incidence of HIV, strategies for reducing transmission, and treatments.

There's something I have to tell you." Anise knew, just by the sound of her boyfriend's voice, that the "something" wasn't good news.

"My herpes is back."

Stunned, Anise tried to absorb all the information packed into this short sentence: She'd had no idea that the man she'd been sleeping with for several months had a sexually transmitted infection (STI).

# Lowering Your Risk of Sexually Transmitted Infections

How did he get it? What else hadn't he told her about his past? What did he mean that it was "back"? Could she have caught it? And, finally, she asked the all-too-human question: How could this have happened to me?

By their very nature, infectious diseases take people by surprise. Some of today's most common and dangerous infectious illnesses spread primarily through sexual contact, and their incidence has skyrocketed. The federal government estimates that 65 million Americans have a sexually transmitted infection (STI). The odds of acquiring an STI in the course of a lifetime are one in four. These diseases cannot be prevented in the laboratory. Only you, by your behavior, can prevent and control them.

All human beings are sexual from birth to death. Whether you are male or female, single or married, straight, gay, lesbian, bisexual, or transgender, sexuality is a normal, natural part of your life. You are just as responsible for your sexual health as for any other aspect of your well-being. To safeguard your sexual health, you need to be aware of and protect yourself from sexually transmitted infections and diseases.

## Sexually Transmitted Infections and Diseases

In medical terms **sexually transmitted infection (STI)** refers to the presence of an infectious agent that can be passed from one sexual partner to another. In public health this term is replacing **sexually transmitted disease (STD)** because sexual infections can be—and often are—transmitted by people who do not have symptoms.

**sexually transmitted infection (STI)** The presence in the human body of an infectious agent that can be passed from one sexual partner to another.

**sexually transmitted disease (STD)** A disease that is caused by a sexually transmitted infection that produces symptoms.

Visit www.cengagebrain.com to access course materials for this text, including the Behavior Change Planner, interactive quizzes, tutorials, and more. See the preface on page xv for details.

## Figure 11.1 How STIs Spread

Most STIs are spread by viruses or bacteria carried in certain body fluids.

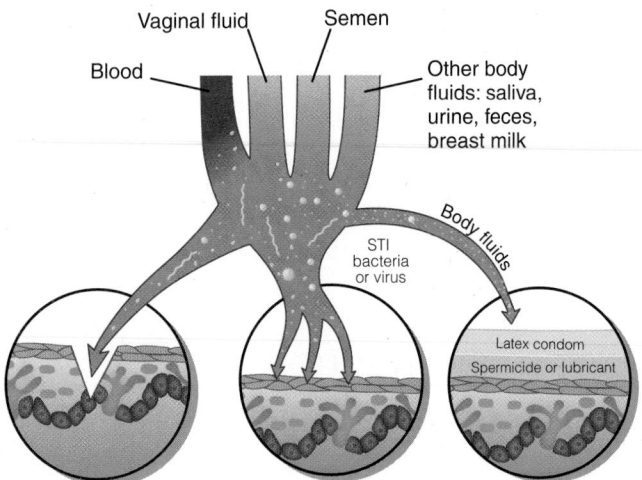

**Tough outer skin** covers the outside of your body, including hands and lips. Viruses and bacteria enter when skin is chapped or through a hangnail, cut, scrape, sore, or needle puncture.

**Fragile inner skin** lines the inside of your vagina or penis, anus, and mouth. Viruses and bacteria can enter through microscopic tears in the skin during sexual contact that involves movement or that lacks lubrication.

**Barrier protection** Latex condoms prevent your partner's body fluids from entering your body. Spermicides kill many STI microbes and reduce friction so condoms are less likely to break.

## STIs and Health

As you learned in this chapter, the odds of acquiring an STI in your lifetime are one in four. Thus, it is in your best interest to be informed about the latest developments regarding STIs. Log on to Global Health Watch, and mouse over Diseases → Infectious Diseases. Choose an STI that you would like to learn more about, and click on it. Scan the Latest News feed, and choose an article to summarize for your online journal entry. Are you doing what you can to ensure that you aren't part of the statistics?

STIs occur in all animals (and even plants) that reproduce sexually. Some people view sexual infections in moral terms. By attaching stigma and shame to STIs, these individuals may not seek treatment and thereby jeopardize their sexual health. However, embarrassment should never justify putting your health at risk.

Remember, STIs can:

- Last a lifetime.
- Put stress on relationships.
- Cause serious medical complications.
- Impair fertility.
- Cause birth defects.
- Lead to major illness and death.

(See Health in the Headlines: STIs and Health.)

According to the CDC, STDs cost the U.S. health-care system an estimated $15.3 billion annually.

Although each STI is distinct, they are all transmitted mainly through:

- Direct sexual contact with someone's symptoms (like genital ulcers) or sexual contact with someone's infected semen, vaginal fluids, blood, and other body fluids.

- Sharing contaminated needles through injectable drug use.

- Maternal transfer (mother to fetus during pregnancy or childbirth).

All STI pathogens like dark, warm, moist body surfaces, particularly the mucous membranes that line the reproductive organs; they hate light, cold, and dryness. Figure 11.1 shows how STIs in body fluids spread from person to person and how a barrier can help prevent their entry.

Table 11.1 lists the common STIs, their transmission, symptoms, and treatment. It is possible to catch or have more than one STI at a time. Curing one doesn't necessarily cure another, and treatments don't prevent another bout with the same STI.

Many STIs, including early HIV infection and gonorrhea in women, may not cause any symptoms. As a result, infected individuals may continue their usual sexual activity without realizing that they're jeopardizing another's well-being.

More Americans are infected with STIs now than at any other time in history. According to the Institute of Medicine, the odds of acquiring an STI during a lifetime are one in four. About 19 million new STIs occur each year in the United States. Young people under age 25 account for nearly half.

Within two years of having sex for the first time, half of teenage girls may acquire an STI. The three most common are chlamydia, gonorrhea, and trichomoniasis; a quarter of the girls infected in a recent study were under age 15.[1] Rates of chlamydia and gonorrhea are consistently highest in the 15- to 24-year age range.[2]

## STIs on Campus

The college years are a prime time for contracting STIs. According to a recent survey, almost nine in ten undergraduates are sexually active, but only about half reported using a condom the last time they had vaginal intercourse or using one mostly or always within the last 30 days. Fewer (31 percent) used condoms the last time they engaged in anal sex; only 4 percent used condoms for oral sex.[3]

Table 11.1 **Common Sexually Transmitted Infections (STIs): Mode of Transmission, Symptoms, and Treatment**

| STI | Transmission | Signs and Symptoms | Treatment |
|---|---|---|---|
| **Human papillomavirus (HPV) (genital warts) (p. 364)** | Spread primarily through vaginal, anal, or oral sex | Cauliflower-like growths in genital and rectal areas | Removal of lesions by laser surgery or chemicals |
| **Herpes simplex (p. 366)** | Genital herpes virus (HSV-2) transmitted by vaginal, anal, or oral sex. Oral herpes virus (HSV-1) transmitted primarily by kissing. | Small, painful red bumps (papules) to the genital region (genital herpes) or mouth (oral herpes). The papules become painful blisters that eventually rupture to form wet, open sores. | No known cure. Treatment may reduce symptoms; acyclovir, famcyclovir, or valacyclovir promote healing and suppress recurrent outbreaks. |
| **Chlamydia (p. 368)** | *Chlamydia trachomatis* bacterium transmitted primarily through sexual contact (can also be spread by fingers from one body site to another) | Men: Watery discharge; pain when urinating<br><br>Women: Usually asymptomatic; sometimes a similar discharge to men's; leading cause of pelvic inflammatory disease (PID) | Antibiotics: doxycycline, azithromycin, ofloxacin, levofloxacin |
| **Gonorrhea ("clap") (p. 370)** | *Neisseria gonorrhoeae* bacterium ("gonococcus") spread through genital, oral-genital, or genital-anal contact | Men: Pus discharge from urethra; burning during urination<br><br>Women: Usually asymptomatic; can lead to PID and sterility in both men and women | Antibiotics: cephalosporins (ceftriaxone or cefixime) |
| **Nongonococcal urethritis (NGU) (p. 370)** | Bacteria, most commonly transmitted through sexual intercourse | Men: Discharge from the penis and irritation during urination<br><br>Women: Mild discharge of pus from the vagina but often no symptoms | A single dose of azithromycin or doxycycline for seven days |
| **Syphilis (p. 371)** | *Treponema pallidum* bacterium ("spirochete") transmitted from open lesions during genital, oral-genital, or genital-anal contact | Primary: Chancre<br>Secondary: Rash<br>Latent: Asymptomatic<br>Late: Irreversible damage to central nervous system, cardiovascular system | Penicillin or other antibiotic |
| **Chancroid (p. 372)** | *Haemophilus ducrevi* bacterium transmitted by sexual interaction | Men: Painful irregular chancre on penis<br>Women: Chancre on labia | Tetracycline |
| **Pubic lice ("crabs") (p. 372)** | *Phthirus pubis* spread easily through body contact or through shared clothing or bedding | Persistent itching; visible lice often located in public hair or other body hairs | 1% permethrin cream for body areas; 1% lindane shampoo for hair |
| **HIV/AIDS (p. 373)** | HIV transmitted in blood and semen, primarily through sexual contact or needle sharing among injection drug users | Asymptomatic at first; opportunistic infections | Combination of three or more antiretroviral drugs (termed highly active antiretroviral therapies, or ART) plus other specific treatment for opportunistic infections and tumors |

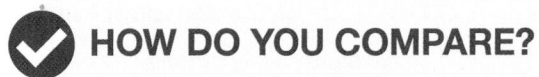

## HOW DO YOU COMPARE?

# PROTECTING YOUR SEXUAL HEALTH

| Students | Percent | Students | Percent |
|---|---|---|---|
| Vaccinated against HPV | 33.2 | Diagnosed with chlamydia | 1.1 |
| Tested for HIV infection | 25.7 | Diagnosed with genital herpes | 0.8 |
| Diagnosed with HPV | 1.9 | Diagnosed with PID | 0.3 |

## HOW DO YOU COMPARE?

What have you done to protect yourself from STIs? Have you been vaccinated against HPV? Have you been tested for HIV (recommended for everyone over age 13)? The incidence of diagnosed STIs on campuses is low, but many individuals are not aware that they have these infections. Write down your feelings about how getting an STI might affect your health and your life in your online journal.

Source: American College Health Association, *American College Health Association-National College Health Assessment II: Reference Group Executive Summary Spring 2010* (Linthicum, MD: American College Health Association, 2010).

White college students, according to the American College Health Association-National College Health Assessment (NCHA), are less likely than African American undergraduates to use condoms for vaginal, oral, and anal sex or to be tested for HIV. Blacks, who reported more sexual partners, were less likely to use hormonal contraceptives and had higher rates of STIs and unintended pregnancy.[4] (See How Do You Compare: Protecting Your Sexual Health.)

Contracting STIs may increase the risk of being infected with HIV. Because college students have more opportunities to have different sexual partners and may use drugs and alcohol more often before sex, they are at greater risk.

Colleges and universities vary in the STI services offered, including screening, diagnosis, and treatment. According to a recent survey, about half of students attend a school where STI screening is available. About half of colleges and universities make condoms available to students—some free in an open display, some free on request, and some for a fee or in vending machines. Larger schools, those with health centers, and those with on-campus housing are more likely to provide STI education and services.

## STIs and Gender

Both men and women can develop STIs, but their risks are not the same. Here is what you need to know about your risks.

### If You Are a Woman

- Keep in mind that your risk of getting an infection is greater than a man's. STIs can be transmitted through breaks in the mucous membranes, and women have more mucosal area exposed and experience more trauma to these tissues during sexual activity than men.

- Don't think you don't have to worry just because you have no symptoms. Symptoms of STIs also tend to be more "silent" in women, so they often go undetected and untreated, leading to potentially serious complications. For instance, pelvic inflammatory disease has no symptoms but puts you at risk of infertility and ectopic pregnancy.

- At your checkup talk to your doctor about whether you should be tested for sexually transmitted infections. You need to ask for these tests, or else they won't be done.

## If You Are a Man

- Involve your partner. Men are more likely to avoid common errors, such as removing condoms before sexual contact ends or slippage during withdrawal, when both partners mutually decide on their use.

- After potential exposure to an STI, give yourself a little extra protection by urinating and washing your genitals with an antibacterial soap.

- At your checkup talk to your doctor about whether you should be tested for sexually transmitted infections. You need to ask for these tests, or else they won't be done.

## STI Risk Factors and Risk Continuum

Various factors put young people at risk of STIs, including:

- **Feelings of invulnerability**, which lead to risk-taking behavior. Even when they are well informed of the risks, adolescents and young adults may remain unconvinced that anything bad can or will happen to them.

- **Multiple partners**. Figure 11.2 illustrates how STI risks increase as relationships become less familiar and exclusive. In surveys of students, a significant number report having had four or more sexual partners during their lifetime.

- **Failure to use condoms**. Among those who reported having had sexual intercourse in the previous three months, fewer than half of the students reported condom use.

  Students who'd had four or more sexual partners were significantly less likely to use condoms than those who'd had fewer partners.

- **Substance abuse**. Individuals who drink or use drugs are more likely to engage in sexually risky behaviors, including sex with partners whose health status and history they do not know, and unprotected intercourse.

  The more alcohol that college students drink or the more marijuana they use, the more likely they are to engage in risky sexual behavior.[5] In a study of young adults of traditional college age in New York City clubs, the majority of those who reported

binge drinking said they had had sex under the influence of alcohol. Almost a third described these encounters as "less safe" because of their drinking.[6]

- **Failure of a partner to be notified and treated**. Although physicians and health officials urge infected individuals to notify all their sexual partners, only an estimated 40 to 60 percent are notified and seek treatment. In surveys, infected individuals have indicated that they would be more likely to inform partners if they could do so via a website with anonymous e-mail and SMS services.[7]

### Figure 11.2 Continuum of Risk for Sexual Relationships and Behaviors

STI risks increase as relationships become less familiar and exclusive and as sexual activities become unprotected and receptive.

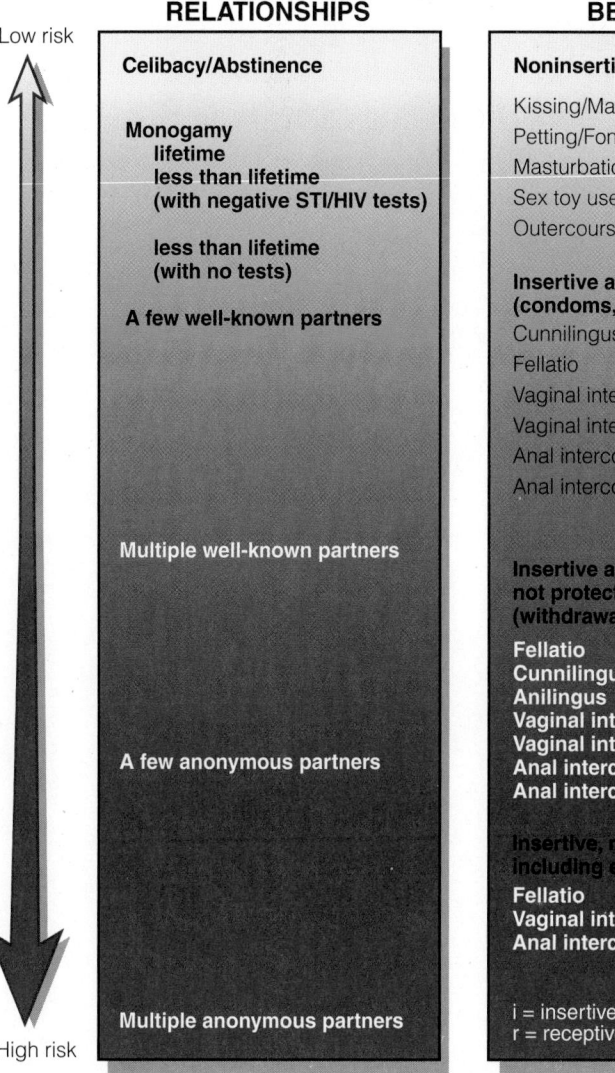

**RELATIONSHIPS**

Low risk

Celibacy/Abstinence

Monogamy
lifetime
less than lifetime
(with negative STI/HIV tests)

less than lifetime
(with no tests)

A few well-known partners

Multiple well-known partners

A few anonymous partners

Multiple anonymous partners

High risk

**BEHAVIORS**

Noninsertive

Kissing/Making out
Petting/Fondling
Masturbation
Sex toy use
Outercourse

Insertive and protected
(condoms, other barriers)
Cunnilingus
Fellatio
Vaginal intercourse (i)
Vaginal intercourse (r)
Anal intercourse (i)
Anal intercourse (r)

Insertive and
not protected
(withdrawal)
Fellatio
Cunnilingus
Anilingus
Vaginal intercourse (i)
Vaginal intercourse (r)
Anal intercourse (i)
Anal intercourse (r)

Insertive, not protected,
including ejaculation
Fellatio
Vaginal intercourse (r)
Anal intercourse (r)

i = insertive partner
r = receptive partner

*Abstain, Be faithful, or use Condoms. Following the ABCs of safer sex doesn't mean you can't have an intimate, loving relationship.*

© iStockphoto.com/Jose Girarte

# The ABCs of Safer Sex

Making smart, healthy choices about sex is the key to preventing sexual illnesses. (See Making Change Happen: The Sexiness of Safer Sex on p. 379, and in *Labs for IPC*.) As you will discover in this chapter, there are many specific steps to take to safeguard your sexual health. However, the three key fundamentals are as simple as A, B, C.

## A Is for Abstain

Abstinence from vaginal and anal intercourse and oral sex is free, available to everyone, extremely effective at preventing both pregnancy and sexually transmitted infections, and has no medical or hormonal side effects. If you decide to abstain only from vaginal or anal penetration, remember that other sexual activity such as oral sex can also expose you to STIs. If you have oral sex, make it safer by using effective barrier methods such as condoms or latex dental dams. (A dental dam is a square piece of latex that can be stretched across the vulva or anus to prevent the transmission of STI.) In the absence of barrier methods, men should avoid ejaculating in their partners' mouths. Also,

- Be aware of sores and discharge or unpleasant odors from your partner's genitals. These are signs to avoid oral sex.

- Don't floss or brush teeth before oral sex. It might tear the lining of the mouth, increasing exposure to viruses.

- Avoid aggressive and deep thrusting in oral sex, which can damage throat tissues and increase susceptibility for throat-based gonorrhea, herpes, and abrasions.

- Remember that oral sex can transmit various STIs, including HPV, herpes, gonorrhea, syphilis, and HIV.

## B Is for Be Faithful

For men and women who are sexually active, a mutually faithful sexual relationship with just one healthy partner is the safest option. Women and men in a committed relationship don't need to worry about getting sexually transmitted infections if:

The CDC has endorsed "expedited partner therapy" (giving medications to the infected person to give to partners) as more effective in cases of gonorrhea, chlamydia, or trichomoniasis. This approach is permissible or potentially allowable in most states but prohibited in Arkansas, Florida, Kentucky, Michigan, Ohio, Oklahoma, South Carolina, Vermont, and West Virginia.[8]

Rate your own sexual health risk by taking the Self Survey, "Assessing Your STI Risk" on page 377.

- Neither partner ever had sex with anyone else.
- Neither partner ever shared needles.
- Neither partner currently has or ever had an STI.

If these criteria fail to apply, two partners should be sure that neither has an STI before giving up on safer-sex practices. Some infections, like HIV, may take years to develop symptoms. The only way to know is by testing.

Of course, a committed relationship remains safe only as long as both partners remain committed. Most women who get HIV from having sex think they are their sex partners' only lover and never suspect that their partners' other lovers are men or women with HIV. (See Health in Action: Telling a Partner You Have an STI.)

## C Is for Condoms

Condoms are the only contraceptive that helps prevent both pregnancy and STIs when used properly and consistently. Male condoms reduce the risk of transmission of an STI by 50 to 80 percent. They are more effective against STIs transmitted by bodily fluids (chlamydia, gonorrhea, HIV, etc.) than those transmitted by skin-to-skin contact (HPV, syphilis, herpes, chancroid). Inexpensive and widely available in pharmacies, supermarkets, and convenience stores, condoms don't require a doctor visit or a prescription.

Most physicians recommend prelubricated, American-made latex or polyurethane condoms. Check the package for FDA approval. Also check the expiration (Exp) or manufacture (MFG) date on the box or individual package to see until when it is safe to use the condom. Make sure the package and the condom appear in good condition. If the package does not state that the condoms are meant to prevent disease, they may not provide adequate protection even if they are the most expensive ones on the shelf. Get the right size. Ill-fitting condoms lead to more problems with slippage and breakage as well as diminished sexual pleasure. Men also may be more likely to remove a condom that doesn't fit well before sex.

Condoms can deteriorate if not stored properly since they are affected by both heat and light. Don't use a condom that has been stored in your

## What to Do If You Have an STI

- **If you suspect that you have an STI, don't feel too embarrassed to get help through a physician's office or a clinic.** Treatment relieves discomfort, prevents complications, and halts the spread of the disease.

- **Following diagnosis, take oral medication** (which may be given instead of or in addition to shots) exactly as prescribed.

- **Try to figure out from whom you got the STI.** Be sure to inform that person, who may not be aware of the problem.

- **If you have an STI, never deceive a prospective partner about it.** Tell the truth—simply and clearly. Be sure your partner understands exactly what you have and what the risks are.

back pocket, your wallet, or the glove compartment of your car. Keep fresh condoms handy at all times. If a condom feels sticky or very dry don't use it; the packaging has probably been damaged.

Although it can be awkward to bring up the subject of condoms, don't let your embarrassment put your health at risk. Discuss using a condom before having sex; don't wait until you're on the brink of a sexual encounter.

See Chapter 10 for instructions on how to put on a condom. Here are some additional guidelines:

- **Use a new condom** each and every time you engage in any form of intercourse.

- **Do not use spermicide containing nonoxynol-9**. According to recent research, nonoxynol-9 without condoms is ineffective against HIV transmission. Even with condoms, it does not protect women from the bacteria that cause gonorrhea and chlamydia.

- **If a condom fails** during vaginal or anal intercourse, remove it carefully. If you continue sexual activity, replace it with a new condom.

# Human Papillomavirus

**Human papillomavirus** (**HPV**) is the most common sexually transmitted infection. According to a recent international study, half of adult men may be infected with HPV.[9] The risk is highest in men who have sex with men and men who have sex with both men and women.

Most people who become infected with HPV do not have any symptoms, and the infection clears on its own. However, HPV infection can cause cervical cancer in women and genital warts and other types of cancers in both sexes.

The biggest risk factor for HPV infection in men is a large number of lifetime sex partners. Men who've had more than 16 sex partners have about three times the HPV risk of those with fewer sex partners and are nearly ten times more likely to contract a potentially cancer-causing strain. Once infected, men who have been circumcised are more likely to have their immune systems "clear" the virus. Circumcised men also are less likely to transmit the virus to female partners.[10]

Of the 100 or more different strains, or types, of HPV, approximately 40 are sexually transmitted. Condoms provide only limited protection. Some "high-risk" HPV strains may lead to cancer of the cervix, vulva, vagina, anus, or penis. If transmitted via oral sex, they increase the risk of mouth and throat cancers.[11] In a recent study, individuals with HPV infections were 32 times more likely to develop such cancers. The risk increases along with the number of oral sex partners.

The "low-risk" types of HPV may cause changes in cervical cells that cause Pap test abnormalities or genital warts. Genital warts are single or multiple growths or bumps, sometimes shaped like cauliflower, that appear in the genital area.

Among women ages 14 to 65 screened for cervical cancer, almost one in four tested positive for HPV. Over half of the women younger than 30 who had abnormal (although not clearly cancerous) cells on their Pap smear had HPV infection. About a third of women with HPV acquire the infection within the year following first intercourse. Almost half of young women with just one male partner may develop HPV over a three-year period. The probability of HPV infection increases with partners who had at least two previous sex partners.

 College students' awareness of HPV and their potential risk is very low. In one study, both sexes saw themselves as not susceptible to HPV. Male students were more likely than female students to think that only women could acquire HPV. In another report, even women with adequate to high levels of knowledge about HPV did not take steps such as using condoms or having regular Pap tests to protect themselves.

## Incidence

Approximately 20 million people in the United States are currently infected with HPV, and 6.2 million Americans get a new HPV infection each year. Worldwide there are more than 440 million individuals with HPV infection. As many as 80 percent of sexually active women acquire HPV by age 50.

Young women who engage in sexual intercourse at an early age are more likely than those with later sexual debuts to become infected with HPV. Their risk also increases if they have multiple sexual partners or a history of a sexually transmitted infection, use drugs, or have partners with multiple sexual partners.

 College-age women are among those at greatest risk of acquiring HPV infection. In various studies conducted in college health centers, 10 to 46 percent of female students (mean age 20 to 22) had positive HPV tests.

## HPV Vaccination

Two vaccines—Gardasil and Cervarix—are currently available to prevent cervical cancer in girls and young women. Both protect against HPV-16 and HPV-18, the two types of HPV that cause most cases of cervical cancer. Gardasil also protects against HPV-6 and HPV-11, which cause most cases of genital warts.

Gardasil is approved for females ages 9 to 26 to protect against cervical cancer and prevent genital warts and for males ages 9 to 26 to prevent genital warts. Cervarix, which does not protect

**human papillomavirus (HPV)** A pathogen that causes genital warts and increases the risk of cervical cancer.

against genital warts, is approved for females ages 10 to 26 to help prevent cervical cancer. Cervarix has not been approved for use in boys or men.

The American Academy of Pediatrics recommends HPV vaccination for all girls at age 11 or 12 and has stated that boys ages 9 to 18 "may" get Gardasil.[12] This vaccine has proven safe and effective in male as well as female recipients.[13] In girls and women who have never been infected with HPV, the vaccine can prevent almost all cases of disease caused by the targeted types of HPV, including cancers of the genitals, cervix, and anus.[14]

Either brand of the vaccine is given in three shots over a six-month period, with the second and third doses administered two and six months after the first dose. Compliance rates for receiving all three doses have been low.[15]

Girls and women ages 13 to 26 who have not been previously immunized or who have not completed the full vaccine series should get vaccinated to catch up on missed doses. Because some groups do not recommend women between ages 19 and 26 receive catch-up doses of this vaccine, talk with your health-care provider if you are in this age group.

There are risks associated with HPV vaccination. Adverse effects, reported in 6.2 percent of patients, include fainting, itchiness, headache, nausea, blood clots, allergic reactions, and death. This is considered within the normal range of a widespread vaccination program for young persons. However, there is controversy about weighing the relative risks and benefits. See Consumer Alert.

In a study of female college students, those who were 18 years old were four times more likely to have received the HPV vaccine than women ages 19 to 26. Those who were aware that HPV causes genital warts were more likely to have received at least one dose of the HPV vaccine. Fewer Asian and African American than white women had been vaccinated.

HPV screening and vaccination are most beneficial for younger women. According to recent research, the rate of newly detected HPV among women over age 42 is significantly lower than among those between ages 18 and 25, and vaccination offers little benefit for women in their forties or older.

## ❶ CONSUMER ALERT

### Should You Get the HPV Vaccine?

Some states are considering legislation to make HPV vaccination mandatory for all girls because the vaccine is most effective when given before a girl becomes sexually active. Some religious groups oppose mandatory immunization because they feel that vaccinating girls against an STI gives them the wrong message about sexual responsibility. Consumer advocates worry about the unknown long-term effects. Others feel that the decision should be made privately by parents in consultation with their pediatricians.

### Facts to Know

- The HPV vaccines, which consist of three shots given over a six-month period, have been extensively tested in thousands of young women worldwide and is considered safe. However, the long-term effects are not known.

- No one yet knows whether a booster shot or shots will be necessary.

- Adverse effects include fainting, nausea, headache, blood clots, allergic reactions, and death. The most common side effects are pain at the injection site and fever.

- An estimated 4,000 women die in the United States and about 274,000 women die internationally annually from cervical cancer. The National Cancer Institute estimates 11,300 new cases of cervical cancer each year.

### Steps to Take

- Talk with your doctor if you are under age 26 and have not yet been vaccinated.

- Check with your insurance provider. Vaccination costs about $400 for the three-shot series. Most insurance companies cover recommended vaccines, but since this one is new, yours may or may not.

- Do *not* get the HPV vaccine if you:
  - Are older than 26 (the vaccine is still being tested in women in this age group).
  - Are pregnant.
  - Have ever had a life-threatening allergic reaction to any component of HPV vaccine.
  - Are moderately to severely ill at the time of vaccination.

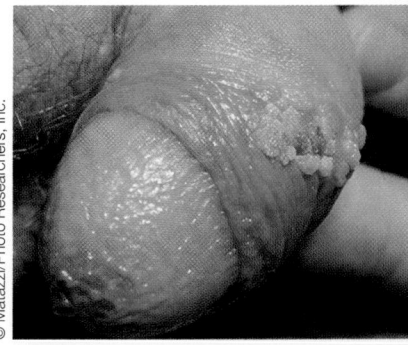
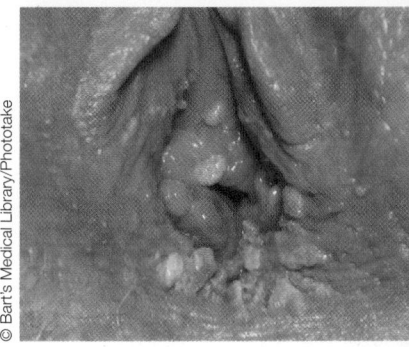

Human papillomavirus, which causes genital warts, is the most common viral STI.

## Signs and Symptoms

Most people with HPV infection do not know they are infected. The virus lives in the skin or mucous membranes and usually cause no symptoms. Some people get visible genital warts or have precancerous changes in the cervix, vulva, anus, or penis. After contact with an infected individual, genital warts may appear within three weeks to 18 months, with an average period of about 3 months.

HPV infection may invade the urethra and cause urinary obstruction and bleeding. It greatly increases a woman's risk of developing a precancerous condition called cervical *intraepithelial neoplasia*, which can lead to cervical cancer. Adolescent girls infected with HPV appear to be particularly vulnerable to developing cervical cancer. It is not known if HPV itself causes cancer or acts in conjunction with cofactors (such as other infections, smoking, or suppressed immunity). A woman's risk of cervical cancer is strongly related to the number of her partner's current and lifetime female partners. Women are five to eleven times as likely to get cervical cancer if their steady sex partner has had 20 or more previous partners.

Most HPV infections are asymptomatic in men, who may unwittingly increase their partners' risk. Men who test positive for HPV typically report significantly more sex partners than those who do not. HPV may also cause genital warts in men and increase the risk of cancer of the penis. People with visible genital warts also may have asymptomatic or subclinical HPV infections that are extremely difficult to treat.

## Diagnosis and Treatment

Most women are diagnosed with HPV after an abnormal Pap test or HPV DNA test. The results of HPV DNA testing can help healthcare providers decide if treatment is necessary to prevent or treat cervical cancer. (See Chapter 15 for a discussion of cervical cancer.) Warning signs for cervical cancer include irregular bleeding or unusual vaginal discharge. Precancerous cervical cells can be destroyed by laser surgery or freezing during a visit to a doctor's office.

No form of therapy has been shown to completely eradicate HPV, nor has any single treatment been uniformly effective in removing warts or preventing their recurrence. CDC guidelines suggest treatments that focus on the removal of visible warts—laser therapy cryotherapy (freezing), and topical applications of podofilox, podophyllin, or trichloroacetic acid—and then eradication of the virus. At least 20 to 30 percent of treated individuals experience recurrence.

# Genital Herpes

Herpes (from the Greek word that means *to creep*) collectively describes some of the most common viral infections in humans. Characteristically, **herpes simplex** causes blisters on the skin or mucous membranes.

Herpes simplex exists in several varieties. *Herpes simplex virus 1 (HSV-1)* can be transmitted by kissing and generally causes cold sores and fever blisters around the mouth. *Herpes simplex virus 2 (HSV-2)* is sexually transmitted and may cause blisters on the penis, inside the vagina, on the cervix, in the pubic area, on the buttocks, on the thighs, or in the mouth and throat (transmitted via oral sex).

About 21 percent of women and 11.5 percent of men have genital herpes, according to a recent CDC report. More than 80 percent do not realize they are infected.[16] HSV transmission occurs through close contact with mucous membranes or abraded skin. Condoms help prevent infection but aren't foolproof.

In the past physicians viewed herpes as an episodic disease with the greatest risk of transmission during flare-up. But as recent research has documented, "classic herpes" that produces acute symptoms is not typical. For many people genital herpes is a chronic, nearly continuously active infection that may produce subtle, varied, and often overlooked symptoms.[17] Most cases are transmitted by sexual partners who are unaware of their infections or do not have symptoms at the time of transmission.[18]

When herpes sores are present, the infected person is highly contagious and should avoid bringing the lesions into contact with someone else's body through touching, sexual interaction, or kissing. However, the herpes virus is present in genital secretions even when patients do

**herpes simplex** A condition caused by one of the herpes viruses and characterized by lesions of the skin or mucous membranes; herpes simplex virus 2 is sexually transmitted and causes genital blisters or sores.

not notice any signs of the disease, and people infected with genital herpes can spread it even between flare-ups when they have no symptoms.

A newborn can be infected with genital herpes while passing through the birth canal, and the frequency of mother-to-infant transmission seems to be increasing.[19] Most infected infants develop typical skin sores, which can be cultured to confirm a herpes diagnosis. Some physicians recommend treatment with acyclovir. Because of the risk to the infant of severe damage and possible death, caesarean delivery may be advised for a woman with active herpes lesions.

## Incidence

At least 50 million people in the United States have genital herpes, but only a minority realize they are infected.[20] About 40 percent of new cases of genital herpes occur in young people ages 15 to 24. An estimated one in five adolescents and adults in this age range have been infected. About one in four women and one in eight men carries the herpes virus.[21]

## Signs and Symptoms

Most people with genital herpes have no symptoms or very mild symptoms that go unnoticed or are not recognized as a sign of infection. The most common is a cluster of blistery sores, usually on the vagina, vulva, cervix, penis, buttocks, or anus. They may last several weeks and go away. They may return in weeks, months, or years.

Other symptoms include: blisters, burning feelings if urine flows over sores, inability to urinate if severe swelling of sores blocks the urethra, itching and pain in the infected area. Severe first episodes of herpes may also cause swollen, tender lymph glands in the groin, throat, and under the arms, fever, chills, headache, and achy flu-like feelings.

The virus that causes herpes never entirely goes away; it retreats to nerves near the lower spinal cord, where it remains for the life of the host. Herpes sores can return without warning weeks, months, or even years after their first occurrence, often during menstruation or times of stress, or with sudden changes in body temperature. Of those who experience HSV recurrence, 10 to 35 percent do so frequently—that is, about six or more times a year. In most people, attacks diminish in frequency and severity over time.

## Diagnosis and Treatment

Testing for the herpes virus has become much more accurate. There are several highly effective antiviral therapies that not only reduce symptoms and heal herpes lesions but also, if taken continuously, significantly reduce the risk of transmission of the virus to sexual partners.[22]

The three antiviral medications approved for the treatment of genital herpes are:

- *Acyclovir.* The oldest antiviral medication for herpes, acyclovir is sold as a generic drug and under the brand name Zovirax®. Available as an ointment and pill, acyclovir has been shown to be safe in persons who have used it continuously (every day) for as long as ten years.

- *Valacyclovir.* Sold as Valtrex®, this medication delivers acyclovir more efficiently so that the body absorbs more of the drug and medication can be taken fewer times during the day.

- *Famcyclovir.* Sold as Famvir®, this drug utilizes penciclovir as its active ingredient to stop HSV. Like valacyclovir, it is well absorb, persists for a long time in the body, and can be taken less frequently than acyclovir.

These antiviral medications are prescribed for initial and recurrent episodes of herpes. In episodic therapy, a person begins taking medication at the first sign of recurrence and continues for several days to hasten the healing or prevent a full outbreak from occurring. In suppressive therapy, people with genital herpes take antiviral medication daily to prevent symptoms. For individuals who have frequent recurrences (six or more per year), suppressive therapy can reduce the number of outbreaks by at least 75 percent. Suppressive therapy may also reduce asymptomatic shedding of HSV.

Various treatments—compresses made with cold water, skim milk, or warm salt water; ice packs; or a mild anesthetic cream—can relieve discomfort. Herpes sufferers should avoid heat, hot baths, or nylon underwear. Some physicians have used laser therapy to vaporize the lesions.

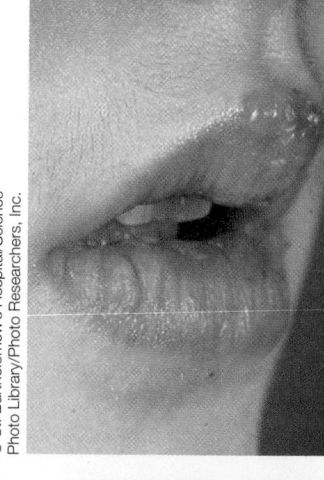

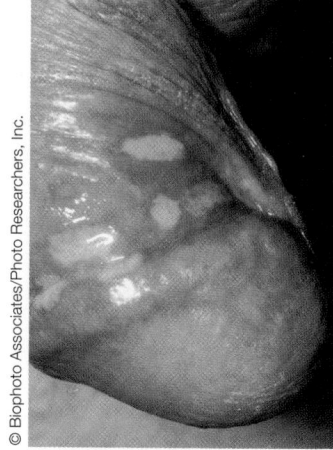

(a) Herpes simplex virus (HSV-1) as a mouth sore; (b) Herpes simplex virus (HSV-2) as a genital sore.

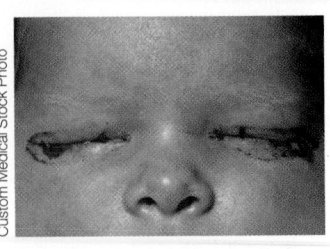

A baby exposed to chlamydial infection in the birth canal during delivery may develop an eye infection. Symptoms include a bloody discharge and swollen eyelids.

**chlamydia** A sexually transmitted infection caused by the bacterium *Chlamydia trachomatis*, often asymptomatic in women, but sometimes characterized by urinary pain; if undetected and untreated, may result in pelvic inflammatory disease (PID).

Clinical trials of an experimental vaccine to protect people from herpes infections are under way.

# Chlamydia

The most widespread sexually transmitted bacterium in the United States is *Chlamydia trachomatis*, which causes more than a million cases of **chlamydia** each year, a number that continues to rise. Almost half of reported cases occur among sexually active young adults between ages 15 and 24.[23] The use of condoms with spermicide can reduce, but not eliminate, the risk of chlamydial infection.

## Incidence

A record number of Americans—some 1.1 million, or 1 in 25 young Americans—are infected with chlamydia.[24] Chlamydia is much more prevalent in young black adults than in young white adults. However, this may be because black and Hispanic women are much more likely to be screened.[25] Women have three times the rate of chlamydia as men.[26] Chlamydial infections are more common in younger than in older women, and they also occur more often in both men and women with gonorrhea.

In a study of almost 800 students who volunteered for screening at ten southern colleges, nearly 10 percent tested positive for chlamydia, with higher rates among black women than white women. Younger students also were more likely to be infected than older ones, possibly because they are more likely to have unprotected intercourse, to engage in sex with multiple partners, and to have partners at higher risk for STDs.[27]

Those at greatest risk of chlamydial infection are individuals 25 years old or younger who engage in sex with more than one new partner within a two-month period and women who use birth control pills or other nonbarrier contraceptive methods. The U.S. Preventive Services Task Force recommends regular screening for chlamydia for all sexually active women under age 25 and for older women with multiple sexual partners, a history of STIs, or inconsistent use of condoms.

## Signs and Symptoms

As many as 75 percent of women and 50 percent of men with chlamydia have no symptoms or symptoms so mild that they don't seek medical attention. Without treatment, up to 40 percent of cases of chlamydia can lead to pelvic inflammatory disease, a serious infection of the woman's fallopian tubes that also can damage the ovaries and uterus. Also, women infected with chlamydia may have three to five times the risk of getting infected with HIV if exposed. Babies exposed to chlamydia in the birth canal during delivery can be born with pneumonia or with an eye infection called conjunctivitis, both of which can be dangerous unless treated early with antibiotics. Symptomless women who are screened and treated for chlamydial infection are almost 60 percent less likely than unscreened women to develop pelvic inflammatory disease. Chlamydia may also be linked to cervical cancer.

When women have symptoms of chlamydia they may experience

- Abdominal pain.
- Abnormal vaginal discharge.
- Bleeding between menstrual periods.
- Cervical or rectal inflammation.
- Low-grade fever.
- Yellowish discharge from the cervix that may have a foul odor.
- Vaginal bleeding after intercourse.
- Painful intercourse.
- Painful urination.
- The urge to urinate more than usual.

When men have symptoms of chlamydia, they may experience

- Pain or burning while urinating.
- Pus or watery or milky discharge from the penis.
- Swollen or tender testicles.
- Rectal inflammation.

Men often don't take these symptoms seriously because the symptoms may appear only early in the day and can be very mild.

Chlamydia, which can spread from a man's urethra to his testicles, can also cause a condition called epididymitis, which can cause sterility. Symptoms include fever, swelling, and extreme pain in the scrotum. Six percent of men with epididymitis develop reactive arthritis, which causes swelling and pain in the joints and can progress and become disabling.

In women and men, chlamydia may cause the rectum to itch and bleed. It can also result in a discharge and diarrhea. If it infects the eyes, it may cause redness, itching, and a discharge. If it infects the throat, it may cause soreness.

## Diagnosis and Treatment

Various antibiotics such as azithromycin and doxycycline kill *Chlamydia*. Some are taken in a single dose; others over several days. Both partners must be treated to avoid reinfections.

The CDC, in its most recent guidelines, recommends that all women with chlamydia be rescreened three to four months after treatment is completed. The reason is that reinfection, which often happens because a patient's sex partners were not treated, increases the risk of pelvic inflammatory disease and other complications. Immediately treating the partners of people infected with gonorrhea or chlamydia can reduce rates of recurrence of these infections.

# Pelvic Inflammatory Disease (PID)

Infection of a woman's fallopian tubes or uterus, called **pelvic inflammatory disease (PID)**, is not actually an STI, but rather a complication of STIs. Ten to 20 percent of initial episodes of PID lead to scarring and obstruction of the fallopian tubes severe enough to cause infertility. Other long-term complications are ectopic pregnancy and chronic pelvic pain. Smoking also may increase the likelihood of PID. Two bacteria—*Gonococcus* (the culprit in gonorrhea) and *Chlamydia*—are responsible for one-half to one-third of all cases of PID. Other organisms are responsible for the remaining cases.

Several studies have shown that women with PID are more likely to have used douches than those without the disease. Consistent condom use may decrease PID risk.

## Incidence

About one in every seven women of reproductive age has PID; half of all adult women may have had it. Each year, about 1 million new cases are reported.

Most cases of PID occur among women under age 25 who are sexually active. *Gonococcus*-caused cases tend to affect poor women; those caused by *Chlamydia* range across all income levels. One-half to one-third of all cases are transmitted sexually, and others have been traced to some IUDs that are no longer on the market.

## Signs and Symptoms

PID is a silent disease that in half of all cases produces no noticeable symptoms as it progresses and causes scarring of the fallopian tubes. Experts are encouraging women with mild symptoms, such as abdominal pain or tenderness, to seek medical evaluation and are encouraging physicians to test these patients for infections.

Other symptoms include fever, vaginal discharge that may have a foul odor, painful intercourse or urination, irregular menstrual bleeding, and, rarely, pain in the right upper abdomen.

## Diagnosis and Treatment

Urine testing is a cost-effective method of detecting gonorrhea and chlamydia in young women and can prevent development of PID. For women with symptoms, a pelvic ultrasound can show whether fallopian tubes are enlarged or an abscess is present. Magnetic resonance imaging (MRI) also can establish a diagnosis of PID and detect other diseases that may be responsible for the symptoms. Treatment consists of antibiotic therapy, usually with at least two antibiotics effective against a wide range of bacteria. A woman's sex partner(s) also should be treated to decrease the risk of reinfection, even if they have no symptoms. PID causes an estimated 15 to 30 percent of all cases of infertility every year and about half of all cases of ectopic pregnancy.

**pelvic inflammatory disease (PID)** An inflammation of the internal female genital tract, characterized by abdominal pain, fever, and tenderness of the cervix.

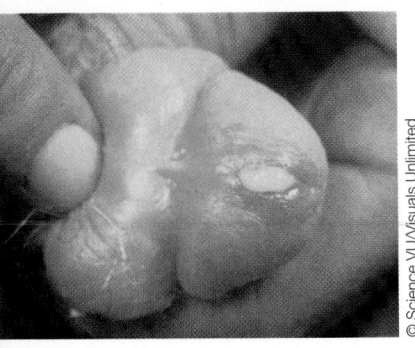

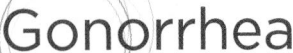

A cloudy discharge is symptomatic of gonorrhea.

# Gonorrhea

**Gonorrhea** (sometimes called "the clap" in street language) is one of the most common STIs in the United States.

## Incidence

An estimated 700,000 new cases occur every year.[28] As with chlamydia, gonorrhea rates are higher in women, particularly those between ages 15 and 24, than in men. Sexual contact, including oral sex, is the primary means of transmission.

## Signs and Symptoms

Most men who have gonorrhea know it. Thick, yellow-white pus oozes from the penis and urination causes a burning sensation. These symptoms usually develop two to nine days after the sexual contact that infected them. Men have a good reason to seek help: It hurts too much not to.

In men, untreated gonorrhea can spread to the prostate gland, testicles, bladder, and kidneys. Among the serious complications are urinary obstruction and sterility caused by blockage of the vas deferens (the excretory duct of the testis).

Women also may experience discharge and burning on urination. However, as many as eight out of ten infected women have no symptoms.

*Gonococcus*, the bacterium that causes gonorrhea, can live in the vagina, cervix, and fallopian tubes for months, even years, and continue to infect the woman's sexual partners. Approximately 5 percent of sexually active American women have positive gonorrhea cultures but are unaware that they are silent carriers.

If left untreated in men or women, gonorrhea spreads through the urinary-genital tract. In women, the inflammation travels from the vagina and cervix, through the uterus, to the fallopian tubes and ovaries. The pain and fever are similar to those caused by stomach upset, so a woman may dismiss the symptoms. Eventually these symptoms diminish, even though the disease spreads to the entire pelvis. Pus may ooze from the fallopian tubes or ovaries into the peritoneum (the lining of the abdominal cavity), sometimes causing serious inflammation. However, this, too, can subside in a few weeks.

*Gonorrhea*, the leading cause of sterility in women, can cause PID. In pregnant women, gonorrhea becomes a threat to the newborn. It can infect the infant's external genitals and can cause a serious form of conjunctivitis. As a preventive step, newborns may have penicillin dropped into their eyes at birth.

In both sexes, gonorrhea can develop into a serious, even fatal, bloodborne infection that can cause arthritis in the joints, attack the heart muscle and lining, cause meningitis, and attack the skin and other organs.

## Diagnosis and Treatment

Although a blood test has been developed for detecting gonorrhea, the tried-and-true method of diagnosis is still a microscopic analysis of cultures from the male's urethra, the female's cervix, and the throat and anus of both sexes.

Because gonorrhea often occurs along with chlamydia, practitioners often prescribe an agent effective against both, such as ofloxacin. Fluoroquinolones are no longer advised for use in its treatment. The CDC now recommends a cephalosporin antibiotic plus azithromycin or doxycyline.[29] Antibiotics taken for other reasons may not affect or cure gonorrhea, because of their dosage or type. And you can't develop immunity to gonorrhea; within days of recovering from one case, you can catch another.

# Nongonococcal Urethritis (NGU)

The term **nongonococcal urethritis (NGU)** refers to any inflammation of the urethra that is not caused by gonorrhea. NGU is the most common STI in men, accounting for 4 to 6 million visits to a physician every year. Three microorganisms—*Chlamydia trachomatis*, *Ureaplasma urealyticum*, and *Mycoplasma genitalium*—are the primary causes; the usual means of transmission is sexual intercourse. Other infectious agents, such as fungi or bacteria, allergic reactions to vaginal secretions, or irritation by soaps or contraceptive foams or gels also may lead to NGU.

In the United States, NGU is more common in men than gonococcal urethritis. The symptoms

**gonorrhea** A sexually transmitted infection caused by the bacterium *Neisseria gonorrhoeae*; symptoms include discharge from the penis; women are generally asymptomatic.

**nongonococcal urethritis (NGU)** Inflammation of the urethra caused by organisms other than the *Gonococcus* bacterium.

in men are similar to those of gonorrhea, including discharge from the penis (usually less than with gonorrhea) and mild burning during urination. Women frequently develop no symptoms or very mild itching, burning during urination, or discharge. Symptoms usually disappear after two or three weeks, but the infection may persist and cause cervicitis or PID in women and, in men, may spread to the prostate, epididymis, or both. Treatment usually consists of doxycycline or azithromycin and should be given to both sexual partners.

# Syphilis

A corkscrew-shaped, spiral bacterium called *Treponema pallidum* causes **syphilis**. This frail microbe dies in seconds if dried or chilled but grows quickly in the warm, moist tissues of the body, particularly in the mucous membranes of the genital tract. Entering the body through any tiny break in the skin, the germ burrows its way into the bloodstream. Sexual contact, including oral sex or intercourse, is a primary means of transmission. Genital ulcers caused by syphilis may increase the risk of HIV infection, while individuals with HIV may be more likely to develop syphilis.

## Incidence

The rate of syphilis in the United States declined by about 90 percent from 1990 through 2000, but has increased every year since, mostly in men. However, syphilis has also been rising in women for the last three years.[30]

## Signs and Symptoms

Syphilis has clearly identifiable stages:

- **Primary syphilis.** The first sign of syphilis is a lesion, or *chancre* (pronounced "shanker"), an open lump or crater the size of a dime or smaller, teeming with bacteria. The incubation period before its appearance ranges from 10 to 90 days; three to four weeks is average. The chancre appears exactly where the bacteria entered the body: in the mouth, throat, vagina, rectum, or penis. Any contact with the chancre is likely to result in infection.

- **Secondary syphilis.** Anywhere from 1 to 12 months after the chancre's appearance, secondary-stage symptoms may appear. Some people have no symptoms. Others develop a skin rash or a small, flat rash in moist regions on the skin; whitish patches on the mucous membranes of the mouth or throat; temporary baldness; low-grade fever; headache; swollen glands; or large, moist sores around the mouth and genitals. These sores are loaded with bacteria; contact with them, through kissing or intercourse, may transmit the infection. Symptoms may last for several days or several months. Even without treatment, symptoms eventually disappear as the syphilis microbes go into hiding.

- **Late and latent syphilis.** Although there are no signs or symptoms, no sores or rashes at this stage, the bacteria are invading various organs inside the body, including the heart and brain. For two to four years, there may be recurring infectious and highly contagious lesions of the skin or mucous membranes. However, syphilis loses its infectiousness as it progresses: After the first two years, a person rarely transmits syphilis through intercourse.

 After four years, even congenital syphilis is rarely transmitted. Until this stage of the disease, however, a pregnant woman can pass syphilis to her unborn child. If the fetus is infected in its fourth month or earlier, it may be disfigured or even die. If infected late in pregnancy, the child may show no signs of infection for months or years after birth, but may then become disabled with the symptoms of tertiary syphilis.

- **Tertiary syphilis.** Ten to 20 years after the beginning of the latent stage, the most serious symptoms of syphilis emerge, generally in the organs in which the bacteria settled during latency. Syphilis that has progressed to this stage has become increasingly rare. Victims of tertiary syphilis may die of a ruptured aorta or of other heart damage, or may have progressive brain or spinal cord damage, eventually leading to blindness, insanity, or paralysis. About a third of those who are not treated during the first three stages of syphilis enter the tertiary stage later in life.

**syphilis** A sexually transmitted infection caused by the bacterium *Treponema pallidum* and characterized by early sores, a latent period, and a final period of life-threatening symptoms, including brain damage and heart failure.

A pubic louse, or "crab."

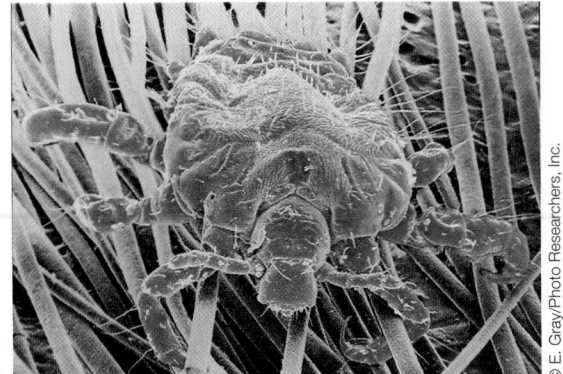

Actual size

© E. Gray/Photo Researchers, Inc.

## Diagnosis and Treatment

Health experts are urging screening with a blood test for syphilis for everyone who seeks treatment for an STI, especially adolescents; for everyone using illegal drugs; and for the partners of these two groups. They also recommend that anyone diagnosed with syphilis be screened for other STIs and be counseled about voluntary testing for HIV.

Penicillin is the drug of choice for treating primary, secondary, and latent syphilis. The earlier treatment begins, the more effective it is. Those allergic to penicillin may be treated with doxycycline, ceftriaxone, or erythromycin. An added danger of not getting treatment for syphilis is an increased risk of HIV transmission.

# Chancroid

A **chancroid** is a soft, painful sore or localized infection caused by the bacterium *Haemophilus ducreyi* and usually acquired through sexual contact. Half of the cases heal by themselves. In other cases, the infection may spread to the lymph glands near the chancroid, where large amounts of pus can accumulate and destroy much of the local tissue. The incidence of this STI, widely prevalent in Africa and tropical and semitropical regions, is rapidly increasing in the United States, with outbreaks in several states, including Louisiana, Texas, and New York. Chancroids, which may increase susceptibility to HIV infection, are believed to be a major factor in the heterosexual spread of HIV. This infection is treated with antibiotics (ceftriaxone, azithromycin, or erythromycin) and can

be prevented by keeping the genitals clean and washing them with soap and water in case of possible exposure.

# Pubic Lice and Scabies

These infections are sometimes, but not always, transmitted sexually. *Pubic lice* (or "crabs") are usually found in the pubic hair, although they can migrate to any hairy areas of the body. Lice lay eggs called nits that attach to the base of the hair shaft. Irritation from the lice may produce intense itching. Scratching to relieve the itching can produce sores. *Scabies* is caused by a mite that burrows under the skin, where they lay eggs that hatch and undergo many changes in the course of their life cycle, producing great discomfort, including intense itching.

Lice and scabies are treated with applications of permethrin cream and lindane shampoo to all the areas of the body where there are concentrations of body hair (genitals, armpits, scalp). You must repeat treatment in seven days to kill any newly developed adults. You must also wash or dry-clean clothing and bedding.

# Trichomoniasis

An estimated 7.4 million new cases of this common curable STI appear each year in men and women. The cause is a single-celled protozoan parasite *Trichomonas vaginalis*, transmitted by vaginal intercourse or vulva-to-vulva contact with an infected partner. Women can acquire this disease from male or female partners; men usually contract it only from infected women.

Most men have no signs or symptoms; some experience irritation inside the penis, mild discharge, or slight burning on urination or ejaculation. Some women develop a frothy, yellow-green vaginal discharge with a strong odor and may experience discomfort during intercourse and urination as well as genital itching and irritation. This inflammation may increase a woman's susceptibility to HIV if she is exposed to the virus.

**chancroid** A soft, painful sore or localized infection usually acquired through sexual contact.

**human immunodeficiency virus (HIV)** A type of virus that causes a spectrum of health problems, ranging from a symptomless infection to changes in the immune system, to the development of life-threatening diseases because of impaired immunity.

**acquired immune deficiency syndrome (AIDS)** The final stages of HIV infection, characterized by a variety of severe illnesses and decreased levels of certain immune cells.

Diagnosis is based on a physical examination and a laboratory test. Treatment consists of a single dose of oral medication, either metronidazole or tinidazole. If untreated, an infected man, even if he has never had symptoms or if his symptoms have gone away, can continue to infect or reinfect partners.

# HIV and AIDS

A few years ago, no one knew about **human immunodeficiency virus** (**HIV**). No one had ever heard of **acquired immune deficiency syndrome** (**AIDS**). Once seen as an epidemic affecting primarily gay men and injection drug users, AIDS has taken on a very different form.

Experts no longer think of AIDS as a single global epidemic. Instead, many regions and countries are experiencing diverse epidemics, some of which remain in their early stages. Sub-Saharan Africa has been the most affected region as measured by HIV/AIDS prevalence rates, followed by the Caribbean. Infection rates continue to rise in Eastern Europe and Asia.

## Incidence

According to the most recent statistics, 33.4 million people are living with HIV/AIDS worldwide. The global HIV/AIDS prevalence rate (the percent of people living with the disease) has leveled off, although the number of people living with the disease continues to increase. An estimated 2.7 million people become newly infected with HIV every year; about 2 million people die of AIDS-related causes. Women comprise half of adults estimated to be living with HIV/AIDS worldwide. Young people under the age of 25 are estimated to account for more than half of all new HIV infections worldwide.[31] However, the incidence of HIV/AIDS in individuals over age 50 is rising.[32]

About 1.1 million people in the United States are living with HIV/AIDS, a number that has grown because those with the disease are living longer. Someone in this country is infected every nine and one-half minutes, with about 56,300 new cases every year. Since the beginning of the epidemic, 617,025 men, women, and children have died of AIDS.[33] Among those at highest risk are:

- **Gay and bisexual men**. Although HIV infection rates have declined among gay and bisexual men, they account for an estimated 53 percent of new HIV infections and constitute the only group for which new infections are on the rise. Younger gay and bisexual men and those of color are at particularly high risk.[34]

- **Black Americans.** Although black Americans represent only 13.5 percent of the population, they account for 50.3 percent of new HIV infections. The rate of HIV diagnosis among black men is eight times that of whites, and the rate for black women is 19 times that of whites.[35]

  Two percent of black Americans are HIV positive, higher than any other group. The AIDS diagnosis rate for blacks is more than nine times that for whites. Blacks also have had the highest age-adjusted death rate due to HIV disease throughout most of the epidemic.[36] The reasons for this discrepancy are complex and include a higher rate of other STDs in black communities, disparities in health care, and poverty.

- **Women.** In 1985 women represented 8 percent of AIDS diagnoses; now they account for 25 percent. According to CDC estimates, almost 280,000 women in the United States are living with HIV or AIDS. Black women make up the largest share of women diagnosed with AIDS (64 percent), compared with 15 percent for whites and 18 percent for Latinas.

  Women are most likely to be infected through heterosexual sex, followed by injection drug use. Mother-to-child transmission of HIV has decreased dramatically because of the use of medicines that significantly reduce the risk of transmission from a woman to her baby.[37]

- **Young adults.** Teens and young adults under the age of 30 continue to be at risk. Those between ages 13 and 20 account for 34 percent of new HIV infections, the largest share of any age group. Most are infected sexually.

## Reducing the Risk of HIV Transmission

HIV/AIDS can be so frightening that some people have exaggerated its dangers, whereas others understate them. The fact is that although no one is immune to HIV, you can reduce the risk if you abstain from sexual activity or remain in a monogamous relationship with an uninfected partner, and do not inject drugs.

If you're not in a long-term monogamous relationship with a partner you're sure is safe, and you're not willing to abstain from sex, there are things you can do to lower your risk of HIV infection. Remember that the risk of HIV transmission depends on sexual behavior, not sexual orientation. Among young men, the prevalence and frequency of sexual risk behaviors are similar regardless of sexual orientation, ethnicity, or age. Homosexual, heterosexual, and bisexual individuals all need to know about the kinds of sexual activity that increase their risk.

*Sexual Transmission* Here's what you should know about sexual transmission of HIV:

- Casual contact does *not* spread HIV infection. You cannot get HIV infection from drinking from a water fountain, contact with a toilet seat, or touching an infected person.

- Compared to other viruses, HIV is extremely difficult to get.

- HIV can live in blood, semen, vaginal fluids, and breast milk.

- Many chemicals, including household bleach, alcohol, and hydrogen peroxide, can inactivate HIV.

- In studies of family members sharing dishes, food, clothing, and frequent hugs with people with HIV infection or AIDS, those who have contracted the virus have shared razor blades or toothbrushes or had other means of blood contact.

- You cannot tell visually whether a potential sexual partner has HIV. A blood test is needed to detect the antibodies that the body produces to fight HIV, thus indicating infection. As noted in Chapter 9, circumcision greatly reduces the risk for HIV infection.

- HIV can be spread in semen and vaginal fluids during a single instance of anal, vaginal, or oral sexual contact between heterosexuals, bisexuals, or homosexuals. The risk increases with the number of sexual encounters with an infected partner.

- Teenage girls may be particularly vulnerable to HIV infection because the immature cervix is easily infected.

- Anal intercourse is an extremely high-risk behavior because HIV can enter the bloodstream through tiny breaks in the lining of the rectum. HIV transmission is much more likely to occur during unprotected anal intercourse than vaginal intercourse.

- Other behaviors that increase the risk of HIV infection include having multiple sexual partners, engaging in sex without condoms or virus-killing spermicides, having sexual contact with persons known to be at high risk (for example, prostitutes or injection drug users), and sharing injection equipment for drugs.

- Individuals are at greater risk if they have an active sexual infection. Sexually transmitted infections, such as herpes, gonorrhea, and syphilis, facilitate transmission of HIV during vaginal or anal intercourse.

- No cases of HIV transmission by deep (French) kissing have been reported, but it could happen. Studies have found blood in the saliva of healthy people after kissing; other lab studies have found HIV in saliva. Social (dry) kissing is safe.

- Oral sex can lead to HIV transmission. The virus in any semen that enters the mouth could make its way into the bloodstream through tiny nicks or sores in the mouth. A man's risk in performing oral sex on a woman is smaller because an infected woman's genital fluids have much lower concentrations of HIV than does semen.

- HIV infection is not widespread among lesbians, although there have been documented cases of possible female-to-female HIV transmission. However, in each instance, one partner had had sex with a bisexual man or male injection drug user or had injected drugs herself.

*Nonsexual Transmission* Efforts to prevent nonsexual forms of HIV transmission have been very effective. Screening the blood supply has reduced the rate of transfusion-associated HIV transmission by 99.9 percent. Treatment with antiretroviral drugs during pregnancy and birth has reduced transmission to newborns by about 90 percent in optimal conditions. Among drug users in some settings, programs that combine addiction treatment and needle exchange reduced the incidence of HIV infection by 30 percent.

## Biological Methods of Preventing HIV Infection

Behavioral methods, such as safer sex practices, remain the primary means of preventing transmission of HIV. However, adding biological approaches may provide greater protection.[38] (See Health on a Budget.)

In initial trials of "pre-exposure prophylaxis" (PrEP), a daily pill called Truvada, which combines two anti-HIV drugs, proved safe and effective in significantly reducing the risk of HIV transmission in high-risk men. The volunteers received condoms and intensive counseling on safe sex practices.[39] Researchers also are studying the use of antiretroviral vaginal gels and topical creams.

## Recognizing and Treating HIV/AIDS

HIV infection refers to a spectrum of health problems that results from immunologic abnormalities caused by the virus when it enters the bloodstream. In theory, the body may be able to resist infection by HIV. In reality, in almost all cases, HIV destroys the cell-mediated immune system, particularly the CD4+ T-lymphocytes (also called *T4 helper cells*). The result is greatly increased susceptibility to various cancers and opportunistic infections (infections that take hold because of the reduced effectiveness of the immune system).

HIV triggers a state of all-out war within the immune system. Almost immediately following infection with HIV, the immune system responds aggressively by manufacturing enormous numbers of CD4+ cells. It eventually is overwhelmed, however, as the viral particles continue to replicate, or multiply. The intense war between HIV and the immune system indicates that the virus itself, not a breakdown in the immune system, is responsible for disease progression.

Shortly after becoming infected with HIV, individuals may experience a few days of flu-like symptoms, which most ignore or attribute to other viruses. Some people develop a more severe mononucleosis-type syndrome. After this stage, individuals may not develop any signs or symptoms of disease for a period ranging from weeks to more than 12 years.

HIV symptoms, which tend to increase in severity and number the longer the virus is in the body, may include any of the following:

- Swollen lymph nodes.
- Fever, chills, and night sweats.
- Diarrhea.
- Weight loss.
- Coughing and shortness of breath.
- Persistent tiredness.
- Skin sores.
- Blurred vision and headaches.
- Development of other infections, such as certain kinds of pneumonia.

HIV infection is associated with a variety of HIV-related diseases, including different cancers and dangerous infections including tuberculosis. HIV-infected individuals may develop persistent

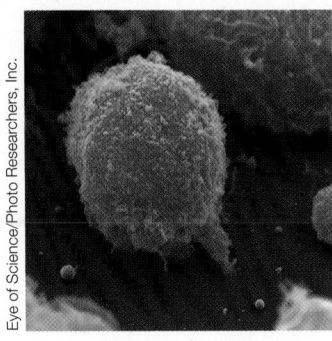

Electron micrograph of a white blood cell being attacked by HIV (*light blue particles*), the virus that causes AIDS.

generalized lymphadenopathy, enlargement of the lymph nodes at two or more different sites in the body. This condition typically persists for more than three months without any other illness to explain its occurrence. Diminished mental function may appear before other symptoms. Tests conducted on infected but apparently healthy men have revealed impaired coordination, problems in thinking, or abnormal brain scans. Psychological problems, including depression, anxiety, and stress, occur "in epidemic proportions" in individuals with HIV, according to recent research, and can affect their behavior (such as taking steps to prevent transmitting the virus) and treatment outcome. HIV also increases the risk of stroke[40] and of bone fractures.[41]

*HIV Testing*   One in five Americans infected with HIV doesn't know it. Anyone receiving routine medical care and testing can be screened for HIV without giving specific informed consent. The goal is to identify the estimated 250,000 Americans who have undiagnosed HIV.

All HIV tests measure antibodies, cells produced by the body to fight HIV infection. A negative test indicates no exposure to HIV. It can take three to six months for the body to produce the telltale antibodies, however, so a negative result may not be accurate, depending on the timing of the test.

HIV testing can be either confidential or anonymous. In confidential testing, a person's name is recorded along with the test results, which are made available to medical personnel and in 32 states, the state health department. In anonymous testing, no name is associated with the test results. Anonymous testing is available in 39 states.

The only home HIV test approved by the FDA, Home Access, is available in drug stores or online for $40 to $50. An individual draws a blood sample by pricking a finger and sends it to a laboratory along with a personal identification number. Results are given over the phone by a trained counselor, usually within several days.

Newly developed blood tests can determine how recently a person was infected with HIV and distinguish between long-standing infections and those contracted within the previous four to six months.

*Diagnosing AIDS*   A diagnosis of AIDS applies to anyone with HIV whose immune system is severely impaired, as indicated by a CD4+ count of less than 200 cells per cubic millimeter of blood, compared to normal CD4+ cell counts in healthy people not infected with HIV of 800 to 1,200 per cubic millimeter of blood. In addition, AIDS is diagnosed in persons with HIV infection who experience recurrent pneumonia, invasive cervical cancer, or pulmonary tuberculosis.

People with AIDS also may experience persistent fever, diarrhea that persists for more than one month, or involuntary weight loss of more than 10 percent of normal body weight. Neurological disease—including dementia (confusion and impaired thinking) and other problems with thinking, speaking, movement, or sensation—may occur. Secondary infectious diseases that may develop in people with AIDS include *Pneumocystis carinii* pneumonia, tuberculosis, or oral candidiasis (thrush). Secondary cancers associated with HIV infection include Kaposi's sarcoma and cancer of the cervix.

*Treatments*   New forms of therapy have been remarkably effective in boosting levels of protective T cells and reducing *viral load*—the amount of HIV in the bloodstream. Starting HIV treatment early, before a patient's immune system is badly weakened, can dramatically improve survival. People with high viral loads are more likely to progress rapidly to AIDS than people with low levels of the virus.

The current "gold-standard" approach to combating HIV is known as ART (Antiretroviral Therapy), which dramatically reduces viral load even though it does not eradicate the virus. This complex regimen uses one of 250 different combinations of three or more antiretroviral drugs, often available in a single tablet. Treatment begins much earlier than in the past, even before moderate immune suppression. This benefits the individual patient and helps prevent HIV transmission to a sexual partner.

Antiretroviral drugs are not available everywhere they are needed. In low- and middle-income countries, only 42 percent of people with AIDS are receiving treatment. Some countries have implemented successful HIV prevention interventions among high-risk populations and scaled up services to prevent mother-to-child transmission. However, others have not, and funding for such services remains inadequate.

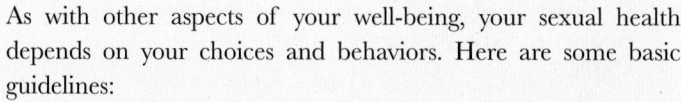

# Protecting Your Sexual Health

As with other aspects of your well-being, your sexual health depends on your choices and behaviors. Here are some basic guidelines:

____ **Talk first**. Get to know your partner. Before having sex, establish a committed relationship that allows trust and open communication. You should be able to discuss past sexual histories and any previous STIs or IV drug use. You should not feel coerced or forced into having sex.

____ **Stay sober**. Alcohol and drugs impair your judgment, make it harder to communicate clearly, and can lead to forgetting or failing to use condoms properly.

____ **Be honest**. If you have an STI, like HPV or herpes, advise any prospective sexual partner. Allow him or her to decide what to do. If you mutually agree on engaging in sexual activity, use latex condoms and other protective measures.

____ **Don't feel you have to have sex** for fear of hurting someone's feelings or fear of being the "only one" who isn't doing it. If you don't want to have sex, be honest, discuss the reasons behind your decision with your partner, and stay true to you.

____ **Respect** everyone's right to make his or her own personal decision—including yours. There is no perfect point in a relationship where sex has to happen. If your partner tells you that he or she is not ready to have sex, respect this decision, discuss the reasons behind it, and be supportive.

____ **Be prepared for a sex emergency**. Consider carrying two condoms with you just in case one breaks or tears. Both men and women are equally responsible for preventing STIs, and both should carry condoms.

____ **Abstinence doesn't mean less affection**. Practicing abstinence—the most effective way to protect against STIs—doesn't mean you can't have an intimate relationship with someone. It just means you don't have vaginal or anal intercourse or oral sex.

____ **Make your sexual health a priority.** Whether you are having sex or not, both men and women need regular check-ups to make sure they are sexually healthy.

**Self Survey**

# Assessing Your STI Risk

This Self Survey looks at your risk of acquiring or transmitting any sexually transmitted infection.

*STI Quiz*

1. **True** or **False**: A person can have an STI and not know it.
2. **True** or **False**: It is normal for women to have some vaginal discharge.
3. **True** or **False**: Once you have had an STI and have been cured, you can't get it again.
4. **True** or **False**: HIV is mainly present in semen, blood, vaginal secretions, and breast milk.
5. **True** or **False**: Chlamydia and gonorrhea can cause pelvic inflammatory disease.
6. **True** or **False**: A pregnant woman who has an STI can pass the disease on to her baby.
7. **True** or **False**: Most STIs go away without treatment, if people wait long enough.
8. **True** or **False**: STIs that aren't cured early can cause sterility.
9. **True** or **False**: Birth control pills offer excellent protection from STIs.
10. **True** or **False**: Condoms can help prevent the spread of STIs.

11. **True** or **False**: If you know your partner, you can't get an STI.

12. **True** or **False**: Chlamydia is the most common bacterial STI.

13. **True** or **False**: A sexually active woman should get an annual Pap test from her doctor.

*Answers*

1. **True** Some of the most common symptoms of an STI infection include abnormal discharge, painful urination, burning, and itching or tingling in the genital area, but it is important to remember that many women and men who have an STI often do not experience any symptoms at all. Chlamydia, for example, often has no symptoms.

2. **True** Normal vaginal discharge has several purposes: cleaning and moistening the vagina and helping to prevent and fight infections. Although it's normal for the color, texture, and amount of vaginal fluids to vary throughout a woman's menstrual cycle, some changes in discharge may indicate a problem.

   If you think you may have a problem, you should see a doctor as soon as possible. First, though, it helps to learn some of the differences between what is normal and abnormal vaginal discharge for you.

3. **False** Having an STI and being cured from it does not mean that your body now has a built-in immunity to the bacteria that causes the infection. You must protect yourself from becoming infected again by using a condom. Remember, it is your body!

4. **True** Although small traces of HIV can be found in tears, saliva, urine, and perspiration, extensive studies have shown that there is not enough of the virus or the virus is not strong enough to be transmitted. Only blood, semen, vaginal secretions, and breast milk have been proven to transmit the HIV virus and hepatitis B. HIV cannot be passed on by casual contact.

5. **True** Many different organisms can cause PID, but most cases are associated with gonorrhea and genital chlamydial infections, two very common STIs. Scientists have found that bacteria normally present in small numbers in the vagina and cervix also may play a role.

6. **True** STIs can be passed from a pregnant woman to the baby before, during, or after the baby's birth. Some STIs (like syphilis) cross the placenta and infect the baby while it is in the uterus (womb). Other STIs (like gonorrhea, chlamydia, hepatitis B, and genital herpes) can be transmitted from the mother to the baby during delivery as the baby passes through the birth canal. HIV can cross the placenta during pregnancy, infect the baby during the birth process, and unlike most other STIs, can infect the baby through breast-feeding.

7. **False** Even if symptoms appear to go away, the infected person will still have the infection and is able to pass the infection on to others until he or she gets treatment. STIs that aren't cured early can cause sterility.

8. **True** If the fallopian tubes are blocked at one or both ends, the egg can't travel through the tubes into the uterus. Blocked tubes may result from pelvic inflammatory disease, which is often caused by untreated STIs.

9. **False** The birth control pill does not protect against sexually transmitted infections. For those having sex, condoms must always be used along with birth control pills to protect against STIs. Abstinence (the decision to not have sex) is the only method that always prevents pregnancy and sexually transmitted infections.

10. **True** Most condoms are made of latex. Those made of lambskin may offer less protection against some sexually transmitted infections, including HIV, so use of latex condoms is recommended. For people who may have an allergic skin reaction to latex, both male and female condoms made of polyurethane are available.

    When properly used, latex and plastic condoms are effective against most STIs. Condoms do not protect against infections spread from sores on the skin not covered by a condom (such as the base of the penis or scrotum).

11. **False** As stated in question number 1, a person can have an STI and not know it. If they can't tell, how can you?

12. **True** The U.S. Centers for Disease Control and Prevention estimates that more than 4 million new cases of chlamydia occur each year. The highest rates of chlamydial infection are in 15- to 19-year-old adolescents regardless of demographics or location.

13. **True** The Pap test is a way to find cell changes on the cervix. Abnormal cells may lead to cancer, so having a Pap test can find and treat them early, before they have time to progress to cancer.

    Although Pap tests do not test for STIs, some STIs such as HPV (human papillomavirus infection) can cause abnormal Pap test results. Certain types of HPV are linked to cancer in both women and men.

*Source: Material taken from The Bacchus Network™ Website, smartersex .org.*

# Making Change Happen

## The Sexiness of Safer Sex

Protecting yourself and your partner doesn't take anything away from the quality of your sex life In fact, it makes it better. Sex involves more than two *bodies*; it involves, engages, and delights two *people*. Protection doesn't mean less affection. You can still have an intimate relationship with someone, and you can still enjoy the pleasures of being together. Safer sex is still sexy—and certainly far sexier than nagging worries about infections that could jeopardize your future sex life. If you're sexually active, read through "The Sexiness of Safer Sex" in *Labs for IPC*. Even if you're not, read through this preview.

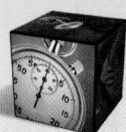

### Get Real

In this stage you rate your sexual safety skills by answering 12 questions, including the following:

- How well do you know your partner(s)? Did you share each other's sexual histories before having sex? Is your partner always open about everything with you? Does your partner keep secrets from you?

- How do you protect yourself and a partner from STIs and, if you are heterosexual, pregnancy?

- Do you use this form of protection every time you have sex?

You also read through a list of sexual behaviors, and check any you've engage in with someone whose sexual history and HIV status you did not know. The list includes safe behaviors, such as computer or phone sex, possibly safe ones such as intercourse with a condom, and unsafe ones, such as intercourse without a condom. On the basis of your answers, you rate your sexual safety skills on a scale from 1 (no risk) to 10 (highest risk). You also get checked for STIs, even if you have no symptoms . . .

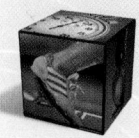

### Get Ready

To prepare, you inform yourself by reading this chapter and going to authoritative websites such as http://www.ashastd.org/ (American Social Health Association) . . .

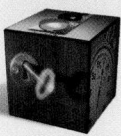

### Get Going

You do one of six exercises in this stage every week. Here is an example:

- **Condom Sense.** Talk with your partner about using a condom before having sex. Don't let embarrassment put your health at risk. Visualize the conversation, and practice the following rebuttals:

| | |
|---|---|
| Don't you trust me? | Trust isn't the point. People can have an STI and not realize it. OR: I trust you but I don't know your last partner. How can I trust that person? |
| Condoms interrupt us just when thing are getting hot. | Not if we put it on together. |
| I don't have a condom with me. | I do. |
| But I love you. | Then you'll help us to protect ourselves. |
| Just this once. | Once is all it takes . . . |

### Lock It In

Make your sexual health a priority. Bring up questions related to STIs with your doctor. If you're a woman under age 26, discuss the pros and cons of getting an HPV vaccination. And be prepared. If you are sexually active and not in an exclusive relationship with a healthy partner, carry condoms with you . . .

# Making This Chapter Work for You

## Review Questions

1. Chlamydial infections
   a. are caused by a virus.
   b. can cause eye infections in men.
   c. usually display no symptoms in women.
   d. are more common in older women.

2. Which statement is *true*?
   a. Gonorrhea is mostly symptomless in men.
   b. Secondary syphilis usually occurs 10 to 20 years after the latent stage.
   c. Pubic lice can be killed with regular shampoo.
   d. African Americans account for a disproportionate share of new AIDS diagnoses.

3. Which of the following statements about HIV transmission is *true*?
   a. Individuals are not at risk for HIV if they are being treated for chlamydia or gonorrhea.
   b. HIV can be transmitted between lesbians.
   c. Heterosexual men who do not practice safe sex are at less risk for contracting HIV than homosexual men who do practice safe sex.
   d. HIV cannot be spread in a single instance of sexual intercourse.

4. A person with AIDS
   a. has a low viral load and a high number of T4 helper cells.
   b. can no longer pass HIV to a sexual partner.
   c. may suffer from secondary infectious diseases and cancers.
   d. will not respond to treatment.

5. Sexually transmitted infections
   a. are the major cause of preventable sterility in the United States.
   b. are declining in incidence on college campuses.
   c. have declined in incidence in developing nations due to improving health standards.
   d. do not increase the risk of being infected with HIV.

6. Viral agents cause all of the following STIs *except*
   a. herpes.
   b. genital warts.
   c. HIV.
   d. chlamydia.

7. Jake is sexually active but doesn't want to use a condom. His other choices to protect himself against STIs include all of these *except*
   a. abstinence.
   b. a sexual relationship with a longtime friend.
   c. a sexual relationship with one STI-free partner.
   d. masturbation only.

8. Which of these activities cannot transmit an STI?
   a. having oral sex
   b. hugging
   c. sharing a needle with a fellow athlete using steroids
   d. sharing a razor

9. Which statement about HPV infection is *false*?
   a. HPV cannot be transmitted through oral sex.
   b. HPV increases a woman's risk of developing cervical cancer.
   c. HPV causes genital warts.
   d. HPV increases a man's risk of cancer of the penis.

10. The herpes simplex virus HSV-2
    a. cannot be transmitted through oral sex.
    b. cannot be transmitted if a condom is used.
    c. can be transmitted even when the infected person shows no symptoms.
    d. can be permanently killed with antiviral medications.

*Answers to these questions can be found on page 672.*

## Critical Thinking

1. Your friend Shayla recently broke up after a five-year relationship with her first boyfriend. How would you counsel Shayla on reentering the dating scene and becoming intimate with a new partner?

2. Tad has told his girlfriend, Kylie, that he has never taken any sexual risks. But when she suggested that they get tested for STIs, he became furious and refused. Now Kylie says she doesn't know what to believe. Could Tad be telling the truth, or is he hiding something? If he is telling the truth, why is Tad so upset? Kylie doesn't want to take any risks, but she doesn't want to lose him either. What would you advise her to say or do? What would you advise Tad to say or do?

3. Have you ever dated someone with an STI? If so, when did you find out about it? How did you feel? Did it affect your sex life? In what way?

4. Any time a person has a blood test, an HIV screening can be performed without asking permission. Do you see this as a violation of privacy or as a good public health practice? Explain.

## Media Menu

Visit www.cengagebrain.com to access course materials and companion resources for this text that will:

- Help you evaluate your knowledge of the material.

- Allow you to prepare for exams with interactive quizzing.

- Use the CengageNOW product to develop a Personalized Learning Plan targeting resources that address areas you should study.

- Coach you through identifying target goals for behavioral change and creating and monitoring your personal change plan throughout the semester using the Behavior Change Planner available in the CengageNOW resource.

## Internet Connections

**www.cdc.gov/std**
**www.cdc.gov/hiv**
These sites at the CDC feature current information, fact sheets, treatment guides, surveillance, and statistics on sexually transmitted infections and HIV/AIDS.

**http://www3.niaid.nih.gov/research/topics**
This site, which is part of the National Institutes of Health, features research on STIs, including basic and clinical research and activities related to vaccine development.

**http://hivinsite.ucsf.edu**
This site, sponsored by the University of California San Francisco School of Medicine, provides statistics, education, prevention, and new developments related to HIV/AIDS.

## Key Terms

The terms listed are used on the page indicated. Definitions of the terms are in the Glossary at the end of the book.

acquired immune deficiency syndrome (AIDS)  372

chanchroid  372

chlamydia  368

gonorrhea  370

herpes simplex  366

human immunodeficiency virus (HIV)  372

human papillomavirus (HPV)  364

nongonococcal urethritis (NGU)  370

pelvic inflammatory disease (PID)  369

sexually transmitted disease (STD)  357

sexually transmitted infection (STI)  357

syphilis  371

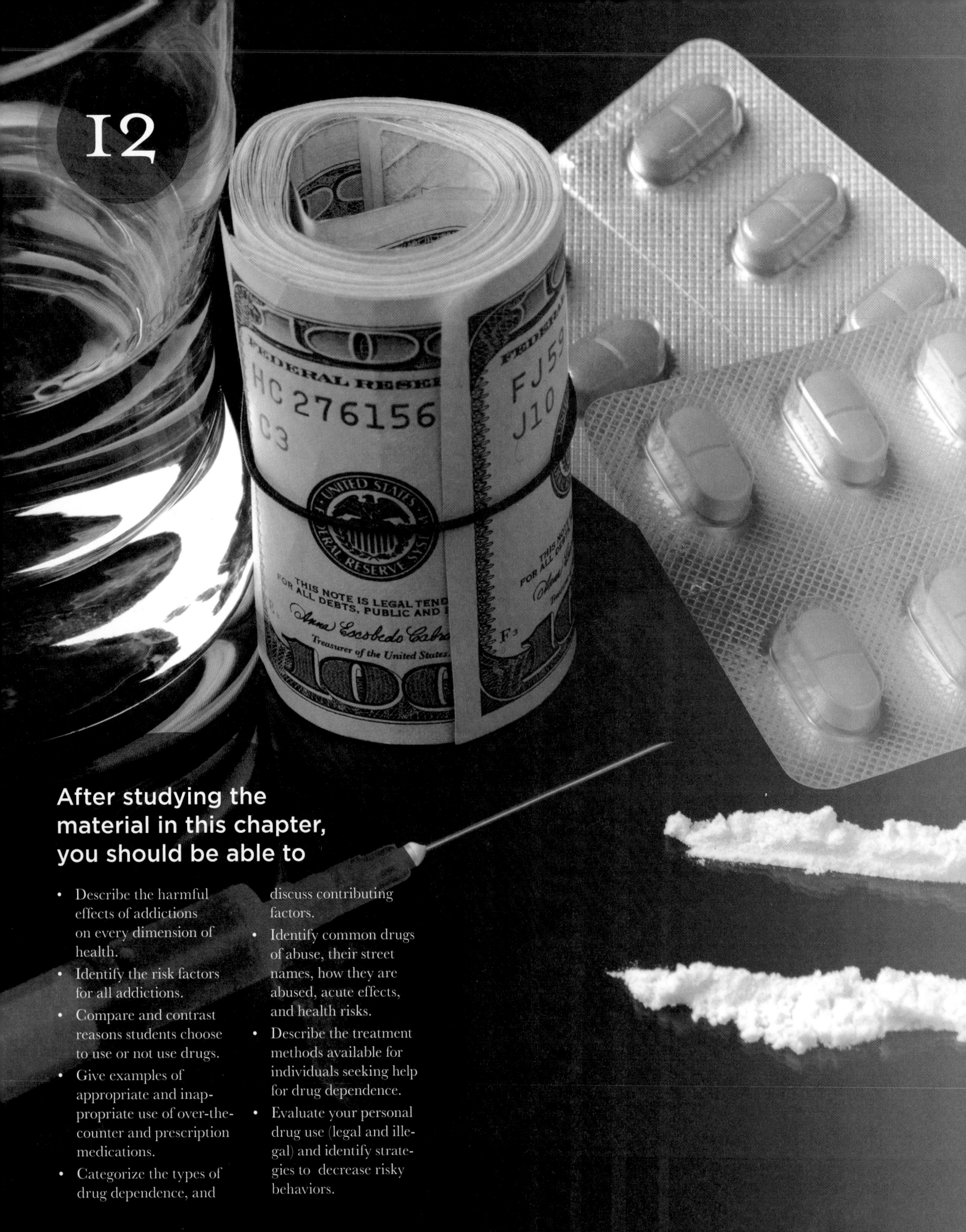

# I2

## After studying the material in this chapter, you should be able to

- Describe the harmful effects of addictions on every dimension of health.
- Identify the risk factors for all addictions.
- Compare and contrast reasons students choose to use or not use drugs.
- Give examples of appropriate and inappropriate use of over-the-counter and prescription medications.
- Categorize the types of drug dependence, and discuss contributing factors.
- Identify common drugs of abuse, their street names, how they are abused, acute effects, and health risks.
- Describe the treatment methods available for individuals seeking help for drug dependence.
- Evaluate your personal drug use (legal and illegal) and identify strategies to decrease risky behaviors.

Navi had too many papers to write and too little time to finish them. One of the guys in his fraternity suggested a prescription stimulant a friend took for an attention deficit disorder. The jolt felt like just what Navi needed. During midterms Navi bought another prescription stimulant from a classmate. As finals approached, he started hoarding stimulants from several people. He popped the final ones to rev up for the last bash of the school

# Avoiding Addictions

year parties. Without realizing it, Navi put himself at risk for drug-related problems—physical, psychological, and legal.

People who try drugs or engage in addictive behaviors don't think they'll ever lose control. Even regular users believe they are smart enough, strong enough, lucky enough not to get caught or hooked. However, over time addictions produce changes in an individual's body, brain, and behavior. In time they can outweigh everything else a person values and holds dearest.

The impact of addictions in college ranges from short-term consequences, such as academic difficulties, to long-term physical and psychological problems. The toll of drug abuse, for instance, includes more than 1,700 deaths, 700,000 assaults, and almost 100,000 sexual attacks and rapes. But knowing the risks isn't enough to keep young people from heading down the dead-end road of addiction. Substance abuse is rising among American teens. In the most recent Monitoring the Future survey of drug, alcohol, and cigarette use, the percentage of high school seniors who used marijuana in the past 30 days was higher than the percentage who smoked cigarettes.[1]

Going beyond warnings, this chapter provides information about and insights into how addictions start, why students use and abuse drugs, the nature and effect of drugs, and the most commonly used, misused, and abused drugs. It also offers practical strategies for preventing, recognizing the signs of, and seeking help for addiction.

## Risky Behaviors

 College is a time when students want to experiment, enjoy, stretch—and take some risks. But there is a difference between the risks of smoking marijuana and the risks of forming a band or trying out for a team. One is an illegal activity that can get you in serious trouble in the short term and cause adverse health consequences in the long run The others impart the thrill that comes with trying something new and mastering a challenge. Are

Visit www.cengagebrain.com to access course materials for this text, including the Behavior Change Planner, interactive quizzes, tutorials, and more. See the preface on page xv for details.

# Develop a Positive Addiction

When you're anxious, bored, restless, or confused, when drugs seem all too appealing as a "quick fix," there are real solutions, "positive addictions" that can help you solve your problems without creating new and bigger ones. A positive addiction—whether it is exercising, mountain climbing, or listening to music—can produce very real "highs," often for very little money. There's a crucial difference between this sort of stimulation and drug dependency: one is real, the other is chemical. With one, you're in control; with the other, drugs are.

Here are some examples:

- **If you feel a need for physical relaxation,** if you want more energy or distraction from physical discomforts, you can turn to athletics, exercise (including walking and hiking), dance, or outdoor hobbies.

- **If you want to stimulate your senses,** enhance sexual stimulation, or magnify the sensations of sight, sound, and touch, train yourself to be more sensitive to nature and beauty. Take time to appreciate the sensations you experience when you're walking in the woods or embracing a person you love. Through activities like sailing or skydiving, you can literally fill up your senses without relying on chemicals.

- **If you want to escape mental boredom,** gain new understanding of the world around you, study better, experiment with your levels of awareness, or indulge your intellectual curiosity, you can challenge your mind through reading, classes, creative games, discussion groups, memory training, or travel.

- **If you're looking for kicks,** adventure, danger, and excitement, sign up for a wilderness survival course. Take up an adventurous sport, like hang gliding or rock climbing. Set a challenging professional or personal goal and direct your energies to meeting it.

you taking risks that don't make sense and that don't add pleasure or passion to your life? Or are you taking risks that empower and inspire you?

The vast majority of college students do not engage in addictive behaviors. However, some do, and the reasons why are complex. According to recent research, the brain's "reward center" responds to both pleasurable and exciting experiences, such as eating chocolate or bungee-jumping, by producing dopamine, a "feel good" chemical in the brain. In individuals with fewer dopamine "auto-receptors," exciting or dangerous activities may trigger higher levels of dopamine than normal, which encourages thrill-seeking behavior.[2] However, biology is not destiny. Although there are promising treatments for addictions (discussed later in this chapter), prevention is the smarter, safer—and far less costly—choice (see Health on a Budget).

## Addictive Behaviors and the Dimensions of Health

Young adults have the highest rates of illicit drug use. Many do not realize that substance abuse and other self-destructive behaviors, such as gambling or compulsive eating, can affect every dimension of health. Some of the harmful effects are:

- **Physical health.** As shown in this and the following chapter, the abuse of alcohol, tobacco, and drugs takes a toll on every organ system in the body, increasing the likelihood of disease, disability, and premature death.

- **Psychological health.** Sometimes people begin abusing substances or engaging in addictive behavior as a way of "self-medicating" symptoms of anxiety or depression. However, alcohol or drugs provide only temporary relief. As abuse continues, shame and guilt increase, and coping with daily stressors becomes more difficult. Depression and anxiety are as likely to be the consequences as the causes of substance abuse.

- **Spiritual health.** Addictive behavior blocks the pursuit of meaning and inner fulfillment. As they rely more and more on a chemical or behavioral escape, individuals lose their sense of self and of connection with others and with a higher power.

- **Social health.** Addictive behavior strains and, in time, severs the ties that bind an individual to family, friends, colleagues, and classmates. The primary relationship in the life of alcoholics or addicts is with a behavior or a drug. They withdraw from others and become increasingly isolated.

- **Intellectual health.** The brain is one of the targets of alcohol and drugs. Under their influence, logic and reasoning break down. Impulses become more difficult to control. Judgment falters. Certain substances, such as ecstasy, can lead to permanent changes in brain chemistry.

- **Environmental health.** The use of some substances, such as tobacco, directly harms the environment. Abusers of alcohol and drugs also pose indirect threats to others because their behavior can lead to injury and damage.

# Gambling on Campus

Problem gambling has become more common among American adults than alcohol dependence. According to recent national surveys, levels of gambling, frequent gambling, and problem gambling increase during the teen years (even though underage gambling is illegal in most states), reach the highest point in the 20s and 30s, and decline after age 70. Men, who are more than twice as likely to be frequent gamblers as women, reach their highest gambling rates in their late teens. Whites are much more likely to report any gambling in the past year than blacks or Asians, but both African Americans and Native Americans report higher levels of frequent gambling.[3]

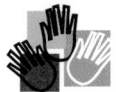 Gambling also is becoming a more serious and widespread problem on college campuses. Many college students buy lottery or scratch tickets, bet on sporting events, or go to casinos. About half of those who gamble at least once a month experience significant problems related to their gambling, including poor academic performance, heavy alcohol consumption, illicit drug use, unprotected sex, and other risky behaviors. An estimated 3 to 6 percent of college students engage in "pathological gambling," which is characterized by "persistent and recurrent maladaptive gambling behavior."

Researchers identified key indicators associated with "pathological" gambling: gambling more than once a month, gambling more than two hours a month, and wagering more than 10 percent of monthly income. A combination of parental gambling problems, gambling frequency, and psychological distress also is associated with college gambling.

College students who gamble say they do so for fun or excitement, to socialize, to win money, or to "just have something to do"—reasons similar to those of adults who gamble. Simply having access to casino machines, ongoing card games, or Internet gambling sites increases the likelihood that students will gamble.

Although most people who gamble limit the time and money they spend, some cross the line and lose control of their gambling "habit." The term *problem gambling* refers to all individuals with gambling-related problems, including mild or occasional ones.

Researchers now view problem or pathological gambling as an addiction that runs in families. Individuals predisposed to gambling because of their family history are more likely to develop a problem if they are regularly exposed to gambling. Alcoholism and drug abuse often occur along with gambling, leading to chaotic lives and greater health risks.

## Risk Factors for Problem Gambling

Among young people (ages 16 to 25) the following behaviors indicate increased risk of problem gambling:

- Being male.
- Gambling at an early age (as young as age 8).
- Having a big win earlier in one's gambling career.
- Consistently chasing losses (betting more to recover money already lost).
- Gambling alone.
- Feeling depressed before gambling.
- Feeling excited and aroused during gambling.
- Behaving irrationally during gambling.
- Having poor grades at school.
- Engaging in other addictive behaviors (smoking, drinking alcohol, illegal drug use).
- Being in a lower socioeconomic class.
- Having parents with a gambling or other addiction problem.
- Having a history of delinquency or stealing money to fund gambling.
- Skipping class to go gambling.

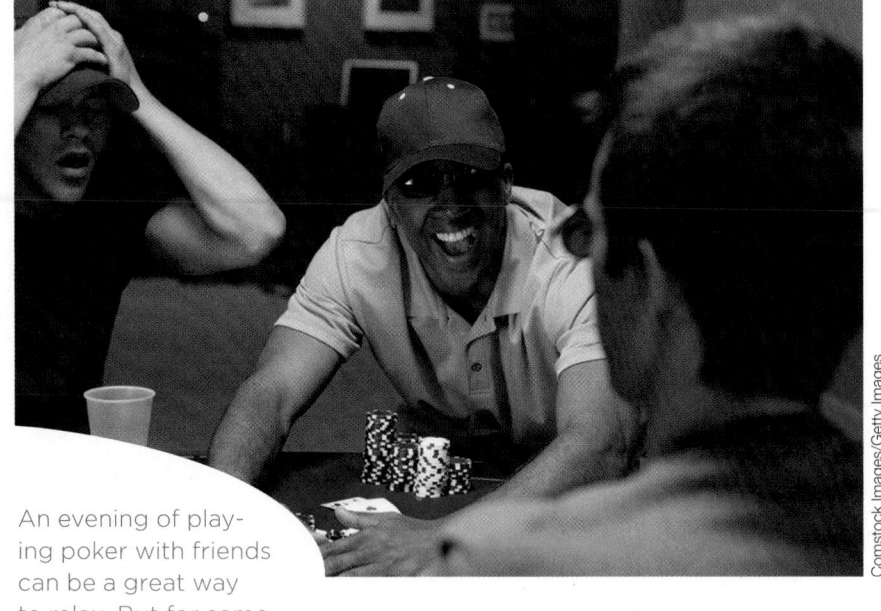

An evening of playing poker with friends can be a great way to relax. But for some college students, gambling can become addictive.

Comstock Images/Getty Images

## Pathological Gamblers

Adult pathological gamblers are more likely to be male, single, nonwhite, and less educated. Women start gambling later than men, but they progress more rapidly to pathological gambling. Genetics and exposure to gambling in childhood are significant influences. More than half of pathological gamblers report at least one first-degree relative with symptoms consistent with gambling problems.

Gamblers typically progress through various stages. In the winning phase, they feel empowered by their winnings and success. Next comes the losing phase, during which gamblers try to win back their losses. This is followed by the desperation phase, during which a gambler may resort to illegal activity, including stealing, to continue gambling. Some gamblers experience a fourth phase, the giving-up phase, where they desperately try to stay afloat in a game even though they realize they can't win.

As many as three-fourths of adult pathological gamblers suffer from depression. They also have high rates of nicotine dependence, alcoholism, and anxiety disorders.[4] An estimated 20 percent suffer from attention-deficit/hyperactivity disorder (ADHD). Even more—30 to 50 percent of pathological gamblers—abuse drugs or alcohol.

No standard or proven treatment exists for pathological gambling, but inpatient treatment centers, self-help groups, cognitive-behavioral psychotherapy, and addiction-based psychotherapy can help.[5]

## Do You Have a Gambling Problem?

- Do you gamble more than once a month?
- Do you wager more than 10 percent of your monthly income?
- Have you ever felt that your gambling or betting was out of control?
- Have you ever gotten into a fight with your family or friends because of gambling or betting?
- Have you ever felt that you lost too much money in gambling or betting?
- Have you ever felt the need to bet more and more money?
- Have you ever had to lie to people important to you about how much you gamble?

Even a single yes answer may indicate a problem. Go online or check with a counselor on campus to find resources, such as a local chapter of Gamblers Anonymous.

# Drug Use on Campus

More than six in ten college students have never used marijuana or other illegal drugs.[6] (See How Do You Compare?, p. 387.) Yet substance abuse remains a serious health risk for the minority of undergraduates who do use drugs.

Marijuana remains the most widely used illicit drug on campus, but the nonmedical use of prescription drugs now outranks other forms of substance abuse. In a recent national survey of college women, 7.8 percent reported that they had used a prescription drug for nonmedical purposes in the past year.[7] According to various national surveys, about 12 percent of college students report that they have misused prescription opioids (discussed later in this chapter) at least once in the past, while 7 percent did so in the last year.[8]

Students who engage only in nonmedical use of prescription pills (dubbed "pill-poppers" in one study) and those who use only illicit drugs ("dopers" in the same study) are similar in some ways and different in others.

Characteristics of illicit drug users:

- Most in late teens and early 20s.
- More likely to be male.
- More likely to be white.
- Lower GPA.
- More likely to be sexually active.
- Less likely to report strong religious values.
- More likely to not be or have never been married.
- Less likely to report good physical or mental health.
- More likely than nonusers to misuse prescription drugs.

Characteristics of users of prescription drugs for nonmedical reasons:

- Unclear if women or men have higher rates.
- More likely to be white.
- Lower GPA.
- Less likely to report good physical or mental health.
- More likely to report knowing a member of the faculty or administration (possibly because of grades and academic performance).

## Why Students Don't Use Drugs

The majority of undergraduates do not use illegal drugs or abuse prescription drugs. What keeps them drug-free? Here are some important factors:

- **Spirituality and religion.** The greater a student's religiosity—a term that encompasses hours spent in prayer, attendance at religious services, and reading spiritual materials—the less likely the student is to use alcohol, illegal drugs, or tobacco. Unfortunately, researchers have noted a drop in students' religiosity during college, along with an increase in their alcohol and marijuana use.
- **Academic engagement.** Illicit drug use is much less common among students who actively participate in classes and feel connected with the subject matter. However, many students report never working closely

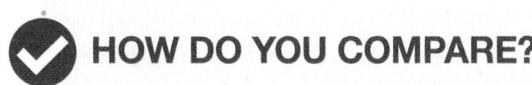

## HOW DO YOU COMPARE?

# STUDENT DRUG USE

|  | Percent |  | Percent |
|---|---|---|---|
| Never used any drug* | **64.2** | Used in the last 30 days | **13.8** |
| Used, but not in last 30 days | **22.0** | Used all 30 days | **1.8** |

*Excluding alcohol, cigarettes, tobacco from a water pipe, and marijuana; including club drugs, methamphetamine, cocaine, other stimulants, sedatives, hallucinogens, anabolic steroids, opiates, inhalants, smokeless tobacco, cigars, other illegal drugs

## HOW DO YOU COMPARE?

Did you know that almost two-thirds of undergraduates have never used drugs? What has been your experience? If you are among the majority, what are the factors that have enabled you to say no to drugs? If you have used drugs, what were your reasons? What role do drugs now play in your life? What has been their impact? Write down your feelings about how drugs might affect your health and your life in your online journal.

Source: American College Health Association, *American College Health Association-National College Health Assessment II: Reference Group Executive Summary Spring 2010* (Linthicum, MD: American College Health Association, 2010).

with a faculty member, never being inspired by an educational experience, or never having an educational or extracurricular experience that motivates them to make an active contribution to a greater goal.

- **Perceived harmfulness.** Although nonmedical use of prescription drugs has increased on college campuses, students—about one in four in a recent survey—who perceived a great risk of harm from repeated or occasional use were the least likely to misuse medications.
- **Athletics.** Although male and female college athletes drink at higher rates than nonathletes, they are less likely to use illegal drugs. One exception is the use of anabolic steroids (discussed in Chapter 8), which college athletes use more than other students.

## Why Students Use Drugs

Various factors influence which students use drugs, including the following:

- **Genetics and family history.** Some college students inherit a genetic or biological predisposition to substance abuse. Researchers have identified specific genes tied to all types of addictions. Some of the genes associated with alcohol dependence are closely linked with addictions to marijuana, nicotine, cocaine, heroin, and other substances. Also, the risk for problem drinking and alcohol abuse is higher among children of substance abusers.

- **Parental attitudes and behavior.** Parents' concerns or expectations influence whether or how much most students drink, smoke, or use drugs. Those who perceive that their parents approve of their drinking, for instance, are more likely to report a drinking-related problem, such as memory loss or missing class. More than one in five underage students report acquiring alcohol from their parents or relatives.

- **Substance use in high school.** Many students start abusing drugs or alcohol well before getting to college. Only 8 percent of undergraduate marijuana users and even fewer cocaine users began their use in college. Misusing prescription drugs before age 16 increases the risk of a substance abuse disorder later in life.

- **Social norms.** College students tend to overestimate drug use on campus. In the American College Health Association National College Health Assessment survey, students reported believing that 8.6 percent of undergraduates had never used marijuana. In fact, 63.2 percent never had. (See Table 12.1.)

- **Positive expectations.** Many students expect a drug to make them feel less stressed or anxious, more relaxed or confident, less shy or inhibited. Among students who use illicit drugs, many say they do so to relieve stress. Others self-medicate, taking drugs to relieve depression or anxiety. Some abuse prescription medications, such as Adderall and Ritalin, because they think these drugs will energize them to study longer or perform better. Even when drugs don't live up to students' expectations, they may continue taking them for some short-term relief or because they have become addicted and cannot stop.

- **Mental health problems.** Students with feelings of hopelessness, sadness, depression, and anxiety as well as those with clinical mental disorders have higher rates of prescription drug abuse and illegal drug use. Students diagnosed with depression in the past school year have higher rates of marijuana, cocaine, alcohol, and tobacco use. Students with a history of ADHD (discussed in Chapter 3) are also more vulnerable to substance abuse. In a recent study, undergraduates with a history of ADHD were more likely to report having used marijuana and other illicit drugs, to begin use at a younger age, and to suffer higher levels of impairment.[9]

- **Social influences.** More than nine in ten students who use illegal drugs were introduced to the habit through friends; most use drugs with friends. Sorority and fraternity members, who tend to socialize more often, are likelier to abuse prescription stimulants, but students who live off campus have higher rates of marijuana and cocaine use.

- **Alcohol use.** Often individuals engage in more than one risky behavior. Researchers have found that those students who report binge drinking are much more likely than other students to report current or past use of marijuana, cocaine, or other illegal drugs.

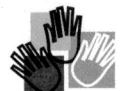

- **Race/ethnicity.** In general, white students have higher levels of alcohol and drug use than do African American students. In a comparison of African American students at predominantly white and predominantly black

Table 12.1 **Marijuana Use on Campus**

| | Percent (%) | | | | | |
| | Actual Use | | | Perceived Use | | |
| | Male | Female | Total | Male | Female | Total |
|---|---|---|---|---|---|---|
| Never used | 59.5 | 65.3 | 63.2 | 9.9 | 7.6 | 8.6 |
| Used, but not in the last 30 days | 19.4 | 20.3 | 19.9 | 11.6 | 9.9 | 10.5 |
| Used 1–9 days | 11.6 | 9.9 | 10.5 | 47.2 | 44.8 | 45.5 |
| Used 10–29 days | 5.3 | 2.9 | 3.8 | 21.8 | 26.7 | 24.9 |
| Used all 30 days | 4.2 | 1.6 | 2.6 | 9.5 | 11.0 | 10.5 |
| *Any use within the last 30 days* | 21.1 | 14.4 | 17.0 | 78.5 | 82.5 | 80.9 |

Source: American College Health Association, *American College Health Association-National College Health Assessment II: Reference Group Executive Summary Spring 2010* (Linthicum, MD: American College Health Association, 2010).

colleges, those at historically black colleges had lower rates of alcohol and drug use than did either white or African American students at white schools. The reason, according to the researchers, may be that these colleges provide a greater sense of self-esteem, which helps prevent alcohol and drug use.

- **Sexual identity.** Gay, lesbian, and bisexual teens may rely on alcohol and marijuana to lessen social anxiety and boost self-confidence when they first come out. However, once they become more involved in the gay community, many are less likely to do so. Nonetheless, lesbians are significantly more likely than heterosexual women to use marijuana, Ecstasy, and other drugs. Gay and bisexual men are significantly less likely than heterosexual men to drink heavily but more likely to use drugs.

# Understanding Drugs and Their Effects

A **drug** is a chemical substance that affects the way you feel and function. In some circumstances, taking a drug can help the body heal or relieve physical and mental distress. In other circumstances, taking a drug can distort reality, undermine well-being, and threaten survival. No drug is completely safe; all drugs have multiple effects that vary greatly in different people at different times. Knowing how drugs affect the brain, body, and behavior is crucial to understanding their impact and making responsible decisions about their use.

*Drug abuse* is the widely used term for the improper use of drugs, but some researchers have broken down the behavior into several categories:

- **Drug abuse** is a pattern of substance use resulting in negative consequences or impairment.
- **Drug dependence** is a pattern of continuing substance use despite cognitive, behavioral, and physical symptoms.
- **Drug misuse** is taking a drug for a purpose or by a person other than that for which

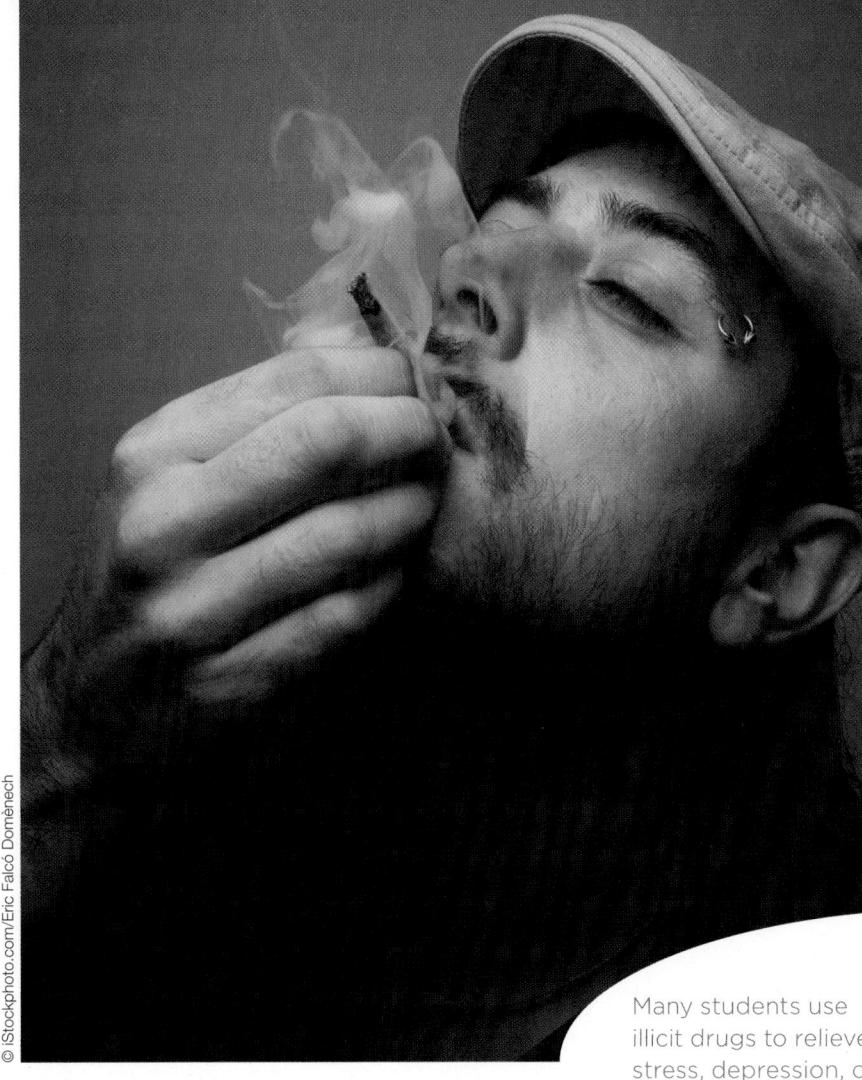

Many students use illicit drugs to relieve stress, depression, or anxiety but end up feeling more stressed, depressed, or anxious.

it was intended or not taking the recommended doses.

- **Drug diversion** is the transfer of a medication from the individual to whom it was prescribed to another person.

Risks are involved with all forms of drug use. Even medications that help cure illnesses or soothe symptoms have side effects and can be misused. Some substances that millions of people use every day, such as caffeine, pose some health risks. Others—like the most commonly used drugs in our society, alcohol and tobacco—can lead to potentially life-threatening problems. With some illicit drugs, any form of use can be dangerous.

Many factors determine the effects a drug has on an individual. These include how the drug enters the body, the dosage, the drug action, and the presence of other drugs in the body—as well as the physical and psychological makeup

**drug** Any substance, other than food, that affects bodily functions and structures when taken into the body.

**drug abuse** The excessive use of a drug in a manner inconsistent with accepted medical practice.

**drug dependence** Continued substance use even when its use causes cognitive, behavioral, and physical symptoms.

**drug misuse** The use of a drug for a purpose (or person) other than that for which it was medically intended.

**drug diversion** The transfer of a drug from the person for whom it was prescribed to another individual.

Figure 12.1 **Routes of Administration of Drugs**

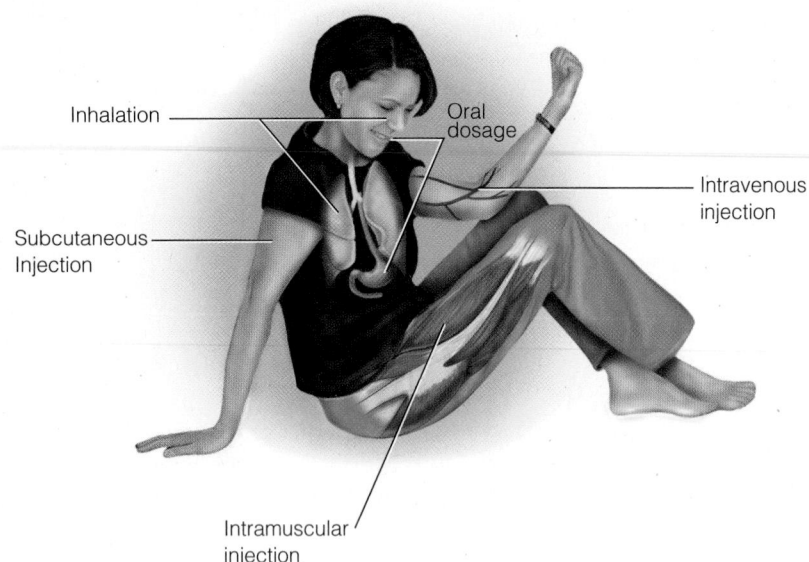

Inhalation

Oral dosage

Subcutaneous Injection

Intravenous injection

Intramuscular injection

moderately fast (within a few minutes); and **subcutaneous** injection, more slowly (within ten minutes).

Injecting drugs is extremely dangerous because many diseases, including hepatitis and infection with human immunodeficiency virus (HIV), can be transmitted by sharing contaminated needles. Injection-drug users who are HIV-positive are a major source of transmission of HIV among heterosexuals (see Chapter 16).

## Dosage and Toxicity

The effects of any drug depend on the amount an individual takes. Increasing the dose usually intensifies the effects produced by smaller doses. Also, the kind of effect may change at different dose levels. For example, low doses of barbiturates may relieve anxiety, while higher doses can induce sleep, loss of sensation, even coma and death.

The dosage level at which a drug becomes poisonous to the body, causing either temporary or permanent damage, is called its **toxicity**. In most cases, drugs are eventually broken down in the liver by special body chemicals called *detoxification enzymes*.

## Individual Differences

Each person responds differently to different drugs, depending on circumstances or setting. The enzymes in the body reduce the levels of drugs in the bloodstream; because there can be 80 variants of each enzyme, every person's body may react differently.

Often drugs intensify the emotional state a person is in. If you're feeling depressed, a drug may make you feel more depressed. A generalized physical problem, such as having the flu, may make your body more vulnerable to the effects of a drug. Genetic differences among individuals also may account for varying reactions.

Personality and psychological attitude also play a role in drug effects. Each user's *mind-set*—his or her expectations or preconceptions about using the drug—affects the experience. Someone who takes a "club drug" (discussed further later in this chapter) to feel more "connected" may feel more sociable simply because that's what he or she expects.

of the person taking the drug and the setting in which the drug is used.

## Routes of Administration

Drugs can enter the body in a number of ways (Figure 12.1). The most common way of taking a drug is by swallowing a tablet, capsule, or liquid. However, drugs taken orally don't reach the bloodstream as quickly as drugs introduced into the body by other means. A drug taken orally may not have any effect for 30 minutes or more.

Drugs can enter the body through the lungs either by inhaling smoke—for example, from marijuana—or by inhaling gases, aerosol sprays, or fumes from solvents or other compounds that evaporate quickly. Young users of such inhalants, discussed later in this chapter, often soak a rag with fluid and press it over their nose. Or they may place inhalants in a plastic bag, put the bag over their nose and mouth, and take deep breaths—a practice called *huffing* and one that can produce serious, even fatal consequences.

Drugs can also be injected with a syringe subcutaneously (beneath the skin), intramuscularly (into muscle tissue, which is richly supplied with blood vessels), or intravenously (directly into a vein). **Intravenous** (IV) injection gets the drug into the bloodstream immediately (within seconds in most cases); **intramuscular** injection,

**intravenous** Into a vein.

**intramuscular** Into or within a muscle.

**subcutaneous** Under the skin.

**toxicity** Poisonousness; the dosage level at which a drug becomes poisonous to the body, causing either temporary or permanent damage.

## Setting

The setting for drug use also influences its effects. Passing around a marijuana joint at a friend's is not a healthy or safe behavior, but the experience of going to a crack house is very different—and entails greater dangers.

## Types of Action

A drug can act *locally*, as novocaine does to deaden pain in a tooth; *generally*, throughout a body system, as barbiturates do on the central nervous system; or *selectively*, as a drug does when it has a greater effect on one specific organ or system than on others, such as a spinal anesthetic. A drug that accumulates in the body because it's taken in faster than it can be metabolized and excreted is called *cumulative*; alcohol is such a drug.

## Interaction with Other Drugs or Alcohol

A drug can interact with other drugs in four different ways:

- An **additive** interaction is one in which the resulting effect is equal to the sum of the effects of the different drugs used.

- A **synergistic** interaction is one in which the total effect of the two drugs taken together is greater than the sum of the effects the two drugs would have had if taken by themselves on separate occasions. Mixing barbiturates and alcohol, for example, has up to four times the depressant effect that either drug has alone.

- A drug can be **potentiating**—that is, one drug can increase the effect of another. Alcohol, for instance, can increase the drowsiness caused by antihistamines (antiallergy medications).

- Drugs can interact in an **antagonistic** fashion—that is, one drug can neutralize or block another drug with opposite effects. Tranquilizers, for example, may counter some of the nervousness and anxiety produced by cocaine.

The danger of mixing alcohol with other drugs cannot be emphasized too strongly. Alcohol and marijuana intensify each other's effects, making driving and many other activities extremely dangerous. Some people who have mixed sedatives or tranquilizers with alcohol never regained consciousness.

## Gender and Drugs

Beginning at a very early age, males and females show different patterns in drug use. Men generally encounter more opportunities to use drugs than women do, but given an opportunity to use drugs for the first time, both genders are equally likely to do so and to progress from initial use to dependence. Vulnerability to some drugs varies with gender. Both are equally likely to become addicted to or dependent on cocaine, heroin, hallucinogens, tobacco, and inhalants. Women are more likely than men to become addicted to or dependent on sedatives and drugs designed to treat anxiety or sleeplessness and less likely than men to abuse alcohol and marijuana.

Males and females may differ in their biological responses to drugs. In studies of animals given the opportunity to self-administer intravenous doses of cocaine or heroin, females began self-administration sooner than males and administered larger amounts of the drugs. Male and female long-term cocaine users showed similar impairment in tests of concentration, memory, and academic achievement following sustained abstinence, even though women in the study had substantially greater exposure to cocaine. Female cocaine users also were less likely than men to exhibit abnormalities of blood flow in the brain's frontal lobes. These findings suggest a gender-related mechanism that may protect women from some of the damage cocaine inflicts on the brain. However, women are more vulnerable to poor nutrition and below-average weight, depression, physical abuse, and if pregnant, preterm labor or early delivery.

# Caffeine and Its Effects

Caffeine, which has been drunk, chewed, and swallowed since the Stone Age, is the most widely used **psychoactive** (mind-affecting)

**additive** Characterized by a combined effect that is equal to the sum of the individual effects.

**synergistic** Characterized by a combined effect that is greater than the sum of the individual effects.

**potentiating** Making more effective or powerful.

**antagonistic** Opposing or counteracting.

**psychoactive** Mind-affecting.

drug in the world. Genetics may determine how much caffeine one craves. Scientists have identified the genes that drive people to consume more—or less—of this stimulant.[10]

Eighty percent of Americans drink coffee, our principal caffeine source—an average of 3.5 cups a day. Coffee contains 100 to 150 milligrams of caffeine per cup; tea, 40 to 100 milligrams; cola, about 45 milligrams. Most medications that contain caffeine are one-third to one-half the strength of a cup of coffee. However, some, such as Excedrin, are very high in caffeine. A "cup" of coffee, according to Table 12.2, contains only 5 ounces, but the smallest size available at most coffee shops is 8 to 12 ounces. You may be ingesting more caffeine than you think.

As a stimulant, caffeine relieves drowsiness, helps in the performance of repetitive tasks, and improves the capacity for work. Caffeine improves performance and endurance during prolonged, exhaustive exercise and, to a lesser degree, enhances short-term, high-intensity athletic performance. Additional benefits include improved concentration, reduced fatigue, and sharpened alertness.

You'll stay more alert, particularly if you are fighting sleep deprivation, if you spread your coffee consumption over the course of the day. For instance, rather than drinking two 8-ounce cups in the morning, try consuming smaller servings of an ounce or two during the course of the day.

In recent decades, some 19,000 studies have examined caffeine's impact on health. Their conclusion: For most people, caffeine poses few serious health risks—and may convey a surprising range of benefits. Drinking up to six cups a day of caffeinated or decaffeinated coffee won't shorten your lifespan and may convey some health benefits, including a lower risk of type 2 diabetes and cardiovascular disease.[11] Caffeine may also protect against Alzheimer's disease, Parkinson's disease, colon cancer, liver cirrhosis, gallstones, and stroke.[12] There is some evidence that coffee may relieve migraines, boost mood, and even prevent cavities. Researchers have found no significant relationship between coffee and tea consumption and the risk of breast cancer.

Despite these positive findings, doctors still advise pregnant women, heart patients, and those at risk for osteoporosis to limit or avoid coffee. High doses of daily caffeine—whether from coffee, tea, caffeinated soda, or hot chocolate—increase the risk of miscarriage. Too much caffeine, particularly in high-powered energy drinks, can be dangerous for everyone.

You can overdose on caffeine and develop symptoms such as restlessness, nervousness, excitement, insomnia, flushed face, increased urination, digestive complaints, muscle twitching, rambling thoughts and speech, rapid heart rate or arrhythmias, periods of inexhaustibility, and physical restlessness. Some people develop these symptoms after as little as 250 milligrams of caffeine a day; others, only with much larger doses. Higher doses may produce ringing in the ears or flashes of light, grand mal seizures, and potentially fatal respiratory failure.

Caffeine withdrawal for those dependent on this substance can cause headaches and other neurological symptoms. Those who must cut back should taper off gradually. One approach is to mix regular and decaffeinated coffee, gradually decreasing the quantity of the former.

Table 12.2 **Caffeine Counts**

| Substance (Typical Serving) | Caffeine (milligrams) |
|---|---|
| No-Doz, one pill | 200 |
| Coffee (drip), one 5-ounce cup | 130 |
| Excedrin, two pills | 130 |
| Espresso, one 2-ounce cup | 100 |
| Energy drink (Red Bull), one can | 80 |
| Instant coffee, one 5-ounce cup | 74 |
| Coca-Cola, 12 ounces | 46 |
| Tea, one 5-ounce cup | 40 |
| Dark chocolate, 1 ounce | 20 |
| Milk chocolate, 1 ounce | 6 |
| Cocoa, 5 ounces | 4 |
| Decaffeinated coffee, one 5-ounce cup | 3 |

# Medications

As many as half of all patients take the wrong medications, in the wrong doses, at the wrong times, or in the wrong ways. Every year these inadvertent errors lead to an estimated 125,000 deaths and more than $8.5 billion in hospital costs. Mistakes occur among people of all ages, both genders, and every race, occupation, level of education, and personality type. Their number one cause: not understanding directions (see Consumer Alert, p. 394).

Doctors occasionally make errors when it comes to prescription drugs. The most frequent are over- or underdosing, omitting information from prescriptions, ordering the wrong dosage form (a pill instead of a liquid, for example), and not recognizing a patient's allergy to a drug.

## Over-the-Counter Drugs

More than half a million health products—remedies for everything from bad breath to bunions—are readily available without a doctor's prescription. This doesn't mean that they're necessarily safe or effective. Indeed, many widely used **over-the-counter (OTC) drugs** pose unsuspected hazards.

Federal regulators have issued warnings for many popular painkillers, including over-the-counter pills like Advil (ibuprofen) and Aleve (naproxin). Their labels cite risks to the heart, stomach, and skin. Tylenol (acetaminophen) and aspirin are generally considered safe for people with temporary pain like headaches and muscle aches. However, aspirin can cause stomach irritation and bleeding. Tylenol and other products containing acetaminophen account for 40 to 50 percent of all acute cases of liver failure, many the result of unintentional overdose. Doctors caution against taking more than eight Tylenol Extra Strength pills (which contain 500 mg per tablet) in a 24-hour period.

Like other drugs, OTC medications can be used improperly, often simply because of a lack of education about proper use. Among those most often misused are the following:

- **Nasal sprays.** Nasal sprays relieve congestion by shrinking blood vessels in the nose.

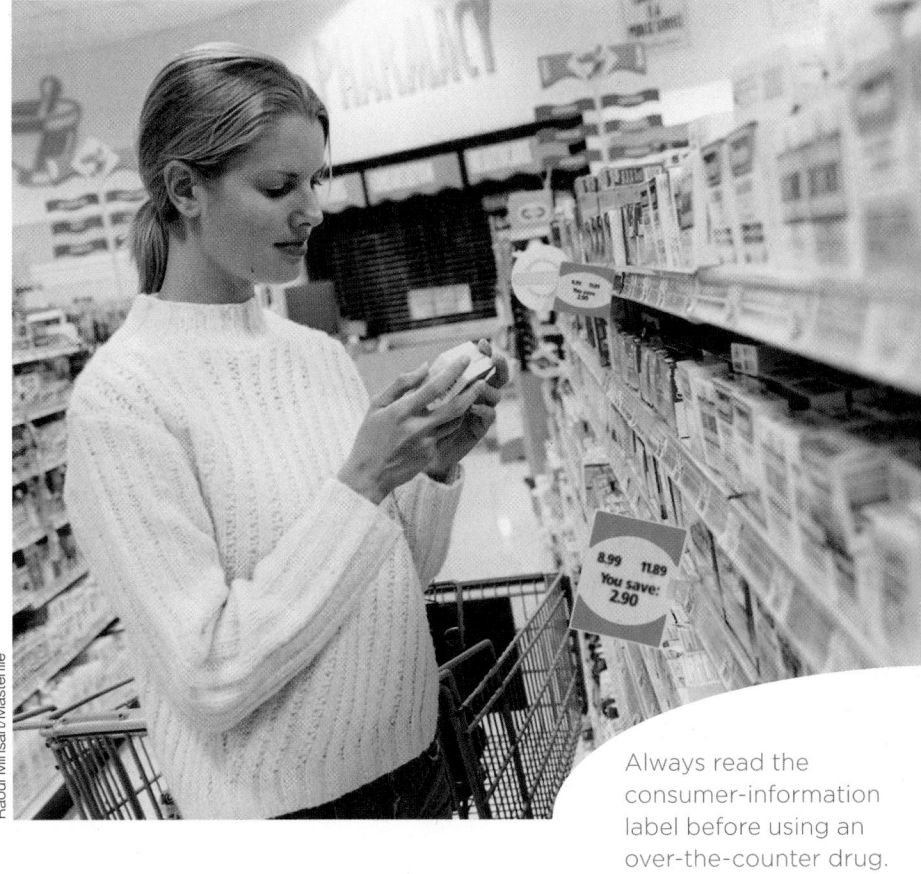

Always read the consumer-information label before using an over-the-counter drug.

If they are used too often or for too many days in a row, the blood vessels widen instead of contracting, and the surrounding tissues become swollen, causing more congestion. To make the vessels shrink again, many people use more spray more often. The result can be permanent damage to nasal membranes, bleeding, infection, and partial or complete loss of smell.

- **Laxatives.** Believing that they must have one bowel movement a day (a common misconception), many people rely on laxatives. Brands that contain phenolphthalein irritate the lining of the intestines and cause muscles to contract or tighten, often making constipation worse rather than better. Bulk laxatives are less dangerous, but regular use is not advised. A high-fiber diet and more exercise are safer and more effective remedies for constipation.

- **Eye drops.** Eye drops make the blood vessels of the eye contract. However, as in the case of nasal sprays, with overuse (several times a day for several weeks), the blood vessels expand, making the eye look redder than before.

**over-the-counter (OTC) drugs** Medications that can be obtained legally without a prescription from a medical professional.

# ❶ CONSUMER ALERT

## Avoid Medication Mistakes

Whenever you get a prescription, be sure to find out from your doctor and pharmacist the name of the drug, what it's supposed to do, and how and when to take it and for how long. Are there foods, drinks, other medications, or activities you should avoid while taking the medication? Ask if the drug causes any side effects and what you should do if any occur.

### Facts to Know

- Popular herbal supplements like gingko biloba and common over-the-counter drugs like aspirin can interact with many prescription drugs to cause serious problems, such as excessive bleeding. Inform your doctor if you take any.
- Don't use a kitchen spoon to dispense liquid medications. Household teaspoons can hold between 3 and 7 milliliters; a prescription "teaspoon" means 5 milliliters. Either measure the dose in the cup or dropper that came with the medicine or ask the pharmacist for a measuring device.
- Don't crush or chew a medicine without checking with your doctor or pharmacist first. Some medications are designed for gradual release rather than all at once and could be harmful if absorbed too quickly.

### Steps to Take

- Keep a record of all your medicines, listing both their brand and generic (chemical) names and the reason you are taking them, and update it regularly. Give a copy of this list to every physician and every pharmacy providing health-care services.
- Always turn on the lights when you take your medication. Familiarize yourself with the imprint on each tablet or capsule so you can recognize each pill. If a refill looks different, check with your pharmacist or doctor before taking it.
- Never take someone else's medications. They could interact with your medications or the dose may be different.
- Always check labels for warnings on interactions with alcohol and instructions on whether or not to take before, with, or after meals.
- Don't take medicine with grapefruit juice, which can interact with more than 200 medications, including cholesterol-lowering statins, sleeping pills, and antianxiety agents.
- Don't leave medicines in a car for prolonged periods. Temperature extremes, along with moisture, light, and oxygen, can affect the potency of many medications.

Check the labels on prescription medications.

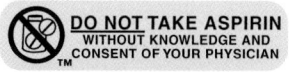 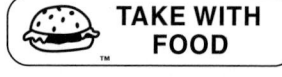
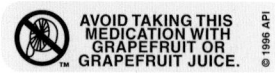 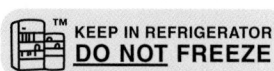
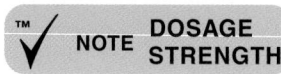 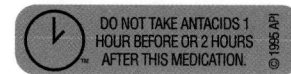

- **Sleep aids.** Although OTC sleeping pills are widely used, there has been little research on their use and possible risks. A national consensus panel on insomnia concluded that they are not effective and cause side effects such as morning-after grogginess. Medications like Tylenol PM and Excedrin PM combine a pain reliever with a sleep-inducing antihistamine, the same ingredient that people take for hay fever or cold symptoms. Although they make people drowsy, they can leave a groggy feeling the next day, and they dry out the nose and mouth.

- **Cough syrup.** Many of the "active" ingredients in over-the-counter cough preparations may be ineffective. Young people may chug cough syrup (called *roboing*, after the OTC medication Robitussin) because they think of dextromethorphan (DXM), a common ingredient in cough medicine, as a "poor man's version" of the popular drug Ecstasy.

- **Painkillers.** Men younger than age 50 who take acetaminophen (the main ingredient in Tylenol) more than two times a week have roughly double the risk of hearing loss compared to men who do not. Men of similar ages who take ibuprofen (the main ingredient in Motrin or Advil) at least twice a week have a nearly two-thirds higher risk of hearing loss. Men who take aspirin twice a week have a one-third higher risk. However, the absolute risk of hearing loss remains small in young and middle-aged men.[13]

## Prescription Drugs

 Most undergraduates have used prescription drugs for medical reasons at some point in their lives. The most widely used ones are pain medications, sedative or anxiety medications, sleeping medications, and stimulant medications. College women use more pain, anxiety, and sleeping pills; college men, more medically prescribed stimulants. (See Table 12.3.)

*Nonadherence* Many prescribed medications aren't taken the way they should be; millions simply aren't taken at all. As many as 70 percent of adults have trouble understanding dosage information and 30 percent can't read standard labels, according to the FDA, which has called for larger, clearer drug labeling. The dangers of nonadherence (not properly taking prescription drugs) include recurrent infections, serious medical complications, and emergency hospital treatment. The drugs most likely to be taken incorrectly are those that treat problems with no obvious symptoms (such as high blood pressure), require complex dosage schedules, treat psychiatric disorders, or have unpleasant side effects.

The most common reason that college students fail to take medicines as directed is forgetting. Others are concerned about cost, or they stop when they feel better.

*Physical Side Effects* Most medications, taken correctly, cause only minor complications. However, no drug is entirely without side effects for all individuals taking it. Serious complications that may occur include heart failure, heart attack, seizures, kidney and liver failure, severe blood disorders, birth defects, blindness, memory problems, and allergic reactions. Even legitimate use of some drugs, such as opioid painkillers, can lead to potentially fatal overdoses.[14]

Allergic reactions to drugs are common. The drugs that most often provoke allergic responses are penicillin and other antibiotics (drugs used to treat infection). Aspirin, sulfa drugs, barbiturates, anticonvulsants, insulin, and local anesthetics can also provoke allergic responses.

*Psychological Side Effects* Dozens of drugs—both over-the-counter and prescription—can cause changes in the way people think, feel, and behave. Unfortunately, neither patients nor their physicians usually connect such symptoms with medications. Doctors may not even mention potential mental and emotional problems because they don't want to scare patients away from what otherwise may be a very effective treatment. What you don't know about a drug's effects on your mind *can* hurt you.

Among the medications most likely to cause psychiatric side effects are drugs for high blood pressure, heart disease, asthma, epilepsy, arthritis, Parkinson's disease, anxiety, insomnia, and depression. Some drugs—such as the powerful hormones called *corticosteroids*, used for asthma,

Table 12.3 **Unauthorized Prescription Drug Use by College Students**

Percentage of college students who reported using prescription drugs that were not prescribed to them within the last 12 months:

|  | Percent (%) | | |
|---|---|---|---|
|  | Male | Female | Total |
| **Antidepressants** | 2.7 | 3.4 | 3.2 |
| **Erectile dysfunction drugs** | 1.4 | 0.8 | 1.0 |
| **Painkillers** | 10.6 | 8.4 | 9.3 |
| **Sedatives** | 4.8 | 4.2 | 4.5 |
| **Stimulants** | 8.0 | 6.4 | 7.0 |
| **Used one or more of the above** | 16.3 | 14.5 | 15.3 |

Source: American College Health Association, *American College Health Association-National College Health Assessment II: Reference Group Executive Summary Spring 2010* (Linthicum, MD: American College Health Association, 2010).

autoimmune diseases, and cancer—can cause different psychiatric symptoms, depending on dosage and other factors. The older you are, the sicker you are, and the more medications you're taking, the greater your risk of developing some psychiatric side effects.

*Drug Interactions* OTC and prescription drugs can interact in a variety of ways. For example, mixing some cold medications with tranquilizers can cause drowsiness and coordination problems, thus making driving dangerous. Moreover, what you eat or drink can impair or completely wipe out the effectiveness of drugs or lead to unexpected effects on the body. For instance, aspirin takes five to ten times as long to be absorbed when taken with food or shortly after a meal than when taken on an empty stomach. If tetracyclines encounter calcium in the stomach, they bind together and cancel each other out.

To avoid potentially dangerous interactions, check the label(s) for any instructions on how or when to take a medication, such as "with a meal." If the directions say that you should take a drug on an empty stomach, take it at least one hour before eating or two or three hours after eating. Don't drink a hot beverage with a medication; the temperature may interfere with the effectiveness of the drug.

Whenever you take a drug, be especially careful of your intake of alcohol, which can change the rate of metabolism and the effects of many different drugs. Because it dilates the blood vessels, alcohol can add to the dizziness sometimes caused by drugs for high blood pressure, angina, or depression. Also, its irritating effects on the stomach can worsen stomach upset from aspirin, ibuprofen, and other anti-inflammatory drugs.

*Generic Drugs*　The **generic** name is the chemical name for a drug. A specific drug may appear on the pharmacist's shelf under a variety of brand names, which may cost more than twice the generic equivalent. About 75 percent of all prescriptions specify a brand name, but pharmacists may—and in some states must—switch to a generic drug unless the doctor specifically tells them not to. Prescriptions filled with generic drugs cost 20 to 85 percent less than their brand-name counterparts.

Generic drugs have the same active ingredients as brand-name prescriptions, but their fillers and binders, which can affect the absorption of a drug, may be different. For some serious illnesses, the generics may not be as effective; some experts recommend sticking with brand names for heart medications, psychiatric drugs, and anticonvulsant drugs (for epilepsy and other seizure disorders).

To determine whether you should buy the generic version of a drug, ask your physician whether it matters if you get a brand-name or generic drug. If it does, ask which brand name is best. Also, find out if switching to a generic or from one generic to another might harm your condition in any way.

*Buying Drugs Online*　Millions of people in the United States purchase prescription medications online. Although some websites fill only faxed prescriptions from medical doctors, others ignore or sidestep traditional regulations and safeguards. Cyberspace distributors often ship pills across state lines without requiring a physical examination by a medical doctor. Instead, a "cyberdoc," who may or may not be qualified or up-to-date in a given specialty, reviews information submitted by a "patient." International pharmacies sometimes sell drugs that are not available or approved in the United States. And patients themselves use bulletin boards and other online resources to sell unused or unwanted medications to each other.

Many individuals turn to the Internet for "lifestyle" drugs such as pills for erectile dysfunction, weight control, and smoking cessation. Customers like the convenience and anonymity of buying drugs online. Although many assume drugs cost less on the Internet, shipping costs tend to drive prices up to the same amount or more than the price at a pharmacy.

The dangers of unregulated distribution of medications have alarmed government agencies and medical groups. The American Medical Association has declared it unethical for physicians to write prescriptions for people they've never met. The National Association of Boards of Pharmacy has developed a seal of approval to help customers determine which sites are legitimate. The FDA and other federal agencies, such as the Federal Trade Commission, which regulates advertising, are trying to find ways to impose some controls.

Consumers have to be wary. Ordering a drug like Accutane, an acne treatment, online may seem harmless. However, without close monitoring by a physician, you could develop complications, such as a bad reaction that aggravates hepatitis or inflames the pancreas. Quality control is another concern. Counterfeit drugs, increasingly sold online, may do little, if any, good and could be harmful. Cyberspace pharmacies provide no information on how the drug was stored or whether its expiration date has passed. In addition, since importing medications without a prescription is against the law, you could find yourself in legal trouble.

# Prescription Drug Abuse on Campus

 One of every five teenagers and adults—about 50 million Americans—have used a prescription drug for a nonmedical purpose. Nonmedical use of any prescription medication is highest among young adults between the ages of 18 and 25, compared with other age groups, and opioid painkillers (discussed later in this chapter) are the most widely misused.[15]

**generic** A consumer product with no brand name or registered trademark.

The abuse of prescription medications on college campuses has increased in the last 15 years. As many as one in five college students misuses or abuses a prescription medication every year. Young adults (between ages 18 and 25) have the highest rates of prescription painkiller abuse of any age group in the country.[16] Only marijuana use is more widespread on campus.

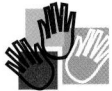College men have higher rates of prescription drug abuse than women. White and Hispanic undergraduates are significantly more likely to abuse medications than are African American and Asian students. Many students taking prescription drugs for medical purposes report being approached by classmates seeking drugs. Undergraduates who misuse or abuse prescription medications are much more likely to report heavy binge drinking and use of illicit drugs. College women who do so are at greater risk for sexual victimization and assault.[17]

Students who abuse prescription drugs may use both stimulants and painkillers. However, most students choose these agents for different reasons. Students who abuse stimulants say they do so to help improve performance at school, to increase alertness, or to enjoy partying more. A much smaller number take stimulants to lose weight or prevent weight gain. Students who abuse prescription painkillers say they do so to relax or get high, although some report taking the drugs to help with depression and anxiety or for chronic pain.

## Prescription Stimulants

The most widely abused prescription drugs are stimulant medications such as Ritalin. Students often view illicit stimulant use as physically harmless and morally acceptable.[18] Many think that stimulants can help them focus, concentrate, and study longer. Yet users of these drugs actually have lower GPAs than nonusers, and there is little evidence that stimulants provide any boost.

In various studies, 5 to 35 percent of college-age individuals have reported nonprescribed use of stimulants, and 16 to 29 percent of students prescribed stimulants for ADHD reported being asked to give, sell, or trade their medications.

Students who are white, are traditional college age (under 24), belong to fraternities or sororities, have lower grade-point averages, and report some symptoms of ADHD are most likely to misuse or pass on stimulants to others. Most illicit users obtain the drugs from friends or peers for free or at a cost of $1 to $5. In a study of 1,550 undergraduates at a large southern university, about four in ten reported illicit stimulant use. These users, along with students with ADHD, reported significantly greater drug use than others.

Although proper medical use of this agent appears safe, misuse or abuse of any stimulant medication can be dangerous, even deadly. When taken in high doses, either orally or nasally, the risk of addiction increases. Physical side effects include cardiorespiratory complications, increased blood pressure, and headache. High doses can trigger panic attacks, aggressive behavior, and suicidal or homicidal impulses. Overdoses can kill.

## Prescription Painkillers

Abuse of prescription painkillers, such as Oxy-Contin and Vicodin, is also widespread on campuses. Students who are members of fraternities and sororities, enrolled at more competitive schools, earning lower grade-point averages, and engaging in substance use and other risky behaviors are more likely to abuse these drugs. Smokers also are more prone to long-term prescription abuse.[19]

Like other addictions, a prescription painkiller "habit" is a treatable brain disease. Recovery usually requires carefully supervised detoxification, appropriate medications (similar to those used for opioid dependence), behavioral therapy, and ongoing support.

# Substance-Use Disorders

People have been using psychoactive chemicals for centuries. Citizens of ancient Mesopotamia and Egypt used opium. More than 3,000 years ago, Hindus included cannabis products in religious ceremonies. For centuries the Inca in South America have chewed the leaves of the coca bush. Yet while drugs existed in most societies, their use was usually limited to small groups. Today millions of people regularly turn to drugs to pick them up, bring them down, alter perceptions, or ease psychological pain.

The word **addiction**, as used by the general population, refers to the compulsive use of a substance, loss of control, negative consequences, and denial. Mental health professionals, who describe drug-related problems in terms of *dependence* and *abuse*, have identified warning signs of a potential problem. (See Health in Action for advice on recognizing substance-use disorders.)

## Dependence

Individuals may develop **psychological dependence** and feel a strong craving for a drug because it produces pleasurable feelings or relieves stress and anxiety. **Physical dependence** occurs when a person develops *tolerance* to the effects of a drug and needs larger and larger doses to achieve intoxication or another desired effect. Individuals who are physically dependent and have a high tolerance to a drug may take amounts many times those that would produce intoxication or an overdose in someone who was not a regular user.

Men and women with a substance dependence disorder may use a drug to avoid or relieve withdrawal symptoms, or they may consume larger amounts of a drug or use it over a longer period than they'd originally intended. They may repeatedly try to cut down or control drug use without success; spend a great deal of time obtaining or using drugs or recovering from their effects; give up or reduce important social, occupational, or recreational activities because of their drug use; or continue to use a drug despite knowledge that the drug is likely to cause or worsen a persistent or recurring physical or psychological problem.

Specific symptoms of dependence vary with particular drugs. Some drugs, such as marijuana, hallucinogens, and phencyclidine, do not cause withdrawal symptoms. The degree of dependence also varies. In mild cases, a person may function normally most of the time. In severe cases, the person's entire life may revolve around obtaining, using, and recuperating from the effects of a drug.

Individuals with drug dependence become intoxicated or high on a regular basis—whether every day, every weekend, or several binges a year. They may try repeatedly to stop using a drug and yet fail, even though they realize their drug use is interfering with their health, family life, relationships, and work.

## Abuse

Some drug users do not develop the symptoms of tolerance and withdrawal that characterize dependence, yet they use drugs in ways that clearly have a harmful effect on them. These individuals are diagnosed as having a *psychoactive substance abuse disorder*. They continue to use drugs despite their awareness of persistent or repeated social, occupational, psychological, or physical problems related to drug use, or they use drugs in dangerous ways or situations (before driving, for instance).

## Intoxication and Withdrawal

**Intoxication** refers to maladaptive behavioral, psychological, and physiologic changes that occur as a result of substance use. **Withdrawal** is the development of symptoms that cause significant psychological and physical distress when an individual reduces or stops drug use. (Intoxication and withdrawal from specific drugs are discussed later in this chapter.)

## Polyabuse

Most users prefer a certain type of drug but also use several others; this behavior is called **polyabuse**. The average user who enters treatment is on five different drugs. The more drugs anyone uses, the greater the chance of side effects, complications, and possibly life-threatening interactions.

## Coexisting Conditions

Mental disorders and substance abuse disorders have a great deal of overlap. Many individuals

**addiction** A behavioral pattern characterized by compulsion, loss of control, and continued repetition of a behavior or activity in spite of adverse consequences.

**psychological dependence** The emotional or mental attachment to the use of a drug.

**physical dependence** The physiological attachment to, and need for, a drug.

**intoxication** Maladaptive behavioral, psychological, and physiologic changes that occur as a result of substance abuse.

**withdrawal** Development of symptoms that cause significant psychological and physical distress when an individual reduces or stops drug use.

**polyabuse** The misuse or abuse of more than one drug.

with substance abuse disorders also have another psychiatric disorder, such as depression. Individuals with such *dual diagnoses* require careful evaluation and appropriate treatment for the complete range of complex and chronic difficulties they face. However, they can benefit from participation in 12-step groups, like Double Trouble in Recovery, that provide treatment for both.

## Causes of Drug Dependence and Abuse

No one fully understands why some people develop drug dependence or abuse disorders, whereas others, who may experiment briefly with drugs, do not. Inherited body chemistry, genetic factors, and sensitivity to drugs may make some individuals more susceptible. These disorders may stem from many complex causes.

*The Biology of Dependence* Scientists now view drug dependence as a brain disease triggered by frequent use of drugs that change the biochemistry and anatomy of neurons and alter the way they work. A major breakthrough in understanding dependence has been the discovery that certain mood-altering substances and experiences—a puff of marijuana, a slug of whiskey, a snort of cocaine, a big win at blackjack—trigger a rise in a brain chemical called **dopamine**, which is associated with feelings of satisfaction and euphoria. This brain chemical or neurotransmitter is one of the crucial messengers that links nerve cells in the brain and its level rises during any pleasurable experience, whether it be a loving hug or a taste of chocolate.

The mechanism governing the rise in dopamine levels is not the same for all drugs. Figure 12.2 shows the one for cocaine. Normally, after dopamine is released from the axon terminal of a neuron and activates dopamine receptors on the adjacent neuron, the dopamine is then transported back to its original neuron by "uptake pumps." Cocaine binds to the uptake pumps and prevents them from transporting dopamine back into the neuron terminal. So more dopamine builds up in the synapse and is free to activate more dopamine receptors.

Addictive drugs have such a powerful impact on dopamine and its receptors that they change the pathways within the brain's pleasure centers.

# Health in Action

## *Recognizing Substance Abuse*

How can you tell if a friend or loved one has a substance-use disorder? Look for the following warning signs:

- **An abrupt change in attitude.** Individuals may lose interest in activities they once enjoyed or in being with friends they once valued.
- **Mood swings.** Drug users may often seem withdrawn or "out of it," or they may display unusual temper flareups.
- **A decline in performance.** Students may start skipping classes, stop studying, or not complete assignments; their grades may plummet.
- **Increased sensitivity.** Individuals may react intensely to any criticism or become easily frustrated or angered.
- **Secrecy.** Drug users may make furtive telephone calls or demand greater privacy concerning their personal possessions or their whereabouts.
- **Physical changes.** Individuals using drugs may change their pattern of sleep, spending more time in bed or sleeping at odd hours. They also may change their eating habits and lose weight.
- **Money problems.** Drug users may constantly borrow money, seem short of cash, or begin stealing.
- **Changes in appearance.** As they become more involved with drugs, users often lose regard for their personal appearance and look disheveled.
- **Defiance of restrictions.** Individuals may ignore or deliberately refuse to comply with deadlines, curfews, or other regulations.
- **Changes in relationships.** Drug users may quarrel more frequently with family members or old friends and develop strong allegiances with new acquaintances, including other drug users.

Various psychoactive chemicals create a craving for more of the same. According to this hypothesis, addicts do not specifically yearn for heroin, cocaine, or nicotine but for the rush of dopamine that these drugs produce. Some individuals, born with low levels of dopamine, may be particularly susceptible to this craving and thus to addiction.

*The Psychology of Vulnerability* Although scientists do not believe there is an addictive personality, certain individuals are at greater risk of drug dependence because of psychological factors, including difficulty controlling impulses, a lack of values that might constrain drug use (whether based in religion, family, or society), low self-esteem, feelings of powerlessness, and depression. The one psychological trait most often linked with drug use is denial. Young people in particular are absolutely

**dopamine** A brain chemical associated with feelings of satisfaction and euphoria.

## Figure 12.2 Dopamine Levels for Cocaine

Within the synapses between adjacent neurons, cocaine binds to the dopamine uptake pumps and thus allows the neurotransmitter dopamine to build up in the synapse and bind to more dopamine receptors.

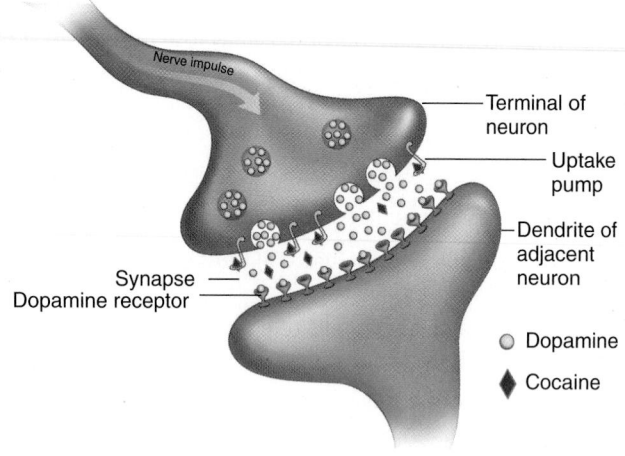

Nerve impulse

Terminal of neuron

Uptake pump

Dendrite of adjacent neuron

○ Dopamine

◆ Cocaine

Synapse
Dopamine receptor

convinced that they will never lose control or suffer in any way as a result of drug use.

Many diagnosed drug users have at least one mental disorder, particularly depression or anxiety. Disorders that emerge in adolescence, such as bipolar disorder, may increase the risk of substance abuse. Many people with psychiatric disorders abuse drugs. Individuals may self-administer drugs to treat psychiatric symptoms; for example, they may take sedating drugs to suppress a panic attack.

***Early Influences*** Teen drug abuse has declined in the last decade, but some teens remain more vulnerable. Young people from lower socioeconomic backgrounds are more likely to use drugs than their more affluent peers, possibly because of economic disadvantage; family instability; a lack of realistic, rewarding alternatives and role models; and increased hopelessness.

Those whose companions are substance abusers are far more likely to use drugs. Peer pressure to use drugs can be a powerful factor for adolescents, although having a drug-using roommate does not increase the odds that a college student will use drugs. The likelihood of drug abuse is also related to family instability, parental rejection, and divorce.

Parents' own attitudes and drug-use history affect their children's likelihood of using marijuana, according to the Substance Abuse and Mental Health Services Administration. Parents who perceive little risk associated with marijuana use have children with similar attitudes, and the children of parents who used marijuana are more likely to try the drug than are children whose parents never used the drug.

## Drugged Driving

Driving under the influence of any substance that acts on the brain can impair motor skills, reaction time, and judgment. Some state laws define "drugged driving" as driving when a drug "renders the driver incapable of driving safely." Other states have "per se" laws, according to which it is illegal to operate a moving vehicle if there is any detectable level of a prohibited drug or its metabolites in a driver's blood.

According to the National Highway Traffic Safety Administration, more than 16 percent of weekend, nighttime drivers test positive for illegal, prescription, or over-the-counter medications. An estimated 10.5 million Americans over age 12 have reported driving under the influence of illicit drugs during the previous year. The rate of drugged driving is highest among young adults ages 18 to 25 (12.8 percent).[20]

*Your Strategies for Prevention*

## How to Say No to Drugs

If people offer you a drug, here are some ways to say no.

- **Let them know you're not interested.** Change the subject. If the pressure seems threatening, just walk away.

- **Have something else to do: "No, I'm going for a walk now."**

- **Be prepared for different types of pressure.** If your friends tease you, tease them back.

- **Keep it simple.** "No, thanks," "No," or "No way" all get the point across.

- **Hang out with people who won't offer you drugs.**

Different drugs affect driving ability in different ways. Here are the facts from the National Institute on Drug Abuse:

- **Alcohol** affects perception, coordination, and judgment, and increases the sedative effects of tranquilizers and barbiturates.

- **Marijuana** affects a wide range of driving skills—including the ability to track (stay in the lane) through curves, brake quickly, and maintain speed and a safe distance between cars—and slows thinking and reflexes. Normal driving skills remain impaired for four to six hours after smoking a single joint.

- **Sedatives, sedative-hypnotics, and antianxiety agents** slow reaction time and interfere with hand–eye coordination and judgment; the greatest impairment is in the first hour after taking the drug. The effects depend on the particular drug: some build up in the body and can impair driving skills the morning after use; others make drivers very sleepy and therefore incapable of driving safely.

- **Amphetamines**, after repeated use, impair coordination. They can also make a driver more edgy and less coordinated and thus more likely to be involved in an accident.

- **Hallucinogens** distort judgment and reality and cause confusion and panic, thus making driving extremely dangerous.

# Common Drugs of Abuse

Table 12.4 describes the common drugs of abuse within these categories: cannabinoids, "club drugs," stimulants, dissociative drugs, hallucinogens, opioids, and other compounds.

## Cannabis

**Marijuana** (pot) and **hashish** (hash)—the most widely used illegal drugs—are derived from the cannabis plant. The major psychoactive ingredient in both is *THC (delta-9-tetrahydrocannabinol)*. Marijuana is the most widely abused substance, with more than 150 million people reporting they've used it at least once in the last year. Some 12 million Americans use cannabis; more than 1 million cannot control this use.

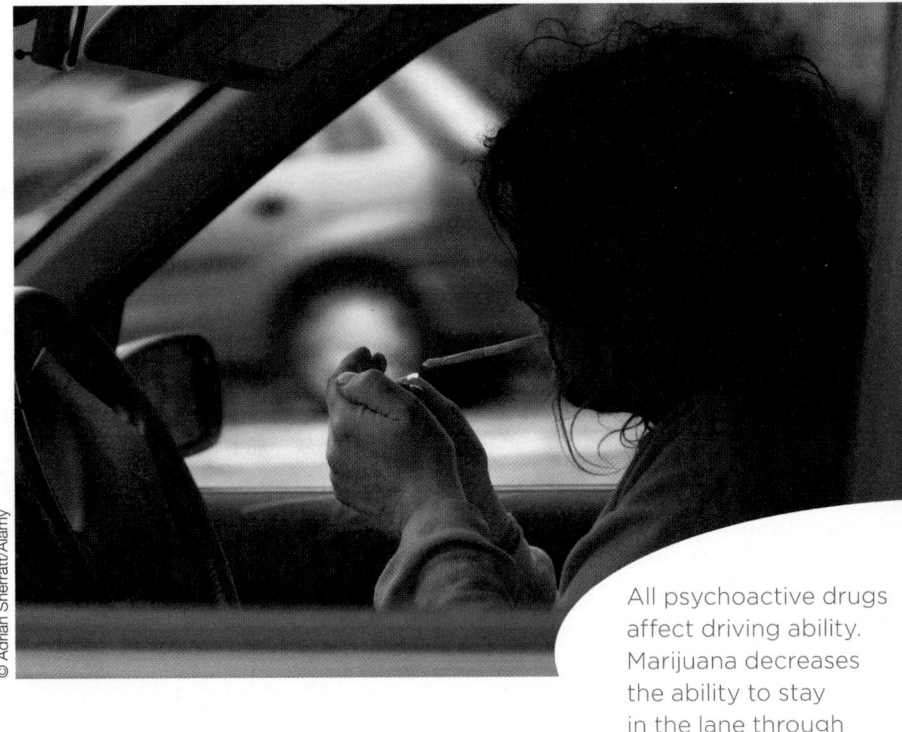

All psychoactive drugs affect driving ability. Marijuana decreases the ability to stay in the lane through curves and slows thinking and reflexes.

Teens and young adults who use marijuana are more likely to develop serious mental health problems. Researchers have documented an association between frequent marijuana use and increased anxiety and depression in young adults, regardless of whether they use other illicit drugs. Teens who use marijuana are more likely to develop psychotic symptoms within ten years.[21]

Some people, particularly advocates for its legalization, argue that marijuana is relatively harmless. However, scientific research has confirmed that long-term use causes many adverse health consequences, including significant brain injury. When used chronically, cannabis can produce dependence, respiratory disease, and psychotic symptoms, especially in vulnerable young adults. It also may interfere with normal brain development in adolescents and young adults. Another recently recognized danger is increased risk of a particularly aggressive form of testicular cancer, the most common cancer in men between ages 15 and 34.

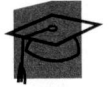 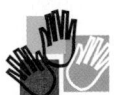 Marijuana use is generally less pervasive than binge drinking (see Chapter 13) on most campuses, although at some schools as many as a third of students report smoking pot. Students who used marijuana in high school are more likely to do so in college. Roommates have very little impact

**marijuana** The drug derived from the cannabis plant, containing the psychoactive ingredient THC, which causes a mild sense of euphoria when inhaled or eaten.

**hashish** A concentrated form of a drug, derived from the cannabis plant, containing the psychoactive ingredient THC, which causes a sense of euphoria when inhaled or eaten.

© Adrian Sherratt/Alamy

## Marijuana

Marijuana, the most widely used illicit drug, continues to make headlines as advocates press for its legalization for medical purposes. To find the latest developments, access Global Health Watch and click on "Addiction." Scroll to "Drugs." Scan the headlines of the newsfeed on your screen, or enter "marijuana" in the search field. Find one recent article related to marijuana, and write a brief comment in your online journal.

on drug use. Men who have not used marijuana before college seem, if anything, turned off rather than turned on by roommates who have smoked pot. Peers have no clear impact on women's marijuana use.

Different types of marijuana have different percentages of THC. Because of careful cultivation, the strength of today's marijuana is much greater than that used in the 1970s. Today a marijuana joint contains 150 mg of THC, compared to 10 mg in the 1960s. Usually, marijuana is smoked in a joint (hand-rolled cigarette) or pipe; it may also be eaten as an ingredient in other foods (as when baked in brownies), though with a less predictable effect.

Marijuana has shown some medical benefits, including boosting appetite in patients who are HIV-positive or undergoing chemotherapy, alleviating cancer and neck pain, reducing pressure on the eyeball in glaucoma patients, and helping people with spasticity (extreme muscle tension) due to multiple sclerosis or injuries. (See Health in the Headlines: Marijuana.)

A growing number of states have passed voter referenda (or legislative actions) making marijuana available to smoke for a variety of medical conditions upon a doctor's recommendation. However, the FDA, after a comprehensive investigation, concluded that "no sound scientific studies supported medical use of marijuana for treatment in the United States, and no animal or human data supported the safety or efficacy of marijuana for general medical use." FDA-approved medications are available as treatment alternatives for many of the proposed uses of smoked marijuana, such as relief of nausea and vomiting induced by chemotherapy. Synthetic versions of the active ingredient in marijuana, developed for medical use, act on the brain like the THC in smoked marijuana but eliminate the need to inhale harmful smoke.

*How Users Feel* The circumstances in which marijuana is smoked, the communal aspects of its use, and the user's experience all can affect the way a marijuana-induced high feels.

In low to moderate doses, marijuana typically creates a mild sense of euphoria, a sense of slowed time (five minutes may feel like an hour), a dreamy sort of self-absorption, and some impairment in thinking and communicating.

Users report heightened sensations of color, sound, and other stimuli, relaxation, and increased confidence. The sense of being stoned peaks within half an hour and usually lasts about three hours. Even when alterations in perception seem slight, it is not safe to drive a car for as long as four to six hours after smoking a single joint.

Some users—particularly those smoking marijuana for the first time or taking a high dose in an unpleasant or unfamiliar setting—experience acute anxiety, which may be accompanied by a panicky fear of losing control. They may believe that their companions are ridiculing or threatening them and experience a panic attack, a state of intense terror.

The immediate physical effects of marijuana include increased pulse rate, bloodshot eyes, dry mouth and throat, slowed reaction times, impaired motor skills, increased appetite, and diminished short-term memory (Figure 12.3). High doses reduce the ability to perceive and to react; all the reactions experienced with low doses are intensified, leading to sensory distortion and, in the case of hashish, vivid hallucinations and LSD-like, psychedelic reactions. The drug remains in the body's fat cells 50 hours or more after use, so people may experience psychoactive effects for several days after use. Drug tests may produce positive results for days or weeks after last use.

*Risks* Marijuana produces a range of effects in different body systems, such as depression, diminished immune responses, and impaired fertility in men. Other risks include damage to the brain, lungs, and heart and to babies born to mothers who use marijuana during pregnancy or while nursing (see Figure 12.3).

**Brain** As brain scans have documented, long-term marijuana use causes significant brain abnormalities, including shrinkage of key structures involved in memory, learning, and emotion, that can lead to memory loss, difficulty learning new information, and psychotic symptoms. Short-term effects include problems with memory and learning; distorted perceptions; difficulty thinking and problem solving; loss of coordination; increased anxiety; and panic attacks. Long-term heavy users of marijuana perform significantly worse on tests of verbal fluency, memory, and coordination than short-term users or nonusers, even after abstaining from pot for more than 24 hours.

Over time, continued heavy marijuana use can disrupt sleep and interfere with students' ability to learn and perform well in school and in challenging careers. Marijuana contributes significantly to accidental death and injury among adolescents, especially through motor vehicle crashes.

**Lungs** Smoking cannabis may cause effects similar to those of smoking tobacco, with many of them appearing at a younger age. They include chronic bronchitis, emphysema, and other lung disorders and increased risk of heart attacks and sudden death. The amount of tar inhaled by marijuana smokers and the level of carbon monoxide absorbed are three to five times greater than among tobacco smokers. The reasons may be that marijuana users inhale more deeply, hold the smoke in the lungs longer, and do not use filters. Smoking a single joint can be as damaging to the lungs as smoking five tobacco cigarettes. Someone who smokes five joints a week may take in as many cancer-causing chemicals as a person who smokes a pack of cigarettes a day.

**Heart** Otherwise healthy people have suffered heart attacks shortly after smoking marijuana. Experiments have also linked marijuana use to elevated blood pressure and decreased oxygen supply to the heart muscle. The risk of heart attack triples within an hour of smoking pot. Smoking marijuana while shooting cocaine can potentially cause deadly increases in heart rate and blood pressure.

**Pregnancy** Babies born to mothers who used marijuana during pregnancy are smaller than those born to mothers who did not use the drug, and the babies are more likely to develop health problems. A nursing mother who uses marijuana passes some of the THC to the baby in her breast milk. This may impair the infant's motor development (control of muscle movement).

*Withdrawal* Marijuana users can develop a compulsive, often uncontrollable craving for the drug. More than 120,000 people enter treatment every year for marijuana addiction. Marijuana withdrawal has proven as difficult as quitting smoking. Stopping after long-term

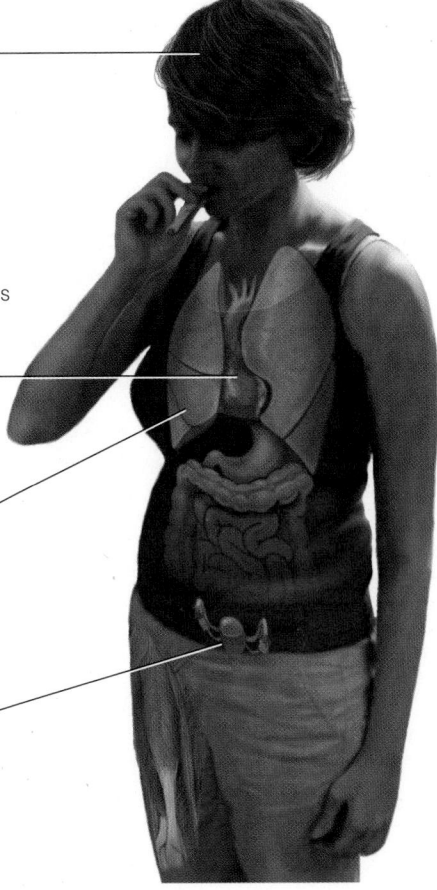

Figure 12.3 **Impact of Marijuana**
Marijuana has negative long-term effects on many systems of the body.

**Negative Long-Term Effects**

**Brain and central nervous system**
• Causes brain abnormalities
• Dulls sensory and cognitive skills
• Impairs short-term memory
• Alters motor coordination
• Causes changes in brain chemistry
• Leads to difficulty in concentration, attention to detail, and learning new complex information
• Increases risk of stroke
• Increases risk of psychotic symptoms
• Causes disturbed sleep

**Cardiovascular system**
• Increases heart rate
• Increases blood pressure
• Decreases blood flow to the limbs

**Respiratory system**
• Damages the lungs (50% more tar than tobacco)
• May cause lung cancer
• May damage throat from inhalation

**Reproductive system**
• In women, may impair ovulation and cause fetal abnormalities if used during pregnancy
• In men, may suppress sexual functioning and may reduce the number, quality, and motility of sperm, possibly affecting fertility

marijuana use can produce *marijuana withdrawal syndrome*, which is characterized by insomnia, restlessness, loss of appetite, and irritability. People who smoke marijuana daily for many years may become aggressive after they stop using it and may relapse to prevent aggression and other symptoms.

## Club Drugs (Designer Drugs)

The National Institute on Drug Abuse identifies a variety of drugs—alcohol, LSD (acid), MDMA (Ecstasy), GHB, GBL, ketamine (Special-K), fentanyl, Rohypnol, and nitrites—as **"club drugs."** They first became popular among teens and young adults at nightclubs, bars, or night-long dances often held in warehouses or other unusual settings. Their use by teenagers has been dropping in recent years.

Young people may take club drugs to relax, energize, and enhance their social interactions,

**club drugs** Illegally manufactured psychoactive drugs that have dangerous physical and psychological effects.

but a large number also experience negative consequences. As many as three in four report side effects such as profuse sweating, hot and cold flashes, tingling or numbness, blurred vision, trouble sleeping, hallucinations, depression, confusion, anxiety, irritability, paranoia, and loss of libido (sex drive). Some also experience difficulty with their usual daily activities and financial and work troubles.

*Ecstasy* **Ecstasy** (E, XTC, X, hug, beans, love drug) is the most common street name for methylenedioxymethamphetamine (MDMA), a synthetic compound with both stimulant and mildly hallucinogenic properties.

 According to various studies, students who take Ecstasy were more likely to use marijuana, binge-drink, smoke cigarettes, have multiple sexual partners, spend more time socializing with friends and less time studying, and consider parties important and religion less important. However, researchers who compared students who used Ecstasy and other illicit drugs with those who used only marijuana have concluded that undergraduates who use Ecstasy may be a subgroup of marijuana users who tend to engage in many risk-taking behaviors. Ecstasy users also think that their peers smoke more marijuana and use more Ecstasy than they actually do.

**How Users Feel** Although it can be smoked, inhaled (snorted), or injected, Ecstasy is almost always taken as a pill or tablet. Its effects begin in 45 minutes and last for three to six hours. Ecstasy pills often contain a variety of other chemicals that increase the danger to users.[22]

MDMA belongs to a family of drugs called *enactogens*, which literally means "touching within." As a mood elevator, it produces a relaxed, euphoric state but does not produce hallucinations. Users of Ecstasy often say they feel at peace with themselves and a sense of connectedness with others. In some settings, they reveal intimate details of their lives (which they may later regret); in other settings, they join in collective rejoicing. Like hallucinogenic drugs, MDMA can enhance sensory experience, but it rarely causes visual distortions, sudden mood changes, or psychotic reactions. Regular users may experience depression and anxiety the week after taking MDMA.

**Risks** Ecstasy is more likely than other stimulants, such as methamphetamine, to kill young, healthy people between the ages of 16 and 24 who are not known to be regular drug users. Researchers theorize that young people's brains, which are still developing in late adolescence and early adulthood, may be more vulnerable to the effects of the drug.

Ecstasy poses risks similar to those of cocaine and amphetamines. These include psychological difficulties (confusion, depression, sleep problems, drug craving, severe anxiety, and paranoia) and physical symptoms (muscle tension, involuntary teeth clenching, nausea, blurred vision, rapid eye movement, faintness, chills, sweating, and increases in heart rate and blood pressure that pose a special risk for people with circulatory or heart disease).

Medical emergencies related to the drug increased 75 percent in recent years. Most of those requiring emergency care were between ages 18 and 29.[23]

Ecstasy can produce nausea, vomiting, and dizziness. When combined with extended physical exertion like dancing, club drugs can lead to hyperthermia (severe overheating), severe dehydration, serious increases in blood pressure, stroke, and heart attack. Without sufficient water, dancers at raves may suffer dehydration and heat stroke, which can be fatal. Individuals with high blood pressure, heart trouble, or liver or kidney disease are in the greatest danger. Several deaths have occurred in teens who suffered brain damage by drinking large amounts of water to counteract the raised body temperature induced by the drug.

MDMA has been implicated in some cases of acute hepatitis, which can lead to liver failure. Even after liver transplantation, the mortality rate for individuals with this condition is 50 percent. Another danger comes from the practice of taking SSRIs (see Chapter 2), which modulate the mood-altering brain chemical serotonin, before Ecstasy. This can cause jaw clenching, nausea, tremors, and, in extreme cases, potentially fatal elevations in body temperature.

Although not a sexual stimulant (if anything, MDMA has the opposite effect), Ecstasy fosters strong feelings of intimacy that may lead to risky sexual behavior. The psychological effects of Ecstasy become less intriguing with repeated

**Ecstasy (MDMA)** A synthetic compound, also known as methylenedioxymethamphetamine, that is similar in structure to methamphetamine and has both stimulant and hallucinogenic effects.

Table 12.4 **Commonly Abused Drugs**

| Substances: Category and Name | Examples of *Commercial and Street Names* | How It's Used | *Acute Effects*/Health Risks |
|---|---|---|---|
| **Cannabinoids** | | | |
| **Marijuana** | Blunt, dope, ganja, grass, herb, joint, bud, Mary Jane, pot, reefer, green, trees, smoke, sinsemilla, skunk, weed | Smoked, swallowed | *Euphoria; relaxation; slowed reaction time; distorted sensory perception; impaired balance and coordination; increased heart rate and appetite; impaired learning, memory; anxiety; panic attacks; psychosis*/cough, frequent respiratory infections; possible mental health decline; addiction |
| **Hashish** | Boom, gangster, hash, hash oil, hemp | Smoked, swallowed | |
| **Club Drugs** | | | |
| **MDMA (methylenedioxy-methamphetamine)** | Ecstasy, Adam, clarity, Eve, lover's speed, peace, uppers | Swallowed, snorted, injected | *MDMA—mild hallucinogenic effects; increased tactile sensitivity; empathic feelings; lowered inhibition; anxiety; chills; sweating; teetch clenching; muscle cramping*/sleep disturbances; depression; impaired memory; hyperthermia; addiction |
| **Flunitrazepam***** | *Rohypnol:* forget-me pill, Mexican Valium, R2, roach, Roche, roofies, roofinol, rope, rophies | Swallowed, snorted | *Flunitrazepam—sedation; muscle relaxation; confusion; memory loss; dizziness; impaired coordination*/addiction |
| **GHB***** | *Gamma-hydroxybutyrate:* G, Georgia home boy, grievous bodily harm, liquid ecstasy, soap, scoop, goop, liquid X | Swallowed | *GHB—drowsiness; nausea; headache; disorientation; loss of coordination; memory loss/ unconsciousness; seizures; coma* |
| **Stimulants** | | | |
| **Cocaine** | *Cocaine hydrochloride:* blow, bump, C, candy, Charlie, coke, crack, flake, rock, snow, toot | Snorted, smoked, injected | *Increased heart rate, blood pressure, body temperature, metabolism; feelings of exhilaration; increased energy, mental alertness; tremors; reduced appetite; irritability; anxiety; panic; paranoia; violent behavior; psychosis*/weight loss, insomnia; cardiac or cardiovascular complications; stroke; seizures; addiction |
| **Amphetamine** | *Biphetamine, Dexedrine:* bennies, black beauties, crosses, hearts, LA turnaround, speed, truck drivers, uppers | Swallowed, snorted, smoked, injected | Also, for cocaine—nasal damage from snorting |
| **Methamphetamine** | *Desoxyn:* meth, ice, crank, chalk, crystal, fire, glass, go fast, speed | Swallowed, snorted, smoked, injected | Also, for methamphetamine—severe dental problems |
| **Dissociative Drugs** | | | |
| **Ketamine** | *Ketalar SV:* cat Valium, K, Special K, vitamin K | Injected, snorted, smoked | *Feelings of being separate from one's body and environment; impaired motor function/ anxiety; tremors; numbness; memory loss; nausea* |
| **PCP and analogs** | *Phencyclidine:* angel dust, boat, hog, love boat, peace pill | Swallowed, smoked, injected | *Also, for ketamine—analgesia; impaired memory; delirium; respiratory depression and arrest; death* |
| **Salvia divinorum** | Salvia, Shepherdess's Herb, Maria Pastora, magic mint, Sally-D | Chewed, swallowed, smoked | *Also, for PCP and analogs—analgesia; psychosis; aggression; violence; slurred speech; loss of coordination; hallucinations* |
| **Dextromethorphan (DXM)** | Found in some cough and cold medications: Robotripping, Robo, Triple C | Swallowed | *Also, or DXM—euphoria; slurred speech; confusion; dizziness; distorted visual perceptions* |

\*\*\*Associated with sexual assaults.

*continued*

Table 12.4 **Commonly Abused Drugs** *(continued)*

| Substances: Category and Name | Examples of *Commercial* and Street Names | How It's Used | *Acute Effects*/Health Risks |
|---|---|---|---|
| **Hallucinogens** | | | |
| **LSD** | *Lysergic acid diethylamide:* acid, blotter, boomers, cubes, microdot, yellow sunshine, blue heaven | Swallowed, absorbed through mouth tissues | *Altered states of perception and feeling; hallucinations; nausea* |
| **Mescaline** | Buttons, cactus, mesc, peyote | Swallowed, smoked | *Also, LSD and mescaline—increased body temperature, heart rate, blood pressure; loss of appetite; sweating; sleeplessness; numbness, dizziness, weakness, tremors; impulsive behavior; rapid shifts in emotion* |
| **Psilocybin** | Magic mushrooms, purple passion, shrooms, little smoke | Swallowed | *Also, for LSD—Flashbacks, Hallucinogen Persisting Perception Disorder*<br><br>*Also for psilocybin—nervousness; paranoia; panic* |
| **Opioids** | | | |
| **Heroin** | *Diacetylmorphine:* smack, horse, brown sugar, dope, H, junk, skag, skunk, white horse, China white; cheese (with OTC cold medicine and antihistamine) | Injected, smoked, snorted | *Euphoria; drowsiness; impaired coordination; dizziness; confusion, nausea; sedation; feeling of heaviness in the body; slowed or arrested breathing/constipation; endocarditis; hepatitis; HIV; addiction; fatal overdose* |
| **Opium** | *Laudanum, paregoric:* big O, black stuff, block, gun, hop | Swallowed, smoked | |
| **Other Compounds** | | | |
| **Anabolic steroids** | *Anadrol, Oxandrin, Durabolin, Depo-Testosterone, Equipoise:* roids, juice, gym candy, pumpers | Injected, swallowed, applied to the skin | *Steroids—no intoxication effects*/hypertension; blood clotting and cholesterol changes; liver cysts; hostility and aggression; acne; in adolescents—premature stoppage of growth; in males—prostate cancer, reduced sperm production, shrunken testicles, breast enlargement; in females—menstrual irregularities, development of beard and other masculine characteristics |
| **Inhalants** | *Solvents (paint thinners, gasoline, glues); gases (butane, propane, aerosol propellants, nitrous oxide); nitrites (isoamyl, isobutyl, cyclohexyl):* laughing gas, poppers, snappers, whippets | Inhaled through nose or mouth | *Inhalants (varies by chemical)—stimulation; loss of inhibition; headache; nausea or vomiting; slurred speech; loss of motor coordination; wheezing/cramps; muscle weakness; depression; memory impairment; damage to cardiovascular and nervous systems; unconsciousness; sudden death* |

**GHB (gamma hydroxybutyrate)** A brain messenger chemical that stimulates the release of human growth hormone; commonly abused for its high and its alleged ability to trim fat and build muscles. Also known as "blue nitro" or the "date rape drug."

**GBL (gamma butyrolactone)** The main ingredient in gamma hydroxybutyrate (GHB); once ingested, GBL converts to GHB and can cause the ingestor to lose consciousness.

use, and the physical side effects become more uncomfortable. Ecstasy poses risks to a developing fetus, including a greater likelihood of heart and skeletal abnormalities and long-term learning and memory impairments in children born to women who used MDMA during pregnancy.

*GHB and GBL* Once sold in health-food stores for its muscle-building and alleged fat-burning properties, **gamma hydroxybutyrate** (GHB, G, Georgia home boy, grievous bodily harm, liquid ecstasy) was banned because of its effects on the brain and nervous system. The main ingredient is **GBL (gamma butyrolactone)**, an industrial solvent often used to strip floors, which converts into GHB once ingested. GHB acts as a sedative while producing feelings of euphoria and heightened sexuality. Because of its amnesic properties, GHB has been used as a "date rape" drug, similar to Rohypnol. Alcohol intensifies its effects, which typically last up to four hours.

Large doses can cause someone to pass out in 15 minutes and fall into a coma within half an hour. Death can occur. Other side effects include nausea, amnesia, hallucinations, decreased heart rate, convulsions, and sometimes blackouts. Long-term use at high doses can lead to a withdrawal reaction: rapid heartbeat, tremor, insomnia, anxiety, and occasionally hallucinations that last a few days to a week.

GHB is addictive. Users who attempt to quit may experience significant withdrawal symptoms, including anxiety, tremors, and insomnia. Most symptoms decrease within one to two weeks of cessation, but severe psychological effects can last for weeks to months.

*Nitrites* Nitrites (amyl, butyl, and isobutyl nitrite) are clear, amber-colored liquids that have had a history of abuse for more than three decades, especially in gay and bisexual men. Popular in dance clubs, they are used recreationally for a high feeling, a slowed sense of time, a carefree sense of well-being, and intensified sexual experiences.

Sold in small glass ampules containing individual doses, nitrites are usually inhaled and rapidly absorbed into the bloodstream. Users feel their physiological and psychological impact in seconds. Acute adverse effects include headache, dizziness, a drop in blood pressure, changes in heart rate, increased pressure within the eye, and skin flushing. Some individuals develop respiratory irritation and cough, sneezing, or difficulty breathing. Chronic use can lead to crusty skin lesions and chemical burns around the nose, mouth, and lips.

*Herbal Ecstasy* Herbal ecstasy, also known as herbal bliss, cloud 9, and herbal X, is a mixture of stimulants such as ephedrine, pseudoephedrine, and caffeine. Sold in tablet or capsule form as a "natural" and safe alternative to Ecstasy, its ingredients vary greatly. Herbal ecstasy can have dangerous and unpleasant side effects, including stroke, heart attack, and a disfiguring skin condition.

## Stimulants

Central nervous system **stimulants** are drugs that increase activity in some portion of the brain or spinal cord. Some stimulants increase motor activity and enhance mental alertness, and some combat mental fatigue. Amphetamine, methamphetamine, caffeine, cocaine, and khat are stimulants. Stimulant medications are used to treat conditions such as ADHD.

*Amphetamine* **Amphetamines** trigger the release of epinephrine (adrenaline), which stimulates the central nervous system. They were once widely prescribed for weight control because they suppress appetite, but they have emerged as a global danger. Amphetamines are sold under a variety of names: amphetamine (brand name Benzedrine, street name bennies), dextroamphetamine (Dexedrine, dex), methamphetamine (Methedrine, meth, speed, crank), and Desoxyn (copilots). Related *uppers* include the prescription drugs methylphenidate (Ritalin), pemoline (Cylert), and phenmetrazine (Preludin). Amphetamines are available in tablet or capsule form.

**How Users Feel** Amphetamines produce a state of hyper-alertness and energy. Users feel confident in their ability to think clearly and to perform any task exceptionally well—although amphetamines do not, in fact, significantly boost performance or thinking. Higher doses make users feel wired: talkative, excited, restless, irritable, anxious, moody.

If taken intravenously, amphetamines produce a characteristic rush of elation and confidence, as well as adverse effects, including confusion, rambling or incoherent speech, anxiety, headache, and palpitations. Individuals may become paranoid; be convinced they are having profound thoughts; feel increased sexual interest; and experience unusual perceptions, such as ringing in the ears, a sensation of insects crawling on their skin, or hearing their name called. Methamphetamine users may feel high and sleepy or may hallucinate and lose contact with reality.

**Risks** Dependence on amphetamines can develop with episodic or daily use. Bingeing—taking high doses over a period of several days—can lead to an extremely intense and unpleasant *crash*, characterized by a craving

**stimulant** An agent, such as a drug, that temporarily relieves drowsiness, helps in the performance of repetitive tasks, and improves capacity for work.

**amphetamine** Any of a class of stimulants that trigger the release of epinephrine, which stimulates the central nervous system; users experience a state of hyper-alertness and energy, followed by a crash as the drug wears off.

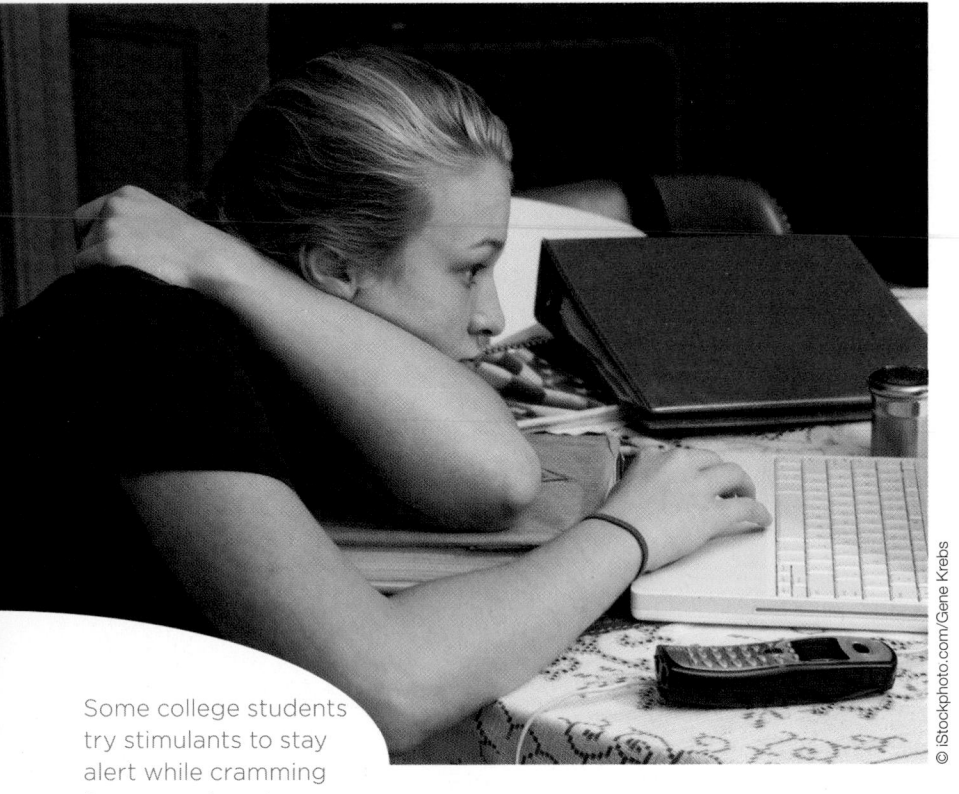

© iStockphoto.com/Gene Krebs

Some college students try stimulants to stay alert while cramming for exams, but these medications do not improve academic performance and can cause harmful effects.

for the drug, shakiness, irritability, anxiety, and depression. Two or more days are required for recuperation.

Amphetamine intoxication may cause the following symptoms:

- Feelings of grandiosity, anxiety, tension, hypervigilance, anger, social hypersensitivity, fighting, jitteriness or agitation, paranoia, and impaired judgment in social or occupational functioning.

- Increased heart rate, dilated pupils, elevated blood pressure, perspiration or chills, and nausea or vomiting.

- Less frequent effects such as speeding up or slowing down of physical movement; muscular weakness; impaired breathing, chest pain, heart arrhythmia; confusion, seizures, impaired movements or muscle tone; or even coma.

- In high doses, a rapid or irregular heartbeat, tremors, loss of coordination, and collapse.

The long-term effects of amphetamine abuse include malnutrition, skin disorders, ulcers, insomnia, depression, vitamin deficiencies, and, in some cases, brain damage that results in speech and thought disturbances. Sexual

dysfunction and impaired concentration or memory also may occur.

**Withdrawal**  When the immediate effects of amphetamines wear off, users experience a *crash* and become shaky, irritable, anxious, and depressed. Amphetamine withdrawal usually persists for more than 24 hours after cessation of prolonged, heavy use. Its characteristic features include fatigue, disturbing dreams, much more or less than usual sleep, increased appetite, and speeding up or slowing down of physical movements. Those who are unable to sleep despite their exhaustion often take sedative-hypnotics (discussed later in this chapter) to help them rest and may then become dependent on them in addition to amphetamines. Symptoms usually reach a peak in two to four days, although depression and irritability may persist for months. Suicide is a major risk.

*Methamphetamine*  Methamphetamine, an addictive stimulant that is less expensive and possibly more addictive than cocaine or heroin, has become America's leading drug problem. More than 12 million Americans have tried methamphetamine, and 1.5 million are regular users, according to federal estimates. Its estimated annual economic cost is $23.4 billion.

Methamphetamine is chemically related to amphetamine, but its effects on the central nervous system are greater. Made in illegal laboratories, street methamphetamine is referred to by many names, such as speed, crystal, fire, glass, meth, and chalk. Methamphetamine hydrochloride, clear chunky crystals resembling ice that can be inhaled by smoking, is called ice, crystal, glass, and tina. Methamphetamine can be snorted, smoked, injected, or ingested orally.

**How Users Feel**  Methamphetamine causes the release of large amounts of dopamine, which creates a sensation of euphoria, increased self-esteem, and alertness. Users also report a marked increase in sexual appetite, which often leads to risky sexual behaviors while under the drug's influence.

Smoking or intravenous injection leads to an intense, pleasurable sensation, called a rush or flash, that lasts only a few minutes. Oral or intranasal use produces a high but not a rush. Users may become addicted quickly, using more methamphetamine more and more frequently.

Despair and suicidal thinking can develop when the stimulant effect wears off.

**Risks** Even small amounts of methamphetamine can increase wakefulness and physical activity, depress appetite, and raise body temperature. Other effects on the central nervous system include irritability, insomnia, confusion, tremors, convulsions, anxiety, paranoia, and aggressiveness.

Methamphetamine increases heart rate and blood pressure and can cause irreversible damage to blood vessels in the brain, producing strokes. Other effects of methamphetamine include respiratory problems, irregular heartbeat, and extreme loss of appetite and weight. During intoxication, the body (and probably brain) temperature rises, sometimes resulting in convulsions. High fevers or collapse of the circulatory system can cause death.

Common psychiatric symptoms are insomnia, irritability, and aggressive behavior. The drug causes intellectual impairment, anxiety, and depression. Chronic users become disorganized and unable to cope with everyday problems. The risk of developing psychotic symptoms—hallucinations and delusions—is very high. They may persist for months or years after use stops.

Another side effect is called meth mouth. In short periods of time, sometimes just months, teeth can turn a grayish-brown, twist, begin to fall out, and take on a peculiar texture. About 40 percent of meth users have serious dental problems.[24] This may be the result of methamphetamine's effects on the metabolic system, plus the huge quantities of sugary soft drinks that users consume for the dry mouth caused by the drug.

Meth users engage in more sex, more carelessly. Meth has become popular among gay and bisexual men, and it has been linked to an increase in unsafe sex practices. Methamphetamine use and needle sharing have been linked to a spike in HIV and hepatitis C infections in gay communities.

Methamphetamine causes abnormalities in brain regions associated with selective attention and in those associated with memory. The brain may recover somewhat after months of abstinence, but problems often remain. Long-term use causes changes in brain chemistry

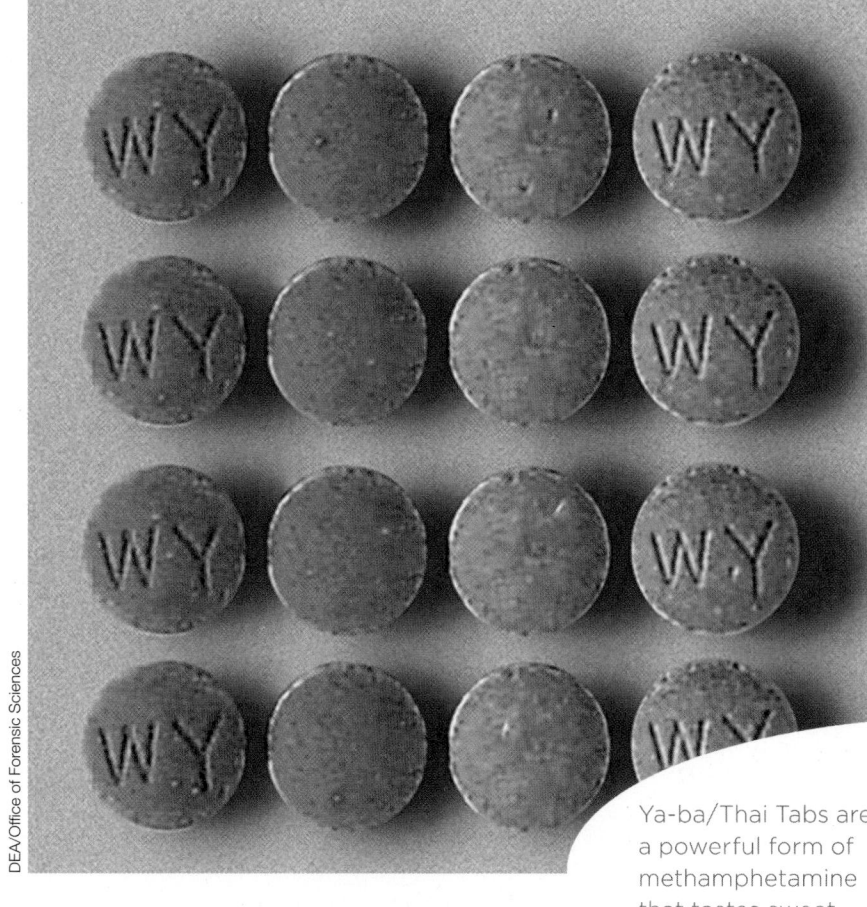

DEA/Office of Forensic Sciences

Ya-ba/Thai Tabs are a powerful form of methamphetamine that tastes sweet.

that may lead to compulsive drug-seeking and make addiction especially hard to overcome. Former methamphetamine addicts may suffer from chronic apathy and anhedonia (inability to experience pleasure) for years.

**The Toll on Society** Law enforcement officials consider methamphetamine their biggest drug problem. Meth-related arrests have soared. Meth addicts are pouring into prisons and recovery centers at an ever-increasing rate. "Meth babies" are crowding the foster-care system. Meth-making operations have been uncovered in all 50 states, with the greatest number in Missouri. Production releases poisonous gases and results in toxic waste that is often dumped down household drains, in a backyard, or at a roadside. The cost of cleaning up the environment is a growing problem for many communities.

Over-the-counter cold medicines (ephedrine and pseudoephedrine) are commonly used in meth production, which is one reason for federal and state restrictions on their sale. As drugstores and retailers have placed nonprescription cold pills behind the pharmacy counter, meth

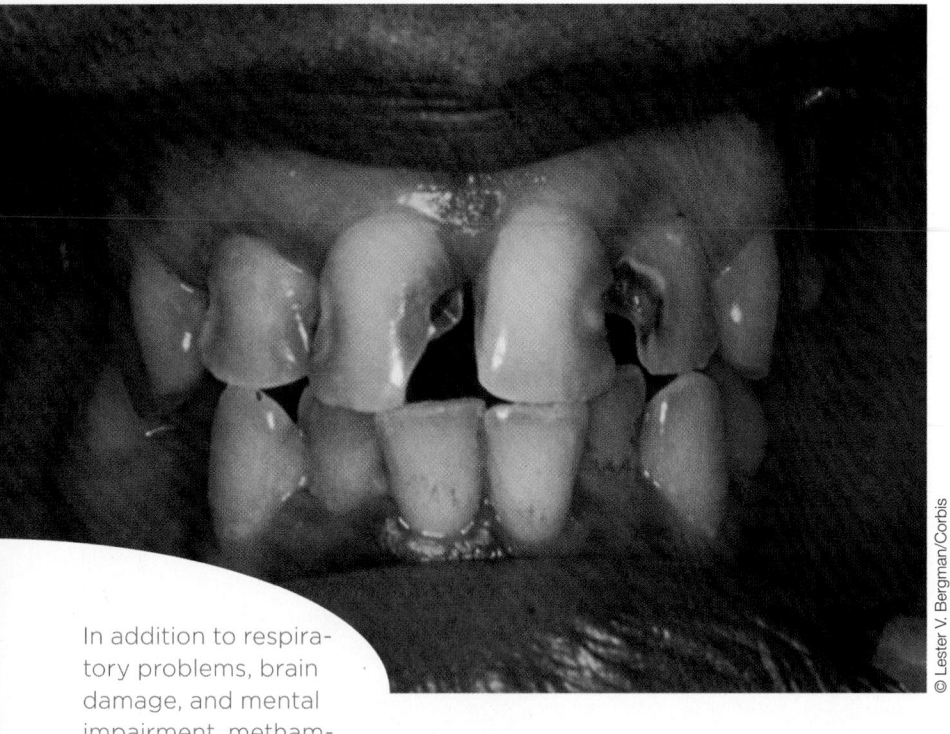

In addition to respiratory problems, brain damage, and mental impairment, methamphetamine damages teeth. This is how "meth-mouth" looks.

**cocaine** A white crystalline powder extracted from the leaves of the coca plant that stimulates the central nervous system and produces a brief period of euphoria followed by a depression.

manufacturing has moved into Mexico, where labs produce hundreds of pounds of meth a year and smuggle it into the United States.

**Withdrawal** Methamphetamine addiction is difficult to treat. As with cocaine, coming off methamphetamine causes intense distress, so users often seek out the drug to relieve their pain. Treatment usually requires the intervention of the patient's family as well as a substance abuse specialist team experienced in treating methamphetamine addiction. Standard substance abuse treatment methods such as education, behavior therapy, individual and family counseling, and support groups may be effective for some. Methamphetamine abusers often use other illicit drugs as well, a problem that can be addressed as part of a comprehensive program.

*Cocaine* **Cocaine** (coke, snow, lady) is a white crystalline powder extracted from the leaves of the South American coca plant. Usually mixed with various sugars and local anesthetics like lidocaine and procaine, cocaine powder is generally inhaled. When sniffed or snorted, cocaine anesthetizes the nerve endings in the nose and relaxes the lung's bronchial muscles.

Cocaine can be dissolved in water and injected intravenously. The drug is rapidly metabolized by the liver, so the high is relatively brief, typically lasting only about 20 minutes. This means that users will commonly inject the drug

repeatedly, increasing the risk of infection and damage to their veins.

Cocaine alkaloid, or *freebase*, is obtained by removing the hydrochloride salt from cocaine powder. *Freebasing* is smoking the fumes of the alkaloid form of cocaine. *Crack*, pharmacologically identical to freebase, is a cheap, easy-to-use, widely available, smokeable, and potent form of cocaine named for the popping sound it makes when burned. Because it is absorbed rapidly into the bloodstream and large doses reach the brain very quickly, it is particularly dangerous. However, its low price and easy availability have made it a common drug of abuse in poor urban areas.

**How Users Feel** A powerful stimulant to the central nervous system, cocaine targets several chemical sites in the brain, producing feelings of soaring well-being and boundless energy. Users feel they have enormous physical and mental ability, yet are also restless and anxious. After a brief period of euphoria, users slump into a depression. They often go on cocaine binges, lasting from a few hours to several days, and consume large quantities of cocaine.

With crack, dependence develops quickly. As soon as crack users come down from one high, they want more crack. Whereas heroin addicts may shoot up several times a day, crack addicts need another hit within minutes. Thus, a crack habit can quickly become more expensive than heroin addiction.

**Risks** Cocaine dependence is an easy habit to acquire. With repeated use, the brain becomes tolerant of the drug's stimulant effects, and users must take more of it to get high. Those who smoke or inject cocaine can develop dependence within weeks. Those who sniff cocaine may not become dependent on the drug for months or years. It is thought that 5 to 20 percent of all coke users—a group as large as the estimated total number of heroin addicts—are dependent on the drug.

The physical effects of acute cocaine intoxication include dilated pupils, elevated or lowered blood pressure, perspiration or chills, nausea or vomiting, speeding up or slowing down of physical activity, muscular weakness, impaired breathing, chest pain, and impaired movements or muscle tone. Prolonged cocaine snorting can result in ulceration of the mucous membrane of

© Lester V. Bergman/Corbis

the nose and damage to the nasal septum (the membrane between the nostrils) severe enough to cause it to collapse.

Although some users initially try cocaine as a sexual stimulant, it does not enhance sexual performance. At low doses, it may delay orgasm and cause heightened sensory awareness, but men who use cocaine regularly have problems maintaining erections and ejaculating. They also tend to have low sperm counts, less active sperm, and more abnormal sperm than nonusers. Both male and female chronic cocaine users tend to lose interest in sex and have difficulty reaching orgasm.

Cocaine use can cause blood vessels in the brain to clamp shut and can trigger a stroke, bleeding in the brain, and potentially fatal brain seizures. Cocaine users can also develop psychiatric or neurological complications (Figure 12.4). Repeated or high doses of cocaine can lead to impaired judgment, hyperactivity, nonstop babbling, feelings of suspicion and paranoia, and violent behavior. The brain never learns to tolerate cocaine's negative effects; users may become incoherent and paranoid and may experience unusual sensations, such as ringing in their ears, feeling insects crawling on the skin, or hearing their name called.

Cocaine can damage the liver and cause lung damage in freebasers. Smoking crack causes bronchitis as well as lung damage and may promote the transmission of HIV through burned and bleeding lips. Some smokers have died of respiratory complications, such as pulmonary edema (the buildup of fluid in the lungs).

Cocaine can trigger the symptoms of a heart attack in young people; the wrong therapeutic responses can be fatal. Cocaine causes the heart rate to speed up and blood pressure to rise suddenly. Its use is associated with many cardiac complications, including arrhythmia (disruption of heart rhythm), angina (chest pain), and acute myocardial infarction (heart attack).

The combination of alcohol and cocaine is particularly lethal. The liver combines the two agents and manufactures cocaethylene, which intensifies cocaine's euphoric effects, while possibly increasing the risk of sudden death. Cocaine users who inject the drug and share needles put themselves at risk for another potentially lethal problem: HIV infection.

Figure 12.4  **Some Effects of Cocaine on the Body**

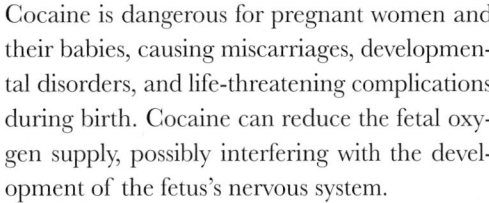

**Central nervous system**
- Repeated use or high dosages may cause severe psychological problems
- Suppresses desire for food, sex, and sleep
- Can cause strokes, seizures, and neurological damage

**Nose**
- Damages mucous membrane

**Cardiovascular system**
- Increases blood pressure by constricting blood vessels
- Causes irregular heartbeat
- Damages heart tissue

**Respiratory system**
- Freebasing causes lung damage
- Overdose can lead to respiratory arrest

**Reproductive system**
- In men, affects ability to maintain erections and ejaculate; also causes sperm abnormalities
- In women, may affect ability to carry pregnancy to term

Cocaine is dangerous for pregnant women and their babies, causing miscarriages, developmental disorders, and life-threatening complications during birth. Cocaine can reduce the fetal oxygen supply, possibly interfering with the development of the fetus's nervous system.

**Withdrawal**  When addicted individuals stop using cocaine, they often become depressed. This may lead to further cocaine use to alleviate depression. Other symptoms of cocaine withdrawal include fatigue, vivid and disturbing dreams, excessive or too little sleep, irritability, increased appetite, and physical slowing down or speeding up. This initial crash may last one to three days after cutting down or stopping the heavy use of cocaine. Some individuals become violent, paranoid, and suicidal.

Symptoms usually reach a peak in two to four days, although depression, anxiety, irritability, lack of pleasure in usual activities, and low-level cravings may continue for weeks. As memories of the crash fade, the desire for cocaine intensifies. For many weeks after stopping, individuals may feel an intense craving for the drug.

**Treatment** Overcoming an addiction to cocaine or other stimulant drug can be challenging. Among the behavioral approaches that have shown the greatest success are:

- Cognitive-behavioral therapy (CBT), which helps patients recognize and avoid drug triggers and learn new ways of coping with them.
- Contingency management, which uses tangible rewards such as vouchers for movies, to encourage abstinence.
- The Matrix Model, which combines a 12-step program, behavioral therapy, family education, and individual counseling.

The FDA has not approved any medications for these addictions, but several drugs have shown promise. These include Antabuse, widely used for alcohol dependence; the muscle relaxant baclofen (Lioresal); the anticonvulsant topiramate (Topamax); and the stimulant modafinil (Provigil), used to treat narcolepsy.

### Khat (Kat, Catha, Chat, Abyssinian Tea)

For centuries people in East Africa and the Arabian peninsula consumed the fresh young leaves of the *Catha edulis shrub* in ways similar to our drinking coffee. Its active ingredients are two controlled substances, cathinone and cathine. Chewing alleviates fatigue and reduces appetite. Compulsive use may result in manic behavior, grandiose illusions, paranoia, and hallucinations.

**Synthetic Stimulants** *Bath salts* and *plant food* are slang terms for powders sold legally online and in drug paraphernalia stores in most states under various names, such as ivory wave, purple wave, red dove, blue silk, zoom, bloom, cloud nine, ocean snow, lunar wave, vanilla sky, white lightning, scarface, and hurricane charlie. Usually these products, marked "not for human consumption" to avoid government regulation, contain various amphetamine-like chemicals, such as methylenedioxypyrovalerone (MDPV), mephedrone, and pyrovalerone, typically swallowed, sniffed, or injected. Snorting and intravenous administration produce the greatest danger.[25]

These chemicals, touted as cocaine substitutes, act in the brain like stimulant drugs and trigger intense cravings not unlike those experienced by methamphetamine users. The medical risks include chest pains, increased blood pressure, increased heart rate, agitation, hallucinations, extreme paranoia, delusions, violent behavior, and death. Emergency room visits related to bath salts have soared in recent years. A common cause of death is suicide. Those who survive suicide attempts may suffer long-term psychiatric symptoms.

Several states, counties, cities, and local municipalities have taken action to ban these products. Nations such as Great Britain and Germany also have taken steps to ban or control MDPV and similar chemicals.

## Depressants

Depressants depress the central nervous system, reduce activity, and induce relaxation, drowsiness, or sleep. They include the benzodiazepines and the barbiturates, the opioids, and alcohol.

### Benzodiazepines and Barbiturates

These depressants are the sedative-hypnotics, also known as anxiolytic or antianxiety drugs. The **benzodiazepines**—the most widely used drugs in this category—are commonly prescribed for tension, muscular strain, sleep problems, anxiety, panic attacks, and anesthesia, and in the treatment of alcohol withdrawal. They include such drugs as chlordiazepoxide (Librium), diazepam (Valium), oxazepam (Serax), lorazepam (Ativan), flurazepam (Dalmane), and alprazolam (Xanax). They differ widely in their mechanism of action, absorption rate, and metabolism, but all produce similar intoxication and withdrawal symptoms.

Rohypnol, a trade name for flunitrazepam—called roofies, rophie, roche, or the forget-me pill—is one of the benzodiazepines that has been of particular concern for the last few years because of its abuse in date rape. When mixed with alcohol, Rohypnol, which is tasteless and odorless, can incapacitate victims and prevent them from resisting sexual assault. It produces "anterograde amnesia," which means individuals may not remember events they experienced while under the effects of the drug. Other adverse effects include decreased blood pressure, drowsiness, visual disturbances, dizziness, confusion, urinary retention, and digestive problems. Rohypnol may be lethal when mixed with alcohol or other depressants.

**benzodiazepines** Antianxiety drugs that depress the central nervous system, reduce activity, and induce relaxation, drowsiness, or sleep; often prescribed to relieve tension, muscular strain, sleep problems, anxiety, and panic attacks; also used as an anesthetic and in the treatment of alcohol withdrawal.

Benzodiazepine sleeping pills have largely replaced the **barbiturates**, which were used medically in the past for inducing relaxation and sleep, relieving tension, and treating epileptic seizures. These drugs are usually taken by mouth in tablet, capsule, or liquid form. When used as a general anesthetic, they are administered intravenously.

**How Users Feel**  Low doses of these drugs may reduce or relieve tension, but increasing doses can cause a loosening of sexual or aggressive inhibitions. Individuals using this class of drugs may experience rapid mood changes, impaired judgment, and impaired social or occupational functioning.

**Risks**  All sedative-hypnotic drugs can produce physical and psychological dependence within two to four weeks. A complication specific to sedatives is *cross-tolerance* (cross-addiction), which occurs when users develop tolerance for one sedative or become dependent on it and develop tolerance for other sedatives as well.

Intoxication with these drugs can produce changes in mood or behavior, such as inappropriate sexual or aggressive acts, mood swings, and impaired judgment. Physical signs include slurred speech, poor coordination, unsteady gait, involuntary eye movements, impaired attention or memory, and stupor or coma.

Taken in combination with alcohol, these drugs have a synergistic effect that can be dangerous or even lethal. For example, an individual's driving ability, already impaired by alcohol, will be made even worse, increasing the risk of an accident. Alcohol in combination with sedative-hypnotics leads to respiratory depression and may result in respiratory arrest and death. Regular users of any of these drugs who become physically dependent should not try to cut down or quit on their own. If they try to quit suddenly, they run the risk of seizures, coma, and death.

**Withdrawal**  Withdrawal from sedative-hypnotic drugs may range from relatively mild discomfort to a severe syndrome with grand mal seizures, depending on the degree of dependence. Withdrawal symptoms include malaise or weakness, sweating, rapid pulse, coarse tremors (of the hands, tongue, or eyelids), insomnia, nausea or vomiting, temporary hallucinations or illusions, physical restlessness, anxiety or irritability, and grand mal seizures. Withdrawal

may begin within two to three days after stopping drug use, and symptoms may persist for many weeks.

*Opioids*  The **opioids** include opium and its derivatives (morphine, codeine, and heroin) and synthetic drugs that have similar sleep-inducing and pain-relieving properties. The opioids come from a resin taken from the seedpod of the Asian poppy. Synthetic opioids, such as meperidine (Demerol), methadone, and propoxyphene (Darvon), are synthesized in a chemical laboratory. Whether natural or synthetic, these drugs are powerful *narcotics*, or painkillers.

Heroin (also known as horse, junk, smack, or downtown), the most widely abused opioid, is illegal in this country. In other nations it is used as a potent painkiller for conditions such as terminal cancer. There are an estimated 600,000 heroin addicts in the United States, with men outnumbering women addicts by three to one. Among people ages 18 to 25, the percentage of heroin users who inject the drug has doubled in the last decade. While the number of young heroin users in major cities has dropped by 50 percent, their numbers have almost tripled in suburban and rural areas.

Heroin users typically inject the drug into their veins. However, individuals who experiment with recreational drugs often prefer *skin-popping* (subcutaneous injection) rather than *mainlining* (intravenous injection); they also may snort heroin as a powder or dissolve it and inhale the vapors. To try to avoid addiction, some users begin by *chipping*, taking small or intermittent doses. Regardless of the method of administration, tolerance can develop rapidly.

Morphine, used as a painkiller and anesthetic, acts primarily on the central nervous system, eyes, and digestive tract. By producing mental clouding, drowsiness, and euphoria, it does not decrease the physical sensation of pain as much as it alters a person's awareness of the pain; in effect, he or she no longer cares about it.

**How Users Feel**  All opioids relax the user. When injected, they can produce an immediate rush (high) that lasts 10 to 30 minutes. For two to six hours thereafter, users may feel indifferent, lethargic, and drowsy; they may slur their words and have problems paying attention, remembering, and going about their normal routine. The primary attractions of heroin are

**barbiturates** Antianxiety drugs that depress the central nervous system, reduce activity, and induce relaxation, drowsiness, or sleep; often prescribed to relieve tension and treat epileptic seizures or as a general anesthetic.

**opioids** Drugs that have sleep-inducing and pain-relieving properties, including opium and its derivatives and nonopioid, synthetic drugs.

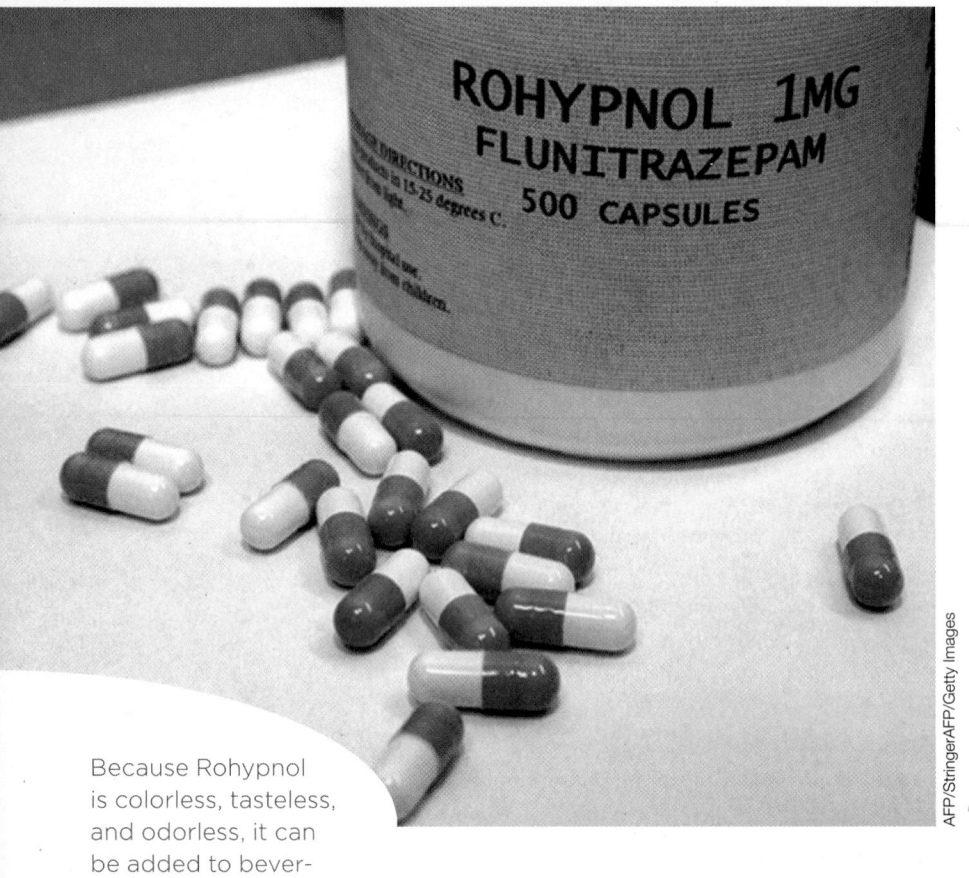

ROHYPNOL 1MG
FLUNITRAZEPAM
500 CAPSULES

AFP/Stringer/AFP/Getty Images

Because Rohypnol is colorless, tasteless, and odorless, it can be added to beverages without your knowledge.

**hallucinogen** A drug that causes hallucinations.

**LSD (lysergic acid diethylamide)** A synthetic psychoactive substance originally developed to explore mental illness.

the euphoria and pain relief it produces. However, some people experience very unpleasant feelings, such as anxiety and fear. Other effects include a sensation of warmth or heaviness, dry mouth, facial flushing, and nausea and vomiting (particularly in first-time users).

**Risks** Addiction is common. Almost all regular users of opioids rapidly develop drug dependence, which can lead to lethargy, weight loss, loss of sex drive, and the continual effort to avoid withdrawal symptoms through repeated drug administration. In addition, they experience anxiety, insomnia, restlessness, and craving for the drug. Users continue taking opioids as much to avoid the discomfort of withdrawal, a classic sign of opioid addiction, as to experience pleasure.

Physical symptoms include constricted pupils (although pupils may dilate from a severe overdose), drowsiness, slurred speech, and impaired attention or memory. Morphine affects blood pressure, heart rate, and blood circulation in the brain. Both morphine and heroin slow down the respiratory system; overdoses can cause fatal respiratory arrest.

Over time, users who inject opioids may develop infections of the heart lining and valves, skin abscesses, and lung congestion. Infections from unsterile solutions, syringes, and shared needles can lead to hepatitis, tetanus, liver disease, and HIV. Depression is common and may be both an antecedent and a risk factor for needle sharing.

Opioid abuse during pregnancy can cause miscarriage, stillbirth, or low birth weight. Babies born to addicted mothers experience withdrawal symptoms after birth.

**Withdrawal** If a regular user stops taking an opioid, withdrawal begins within 6 to 12 hours. The intensity of the symptoms depends on the degree of the addiction; they may grow stronger for 24 to 72 hours and gradually subside over a period of 7 to 14 days, though some symptoms, such as insomnia, may persist for several months. Individuals may develop craving for an opioid, irritability, nausea or vomiting, muscle aches, runny nose or eyes, dilated pupils, sweating, diarrhea, yawning, fever, and insomnia. Opioid withdrawal usually is not life-threatening.

## Hallucinogens

The drugs known as **hallucinogens** produce vivid and unusual changes in thought, feeling, and perception. Hallucinogens do not produce dependence in the same way as cocaine or heroin. Individuals who have an unpleasant experience after trying a hallucinogen may stop using the drug completely without suffering withdrawal symptoms. Others continue regular or occasional use because they enjoy the effects.

**LSD (lysergic acid diethylamide**, acid) was initially developed as a tool to explore mental illness. It became popular in the 1960s and resurfaced among teenagers in the 1990s. LSD is taken orally, either blotted onto pieces of paper that are held in the mouth or chewed along with another substance, such as a sugar cube. Peyote (whose active ingredient is mescaline) is another hallucinogen, but it is much less commonly used in this country.

## Dissociative Drugs

Drugs such as PCP (phencyclidine) and ketamine, initially developed as general anesthetics for surgery, distort perceptions of sight and sound and produce feelings of dissociation or detachment from the environment and self. They alter distribution of the neurotransmitter glutamate, which is involved in perception of pain, responses to the environment, and memory, in the brain.

Because these mind-altering effects are not hallucinations, scientists refer to PCP and ketamine as "dissociative anesthetics." High doses of dextromethorphan, a widely available cough suppressant, and the herb salvia can produce effects similar to those of PCP and ketamine.

*Ketamine*  Ketamine—called K, Special-K, and vitamin K—is an anesthetic used by veterinarians. When cooked, dried, and ground into powder for snorting, ketamine blocks chemical messengers in the brain that carry sensory input. As a result, the brain fills the void with hallucinations. Users may report an "out-of-body" experience with distorted perceptions of time and space. The effects typically begin within 30 minutes and last for approximately two hours.

Ketamine has become common in club scenes and has been used as a date rape drug. Low doses can cause impaired attention and memory, anxiety, agitation, paranoia, and vomiting. Higher doses can cause delirium, amnesia, impaired motor function, high blood pressure, depression, and potentially deadly breathing problems. Repeated ketamine use can be addictive and even a single use can occasionally produce audiovisual "flashbacks," similar to those described by phencyclidine (PCP) users, and long-term memory loss.

*PCP*  PCP (**phencyclidine**, brand name Sernyl; street names angel dust, peace pill, lovely, and green) is an illicit drug manufactured as a tablet, capsule, liquid, flake, spray, or crystal-like white powder that can be swallowed, smoked, sniffed, or injected. Sometimes it is sprinkled on crack, marijuana, tobacco, or parsley, and smoked. A fine-powdered form of PCP can be snorted or injected.

PCP use peaked in the 1970s, but it remains a popular drug of abuse in both inner-city ghettos and suburban high schools. Users often think that the PCP they take together with another illegal psychoactive substance, such as amphetamines, coke, or hallucinogens, is responsible for the highs they feel, so they seek it out specifically.

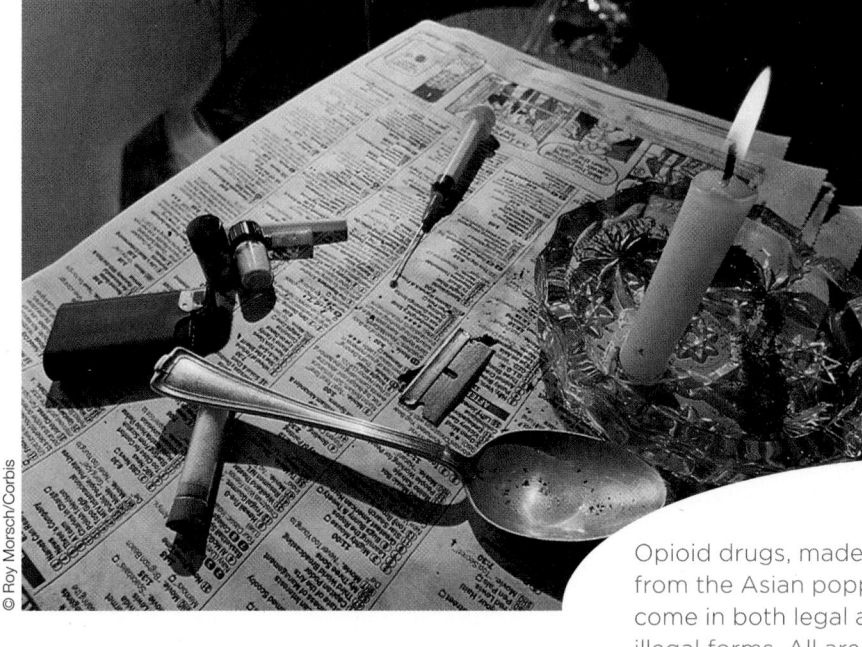

© Roy Morsch/Corbis

Opioid drugs, made from the Asian poppy, come in both legal and illegal forms. All are highly addictive.

The effects of PCP are utterly unpredictable. It may trigger violent behavior or irreversible psychosis the first time it is used, or the twentieth time, or never. In low doses, PCP produces changes—from hallucinations or euphoria to feelings of emptiness or numbness—similar to those produced by other psychoactive drugs. Higher doses may produce a stupor that lasts several days, increased heart rate and blood pressure, skin flushing, sweating, dizziness, and numbness.

Some people experience repetitive motor movements (such as facial grimacing), hallucinations, and paranoia. Suicide is a definite risk. Intoxication typically lasts four to six hours, but some effects can linger for several days. Delirium may occur within 24 hours of taking PCP or after recovery from an overdose and can last as much as a week.

*Salvia*  Salvia (*Salvia divinorum*) is an herb grown in southern Mexico and Central and South America. Its main active ingredient, salvinorin A, activates kappa opioid receptors that differ from those activated by the more commonly known opioids, such as heroin and morphine. Traditionally ingested by chewing fresh leaves or drinking their extracted juices, *S. divinorum* when dried can also be smoked as a joint, consumed in water pipes, or vaporized and inhaled.

People who abuse salvia generally experience hallucinations or "psychotomimetic" episodes

**PCP (phencyclidine)** A synthetic psychoactive substance that produces effects similar to other psychoactive drugs when swallowed, smoked, sniffed, or injected, but also may trigger unpredictable behavioral changes.

**salvia** An herb with hallucinogenic properties when smoked or inhaled.

(a transient experience that mimics a psychosis) that occur in less than a minute and last less than 30 minutes. They include psychedelic-like changes in visual perception, mood and body sensations, emotional swings, feelings of detachment, and a greatly altered perception of external reality and the self. The long-term effects of salvia abuse have not been investigated systematically.

The Drug Enforcement Agency has listed salvia as a drug of concern and is considering classifying it as a drug with high potential for abuse, like LSD or marijuana.

## Inhalants

**Inhalants** or *delerians* are chemicals that produce vapors with psychoactive effects. The most commonly abused inhalants are solvents, aerosols, model-airplane glue, cleaning fluids, and petroleum products like kerosene and butane. Some anesthetics and nitrous oxide (laughing gas) are also abused.

Young people who have been treated for mental health problems, have a history of foster care, or already abuse other drugs have an increased risk of abusing or becoming dependent on inhalants. In addition, adolescents who first begin using inhalants at an early age are more likely to become dependent on them. Approximately 11 percent of adolescents nationwide report having used inhalants in their lifetime. Teens with inhalant use disorders report coexisting multiple drug abuse and dependence, mental health treatment, and delinquent behaviors. Only alcohol is a more widely used intoxicant among preteens and teens. More 12-year-olds admit to sniffing potentially deadly inhalants than to smoking marijuana.[26]

Inhalants very rapidly reach the lungs, bloodstream, and other parts of the body. At low doses, users may feel slightly stimulated; at higher doses, they may feel less inhibited. Intoxication often occurs within five minutes and can last more than an hour. Inhalant users do not report the intense rush associated with other drugs; nor do they experience the perceptual changes associated with LSD. However, inhalants interfere with thinking and impulse control, so users may act in dangerous or destructive ways.

**inhalants** Substances that produce vapors having psychoactive effects when sniffed.

Often there are visible external signs of use: a rash around the nose and mouth; breath odors; residue on face, hands, and clothing; redness, swelling, and tearing of the eyes; and irritation of throat, lungs, and nose that leads to coughing and gagging. Nausea and headache also may occur.

Regular use of inhalants leads to tolerance, so the sniffer needs more and more to attain the desired effects. Younger children who use inhalants several times a week may develop dependence. Older users who become dependent may use the drugs many times a day.

Although some young people believe inhalants are safe, this is far from true. Inhalation of butane from cigarette lighters displaces oxygen in the lungs, causing suffocation. Users also can suffocate while covering their heads with a plastic bag to inhale the substance or from inhaling vomit into their lungs while high. The effects of inhalants are unpredictable, and even a single episode can trigger asphyxiation or cardiac arrhythmia, leading to disability or death. Abusers also can develop difficulties with memory and abstract reasoning, problems with coordination, and uncontrollable movements of the extremities.

# Treating Substance Dependence and Abuse

An estimated 6.1 million Americans are in need of drug treatment, but the majority—some 5 million—never get treatment. The most difficult step for a drug user is to admit that he or she *is* in fact an addict. If drug abusers are not forced to deal with their problem through some unexpected trauma, such as being fired or going bankrupt, those who care—family, friends, coworkers, doctors—may have to confront them and insist that they do something about their addiction. Often this *intervention* can be the turning point for addicts and their families. Treatment has proved equally successful for young people and for older adults.

Some universities offer interventions for students who violate college substance abuse policies. *Motivational interviewing*, a brief intervention in which counselors express empathy to support personal change, has proved effective in reducing alcohol and drug consumption.

Treatment may take place in an outpatient setting, a residential facility, or a hospital. Increasingly, treatment thereafter is tailored to address coexisting or dual diagnoses. A personal treatment plan may consist of individual psychotherapy, marital and family therapy, medication, and behavior therapy. Once an individual has made the decision to seek help for substance abuse, the first step usually is detoxification, which involves clearing the drug from the body.

Controlled and supervised withdrawal within a medical or psychiatric hospital may be recommended if an individual has not been able to stop using drugs as an outpatient or in a residential treatment program. Detoxification is most likely to be complicated in a polysubstance abuser, who may require close monitoring and treatment of potentially fatal withdrawal symptoms. Other reasons for inpatient treatment include lack of psychosocial support for maintaining abstinence and the absence of a drug-free living environment. Restrictions on insurance coverage may limit the number of days of inpatient care. Increasingly, once individuals complete detoxification, they continue treatment in residential programs or as outpatients.

Anti-addiction medications that target neurotransmitters in the brain are becoming safer and more effective. With treatment, substance abusers are less prone to relapse. If they do return to drug use, their relapses tend to be shorter and less frequent.

The aim of chemical dependence treatment is to help individuals establish and maintain their recovery from alcohol and drugs of abuse. Recovery is a dynamic process of personal growth and healing in which the drug user makes the transition from a lifestyle of active substance use to a drug-free lifestyle.[27]

## Principles of Drug Addiction Treatment

More than three decades of scientific research show that treatment can help drug-addicted individuals stop drug use, avoid relapse, and successfully recover their lives. Based on this research, NIDA has developed fundamental principles that characterize effect drug abuse treatment. They include the following:

- **Addiction is a complex but treatable disease that affects brain function and behavior.** Drugs alter the brain's structure and how it functions, resulting in changes that persist long after drug use has ceased. This may help explain why abusers are at risk for relapse even after long periods of abstinence.

- **No single treatment is appropriate for everyone.** Matching treatment settings, interventions, and services to an individual's particular problems and needs is critical to his or her ultimate success.

- **Treatment needs to be readily available.** Because drug-addicted individuals may be uncertain about entering treatment, taking advantage of available services the moment people are ready for treatment is critical.

- **Effective treatment attends to multiple needs of the individual, not just his or her drug abuse.** To be effective, treatment must address the individual's drug abuse and any associated medical, psychological, social, vocational, and legal problems.

- **Remaining in treatment for an adequate period of time is critical.** The appropriate duration for an individual depends on the type and degree of his or her problems and needs. Research indicates that most addicted individuals need at least three months in treatment to significantly reduce or stop their drug use and that the best outcomes occur with longer durations of treatment.

- **Counseling—individual and/or group—and other behavioral therapies are the most commonly used forms of drug abuse treatment.** Behavioral therapies vary in their focus and may involve addressing a patient's motivations to change, building skills to resist drug use, replacing drug-using activities with constructive and rewarding activities, improving problem-solving skills, and facilitating better interpersonal relationships.

- **Medications are an important element of treatment for many patients, especially when combined with counseling and other behavioral therapies.** For example, methadone and buprenorphine are effective in helping individuals addicted to heroin or other opioids stabilize their lives and reduce their illicit drug use.

- **Many drug-addicted individuals also have other mental disorders.** Drug abuse and addiction—both of which are mental disorders—often co-occur with other mental illnesses. When these problems co-occur, treatment should address both (or all), including the use of medications as appropriate.

- **Medically assisted detoxification is only the first stage of addiction treatment and by itself does little to change the long-term drug abuse.** Although medically assisted detoxification can safely manage the acute physical symptoms of withdrawal, detoxification alone is rarely sufficient to help addicted individuals achieve long-term abstinence. Thus, patients should be encouraged to continue drug treatment following detoxification.

- **Treatment does not need to be voluntary to be effective.** Sanctions or enticements from family, the employment setting, and/or the criminal justice system can significantly increase treatment entry, retention rates, and the ultimate success of drug treatment interventions.

- **Drug use during treatment must be monitored continuously, as lapses during treatment do occur.** Knowing their drug use is being monitored can be a powerful incentive for patients and can help them withstand urges to use drugs.

## 12-Step Programs

Since its founding in 1935, Alcoholics Anonymous (AA)—the oldest, largest, and most successful self-help program in the world—has spawned a worldwide movement. As many as 200 different recovery programs are based on the spiritual **12-step program** of AA. Participation in 12-step programs for drug abusers, such as Substance Anonymous, Narcotics Anonymous, and Cocaine Anonymous, is of

fundamental importance in promoting and maintaining long-term abstinence.

The basic precept of 12-step programs is that members have been powerless when it comes to controlling their addictive behavior on their own. These programs don't recruit members. The desire to stop must come from the individual, who can call the number of a 12-step program, listed in the telephone book, and find out when and where the next nearby meeting will be held. A representative may offer to send someone to the caller's house to talk about the problem and to escort him or her to the next meeting.

Meetings of various 12-step programs are held daily in almost every city in the country. (Some chapters, whose members often include the disabled or those in remote areas, meet via Internet chat rooms or electronic bulletin boards.) There are no dues or fees for membership. Many individuals belong to several programs because they have several problems, such as alcoholism, substance abuse, and pathological gambling. All have only one requirement for membership: a desire to stop an addictive behavior.

To get the most out of a 12-step program:

- Try out different groups until you find one you like and in which you feel comfortable.

- Once you find a group in which you feel comfortable, go back several times (some recommend a minimum of six meetings) before making a final decision on whether to continue.

- Keep an open mind. Listen to other people's stories and ask yourself if you've had similar feelings or experiences.

- Accept whatever feels right to you and ignore the rest. One common saying in 12-step programs is, "Take what you like and leave the rest."

## Relapse Prevention

The most common clinical course for substance abuse disorders involves a pattern of multiple relapses over the course of a lifespan. It is important for individuals with these problems and their families to recognize this fact. When relapses do occur, they should be viewed as neither a mark of defeat nor evidence of moral weakness. While painful, they do not erase the progress that has been achieved and ultimately

**12-step programs** Self-help group programs based on the principles of Alcoholics Anonymous.

may strengthen self-understanding. They can serve as reminders of potential pitfalls to avoid in the future.

One key to preventing relapse is learning to avoid obvious cues and associations that can set off intense cravings. This means staying away from the people and places linked with past drug use. Some therapists use conditioning techniques to give former users some sense of control over their urge to use the drug. The theory behind this approach, which is called *extinction* of conditioned behavior, is that with repeated exposure—for example, to videotapes of dealers selling crack cocaine—the arousal and craving will diminish. While this technique by itself cannot ward off relapses, it does seem to enhance the overall effectiveness of other therapies.

Another important lesson that therapists emphasize is that every lapse does not have to lead to a full-blown relapse. Users can turn to the skills acquired in treatment—calling people for support or going to meetings—to avoid a major relapse. Ultimately, users must learn much more than how to avoid temptation; they must examine their entire view of the world and learn new ways to live in it without turning to drugs. This is the underlying goal of the recovery process.

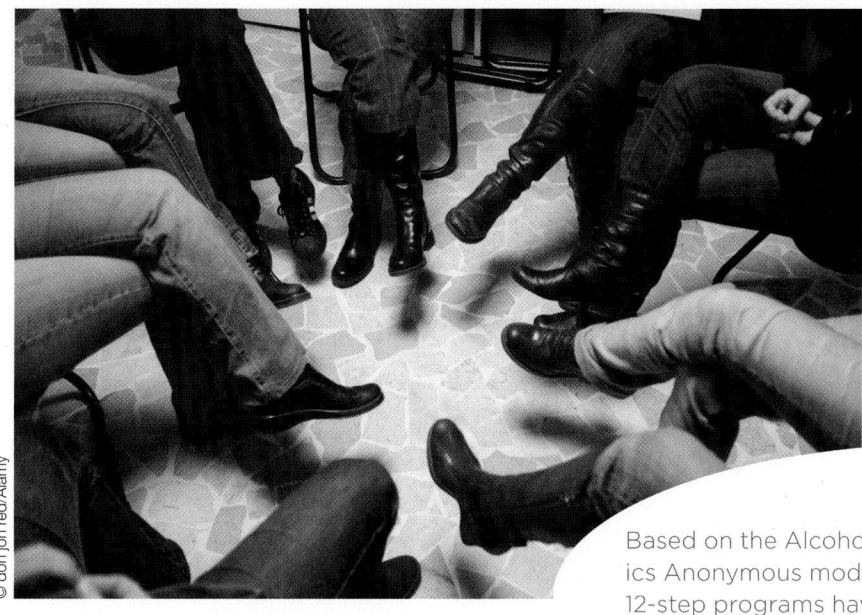

© don jon red/Alamy

Based on the Alcoholics Anonymous model, 12-step programs have helped many people overcome addiction. The one requirement for membership is a desire to end a pattern of addictive behavior.

# Choosing an Addiction-Free Lifestyle

People with substance abuse disorders and addictive behaviors lose control of their choices and their lives. Their compulsion to gamble or to use a drug seems irresistible. You, in contrast, have a choice. You can create a life and a lifestyle with no need and no room for reliance on a substance or a self-destructive behavior. Check those that you have already implemented. Are there others you plan to incorporate into your life?

____ **Set goals for yourself.** Think about who you want to become, what you'd like to do, the future you wish for yourself. Focus on what it will take—years of education, perhaps, or specialized training—to achieve these goals. Understand that drugs can only get in the way and diminish your potential.

____ **Participate in drug-free activities.** If you're bored or unfocused, drugs may appeal to you simply as something to do. Take charge of your time. Play a sport. Work out at the gym. Join a club. Volunteer. Start a blog.

____ **Educate yourself.** Much of the information that young people hear from friends, particularly drug-using friends, is wrong. Drugs that are used as medicines are not safe for recreational use. The fact that many people at a party or club are having fun doesn't mean that some aren't endangering their brains and their lives by taking club drugs. Get the facts for yourself from sites such as those on page 423.

____ **Choose friends with a future.** The world of drug users shrinks. Nothing matters more than the next hit, the next high, the next fix. Losing all sense of tomorrow, they focus on getting through the day with the help of drugs. Are these the people you want to spend time with? Choose friends who can broaden your world with new ideas, ambitious plans, and great dreams for tomorrow.

If you think you may have a problem with drugs, take the Self Survey "Do You Have a Substance-Use Disorder?" and read the Health Action Plan in *Your Personal Wellness Guide.*

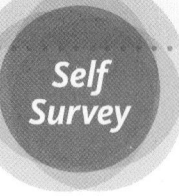

Self
Survey

# Do You Have a Substance-Use Disorder?

Check the statements that apply to you.

- Use more of an illegal drug or a prescription medication or use a drug for a longer period of time than you desire or intend. ____
- Try, repeatedly and unsuccessfully, to cut down or control drug use. ____
- Spend a great deal of time doing whatever is necessary in order to get drugs, taking them, or recovering from their use. ____
- Be so high or feel so bad after drug use that you often cannot work or fulfill other responsibilities. ____
- Give up or cut back on important social, work, or recreational activities because of drug use. ____
- Continue to use drugs even though you realize that they are causing or worsening physical or mental problems. ____
- Use a lot more of a drug in order to achieve a "high" or desired effect or feel fewer such effects than in the past. ____

- Use drugs in dangerous ways or situations. ____
- Have repeated drug-related legal problems, such as arrests for possession. ____
- Continue to use drugs, even though the drug causes or worsens social or personal problems, such as arguments with a spouse. ____
- Develop hand tremors or other withdrawal symptoms if you cut down or stop drug use. ____
- Take drugs to relieve or avoid withdrawal symptoms. ____

The more blanks that you (or someone close to you) checks, the more reason you have to be concerned about drug use. The most difficult step for anyone with a substance-use disorder is to admit that he or she has a problem. Sometimes a drug-related crisis, such as being arrested or fired, forces individuals to acknowledge the impact of drugs. If not, those who care—family, friends, boss, physician—may have to confront them and insist that they do something about it. This confrontation, planned beforehand, is called an *intervention* and can be the turning point for drug users and their families.

# Making Change Happen

## Don't Go There

The use of illegal drugs can lead to terrible, life-changing consequences for you and your family. Legal drugs, when used for reasons other than those for which they were prescribed, can be even stronger and more deadly. Drugs interfere with learning and education by making it more difficult to pay attention, concentrate, and remember. They create problems for and with people who love you. Drugs produce short- and long-term side effects that can range from mood changes to potentially fatal abnormalities in your breathing and heart rate. Most important, drugs can steal control of your life and your future—or can steal life itself.

But there are other, perhaps less obvious, reasons not to go down the path of drug use or other compulsive behaviors. For one thing, there is no need to. As you'll learn in "Don't Go There" in *Labs for IPC*, you can experience the sensations drugs can offer in other ways yet remain in charge and in control. Here's a preview.

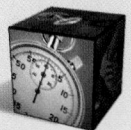

### Get Real
In this stage you complete an inventory of your drug-related behaviors by means of a checklist with 26 items, including the following three:

__ • Used marijuana.

__ • Felt that you could not control or stop using a particular drug.

__ • Took any medicine, including painkillers and stimulants, for a reason other than that for which it was prescribed.

The more checks you see, the greater your risk of losing control of your life to a compulsive behavior or a substance of abuse . . .

In another exercise, you answer the question "What if?" by writing brief essays that begin with three different phrases, including:

• "As long as I stuck to prescription meds, I was sure I'd be able to stop whenever I wanted. But . . ."

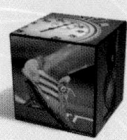

### Get Ready
In this stage you list all the advantages and benefits that your compulsive substance use has brought you. You might mention things such as:

• It made me feel that I fit in with a certain group.

• It was a way to blow off steam and relax . . .

You then list the disadvantages and negative consequences you've experienced as a result of your compulsive substance use, such as:

• Being unable to afford other things because of money spent on drugs or gambling.

• Side effects from drugs, which can include elevated blood pressure, heart rate, and breathing problems . . .

You also start tracking compulsive behavior or substance use by recording every time you engage in the behavior (such as gambling), when, how long, how much you gamble . . .

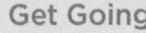

### Get Going
This stage consists of five steps, including the following three:

• Consciously choosing an alternative behavior rather than your drug or escape of choice the next time you're stressed out or feeling lonely, down, or anxious . . .

• Quitting for 90 days. If you claim you can stop any time, prove it . . . Just stop. Yes, stop. And don't go back to your drug use or compulsive behavior for three consecutive months.

• Creating positive diversions, noncompulsive, nonchemical ways of achieving physical relaxation, sensory stimulation, greater creativity . . .

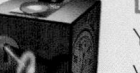

### Lock It In
You continue self-monitoring to prove to yourself that you really are in the driver's seat regarding your use of drugs, alcohol, and other addictive substances and behaviors. You also keep expanding your repertoire of positive activities and coping skills . . .

# Making This Chapter Work for You

## Review Questions

1. Individuals with substance-use disorders
   a. are usually not physically dependent on their drug of choice.
   b. have a compulsion to use one or more addictive substances.
   c. require less and less of the preferred drug to achieve the desired effect.
   d. suffer withdrawal symptoms when they use the drug regularly.

2. Which of the following statements about club drugs is *true*?
   a. Club drugs can produce many unwanted effects, including hallucinations and paranoia.
   b. Most club drugs do not pose the same health dangers as "hard" drugs such as heroin.
   c. MDMA is the street name for Ecstasy.
   d. When combined with extended physical exertion, club drugs can lead to hypothermia (lowered body temperature).

3. Which of the following statements about marijuana is *false*?
   a. People who have used marijuana may experience psychoactive effects for several days after use.
   b. Marijuana has shown some effectiveness in treating chemotherapy-related nausea.
   c. Unlike long-term use of alcohol, regular use of marijuana does not have any long-lasting health consequences.
   d. Depending on the amount of marijuana used, its effects can range from a mild sense of euphoria to extreme panic.

4. Which of the following statements about drugs is *false*?
   a. Toxicity is the dosage level of a prescription.
   b. Drugs can be injected into the body intravenously, intramuscularly, or subcutaneously.
   c. Drug misuse is the taking of a drug for a purpose other than that for which it was medically intended.
   d. An individual's response to a drug can be affected by the setting in which the drug is used.

5. The opioids
   a. are not addictive if used in a prescription form such as codeine or Demerol.
   b. produce an immediate but short-lasting high and feeling of euphoria.
   c. include morphine, which is typically used for cough suppression.
   d. are illegal in the United States, although they are allowed in other countries to help control severe pain.

6. Which of the following statements about drug dependence treatment is *false*?
   a. Chemical dependence treatment programs usually involve medications to alleviate withdrawal symptoms.
   b. Detoxification is usually the first step in a drug treatment program.
   c. Relapses are not uncommon for a person who has undergone drug treatment.
   d. The 12-step recovery program associated with Alcoholics Anonymous has been shown to be ineffective with individuals with drug dependence disorders.

7. To help ensure that an over-the-counter or prescription drug is safe and effective:
   a. take smaller dosages than indicated in the instructions.
   b. test your response to the drug by borrowing a similar medication from a friend.
   c. ask your doctor or pharmacist about possible interactions with other medications.
   d. buy all of your medications online.

8. Cocaine dependence can result in all of the following *except*
   a. stroke.
   b. paranoia and violent behavior.
   c. heart failure.
   d. enhanced sexual performance.

9. Amphetamine is very similar to which of the following in its effects on the central nervous system?
   a. marijuana
   b. heroin
   c. cocaine
   d. alcohol

10. Prescription drug abuse on college campuses
    a. is not a problem.
    b. is higher among college women than college men.
    c. is more widespread than the use of marijuana.
    d. is more widespread than the use of Ecstasy, cocaine, and meth.

*Answers to these questions can be found on page 672.*

## Critical Thinking

1. Suppose that a close friend is using amphetamines to keep her energy levels high so that she can continue to attend school full-time and hold down a job to pay her school expenses. You fear that she is developing a substance abuse disorder. What can you do to help her realize the dangers of her behavior? What resources are available at your school or in your community to help her deal with both her drug problem and her financial needs?

2. Some Web enthusiasts oppose any kind of government regulations on the Internet. Do you agree or disagree? How would you address the problems associated with distributing drugs online, including the sale of counterfeit drugs?

## Media Menu

Visit www.cengagebrain.com to access course materials for this text, including the Behavior Change Planner, interactive quizzes, tutorials, and more.

## Internet Connections

**www.nida.nih.gov**
This government site—a virtual clearinghouse of information for students, parents, teachers, researchers, and health professionals—features current treatment and research, as well as a comprehensive database on common drugs of abuse. The science of drug abuse and addictions is discussed with a focus on the major illegal drugs in use, with additional resources on drug testing, treatment research, and trends/statistics.

**www.drugfree.org**
This site features current resources and photographs on a wide spectrum of drugs, including performance-enhancing drugs, club drugs, and commonly abused prescription drugs. The drug guide even allows you to search for a drug using its slang name.

**www.clubdrugs.org**
This site is a service of the National Institute on Drug Abuse to provide information on club drugs.

**www.factsontap.org**
Facts on Tap is one of the programs of Phoenix House, the largest nonprofit alcohol and drug abuse treatment and prevention facility in the United States.

## Key Terms

The terms listed are used on the page indicated. Definitions of the terms are in the Glossary at the end of the book.

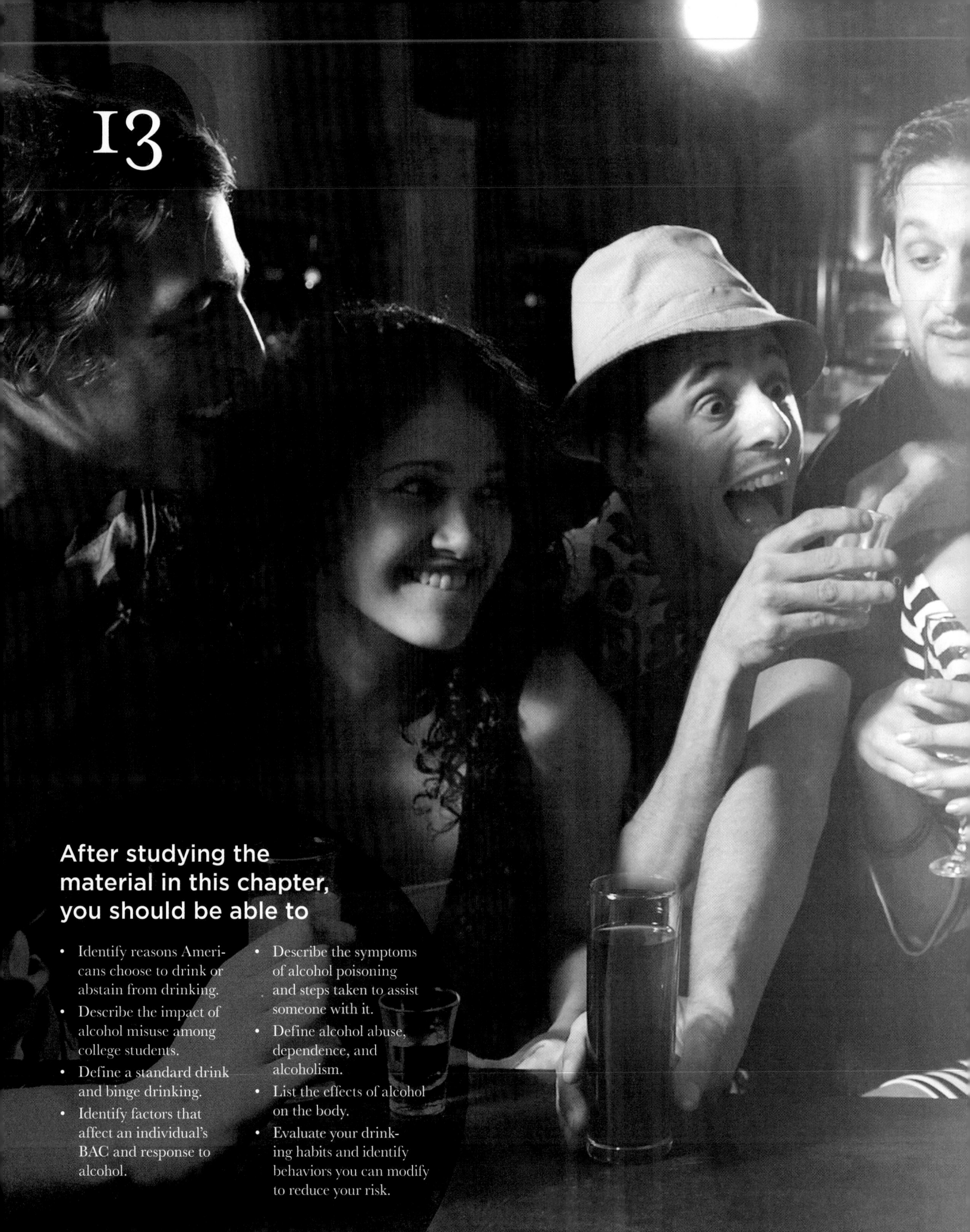

# 13

## After studying the material in this chapter, you should be able to

- Identify reasons Americans choose to drink or abstain from drinking.
- Describe the impact of alcohol misuse among college students.
- Define a standard drink and binge drinking.
- Identify factors that affect an individual's BAC and response to alcohol.

- Describe the symptoms of alcohol poisoning and steps taken to assist someone with it.
- Define alcohol abuse, dependence, and alcoholism.
- List the effects of alcohol on the body.
- Evaluate your drinking habits and identify behaviors you can modify to reduce your risk.

It was just another Friday night at the frat house. The drinking started early and usually didn't stop until dawn. One of the brothers, a popular easy-going guy named Ryan—not usually much of a drinker—was celebrating a big birthday: his twenty-first. Egged on by the hooting crowd, Ryan bolted down one drink after another, after another, after another.

# Alcohol

By the time Ryan reached 12 drinks, he was slurring his words. As he kept chugging drinks, his face looked flushed; he started sweating heavily. When Ryan lurched to his feet, he swayed unsteadily for a few moments and then collapsed. At first everyone laughed. Then two of his buddies tried to revive him. They couldn't.

"He's not breathing!" one of them shouted. Someone called 911, and paramedics rushed Ryan to the nearest hospital. His blood-alcohol concentration was several times above the legal limit. Despite intensive efforts by the medical team, nothing helped. Ryan's twenty-first birthday was his last.

As Ryan's tragic death shows, alcohol, when not used responsibly, can take an enormous toll. Alcohol and tobacco are the most widely used mind-altering substances in the world. Each dangerous in itself, drinking and smoking tend to go together. The more individuals smoke and drink, the less likely they are to eat a nutritious diet and follow a healthy lifestyle.

Even if you never drink to excess, you live with the consequences of others' drinking. That's why it's important for everyone to know about the very real dangers of alcohol abuse. This chapter provides information that can help you understand, avoid, and change behaviors that could destroy your health, happiness, and life.

## Drinking in America

Alcohol is the most widely used drug in the world. No medical conditions, other than heart disease, cause more disability and premature death than alcohol-related problems. No mental or medical disorders touch the lives of more families. No other form of disability costs individuals, employers, and the government more for treatment, injuries, reduced worker productivity, and property damage. The costs in emotional pain and in lost and shattered lives because of irresponsible drinking are beyond measure.

Many Americans drink alcohol; most do not misuse or abuse it. According to the most recent statistics available from the National Institute

Visit www.cengagebrain.com to access course materials for this text, including the Behavior Change Planner, interactive quizzes, tutorials, and more. See the preface on page xv for details.

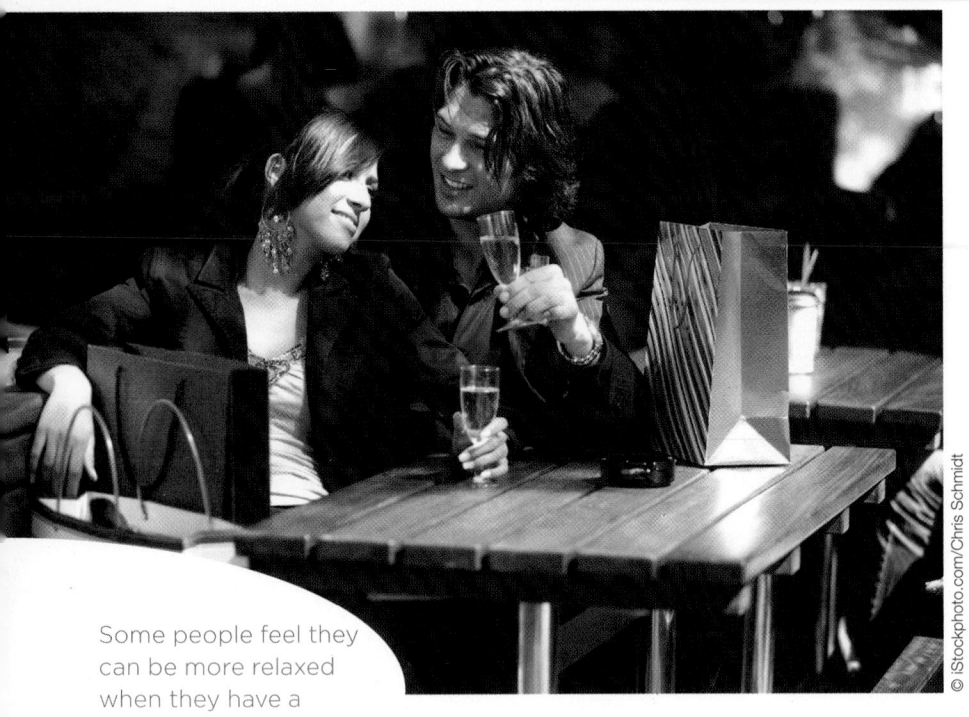

Some people feel they can be more relaxed when they have a drink. However, alcohol lowers inhibitions and can lead to behavior that one or both people regret later.

on Alcohol Abuse and Alcoholism, 52 percent of adults over age 18 are current regular drinkers; 13 percent are infrequent drinkers; 6 percent are former regular drinkers; 9 percent are former infrequent drinkers; and 20 percent are lifetime abstainers.[1]

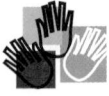 White men and women are more likely to drink than other adults. Seventy percent of white men say they drink, compared to 57 percent of black men, 55 percent of Asian men, and 58 percent of American Indian or Alaska Native men. Among women, 59 percent of white women drink, compared with 40 percent for blacks, 32 percent for Asians, and 45 percent for American Indian or Alaska Natives.[2]

The current alcohol-use rate for blacks age 18 and older is significantly lower than the national adult average (44 percent versus 55 percent). Blacks also have a lower rate of binge drinking than other Americans (22 percent versus 26 percent).[3]

Nearly three-quarters of Americans with graduate degrees drink, compared to 44 percent of those with less than a high school education. Richer people also drink more than poor ones. Among families with incomes below the poverty level, 45 percent drink, compared with 73 percent of those with incomes four or more times greater.[4]

The median age of first alcohol use is 15. Drinking typically increases in the late teens, peaks in the early 20s, and decreases as people age. The median age of onset for alcohol-use disorders is 19 to 20.

# Why People Don't Drink

More Americans are choosing not to drink, and alcohol consumption is at its lowest level in decades. About a quarter of adults—31 percent of women and 18 percent of men—report drinking no alcohol in the last year.

With fewer people drinking alcohol, nonalcoholic beverages have grown in popularity. They appeal to drivers, boaters, individuals with health problems that could worsen with alcohol, those who are older and can't tolerate alcohol, anyone taking medicines that interact with alcohol (including antibiotics, antidepressants, and muscle relaxers), and everyone interested in limiting alcohol intake. Under federal law, these drinks can contain some alcohol but a much smaller amount than regular beer or wine. Nonalcoholic beers and wines on the market also are lower in calories than alcoholic varieties.

Certain people should not drink at all. These include:

- Anyone younger than age 21. Underage drinking (discussed later in this chapter) poses many medical, behavioral, and legal dangers.

- Anyone who plans to drive, operate motorized equipment, or engage in other activities that require alertness and skill (including sports and recreational activities).

- Women who are pregnant or trying to become pregnant.

- Individuals taking certain over-the-counter or prescription medications. (See Consumer Alert, p. 445.)

- People with medical conditions that can be made worse by drinking.

- Recovering alcoholics.

## Why People Drink

The most common reason people drink alcohol is to relax. Because it depresses the central nervous system, alcohol can make people feel less tense. Some psychologists theorize that men engage in *confirmatory drinking*; that is, they drink to reinforce the image of masculinity associated with alcohol consumption. Both genders may engage in *compensatory drinking*, consuming alcohol to heighten their sense of masculinity or femininity.

Here are some other reasons why men and women drink:

- **Social ease.** When people use alcohol, they may seem bolder, wittier, sexier. At the same time, they become more relaxed and seem to enjoy each other's company more. Because alcohol lowers inhibitions, some people see it as a prelude to seduction.

- **Role models.** Athletes, some of the biggest celebrities in our country, have a long history of appearing in commercials for alcohol. Many advertisements feature glamorous men and women holding or sipping alcoholic beverages.

- **Advertising.** Brewers and beer distributors spend multimillions of dollars every year promoting the message: If you want to have fun, have a drink. Young people may be especially responsive to such sales pitches.

- **Relationship issues.** Single, separated, or divorced men and women drink more and more often than married ones.

Individuals with drinking problems often turn to alcohol for other reasons, including:

- **Psychological factors.** Both men and women may drink to compensate for feelings of inadequacy. Yet women who tend to ruminate or mull over bad feelings may find that alcohol increases this tendency and makes them feel more distressed.

- **Self-medication.** More so than men, some women feel it's permissible to use alcohol as if it were a medicine. As long as they're taking it for a reason, it seems acceptable to them.

- **Childhood traumas.** Female alcoholics often report that they were physically or sexually abused as children or suffered great distress because of poverty or a parent's death.

- **Depression.** Women are more likely than men to be depressed prior to drinking and to suffer from both depression and a drinking problem at the same time.

- **Inherited susceptibility.** In both women and men, genetics accounts for 50 to 60 percent of a person's vulnerability to a serious drinking problem.

# Drinking on Campus

 Young adults are the most frequent users of alcohol in the United States, and college students consume more alcohol more often and more dangerously than nonstudents the same age. (See How Do You Compare?) Many health experts consider the use and abuse of alcohol as the primary health concern for college students.

About one in three students increases alcohol use and encounters more related problems throughout the college years; a third do not change previous patterns; and a third decrease drinking.[5] But alcohol can affect every aspect of a student's life. Nearly 160,000 freshmen drop out of college after their first year for alcohol- or drug-related reasons, according to the CORE Institute, which surveys drinking practices on campuses. College drinking is responsible for an estimated 1,700 annual alcohol-related deaths, 599,000 injuries, more than 696,000 physical attacks, and more than 97,000 sexual assaults.[6]

In the preliminary findings of an ongoing study of binge drinking and college students, alcohol significantly lowered GPAs in the first year of college. The undergraduates who binged showed significantly higher levels of both depression and anxiety; those who drank but did not binge demonstrated the greatest impulsivity; and those who binged within the 30 days prior to testing made significantly more errors on a test of spatial working memory.[7]

Although the percentage of students who drink hasn't changed much over the years, drinking on campus has. At many schools, students' social lives revolve around parties, games, and

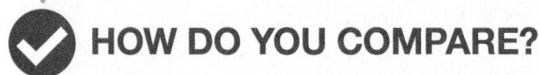
# STUDENT DRINKING

| Alcohol Consumption | Percent (%) | | | | | |
| --- | --- | --- | --- | --- | --- | --- |
| | Actual Use | | | Perceived Use | | |
| | Male | Female | Total | Male | Female | Total |
| Never used | 21.5 | 20.4 | 20.9 | 4.2 | 2.9 | 3.5 |
| Used, but not in the last 30 days | 12.2 | 14.8 | 13.9 | 2.4 | 1.8 | 2.0 |
| Used 1–9 days | 47.1 | 51.6 | 49.7 | 39.2 | 32.7 | 35.0 |
| Used 10–29 | 17.3 | 12.6 | 14.3 | 40.7 | 46.7 | 44.4 |
| Used all 30 days | 1.9 | 0.6 | 1.1 | 13.4 | 15.9 | 15.1 |
| Any use within the last 30 days | 66.3 | 64.8 | 65.2 | 93.3 | 95.3 | 94.4 |

## HOW DO YOU COMPARE?

As the figures above show, most undergraduates overestimate the number of students who drink—and drink frequently—and underestimate the number who don't drink often at all. How do your perceptions and actual behavior compare? What role does alcohol play in your life? Describe its impact on you, your choices, and your behavior in your online journal.

Source: American College Health Association, *American College Health Association-National College Health Assessment II: Reference Group Executive Summary Spring 2010* (Linthicum, MD: American College Health Association, 2010).

bar crawls. More students drink simply to get drunk and drink more per drinking episode.

Overall, students drink more heavily on weekends than weekdays and at the beginning of each semester or quarter than during final exam periods. The highest drinking days include Halloween, New Year's Eve, and St. Patrick's Day.[8]

In a recent study that followed undergraduates for 70 days, students drank the most on weekends, with Fridays and Saturdays accounting for 60 percent of all drinks consumed and Thursdays or an additional 17 percent. The odds of drinking heavily, drinking enough to stumble around, and drinking enough to pass out were also greater on weekend days. Male undergraduates, those who started drinking at an early age, members of the Greek system, and those motivated by a desire to socialize and have fun were more likely to drink on weekdays as well as weekends.[9]

Alcohol consumption especially soars on "game days," when a significant number of students engage in "extreme ritualistic alcohol consumption," which is defined as consuming ten or more drinks on the same day for a male and eight or more for a female. In a recent study, about 16 percent of students—twice as many men as women—engaged in this level of drinking on game days.[10]

More college women drink, and they drink more than in the past. College women who drink are at much greater risk of unwanted sexual activity. In one study more than one in five reported some type of sexual assault.

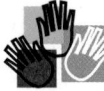 College men drink more, more often, and more intensely than women. Caucasians drink more than African or Asian Americans. Fraternity and sorority members, athletes, and vigorous exercisers also use more alcohol more often than other students. The students who drink the least are those attending two-year institutions, religious schools, commuter schools, and historically black colleges and universities.

## Why Students Don't Drink

According to the National College Health Assessment, 21 percent of students report never using alcohol. Students who don't drink give various reasons for their choice, including not having access to alcohol, parental or peer pressure, being underage, costs, religious reasons, and not liking the taste.[11]

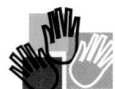 African American students are more likely than white undergraduates to abstain and to report never having had an alcoholic drink or not having a drink in the past 30 days. They also drink less frequently and consume fewer drinks per occasion than whites.

Spiritual and religious values also influence drinking on campus. In a recent study, students at a religious college were four times less likely to be moderate or heavy drinkers compared with those at a public university. Students with the least tendency toward religious beliefs were 27 times more likely to be heavy drinkers than those with greater religiosity.[12]

Character virtues also correlate with drinking choices. Temperance, which psychologists define as a combination of forgiveness, humility, prudence, and self-regulation, is associated with sexual abstinence, less risky drinking, and fewer negative consequences from drinking. Other character traits, including wisdom and courage, do not seem linked to a particular drinking pattern.[13]

## Why Students Drink

Undergraduates have always turned to alcohol for the same reasons. Away from home, often for the first time, many are excited by and apprehensive about their newfound independence. When new pressures seem overwhelming, when they feel awkward or insecure, when they just want to let loose and have a good time, they reach for a drink.

The following list summarizes the most common influences on student drinking.

- **Social norms.** Compared with other factors, such as race, gender, year in school, and fraternity/sorority membership, social norms (discussed in Chapter 1) have the strongest association with how much college students drink. Students' perceptions of how much their peers, particularly those closest to them, drink have more influence on their own drinking than do parents or resident advisors. Yet, students generally overestimate how much and how often their classmates drink.

- **Party schools.** Colleges and universities in the Northeast, those with a strong Greek system, and those where athletics predominate have higher drinking rates than others. Students who drank heavily before college are more likely to join a fraternity or sorority, and the environment in many Greek organizations fosters continued drinking. Students who never join or who drop out of a fraternity or sorority report less risky drinking behavior.

- **Living arrangements.** Drinking rates are highest among students living in fraternity and sorority houses, followed by those in on-campus housing (dormitories, residence halls) and off-campus apartments or houses. Students living at home with their families drink the least.

- **Celebrations.** A twenty-first birthday poses a common and serious risk. In a study of some 2,500 college drinkers, four in five reported drinking to celebrate their twenty-first birthdays, 12 percent (men and women) reported having 21 drinks, and about half drank more than they ever had before.[14] Tailgating parties, big game rallies, Halloween bonfires, and other events fueled by "fun" also become occasions for drinking. The most notorious celebratory drinking occurs during Spring Break.

- **Participation in sports.** College athletes drink more often and more heavily than non-athletes. They may be at greater risk because many are younger than 21, belong to Greek organizations, have lower GPAs, or spend more time socializing than other students. Individual sports also matter. Male hockey and female soccer players drink the most; male basketball players and cross-country or track athletes of both sexes, the least. Female athletes may drink more than other college women because they are following the male athletic model of taking the lead, not just on the field, but also at the party or bar.

- **Coping.** Students turn to alcohol to cope with everyday problems and personal issues. Those with symptoms of depression who lack skills to cope with daily problems, particularly males, are more likely to drink than others. Students who feel angry, hostile,

# Drink Less, Save More

Yet another good reason to control how much you drink is economic. The less spending money that college students have, the less they drink—and the less likely they are to get drunk and to suffer alcohol-related negative consequences. Here are some simple ways to spend less on alcohol:

- **Pace yourself.** Start with a soft drink and have a nonalcoholic drink every second or third drink.

- **Stay busy.** You will drink less if you play pool or dance rather than just sitting and drinking.

- **Try low-alcohol alternatives,** such as light beers and low- or no-alcohol wines.

- **Have alcohol-free days.** Don't drink at all at least two days a week.

- **Drink slowly.** Take sips and not gulps. Put your glass down between sips.

- **Avoid salty snacks.** Salty foods like chips or nuts make you thirsty so you drink more.

- **Have one drink at a time.** Don't let people top up your drinks. It makes it harder to keep track of how much alcohol you're consuming.

## Alcohol Expectancy

According to expectancy theory, an individual's belief, rational or not, that a certain behavior or experience will have a particular effect, positive or negative, increases the probability of this effect. As many studies have shown, expectancy influences how much and how often individuals drink. College women generally expect positive social experiences when drinking alcohol; young adult men expect sexual arousal and more aggressive behavior.[16]

Many college students drink because they believe "liquid courage" will make them feel better—more at ease, less stressed, more sociable, less self-conscious.[17] The behaviors most commonly reported by students when they drink reflect these expectations: flirting, dancing, telling jokes, and laughing harder or more frequently.

## Defensive Drinking

In the most recent ACHA survey, the vast majority of students—97 percent—reported using at least one behavioral strategy to control their drinking and prevent alcohol-related problems. The most popular strategies were staying with the same group of friends throughout an event, choosing a designated driver, eating before and/or while drinking, sticking with only one form of alcohol, and deciding in advance not to exceed a set number of drinks.[18] The more that students rely on protective behavioral strategies, the less alcohol they consume and the fewer alcohol-related problems they encounter.[19] (For additional strategies, see Health on a Budget.)

## High-Risk Drinking on Campus

The most common types of student high-risk drinking are binge drinking, predrinking, underage drinking, binge drinking combined with disordered eating, and consumption of caffeinated alcoholic beverages.

*Binge Drinking*   According to the National Institute of Alcohol Abuse and Alcoholism, a **binge** is a pattern of drinking alcohol that brings blood alcohol concentration (BAC) (discussed later in this chapter) to 0.08 gram-percent or above. For a typical adult man, this

nervous, guilty, or ashamed are more likely to drink in their dorm rooms and apartments than those who report positive moods. Students who score high in social anxiety report heavier drinking, even after a basic intervention designed to reduce alcohol consumption.[15]

**Parental approval.** Students who believe that their parents approve of drinking are more likely to drink and to report a drinking-related problem. This relationship is even stronger in younger students and those who perceive that their mothers approve of drinking.

**First-year transition.** Some students who drank less in high school than classmates who weren't headed for college start drinking, and drinking heavily, in college—often during their first six weeks on campus and peaking during school breaks. Alcohol consumption declines over the course of an undergraduate education, but a substantial number of students continue to drink heavily through their third year.

**binge** For a man, having five or more alcoholic drinks at a single sitting; for a woman, having four drinks or more at a single sitting.

pattern corresponds to consuming five or more drinks in about two hours; for a woman, four or more drinks.

In a recent study, binge drinkers consumed an average of eight drinks during their most recent drinking episode. Men consumed more drinks than women, and those between ages 18 and 34 drank more than older binge drinkers.[20]

Colleges vary widely in their binge-drinking rates—from 1 percent to more than 70 percent. The federal government has set a goal of cutting the current binge-drinking rate of 40 percent among college students in half as a goal for *Healthy People 2010–2020*. How do you think your campus compared?

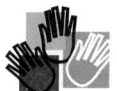 **Who Binge-Drinks in College?** An estimated four in ten college students drink at binge levels or greater. They consume 91 percent of all alcohol that undergraduates report drinking. (See Table 13.1.) Hundreds of studies have created a portrait of who they are and how they differ from others. Here are some of their characteristics.

- More likely to be male than female, although one in three women—up from one in four—reports binge drinking.
- More likely to be white than any other ethnic or racial group (least likely to be African American women).[21]
- More likely to be under age 24 than older.
- More likely to be enrolled in four-year colleges than two-year ones.
- More likely to live in states with fewer alcohol control policies.
- More likely to be involved in athletics and socialize frequently.
- More likely to be in a fraternity or sorority.
- More likely to be dissatisfied with their bodies, not exercise, eat poorly, and go on unhealthy diets.
- More likely to put themselves or others at risk by driving after drinking.
- Much more likely to miss classes or fall behind in schoolwork.
- More likely to abuse other substances, including nicotine, marijuana, cocaine, and LSD.
- Much more likely to engage in vandalism, be injured or hurt, engage in unplanned or

## Table 13.1  Binge Drinking on Campus

Reported number of drinks consumed the last time students "partied" or socialized (only students reporting one or more drinks were included):

| Number of Drinks | Percent (%) | | |
| --- | --- | --- | --- |
| | Male | Female | Total |
| 4 or fewer | 30.1 | 45.6 | 39.8 |
| 5 | 7.3 | 8.9 | 8.3 |
| 6 | 6.9 | 6.2 | 6.4 |
| 7 or more | 28.6 | 12.0 | 18.0 |

Reported number of times college students consumed five or more drinks in a sitting within the last two weeks:

| | Percent (%) | | |
| --- | --- | --- | --- |
| | Male | Female | Total |
| N/A don't drink | 22.3 | 21.7 | 22.0 |
| None | 34.2 | 48.0 | 42.9 |
| 1–2 times | 25.7 | 21.6 | 23.0 |
| 3–5 times | 13.6 | 7.3 | 9.6 |
| 6 or more times | 4.2 | 1.4 | 2.5 |

Source: American College Health Association, *American College Health Association-National College Health Assessment II: Reference Group Executive Summary Spring 2010* (Linthicum, MD: American College Health Association, 2010).

unprotected sexual activity, or get in trouble with campus police.

**Why Students Binge-Drink** Young people who came from, socialized within, or were exposed to "wet" environments—settings in which alcohol is cheap and accessible and drinking is prevalent—are more likely to engage in binge drinking. Students who report drinking at least once a month during their final year of high school are over three times more likely to binge-drink in college than those who drank less frequently in high school.

The factors that most influence students to binge-drink are:

- **Low price for alcohol.** Beer, which is cheap and easy to obtain, is the beverage of choice among binge drinkers.
- **Easy access to alcohol.** In one study, the density of alcohol outlets (such as bars) near campus affected the drinking of students.
- **Attending a school** or living in a residence with many binge drinkers.

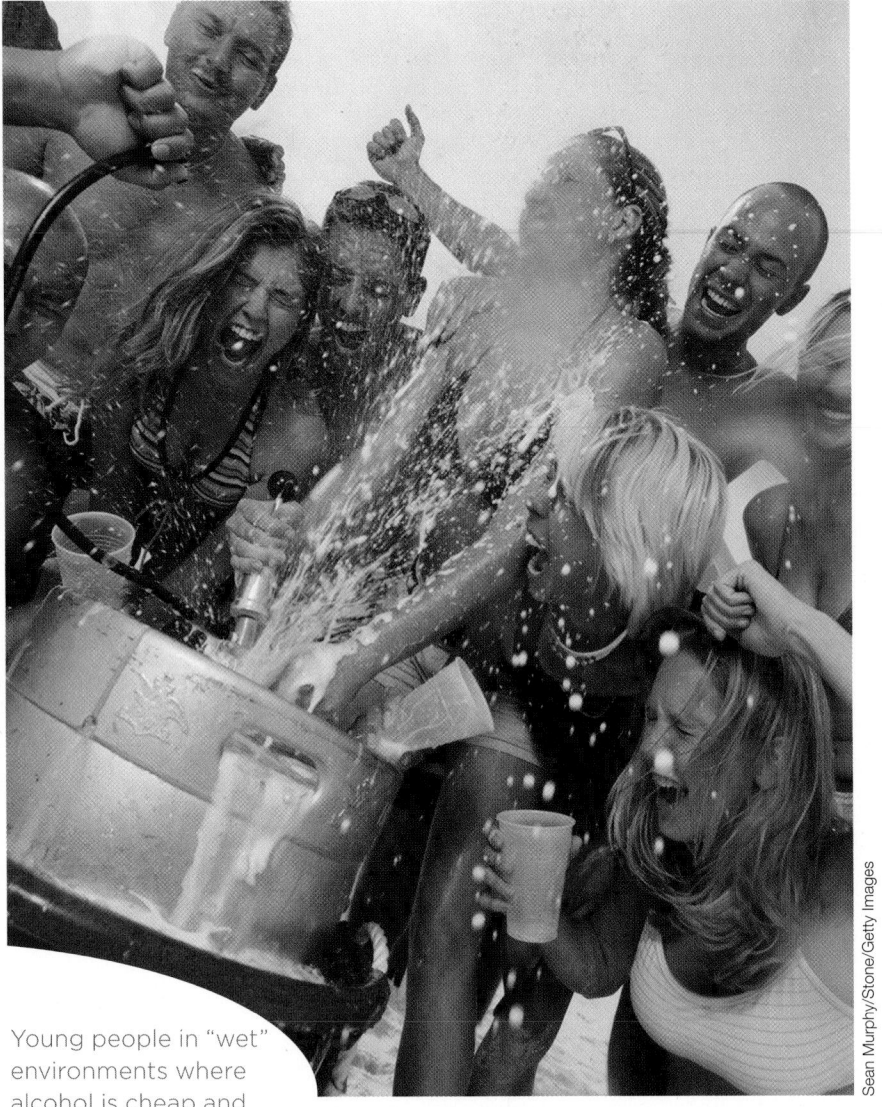

Young people in "wet" environments where alcohol is cheap and accessible are more likely to engage in binge drinking.

the first time very soon after they arrive on campus. Binges become less common in their subsequent years at school and almost always end with education. Real life, one educator notes, is "a strong disincentive" to this type of drinking.

**Drinking Games** Two-thirds of college students engage in drinking games that involve binge drinking.[22] All share a common theme: becoming intoxicated in a short period of time. Men are more likely to participate than women and to consume larger amounts of alcohol.[23] Players, who don't monitor or regulate how much they're drinking, are at risk of extreme intoxication. Drinking games have been implicated in alcohol-related injuries and deaths from alcohol poisoning.

*Predrinking/Pregaming* Drinking before going out has become increasingly common on college campuses, where **predrinking** (also called pregaming, preloading, or front-loading) is announced and celebrated in text messages, e-mails, blogs, YouTube videos, and Facebook entries.

In a recent study at ten Pennsylvania colleges, almost two thirds—64 percent—of undergraduates reported pregaming and consumed an average of 4.9 drinks during their last pre-event drinking episode. Social norms and assumptions about others' drinking patterns influenced this drinking pattern. Undergraduates who estimated that the average student pregamed three or more times in the last two weeks were more likely to drink before an event and to drink heavily.[24]

Predrinkers consistently report much higher alcohol consumption during the evening and more negative consequences, such as getting into a fight, being arrested, or being referred to a university's mandatory alcohol intervention program.

**Why Is Predrinking Popular?** College students predrink for a variety of reasons, including:

- **Economic.** Many say they want to avoid paying for expensive drinks at a bar, although most end up drinking just as much if not more than they do when they don't drink beforehand.[25] (For better ways to save money on booze, see Health on a Budget on p. 430.)

- **Belief** that close friends were likely to binge.
- **Drinking games**—such as beer pong or drinking whenever a certain phrase is mentioned in a song or on a TV program—can result in high levels of intoxication in a short period of time.
- **Parents who drank** or did not disapprove of their children drinking.
- **Recreational drinking** before age 16.

Some educators view bingeing as a product of the college environment. More students binge-drink at the beginning of the school year and then cut back as the semester progresses and academic demands increase. Binge drinking also peaks following exam times, during home football weekends, and during Spring Break. Many new students engage in binge drinking for

**predrinking** Consuming alcoholic beverages, usually with friends, before going out to bars or parties; also called pre-gaming, pre-loading, or front-loading.

- **Intoxication.** A growing number of students seem to want to get drunk as quickly as possible.

- **Socializing.** Predrinking gives students a chance to chat with their friends, which often isn't possible in noisy, crowded clubs or bars.

- **Anxiety reduction.** By drinking before meeting strangers, students say they feel less shy or self-conscious.

- **Group bonding.** Young men may use predrinking as what one researcher calls "a collective ritual of confidence building to prepare themselves for subsequent interactions with the opposite sex."

**The Perils of Predrinking** When students get together to drink before a game or a night out, they usually consume large quantities of alcohol quite rapidly. In part that's because they're drinking in places without restraints on how much they can drink. Various studies have shown that students drink more and have higher blood-alcohol concentrations on days when they predrink. They also are at greater risk of blackouts, passing out, hangovers, and alcohol poisoning.

In addition to drinking more alcohol, predrinkers are more likely to use other drugs, such as marijuana and cocaine. The combined effects of these substances further increase the risk of injury, violence, or victimization.

*Underage Drinking on Campus* Each year, approximately 5,000 young people under the age of 21 die as a result of underage drinking. This figure includes about 1,900 deaths from motor vehicle crashes, 1,600 as a result of homicides, 300 from suicide, as well as hundreds from other injuries such as falls, burns, and drownings. Students under age 21 drink less often than older students, but tend to drink more heavily and to experience more negative alcohol-related consequences. More underage students report drinking "to get drunk" and drinking at binge levels when they consumed alcohol.

Underage college students are most likely to drink if they can easily obtain cheap alcohol, especially beer. They tend to drink in private settings, such as dorms and fraternity parties, and to experience such drinking-related consequences as doing something they regretted, forgetting where they were or what they did,

*Your Strategies for Prevention*

## How to Manage Predrinking and Drinking without Getting Drunk

Here are some strategies students frequently use:

- Eat before and/or during drinking.

- Keep track of how many drinks you're having.

- Avoid drinking games.

- Decide in advance how many drinks to have.

- Alternate alcoholic and nonalcoholic beverages.

- Limit yourself to no more than one drink an hour.

- Have a friend let you know when you've had enough.

- Choose not to drink.

causing property damage, getting into trouble with police, and being hurt or injured. The drinking behavior of underage students also depends on their living arrangements. Those in controlled settings, such as their parents' home or a substance-free dorm, are less likely to binge-drink. Students living in fraternities or sororities are most likely to binge-drink, regardless of age.

*Binge Drinking and Disordered Eating* The combination of two risky behaviors—disordered eating and heavy drinking—poses special dangers to students. As discussed in Chapter 7, disordered eating can range from excessive concern about weight to binge eating to extreme weight-control methods, such as purging. In some studies, as many as 60 percent of college women reported binge eating and purging, while 9 percent of college men reported some form of disordered eating. In a recent report, 63 percent of female students and 83 percent of males engaged in binge drinking; 48 percent also reported binge eating.[26] In women, the combination of these behaviors increases the risk of many negative consequences, including blackouts, unintended sexual activity, and forced sexual intercourse.

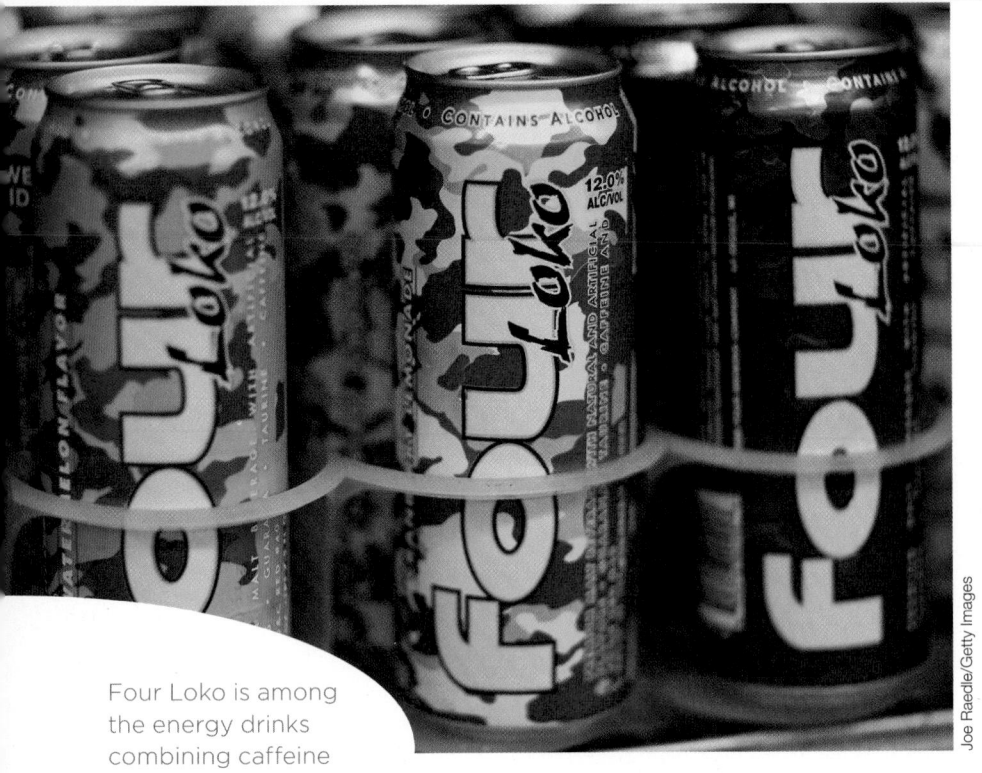

Four Loko is among the energy drinks combining caffeine and alcohol that have been banned at certain colleges.

Joe Raedle/Getty Images

Some students restrict calories from food prior to planned drinking—some to avoid weight gain; others, to enhance the effects of alcohol. The popular media have created the term "drunkorexia" to describe this risky behavior, but it is not an official psychiatric term.

In a recent study at a southeastern university, 14 percent of male and female students reported restricting calories prior to planned drinking—6 percent to avoid weight gain and 10 percent to enhance alcohol's effects. The students who engaged in binge drinking frequently were most likely to cut back on calories before drinking.

***Caffeinated Alcoholic Beverages*** Caffeinated alcoholic beverages (CABs) are pre-mixed beverages that combine alcohol, caffeine, and other stimulants. Often malt- or distilled-spirits-based, they usually have a higher alcohol content (5 to 12 percent) than beer (4 to 5 percent). Because CABs may have higher alcohol content than beer, some states have classified CABs as liquor, thereby limiting the locations where these beverages can be sold.

Like energy drinks (discussed in Chapter 5), CABs—sometimes dubbed "blackout in a can"—have surged in popularity among teens and young adults. The FDA and local authorities have banned some brands, but young people continue to combine energy drinks such as Red Bull with vodka or other forms of alcohol. The caffeine in these drinks may mask the depressant effects of alcohol, but it has no effect on the metabolism of alcohol by the liver and thus does not reduce breath alcohol concentrations or reduce alcohol-related risks.

Drinkers who consume alcohol mixed with energy drinks are three times more likely to reach the breath alcohol levels associated with binge drinking than are those who do not report mixing alcohol with energy drinks. They also are about twice as likely as other drinkers to report being taken advantage of sexually, taking advantage of someone else sexually, and driving or getting into a car with a driver under the influence of alcohol.[27]

## Why Students Stop Drinking

Only 1 percent of students ages 18 to 24 receive treatment for alcohol or drug abuse. Nonetheless, as many as 22 percent of alcohol-abusing college students "spontaneously" reduce their drinking as they progress through college. Unlike older adults, who often hit bottom before they change their drinking behaviors, many college students go through a gradual process of reduced drinking. Researchers refer to this behavioral change as early cessation, natural reduction, natural recovery, or spontaneous recovery.

As with other behavioral changes, individuals must be ready to change their drinking patterns. In a recent study, students who binged frequently, who experienced more alcohol-related interpersonal and academic problems, who did not also use marijuana, and who lived in a residence hall where binge drinking was the norm showed a greater readiness to change.[28]

Why do students say they stop heavy drinking? One common response: "It was just getting old." Some describe more specific reasons why alcohol lost its appeal, including vomiting, urinating in hallways, being physically fondled, sexual assault, violence, accidents, injuries, unprotected intercourse, and emergency room visits. Vicarious experiences, such as a roommate's arrest for driving under the influence or a sorority sister's date rape, have a powerful impact.

# Alcohol-Related Problems on Campus

As many as 10 to 30 percent of college students experience some negative consequences of drinking.

In the National College Health Assessment, 35 percent of students who drank did something they later regretted; 31 percent forgot who they were with or what they did. Men were more likely than women to injure themselves, have unprotected sex, get involved in a fight, or physically injure another person. Women were more likely to have someone use force or threat of force to have sex with them. (See Table 13.2.) Students who drink heavily also are much more likely to abuse prescription drugs (see Chapter 12).

*Consequences of Drinking*  Among the other problems linked to drinking are:

- **Atypical behavior.** Under the influence of alcohol, students behave in ways they normally wouldn't. Male heavy drinkers are more prone to behave in ways that are considered "antisocial," or contrary to the standards of our society, such as forcing or trying to force unwanted sexual contact, driving drunk, exposing themselves, or having sex with a stranger.

- **Academic problems.** The more that students drink, the more likely they are to fall behind in schoolwork, miss classes, have lower GPAs, and face suspensions. In general, students with an A average have three to four drinks per week, while students with D or F averages drink almost ten drinks a week. (See Figure 13.1.)

- **Risky sexual behavior.** About one in five college students reports engaging in unplanned sexual activity, including having sex with someone they just met and having unprotected sex.[29]

- **Sexual assault.** In a recent survey, almost 20 percent of undergraduate women reported some type of completed sexual assault since entering college. Most occurred after women voluntarily consumed alcohol; a few after they were unknowingly given a drug in their drinks.[30]

Alcohol increases the risk of violence among couples, especially violence both to and by the female partner. In a recent analysis, 30 percent

of couples who reported violent behavior said they had used alcohol before or during the episode.[31] In a study of college students, heavy drinking was associated with dating violence by men in their freshman year. Among women, heavy drinking in their sophomore year predicted dating violence in their junior year.[32]

## Table 13.2 **Consequences of Drinking**

College students who drank alcohol reported the following consequences occurring in the last 12 months as a result of their own drinking:*

|  | Percent (%) | | |
|---|---|---|---|
|  | Male | Female | Total |
| Did something you later regretted | 35.0 | 34.5 | 34.7 |
| Forgot where you were or what you did | 33.3 | 30.0 | 31.2 |
| Got in trouble with the police | 5.9 | 3.0 | 4.1 |
| Had sex with someone without giving your consent | 2.0 | 2.4 | 2.3 |
| Had sex with someone without getting her or his consent | 0.9 | 0.3 | 0.6 |
| Had unprotected sex | 19.2 | 16.1 | 17.3 |
| Physically injured yourself | 18.2 | 15.5 | 16.6 |
| Physically injured another person | 4.5 | 1.8 | 2.9 |
| Seriously considered suicide | 1.9 | 1.6 | 1.7 |
| Reported one or more of the above | 53.5 | 49.8 | 51.1 |

*Students responding "N/A, don't drink" were excluded from this analysis.

Source: American College Health Association, American College Health Association-National College Health Assessment II: Reference Group Executive Summary Spring 2010 (Linthicum, MD: American College Health Association, 2010).

## Figure 13.1 **Alcohol and Academic Success**

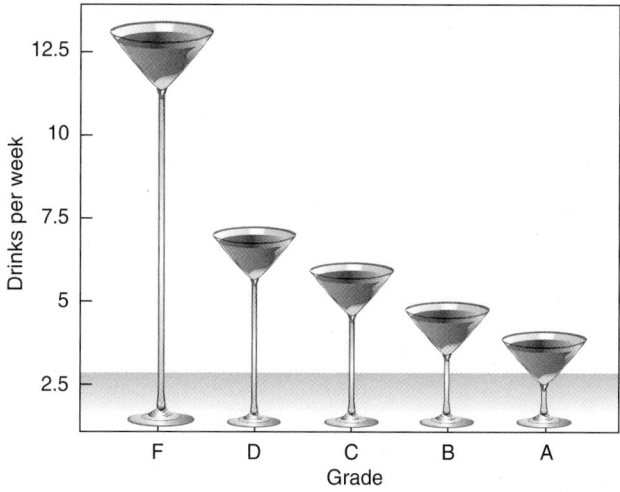

Source: Core Institute and SIU's Core Institute and SDSU's eCHECKUP TO GO, http://core.siuc.edu and http://www.echeckuptogo.com.

- **Unintentional injury.** More than 30 percent of college drinkers have been hurt or injured as a result of drinking. They also are more likely to cause injury to others, to have a car accident, to suffer burns, and to suffer a fall serious enough to require medical attention.

- **Consequences beyond college.** Alcohol-related convictions, including carrying a false I.D. or driving under the influence of alcohol, remain on an individual's criminal record and could affect a student's graduate school and professional opportunities.

- **Illness and death.** Many students suffer short-term health consequences of drinking, such as headaches and hangovers. Heavy alcohol use in college students is associated with immunological problems and digestive and upper respiratory disorders. Even moderate drinking can contribute to infertility in women. Longer-term consequences of heavy drinking include liver disease, stroke, heart disease, and certain types of cancer. About 300,000 of today's college students will eventually die from alcohol-related causes, including drunk-driving accidents, cirrhosis of the liver, various cancers, and heart disease.

 ***Drinking and Driving*** Drunk driving is the most frequently committed crime in the United States. In the ACHA survey, 27 percent of students reported driving after having had any alcohol; 3 percent drove after five or more drinks. In a recent study, traditional-age undergraduates typically increased how often and how much they drank from ages 18 to 21 and then decreased the amount they drank on any one occasion from ages 21 to 23. Driving after drinking increased across this entire age range, with the biggest jump between ages 21 and 23.[33]

Alcohol impairs driving-related skills regardless of the age of the driver or the time of day it is consumed. However, younger drinkers and drivers are at greatest risk. Underage drinkers are more likely to drive after drinking, to ride with intoxicated drivers, and to be injured after drinking—at least in part because they believe that people can drive safely and legally after drinking.[34]

Although most drunk drivers are men, more young women than ever before are driving drunk and getting into fatal car accidents. More young women than men involved in deadly crashes had high blood-alcohol levels, according to a recent analysis of data from the National Highway Traffic Safety Administration.[35]

Of the 5,000 alcohol-related deaths among 18- to 24-year-olds, 80 percent were caused by alcohol-related traffic accidents. A young person dies in an alcohol-related traffic crash an average of once every three hours.[36] Since states began setting the legal drinking age at 21, the National Highway Safety Board estimates that over 26,000 lives have been saved.[37]

Safety groups also attribute the decline in alcohol-related deaths to enforcement tools like sobriety checkpoints and to the states' adoption of a uniform drunken-driving standard of a BAC of 0.08 percent.

In the last two decades, families of the victims of drunk drivers have organized to change the way the nation treats its drunk drivers. Because of the efforts of MADD (Mothers Against Drunk Driving), SADD (Students Against Destructive Decisions), and other lobbying groups, cities, counties, and states are cracking down on drivers who drink. Since courts have held establishments that serve alcohol liable for the consequences of allowing drunk customers to drive, many bars and restaurants have joined the campaign against drunk driving.

To prevent drunk-driving disasters, take the following steps:

- When going out in a group, always designate one person who won't drink at all to serve as the driver.

- Never get behind the wheel if you've had more than two drinks within two hours, especially if you haven't eaten.

- Never let intoxicated friends drive home. Call a taxi, drive them yourself, or arrange for them to spend the night in a safe place.

**"Secondhand" Drinking Problems**
Heavy alcohol use can endanger both drinkers and others. Secondhand problems caused by other's alcohol use include loss of sleep, interruption of studies, assaults, vandalism, and unwanted sexual advances. Students living on

campuses with high rates of binge drinking are two or more times as likely to experience these secondhand effects as those living on campuses with low rates. In one study, nearly three-quarters of campus rapes happened when the victims were so intoxicated that they were unable to consent or refuse.

## How Schools Are Sobering Up

The National Institute on Alcohol Abuse and Alcoholism has studied interventions that effectively deal with college drinking problems. Programs that address alcohol-related attitudes and behaviors, use survey data to counter students' misconceptions about their fellow students' drinking practices, and increase students' motivation to change their drinking habits have proved effective.[38]

- **Social norms.** This approach, which communicates actual facts about drinking behavior to dispel myths, is simple, cost-efficient, and effective. Its positive message is that most students on virtually every campus believe in and practice safety, responsibility, and moderation, rather than excess drinking.

- **Motivational enhancement.** This non-judgmental, supportive approach to personal change also has proved beneficial. In brief interventions, specially trained counselors help build students' self-efficacy, in this case, their belief in their ability to change their drinking behavior.

- **Challenging alcohol expectancy.** As already noted, students who expect alcohol to affect them in specific ways (such as being more at ease socially or more sexually aroused) are more likely to experience such effects. Challenging the validity of such expectations has proven particularly effective as a group intervention for male students, but less so for women.[39]

- **Freshman education.** Since first-year students are at particular risk for alcohol-related problems, some schools focus on incoming freshmen with interventions that include self-surveys, group discussions about normal drinking behavior, and practical strategies for high-risk situations.

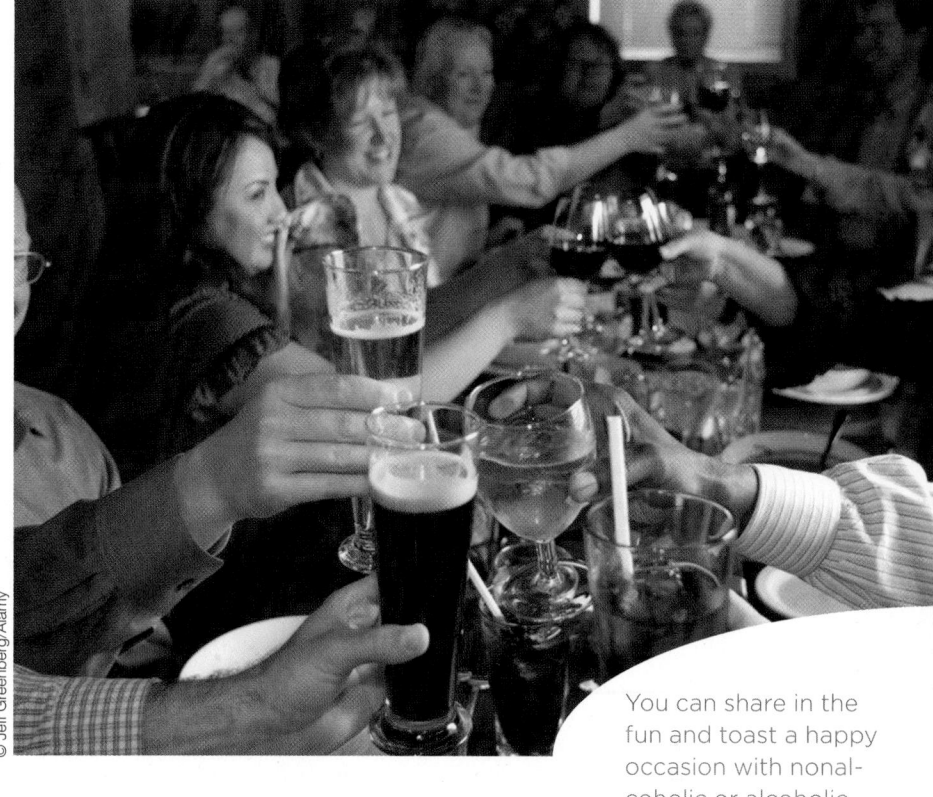

© Jeff Greenberg/Alamy

You can share in the fun and toast a happy occasion with nonalcoholic or alcoholic beverages.

- **"E-interventions."** Electronically based interventions including text messages, e-mails, and podcasts have become increasingly popular. Web-based interventions, such as The Alcohol e-CheckUpToGo (e-Chug), have shown promise in reducing alcohol-related problems among first-year students.

- **Alcohol policies.** University alcohol policies include campus alcohol bans, no alcohol at university-sponsored events, prohibition of beer kegs, limits on the maximum number of drinks served per student, and dry sorority and fraternity initiation activities. Studies suggest that students who attend schools that ban alcohol are less likely to engage in heavy binge drinking, more likely to abstain from using alcohol, and less likely to experience the secondhand effects of drinking.

Some college presidents and administrators have recommended lowering the minimum legal drinking age to 18 to reduce binge drinking by underage students. Critics point out that this approach might just shift the problem to high schools and might have a minimal impact on risky drinking on campus.[40] (See Health in the Headlines: Campus Drinking.)

### Health in the Headlines

## Campus Drinking

Many schools are confronting the serious issues related to student drinking by setting up programs and changing their policies. To learn more about these approaches, access the Addiction portal of Global Health Watch (found under Health and Wellness), click on "alcoholism" and scan the latest news about student drinking and college alcohol policies. How does your school compare—both in terms of alcohol-related problems and in campus initiatives to prevent dangerous drinking? If you use alcohol, how have drinking programs and policies affected your alcohol consumption? Record your observations in your online journal.

Figure 13.2 **How Many Standard Drinks Are You Drinking?**

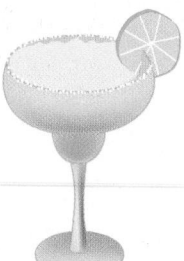

**Margarita:**

1½ oz. tequila (80 proof) = 1.5 oz. × 40 percent alcohol = 0.6 oz. alcohol

¾ oz. triple sec (60 proof) = 0.75 oz. × 30 percent alcohol = 0.23 oz. alcohol

Splash of sour mix

0.83 oz. alcohol = 1½ drinks

Dash of lime juice

Salt for the rim

**Malt liquor:**

16 oz. × 6.4 percent alcohol = 1 oz. alcohol = 2 drinks

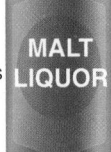

# Understanding Alcohol

Pure alcohol is a colorless liquid obtained through the fermentation of a liquid containing sugar. **Ethyl alcohol**, or *ethanol*, is the type of alcohol in alcoholic beverages. Another type—methyl, or wood, alcohol—is a poison that should never be drunk. Any liquid containing 0.5 to 80 percent ethyl alcohol by volume is an alcoholic beverage. However, different drinks contain different amounts of alcohol.

The types of alcohol consumed vary around the world. Beer accounts for most of the alcohol consumed in the United States. People in southern European countries such as France, Spain, Italy, and Portugal prefer wine.

Do you know what a "drink" is? Most students—particularly freshmen, sophomores, and women—don't.[41] In one experiment undergraduates defined a "drink" as one serving, regardless of how big it was or how much alcohol it contained. In fact, one standard drink can be any of the following:

- **One bottle or can** (12 ounces) of beer, which is 5 percent alcohol.
- **One glass** (4 or 5 ounces) of table wine, such as burgundy, which is 12 percent alcohol.
- **One small glass** (2½ ounces) of fortified wine, which is 20 percent alcohol.
- **One shot** (1 ounce) of distilled spirits (such as whiskey, vodka, or rum), which is 50 percent alcohol.

All of these drinks contain close to the same amount of alcohol—that is, if the number of ounces in each drink is multiplied by the percentage of alcohol, each drink contains the equivalent of approximately ½ ounce of 100 percent ethyl alcohol.

Drinks at college parties vary greatly in their alcoholic content. It may be impossible for students to monitor their alcohol intake simply by counting the number of drinks they have. In one study, when asked to pour a liquid into cups of various sizes to reflect what they perceived to be one beer, one shot, or the amount of liquor in one mixed drink, undergraduates overpoured beer by 25 percent, shots by 26 percent, and mixed drinks by 80 percent.

The words *bottle* and *glass* also can be deceiving. Drinking a 16-ounce bottle of malt liquor, which is 6.4 percent alcohol, is not the same as drinking a 12-ounce glass of light beer (3.2 percent alcohol): The malt liquor contains 1 ounce of alcohol and is the equivalent of two drinks. Two bottles of high-alcohol wines (such as Cisco), packaged to resemble much less powerful wine coolers, can lead to alcohol poisoning, especially in those who weigh less than 150 pounds.

With distilled spirits (such as bourbon, scotch, vodka, gin, and rum), alcohol content is expressed in terms of **proof**, a number that is twice the percentage of alcohol: 100-proof bourbon is 50 percent alcohol; 80-proof gin is 40 percent alcohol. Many mixed drinks are equivalent to one and a half or two standard drinks; for instance, see the margarita in Figure 13.2.

**ethyl alcohol** The intoxicating agent in alcoholic beverages; also called ethanol.

**proof** The alcoholic strength of a distilled spirit, expressed as twice the percentage of alcohol present.

# Blood-Alcohol Concentration

The amount of alcohol in your blood at any given time is your **blood-alcohol concentration (BAC)**. It is expressed in terms of the percentage of alcohol in the blood and is often measured from breath or urine samples.

Law enforcement officers use BAC to determine whether a driver is legally drunk. All the states have followed the recommendation of the federal Department of Transportation to set 0.08 percent—the BAC that a 150-pound man would have after consuming about three mixed drinks within an hour—as the threshold at which a person can be cited for drunk driving (Figure 13.3).

Using a formula for blood-alcohol concentration developed by highway transportation officials, researchers calculate that when college students drink, their typical BAC is 0.079, dangerously close to the legal limit.

A BAC of 0.05 percent indicates approximately 5 parts alcohol to 10,000 parts other blood components. Most people reach this level after consuming one or two drinks and experience all the positive sensations of drinking—relaxation, euphoria, and well-being—without feeling intoxicated. If they continue to drink past the 0.05 percent BAC level, they start feeling worse rather than better, gradually losing control of speech, balance, and emotions. At a BAC of 0.2 percent, they may pass out. At a BAC of 0.3 percent, they could lapse into a coma; at 0.4 percent, they could die.

Many factors affect an individual's BAC and response to alcohol, including the following:

- **How much and how quickly you drink.** The more alcohol you put into your body, the higher your BAC. If you chug drink after drink, your liver, which metabolizes about $\frac{1}{2}$ ounce of alcohol an hour, won't be able to keep up—and your BAC will soar.
- **What you're drinking.** The stronger the drink, the faster and harder the alcohol hits. Straight shots of liquor and cocktails such as martinis will get alcohol into your bloodstream faster than beer or table wine. Beer and wine not only contain lower concentrations of alcohol, but they also contain nonalcoholic substances that slow the rate of **absorption** (passage of the alcohol into your body tissues). If the drink contains water, juice, or milk, the rate of absorption will be slowed. However, carbon dioxide—whether in champagne, ginger ale, or a cola—whisks alcohol into your bloodstream. Also, the alcohol in warm drinks—such as a hot rum toddy or warmed sake—moves into your bloodstream more quickly than the alcohol in chilled wine or scotch on the rocks.

- **Your size.** If you're a large person (whether due to fat or to muscle), you'll get drunk more slowly than someone smaller who's drinking the same amount of alcohol at the same rate. Heavier individuals have a larger water volume, which dilutes the alcohol they drink.

- **Your gender.** Women have lower quantities of a stomach enzyme that neutralizes alcohol, so one drink for a woman has the impact that two drinks have for a man. Hormone levels also affect the impact of alcohol. Women are more sensitive to alcohol just before menstruation, and birth control pills and other forms of estrogen can intensify alcohol's impact.

- **Your age.** The same amount of alcohol produces higher BACs in older drinkers, who have lower volumes of body water to dilute the alcohol than younger drinkers do. People over 50 may become impaired after only one or two drinks.

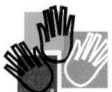 **Your race.** Many members of certain ethnic groups, including Asians and Native Americans, are unable to break down alcohol as quickly as Caucasians. This can result in higher BACs, as well as uncomfortable reactions, such as flushing and nausea, when they drink.

- **Other drugs.** Some common medications—including aspirin, acetaminophen (Tylenol), and ulcer medications—can cause blood-alcohol levels to increase more rapidly. Individuals taking these drugs can be over the legal limit for blood-alcohol concentration after as little as a single drink.

- **Family history of alcoholism.** Some children of alcoholics don't develop any of the usual behavioral symptoms that indicate

**blood-alcohol concentration (BAC)** The amount of alcohol in the blood, expressed as a percentage.

**absorption** The passage of substances into or across membranes or tissues.

## Figure 13.3 Alcohol Impairment Chart

Source: Adapted from data supplied by the Pennsylvania Liquor Control Board.

| Men | Approximate blood alcohol percentage | | | | | | | | |
|---|---|---|---|---|---|---|---|---|---|
| | Body weight in pounds | | | | | | | | |
| **Drinks** | 100 | 120 | 140 | 160 | 180 | 200 | 220 | 240 | |
| 0 | .00 | .00 | .00 | .00 | .00 | .00 | .00 | .00 | Only safe driving limit |
| 1 | .04 | .03 | .03 | .02 | .02 | .02 | .02 | .02 | Impairment begins |
| 2 | .08 | .06 | .05 | .05 | .04 | .04 | .03 | .03 | Driving skills significantly affected |
| 3 | .11 | .09 | .08 | .07 | .06 | .06 | .05 | .05 | |
| 4 | .15 | .12 | .11 | .09 | .08 | .08 | .07 | .06 | Possible criminal penalties |
| 5 | .19 | .16 | .13 | .12 | .11 | .09 | .09 | .08 | |
| 6 | .23 | .19 | .16 | .14 | .13 | .11 | .10 | .09 | |
| 7 | .26 | .22 | .19 | .16 | .15 | .13 | .12 | .11 | |
| 8 | .30 | .25 | .21 | .19 | .17 | .15 | .14 | .13 | Legally intoxicated |
| 9 | .34 | .28 | .24 | .21 | .19 | .17 | .15 | .14 | Criminal penalties |
| 10 | .38 | .31 | .27 | .23 | .21 | .19 | .17 | .16 | |

Subtract 0.01 percent for each 40 minutes of drinking.
One drink is 1.25 oz. of 80 proof liquor, 12 oz. of beer, or 5 oz. of table wine.

| Women | Approximate blood alcohol percentage | | | | | | | | | |
|---|---|---|---|---|---|---|---|---|---|---|
| | Body weight in pounds | | | | | | | | | |
| **Drinks** | 90 | 100 | 120 | 140 | 160 | 180 | 200 | 220 | 240 | |
| 0 | .00 | .00 | .00 | .00 | .00 | .00 | .00 | .00 | .00 | Only safe driving limit |
| 1 | .05 | .05 | .04 | .03 | .03 | .03 | .02 | .02 | .02 | Impairment begins |
| 2 | .10 | .09 | .08 | .07 | .06 | .05 | .05 | .04 | .04 | Driving skills significantly affected |
| 3 | .15 | .14 | .11 | .10 | .09 | .08 | .07 | .06 | .06 | |
| 4 | .20 | .18 | .15 | .13 | .11 | .10 | .09 | .08 | .08 | Possible criminal penalties |
| 5 | .25 | .23 | .19 | .16 | .14 | .13 | .11 | .10 | .09 | |
| 6 | .30 | .27 | .23 | .19 | .17 | .15 | .14 | .12 | .11 | |
| 7 | .35 | .32 | .27 | .23 | .20 | .18 | .16 | .14 | .13 | Legally intoxicated |
| 8 | .40 | .36 | .30 | .26 | .23 | .20 | .18 | .17 | .15 | Criminal penalties |
| 9 | .45 | .41 | .34 | .29 | .26 | .23 | .20 | .19 | .17 | |
| 10 | .51 | .45 | .38 | .32 | .28 | .25 | .23 | .21 | .19 | |

Subtract 0.01 percent for each 40 minutes of drinking.
One drink is 1.25 oz. of 80 proof liquor, 12 oz. of beer, or 5 oz. of table wine.

| .01–.06 BAC | .06–.10 BAC | .11–.20 BAC | .21–.29 BAC | .30–.39 BAC | .40+ BAC |
|---|---|---|---|---|---|
| Relaxation, sense of well-being, loss of inhibition, lowered alertness | Blunted feelings, disinhibition, extroversion, reduced sexual pleasure | Emotional swings, anger, sadness, boisterous | Stupor, impaired sensations | Not responsive, slowed heart rate, breathing, risk of death | Not responsive, death |
| Some impact on thought, judgment, coordination, concentration | Impaired reflexes, reasoning, depth perception, distance acuity, peripheral vision, glare recovery | Impaired reaction time, gross motor control, staggering, slurred speech | Severe motor impairment, memory blackouts | | |

someone is drinking too much. It's not known whether this behavior is genetically caused or is a result of growing up with an alcoholic.

- **Eating.** Food slows the absorption of alcohol by diluting it, by covering some of the membranes through which alcohol would be absorbed, and by prolonging the time the stomach takes to empty.

- **Expectations.** In various experiments, volunteers who believed they were given alcoholic beverages but were actually given nonalcoholic drinks acted as if they were guzzling the real thing and became more talkative, relaxed, and sexually stimulated.

- **Physical tolerance.** If you drink regularly, your brain becomes accustomed to a certain level of alcohol. You may be able to look and behave in a seemingly normal fashion, even though you drink as much as would normally intoxicate someone your size. However, your driving ability and judgment will still be impaired.

Once you develop tolerance, you may drink more to get the desired effects from alcohol. In some people, this can lead to abuse and alcoholism. On the other hand, after years of drinking, some people become exquisitely sensitive to alcohol. Such reverse tolerance means that they can become intoxicated after drinking only a small amount of alcohol.

## Moderate Alcohol Use

Many people describe themselves as "light" or "moderate" drinkers. However, these are not scientific terms. It is more precise to think in terms of the amount of alcohol that seems safe for most people. The federal government's Dietary Guidelines for Americans recommend no more than one drink a day for women and no more than two drinks a day for men. The American Heart Association (AHA) advises that alcohol account for no more than 15 percent of the total calories consumed by an individual every day, up to an absolute maximum of 1.75 ounces of alcohol a day—the equivalent of three beers, two mixed drinks, or three and a half glasses of wine.

Moderate alcohol use has been linked with some positive health benefits, including lower risks of heart disease. In addition, middle-aged women who report light to moderate drinking are less likely to put on excessive weight over time.[42] However, even occasional binges of four to five drinks a day can undo alcohol's positive effects.

The benefits of alcohol also are related to age. Below age 40 drinking at all levels is associated with an increased risk or death. Among people older than 50 or 60, moderate drinkers have the lowest risk of death.[43]

Using a mathematical model, researchers have determined that alcohol-related problems occur at every drinking level, including just two drinks, but increase fivefold at three drinks and more gradually thereafter.[44] Individuals who drink heavily have a higher mortality rate than those who have two or fewer drinks a day. However, the boundary between moderate and heavy drinking isn't the same for everyone. For some people, the upper limit of safety is zero: Once they start, they can't stop.

## Intoxication

If you drink too much, the immediate consequence is that you get drunk—or, more precisely, intoxicated. Alcohol intoxication, which can range from mild inebriation to loss of consciousness, is characterized by at least one of the following signs: slurred speech, poor coordination, unsteady gait, abnormal eye movements, impaired attention or memory, stupor, or coma.

Medical risks of intoxication include falls, hypothermia in cold climates, and increased risk of infections because of suppressed immune function. Time and a protective environment are the recommended treatments for alcohol intoxication. Also follow these guidelines:

- Continually monitor the intoxicated person.

- If the person is "out," check breathing, waking the person often to be sure he or she is not unconscious.

- Do not force the person to walk or move around.

- Do not allow the person to drive a car or ride a bicycle.

- Do not give the person food, liquid (including coffee), medicines, or drugs to sober the person up.

- Do not give the person a cold shower; the shock of the cold could cause unconsciousness.

## Alcohol Poisoning

Because federal law requires colleges to publish all student deaths, the stories of young lives ended by alcohol poisoning have gained national attention. Yet many students remain unaware that alcohol, in large enough doses, can and does kill.

Alcohol depresses nerves that control involuntary actions, such as breathing and the gag reflex (which prevents choking). A fatal dose of alcohol will eventually suppress these functions. Because alcohol irritates the stomach, people who drink an excessive amount often vomit. If intoxication has led to a loss of consciousness, a drinker is in danger of choking on vomit, which can cause death by asphyxiation. Blood-alcohol concentration can rise even after a drinker has passed out because alcohol in the stomach and intestine continues to enter the bloodstream and circulate throughout the body.

The signs of alcohol poisoning include:

- Mental confusion, stupor, coma, or person cannot be roused.
- Vomiting.
- Seizures.
- Slow breathing (fewer than eight breaths per minute).
- Irregular breathing (ten seconds or more between breaths).
- Hypothermia (low body temperature), bluish skin color, paleness.

Alcohol poisoning is a medical emergency requiring immediate treatment. Black coffee, a cold shower, or letting a person "sleep it off" does not help. Without medical treatment, breathing slows, becomes irregular, or stops. The heart beats irregularly. Body temperature falls, which can cause cardiac arrest. Blood sugar plummets, which can lead to seizures. Vomiting creates severe dehydration, which can cause seizures, permanent brain damage, or death. Even if the victim lives, an alcohol overdose can result in irreversible brain damage.

Rapid binge drinking is especially dangerous because the victim can ingest a fatal dose before becoming unconscious. If you suspect alcohol poisoning, call 911 for help. Don't try to guess the level of drunkenness. Tell emergency medical technicians the symptoms and, if you know, how much alcohol the victim drank. Prompt action may save a life. Here's what to do:

- If the person is breathing less than twelve times per minute or stops breathing for periods of ten seconds or more, **call 911**.
- If the person is asleep and you are unable to wake him or her up, **call 911**.
- Look at the person's skin. If it is cold, clammy, pale, bluish in color, **call 911**.
- Stay with a person who is vomiting. Try to keep him or her sitting up. If the person must lie down, keep him on his side with head turned to the side. Watch for choking; if the person begins to choke, **call 911**.

# The Impact of Alcohol on the Body

Unlike food or drugs in tablet form, alcohol is directly and quickly absorbed into the bloodstream through the stomach walls and upper intestine. The alcohol in a typical drink reaches the bloodstream in 15 minutes and rises to its peak concentration in about an hour. The bloodstream carries the alcohol to the liver, heart, and brain (Figure 13.4).

Most of the alcohol you drink can leave your body only after metabolism by the liver, which converts about 95 percent of the alcohol to carbon dioxide and water. The other 5 percent is excreted unchanged, mainly through urination, respiration, and perspiration.

Alcohol is a diuretic, a drug that speeds up the elimination of fluid from the body, so drink water when you drink alcohol to maintain your fluid balance. And alcohol lowers body temperature, so you should never drink to get or stay warm.

## Digestive System

Alcohol reaches the stomach first, where it is partially broken down. The remaining alcohol is absorbed easily through the stomach tissue into the bloodstream. In the stomach, alcohol triggers the secretion of acids, which irritate the stomach lining. Excessive drinking at one sitting

## Figure 13.4 **The Effects of Alcohol Abuse on the Body**

Alcohol has a major effect on the brain, damaging brain cells, impairing judgment and perceptions, and often leading to accidents and altercations. Alcohol also damages the digestive system, especially the liver.

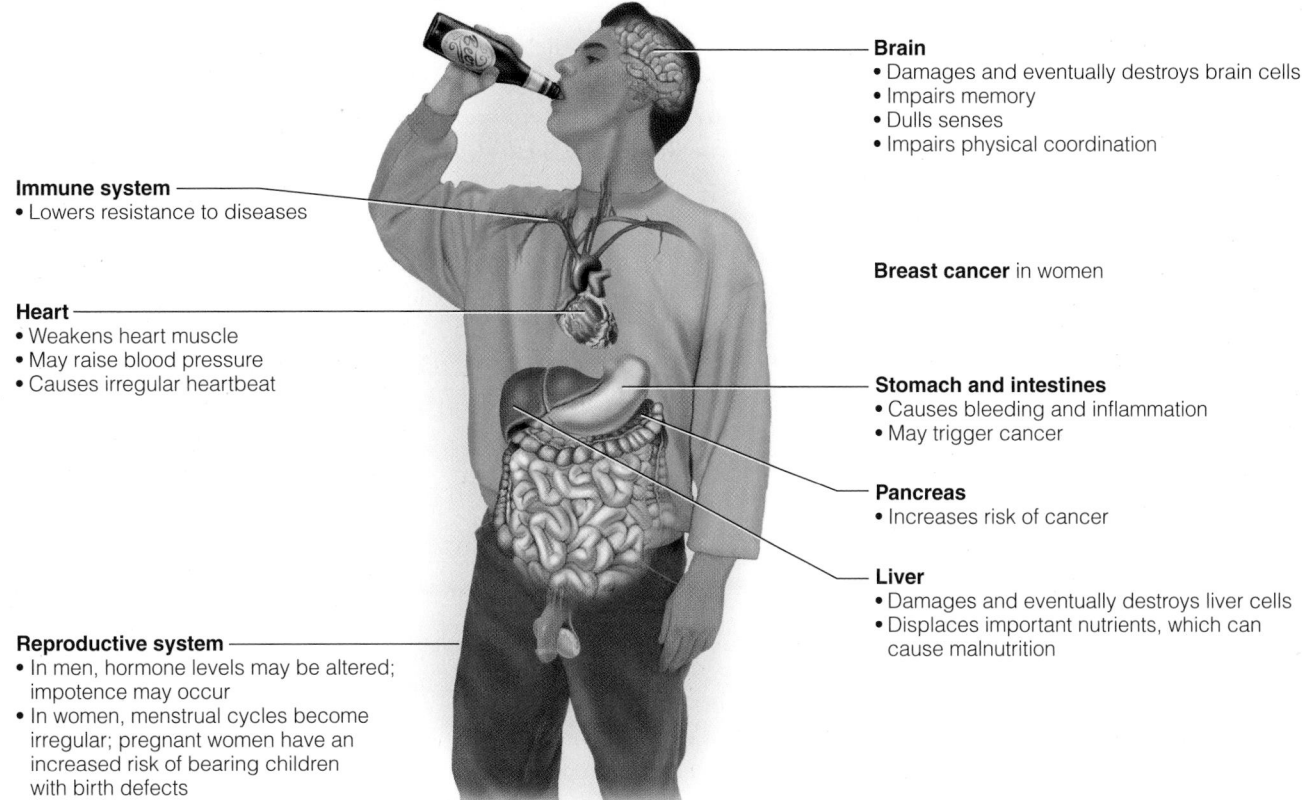

**Immune system**
• Lowers resistance to diseases

**Heart**
• Weakens heart muscle
• May raise blood pressure
• Causes irregular heartbeat

**Reproductive system**
• In men, hormone levels may be altered; impotence may occur
• In women, menstrual cycles become irregular; pregnant women have an increased risk of bearing children with birth defects

**Brain**
• Damages and eventually destroys brain cells
• Impairs memory
• Dulls senses
• Impairs physical coordination

**Breast cancer** in women

**Stomach and intestines**
• Causes bleeding and inflammation
• May trigger cancer

**Pancreas**
• Increases risk of cancer

**Liver**
• Damages and eventually destroys liver cells
• Displaces important nutrients, which can cause malnutrition

may result in nausea; chronic drinking may result in peptic ulcers (breaks in the stomach lining) and bleeding from the stomach lining.

The alcohol in the bloodstream eventually reaches the liver. The liver, which bears the major responsibility of fat metabolism in the body, converts this excess alcohol to fat. After a few weeks of four or five drinks a day, liver cells start to accumulate fat. Alcohol also stimulates liver cells to attract white blood cells, which normally travel throughout the bloodstream engulfing harmful substances and wastes. If white blood cells begin to invade body tissue, such as the liver, they can cause irreversible damage. More than 2 million Americans have alcohol-related liver diseases, such as alcoholic hepatitis and cirrhosis of the liver.

## Weight and Waists

At 7 calories per gram, alcohol has nearly as many calories as fat (9 calories per gram) and significantly more than carbohydrates or protein (which have 4 calories per gram). Since a

standard drink contains 12 to 15 grams of alcohol, the alcohol in a single drink adds about 100 calories to your daily intake. A glass of wine contains as many calories as some candy bars; you would have to walk a mile to burn them off. In addition to being a calorie-dense food, alcohol stimulates the appetite so you're likely to eat more. Obesity plus daily drinking boosts the risks of liver disease in men and women.[45]

## Cardiorespiratory System

Alcohol gets mixed reviews regarding its effects on the cardiorespiratory system.

 According to the American Heart Association, college students who drink excessively may double their levels of C-reactive protein (CRP), a biological marker for inflammation associated with a higher chance of cardiorespiratory problems. Although the long-term impact is unknown, researchers caution that high CRP levels could predict future risk of heart disease.[46] However, several studies have shown that people who drink moderate amounts of alcohol have lower mortality rates after a heart attack, as well as a lower risk of heart attack compared to abstainers and heavy drinkers.

Some cardiologists contend that the benefits of moderate drinking may be overstated, especially because of alcohol's contribution to the epidemic of obesity around the world. Consumption of two or more drinks per day may increase a person's risk of pancreatic cancer by about 22 percent. Heavier drinking triggers the release of harmful oxygen molecules called free radicals, which can increase the risk of heart disease, stroke, and cirrhosis of the liver. Alcohol use can weaken the heart muscle directly, causing a disorder called cardiomyopathy. The combined use of alcohol and other drugs, including tobacco and cocaine, greatly increases the likelihood of damage to the heart.

## Cancer

Overall past and current drinking may contribute to about 10 percent of all cancer cases in men and 3 percent in women. Alcohol consumption has been more specifically implicated as a cause of cancers of the oral cavity, pharynx, larynx, esophagus, liver, colon-rectum, and female breast. The risk increases above the recommended upper limit of two drinks a day for men and one drink for women.[47]

## Brain and Behavior

At first when you drink, you feel up. In low dosages, alcohol affects the regions of the brain that inhibit or control behavior, so you feel looser and act in ways you might not otherwise. However, you also experience losses of concentration, memory, judgment, and fine motor control; and you have mood swings and emotional outbursts.

Moderate amounts of alcohol can have disturbing effects on perception and judgment, including the following:

- **Impaired perceptions.** You're less able to adjust your eyes to bright lights because glare bothers you more. Although you can still
- hear sounds, you can't distinguish between them or judge their direction well.

- **Dulled smell and taste.** Alcohol itself may cause some vitamin deficiencies, and the poor eating habits of heavy drinkers result in further nutrition problems.
- **Diminished sensation.** On a freezing winter night, you may walk outside without a coat and not feel the cold.
- **Altered sense of space.** You may not realize, for instance, that you have been in one place for several hours.
- **Impaired motor skills.** Writing, typing, driving, and other abilities involving your muscles are impaired. This is why law enforcement officers sometimes ask suspected drunk drivers to touch their nose with a finger or to walk a straight line. Drinking large amounts of alcohol impairs reaction time, speed, accuracy, and consistency, as well as judgment.
- **Impaired sexual performance.** While drinking may increase your interest in sex, it may also impair sexual response, especially a man's ability to achieve or maintain an erection. As Shakespeare wrote, "It provokes the desire, but it takes away the performance."

Moderate and heavy drinkers show signs of impaired intelligence, slowed-down reflexes, and difficulty remembering. Because alcohol is a central nervous system depressant, it slows down the activity of the neurons in the brain, gradually dulling the responses of the brain and nervous system. One or two drinks act as a tranquilizer or relaxant. Additional drinks result in a progressive reduction in central nervous system activity, leading to sleep, general anesthesia, coma, and even death.

Heavy alcohol use may pose special dangers to the brains of drinkers at both ends of the age spectrum. Adolescents who drink regularly show impairments in their neurological and cognitive functioning. Elderly people who drink heavily appear to have more brain shrinkage, or atrophy, than those who drink lightly or not at all. In general, moderate drinkers have healthier brains and a lower risk of dementia than those who don't drink and those who drink to excess.

## Interaction with Other Drugs

Alcohol can interact with other drugs—prescription and nonprescription, legal and illegal. Of the 100 most frequently prescribed drugs, more than half contain at least one ingredient that interacts adversely with alcohol. Because alcohol and other psychoactive drugs may work on the same areas of the brain, their combination can produce an effect much greater than that expected of either drug by itself. For example, the liver combines alcohol and cocaine to produce cocaethylene, which intensifies the drug's effects and may increase the risk of sudden death. Alcohol is particularly dangerous when combined with other depressants and antianxiety medications. (See Consumer Alert.)

## Immune System

Chronic alcohol use can inhibit the production of both white blood cells, which fight off infections, and red blood cells, which carry oxygen to all the organs and tissues of the body. Alcohol may increase the risk of infection with human immunodeficiency virus (HIV) by altering the judgment of users so that they more readily engage in activities such as unsafe sex that put them in danger. If you drink when you have a cold or the flu, alcohol interferes with the body's ability to recover. It also increases the chance of bacterial pneumonia in flu sufferers.

## Increased Risk of Dying

Alcohol kills. Alcohol is responsible for 100,000 deaths each year and is the third leading cause of

## ❶ CONSUMER ALERT

### Alcohol and Drug Interactions

| Drug | Possible Effects of Interaction |
|---|---|
| Allergy, cold, flu medicines (Allegra, Benadryl, Claritin, Dimetapp, Sudafed, Tylenol Cold & Flu) | Drowsiness, dizziness, increased risk for overdose. |
| Analgesics (painkillers) | |
|   Narcotic (Codeine, Demerol, Percodan, Vicodin) | Increase in central nervous system depression, possibly leading to respiratory failure and death. |
|   Nonnarcotic (aspirin, acetaminophen, ibuprofen) | Irritation of stomach resulting in bleeding and increased susceptibility to liver damage. |
| Antabuse (disulfiram: an aid to quit drinking) | Nausea, vomiting, headache, high blood pressure, and erratic heartbeat. |
| Antianxiety drugs (Valium, Librium, Ativan, Xanax) | Increase in central nervous system depression; decreased alertness and impaired judgment. |
| Antidepressants (Prozac, Zoloft, Celexa, Lexapro, Paxil, Wellbutrin, Luvox, and others) | Increase in central nervous system depression; certain antidepressants in combination with red wine could cause a sudden increase in blood pressure. |
| Antihistamines (Actifed, Dimetapp, and other cold medications) | Increase in drowsiness; decrease in ability to drive. |
| Antibiotics | Nausea, vomiting, headache; some medications rendered less effective. |
| Central nervous system stimulants (caffeine, Dexedrine, Ritalin) | Stimulant effects of these drugs may reverse depressant effect of alcohol but do not decrease its intoxicating effects. |
| Cocaine | Intensification of cocaine's effects; increased risk of sudden death. |
| Sedatives (Dalmane, Nembutal, Quaalude) | Increase in central nervous system depression, possibly leading to coma, respiratory failure, and death. |

death after tobacco and improper diet and lack of exercise. The leading alcohol-related cause of death is injury. Alcohol plays a role in almost half of all traffic fatalities, half of all homicides, and a quarter of all suicides. The second leading cause of alcohol-related deaths is cirrhosis of the liver, a chronic disease that causes extensive scarring and irreversible damage. In addition, as many as half of patients admitted to hospitals and 15 percent of those making office visits seek or need medical care because of the direct or indirect effects of alcohol.

Young drinkers—teens and those in their early 20s—are at highest risk of dying from injuries, mostly car accidents. Older drinkers over age 50 face the greatest danger of premature death from cirrhosis of the liver, hepatitis, and other alcohol-linked illnesses.

Most studies of the relationship between alcohol consumption and death from all causes show that moderate drinkers—those who consume approximately seven drinks per week—have a lower risk of death than abstainers, while heavy drinkers have a higher risk than either group. In one ten-year study, never-drinkers showed no elevated risk of dying, while consistent heavier drinkers were at higher risk of dying of any cause than other men.

# Alcohol, Gender, and Race

Experts in alcohol treatment are increasingly recognizing racial and ethnic differences in risk factors for drinking problems, patterns of drinking, and most effective types of treatment.

## Gender

In general, men drink more frequently, consume a larger quantity of alcohol per drinking occasion, and report more problems related to drinking. More than half of women drink: They drink alone more often, binge less, have more regular drinking patterns, and drink smaller quantities than men.

The bodies of men and women respond to alcohol in different ways. Because they have a far smaller quantity of a protective enzyme in the stomach to break down alcohol before it's absorbed into the bloodstream, women absorb about 30 percent more alcohol into their bloodstream than men—see Table 13.3. The alcohol travels through the blood to the brain, so women become intoxicated much more quickly. And because there's more alcohol in the bloodstream to break down, the liver may also be adversely affected. In alcoholic women, the stomach seems to completely stop digesting alcohol, which may explain why female alcoholics are more likely to suffer liver damage than men.

An estimated 15 percent of women drink alcohol while pregnant, most having one drink or less per day. Even light consumption of alcohol can lead to **fetal alcohol effects (FAE)**: low birth weight, irritability as newborns, and permanent mental impairment. A few drinking binges of four or more drinks a day during pregnancy may significantly increase the risk of childhood mental health and learning problems.

The babies of women who consume three or more ounces of alcohol (the equivalent of six or seven cocktails) are at risk of more severe problems. One of every 750 newborns has a cluster of physical and mental defects called

**fetal alcohol effects (FAE)** Milder forms of FAS, including low birth weight, irritability as newborns, and permanent mental impairment as a result of the mother's alcohol consumption during pregnancy.

Table 13.3 **How Alcohol Discriminates**

| | Women ♀ | Men ♂ |
|---|---|---|
| Ability to Dilute Alcohol | Average total body water: 52% | Average total body water: 61% |
| Ability to Metabolize Alcohol | Women have a smaller quantity of dehydrogenase, an enzyme that breaks down alcohol. | Men have a larger quantity of dehydrogenase, which allows them to break down the alcohol they take in more quickly. |
| Hormonal Factors, Part 1 | Premenstrual hormonal changes cause intoxication to set in faster during the days right after a woman gets her period. | Their susceptibility to getting drunk does not fluctuate dramatically at certain times of the month. |
| Hormonal Factors, Part 2 | Alcohol increases estrogen levels. Birth control pills or other medicines with estrogen increase intoxication. | Alcohol also increases estrogen levels in men. Chronic alcoholism has been associated with loss of body hair and muscle mass, development of swollen breasts and shrunken testicles, and impotence. |

Source: www.factsontap.org/factsontap/risky/discrimination.htm.

**fetal alcohol syndrome (FAS)**: small head, abnormal facial features, jitters, poor muscle tone, sleep disorders, sluggish motor development, failure to thrive, short stature, delayed speech, mental retardation, and hyperactivity.

Alcohol interferes with male sexual function and fertility through direct effects on testosterone and the testicles. In half of alcoholic men, increased levels of female hormones lead to breast enlargement and a feminine pubic hair pattern. Damage to the nerves in the penis by heavy drinking can lead to impotence. In women who drink heavily, a drop in female hormone production may cause menstrual irregularity and infertility.

## Race

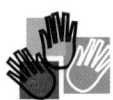

***African American Community*** Overall, African Americans consume less alcohol per person than whites, yet twice as many blacks die of cirrhosis of the liver each year. In some cities, the rate of cirrhosis is ten times higher among African American than white men. Alcohol also contributes to high rates of hypertension, esophageal cancer, and homicide among African American men.

***Hispanic Community*** The various Hispanic cultures tend to discourage any drinking by women but encourage heavy drinking by men as part of machismo, or feelings of manhood. Hispanic men have higher rates of alcohol use and abuse than the general population and suffer a high rate of cirrhosis. Moreover, American-born Hispanic men drink more than those born in other countries.

Few Hispanics with severe alcohol problems enter treatment, partly because of a lack of information, language barriers, and poor community-based services. Hispanic families generally try to resolve problems themselves, and their cultural values discourage the sharing of intimate personal stories, which characterizes Alcoholics Anonymous and other support groups. Churches often provide the most effective forms of help.

***Native American Community*** European settlers introduced alcohol to Native Americans. Because of the societal and physical problems resulting from excessive drinking, at

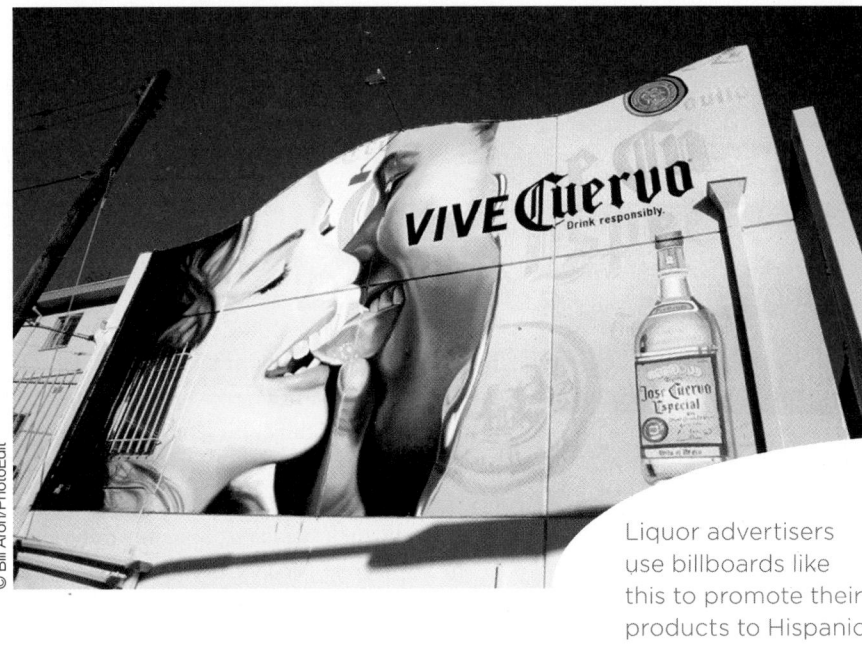

Liquor advertisers use billboards like this to promote their products to Hispanic Americans.

the request of tribal leaders, the U.S. Congress in 1832 prohibited the use of alcohol by Native Americans. Many reservations still ban alcohol use, so Native Americans who want to drink may have to travel long distances to obtain alcohol, which may contribute to the high death rate from hypothermia and pedestrian and motor-vehicle accidents among Native Americans. (Injuries are the leading cause of death among this group.)

Certainly, not all Native Americans drink, and not all who drink do so to excess. However, they have three times the general population's rate of alcohol-related injury and illness. Cirrhosis of the liver is the fourth leading cause of death among this cultural group. While many Native American women don't drink, those who do have high rates of alcohol-related problems, which affect both them and their children. Their rate of cirrhosis of the liver is 36 times that of white women. In some tribes, 10.5 out of every 1,000 newborns have fetal alcohol syndrome, compared with 1 to 3 out of 1,000 in the general population.

***Asian American Community*** Asian Americans tend to drink very little or not at all, in part because of an inborn physiological reaction to alcohol that causes facial flushing, rapid heart rate, lowered blood pressure, nausea, vomiting, and other symptoms. A very high percentage of women of all Asian American nationalities abstain completely. Some

**fetal alcohol syndrome (FAS)** A cluster of physical and mental defects in the newborn, including low birth weight, smaller-than-normal head circumference, intrauterine growth retardation, and permanent mental impairment caused by the mother's alcohol consumption during pregnancy.

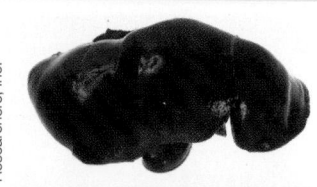

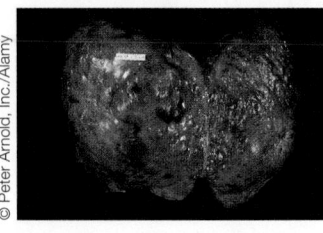

Martin M. Rotker/Photo Researchers, Inc.

© Peter Arnold, Inc./Alamy

A normal liver (top) compared to one with cirrhosis.

sociologists have expressed concern, however, that as Asian Americans become more assimilated into American culture, they'll drink more—and possibly suffer very adverse effects from alcohol.

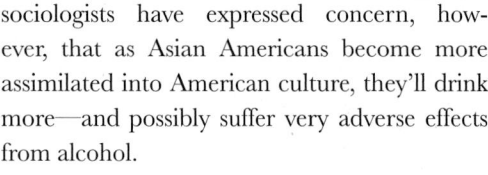

# Alcohol Problems

By the simplest definition, problem drinking is the use of alcohol in any way that creates difficulties, potential difficulties, or health risks for an individual. Like alcoholics, problem drinkers are individuals whose lives are in some way impaired by their drinking. The only difference is one of degree. Alcohol becomes a problem, and a person becomes an alcoholic, when the drinker can't "take it or leave it." He or she spends more and more time anticipating the next drink, planning when and where to get it, buying and hiding alcohol, and covering up secret drinking. As many as one in six adults in the United States may have a problem with drinking.

**Alcohol abuse** involves continued use of alcohol despite awareness of social, occupational, psychological, or physical problems related to drinking, or drinking in dangerous ways or situations (before driving, for instance). A diagnosis of alcohol abuse is based on one or more of the following occurring at any time during a 12-month period:

- A failure to fulfill major role obligations at work, school, or home (such as missing work or school).
- The use of alcohol in situations in which it is physically hazardous (such as before driving).
- Alcohol-related legal problems (such as drunk-driving arrests).
- Continued alcohol use despite persistent or recurring social or interpersonal problems caused or exacerbated by alcohol (such as fighting while drunk).

**Alcohol dependence** is a separate disorder in which individuals develop a strong craving for alcohol because it produces pleasurable feelings or relieves stress or anxiety. Over time they experience physiological changes that lead to *tolerance* of its effects; this means that they must

consume larger and larger amounts to achieve intoxication. If they abruptly stop drinking, they suffer *withdrawal*, a state of acute physical and psychological discomfort. A diagnosis of alcohol dependence is based on three or more of the following symptoms occurring during any 12-month period:

- Tolerance, as defined by either a need for markedly increased amounts of alcohol to achieve intoxication or desired effect, or a markedly diminished effect with continued drinking of the same amount of alcohol as in the past.
- Withdrawal, including at least two of the following symptoms: sweating, rapid pulse, or other signs of autonomic hyperactivity; increased hand tremor; insomnia; nausea or vomiting; temporary hallucinations or illusions; physical agitation or restlessness; anxiety; or grand mal seizures.
- Drinking to avoid or relieve the symptoms of withdrawal.
- Consuming larger amounts of alcohol, or drinking over a longer period than was intended.
- Persistent desire or unsuccessful efforts to cut down or control drinking.
- A great deal of time spent in activities necessary to obtain alcohol, drink it, or recover from its effects.
- Important social, occupational, or recreational activities given up or reduced because of alcohol use.
- Continued alcohol use despite knowledge that alcohol is likely to cause or exacerbate a persistent or recurring physical or psychological problem.

 About a third of college students meet the diagnostic criteria for alcohol abuse, while 6 percent qualify for a diagnosis of alcohol dependence.[48] Although many students reduce their alcohol consumption after college, others continue to drink heavily and face increased risk of alcohol-use disorders and alcohol-related problems and medical risks. (See Self Survey: Do You Have a Drinking Problem? to assess your drinking status.)

**Alcoholism**, as defined by the National Council on Alcoholism and Drug Dependence and

**alcohol abuse** Continued use of alcohol despite awareness of social, occupational, psychological, or physical problems related to its use, or use of alcohol in dangerous ways or situations, such as before driving.

**alcohol dependence** Development of a strong craving for alcohol due to the pleasurable feelings or relief of stress or anxiety produced by drinking.

**alcoholism** A chronic, progressive, potentially fatal disease characterized by impaired control of drinking; a preoccupation with alcohol; continued use of alcohol despite adverse consequences; and distorted thinking, most notably denial.

the American Society of Addiction, is a primary, chronic disease in which genetic, psychosocial, and environmental factors influence its development and manifestations. The disease is often progressive and fatal. Its characteristics include an inability to control drinking; a preoccupation with alcohol; continued use of alcohol despite adverse consequences; and distorted thinking, most notably denial. Like other diseases, alcoholism is not simply a matter of insufficient willpower but a complex problem that causes many symptoms, can have serious consequences, yet can improve with treatment.

## Causes of Alcohol Dependence and Abuse

Although the exact cause of alcohol dependence and abuse is not known, certain factors—including biochemical imbalances in the brain, heredity, cultural acceptability, and stress—all seem to play a role. They include the following:

- **Genetics.** Scientists have not yet identified conclusively a specific gene that puts people at risk for alcoholism. However, epidemiological studies have shown evidence of heredity's role. Studies of twins suggest that heredity accounts for two-thirds of the risk of becoming alcoholic in both men and women.

- **Stress and traumatic experiences.** Many people start drinking heavily as a way of coping with psychological problems.

- **Parental alcoholism.** According to researchers, alcoholism is four to five times more common among the children of alcoholics, who may be influenced by the behavior they see in their parents.

- **Drug abuse.** Alcoholism is also associated with the abuse of other psychoactive drugs, including marijuana, cocaine, heroin, amphetamines, and various antianxiety medications.

## Medical Complications of Alcohol Abuse and Dependence

As previously discussed, excessive alcohol use adversely affects virtually every organ system

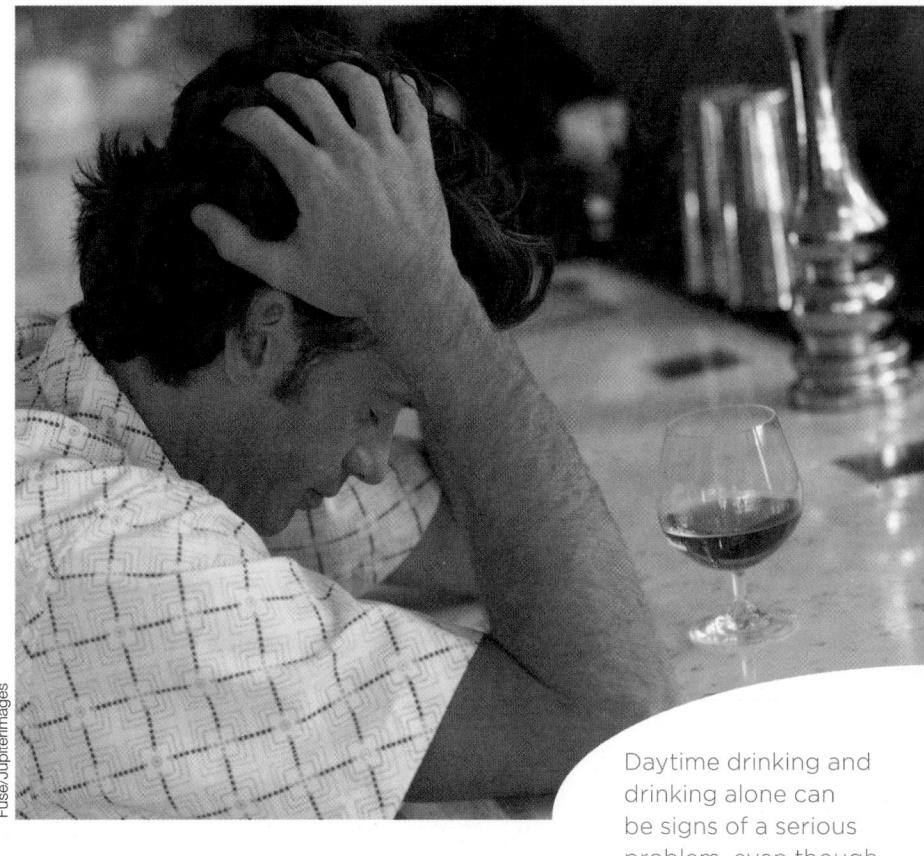

Fuse/Jupiterimages

Daytime drinking and drinking alone can be signs of a serious problem, even though the drinker may otherwise appear to be in control.

in the body, including the brain, the digestive tract, the heart, muscles, blood, and hormones (look back at Figure 13.4, page 443). In addition, because alcohol interacts with many drugs, it can increase the risk of potentially lethal overdoses and harmful interactions. A summary of the major risks and complications follows:

- **Liver disease.** Chronic heavy drinking can lead to alcoholic hepatitis (inflammation and destruction of liver cells) and in the 15 percent of people who continue drinking beyond this stage, cirrhosis (irreversible scarring and destruction of liver cells). The liver eventually may fail completely, resulting in coma and death.

- **Cardiorespiratory disease.** Heavy drinking can weaken the heart muscle (causing cardiac myopathy), elevate blood pressure, and increase the risk of stroke.

- **Cancer.** Heavy alcohol use may contribute to cancer of the liver, stomach, and colon, as well as malignant melanoma, a deadly form of skin cancer.

- **Brain damage.** Long-term heavy drinkers may suffer memory loss and be unable

## How to Recognize the Warning Signs of Alcoholism

- Experiencing the following symptoms after drinking: frequent headaches, nausea, stomach pain, heartburn, gas, fatigue, weakness, muscle cramps, irregular or rapid heartbeats.

- Needing a drink in the morning to start the day.

- Denying any problem with alcohol.

- Doing things while drinking that are regretted afterward.

- Experiencing dramatic mood swings, from anger to laughter to anxiety.

- Having sleep problems.

- Experiencing depression and paranoia.

- Forgetting what happened during a drinking episode.

- Changing brands or going on the wagon to control drinking.

- Having five or more drinks a day.

to think abstractly, recall names of common objects, and follow simple instructions. Chronic brain damage resulting from alcohol consumption is second only to Alzheimer's disease as a cause of cognitive deterioration in adults.

- **Vitamin deficiencies.** Alcoholism is associated with vitamin deficiencies, especially of thiamin ($B_1$). Lack of thiamin may result in Wernicke-Korsakoff syndrome, which is characterized by disorientation, memory failure, hallucinations, and jerky eye movements, and can be disabling enough to require lifelong custodial care.

- **Digestive problems.** Alcohol triggers the secretion of acids in the stomach that irritate the mucous lining and cause gastritis. Chronic drinking may result in peptic ulcers (breaks in the stomach lining) and bleeding from the stomach lining.

**detoxification** The supervised removal of a poisonous or harmful substance (such as a drug) from the body; a therapy for alcoholics in which they are denied alcohol in a controlled environment.

# Alcoholism Treatments

An estimated 8 million adults in the United States have alcohol dependence. Only a minority ever undergo treatment for alcohol-related problems. Until recent years, the only options for professional alcohol treatment were, as one expert puts it, "intensive, extensive, and expensive," such as residential programs at hospitals or specialized treatment centers. Today individuals whose drinking could be hazardous to their health may choose from a variety of approaches, including medication, behavioral therapy, or both. Treatment that works well for one person may not work for another. As research into the outcomes of alcohol treatments has grown, more attempts have been made to match individuals to approaches tailored to their needs and more likely to help them overcome their alcohol problems.[49]

Men and women who have seriously remained sober for more than a decade credit a variety of approaches, including Alcoholics Anonymous (AA), individual psychotherapy, and other groups, such as Women for Sobriety. There is no one sure path to sobriety—a wide variety of treatments may offer help and hope to those with alcohol-related problems. Genetics may predict the success of specific therapies in helping individuals overcome alcohol dependence.[50]

## Detoxification

The first phase of treatment for alcohol dependence focuses on **detoxification**, the gradual withdrawal of alcohol from the body. For 90 to 95 percent of alcoholics, withdrawal symptoms are mild to moderate. They include sweating; rapid pulse; elevated blood pressure; hand tremor; insomnia; nausea or vomiting; malaise or weakness; anxiety; depressed mood or irritability; headache; and temporary hallucinations or illusions. Withdrawal can be life-threatening when accompanied by medical problems, such as grand mal seizures, pneumonia, liver failure, or gastrointestinal bleeding. The standard treatment is a safer sedative, such as Valium or Ativan, with a gradual reduction in the dose.

Alcohol withdrawal delirium, commonly known as **delirium tremens**, or **DTs**, is most common in chronic heavy drinkers who also suffer from a physical illness, fatigue, depression, or malnutrition. Delirium tremens are characterized by agitated behavior, delusions, rapid heart rate, sweating, vivid hallucinations, trembling hands, and fever. The symptoms usually appear over several days after heavy drinking stops. Individuals frequently report terrifying visual hallucinations, such as seeing insects all over their bodies. With treatment, most cases subside after several days, although delirium tremens has been known to last as long as four or five weeks. In some cases, complications such as infections or heart arrhythmias prove fatal.

## Medical Treatments

Antianxiety and antidepressive drugs are sometimes used in early treatment for alcoholism, especially for those with underlying mental disorders. Four drugs—disulfiram, naltrexone, acamprosate, and topiramate—are approved to reduce the persistent craving for alcohol. Vitamin supplements, especially thiamin and folic acid, can help overcome some of the nutritional deficiencies linked with alcoholism.[51]

The drug disulfiram (Antabuse), given to deter drinking, causes individuals to become nauseated and acutely ill when they consume alcohol. Antabuse interrupts the removal of acetaldehye by the liver, so this toxic substance accumulates and causes nausea or vomiting. If individuals taking Antabuse drink at all or consume foods with alcoholic content, they become extremely ill. They must avoid foods cooked or marinated in wine and cough syrup preparations containing alcohol. Some individuals have reactions to the alcohol in after-shave lotion. A large amount of alcohol can make them dangerously ill; fatalities have occurred. Side effects are usually mild and include drowsiness, bad breath, skin rash, and temporary impotence. Because Antabuse does not reduce cravings for alcohol, psychotherapy and support groups remain a necessary part of treatment.

## Inpatient or Residential Treatment

In the past, 28-day treatment programs in a medical or psychiatric hospital or a residential facility were the cornerstone of early recovery treatment. According to outcome studies, inpatient treatment was effective, with as many as 70 percent of "graduates" remaining abstinent or stable, nonproblem drinkers for five years after. However, because of cost pressures from the insurance industry, the length of stay has been reduced, and there's been increasing emphasis on outpatient care.

## Outpatient Treatment

Outpatient treatment may involve group therapy, individual supportive therapy, marital or family therapy, regular attendance at Alcoholics Anonymous (AA) or another support group, brief interventions, and relapse prevention. According to outcome studies, intensive outpatient treatment at a day hospital (with individuals returning home every evening) are as effective as inpatient care. Outpatient therapy continues for at least a year, but many individuals continue to participate in outpatient programs for the rest of their lives.

*Brief Interventions* These methods include individual counseling, group therapy, and training in specific skills—such as assertiveness—all packed into a six- to eight-week period. Offered at a growing number of centers, brief interventions may be most helpful for problem drinkers who are not physically dependent on alcohol. They have proved effective in reducing alcohol consumption up to one year compared with no intervention or standard care. However, at ten years, there is no difference in alcohol consumption among those who had a brief intervention and those who did not. This indicates the need for follow-up advice and counseling.

According to a recent review, Internet-based interventions can be more effective than simply providing printed materials in helping some alcoholics drink a little less.[52] However, follow-up with a counselor has proven more effective in reducing weekly drinking frequency and alcohol consumption.[53]

*Moderation Training* Highly controversial, this approach uses cognitive-behavioral techniques, such as keeping a diary to chart drinking patterns and learning "consumption management" techniques, such as never having more than one drink an hour.

**delirium tremens (DTs)** The delusions, hallucinations, and agitated behavior following withdrawal from long-term chronic alcohol abuse.

Treatment programs in other countries, such as Great Britain and Canada, have long offered moderation training for problem drinkers who consume too much alcohol. However, most experts agree that the best—and perhaps only—hope for recovery for chronic alcoholics who are physically dependent on alcohol is complete abstinence.

*12-Step Self-Help Programs* The best-known and most commonly used self-help program for alcohol problems is Alcoholics Anonymous (AA), which was founded more than 60 years ago and which has grown into an international organization that includes 2 million members and 185,000 groups worldwide. Acknowledging the power of alcohol, AA offers support from others struggling with the same illness, from a sponsor available at any time of the day or night, and from fellowship meetings that are held every day of the year. Because anonymity is a key part of AA, it has been difficult for researchers to study its success, but it is generally believed to be a highly effective means of overcoming alcoholism and maintaining abstinence. Its 12 steps, which emphasize honesty, sobriety, and acknowledgment of a "higher power," have become the model for self-help groups for other addictive behaviors, including drug abuse (discussed in Chapter 12) and compulsive eating.

The average age of entry into AA is 30; about 60 percent of the members are men. Members encompass a wide range of ages, occupations, nationalities, and socioeconomic classes. People generally attend 12-step meetings every day when they first begin recovery; most programs recommend 90 meetings in 90 days. Many people taper off to one or two meetings a week as their recovery progresses. No one knows exactly how 12-step programs help people break out of addictions. Some individuals stop their drinking, or other destructive behavior, simply on the basis of the information they get at meetings. Others bond to the group and use it as a social support and refuge while they explore and release their inner feelings—a process similar to what happens in psychotherapy.

Many individuals recovering from substance abuse—as many as one in ten Americans, by some estimates—will attend a 12-step meeting in their lifetime. For many with alcohol-related problems, AA is the first and only treatment they receive. Does AA work? Some studies have found that fewer than 1 in 30 people remain in AA after one year, although this may be because many are coerced to make their initial visits. However, continued AA attendance is modestly associated with abstinence and improved social functioning. According to the "helper theory principle," when people with a condition help others with a similar problem, they also help themselves. This principle, fundamental to AA, may contribute to their continuing sobriety.[54]

Spirituality is another key and controversial component of AA, with 11 of its 12 steps explicitly referring to the importance of God or a higher power for recovery. Yet both spiritually oriented and atheistic individuals benefit equally from AA programs. In a ten-year study, individuals involved with AA reported significantly larger gains in religious practices, such as prayer, compared with those without such exposure. Individuals who maintain consistent AA membership reported the greatest increases in "God consciousness" and religious practices.

*Harm Reduction Therapy* This controversial approach aims to help substance abusers reduce the negative impact of alcohol or drugs on their lives. Its fundamental principles include the following:

- While absolute abstinence may be preferable for many or most substance abusers, very few achieve it. Even these few will take time to reach this point and may relapse periodically.

- The field of medicine accepts and practices other types of treatments that preserve health and well-being even when people fail to comply with all recommended behaviors.

- Therapists cannot make judgments for clients, even though they should present accurate information and may even express their own beliefs.

- There are many shades of improvement in every kind of therapy. If a certain level of improvement is all a person is capable of reaching, that person should be encouraged.

*Alternatives to AA* Secular Organizations for Sobriety (SOS) was founded in 1986 as an alternative for people who couldn't accept the spirituality of AA. Like AA, SOS holds confidential meetings, celebrates sobriety anniversaries, and views recovery as a one-day-at-a-time process.

Rational Recovery, which also emphasizes anonymity and total abstinence, focuses on the self rather than spirituality. Members use reason instead of prayer and learn to control the impulse to drink by learning how to control the emotions that lead them to drink.

## Recovery

Recovery from alcoholism is a lifelong process of personal growth and healing. The first two years are the most difficult, and relapses are extremely common. By some estimates, more than 90 percent of those recovering from substance use will use alcohol or drugs in any one 12-month period after treatment. However, approximately 70 percent of those who get formal treatment stop drinking for prolonged periods. Even without treatment, 30 percent of alcoholics are able to stop drinking for long periods. Those most likely to remain sober after treatment have the most to lose by continuing to drink: they tend to be employed, married, and upper-middle class. Recovering alcoholics who help other alcoholics stay sober are better able to maintain their own sobriety.

Most recovering alcoholics experience urges to drink, especially during early recovery when they are likely to feel considerable stress. These urges are a natural consequence of years of drinking and diminish with time. Mood swings are common during recovery, and individuals typically describe themselves as alternately feeling relieved or elated and then discouraged or tearful. Such disconcerting ups and downs also decrease over time. Patience—learning to take "one day at a time"—is crucial.[55]

Increasingly, treatment programs focus on **relapse prevention**, which includes the development of coping strategies and learning techniques that make it easier to live with alcohol cravings and rehearsal of various ways of saying "no" to offers of a drink. According to outcomes research, social skills training—a combination of stress management therapy, assertiveness and communication skills training, behavioral self-control training, and behavioral marital therapy—has proved effective in decreasing the duration and severity of relapses after one year in a group of alcoholics. A new approach to relapse behavior, "Mindfulness-Based-Relapse Prevention" teaches clients meditation techniques as a way of coping with cravings and high-risk relapse situations.

# Alcoholism's Impact on Relationships

Alcoholism shatters families and creates unhealthy patterns of communicating and relating. Separation and divorce rates are high among alcoholics.

Having a heavy drinker—a friend, family member, or colleague—in your life can put your own health and well-being at risk. In a recent study, those linked with a heavy drinker reported more symptoms such as chronic pain, anxiety, and depression.[56]

## Growing Up with an Alcoholic Parent

An estimated 28 million children in the United States (or one of every four) are living in a household with an alcoholic adult. Parental alcoholism increases the likelihood of childhood ADHD, conduct disorder, and anxiety disorders. The experience often leads youngsters to play certain roles: The adjuster or "lost child" does whatever the parent says. The responsible child, or "family hero," typically takes over many household tasks and responsibilities. The acting-out child, or "scapegoat," shows his or her anger early in life by causing problems at home or in school and taking on the role of troublemaker. The "mascot" disrupts tense situations by focusing attention on himself or herself, often by clowning. Regardless of which roles they assume, the children of alcoholics are prone to learning disabilities, eating disorders, and addictive behavior.

Numerous studies have linked parental drinking to child abuse and neglect. Children of women who are problem drinkers have twice the risk of serious injury as children of mothers who don't drink. Children with two parents who are problem drinkers are at even higher risk. As teenagers, children of alcoholics are more likely to report early sexual intercourse and face a greater risk of adolescent pregnancy.

**relapse prevention** An alcohol recovery treatment method that focuses on social skills training to develop ways of preventing or minimizing a relapse.

# Health in Action

## If Someone Close to You Drinks Too Much

- **Try to remain calm, unemotional, and factually honest in speaking about the drinker's behavior.** Include the drinker in family life.

- **Discuss the situation with someone you trust: a member of the clergy, social worker, friend, or someone who has experienced alcoholism directly.**

- **Never cover up or make excuses for the drinker, or shield him or her from the consequences of drinking.** Assuming the drinker's responsibilities undermines his or her dignity and sense of importance.

- **Refuse to ride with the drinker if he or she is driving while intoxicated.**

- **Encourage new interests and participate in leisure-time activities that the drinker enjoys.**

- **Try to accept setbacks and relapses calmly.**

In addition to focusing on your friend or family member, take time to sort through your own feelings about the situation. Record your observations and concerns in your online journal.

## Adult Children of Alcoholics

Growing up with an alcoholic parent can have a long-lasting effect. Adult children of alcoholics are at risk for many problems. Some try to fill the emptiness inside with alcohol, drugs, or addictive habits. Others find themselves caught up in destructive relationships that repeat the patterns of their childhood. They are likely to have difficulty solving problems, identifying and expressing their feelings, trusting others, and being intimate. In addition to their own increased risk of addictive behavior, they are likely to marry individuals with some form of addiction and keep on playing out the roles of their childhood. They may feel inadequate, not know how to set limits or recognize normal behavior, be perfectionistic, and want to control all aspects of their lives. However, not all adult children are alike or necessarily suffer from psychological problems or face an increased risk of substance abuse themselves.

Because the impact of alcoholism can be so enduring, support groups—such as Adult Children of Alcoholics, Children of Alcoholics, and Adult Children of Dysfunctional Families—have spread throughout the country in the last decade. These organizations provide adult children of alcoholics a mutually supportive group setting in which to discuss their childhood experiences with alcoholic parents and the emotional consequences they carry into adult life. Through such groups or other forms of therapy, individuals may learn to move beyond anger and blame, see the part they themselves play in their current state of unhappiness, and create a future that is healthier and happier than their past. (See Health in Action.)

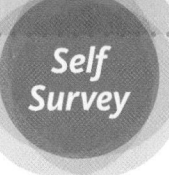

## Build Your Future

# Take Charge of Alcohol

If you use alcohol, develop a defensive drinking program. Check the steps that you have taken or will take in the future to stay in control of your alcohol intake.

_____ Finding alternative ways to soothe stress. Daily sessions of meditation have proven effective in helping high-risk student drinkers relax.

_____ Setting a limit on how many drinks you're going to have ahead of time—and sticking to it.

_____ When you're mixing a drink, measuring the alcohol.

_____ Alternating nonalcoholic and alcoholic drinks.

_____ Drinking slowly; not guzzling.

_____ Eating before and while drinking.

_____ Avoiding tasks that require skilled reactions during or after drinking.

_____ Not encouraging or reinforcing others' irresponsible behavior.

_____ Checking out community resources. Are there chapters of AA and Al-Anon on campus? Find out more about the BACCHUS (Boost Alcohol Consciousness Concerning the Health of University Students) network, including programs in your area. Do these groups offer volunteer opportunities that interest you?

_____ Talking to your dormmates, fraternity brothers, sorority sisters, or roommates about steps you could take collectively, such as restricting drinking in rooms or setting up a "Seize the Keys" policy to prevent drunk driving.

## Self Survey

# Do You Have a Drinking Problem?

This self-assessment, the Michigan Alcoholism Screening Test (MAST), is widely used to identify potential problems. This test screens for the major psychological, sociological, and physiological consequences of alcoholism.

Answer Yes or No to the following questions, and add up the points shown in the right column for your answers.

| | Yes | No | Points |
|---|---|---|---|
| 1. Do you enjoy a drink now and then? | _____ | _____ | (0 for either) |
| 2. Do you think that you're a normal drinker? (By normal, we mean that you drink less than or as much as most other people.) | _____ | _____ | (2 for no) |
| 3. Have you ever awakened the morning after some drinking the night before and found that you couldn't remember part of the evening? | _____ | _____ | (2 for yes) |
| 4. Does your wife, husband, a parent, or other near relative ever worry or complain about your drinking? | _____ | _____ | (1 for yes) |
| 5. Can you stop drinking without a struggle after one or two drinks? | _____ | _____ | (2 for no) |
| 6. Do you ever feel guilty about your drinking? | _____ | _____ | (1 for yes) |
| 7. Do friends or relatives think that you're a normal drinker? | _____ | _____ | (2 for no) |
| 8. Do you ever try to limit your drinking to certain times of the day or to certain places? | _____ | _____ | (0 for either) |
| 9. Have you ever attended a meeting of Alcoholics Anonymous? | _____ | _____ | (2 for yes) |
| 10. Have you ever gotten into physical fights when drinking? | _____ | _____ | (1 for yes) |
| 11. Has your drinking ever created problems for you and your wife, husband, a parent, or other relative? | _____ | _____ | (2 for yes) |

12. Have your wife, husband, or other family members ever gone to anyone for help about your drinking?  _____  _____  (2 for yes)

13. Have you ever lost friends because of your drinking?  _____  _____  (2 for yes)

14. Have you ever gotten into trouble at work or school because of your drinking?  _____  _____  (2 for yes)

15. Have you ever lost a job because of your drinking?  _____  _____  (2 for yes)

16. Have you ever neglected your obligations, your family, or your work for two or more days in a row because of drinking?  _____  _____  (2 for yes)

17. Do you drink before noon fairly often?  _____  _____  (1 for yes)

18. Have you ever been told you have liver trouble? Cirrhosis?  _____  _____  (2 for yes)

19. After heavy drinking, have you ever had delirium tremens (DTs) or severe shaking, or heard voices or seen things that weren't actually there?  _____  _____  (2 for yes*)

20. Have you ever gone to anyone for help about your drinking?  _____  _____  (5 for yes)

21. Have you ever been in a hospital because of your drinking?  _____  _____  (5 for yes)

22. Have you ever been a patient in a psychiatric hospital or on a psychiatric ward of a general hospital where drinking was part of the problem that resulted in hospitalization?  _____  _____  (2 for yes)

23. Have you ever been seen at a psychiatric or mental health clinic or gone to any doctor, social worker, or clergyman for help with any emotional problem where drinking was part of the problem?  _____  _____  (2 for yes)

24. Have you ever been arrested for drunk driving, driving while intoxicated, or driving under the influence of alcoholic beverages?  _____  _____  (2 for yes)

25. Have you ever been arrested, or taken into custody, even for a few hours, because of drunken behavior?  _____  _____  (2 for yes)

   (If Yes, how many times?)  _____**

*Five points for delirium tremens
**Two points for each arrest

## Scoring

In general, five or more points places you in an alcoholic category; four points suggests alcoholism; three or fewer points indicates that you're *not* an alcoholic.

# *Making Change Happen*

## Your Alcohol Audit

We have no objection to drinking. What does concern us is drinking without thinking. When you drink without thinking, you give up control and turn your life over to alcohol. And when you lose control, you lose. You can end up a hapless spectator or a victim of consequences you never intended. A third of students report doing something they later regretted as a result of their drinking. "Your Alcohol Audit" in *Labs for IPC* can help you avoid this experience—ever or again. If just thinking about drinking makes you uneasy, definitely read the following and do this lab. The feeling is a red flag you shouldn't ignore.

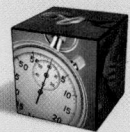

### Get Real

In this section, you analyze your drinking by answering 12 questions, including the following three:

- When did you last have a drink? How many drinks did you have? Why did you choose to drink?

- How often do you drink? When do you drink? Where?

- Have you ever failed to do what was expected of you because of drinking? How often?

On a scale of 1 (no reason for concern) to 10 (I have a drinking problem), you rate your concern about the role of alcohol in your life.

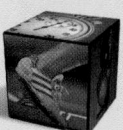

### Get Ready

In this stage, you research alcoholism in your family, going back to your grandparents. If drinking problems run in your family, you need to think about drinking even more carefully than other students. You also list what you see as the advantages of drinking (such as feeling less socially anxious) and then its negative consequences (such as headaches, hangovers, or blowing a test because you were too wasted to study).

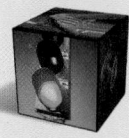

### Get Going

In this stage you set a drinking quota and write in your *IPC Journal*:

"My limit is _____ drink(s) whenever I drink."

You keep to this limit through a variety of strategies, including the following:

- When "No" Isn't Enough

Being with people who are drinking doesn't mean you have to drink as much as they do. Here are some effective ways to get your message across. Rehearse the following two examples before you go out:

| | |
|---|---|
| "Just have one beer." | "I have a bet with someone (no need to say it's you) to see how long I can go without drinking." OR "I can't stop at one, and I'm not going there tonight." |
| "Why aren't you drinking?" | "I've got practice/work/a job interview/whatever first thing tomorrow." |

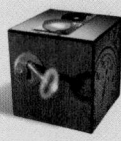

### Lock It In

Responsible drinking requires attention. Among other steps, you continue your alcohol audit for the rest of the term by using this format:

| Day of Week | Number of Drinks | Type of Drinks | Place Consumed |
|---|---|---|---|
| Monday | | | |
| Tuesday | | | |
| Wednesday | | | |
| Thursday | | | |
| Friday | | | |
| Saturday | | | |
| Sunday | | | |

Check how the amounts recorded compare with the goal you set at the beginning of the "Get Going" section.

# Making This Chapter Work for You

## Review Questions

1. Which of the following statements about the effects of alcohol on the body systems is *true*?
   a. In most individuals, alcohol sharpens the responses of the brain and nervous system, enhancing sensation and perception.
   b. Moderate drinking may have a positive effect on the cardiorespiratory system.
   c. French researchers have found that drinking red wine with meals may have a positive effect on the digestive system.
   d. The leading alcohol-related cause of death is liver damage.

2. Racial and ethnic patterns related to alcohol use include which of the following?
   a. Asian American women tend to have higher rates of alcoholism than Asian American men.
   b. Alcohol-related deaths are highest as a percentage of population among Native Americans.
   c. White Americans tend to have higher rates of cirrhosis of the liver than African Americans or Native Americans.
   d. The Hispanic culture discourages men from drinking because heavy drinking indicates a lack of machismo.

3. Alcoholism
   a. is considered a chronic disease with genetic, psychosocial, and environment components.
   b. is characterized by a persistent lack of willpower.
   c. may be classified as either Type A, which affects people who are high-strung, or Type B, which affects people who are more mild mannered.
   d. is easily controlled by avoiding exposure to social situations where drinking is common.

4. Which of the following statements about alcohol abuse and dependence is *false*?
   a. Alcohol dependence involves a persistent craving for and an increased tolerance to alcohol.
   b. An individual may have a genetic predisposition for developing alcoholism.
   c. Alcoholics often abuse other psychoactive drugs.
   d. Alcohol abuse and alcohol dependence are different names for the same problem.

5. Health risks of alcoholism include all of the following *except*
   a. hypertension.
   b. lung cancer.
   c. peptic ulcers.
   d. hepatitis.

6. Which of the following statements about alcoholism treatment is *true*?
   a. Inpatient treatment has been shown to be more effective than outpatient treatment.
   b. Alcoholism can be cured by detoxifying or ridding the body of all traces of alcohol.
   c. Antabuse is a medication given to alcoholics with underlying mental disorders.
   d. A combination of medical, behavioral, and self-help approaches may be necessary to treat alcohol abuse and dependence.

7. Which of the following statements about drinking on college campuses is *true*?
   a. The federal government has a goal to reduce the binge-drinking rate among college students to 20 percent.
   b. The number of women who binge-drink has decreased.
   c. Because of peer pressure, students in fraternities and sororities tend to drink less than students in dormitories.
   d. Students who attend two-year institutions tend to binge-drink when alcohol is available.

8. Responsible drinking includes which of the following behaviors?
   a. Avoid eating while drinking because eating speeds up absorption of alcohol.
   b. Limit alcohol intake to no more than four drinks in an hour.
   c. Take aspirin while drinking to lower your risk of a heart attack.
   d. Socialize with individuals who limit their alcohol intake.

9. Which of these is a standard drink?
   a. a margarita
   b. a 12-oz regular beer
   c. a double martini
   d. a 16-oz can of malt liquor

10. An individual's response to alcohol depends on all of the following *except*
   a. the rate at which the drink is absorbed into the body's tissues.
   b. the blood-alcohol concentration.
   c. socioeconomic status.
   d. gender and race.

*Answers to these questions can be found on page 672.*

## Critical Thinking

1. Driving home from a friend's twenty-first birthday party, 18-year-old Rick has had too much to drink. As he crosses the dividing line on the two-lane road, the driver of an oncoming car—a young mother with two young children in the backseat—swerves to avoid an accident. She hits a concrete wall and dies instantly, but her children survive. Rick has no record of drunk driving. Should he go to prison? Is he guilty of manslaughter? How would you feel if you were the victim's husband? If you were Rick's friend?

2. Have you ever been around people who have been intoxicated when you have been sober? What did you think of their behavior? Were they fun to be around?

Was the experience not particularly enjoyable, boring, or difficult in some way? Have you ever been intoxicated? How do you behave when you are drunk? Do you find the experience enjoyable? What do the people around you think of your actions when you are drunk?

3. What effects has alcohol use had in your life? Try making a list of the positive and negative effects your own alcohol use has had. Be specific. If you continue to drink at your current rate, what positive and negative effects do you think it will have on your future? What effects have other people's drinking had on your life? List family members and friends who drink regularly and how their drinking has affected you.

## Media Menu

Visit www.cengagebrain.com to access course materials and companion resources for this text that will:

- Help you evaluate your knowledge of the material.
- Allow you to prepare for exams with interactive quizzing.

- Use the CengageNOW product to develop a Personalized Learning Plan targeting resources that address areas you should study.
- Coach you through identifying target goals for behavioral change and creating and monitoring your personal change plan throughout the semester using the Behavior Change Planner available in the CengageNOW resource.

## Internet Connections

**www.factsontap.org**
This excellent site is geared to college students. Sections include Alcohol & Student Life, Alcohol & Sex, Alcohol & Your Body.

**www.collegedrinkingprevention.gov**
This website, sponsored by the National Institute of Alcohol Abuse and Alcoholism, focuses on the college alcohol culture with information for students, parents, college health administrators, and more. The site also features information about alcohol abuse prevention, college alcohol policies, research topics, and factual

information about the consequences of alcohol abuse and alcoholism.

**www.al-anon.alateen.org**
This site provides information and referrals to local Al-Anon and Alateen groups. It also includes a self-quiz to determine if you are affected by someone who has an alcohol problem.

**www.nacoa.org**
This association provides information about and for children of alcoholics. The website contains numerous links to relevant support groups.

## Key Terms

The terms listed are used on the page indicated. Definitions of the terms are in the Glossary at the end of the book.

absorption   439

alcohol abuse   448

alcohol dependence   448

alcoholism   448

binge   430

blood-alcohol concentration (BAC)   439

delirium tremens (DTs)   451

detoxification   450

ethyl alcohol   438

fetal alcohol effects (FAE)   446

fetal alcohol syndrome (FAS)   447

predrinking   432

proof   438

relapse prevention   453

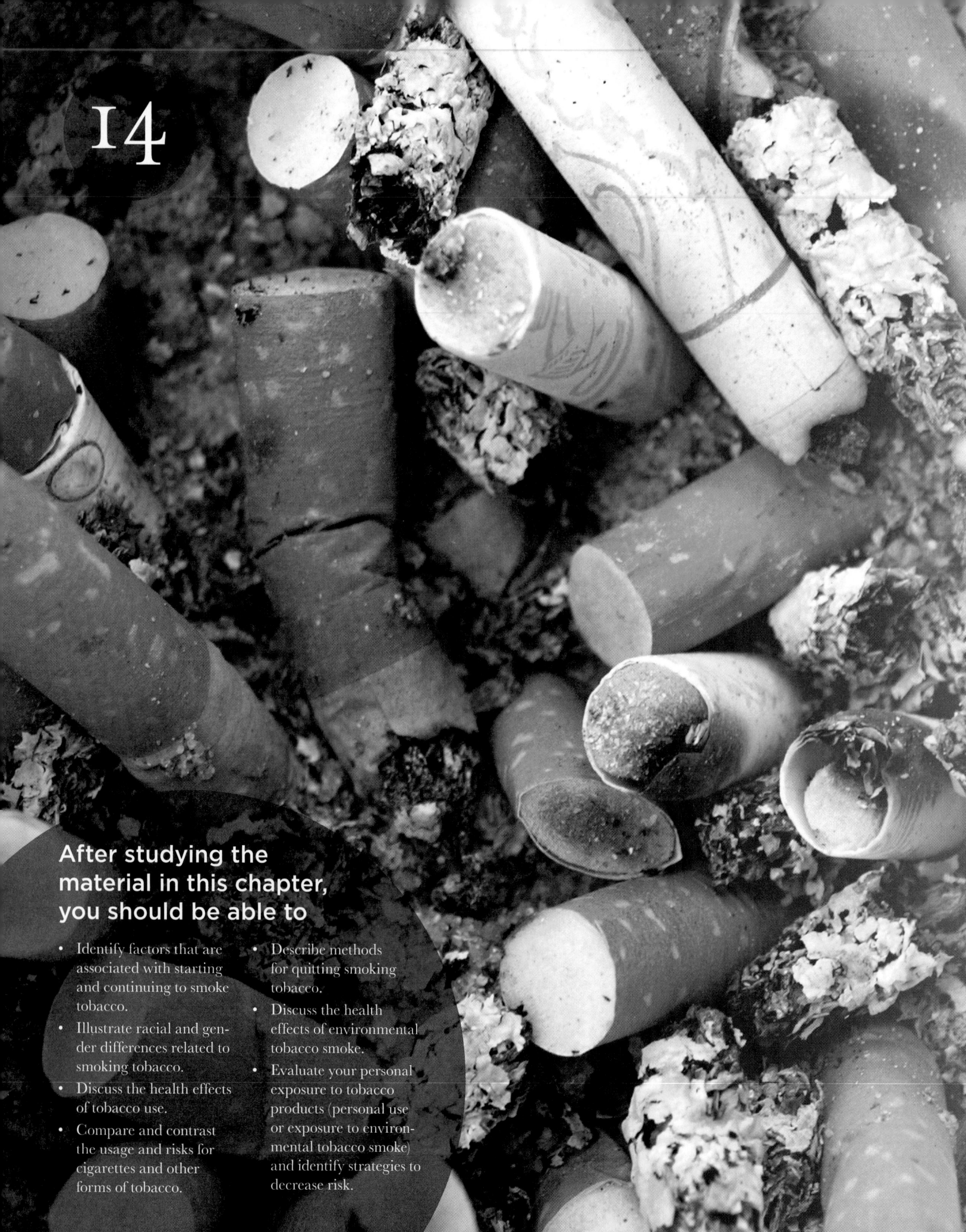

14

## After studying the material in this chapter, you should be able to

- Identify factors that are associated with starting and continuing to smoke tobacco.

- Illustrate racial and gender differences related to smoking tobacco.

- Discuss the health effects of tobacco use.

- Compare and contrast the usage and risks for cigarettes and other forms of tobacco.

- Describe methods for quitting smoking tobacco.

- Discuss the health effects of environmental tobacco smoke.

- Evaluate your personal exposure to tobacco products (personal use or exposure to environmental tobacco smoke) and identify strategies to decrease risk.

Marissa didn't really want her first cigarette. Her tent mate at camp had snatched one from a counselor's pack, and the two of them had climbed to a remote rock to share it. Marissa hated everything about her first drag: the taste, the smell, the horrible burning in her throat and lungs. But she loved feeling more grown-up and sophisticated than other seventh graders. By the time she reached high school, Marissa would sneak off to smoke with friends at least once a week. By graduation, she was smoking daily.

# Tobacco

As a college freshman, Marissa discovered that she was part of an unpopular minority. Even though her dorm didn't ban smoking, her roommate declared their room a smoke-free zone. Her college didn't allow smoking in any classrooms or public areas. And many of her new friends reacted as if smoking was a sign of impaired intelligence. Marissa has decided to quit, but she's discovered that nicotine dependence is very difficult to overcome. "I just wish I'd never started smoking in the first place," she says.

Despite overwhelming evidence of tobacco's dangers, smoking remains widespread. Some 12 million cigarettes are smoked around the world every minute of every day. An estimated 6.3 trillion cigarettes are produced annually—more than 900 cigarettes for every man, woman, and child on the planet.

This chapter discusses smoking around the world, in America, and on campus. It provides information on the effects of tobacco on the body, tobacco dependence, quitting smoking, smokeless tobacco, and environmental tobacco smoke. This information may help you to breathe easier today—and may help ensure cleaner air for others to breathe tomorrow.

## Smoking in America

The total number of smokers is increasing as the world population continues to climb. Male smoking is declining slowly, but female smoking, especially in some developing countries, is increasing. Although cigarettes are expensive in the poorest countries, their citizens are the heaviest smokers.

Despite widespread awareness of the dangers of tobacco, smoking continues to kill more people than AIDS, alcohol, drug abuse, car crashes,

Visit www.cengagebrain.com to access course materials for this text, including the Behavior Change Planner, interactive quizzes, tutorials, and more. See the preface on page xv for details.

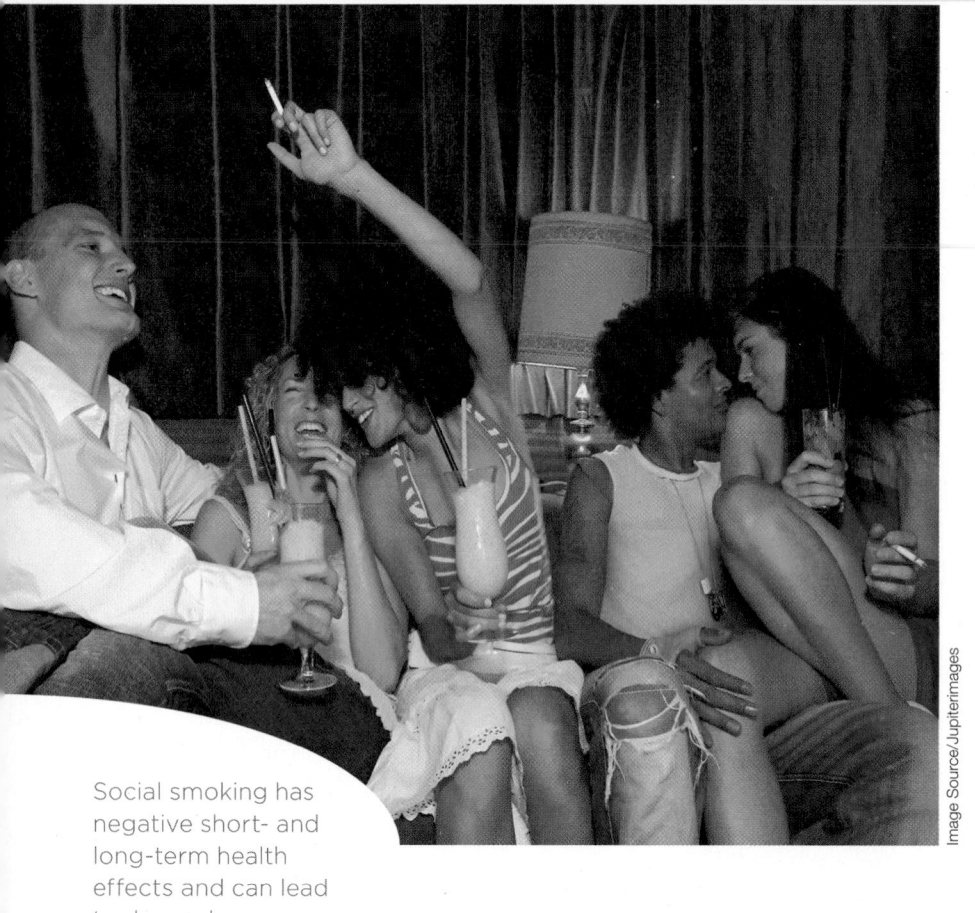

Social smoking has negative short- and long-term health effects and can lead to dependence.

Utah. Native Americans have the highest smoking rates, while Asians and Hispanics have the lowest. Individuals with undergraduate and graduate degrees are least likely to smoke.

One study indicates that cigarette smokers have lower IQs than nonsmokers, and the more a person smokes, the lower his or her IQ. On average, young men who smoked a pack or more of cigarettes a day had IQ scores 7.5 points lower than nonsmokers.

There are now more former smokers than active smokers in the United States, and more than half the population lives where smoking is prohibited in workplaces.

## Why People Start Smoking

 Most people are aware that an enormous health risk is associated with smoking, but many don't know exactly what that risk is or how it might affect them.

The two main factors linked with the onset of a smoking habit are age and education. The majority of white men with less than a high school education are current or former daily cigarette smokers. White women with a similar educational background are also very likely to smoke or to have smoked every day. Hispanic men and women without a high school education are less likely to be or become daily smokers.

The following factors are associated with reasons for smoking.

***Limited Education*** People who have graduated from college are much less likely to smoke than high school graduates; those with fewer than 12 years of education are more likely to smoke. An individual with 8 years or less of education is 11 times more likely to smoke than someone with postgraduate training.

***Underestimation of Risks*** Young people who think the health risks of smoking are fairly low are more likely than their peers to start smoking. In a two-year study, teenagers who thought they had little chance of developing either short-term problems—such as a higher risk of colds or a chronic cough—or long-term problems—such as heart disease, cancer, and respiratory diseases—were three to four times more likely to start smoking.

## Health in the Headlines

### A Global Threat

Tobacco is one of the leading causes of disease and death around the world. To gain a global perspective on tobacco and the ways that various nations are responding to this health threat, go to the "Addiction" portal of Global Health Watch (found under Health and Wellness), click on "Tobacco" and scan the latest news. You will probably see reports from different continents and countries. Select two examples and write a brief description in your online journal.

murders, suicides, and fires combined. The worldwide death toll is 6 million people a year and is expected to climb to 8 million by 2030. (See Health in the Headlines.)

Since 1965 smoking prevalence has decreased from 40 percent to about 20 percent across the nation, with the greatest declines in smoking and in lung cancer in the state of California. High-intensity smoking (defined as 20 or more cigarettes a day) has dropped most dramatically.[1] According to the Centers for Disease Control and Prevention (CDC), some 43 million men and women smoke. The more and the longer they smoke, the greater their risks of heart disease, respiratory problems, several types of cancer, and a shortened lifespan. An estimated 400,000 individuals die prematurely in the United States due to tobacco use each year.

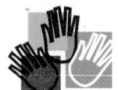 The groups with the lowest smoking rates include women with undergraduate or graduate degrees, men with graduate degrees, Hispanic and Asian women, people over age 65, and the residents of

**Adolescent Experimentation and Rebellion** For teenagers, smoking may be a coping mechanism for dealing with boredom and frustration; a marker of the transition into high school or college; a bid for adult status; a way of gaining admission to a peer group; or a way to have fun, reduce stress, or boost energy. The teenagers most likely to begin smoking are those least likely to seek help when their emotional needs are not met. They might smoke as a means of gaining social acceptance or to self-medicate when they feel helpless, lonely, or depressed. Depressed teens are more susceptible to cigarette ads than their counterparts. For example, they are more likely to have a favorite cigarette ad or own clothing with cigarette logos.

**Stress** In studies that have analyzed the impact of life stressors, depression, emotional support, marital status, and income, researchers have concluded that an individual with a high stress level is approximately 15 times more likely to be a smoker than a person with low stress. About half of smokers identify workplace stress as a key factor in their smoking behavior.

**Parental Role Models** Children who start smoking are 50 percent more likely than youngsters who don't smoke to have at least one smoker in their family. A mother who smokes seems a particularly strong influence on making smoking seem acceptable. The majority of youngsters who smoke say that their parents also smoke and are aware of their own tobacco use.

**Addiction** Nicotine addiction is as strong or stronger than addiction to drugs such as cocaine and heroin. The first symptoms of nicotine addiction can begin within a few days of starting to smoke and after just a few cigarettes, particularly in teenagers. Smoking a single cigarette before age 11 increases the odds of becoming dependent on nicotine. (See Self Survey: "Are You Addicted to Nicotine?" at the end of this chapter.)

**Genetics** Researchers speculate that genes may account for about 50 percent of smoking behavior, with environment playing an equally important role. Studies have shown that identical twins, who have the same genes, are more likely to have matching smoking profiles than fraternal twins. If one identical twin is a heavy smoker, the other is also likely to be; if one smokes only occasionally, so does the other.

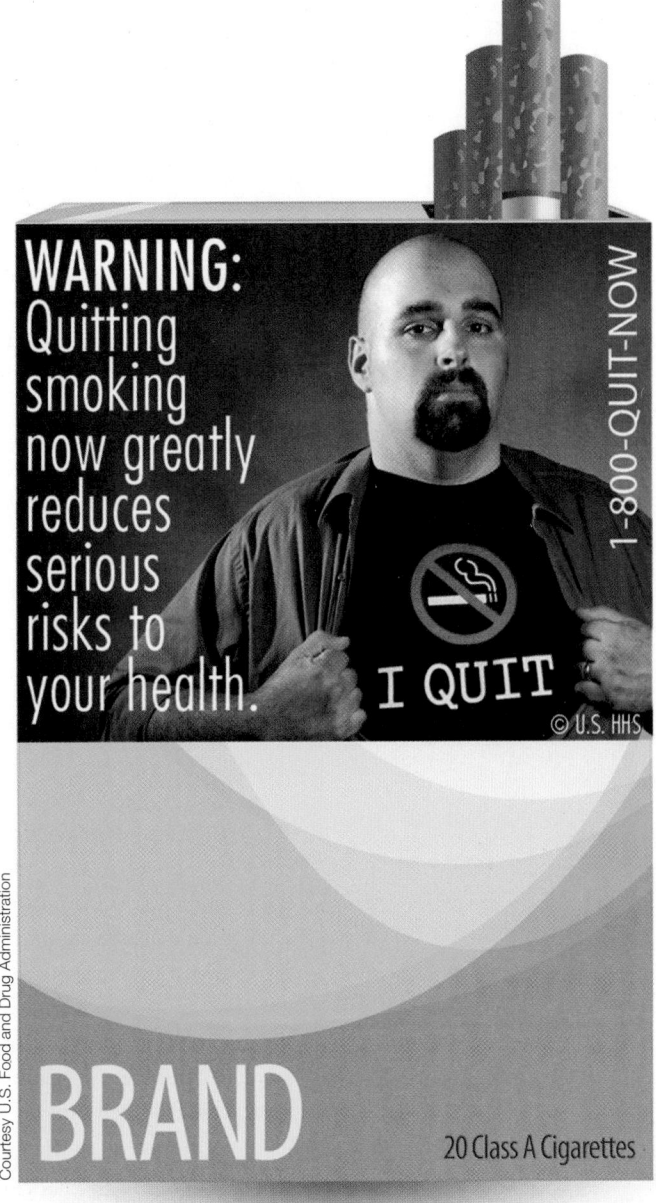

Courtesy U.S. Food and Drug Administration

Some cigarette labels warn of the dangers of smoking; others emphasize the benefits of quitting.

According to NIDA research, genetic factors play a more significant role for initiation of smoking in women than in men, but they play a less significant role in smoking persistence for women.

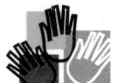 **Weight Control** Concern about weight is a significant risk factor for smoking among young women. Daily smokers are two to four times more likely to fast, use diet pills, and purge to control their weight than nonsmokers. Although black girls smoke at substantially lower rates than white girls, the common factor in predicting daily smoking among all girls, regardless of race, is concern with weight.

*Health on a Budget*

# The Toll of Tobacco

Whether or not you smoke, you indirectly pay the price of tobacco use around the world:

| | |
|---|---|
| Global economic cost | $500 billion |
| U.S. economic cost | $193 billion |
| Annual global number of tobacco-caused deaths | 6 million |
| Annual number of premature deaths due to tobacco in the U.S. | 443,000 |
| Property damage in fires caused by smoking, globally | $27 billion |
| Injuries in fires caused by smoking, globally | 60,000 |
| Deaths in fires caused by smoking, globally | 17,300 |
| Deaths caused by secondhand smoke in the U.S. | 3,000 |

Source: www.tobaccoatlas.org

*Aggressive Marketing* Cigarette companies spend billions of dollars each year on advertisements and promotional campaigns, with manufacturers targeting ads especially at teens, minorities, and the poor. Many ads create an association between cigarettes and alcohol, linking the act of smoking with lifestyles that involve drinking—a combination that public health officials describe as "alarming" because of the health risks posed by these two behaviors.

*Media Messages* Many cigarette advertisements exploit themes that are especially meaningful to teens, such as masculinity for boys and thinness for girls, and social acceptance for both. In a recent study, young people who had never smoked were more likely to start within months of viewing cigarette ads.[2] Among smokers, merely seeing a character in a movie light up triggers a craving for a cigarette, according to brain imaging studies.[3]

*Deceptive Labels* As many as a fifth of smokers wrongly believe that some cigarettes "could be less harmful than others" because of the wording that appears on labels.[4] Many countries have banned words such as "light," "mild," or "low-tar," but consumers often assume that descriptions such as "silver" or "gold" imply that certain brands pose fewer risks. This is not the case. (See "Consumer Alert.")

## ❶ CONSUMER ALERT

### "Safer" Cigarettes

Tobacco companies are producing low-tar and "lower-risk" cigarettes that they claim reduce secondhand smoke or have fewer carcinogens and less nicotine. These brands claim to use genetic engineering or a chemical process to remove major carcinogens.

### Facts to Know

- Low-tar, "lite" cigarettes impair blood flow just as severely as regular cigarettes.

- So-called safer cigarettes may actually lead to increased addiction. In one experiment, smokers puffed on their own brand and then on a so-called safer cigarette brand called Advance. While Advance cigarettes supposedly contain less of a type of cancer-causing substance called nitrosamines, they delivered 25 percent more nicotine into the blood than the smokers' own brands.

- Other cigarettes deliver less nicotine and boost smokers' heart rates and carbon monoxide levels less than traditional cigarettes. However, they aren't as satisfying to smokers, who may smoke more of them.

### Steps to Take

- Don't believe claims that any cigarette is safe or "safer."

- Do the truly safe thing: Stop smoking.

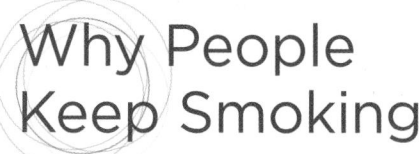

# Why People Keep Smoking

Whatever the reasons for lighting up that first cigarette, very different factors keep cigarettes burning pack after pack, year after year. In national polls, 7 in 10 smokers say that they want to quit but can't. The reason isn't a lack of willpower. Medical scientists have recognized tobacco dependence as an addictive disorder that may be more powerful than heroin dependence and that may affect more than 90 percent of all smokers.

## Pleasure

According to the American Cancer Society, 9 in 10 regular smokers find smoking pleasurable. Nicotine—the addictive ingredient in tobacco—is the reason. Researchers have shown that nicotine reinforces and strengthens the desire to smoke by acting on brain chemicals that influence feelings of well-being. This drug also can improve memory, help in performing certain tasks, reduce anxiety, dampen hunger, and increase pain tolerance.

## Mental Disorders

Individuals with mental disorders are twice as likely to smoke as others, and people with mental illness may account for nearly one-half of the tobacco market in the United States. Heavy smoking also is linked with an almost elevenfold risk of anxiety disorders in early adulthood.

Smokers with a history of depression are about half as likely to quit as others. Even after a recovery from major depression, smokers often continue to report some symptoms of depression. Smokers who are depressed tend to smoke more cigarettes than other smokers, are less successful in their efforts to stop smoking, and are more prone to depression after quitting. The longer people smoke, the more likely they are to develop symptoms of depression and anxiety.

## Fear of Weight Gain

Smokers burn up an extra 100 calories a day—the equivalent of walking a mile—probably because nicotine increases metabolic rate. Once they start smoking, many individuals say they cannot quit because they fear they'll gain weight. The CDC estimates that women who stop smoking gain an average of 8 pounds, while men put on an average of 6 pounds. One in eight women and one in ten men who stop smoking put on 29 pounds or more. The reasons for this weight gain include nicotine's effects on metabolism as well as emotional and behavioral factors, such as the habit of frequently putting something into one's mouth. Yet as a health risk, smoking a pack and a half to two packs a day is a greater danger than carrying 60 pounds of extra weight.

Weight gain for smokers who quit is not inevitable. Aerobic exercise helps increase metabolic rate, and limiting alcohol and foods high in sugar and fat can help smokers control their weight as they give up cigarettes.

## Dependence

Nicotine has a much more powerful hold on smokers than alcohol does on drinkers. Whereas about 10 percent of alcohol users lose control of their intake of alcohol and become alcoholics, as many as 80 percent of all heavy smokers have tried to cut down on or quit smoking but cannot overcome their dependence.

 About 8 percent of full-time college students meet the diagnostic criteria for past-30-day nicotine dependence, much lower than the rate of the general population (15 percent).

Nicotine causes dependence by at least three means:

- It provides a strong sensation of pleasure.
- It leads to fairly severe discomfort during withdrawal.
- It stimulates cravings long after obvious withdrawal symptoms have passed.

Few drugs act as quickly on the brain as nicotine does. It travels through the bloodstream to the brain in seven seconds—half the time it takes for heroin injected into a blood vessel to reach the brain. And a pack-a-day smoker gets 200 hits of nicotine a day—73,000 a year.

After a few years of smoking, the most powerful incentive for continuing to smoke is to avoid the discomfort of withdrawal. Generally, 10 cigarettes a day will prevent withdrawal effects. For many who smoke heavily, signs of withdrawal, including changes in mood and performance, occur within two hours after smoking their last cigarette. Smokeless tobacco users also get constant doses of nicotine. However, absorption of nicotine by the lungs is more likely to lead to dependence than absorption through the linings of the nose and mouth. As with other drugs of abuse, continued nicotine intake results in tolerance (the need for more of a drug to maintain the same effect), which is why only 2 percent of all smokers smoke just a few cigarettes a day, or smoke only occasionally.

# STUDENT SMOKING

| | | Percent (%) | | | | |
|---|---|---|---|---|---|---|
| | | Actual Use | | | Perceived Use | |
| Cigarette | Male | Female | Total | Male | Female | Total |
| Never used | 62.7 | 68.6 | 66.4 | 8.2 | 5.8 | 6.8 |
| Used, but not in the last 30 days | 18.1 | 17.4 | 17.6 | 12.0 | 9.8 | 10.6 |
| Used 1–9 days | 9.8 | 7.1 | 8.1 | 39.0 | 33.9 | 35.7 |
| Used 10–29 days | 3.6 | 2.3 | 2.7 | 21.6 | 23.5 | 22.7 |
| Used all 30 days | 5.8 | 4.7 | 5.2 | 19.3 | 27.0 | 24.2 |
| Any use within the last 30 days | 19.2 | 14.0 | 16.0 | 79.8 | 84.4 | 82.7 |

## HOW DO YOU COMPARE?

The gap between the actual percentage of students who have never smoked cigarettes and the perceived number is huge: 66 percent versus 6.8 percent. If you are among the majority of nonsmokers, what has helped you say no to tobacco? If you smoked in the past, what were your reasons for starting? If you still smoke, what keeps you lighting up? Write down your reflections on tobacco in your online journal.

Source: American College Health Association, *American College Health Association-National College Health Assessment II: Reference Group Executive Summary Spring 2010* (Linthicum, MD: American College Health Association, 2010).

## Use of Other Substances

Many smokers also drink or use drugs. According to the Addiction Research Foundation in Canada, tobacco smokers say cigarettes are harder to abandon than other drugs, even when they find them less pleasurable than their preferred drug of abuse. Individuals who drink excessively also find their cigarette habit a hard one to break.

## Tobacco Use on Campus

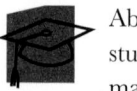

About one in every four to five students currently smokes, but a majority—66 percent—have never smoked.[5] (See How Do You Compare?) Many students who had never tried smoking may experiment with cigarettes in college. However, eight in ten college smokers started smoking before age 18. They report smoking on twice as many days and smoke nearly four times as many cigarettes as those who began smoking at an older age.

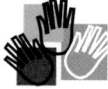

White students have the highest smoking rates, followed by Hispanic, Asian, and African American students. Although black students are least likely to smoke, more are doing so than in the past. Smoking rates remain consistently lower at predominantly black colleges and universities, however. About equal percentages of college men and women smoke although women are somewhat more likely than men to report smoking daily.

Many college students say they smoke as a way of managing depression or stress. Studies consistently link smoking with depression and low life satisfaction. Smokers are significantly more likely to have higher levels of perceived stress than nonsmokers. In one study, students who had been diagnosed or treated for depression were seven times as likely as other students to use tobacco. The more depressed students, particularly women, are the more likely they are to use nicotine as a form of self-medication.[6]

Male students who smoke are more likely to say that smoking makes them feel more masculine and less anxious. More than half of female smokers feel that smoking helps them control their weight, although only 3 percent say it is their primary reason for smoking. Overweight female students are more likely to smoke to lose weight and to see weight gain as a barrier to quitting.

Students can and do change their smoking behavior. In one study, over the course of four years of college, about half of students who smoked every few days, every few weeks, or every few months quit, as did 13 percent of daily smokers. More than a quarter of daily smokers cut back. On the other hand, 12 percent of nonsmokers took up the habit, and most daily smokers continued to smoke through the end of college.

## Social Smoking

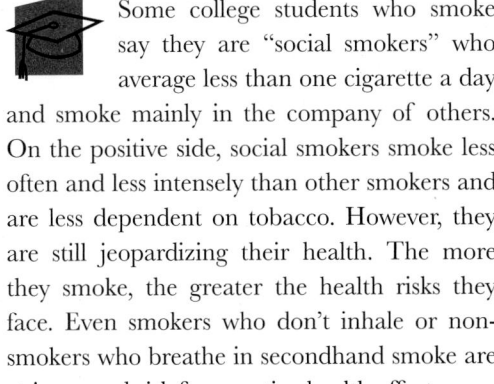 Some college students who smoke say they are "social smokers" who average less than one cigarette a day and smoke mainly in the company of others. On the positive side, social smokers smoke less often and less intensely than other smokers and are less dependent on tobacco. However, they are still jeopardizing their health. The more they smoke, the greater the health risks they face. Even smokers who don't inhale or nonsmokers who breathe in secondhand smoke are at increased risk for negative health effects.

In research studies, smoking less than a pack a week of cigarettes has proved to damage the lining of blood vessels and to increase the risk of heart disease as well as of cancer. In women taking birth control pills, even a few cigarettes a week can increase the likelihood of heart disease, blood clots, stroke, liver cancer, and gallbladder disease. Pregnant women who smoke only occasionally still run a higher risk of giving birth to unhealthy babies. Another risk is addiction. Social smokers are less motivated to quit and make fewer attempts to do so. Many end up smoking more cigarettes for many more years than they intended.

## College Tobacco-Control Policies

A growing number of colleges are stamping out smoking on campus. More than 140 schools are completely smoke-free; an additional 30 have banned smoking everywhere but in designated outdoor areas. At least 500 campuses have smoke-free policies in residential housing.

Several national health organizations, including the American College Health Association and the National Center on Addiction and Substance Abuse, have recommended that colleges ban smoking in and around all campus buildings, including student housing, and prohibit the sale, advertisement, and promotion of tobacco products on campus. Universities that have banned smoking from designated residence halls report decreased damage to the buildings, increased retention of students, and improved enforcement of marijuana policies. In general, schools in the West have done the most to implement tobacco policies. Those in the South, particularly in the major tobacco-growing states, have done the least.

# Smoking, Gender, and Race

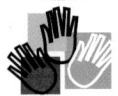 Almost 1 billion men in the world smoke—about 35 percent of men in developed countries and 50 percent of men in developing countries. In all but four countries, one in every four adults currently smokes.[7] Male smoking rates are slowly declining, but tobacco still kills about 5 million men every year. In general, higher-educated men are abandoning tobacco addiction, while poorer, less-educated men continue to smoke.[8]

High nicotine intake may affect male hormones, including testosterone. Smoking also can reduce blood flow to the penis, impairing a man's sexual performance and increasing the likelihood of erectile dysfunction.

Smoking is a risk factor for developing rheumatoid arthritis for men, but not for women. Women who smoke are more likely to develop osteoporosis, a bone weakening disease. On average, girls who begin smoking during adolescence continue smoking for 20 years, four years longer than boys. Women are at greater risk for developing smoking-related illnesses compared with men who smoke the same amount. Lung cancer now claims more women's lives than breast cancer. As discussed later in this chapter, both active and passive smoking increase a woman's risk of breast cancer. In men, cigarette smoking increases the risk of aggressive prostate cancer.

About 250 million women in the world are daily smokers—22 percent of women in developed countries and 9 percent of women in low- and middle-resource countries. Cigarette smoking among women is declining in the United States, but in several southern, central, and eastern European countries, cigarette smoking rates among women are either stable or increasing.

According to the U.S. Surgeon General, women account for 39 percent of smoking-related deaths each year, a proportion that has doubled since 1965. Each year, American women lose an estimated 2.1 million years of life due to premature deaths attributable to smoking. If she smokes, a woman's annual risk of dying more than doubles after age 45 compared with a woman who has never smoked.

Smoking directly affects women's reproductive organs and processes. Women who smoke are less fertile and experience menopause one or two years earlier than women who don't smoke. Smoking also greatly increases the possible risks associated with taking oral contraceptives.

Women who smoke during pregnancy increase their risk of miscarriage and pregnancy complications, including bleeding, premature delivery, and birth defects such as cleft lip or palate. Smoking narrows the blood vessels and reduces blood flow to the fetus, resulting in lower birth weight, shorter length, smaller head circumference, and possibly lower IQ. Youngsters whose mothers smoked during pregnancy also tend to have problems with hyperactivity, inattention, and impulsivity. Some of these behavior problems persist through the teenage years and even into adulthood. At ages 16 to 18, children exposed to prenatal smoking have higher rates of conduct disorder, substance use, and depression than others.

Cigarette smoking is a major cause of disease and death in all population groups. However, tobacco use varies within and among racial and ethnic minority groups. Among adults, Native Americans and Alaska Natives have the highest rates of tobacco use. African American and Southeast Asian men also have a high smoking rate. Asian American and Hispanic women

have the lowest rates of smoking. Tobacco use is significantly higher among white college students than among Hispanic, African American, and Asian American students.

Tobacco is the substance most abused by Hispanic youth, whose smoking rates have soared in the last ten years. In general, smoking rates among Hispanic adults increase as they adopt the values, beliefs, and norms of American culture. Recent declines in the prevalence of smoking have been greater among Hispanic men with at least a high school education than among those with less education.

# Tobacco's Immediate Effects

Tobacco, an herb that can be smoked or chewed, directly affects the brain. While its primary active ingredient is nicotine, tobacco smoke contains almost 400 other compounds and chemicals, including gases, liquids, particles, tar, carbon monoxide, cadmium, pyridine, nitrogen dioxide, ammonia, benzene, phenol, acrolein, hydrogen cyanide, formaldehyde, and hydrogen sulfide.

## How Nicotine Works

A colorless, oily compound, **nicotine** is poisonous in concentrated amounts. If you inhale while smoking, 90 percent of the nicotine in the smoke is absorbed into your body. Even if you draw smoke only into your mouth and not into your lungs, you still absorb 25 to 30 percent of the nicotine. The FDA has concluded that nicotine is a dangerous, addictive drug that should be regulated. Yet in recent years tobacco companies have increased the levels of addictive nicotine by an average of 1.6 percent per year.

Faster than an injection, smoking speeds nicotine to the brain in seconds (Figure 14.1). Nicotine affects the brain in much the same way as cocaine, opiates, and amphetamines, triggering the release of dopamine, a neurotransmitter associated with pleasure and addiction, as well as other messenger chemicals. Because nicotine acts on some of the same brain regions

**nicotine** The addictive substance in tobacco; one of the most toxic of all poisons.

stimulated by interactions with loved ones, smokers subconsciously come to regard cigarettes as a friend that they turn to when they're stressed, sad, or mad.

Nicotine may enhance smokers' performance on some tasks but leaves other mental skills unchanged. Nicotine also acts as a sedative. How often you smoke and how you smoke determine nicotine's effect on you. If you're a regular smoker, nicotine will generally stimulate you at first, then tranquilize you. Shallow puffs tend to increase alertness because low doses of nicotine facilitate the release of the neurotransmitter *acetylcholine*, which makes the smoker feel alert. Deep drags, on the other hand, relax the smoker because high doses of nicotine block the flow of acetylcholine.

Nicotine stimulates the adrenal glands to produce adrenaline, a hormone that increases blood pressure, speeds up the heart rate by 15 to 20 beats a minute, and constricts blood vessels (especially in the skin). Nicotine also inhibits the formation of urine, dampens hunger, irritates the membranes in the mouth and throat, and dulls the taste buds so foods don't taste as good as they would otherwise.

Nicotine withdrawal usually begins within hours. Symptoms include craving, irritability, anxiety, restlessness, and increased appetite.

## Tar and Carbon Monoxide

As it burns, tobacco produces **tar**, a thick, sticky dark fluid made up of several hundred different chemicals—many of them poisonous, some of them *carcinogenic* (enhancing the growth of cancerous cells). As you inhale tobacco smoke, tar and other particles settle in the forks of the branchlike bronchial tubes in your lungs, where precancerous changes are apt to occur. In addition, tar and smoke damage the mucus and the cilia in the bronchial tubes, which normally remove irritating foreign materials from your lungs.

Smoke from cigarettes, cigars, and pipes also contains **carbon monoxide**, the deadly gas that comes out of the exhaust pipes of cars, in levels 400 times those considered safe in industry. Carbon monoxide interferes with the ability of the hemoglobin in the blood to carry oxygen, impairs normal functioning of the nervous

Figure 14.1 **The Immediate Effects of Nicotine on the Body**

The primary active ingredient in tobacco is nicotine, a fast-acting and potent drug.

Sources: American Cancer Society, National Cancer Institute.

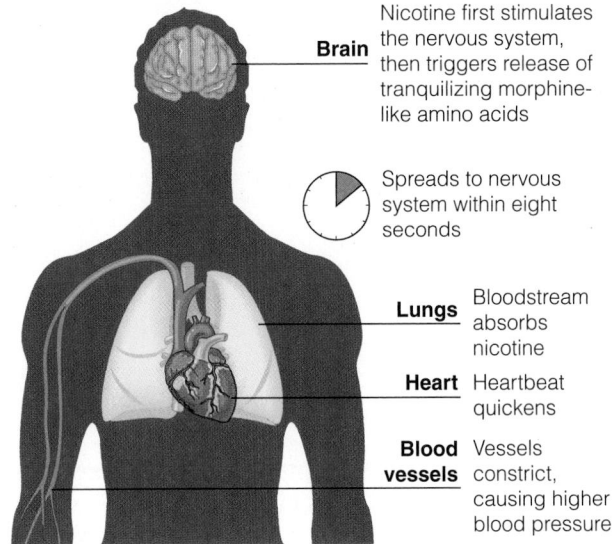

Brain — Nicotine first stimulates the nervous system, then triggers release of tranquilizing morphine-like amino acids

Spreads to nervous system within eight seconds

Lungs — Bloodstream absorbs nicotine

Heart — Heartbeat quickens

Blood vessels — Vessels constrict, causing higher blood pressure

system, and is at least partly responsible for the increased risk of heart attacks and strokes in smokers.

# Health Effects of Cigarette Smoking

Figure 14.2 shows a summary of the physiological effects of tobacco and the other chemicals in tobacco smoke. If you're a smoker who inhales deeply and started smoking before the age of 15, you're trading a minute of future life for every minute you now spend smoking. Smoking's effect on your chance of dying is similar to adding five to ten years to your age. A 55-year-old man or woman who smokes has about the same risk of dying in the next decade as a 65-year-old who never smoked. Smoking is responsible for 64 percent of deaths in current smokers and 28 percent in past smokers.

A cigarette smoker is 10 times more likely to develop lung cancer than a nonsmoker and 20 times more likely to have a heart attack. Heavy smoking, as well as secondhand smoke

**tar** A thick, sticky dark fluid produced by the burning of tobacco, made up of several hundred different chemicals, many of them poisonous, some of them carcinogenic.

**carbon monoxide** A colorless, odorless gas produced by the burning of gasoline or tobacco; displaces oxygen in the hemoglobin molecules of red blood cells.

## Figure 14.2  Some Effects of Smoking on the Body

Smoking harms the respiratory system and the cardiorespiratory system. The leading cause of death for smokers is heart attack.

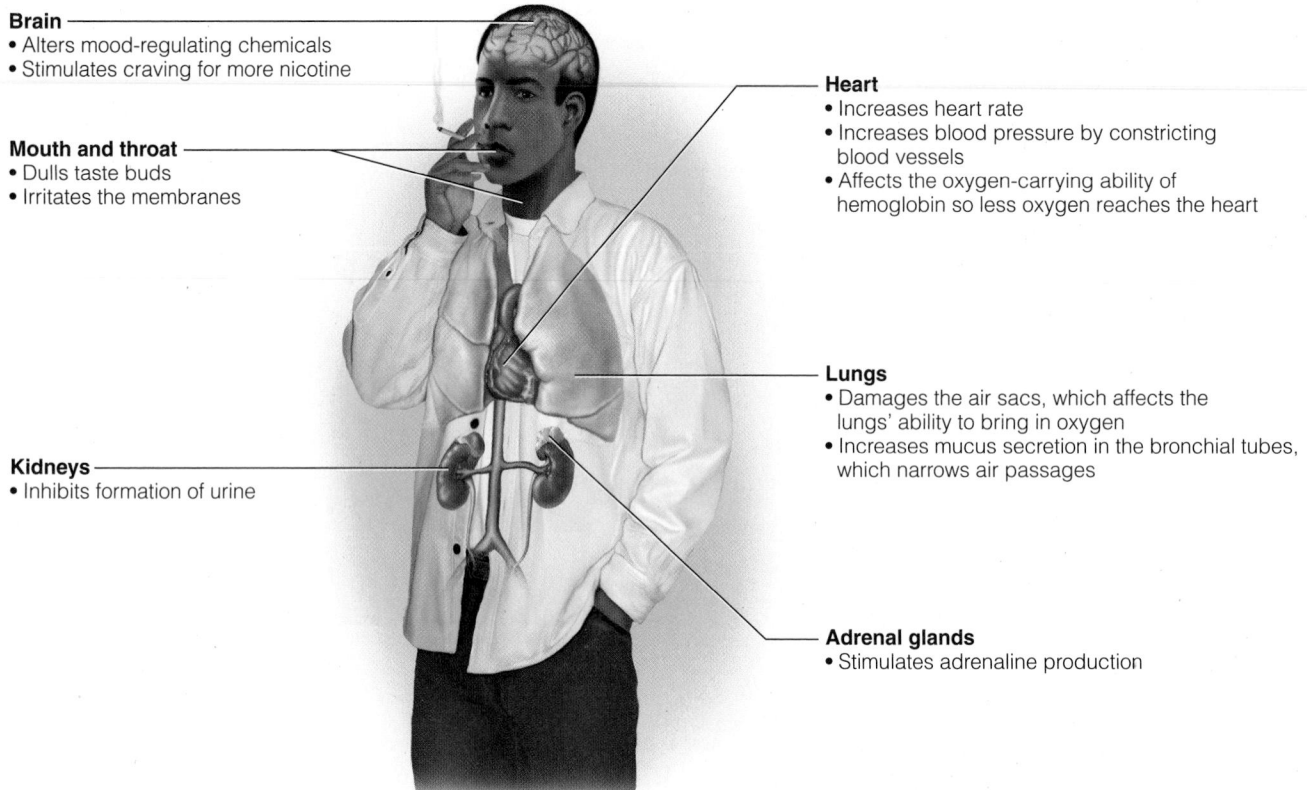

**Brain**
- Alters mood-regulating chemicals
- Stimulates craving for more nicotine

**Mouth and throat**
- Dulls taste buds
- Irritates the membranes

**Kidneys**
- Inhibits formation of urine

**Heart**
- Increases heart rate
- Increases blood pressure by constricting blood vessels
- Affects the oxygen-carrying ability of hemoglobin so less oxygen reaches the heart

**Lungs**
- Damages the air sacs, which affects the lungs' ability to bring in oxygen
- Increases mucus secretion in the bronchial tubes, which narrows air passages

**Adrenal glands**
- Stimulates adrenaline production

(discussed later in this chapter), can increase a woman's risk of breast cancer.[9] Daily smokers also are more likely to have suicidal thoughts or attempt suicide, although the reasons are not clear (see Chapter 2).

## Health Effects on Students

 Although little research has focused specifically on college students, young people who smoke are less physically fit and suffer diminished lung function and growth. Young smokers frequently report symptoms such as wheezing, shortness of breath, coughing, and increased phlegm. They also are more susceptible to respiratory diseases. Young smokers are three times more likely to have consulted a doctor or mental health professional because of an emotional or psychological problem and almost twice as likely to develop symptoms of depression. Frequent smoking also has been linked to panic attacks and panic disorder in young people.

Long-term health consequences of smoking in young adulthood include dental problems, lung disorders (including asthma, chronic bronchitis, and emphysema), heart disease, and cancer. Young women who smoke may develop menstrual problems, including irregular periods and painful cramps. If they use oral contraceptives, they are at increased risk of heart disease or stroke.

## Heart Disease and Stroke

The toxic chemicals in tobacco signal the heart to beat faster and harder. Blood vessels constrict, forcing blood to travel through a narrower space. Blood pressure increases—temporarily at first. Over time, smokers develop chronic high blood pressure. Smoking increases harmful cholesterol (LDL) and lowers beneficial cholesterol (HDL). It also leads to the buildup of plaque, or fatty deposits within the arteries; hardening of the arteries; and greater risk of blood clots. Both current and former smokers run a higher risk for an abnormal heart rhythm.

Although a great deal of publicity has been given to the link between cigarettes and lung cancer, heart attack is actually the leading cause of death for smokers. Smoking doubles the risk of heart disease and increases the risk of sudden death two to four times. The effect of smoking on risk of heart attack is greater in younger smokers. The number of cigarettes smoked daily may have a greater impact on the cardiovascular system than total years of smoking.[10]

Smokers who suffer heart attacks have only a 50 percent chance of recovering. Smokers have a 70 percent higher death rate from heart disease than nonsmokers, and those who smoke heavily have a 200 percent higher death rate.

The federal Office of the Surgeon General blames cigarettes for one of every ten deaths attributable to heart disease. Smoking is more dangerous than the two most notorious risk factors for heart disease: high blood pressure and high cholesterol. If smoking is combined with one of these, the chances of heart attack are four times greater. Women who smoke and use oral contraceptives have a ten times higher risk of suffering heart attacks than women who do neither.

In addition to contributing to heart attacks, cigarette smoking increases the risk of stroke two to three times in men and women, even after other risk factors are taken into account.

Even people who have smoked for decades can reduce their risk of heart attack if they quit smoking. However, studies indicate some irreversible damage to blood vessels. Progression of atherosclerosis (hardening of the arteries) among former smokers continues at a faster pace than among those who never smoked.

## Lung Cancer

Smoking is linked to at least ten different cancers and accounts for 30 percent of all deaths from cancer. Smoking is the cause of more than 80 percent of all cases of lung cancer. The more people smoke, the longer they smoke, and the earlier they start smoking, the more likely they are to develop lung cancer.

Smoking causes about 130,000 lung cancer deaths each year. Smokers of two or more packs a day have lung cancer mortality rates 15 to 25 times greater than nonsmokers. If smokers stop smoking before cancer has started, their lung tissue tends to repair itself, even if there were already precancerous changes. However, their risk is never as low as that of individuals who never smoked.[11] In a recent study, a significant percentage (about one in five) of patients diagnosed with lung cancer continued to smoke even though doing so could jeopardize their recovery.[12]

Chemicals in cigarette smoke and other environmental pollutants switch on a particular gene in the lung cells of some individuals. This gene produces an enzyme that helps manufacture powerful carcinogens, which set the stage for cancer. The gene seems more likely to be activated in some people than in others, and people with this gene are at much higher risk of developing lung cancer. However, smokers without the gene still remain at risk, because other chemicals and genes also may be involved in the development of lung cancer.

Smokers who are depressed are more likely to get cancer than nondepressed smokers. Although researchers don't know exactly how smoking and depression may work together to increase the risk of cancer, one possibility is that stress and depression cause biological changes that lower immunity, such as a decline in natural killer cells that fight off tumors.

## Respiratory Diseases

Smoking quickly impairs the respiratory system, including the cough reflex, a vital protective response. Even some teenage smokers show signs of respiratory difficulty—breathlessness, chronic cough, excess phlegm production—when compared with nonsmokers of the same age. Cigarette smokers are up to 18 times more likely than nonsmokers to die of noncancerous diseases of the lungs.

Cigarette smoking is the major cause of chronic obstructive pulmonary disease (COPD), which includes emphysema and chronic bronchitis. COPD is characterized by progressive limitation of the flow of air into and out of the lungs. In emphysema, the limitation of air flow is the result of disease changes in the lung tissue, affecting the bronchioles (the smallest air passages) and the walls of the alveoli (the tiny air sacs of the lung). Eventually, many of the air sacs are destroyed, and the lungs become much

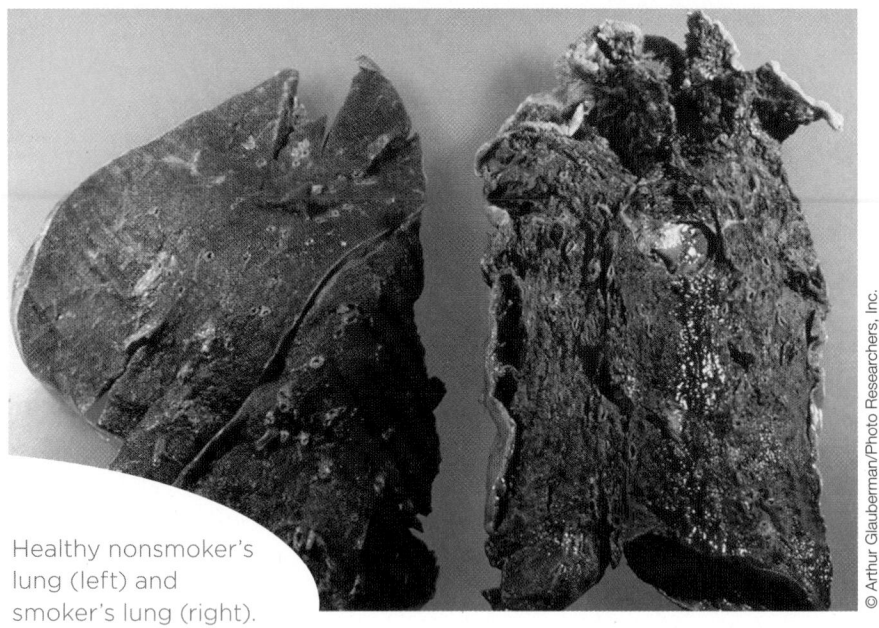

Healthy nonsmoker's lung (left) and smoker's lung (right). Healthy lungs are pink, with a smooth but porous texture. A smoker's lungs show obvious signs of impairment. Bronchial tubes are inflamed, air passages are constricted, and tar coats the bronchial tubes.

© Arthur Glauberman/Photo Researchers, Inc.

primarily because of respiratory illnesses. The link between smoking and asthma has proven stronger than suspected, and individuals with asthma are much more likely to have a history of nicotine dependence.[13] In addition, each year cigarette-ignited fires claim thousands of lives.

Smoking is an independent risk factor for high-frequency hearing loss and also adds to the danger of hearing loss for those exposed to noise. Cigarette smoking also may increase the likelihood of anxiety, panic attacks, and social phobias.

less able to bring in oxygen and remove carbon dioxide. As a result, the heart has to work harder to deliver oxygen to all organs of the body.

In chronic bronchitis, the bronchial tubes in the lungs become inflamed, thickening the walls of the bronchi, and the production of mucus increases. The result is a narrowing of the air passages. Smoking is more dangerous than any form of air pollution, at least for most Americans, but exposure to both air pollution and cigarettes is particularly harmful.

## Other Smoking-Related Problems

Smokers are more likely than nonsmokers to develop gum disease, and they lose significantly more teeth. Even those who quit have worse gum problems than people who never smoked at all. Smoking may also contribute to the loss of teeth and teeth-supporting bone, even in individuals with good oral hygiene.

Cigarette smoking is associated with stomach and duodenal ulcers; mouth, throat, and other types of cancer; and cirrhosis of the liver. Smoking may worsen the symptoms or complications of allergies, diabetes, hypertension, peptic ulcers, and disorders of the lungs or blood vessels. Some men who smoke ten cigarettes or more a day may experience erectile dysfunction. Cigarette smokers also tend to miss work one-third more often than nonsmokers,

# Other Forms of Tobacco

Two percent of Americans smoke cigars; 2 percent use smokeless tobacco. Ingesting tobacco may be less deadly than smoking cigarettes, but it is dangerous. Smoking cigars, clove cigarettes, and pipes and chewing or sucking on smokeless tobacco all put the user at risk of cancer of the lip, tongue, mouth, and throat, as well as other diseases and ailments. Despite claims of lower risk, "safer" cigarettes still jeopardize smokers' health.

## Cigars

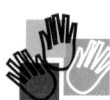

Cigar use has declined in the last few years. However, after cigarettes, cigars are the tobacco product most widely used by college students. About 16 percent of college men (and 4 percent of women) smoke cigars. White and African American students are more likely to smoke cigars than Hispanic or Asian American students.

Even though cigar smokers may not inhale, a byproduct of nicotine called continine builds up in their blood.[14] Cigars can cause cancer of the lung and the digestive tract. The risk of death related to cigars approaches that of cigarettes, depending on the number of cigars smoked and the amount of cigar smoke inhaled.

Neither pipes nor cigars are "healthier" alternatives to cigarettes. "Inhalation of tobacco smoke by any means is deleterious," concluded researchers who found that both pipes and cigars raise blood levels of cotinine.[15]

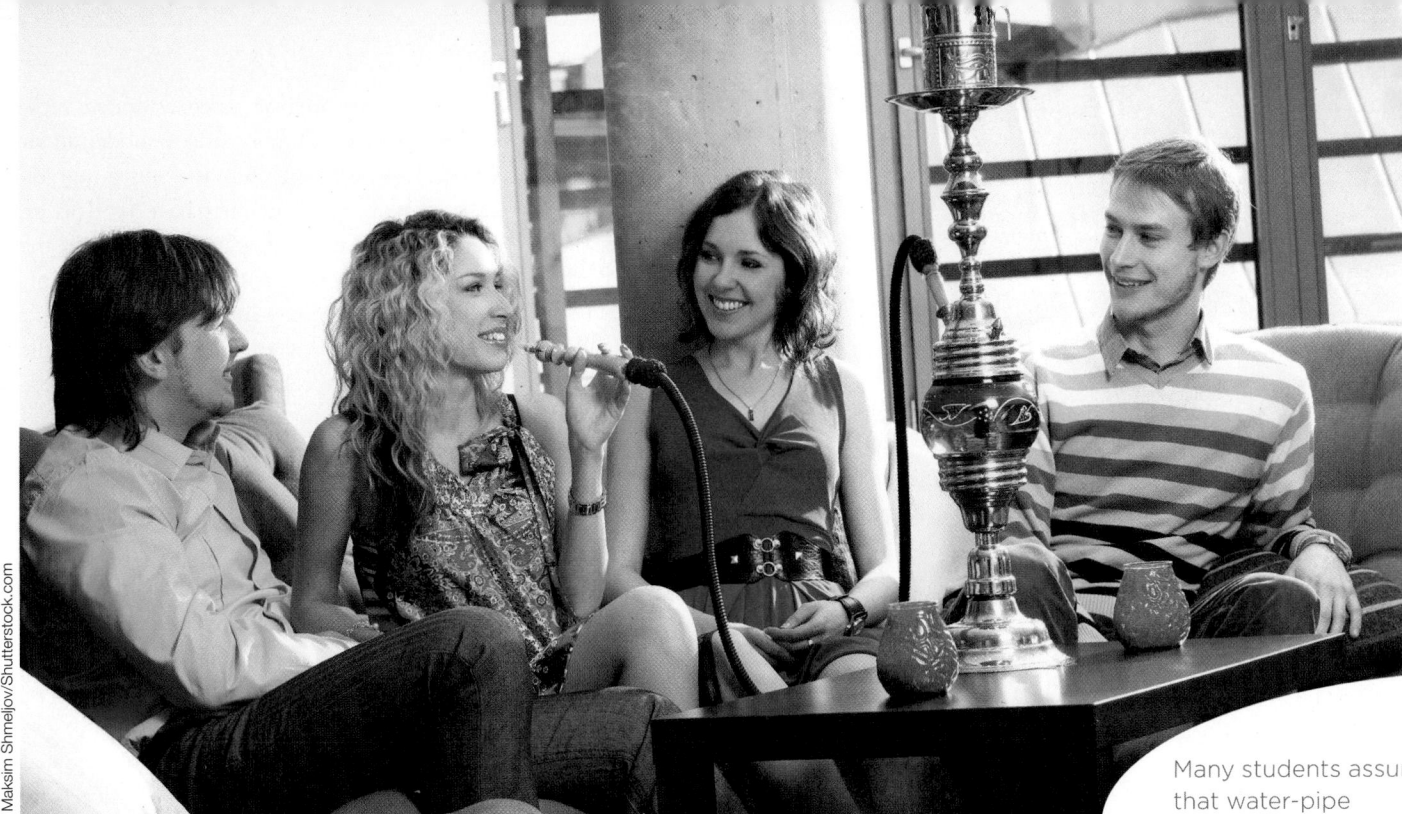

Many students assume that water-pipe smoking is safer than cigarette smoking, but the risks are similar.

# Water Pipes (Hookahs)

A water pipe (known by different terms, such as hookah, narghile, arghile, and hubble-bubble, in different parts of the world) involves the passage of smoke through water prior to inhalation. Although also used to smoke other substances, including marijuana and hashish, water pipes are most often used with flavored tobacco, made by mixing shredded tobacco with honey or molasses and dried fruit. This mix is most commonly called shisha in the United States.

According to the ACHA's National College Health Assessment, about 31 percent of college students have smoked tobacco from a water pipe (see Table 14.1). As with conventional cigarettes, students overestimate their peers' use of hookahs.[16]

Many students assume that water-pipe smoking is safer than cigarette smoking, but the existing research indicates that the risks are similar. In a recent meta-analysis, water-pipe smoking was significantly associated with lung cancer, respiratory illnesses, low birth weight, and periodontal disease. Mainstream water-pipe smoke (the smoke inhaled by a user) contains large amounts of carcinogens, hydrocarbons, and heavy metals, including 36 times the amount of tar in cigarette smoke.[17]

Water-pipe smoking usually occurs in a group setting. Commercial water-pipe venues, offering ready-to-smoke water pipes, have proliferated in many college towns. Students who use water pipes tend to be younger, male, and white. They also are more likely than other undergraduates to perceive water-pipe tobacco smoking as less harmful and less addictive than cigarette smoking.

Table 14.1 **Tobacco from a Water Pipe (Hookah)**

| | Percent (%) | | | | | |
|---|---|---|---|---|---|---|
| | **Actual Use** | | | **Perceived Use** | | |
| | Male | Female | Total | Male | Female | Total |
| Never used | 64.3 | 72.1 | 69.2 | 15.4 | 12.7 | 13.8 |
| Used, but not in the last 30 days | 25.0 | 21.3 | 22.6 | 20.4 | 18.1 | 18.9 |
| Used 1–9 days | 9.3 | 6.0 | 7.2 | 49.5 | 51.2 | 50.5 |
| Used 10–29 days | 1.1 | 0.5 | 0.7 | 10.3 | 13.4 | 12.3 |
| Used all 30 days | 0.4 | 0.1 | 0.2 | 4.4 | 4.5 | 4.5 |
| Any use within the last 30 days | 10.7 | 6.6 | 8.1 | 64.2 | 69.1 | 67.3 |

Source: American College Health Association, *American College Health Association-National College Health Assessment II: Reference Group Executive Summary Spring 2010* (Linthicum, MD: American College Health Association, 2010).

## Pipes

Many cigarette smokers switch to pipes to reduce their risk of health problems. But former cigarette smokers may continue to inhale, even though pipe smoke is more irritating to the respiratory system than cigarette smoke. People who have smoked only pipes and who do not inhale are less likely to develop lung and heart disease than cigarette smokers. However, they are likely to suffer respiratory problems and to develop—and die of—cancer of the mouth, larynx, throat, and esophagus.[18]

## Bidis

Skinny, sweet-flavored cigarettes called **bidis** (pronounced "beedees") have become a smoking fad among teens and young adults. For centuries, bidis were popular in India, where they are known as the poor man's cigarette and sell for less than five cents a pack. They look strikingly like clove cigarettes or marijuana joints and are available in flavors like grape, strawberry, and mandarin orange. Bidis are legal for adults and even minors in some states and are sold on the Internet as well as in stores.

Although bidis contain less tobacco than regular cigarettes, their unprocessed tobacco is more potent. Smoke from bidis has about three times as much nicotine and carbon monoxide and five times as much tar as smoke from regular filtered cigarettes. Because bidis are wrapped in nonporous brownish leaves, they don't burn as easily as cigarettes, and smokers have to inhale harder and more often to keep them lit. In one study, smoking a single bidi required 28 puffs, compared to 9 puffs for cigarettes.

## Clove Cigarettes

Sweeteners have long been mixed with tobacco, and clove, a spice, is the latest ingredient to be added to the recipe for cigarettes. Clove cigarettes typically contain two-thirds tobacco and one-third clove. Consumers of these cigarettes are primarily teenagers and young adults.

Many users believe that clove cigarettes are safer because they contain less tobacco, but this isn't necessarily the case. The CDC reports that people who smoke clove cigarettes may be at risk of serious lung injury.

**bidis** Skinny, sweet-flavored cigarettes.

Clove cigarettes deliver twice as much nicotine, tar, and carbon monoxide as moderate-tar American brands. Eugenol, the active ingredient in cloves (which dentists have used as an anesthetic for years), deadens sensation in the throat, allowing smokers to inhale more deeply and hold smoke in their lungs for a longer time. Chemical relatives of eugenol can produce the kind of damage to cells that may lead to cancer.

## Smokeless Tobacco

An estimated 3 percent of adults in the United States use smokeless tobacco products (sometimes called "spit").[19] Use of chewing tobacco by teenage boys, particularly in rural areas, has surged 30 percent in the last decade. About 9 percent of college men (and 0.4 percent of women) are smokeless tobacco users. These substances include snuff, finely ground tobacco that can be sniffed or placed inside the cheek and sucked, and chewing tobacco, tobacco leaves mixed with flavoring agents such as molasses. With both, nicotine is absorbed through the mucous membranes of the nose or mouth.

Smokeless tobacco causes a user's heart rate, blood pressure, and epinephrine (adrenaline) levels to jump. In addition, it can cause cancer and noncancerous oral conditions and lead to nicotine addiction and dependence. People who use smokeless tobacco, or "snuff," become just as hooked on nicotine as cigarette smokers—if not more. Those who both smoke and use snuff may be especially nicotine dependent.[20]

Powerful carcinogens in smokeless tobacco include nitrosamines, polycyclic aromatic hydrocarbons, and radiation-emitting polonium. Its use can lead to the development of white patches on the mucous membranes of the mouth, particularly on the site where the tobacco is placed. Most lesions of the mouth lining that result from the use of smokeless tobacco dissipate six weeks after the use of the tobacco product is stopped. However, when first found, about 5 percent of these lesions are cancerous or exhibit changes that progress to cancer within ten years if not properly treated. Cancers of the lip, pharynx, larynx, and esophagus have all been linked to smokeless tobacco. Nicotine replacement with gum or patches decreases cravings for smokeless tobacco and helps with short-term abstinence.

However, it does not improve long-term abstinence. Behavioral approaches are more effective for long-term quitting.

# Quitting

The U.S. Public Health Service's most recent guidelines for treating tobacco use and dependence recognize tobacco dependence as "a chronic disease that often requires repeated intervention and multiple attempts to quit. Effective treatments exist, however, that can significantly increase rates of long-term abstinence."

More than 70 percent of the 45 million smokers in the United States say they want to quit; approximately 44 percent try to quit each year. Yet only 4 to 7 percent succeed in any given year.

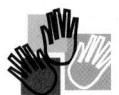 About half of whites who have smoked were able to kick the habit, compared with 45 percent of Asian Americans, 43 percent of Hispanics, and 37 percent of African Americans. About eight in ten African Americans choose menthol cigarettes, compared with just one-quarter of adults of other races, which may make quitting harder. According to recent research, menthol smokers smoke fewer cigarettes per day than smokers of regular cigarettes but may be inhaling as much if not more nicotine, which creates a stronger addiction. Menthol smokers may be "twice-addicted"—both to the menthol, which makes it easier to inhale, and to the tobacco.[21]

Men and women with college and graduate degrees were much more likely to quit successfully than high school dropouts. Quitting eliminates the excess risk of dying from heart disease fairly quickly; after 20 smoke-free years the risk of smoking-related cancers drops to that of someone who never smoked.

Compared with men, women seem to have a higher behavioral dependence on cigarettes. For them, wearing a nicotine patch or chewing nicotine gum does not substitute for the "hand-to-mouth" behaviors associated with smoking, such as lighting a cigarette, inhaling, and handling the cigarette. Some investigators have found that women are more likely to quit successfully when they receive a combination of nicotine replacement and the use of a device like the Nicotine Inhaler to substitute for smoking behaviors.

 While counseling and medication are each beneficial, the combination is more effective than either alone. In a study of community college students, a computer-assisted interactive smoking cessation program helped 17 percent stop. One campus-based program that employed peer facilitators to help smokers quit and avoid relapse reported a success rate of 88 percent. Being "in the group" was the single most powerful contributor to quitting, and participants said their sense of connectedness helped them quit and stay smoke-free.

Nicotine withdrawal symptoms can behave like characters in a bad horror movie: Just when you think you've killed them, they're back with a vengeance. In recent studies, some people who tried to quit smoking reported a small improvement in withdrawal symptoms over two weeks, but then their symptoms leveled off and persisted. Others found that their symptoms intensified rather than lessened over time. For reasons scientists cannot yet explain, former smokers who start smoking again put their lungs at even greater jeopardy than smokers who never quit.

Once a former smoker takes a single puff, the odds of a relapse are 80 to 85 percent. Smokers are most likely to quit in the third, fourth, or fifth attempt. But thanks to new products and programs, it may be easier now than ever before to become an ex-smoker.

## Quitting on Your Own

More than 90 percent of former smokers quit on their own—by throwing away all their cigarettes, by gradually cutting down, or by first switching to a less potent brand. One characteristic of successful quitters is that they see themselves as active participants in health maintenance and take personal responsibility for their own health. Physically active smokers have greater success quitting, possibly because participating in one healthy behavior, such as exercise, leads to adoption of other positive behaviors. Often they experiment with a variety of strategies, such as learning relaxation techniques. In women, exercise has proved especially effective for quitting and avoiding weight gain. Making a home a smoke-free zone also increases a smoker's likelihood of successfully quitting.

## Virtual Support

Electronic communications via cell phones, e-mails, text messages, blogs, and social networking sites may be particularly effective in helping young smokers quit. In the few research studies that have been done, these approaches generally resulted in higher quit rates—but only if continued over time. Short text messages can help individuals track their smoking urges and provide encouragement in resisting them.[22] Other options include "apps" for smart phones and online support groups.

## Stop-Smoking Groups

Joining a support group doubles your chances of quitting for good. The American Cancer Society's FreshStart program runs about 1,500 stop-smoking clinics, each with about 8 to 18 members meeting for eight 2-hour sessions over four weeks. Instructors explain the risks of smoking, encourage individuals to think about why they smoke, and suggest ways of unlearning their smoking habit. A quitting day is set for the third or fourth session.

The American Lung Association's Freedom from Smoking program consists of eight 1- to 2-hour sessions over seven weeks. The approach is similar to the American Cancer Society's, but smokers keep diaries and team up with buddies. Ex-smokers serve as advisers on quitting day. Both groups estimate that 27 or 28 percent of their participants successfully stop smoking.

Stop-smoking classes are also available through science departments and student health services on many college campuses, as well as through community public health departments. The Seventh-Day Adventists sponsor a four-week Breathe Free Plan, in which smokers commit themselves to clean living (no smoking, alcohol, tea, or coffee, along with a balanced diet and regular exercise).

Many businesses sponsor smoking-cessation programs for employees, which generally follow the approaches of professional groups. Motivation may be even higher in these programs than in programs outside the workplace because some companies offer attractive incentives to participants, such as lower rates on their health insurance.

Some smoking-cessation programs rely primarily on **aversion therapy**, which provides a negative experience every time a smoker has a cigarette. This may involve taking drugs that make tobacco smoke taste unpleasant, undergoing electric shocks, having smoke blown at you, or rapid smoking (the inhaling of smoke every six seconds until you're dizzy or nauseated).

Nicotine Anonymous, a nonprofit organization based on the 12 steps to recovery developed by Alcoholics Anonymous, acknowledges the power of nicotine and provides support to help smokers, chewers, and dippers live free of nicotine. New members are encouraged to abstain from using nicotine "one day at a time" and to attend meetings regularly. In addition to local meetings, NicA offers online support and networking, which puts people in touch with others in their region who share their desire to quit using nicotine.

## Nicotine Replacement Therapy (NRT)

This approach uses a variety of products that supply low doses of nicotine in a way that allows smokers to taper off gradually over a period of months. Nicotine replacement therapies include nonprescription products (nicotine gum, lozenges, nicotine-free cigarettes, and nicotine patches) and prescription products (nicotine nasal spray and nicotine inhaler). The nasal spray, dispensed from a pump bottle, delivers nicotine to the nasal membranes and reaches the bloodstream faster than any other nicotine replacement therapy product. The inhaler delivers nicotine into the mouth and enters the bloodstream much more slowly than the nicotine in cigarettes.

Smokers who use NRT are 1.5 to 2 times more likely to quit. Because nicotine is a powerful, addictive substance, using nicotine replacements for a prolonged period is not advised. Pregnant women and individuals with heart disease shouldn't use them.

The most effective approaches combine medication—nicotine patches or Zyban, for instance—with psychological intervention. Each doubles a person's chance of quitting successfully.

Nicotine replacement therapy has proved more beneficial for men than for women—particularly

**aversion therapy** A treatment that attempts to help a person overcome a dependence or bad habit by making the person feel disgusted or repulsed by that habit.

with higher doses of nicotine. Men who receive more nicotine achieve a higher quit rate than men getting lower doses.

For women, the nicotine "dose" does not have an impact on successful quitting. They are no more likely to stop smoking with high doses than with lower ones, indicating that they may be less dependent on nicotine than men.

*Nicotine Gum* Nicotine gum (now available in generics as well) contains a nicotine resin that's gradually released as the gum is chewed. Absorbed through the mucous membrane of the mouth, the nicotine doesn't produce the same rush as a deeply inhaled drag on a cigarette. However, the gum maintains enough nicotine in the blood to diminish withdrawal symptoms.

Although this gum is lightly spiced to mask nicotine's bitterness, many users say that it takes several days to become accustomed to its unusual taste. Its side effects include mild indigestion, sore jaws, nausea, heartburn, and stomachache. Also, because nicotine gum is heavier than regular chewing gum, it may loosen fillings or cause problems with dentures. Drinking coffee or other beverages may block absorption of the nicotine in the gum; individuals trying to quit smoking shouldn't ingest any substance immediately before or while chewing nicotine gum.

Most people use nicotine gum as a temporary crutch and gradually taper off until they can stop chewing it relatively painlessly. However, 5 to 10 percent of users transfer their dependence from cigarettes to the gum. When they stop using nicotine gum, they experience withdrawal symptoms, although the symptoms tend to be milder than those prompted by quitting cigarettes. Intensive counseling to teach smokers coping methods can greatly increase success rates.

*Nicotine Patches* Nicotine transdermal delivery system products, or patches, provide nicotine, their only active ingredient, via a patch attached to the skin by an adhesive. Like nicotine gum, the nicotine patch minimizes withdrawal symptoms, such as intense craving for cigarettes. Nicotine patches help nearly 20 percent of smokers quit entirely after six weeks, compared with 7 percent on a placebo patch. Some insurance programs pay for patch therapy. Nicotine patches, which cost between $3.25

© AJPhoto/Photo Researchers, Inc.

Nicotine gum, when chewed, gradually releases a nicotine resin and helps some smokers quit.

and $4 each, are replaced daily during therapy programs that run between 6 and 16 weeks. Extended use for 24 weeks rather than the standard eight provides added benefit.[23]

Some patches deliver nicotine around the clock and others for just 16 hours (during waking hours). Those most likely to benefit from nicotine patch therapy are people who smoke more than a pack a day, are highly motivated to quit, and participate in counseling programs. While using the patch, 37 to 77 percent of people are able to abstain from smoking. When combined with counseling, the patch can be about twice as effective as a placebo, enabling 26 percent of smokers to abstain for six months.

Patch wearers who smoke or use more than one patch at a time can experience a nicotine overdose; some users have even suffered heart attacks. Occasional side effects include redness,

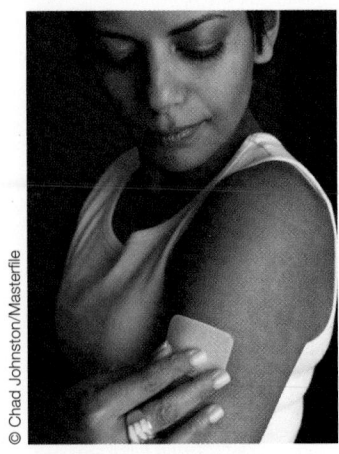

A nicotine patch releases nicotine through the skin in measured amounts, which are gradually decreased over time.

itching, or swelling at the site of the patch application; insomnia; dry mouth; and nervousness.

*Nicotine Inhaler*  Available only by prescription, the Nicotine Inhaler consists of a mouthpiece and a cartridge containing a nicotine-impregnated plug. The smoker inhales through the mouthpiece, using either shallow or deep puffs. The inhaled air becomes saturated with nicotine, which is absorbed mainly through the tissues of the mouth. The inhaler releases less nicotine per puff than a cigarette and does not contain a cigarette's harmful tars, carbon monoxide, and smoke. Treatment is recommended for 3 months with a gradual reduction over the next 6 to 12 weeks. Total treatment should not exceed 6 months.

## Medications

Another alternative to the patch is *bupropion*, a drug initially developed to treat depression, that is marketed in a slow-release form for nicotine addiction as Zyban. In studies that have combined Zyban with nicotine replacement and counseling, 40 to 60 percent of those treated have remained smoke-free for at least a year after completing the program. This success rate is much higher than the 10 to 26 percent reported among smokers who try to quit by using nicotine replacement alone. For women, combining medication with behavioral therapy to address weight issues has proven effective.[24] The combination of Zyban and nicotine replacement also prevented the initial weight gain that often accompanies quitting. Another medication used to treat nicotine addiction is varenicline (Chantix), which may be more effective if taken for a month rather than a week prior to quitting.[25]

## Other Ways to Quit

Hypnosis may help some people quit smoking. Hypnotherapists use their techniques to create an atmosphere of strict attention and give smokers in a mild trance positive suggestions for breaking their cigarette habit.

Acupuncture, in which a circular needle or staple is inserted in the flap in front of the opening to the ear, has also had some success. When smokers feel withdrawal symptoms, they gently move the needle or staple, which may increase the production of calming chemicals in the brain.

Since 1976, a November day has been set aside in the United States for the annual Great American Smoke-Out, an idea promoted by the American Cancer Society to encourage smokers to give up cigarettes for 24 hours.

## Quitting and the Risks Associated with Smoking

Not smoking another cigarette is a gift to your body and your life. (See Table 14.2.) It is not a guarantee that there will be no consequences of the cigarettes you've already smoked. (See "Health in Action.")

Within a year of quitting, an ex-smoker's risk of heart disease drops to half that of active smokers. After 15 years, it approaches that of people who've never smoked. This is great news because the risk of dying prematurely from heart disease is far greater than that of dying from cancer.

The risk of lung cancer from smoking fades more slowly, perhaps because of permanent DNA damage to lung cells. Even 10 to 15 years after quitting, an ex-smoker is several times more likely to die of lung cancer than someone who has never smoked. Former smokers are also more vulnerable to the effects of secondhand

Table 14.2 **Why Quit?**

**Quitting is the smartest choice a smoker can make—and keeps paying off far into the future. Consider these facts:**

- **20 minutes after quitting:** Your heart rate and blood pressure drop.
- **12 hours after quitting:** The carbon monoxide level in your blood drops to normal.
- **2 weeks to 3 months after quitting:** Your circulation improves and your lung function increases.
- **1 to 9 months after quitting:** Coughing and shortness of breath decrease; cilia (tiny hairlike structures that move mucus out of the lungs) regain normal function, increasing the ability to handle mucus, clean the lungs, and reduce the risk of infection.
- **1 year after quitting:** Your excess risk of coronary heart disease is half that of a smoker's.
- **5 years after quitting:** Your stroke risk is reduced to that of a nonsmoker.
- **10 years after quitting:** The lung cancer death rate is about half that of a continuing smoker's. Your risk of cancer of the mouth, throat, esophagus, bladder, cervix, and pancreas also decreases.
- **15 years after quitting:** Your risk of coronary heart disease is that of a nonsmoker's.

Source: American Cancer Society.

smoke in the workplace, even if they haven't lit up for the last ten years.

Does the lung cancer risk ever go away? That may depend partly on how old you are when you quit. Women who quit before age 30 are no more likely to die from lung cancer than those who never smoked. However, a study of American veterans started in the 1950s showed that, even 40 years later, former smokers had a 50 percent greater chance of dying from lung cancer than lifetime nonsmokers.

While quitting sooner is better than later, later is better than never. Even smokers who quit in their sixties significantly reduce their lung cancer risk—and add several years to their life expectancy.

# Environmental Tobacco Smoke

Maybe you don't smoke—never have, never will. That doesn't mean you don't have to worry about the dangers of smoking, especially if you live or work with people who smoke. **Environmental tobacco smoke**, or secondhand cigarette smoke, the most hazardous form of indoor air pollution, ranks behind cigarette smoking and alcohol as the third-leading preventable cause of death.

On average, a smoker inhales what is known as **mainstream smoke** eight or nine times with each cigarette, for a total of about 24 seconds. However, the cigarette burns for about 12 minutes, and everyone in the room (including the smoker) breathes in what is known as **sidestream smoke**.

According to the American Lung Association, incomplete combustion from the lower temperatures of a smoldering cigarette makes sidestream smoke dirtier and chemically different from mainstream smoke. It has twice as much tar and nicotine, five times as much carbon monoxide, and 50 times as much ammonia. And because the particles in sidestream smoke are small, this mixture of irritating gases and carcinogenic tar reaches deeper into the lungs and poses a greater threat to infants and children. If you're a nonsmoker sitting next to

## Health in Action

### Kicking the Habit
Here's a six-point program to help you or someone you love quit smoking. (Caution: Don't undertake the quit-smoking program until you have a two- to four-week period of relatively unstressful work and study schedules or social commitments.)

1. **Identify your smoking habits**. Keep a daily diary (a piece of paper wrapped around your cigarette pack with a rubber band will do) and record the time you smoke, the activity associated with smoking (after breakfast, in the car), and your urge for a cigarette (desperate, pleasant, or automatic). For the first week or two, don't bother trying to cut down; just use the diary to learn the conditions under which you smoke.
2. **Get support.** It can be tough to go it alone. Phone your local chapter of the American Cancer Society or Nicotine Anonymous or otherwise get the names of some ex-smokers who can give you support.
3. **Begin by tapering off.** For a period of one to four weeks, aim at cutting down to, say, 12 or 15 cigarettes a day; or change to a lower-nicotine brand and concentrate on not increasing the number of cigarettes you smoke. As indicated by your diary, begin by cutting out those cigarettes you smoke automatically. In addition, restrict the times you allow yourself to smoke. Throughout this period, stay in touch, once a day or every few days, with your ex-smoker friend(s) to discuss your problems.
4. **Set a quit date.** At some point during the tapering-off period, announce to everyone—friends, family, and ex-smokers—when you're going to quit. Do it with flair. Announce it to coincide with a significant date, such as your birthday or anniversary.
5. **Stop.** A week before Q-day, smoke only five cigarettes a day. Begin late in the day, say after 4:00 p.m. Smoke the first two cigarettes in close succession. Then, in the evening, smoke the last three, also in close succession, about 15 minutes apart. Focus on the negative aspects of cigarettes, such as the rawness in your throat and lungs. After seven days, quit and give yourself a big reward on that day, such as a movie or a fantastic meal or new clothes.
6. **Follow up.** Stay in touch with your ex-smoker friend(s) during the following two weeks, particularly if anything stressful or tense occurs that might trigger a return to smoking. Think of the person you're becoming—the very person cigarette ads would have you believe smoking makes you. Now that you're quitting smoking, you're becoming healthier, sexier, more sophisticated, more mature, and better looking—and you've earned it!

As you go through this process, record your physical and psychological reactions in your online journal.

Sources: American Cancer Society, National Cancer Institute.

someone smoking seven cigarettes an hour, even in a ventilated room, you'll take in almost twice the maximum amount of carbon monoxide set for air pollution in industry—and it will take hours for the carbon monoxide to leave your body.

Even a little secondhand smoke is dangerous. As a cancer-causing agent, secondhand smoke may be twice as dangerous as radon gas and more than a hundred times more hazardous than

**environmental tobacco smoke** Secondhand cigarette smoke; the third-leading preventable cause of death.

**mainstream smoke** The smoke inhaled directly by smoking a cigarette.

**sidestream smoke** The smoke emitted by a burning cigarette and breathed by everyone in a closed room, including the smoker; contains more tar and nicotine than mainstream smoke.

Secondhand smoke also may increase the risk of cancer of the nasal sinus cavity and of the pharynx in adults and leukemia, lymphoma, and brain tumors in children.

Exposure to tobacco smoke irritates the airways and contributes to respiratory diseases such as asthma. Because of its toxic effects on the heart and blood vessels, it may increase the risk of heart disease by an estimated 25 to 30 percent. In the United States secondhand smoke is thought to cause about 46,000 heart disease deaths a year.[27] According to a recent study, people exposed to secondhand smoke may face a significantly greater risk of developing Alzheimer's disease or other dementias.[28]

Children are particularly vulnerable to secondhand smoke, beginning before birth.[29] Prenatal exposure to tobacco can have significant effects that may extend from infancy into adulthood. A mother's smoking during pregnancy affects a child's growth, cognitive development, and behavior both before and after birth. Birthweight decreases in direct proportion to the number of cigarettes smoked. The babies of teenage mothers who smoke have lower birthweight, length, head circumference, and chest circumference. As they grow, children of smokers tend to be shorter and weigh less than children of nonsmokers.

Even if their mothers don't smoke, children exposed to secondhand smoke before birth also are likely to weigh less and to perform more poorly on tests of speech, language skills, intelligence, and visual-spatial abilities and to develop behavior problems. These youngsters perform at a level between that of children of active smokers and children of nonsmokers.

Exposure to smoke after birth increases the risk of sudden infant death syndrome (SIDS) and is associated with lower IQ scores and deficits in cognitive development.

Children who breathe environmental tobacco smoke suffer from more asthma, wheezing, and bronchitis than children in smoke-free homes. They also face increased risk of lung cancer, heart disease, and stroke. African American children may be more susceptible to the toxins in secondhand smoke.

The negative effects of early exposure to environmental tobacco smoke persist even after

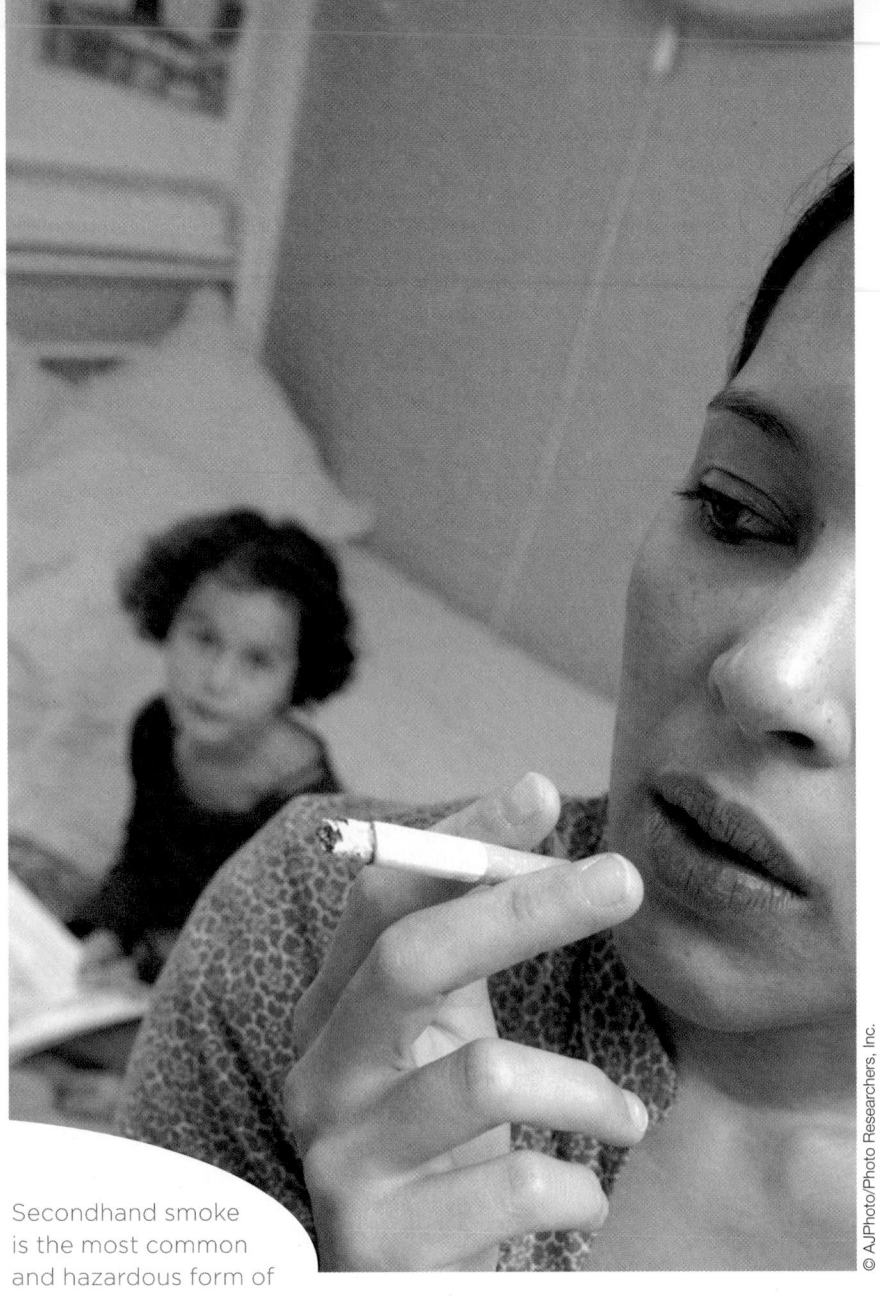

Secondhand smoke is the most common and hazardous form of indoor air pollution.

© AJPhoto/Photo Researchers, Inc.

outdoor pollutants regulated by federal law. Secondhand smoke also increases the sick leave rates among employees.

## Health Effects of Secondhand Smoke

Environmental tobacco smoke is both dangerous and deadly. A proven culprit in the development of lung cancer, it leads to an estimated 3,000 deaths among adult nonsmokers every year. The Surgeon General estimates that living with a smoker increases a nonsmoker's chances of developing lung cancer by 20 to 30 percent. Both smoking and secondhand smoke increase a post menopausal woman's risk of breast cancer.[26]

youngsters leave home. In recent research at Ohio State University, college students who grew up in a smoker's household had higher resting heart rates and blood pressure at rest and during psychological stress than those who grew up in smoke-free homes. Teen exposure to cigarette smoke increases the risk of metabolic syndrome (discussed in Chapter 15).

## Thirdhand Smoke

Thirdhand smoke is the nicotine residue that is left behind on furniture, walls, and carpeting after a cigarette has been smoked in a room. According to scientists, particulates made up of ozone and nicotine can become airborne a second time and, because they are so small, easily penetrate into the deepest parts of the lung. Over time, they could contribute to breathing problems like asthma or possibly even cancer. Because ozone can continue to pull nicotine off surfaces and back into the air for months, exposure to thirdhand smoke may continue long after smoking in the area has ceased. The danger may be greatest to infants, children, pregnant women, and the elderly.[30]

***Tobacco Control Policies*** More than three decades after U.S. government health authorities began to warn of the dangers of cigarette smoking, tobacco remains a politically hot topic. However, a majority of people support tobacco control strategies, including creation of smoke-free environments, an increase in cigarette excise taxes, more funds to prevent people from smoking and to help smokers quit, and restriction of youth access to tobacco.

The Family Smoking Prevention and Tobacco Control Act, signed into law in 2009, allows the FDA to forbid advertising geared toward children, to lower the amount of nicotine in tobacco products, to ban sweetened cigarettes that appeal to young people, and to prohibit labels like "light" and "low tar."

Policy initiatives, such as bans on smoking in public places, have proven beneficial for smokers and everyone in their vicinity. Nonsmokers

Figure 14.3 **Nonsmoker's Bill of Rights**

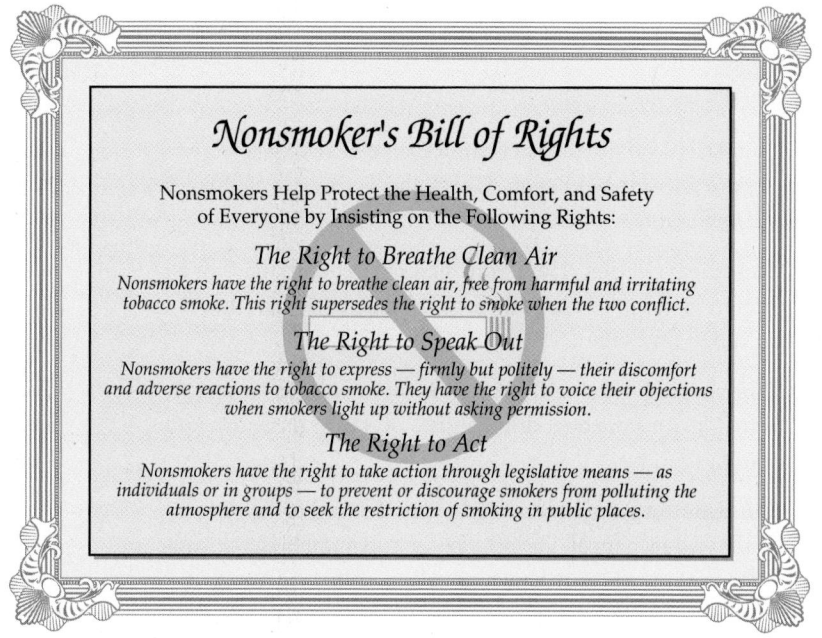

are exposed to less secondhand smoke, while smokers tend to smoke less and are more likely to quit. In regions where smoking bans have been mandated by law, employees, customers, and business owners report high compliance and satisfaction with the results.[31]

## The Fight for Clean Air

Nonsmokers, realizing that their health is being jeopardized by environmental tobacco smoke, have increasingly turned to legislative and administrative measures to clear the air and protect their rights (Figure 14.3). Most states now have some restrictions on smoking in bars, restaurants, and workplaces. Nationally, the airlines have banned smoking on domestic flights. Many institutions, including medical centers and some universities, no longer allow smoking on their premises. States that have launched comprehensive antismoking programs, including higher cigarette taxes and a media campaign, have lowered smoking prevalence and secondhand smoke levels.

# Becoming Smoke-Free

If you smoke—even just a few cigarettes a few times a week—you are at risk of nicotine addiction. Check the steps you will take to get back into control:

_____ **Delaying tactics.** Have your first cigarette of the day 15 minutes later than usual, then 15 minutes later than that the next day, and so on.

_____ **Distracting yourself.** When you feel a craving for a cigarette, talk to someone, drink a glass of water, or get up and move around.

_____ **Establishing nonsmoking hours.** Instead of lighting up at the end of a meal, for instance, get up immediately, brush your teeth, wash your hands, or take a walk.

_____ **Never smoking two packs of the same brand in a row.** Buy cigarettes only by the pack, not by the carton.

_____ **Making it harder to get to your cigarettes.** Lock them in a drawer, wrap them in paper, or leave them in your coat or car.

_____ **Changing the way you smoke.** Smoke with the hand you don't usually use. Smoke only half of each cigarette.

_____ **Stopping completely for just one day at a time.** Promise yourself 24 hours of freedom from cigarettes; when the day's over, make the same commitment for one more day. At the end of any 24-hour period, you can go back to smoking and not feel guilty.

_____ **Spending more time in places where you can't smoke.** Take up bike riding or swimming. Shower often. Go to movies or other places where smoking isn't allowed.

_____ **Going cold turkey.** If you're a heavily addicted smoker, try a decisive and complete break. Smokers who quit completely are less likely to light up again than those who gradually decrease their daily cigarette consumption, switch to low-tar and low-nicotine brands, or use special filters and holders.

If these tactics don't work, talk to your doctor about nicotine replacement options or prescription medications.

# Are You Addicted to Nicotine?

| | Yes | No |
|---|---|---|
| 1. Do you smoke every day? | _____ | _____ |
| 2. Do you smoke because of shyness and to build up self-confidence? | _____ | _____ |
| 3. Do you smoke to escape from boredom and worries or while under pressure? | _____ | _____ |
| 4. Have you ever burned a hole in your clothes, carpet, furniture, or car with a cigarette? | _____ | _____ |
| 5. Have you ever had to go to the store late at night or at another inconvenient time because you were out of cigarettes? | _____ | _____ |
| 6. Do you feel defensive or angry when people tell you that your smoke is bothering them? | _____ | _____ |
| 7. Has a doctor or dentist ever suggested that you stop smoking? | _____ | _____ |
| 8. Have you ever promised someone that you would stop smoking, then broken your promise? | _____ | _____ |
| 9. Have you ever felt physical or emotional discomfort when trying to quit? | _____ | _____ |
| 10. Have you ever successfully stopped smoking for a period of time, only to start again? | _____ | _____ |
| 11. Do you buy extra supplies of tobacco to make sure you won't run out? | _____ | _____ |
| 12. Do you find it difficult to imagine life without smoking? | _____ | _____ |
| 13. Do you choose only those activities and entertainments during which you can smoke? | _____ | _____ |
| 14. Do you prefer, seek out, or feel more comfortable in the company of smokers? | _____ | _____ |
| 15. Do you inwardly despise or feel ashamed of yourself because of your smoking? | _____ | _____ |

16. Do you ever find yourself lighting up without having consciously decided to? ＿＿＿＿ ＿＿＿＿

17. Has your smoking ever caused trouble at home or in a relationship? ＿＿＿＿ ＿＿＿＿

18. Do you ever tell yourself that you can stop smoking whenever you want to? ＿＿＿＿ ＿＿＿＿

19. Have you ever felt that your life would be better if you didn't smoke? ＿＿＿＿ ＿＿＿＿

20. Do you continue to smoke even though you are aware of the health hazards posed by smoking? ＿＿＿＿ ＿＿＿＿

If you answered Yes to one or two of these questions, there's a chance that you are addicted or are becoming addicted to nicotine. If you answered Yes to three or more of these questions, you are probably already addicted to nicotine.

Source: *Nicotine Anonymous World Services, San Francisco.*

## *Making Change Happen*

### Butt Out

Stained teeth. Bad breath. Premature wrinkles. Gum disease. Yellow fingernails. No one starts smoking to acquire any of these, but they come with the territory—along with far more serious health consequences. Maybe you don't think of yourself as a smoker because you only smoke at parties, or during finals, or with particular friends. Maybe you've cut back or are thinking about quitting.

If you smoke at all—a cigarette a week or a pack a day, in social settings or anywhere you can—do the "Butt Out" lab in *Labs for IPC*. There is nothing more important that you can do for yourself, your health, and your future than to quit.

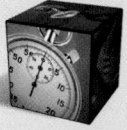

**Get Real**

In this stage you answer a series of questions in your *IPC Journal*, including the following:

 • Describe your smoking style:

• Where do you smoke?

• When do you smoke?

• With whom do you smoke?

• How do you smoke (light one cigarette after another, smoke between sips of coffee or beer, smoke before meals to kill your appetite, etc.)?

You also write a story called "My Smoking History," using only the past tense and the phrase "chose to smoke" rather than the word "smoked."

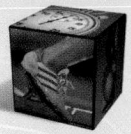

**Get Ready**

In this stage, you list all the reasons you decided to quit. For example:

 • No more coughing.

• No more complaints from my partner about how I smell or taste.

• Save money.

You print out your list, and read it at the beginning and end of every day. You also read pages 475–478 in this chapter and decide on a quit plan. You check out any campus-based programs and make the necessary appointments and arrangements . . .

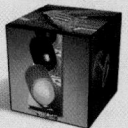

**Get Going**

You start the morning by saying, "I am not a smoker." Be sure to repeat this mantra morning and night and as often as possible during the day. Make this statement even if you are tapering down your tobacco use and continuing to smoke. In time you will find it easier not to smoke because you see yourself as a nonsmoker.

Additional steps include:

• Staying out of smoking zones.

• Dealing with nicotine withdrawal.

• Talking back to yourself when a rationalization for smoking pops into your mind. For example, if you think, "You've got to die of something," your response would be, "I don't have to get a terrible disease and die years ahead of my time in pain."

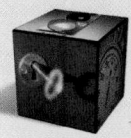

**Lock It In**

*Staying* quit is the final, and most important, stage of the butt-out process. This stage provides proven strategies, including the following:

• **Rehearse.** If you used to smoke at parties, visualize yourself going to the party with a nonsmoker friend. See yourself steering away from the smokers outside. Visualize yourself saying, "No, thank you. I don't smoke . . ."

## Review Questions

1. Which of the following statements is *false*?
   a. Using chewing tobacco can lead to lesions on the mucous membranes of the mouth.
   b. Bidis come in several flavors.
   c. The active ingredient in cloves lowers sensation in the throat, so clove-cigarette smokers inhale more deeply.
   d. Smoking cigars is safe if you don't inhale.

2. Quitting smoking
   a. usually results in minor withdrawal symptoms.
   b. will do little to reverse the damage to the lungs and other parts of the body.
   c. can be aided by using nicotine replacement products.
   d. is best done by cutting down on the number of cigarettes you smoke over a period of months.

3. Ways to help yourself quit include all of the following *except*
   a. join a support group.
   b. make your home a smoke-free zone.
   c. try acupuncture.
   d. switch to bidis.

4. Secondhand tobacco smoke is
   a. the smoke inhaled by a smoker.
   b. more hazardous than outdoor pollution as a cancer-causing agent.
   c. less hazardous than mainstream smoke.
   d. less likely to cause serious health problems in children than in adults.

5. Which of the following statements about smoking is *false*?
   a. Smoking behavior may have a genetic component.
   b. People who graduate college are less likely to smoke than those who complete only high school.
   c. Most regular smokers enjoy smoking.
   d. Nicotine addiction doesn't take hold until six months after a person starts smoking.

6. Tobacco use on college campuses
   a. is higher among black students.
   b. continues to increase despite no-smoking policies by all schools.
   c. is less than that of same-age peers who aren't in school.
   d. is most often in the form of smokeless tobacco.

7. Which of the following statements is *false*?
   a. People pursuing a graduate degree are more likely to begin smoking than those entering as undergraduates.
   b. Children are 50 percent more likely to smoke if at least one parent smokes.
   c. People who think they have little chance of developing short-term problems are more likely to smoke.
   d. Nicotine addiction is as strong or stronger than addiction to cocaine.

8. Women smokers
   a. are more likely to die from breast cancer than lung cancer.
   b. are less fertile than nonsmokers.
   c. are less likely to develop osteoporosis.
   d. bear children with fewer birth defects.

9. Which of the following statements about tobacco and its components is *true*?
   a. Nicotine affects the central nervous system in eight seconds.
   b. Tobacco stimulates the kidneys to form urine.
   c. Carbon monoxide contained in tobacco smoke is an addictive substance.
   d. The tar in burning tobacco impairs oxygen transport in the body.

10. Cigarette smokers
    a. are more likely to die of lung cancer than heart disease.
    b. usually develop lung problems after years of tobacco use.
    c. have two to three times the risk of suffering a stroke than nonsmokers.
    d. may completely reverse the damage to their blood vessels if they quit smoking.

*Answers to these questions can be found on page 672.*

## Critical Thinking

1. Has smoking become unpopular among your friends or family? What social activities continue to be associated with smoking? Can you think of any situation in which smoking might be frowned upon?

2. How would you motivate someone you care about to stop smoking? What reasons would you give for them to stop? Describe your strategy.

3. According to the chapter, environmental tobacco smoke is even more dangerous than mainstream smoke. If you're a nonsmoker, how would you react to someone who's smoking in the same room you occupy? Define the rights of smokers and nonsmokers.

## Media Menu

Visit www.cengagebrain.com to access course materials and companion resources for this text that will:

- Help you evaluate your knowledge of the material.

- Allow you to prepare for exams with interactive quizzing.

- Use the CengageNOW product to develop a Personalized Learning Plan targeting resources that address areas you should study.

- Coach you through identifying target goals for behavioral change and creating and monitoring your personal change plan throughout the semester using the Behavior Change Planner available in the CengageNOW resource.

## Internet Connections

**www.cdc.gov/tobacco**
This comprehensive feature on the Centers for Disease Control and Prevention (CDC) website provides educational information, research, a report from the U.S. Surgeon General, tips on how to quit, and much more.

**http://joechemo.org**
Based on the character Joe Chemo, an antismoking parody of Joe Camel, this site is highly interactive and allows visitors to test their "Tobacco IQ," get a personalized "Smoke-o-Scope," and send free Joe Chemo

e-cards. There is also extensive information for teachers, antismoking activists, health-care providers, journalists, and smokers who wish to quit.

**www.tobaccofacts.org**
This excellent site provides access to many facts and resources regarding tobacco use.

**www.tobacco.neu.edu**
This site provides current information on tobacco-related litigation and legislation.

## Key Terms

The terms listed are used on the page indicated. Definitions of the terms are in the Glossary at the end of the book.

| | | |
|---|---|---|
| aversion therapy 476 | environmental tobacco smoke 479 | sidestream smoke 479 |
| bidis 474 | mainstream smoke 479 | tar 469 |
| carbon monoxide 469 | nicotine 468 | |

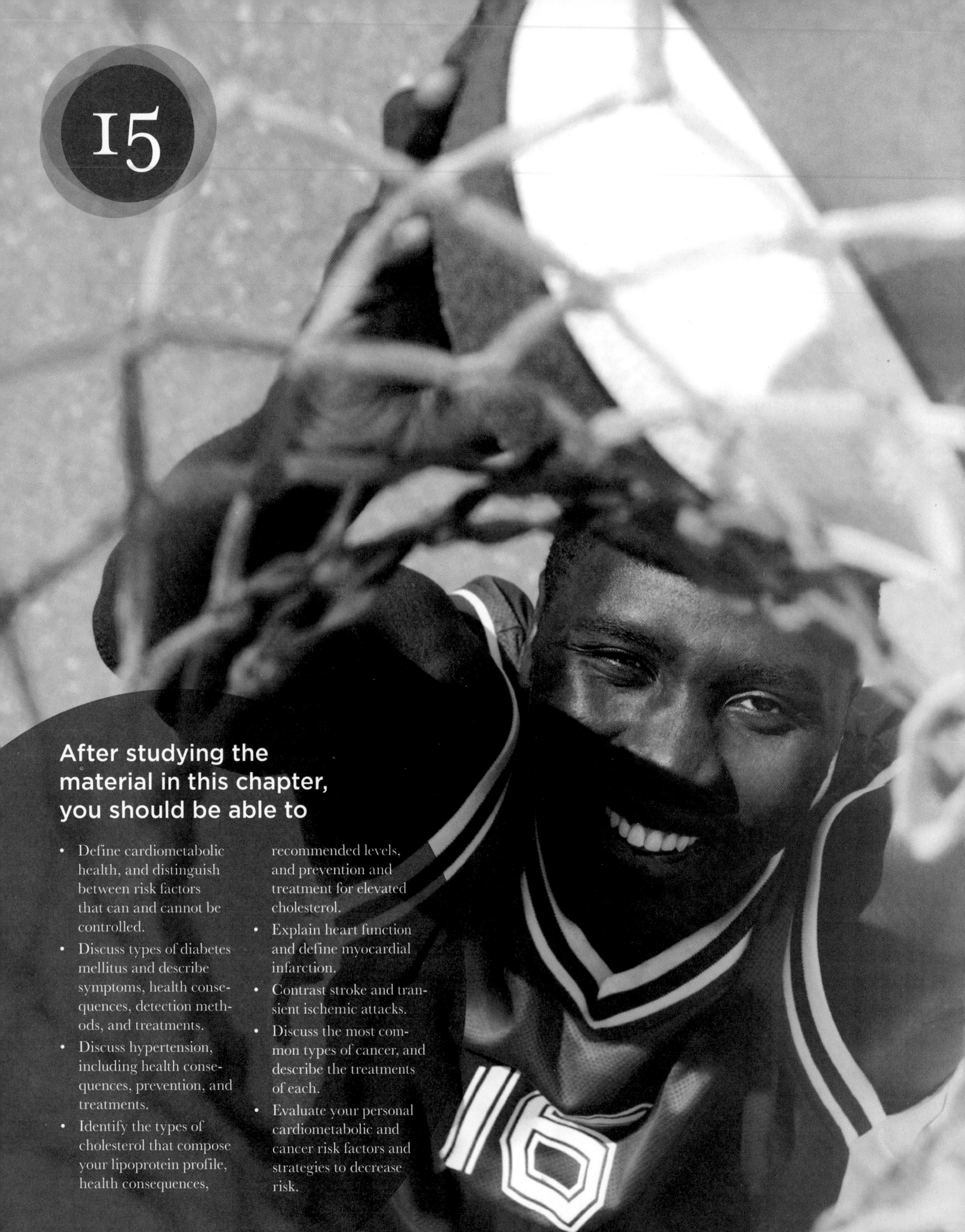

# 15

## After studying the material in this chapter, you should be able to

- Define cardiometabolic health, and distinguish between risk factors that can and cannot be controlled.

- Discuss types of diabetes mellitus and describe symptoms, health consequences, detection methods, and treatments.

- Discuss hypertension, including health consequences, prevention, and treatments.

- Identify the types of cholesterol that compose your lipoprotein profile, health consequences,

recommended levels, and prevention and treatment for elevated cholesterol.

- Explain heart function and define myocardial infarction.

- Contrast stroke and transient ischemic attacks.

- Discuss the most common types of cancer, and describe the treatments of each.

- Evaluate your personal cardiometabolic and cancer risk factors and strategies to decrease risk.

Chris never forgot the terror he felt when his dad had his first heart attack. Only ten, he couldn't understand why this towering giant of a man had fallen to the ground, his face twisted in pain, his fist pressed against his chest. His father seemed different when he came home from the hospital, as if something had gone out of him. But his face would still light up with an impish grin, especially when he'd sneak a cigarette and wink at Chris

# Preventing Major Disease

so he wouldn't tell his mother. The second heart attack came four years later. This time Chris's dad didn't come home.

Chris promised his mother that he'd take better care of his heart. He wouldn't smoke; he'd watch his blood pressure and weight; he'd keep tabs on his diet; he'd exercise regularly. Chris didn't forget these promises as time passed. But like many college students, he felt invincible. He was shocked when a sports physical revealed that his blood pressure was high and his levels of the most dangerous type of cholesterol were elevated. But he also felt lucky: "I got my wake-up call," he explains. "And I'm not going to ignore it."

As Chris realizes, it's never too soon, or too late, to start protecting your health and your future. Whether or not you will get a serious disease at some time in your life may seem to be a matter of odds. Genetic tendencies, environmental factors, and luck affect your chances of having to face many health threats. However, often you can prevent or delay major illnesses, such as heart disease, for years, even decades.

The time to start protecting your health is now. People mistakenly think of heart disease, cancer, and other disorders as illnesses of middle and old age. But the events leading up to these diseases often begin in childhood, progress in adolescence, and become a health threat to men in their 30s and 40s and to women in their 40s and 50s. This chapter provides the information about the risk factors, silent dangers, and medical advances that can improve your chances of a healthier, longer life.

## The Power of Prevention

Young people often feel immune to such serious diseases, but illness can strike anyone. Regardless of your age, being in tune with your body is one of the best ways to safeguard your health.

More Americans are developing chronic illnesses such as diabetes and high blood pressure, often having more than three such conditions

Visit www.cengagebrain.com to access course materials for this text, including the Behavior Change Planner, interactive quizzes, tutorials, and more. See the preface on page xv for details.

# Lowering Your Cardiometabolic Risks

Yes, advances in treatment can help if you eventually develop a cardiometabolic condition. But changes in lifestyle can do even more: To make healthy changes, select some of the behavioral modifications that require little or no expense to follow.

## Changes You Can Make Today

- Eat a good breakfast: whole-grain cereal, juice, yogurt, and so forth.

- Take a walk after lunch.

- Skip dessert at dinner.

- Eat one more serving of vegetables.

- Eat one more piece of fruit.

- Drink one more glass of water.

- Take the stairs for one or two flights rather than riding the elevator in your dorm or classroom building.

- Get seven to eight hours of sleep tonight.

- Don't smoke.

## Changes You Can Make This Term

- **Block out time for exercise on your calendar.** Try for at least 30 minutes of physical activity most days.

- **If you haven't had your lipoproteins checked within the last year, schedule a test.**

- **If you don't know your blood pressure, find out what it is.**

- **Make a list of stress-reducing activities, such as meditation or listening to music.** Select two or three to try every week.

- **Learn your family history.** Inheriting a predisposition to high blood pressure, diabetes, or heart disease means that you need extra preventive care.

- **Develop and use a support system of friends and family members.** Identify individuals you can talk to, work out with, or call.

**cardiometabolic** Referring to the heart and to the biochemical processes involved in the body's functioning.

at a time—a financial as well as a physiological burden. Many chronic problems begin early in life. One in five children and teens in the United States has high cholesterol.[1] More than a third of youngsters over age six are overweight. Obese children are twice as likely to die before age 55 as normal-weight youngsters.[2] An estimated one in four college students already has at least one risk factor, such as excess weight or physical inactivity, that increases the risk of conditions affecting the heart and metabolism. The habits you develop now—regular exercise, sensible

eating, responsible drinking, getting regular checkups—can keep you healthy for decades to come. (See How Do You Compare? p. 489.)

Deaths from the number-one killer of Americans—heart disease—have dropped 30 percent since 1996.[3] Despite the gains that have been made, more people are still dying of illnesses than should be, many at young ages. "Everything is coming together in the worst way—obesity, inactivity, smoking," says Dr. Clyde Yancy, president of the American Heart Association. "In our younger group, instead of seeing improvement, it is getting worse."[4]

Simple lifestyle changes could reduce cardiovascular deaths by another 20 percent. However, many Americans are ignoring the basic rules for preventing cardiovascular disease, such as keeping their weights and their waistlines under control. (See Health on a Budget.)

# Your Cardiometabolic Health

In recent years medical scientists in the United States and Canada have focused on the complex connections between various risk factors, symptoms, and diseases.[5] Physical inactivity, for instance, increases the risk of obesity, which in turn leads to greater risk of many diseases. This new awareness has led to a focus on **cardiometabolic** health. "Cardio" refers to the heart and blood vessels of the cardiovascular system; "metabolic," to the biochemical processes involved in the body's functioning.

## Cardiometabolic Risk Factors

Specific risk factors determine your cardiometabolic health. Once you understand your risk, you can start making changes to lower your odds of developing metabolic syndrome, diabetes, and heart disease.

Reducing as many risk factors as possible, rather than just focusing on one such as cholesterol, is more effective in preventing a heart attack.[6]

**Risk Factors You Can Control** The choices you make and the habits you follow can have a significant impact on whether or not you remain healthy. Avoid the following potential risks for the sake of your cardiometabolic health.

**Overweight/Obesity** Excess weight, an increasingly common and dangerous cardiometabolic risk factor in both men and women, undermines good health. The higher your BMI (Body Mass Index, discussed in Chapter 8) during adolescence, according to a recent study, the greater your risk of type 2 diabetes and heart disease in the future.[7] Even teens with a BMI in the high "normal" range face an increased likelihood of health problems. Overweight teens who lose weight and keep their BMI within a healthy range as adults can eliminate the danger of diabetes, but being obese at any age endangers cardiovascular health.[8] Obese adult men are at dramatically higher risk of dying from a heart attack regardless of whether they have any other risk factors.[9]

**Waist Circumference** Doctors had believed that apple-shaped people who carry most of their excess weight around their waists are at greater risk of cardiometabolic conditions than are pear-shaped individuals who carry most of their excess weight below their waist. The more visceral (abdominal) fat that you have, the more resistant your body's cells become to the effects of your own insulin. However, recent research suggests that fat alone, regardless of where it is stored, boosts the likelihood of heart attack or stroke. Subcutaneous fat (located under the skin) as well as visceral fat pose dangers to cardiometabolic health.[10]

A measurement of more than 40 inches in men and more than 35 inches in women indicates increased health risks. A "pot belly" raises risk even when a person's weight is normal. Rather than waist circumference alone, the ratio of waist to height may be a more precise indicator of risk.[11]

**Physical Inactivity** As discussed in Chapter 8, about one-quarter of U.S. adults are sedentary and another third are not active enough to reach a healthy level of fitness. The risk for cardiometabolic conditions is higher for people who are inactive compared with those who engage in regular physical activity.

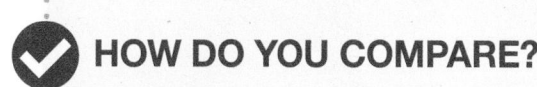
Fitness may be more important than overweight or obesity per se for women's cardiometabolic risk. A minimum of 30 minutes a day of moderate activity at least five days a week can lift a woman from the "low-fitness category" and lessen her cardiometabolic risk.

The greater the exercise "dose," the more benefits it yields. In studies that compared individuals of different fitness levels, the least fit were at much greater risk of dying. In men, more rigorous exercise, such as jogging, produces greater protection against heart disease and boosts longevity.

**Tobacco Use** Smoking may be the single most significant risk factor for cardiometabolic conditions. Each year smoking causes more than 250,000 deaths from cardiovascular disease—far more than it causes from cancer and lung disease. Smokers who have heart attacks are more likely to die from them than are nonsmokers. Smoking is the major risk factor for *peripheral arterial disease*, in which the vessels that carry blood to the leg and arm muscles become hardened and clogged.

Both active and passive smoking accelerate the process by which arteries become clogged and increase the risk of heart attacks and strokes.

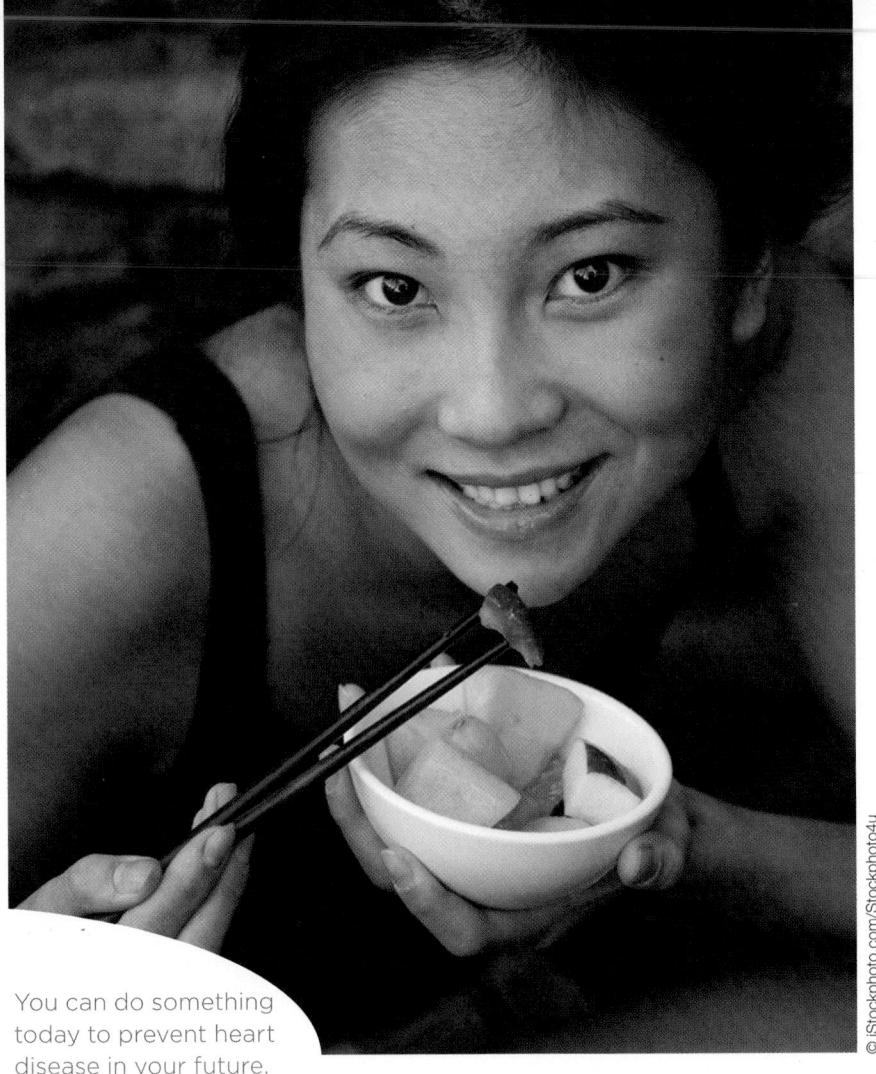

You can do something today to prevent heart disease in your future. Eat some fruit.

**systolic blood pressure**
Highest blood pressure when the heart contracts.

**diastolic blood pressure**
Lowest blood pressure between contractions of the heart.

**hypertension** High pressure occurring when the blood exerts excessive pressure against the arterial walls.

**cholesterol** An organic substance found in animal fats; linked to cardiovascular disease, particularly atherosclerosis.

**lipoprotein** A compound in blood that is made up of proteins and fat; a high-density lipoprotein (HDL) picks up excess cholesterol in the blood; a low-density lipoprotein (LDL) carries more cholesterol and deposits it on the walls of arteries.

Overall, nonsmokers exposed to environmental tobacco smoke are at a 25 percent higher relative risk of developing coronary heart disease than nonsmokers not exposed to environmental tobacco smoke.

**High Blood Glucose** As discussed in greater detail on page 493, your stomach and digestive system break down the food you eat into glucose, a type of sugar. The hormone insulin acts like a key, letting glucose into cells and providing energy. "Insulin resistant" cells no longer respond well to insulin, and then glucose, unable to enter the cells, builds up in the bloodstream. Frequent thirst, blurry vision, weakness, unexplained weight loss, or unusual hunger can be signs of high blood glucose. A simple blood test will tell you if your glucose levels are too high. Here is what the readings mean:

| | |
|---|---|
| Healthy blood glucose | Under 100 |
| Prediabetes | 100–125 |
| Diabetes | More than 125 |

## High Blood Pressure (Hypertension)

Blood pressure is a result of the contractions of the heart muscle, which pumps blood through your body, and the resistance of the walls of the vessels through which the blood flows. Each time your heart beats, your blood pressure goes up and down within a certain range. It's highest when the heart contracts; this is called **systolic blood pressure**. It's lowest between contractions; this is called **diastolic blood pressure**. A blood pressure reading consists of the systolic measurement "over" the diastolic measurement, recorded in millimeters of mercury (mm Hg).

High blood pressure, or **hypertension**, occurs when the artery walls become constricted so that the force exerted as the blood flows through them is greater than it should be. Physicians see blood pressure as a continuum: The higher the reading, the greater the risk of stroke and heart disease.

As a result of the increased work in pumping blood, the heart muscle of a person with hypertension can become stronger and also stiffer. This stiffness increases resistance to filling up with blood between beats, which can cause shortness of breath with exertion. Hypertension can also act on the kidney arteries, which can lead to kidney failure in some cases. In addition, hypertension accelerates the development of plaque buildup within the arteries. Especially when combined with obesity, smoking, high cholesterol levels, or diabetes, hypertension increases the risks of cardiovascular problems several times. However, you can control high blood pressure through diet, exercise, and, if necessary, medication.

**Lipoprotein Levels** **Cholesterol** is a fatty substance found in certain foods and also manufactured by the body. Figure 15.1 shows food sources of cholesterol. The measurement of cholesterol in the blood is one of the most reliable indicators of the formation of plaque, the sludgelike substance that builds up on the inner walls of arteries. You can lower blood cholesterol levels by cutting back on high-fat foods and exercising more, thereby reducing the risk of a heart attack.

**Lipoproteins** are compounds in the blood that are made up of proteins and fat. The different types are classified by their size or density. The heaviest are *high-density lipoproteins*, or HDLs, which have the highest proportion of protein. These "good guys," as some cardiologists refer to them, pick up excess cholesterol in the blood and carry it back to the liver for removal from the body. An HDL level of 40 mg/dL or lower substantially increases the risk of heart disease. (Cholesterol levels are measured in milligrams of cholesterol per deciliter of blood—mg/dL.) The average HDL for men is about 45 mg/dL; for women, it is about 55 mg/dL.

Low-density lipoproteins, or LDLs, and very low-density lipoproteins (VLDLs) carry more cholesterol than HDLs and deposit it on the walls of arteries—they're the "bad guys." The higher your LDL cholesterol, the greater your risk for heart disease. If you are at high risk of heart disease, any level of LDL higher than 100 mg/dL may increase your danger.

**Triglycerides** are fats that flow through the blood after meals and have been linked to increased risk of coronary artery disease, especially in women. Triglyceride levels tend to be highest in those whose diets are high in calories, sugar, alcohol, and refined starches. High levels of these fats may increase the risk of obesity, and cutting back on these foods can reduce high triglyceride levels.

Figure 15.2 summarizes the factors to ask your doctor about at your next checkup.

### Risk Factors You Can't Control

**Family History** Certain cardiometabolic risk factors, such as abnormally high blood levels of lipids, can be passed down from generation to generation. Although you can't rewrite your family history, individuals with an inherited vulnerability can lower the danger by changing the risk factors within their control. Your cardiometabolic health depends to a great extent on your behavior, including the decisions you make about the foods you eat or the decision not to smoke.

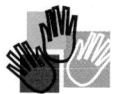 **Race and Ethnicity** Cardiometabolic risk factors occur at higher rates among ethnic minority populations such as African Americans, Hispanic Americans, and Native Americans. For reasons that aren't entirely clear, people of some races are more likely to develop diabetes. Blacks and Hispanics have double the rate than those for whites. The incidence is even higher among

Figure 15.1  **Cholesterol in Our Food**

Food sources of cholesterol in the U.S. diet. Percentages indicate the proportion of cholesterol each type of food contributes to the diet.

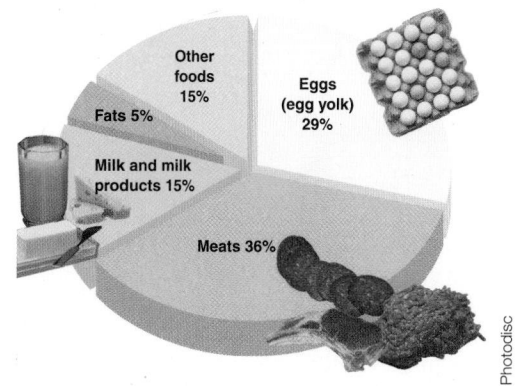

Other foods 15%
Fats 5%
Eggs (egg yolk) 29%
Milk and milk products 15%
Meats 36%

Photodisc

Figure 15.2  **Checkup Chart**

Adapted from CheckUpAmerica.org.

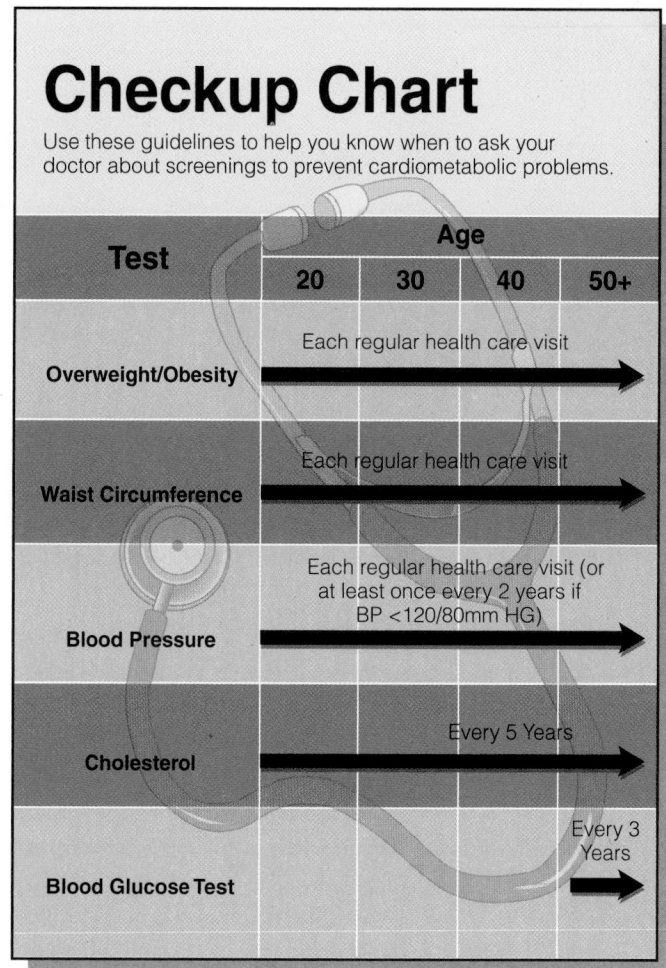

# Checkup Chart

Use these guidelines to help you know when to ask your doctor about screenings to prevent cardiometabolic problems.

| Test | Age | | | |
|---|---|---|---|---|
| | 20 | 30 | 40 | 50+ |
| Overweight/Obesity | Each regular health care visit → | | | |
| Waist Circumference | Each regular health care visit → | | | |
| Blood Pressure | Each regular health care visit (or at least once every 2 years if BP <120/80mm HG) → | | | |
| Cholesterol | | Every 5 Years → | | |
| Blood Glucose Test | | | | Every 3 Years → |

**triglyceride** A fat that flows through the blood after meals and is linked to increased risk of coronary artery disease.

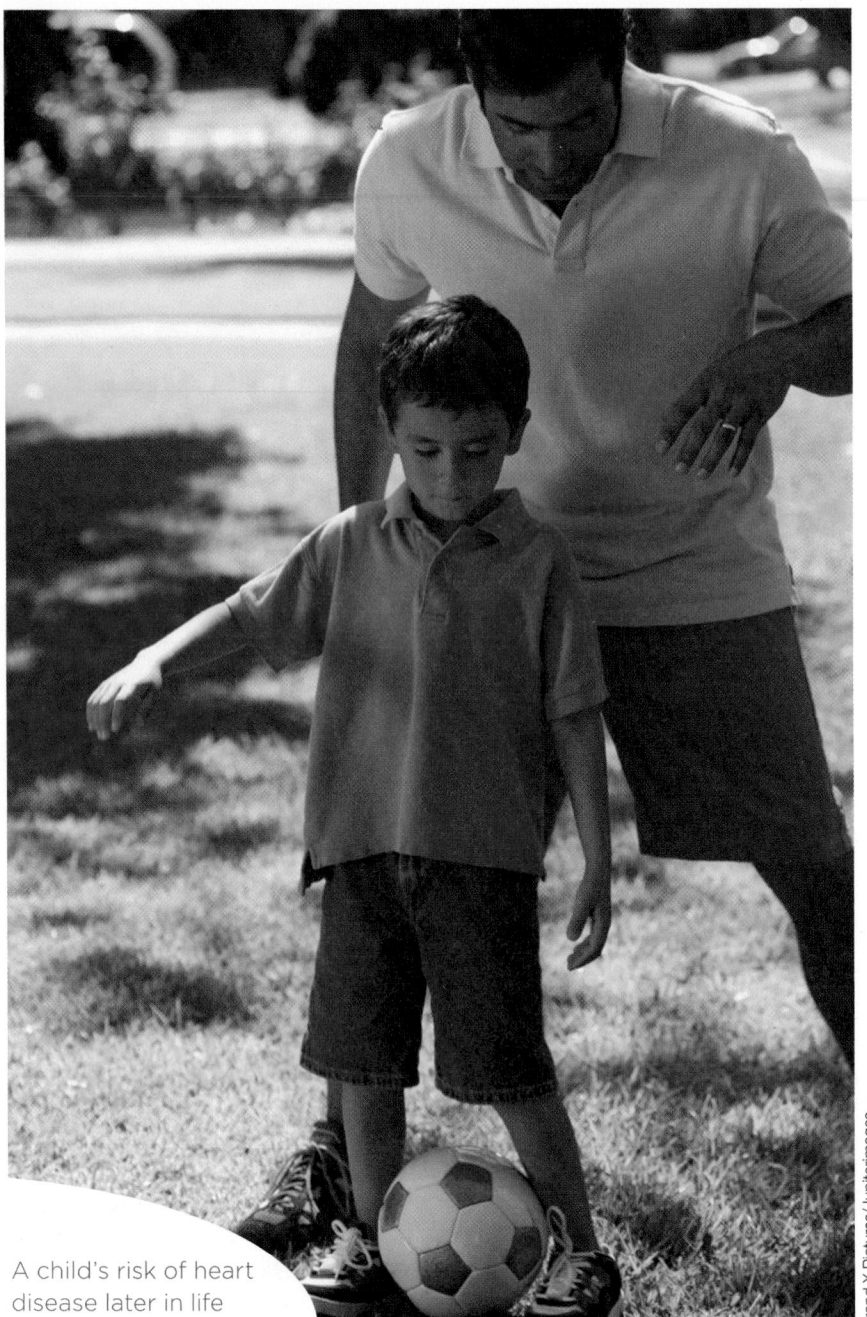

A child's risk of heart disease later in life depends on many factors, including family history, diet, and physical activity.

**metabolic syndrome** A cluster of disorders of the body's metabolism that make diabetes, heart disease, or stroke more likely.

risk factor for members of this minority group, who are less likely to receive medical treatments or undergo corrective surgery. Family history, lifestyle, diet, and stress may also play a role, starting early in life. However, researchers have found no single explanation for why African American youngsters, like their parents, tend to have higher blood pressure than white children.

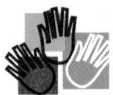 Black women are twice as likely as white women to suffer heart attacks and to die from heart disease. Common cardiometabolic risk factors—high blood pressure, diabetes, and high cholesterol—account for this increased jeopardy. In addition, black women are less likely to receive common medications, such as cholesterol-lowering drugs, to lower their risk.

**Age** Cardiometabolic risk factors increase as people get older, especially past the age of 45. This may be because many individuals tend to exercise less, lose muscle mass, and gain weight as they age. However, cardiometabolic conditions are also increasing dramatically among younger people.

# Metabolic Syndrome

**Metabolic syndrome**, once called Syndrome X or insulin-resistant syndrome, is not a disease but a cluster of disorders of the body's metabolism—including high blood pressure, high insulin levels, abdominal obesity, and abnormal cholesterol levels—that make a person more likely to develop diabetes, heart disease, or stroke. Each of these conditions is by itself a risk factor for other diseases. In combination, they dramatically boost the chances of potentially life-threatening illnesses.

This dangerous syndrome has become so widespread that health officials describe it as an epidemic that affects one in four Americans, especially Hispanic men and women.

 College-age men and women who maintain their weight as they get older are much less likely to develop metabolic syndrome. About one in four undergraduates already has one risk factor for

American Indians. Among the Pima Indians of Arizona, half of all adults have type 2 diabetes, one of the highest rates of diabetes in the world. Nearly four in every ten black adults have cardiovascular disease. Among Hispanic Americans, nearly three in ten have cardiovascular disease.

African Americans are twice as likely to develop high blood pressure as whites. African Americans also suffer strokes at an earlier age and of greater severity. Poverty may be an unrecognized

Brand X Pictures/Jupiterimages

metabolic syndrome. Young adults with metabolic syndrome are more likely than others their age to have thicker neck arteries, an indicator of atherosclerosis, the buildup of fatty plaques in arteries. Because retired professional football players have increased rates of metabolic syndrome and atherosclerosis, health professionals have called for regular screening of athletes, beginning in high school and college. An all-too-common culprit for young people is consumption of sugary soft drinks, which, according to a recent report by the American Heart Association, contribute to 130,000 new cases of diabetes and 14,000 new cases of heart disease every year.[12] Watching television compounds the risk. Every hour you spend watching TV may increase your risk of an early death from cardiovascular disease by as much as 18 percent.[13] However, losing 7 to 10 percent of your initial body weight may reverse the symptoms of metabolic syndrome.

Three or more of the following characteristics indicate metabolic syndrome:

- **A larger-than-normal waist measurement**—40 inches or more in men and 35 inches or more in women (for Asians and individuals with a genetic predisposition to diabetes, 37 to 39 inches in men and 31 to 35 inches in women).
- **A higher-than-normal triglyceride level**—150 mg/dL or more.
- **A lower-than-normal high-density lipoprotein (HDL) level**—less than 40 mg/dL in men or 50 mg/dL in women.
- **A higher-than-normal blood pressure**—130 mm Hg systole over 85 mm Hg diastole (130/85), or higher.
- **A higher-than-normal fasting blood sugar**—110 mg/dL or higher.

People with three factors of metabolic syndrome are nearly twice as likely to have a heart attack or stroke and more than three times more likely to develop heart disease than those with none.

Men with four or five characteristics of the syndrome have nearly four times the risk of heart attack or stroke and more than 24 times the risk of diabetes.

According to a review of 35 clinical trials, eating a Mediterranean diet, high in fresh produce, olive oil, and fish (discussed in Chapter 6), may prevent or even reverse metabolic syndrome.[14]

## Insulin Resistance

In a healthy body, the digestive system breaks food down into glucose, which then travels in the bloodstream to cells throughout the body. As the blood glucose level rises after a meal, the pancreas releases insulin to help cells take in the glucose. Insulin resistance is a condition in which the body produces insulin but does not use it properly.

When muscle, fat, and liver cells do not respond properly to insulin, the pancreas tries to keep up with the increased demand for insulin by producing more, but eventually it cannot. Excess glucose builds up in the bloodstream, setting the stage for diabetes. Many people with insulin resistance have high levels of both glucose and insulin circulating in their blood at the same time.

Insulin resistance increases the chance of developing type 2 diabetes and heart disease. Excess weight and lack of physical activity, along with genetic factors, contribute to insulin resistance.

## Prediabetes

Prediabetes—sometimes called impaired fasting glucose or impaired glucose tolerance—is a condition in which blood glucose levels are higher than normal but not high enough for a diagnosis of diabetes. According to the most recent estimates from the CDC, more than a third of adults in the United States—an estimated 79 million men and women—have prediabetes, although more than 90 percent are not aware of it. Among Americans age 65 or older, half may have prediabetes.[15]

## Risk Factors

Several factors—some of which you can control—increase your risk for prediabetes and diabetes.

- Overweight or obese.
- Age 60 or older.
- Physically inactive.
- Parent or sibling with diabetes.

## Diabetes

More than a third of Americans have prediabetes and are at risk of developing diabetes mellitus. To understand more about this major health threat, go to Global Health Watch, click on "Diseases" and then on "Major Diseases." You will find "Diabetes" on the drop-down menu to the right. Read through the headlines under "Latest News" and summarize one article in your online journal.

**diabetes mellitus** A disease in which the inadequate production of insulin leads to failure of the body tissues to break down carbohydrates at a normal rate.

- Family background that is African American, Alaska Native, American Indian, Asian American, Hispanic/Latino, or Pacific Islander.
- Exercising fewer than three times a week.
- Giving birth to a baby weighing more than nine pounds or being diagnosed with diabetes during pregnancy.
- High blood pressure—140/90 or above—or being treated for high blood pressure.
- HDL, or "good," cholesterol level below 35 mg/dL or a triglyceride level above 250 mg/dL.
- Impaired fasting glucose (IFG) or impairing glucose tolerance (IGT) on previous testing.
- Other conditions associated with insulin resistance, such as severe obesity.
- History of cardiovascular disease.[16]

Insulin resistance and prediabetes usually do not cause symptoms. Some people develop dark rings or patches of skin on the neck, elbows, knees, knuckles, and armpits. Most people with prediabetes develop type 2 diabetes (discussed in the following pages) within ten years, unless they lose at least 5 percent of their body weight by making changes in their diet and level of physical activity.

Long-term damage to the body, especially the heart and circulatory system, may occur during prediabetes. If people with prediabetes take action to manage their blood glucose, they can delay or prevent these harmful effects. Diets rich in cereal fiber, magnesium, calcium, and Vitamin D may help. Lifestyle changes also have shown promise.

# Diabetes Mellitus

About 12 percent of people in the United States have **diabetes mellitus**, a disease in which the body doesn't produce or respond properly to insulin. In those with diabetes, the pancreas, which produces insulin (the hormone that regulates carbohydrate and fat metabolism) doesn't function as it should. When the pancreas either stops producing insulin or doesn't produce sufficient insulin to meet the body's needs, almost every body system can be damaged. (See Figure 15.3.)

Worldwide an estimated 280 million people—6.4 percent of the people living on the planet—have diabetes. Nearly 26 million American have diabetes; an estimated 1.9 million receive new diagnoses every year.[17] The CDC projects that up to a third of Americans could have diabetes by 2050 if they continue to gain weight and avoid exercise. (See "Health in the Headlines.") However, nearly 90 percent of adult diabetics

## Figure 15.3  How Diabetes Affects the Body

Diabetes affects almost every organ system of the body in complex and often subtle ways.

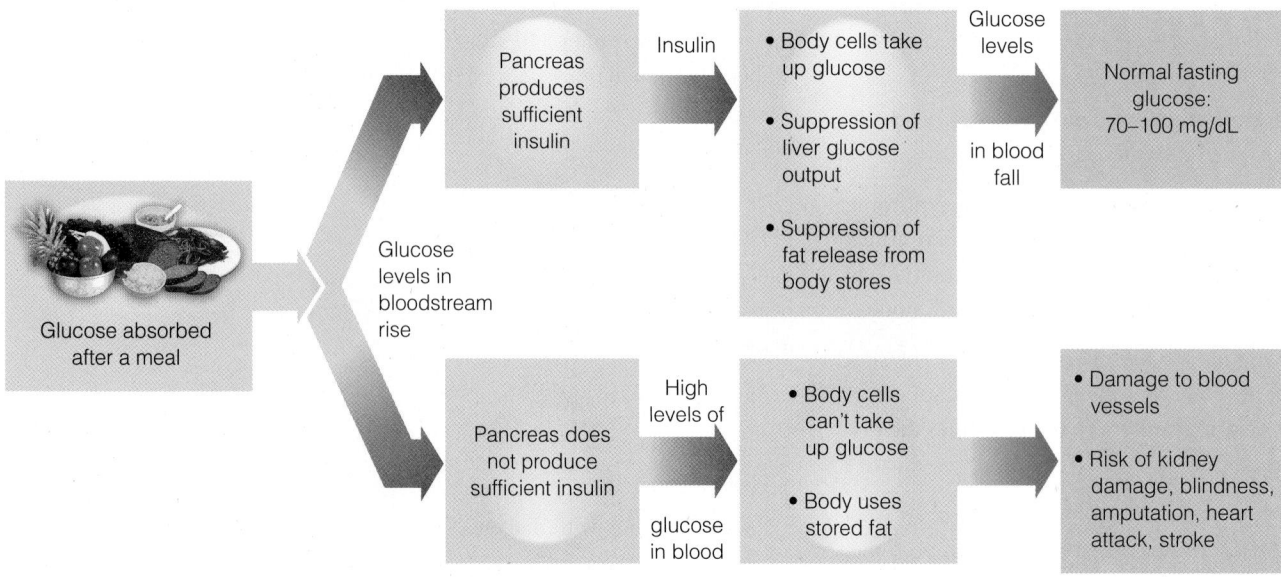

do not meet the recommended healthy levels for blood sugar, blood pressure, and cholesterol.[18] This puts them at risk of an early death from heart disease or of significant complications of untreated diabetes, such as blindness and chronic kidney disease.

About 8.5 percent of Americans overall have diabetes, but the rate is much higher—11 percent or greater—in 15 states, mostly in the South. People living in this so-called diabetes belt are more likely to become obese, sedentary, and less educated than in the country as a whole.[19] Racial and ethnic minorities around the country also have higher rates: 16 percent for American Indians/Alaska Natives, 13 percent for blacks, 12 percent for Hispanics, and 8 percent for Asian Americans, compared with 7 percent for whites.

Diabetes shortens life expectancy by an average of 8 years—7.8 years for men, 8.4 years for women. The risk of premature death among people with diabetes is about twice that of people without the disease. Obesity, diabetes, and heart disease also can work together to speed dementia and other brain disorders, such as cognitive impairment.

In addition to increasing the risk of dying from heart attack or stroke, untreated or uncontrolled diabetes also ups the danger of dying from many cancers by 25 percent and heightens the likelihood of death from infection and kidney and liver disease.[20]

According to the American Diabetes Association, the total economic cost of diabetes is more than $132 billion a year. Diabetes accounts for $1 of every $10 spent on health care in the United States. An estimated 48 million Americans may develop diabetes by 2050.

## Understanding Diabetes

Glucose is the primary form of sugar that the body cells use for energy. When a person without diabetes eats a meal, the level of glucose in the blood rises, triggering the production and release of insulin by special cell clusters in the pancreas. Insulin enhances the movement of glucose into various body cells, bringing down the level of glucose in the blood. In those who have diabetes, however, insulin secretion is either nonexistent or deficient. Without sufficient insulin, the glucose in the blood is unable to enter most body cells, so the cells' energy needs aren't met. The levels of glucose in the blood rise higher and higher after each meal. This unused glucose eventually passes through the kidneys, which are unable to process the excessive glucose, and out of the body in urine.

Deprived of the fuel it needs, the body begins to break down stored fat as a source of energy. This process produces weak acids, called ketones. A buildup of ketones leads to ketoacidosis, an upheaval in the body's chemical balance that brings on nausea, vomiting, abdominal pain, lethargy, and drowsiness. Severe ketoacidosis can lead to coma and eventual death.

Before the development of insulin injections, diabetes was a fatal illness. Today diabetics can have normal lifespans. However, diabetes still can lead to devastating complications. Uncontrolled glucose levels slowly damage blood vessels throughout the body; thus, individuals who become diabetic early in life may face devastating complications even before they reach middle age. Diabetes is the number one cause of blindness, nontraumatic amputations, and kidney failure, and diabetes increases by two or three times the risk of heart attack or stroke.

The risk of heart attack increases the longer a man has diabetes. In a recent study, men who have had type 2 diabetes for a decade or more face the same risk as those who have already had a prior heart attack.[21]

## Types of Diabetes

Diabetes includes several conditions in which the body has difficulty controlling levels of glucose in the bloodstream. After an overnight fast, most people have blood glucose levels between 70 and 100 milligrams of glucose per deciliter of blood (mg/dL). This is considered normal. If your fasting blood glucose level is between 101 and 125 mg/dL, you have prediabetes. If your fasting blood glucose is consistently 126 mg/dL or higher, you have diabetes.

- **Type 1 diabetes.** In this form of diabetes (once called juvenile-onset or insulin-dependent diabetes), the body's immune system attacks the insulin-producing beta cells in the pancreas and destroys them. The pancreas then produces little or no insulin and therefore blood glucose cannot enter the cells to be used for energy. Type 1 diabetes develops most often in young people but can appear in adults. Individuals with type 1 diabetes require insulin therapy because their own bodies no longer supply this vital hormone.

- **Type 2 diabetes.** In type 2 diabetes (once called adult-onset or non-insulin-dependent diabetes), either the pancreas does not make enough insulin or the body is unable to use insulin correctly. Type 2 diabetes is becoming more common in children and teenagers because of the increase in obesity in the young.

- **Gestational diabetes.** Women who get diabetes while they are pregnant are more likely to have a family history of diabetes, especially on their mothers' side; they are at greater risk of developing diabetes later in life.

Although type 1 and type 2 diabetes have different causes, two factors are important in both: an inherited predisposition to the disease and something in the environment that triggers diabetes. Genes alone are not enough. In most cases of type 1 diabetes, people need to inherit risk factors from both parents and to experience some environmental trigger, which might involve prenatal nutrition, a virus, or an unknown agent.

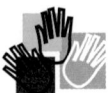 In type 2 diabetes, family history is one of the strongest risk factors for getting the disease, but only in Westernized countries. African Americans, Mexican Americans, and Native Americans have the highest rates, but people who live in less developed nations tend not to get type 2 diabetes, no matter how high their genetic risk.

Excess weight, especially around the waistline, is the major and most controllable risk factor for type 2 diabetes. Losing weight greatly reduces this risk and, in individuals with the disease, can help get blood sugar under control. Researchers also have found a complex relationship between depression and type 2 diabetes. Individuals with depressive symptoms are somewhat more likely to develop the disorder, while people being treated for type 2 diabetes have higher odds of becoming depressed.

Diabetic women who become pregnant face higher risks of miscarriage and babies with serious birth defects; however, precise control of blood sugar levels before conception and in early pregnancy can lower the likelihood of these problems.

The Diabetes Prevention Program (DPP), a landmark study sponsored by the National Institutes of Health, found that people at increased risk for type 2 diabetes can prevent or delay the onset of the disease by taking the following steps:

- Exercise 30 minutes on at least five days of the week.

- If you're overweight or obese, lose weight. Aim to lose 5 to 7 percent of your initial weight.

- Eat a diet rich in complex carbohydrates (bread and other starches) and high-fiber foods and low in sodium and fat.

- Eat fruits and vegetables that are rich in antioxidants, substances that prevent oxygen damage to cells.

- If your doctor advises, take medications, such as metformin (Glucophage), to help lower your blood sugar.

## Diabetes Signs and Symptoms

About a third of individuals with type 2 diabetes do not realize they have the illness. If you have risk factors for the disease, watch for the following warning signs:

- **Increased thirst and frequent urination.** Excess glucose circulating in your body draws water from your tissues, making you feel dehydrated. Drinking water and other beverages to quench thirst leads to more frequent urination.

- **Flu-like symptoms.** Type 2 diabetes can sometimes feel like a viral illness, with such symptoms as extreme fatigue and weakness. When glucose, your body's main fuel, doesn't reach cells, you may feel tired and weak.

- **Weight loss or weight gain.** Because your body is trying to compensate for lost fluids and glucose, you may eat more than usual and gain weight, or the opposite may occur. Although eating more than normal, you may lose weight because your muscle tissues don't get enough glucose to generate growth and energy.

- **Blurred vision.** High levels of blood glucose pull fluid from body tissues, including the lenses of the eyes, which affects ability to focus. Vision should improve with treatment of diabetes.

- **Slow-healing sores or frequent infections.** Diabetes affects the body's ability to heal and fight infection. Bladder and vaginal infections can be a particular problem for women.

- **Nerve damage (neuropathy).** Excess blood glucose can damage the small blood vessels to your nerves, leading to symptoms such as tingling and loss of sensation in hands and feet.

- **Red, swollen, tender gums.** Diabetes increases the risk of infection in your gums and in the bones that hold your teeth in place.

## Detecting Diabetes

To identify individuals with this disease as early as possible, the American Diabetes Association now recommends screening every three years for all men and women beginning at age 45. The American College of Endocrinology recommends screening at age 30 for individuals at risk, including those who are overweight, sedentary, have a family history of diabetes, or have high blood pressure or heart disease.

Tests that can detect diabetes include:

- **Random blood sugar test.** Because you don't necessarily fast for this test, your blood glucose may be high because you've just eaten. Even so, it shouldn't be higher than 200 mg/dL.

- **Fasting blood glucose test.** In general, glucose is lowest after an overnight fast. That's why the preferred way to test your blood sugar is after you've fasted overnight or for at least eight hours.

- **Glucose challenge test.** Often used to screen pregnant women for gestational diabetes, this test measures glucose before drinking eight ounces of an extremely sweet liquid after fasting for six hours, then every hour for a three-hour period. If your blood sugar rises more than expected and doesn't return to normal by the third hour, you likely have diabetes.

## Diabetes Management

Unlike many other medical conditions, patients must take charge of their diabetes and monitor their blood glucose regularly to prevent or delay the serious complications of the disease. Diabetes educators teach patients a new set of ABCs: Manage your **A1c** (blood glucose or sugar), **B**lood pressure, and **C**holesterol:

- **A** is for the **A1c test.** This test measures the amount of glucose attached to hemoglobin molecules, the iron-rich molecules in red blood cells that deliver oxygen to the body. The higher your blood glucose levels, the more hemoglobin molecules you will have with glucose attached—and the greater the risk of damage to eyes, kidneys, and feet. In general, the life cycle of a red blood cell is 75 to 90 days, which is why the A1c test shows average blood glucose levels for the past two to three months. The American Diabetes Association recommends a goal for A1c of less than 7 percent. The American College of Endocrinology recommends a goal of 6.5 percent. (Normal A1c levels are below 6.) Individuals with diabetes should have their A1c levels checked at least twice a year.

- **B** is for **blood pressure.** As discussed on page 501, the goal for most people is 115/75. High blood pressure can cause heart attack, stroke, and kidney disease.

- **C** is for **cholesterol.** The LDL goal for most people is less than 160 mg/dL (see Table 15.2 on page 503). Bad cholesterol, or LDL, can build up and clog your blood vessels.

## Treatment

The goal for diabetics is to keep blood sugar levels as stable as possible to prevent complications, such as kidney damage.[22] Home glucose monitoring, including new continuous glucose monitors, allows diabetics to check their blood sugar levels as many times a day as necessary and to adjust their diet or insulin doses as appropriate.

Types of insulin differ in how long it takes to start working after injection (onset), when it works hardest (peak), and how long it lasts in the body (duration). Individuals with diabetes may use different types in various combinations, depending on time of day and timing of meals. New insulin inhalers offer an alternative to injections for those with type 2 diabetes.

Those with type 1 diabetes require daily doses of insulin via injections, an insulin infusion pump, or oral medication. Those with type 2 diabetes often can control their disease through a well-balanced diet, exercise, and weight management. However, insulin therapy may be needed to keep blood glucose levels near normal or normal, thereby reducing the risk of damage to the eyes, nerves, and kidneys. New medications help control weight and lower blood pressure and cholesterol.

Medical advances hold out bright hopes for diabetics. Laser surgery, for instance, is saving eyesight. Bypass operations are helping restore blood flow to the heart and feet. Dialysis machines and kidney and pancreas transplants save many lives.

The number of Americans receiving treatment for diabetes has doubled to about 19 million (some 8.5 percent of the population) since 2007. During this period, the costs of diabetes treatment increased from $18.5 billion to $40.8 billion.[23]

## Can Diabetes Be Cured?

In most cases, diabetes requires lifelong management and treatment. However, a cure for some patients no longer seems impossible.[24] About 400 to 500 pancreas transplants are performed in the United States every year; when successful they normalize glucose levels, thereby curing diabetes. However, only about half of these transplants continue to function for ten years.

Gastric bypass surgery (which limits the amount of food a person can ingest) for extremely obese individuals has led to lasting remission of diabetes, sometimes even before a patient loses weight. (See Chapter 6.) Scientists do not yet know how bypass surgery "cures" diabetes, but it may affect chemicals involved in insulin resistance. Some surgeons are advocating this approach for all diabetics with body mass indexes (BMIs) over 50; others, as an option for those with BMIs over 35.[25]

Among other promising approaches are the use of stem cells to "rejuvenate" the pancreas, antibodies to block the autoimmune response of type 1 diabetes, and a more sophisticated artificial pancreas to monitor and manage glucose levels.[26]

# Hypertension

Blood pressure refers to the force of blood against the walls of arteries. When blood pressure remains elevated over time—a condition called hypertension—it forces the heart to pump harder than is healthy. Because the heart must force blood into arteries that are offering increased resistance to blood flow, the left side of the heart becomes enlarged. If untreated, high blood pressure can cause a variety of cardiovascular complications, including heart attack and stroke—two of the three leading causes of death among U.S. adults—as well as kidney failure and blindness (Figure 15.4).

In a young person even mild hypertension can cause organs such as the heart, brain, and kidneys to start to deteriorate. By age 50 or 60, the damage may be irreversible.

## Who Is at Risk?

According to a recent report by the World Health Organization, about 1 billion people worldwide have hypertension, which causes one in every eight deaths globally, making it the third leading killer in the world.[27] In the United States, high blood pressure is responsible for about a third of cardiovascular problems like heart attack or stroke and a quarter of all premature deaths.

 About a third of adults age 18 and older in the United States—some 65 million men and women—have high blood pressure. Hypertension is responsible for roughly one in six deaths among adults every year.

Blood pressure has increased among children and adolescents as well as adults, with the highest rates among black and Mexican American children. The primary culprit is the increase in obesity in the young. No one knows why African Americans are more vulnerable, although some speculate that overweight or dietary factors may contribute.

## Figure 15.4 Consequences of High Blood Pressure

If left untreated, elevated blood pressure can damage blood vessels in several areas of the body and lead to serious health problems.

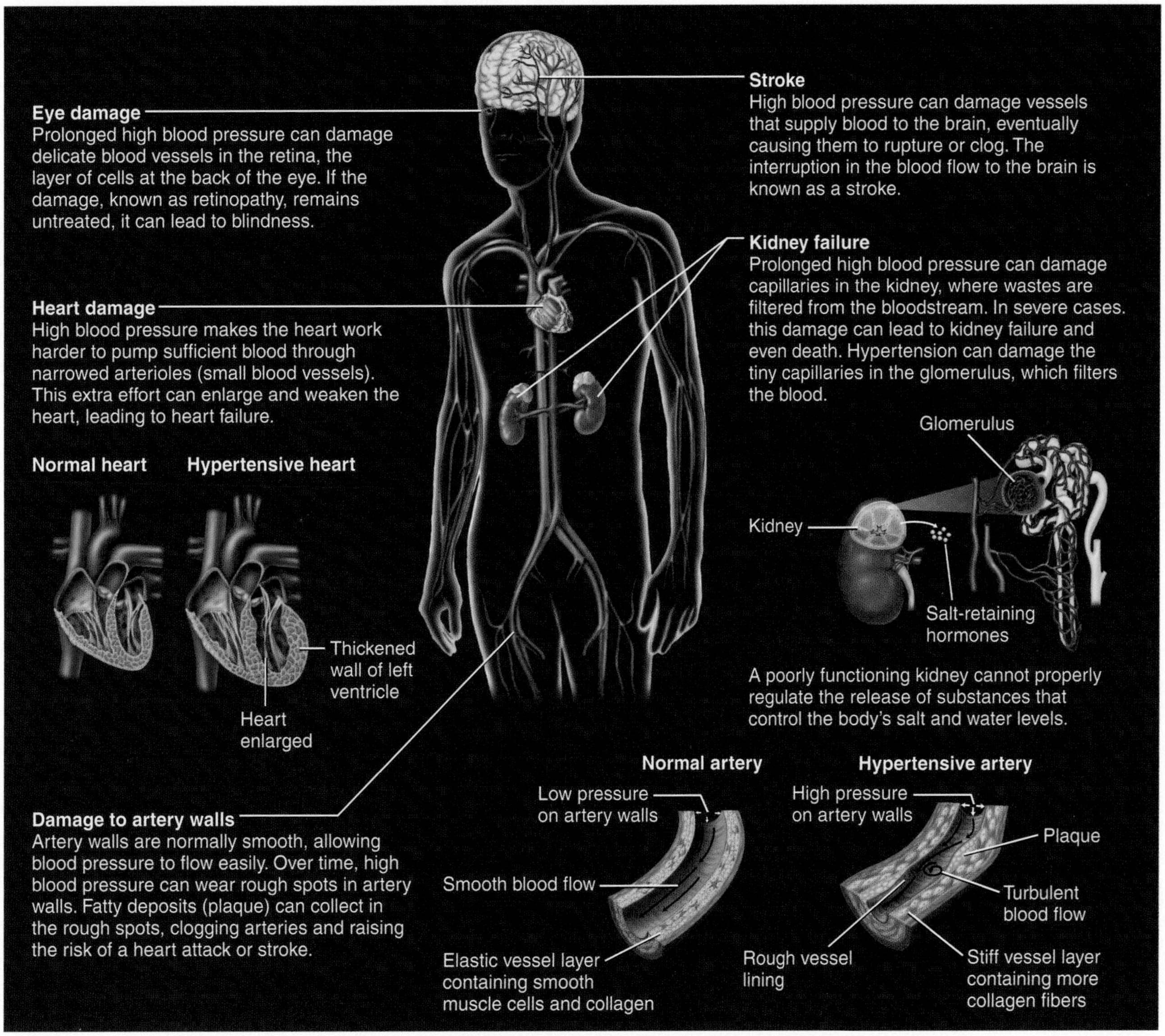

**Eye damage**
Prolonged high blood pressure can damage delicate blood vessels in the retina, the layer of cells at the back of the eye. If the damage, known as retinopathy, remains untreated, it can lead to blindness.

**Stroke**
High blood pressure can damage vessels that supply blood to the brain, eventually causing them to rupture or clog. The interruption in the blood flow to the brain is known as a stroke.

**Heart damage**
High blood pressure makes the heart work harder to pump sufficient blood through narrowed arterioles (small blood vessels). This extra effort can enlarge and weaken the heart, leading to heart failure.

**Kidney failure**
Prolonged high blood pressure can damage capillaries in the kidney, where wastes are filtered from the bloodstream. In severe cases. this damage can lead to kidney failure and even death. Hypertension can damage the tiny capillaries in the glomerulus, which filters the blood.

**Normal heart** **Hypertensive heart**

Thickened wall of left ventricle

Heart enlarged

Glomerulus

Kidney

Salt-retaining hormones

A poorly functioning kidney cannot properly regulate the release of substances that control the body's salt and water levels.

**Normal artery** **Hypertensive artery**

Low pressure on artery walls

High pressure on artery walls

Plaque

Smooth blood flow

Turbulent blood flow

**Damage to artery walls**
Artery walls are normally smooth, allowing blood pressure to flow easily. Over time, high blood pressure can wear rough spots in artery walls. Fatty deposits (plaque) can collect in the rough spots, clogging arteries and raising the risk of a heart attack or stroke.

Elastic vessel layer containing smooth muscle cells and collagen

Rough vessel lining

Stiff vessel layer containing more collagen fibers

---

Different races also suffer different consequences of high blood pressure. An African American with the same elevated blood pressure reading as a Caucasian faces a greater risk of stroke, heart disease, and kidney problems.

 Family history also plays a role. "If you study healthy college students with normal blood pressures, those who have one parent with hypertension will have blood pressure that's a little higher than average," notes Rose Marie Robertson, M.D., of the American Heart Association. "If two parents have high blood pressure, their levels will be a little higher, and they're destined to go higher still. If your parents have high blood pressure, have yours checked regularly."[28]

Men and women are equally likely to develop hypertension, but in women blood pressure tends to rise around the time of menopause. A larger proportion of middle-aged women than men have high systolic blood pressure, which puts their hearts in greater danger.[29]

For individuals who smoke, are overweight, don't exercise, or have high cholesterol levels, hypertension multiplies the risk of heart disease and stroke. Overweight people with high blood pressure have twice the risk of dying of a heart attack or stroke as those with normal blood pressure. At ultrahigh risk are people with diabetes or kidney disease.

## What Is a Healthy Blood Pressure?

Current guidelines (Table 15.1) categorize a reading of 120-139/80-89 as **prehypertension**, a condition that is likely to worsen in time. A healthy reading is 115/75 mm Hg. Once blood pressure rises above this threshold, the risk of cardiovascular disease may increase.

 In healthy adults, blood pressure screening should begin at age 21, with repeat evaluations at least every two years, or more often depending on your current health, medical history, and risk factors for cardiovascular disease. According to the National College Health Assessment survey, about nine in ten students have done so.

To get an accurate blood pressure reading, you should visit the doctor's office at least twice and have your blood pressure taken two or more

**prehypertension** A condition of slightly elevated blood pressure, which is likely to worsen in time.

Table 15.1 **What Your Blood Pressure Reading Means**

| Normal Results |
|---|
| In adults, the systolic pressure should be less than 120 mm Hg and the diastolic pressure should be less than 80 mm Hg. |
| **What Abnormal Results Mean** |
| **Prehypertension** |
| Top number is consistently 120 to 139 or the bottom number reads 80 to 89. |
| **Stage 1: Mild hypertension** |
| Top number is consistently 140 to 159 or the bottom number reads 90 to 99. |
| **Stage 2: Moderate-to-severe hypertension** |
| Top number is consistently 160 or over or the bottom number reads 100 or over. |
| **Low blood pressure (hypotension)** |
| Top number reading lower than 90 or pressure 25 mm Hg lower than usual. |
| Blood pressure readings may be affected by many different conditions, including cardiovascular disorders; neurological conditions; kidney and urological disorders; psychological factors such as stress, anger, or fear; various medications; and "white coat hypertension," which may occur if the medical visit itself produces extreme anxiety. |

Source: National Institute of Medicine National Institutes of Health.

times while you're seated. The average of those measurements determines how your blood pressure is classified.

The current guidelines classify hypertension into two categories:

- **Stage 1.** This consists of a systolic pressure ranging from 140 to 159 or a diastolic pressure ranging from 90 to 99.
- **Stage 2.** The most severe form of hypertension occurs with a systolic pressure of 160 or higher or a diastolic reading of 100 or higher.

Only one of the numbers—the top or bottom—needs to be high to meet these criteria. In people over age 50, systolic pressure is more important than diastolic. If it rises to 140 mm Hg or higher, doctors advise treatment regardless of the diastolic pressure.

## Lowering High Blood Pressure

Lifestyle changes are a first-line weapon in the fight against high blood pressure. Rather than making a single change, a combination of behavioral changes, including losing weight, eating heart-healthy foods, reducing sodium, and exercising more, yields the best results. A low-carbohydrate diet (discussed in Chapter 6) may be most effective for lowering blood pressure.

Too much sodium and too little potassium boost blood pressure in people who are sensitive to salt. The American Medical Association is calling for food makers and restaurants to cut the sodium content of food by 50 percent by 2016. For a healthful diet, aim for less than 1.5 grams of sodium a day, and at least 4.7 grams of potassium. The lower the amount of sodium in the diet, the lower the blood pressure for both those with and those without hypertension and for both genders and all racial and ethnic groups. However, reducing dietary sodium has an even greater effect on blood pressure in blacks than whites, and in women than men.

The National Heart, Lung and Blood Institute has developed what is known as the DASH diet. Following DASH, which stands for Dietary Approaches to Stop Hypertension, has proved as effective as drug therapy in lowering blood

## How to Lower Your Blood Pressure

- **Get moving.** Regular exercise can lower blood pressure by 10 points, prevent the onset of high blood pressure, or let you reduce your dosage of blood pressure medications.

- **Eat your way to better blood pressure.** Choose more fruits, vegetables, low-fat dairy products, whole grains, poultry, fish, and nuts. Cut down on red meat, sweets, sugar-containing beverages, and saturated fat and cholesterol.

- **Lose ten.** Shedding 10 percent of your current weight—or even ten pounds—can make a big difference.

- **Don't smoke.** A single cigarette can cause a 20-point spike in systolic blood pressure. Don't light up. See Chapter 6 for tips on quitting.

- **Hold the salt.** If you're salt sensitive, you may be spiking your blood pressure as you spice your food.

- **Stick with your medications.** If your doctor has prescribed medication to lower your blood pressure, take it conscientiously. Your future health may depend on it.

pressure. An additional benefit: The DASH diet also lowers harmful blood fats, including cholesterol and low-density lipoprotein, and the amino acid homocysteine (one of the new suspects in heart disease risk).

Too much sodium and too little potassium boost blood pressure in people who are sensitive to salt. The American Medical Association is calling for food makers and restaurants to cut the sodium content of food by 50 percent by 2016. For a healthful diet, aim for less than 1.5 grams of sodium a day, and at least 4.7 grams of potassium. The lower the amount of sodium in the diet, the lower the blood pressure for both those with and those without hypertension and for both genders and all racial and ethnic groups. However, reducing dietary sodium has an even greater effect on blood pressure in blacks than whites, and in women than men.

**Medications**    Making healthy lifestyle modifications can help reduce Stage 1 hypertension, but most people also require a medication. Drugs for lowering blood pressure come in a range of regimens (once a day to several times a day) with a range of effects on other conditions, interactions with other drugs, and potential side effects.

Medications to lower blood pressure have proven beneficial for individuals who have cardiovascular disease, but the scientific jury is out for those who do not because of the long-term costs and possible adverse effects. The current recommendation for those with blood pressure under 140/90 mm Hg is to lower blood pressure through lifestyle modifications, including dietary changes and regular exercise.[30] Some of the medicines used to treat high blood pressure are:

- Alpha blockers
- Angiotensin-converting enzyme (ACE) inhibitors
- Angiotension receptor blockers (ARBs)
- Beta-blockers
- Calcium channel blockers
- Central alpha agonists
- Diuretics
- Renin inhibitors, including aliskiren (Tekturna)
- Vasodilators

If your blood pressure is very high, you may need additional medications. Those with Stage 2 hypertension typically need at least two types of high blood pressure medications (antihypertensives) to reduce blood pressure to a safer level. The goal for most people with hypertension is to reduce blood pressure to below 140/90 mm Hg.

About 20 to 30 percent of people with high blood pressure have "resistant hypertension," which means that their blood pressure remains elevated despite taking three medications to lower it. In addition to medical conditions and certain medications, lifestyle factors, including excess weight, salt intake, and alcohol consumption, can contribute to this problem. New guidelines from the American Heart Association recommend weight loss, reduced salt, and decreased alcohol.[31]

Only about one-third of people with hypertension have it effectively controlled—below 140/90 mm Hg. Reducing systolic blood pressure 12 mm Hg for ten years can prevent one death in every 11 people treated for hypertension. In those with existing cardiovascular disease or organ damage, such as kidney disease, that reduction has an even bigger benefit, preventing one death in every nine people treated.

# Your Lipoprotein Profile

Medical science has changed the way it views and targets the blood fats that endanger the healthy heart. In the past, the focus was primarily on total cholesterol in the blood. The higher this number was, the greater the risk of heart disease. The NHLBI's National Cholesterol Education Program has recommended more comprehensive testing, called a *lipoprotein profile*, for all individuals age 20 or older.

This blood test, which should be performed after a 9- to 12-hour fast and repeated at least once every five years, provides readings of:

- **Total cholesterol.**
- **LDL (bad) cholesterol**, the main culprit in the buildup of plaque within the arteries.
- **HDL (good or *healthy*) cholesterol**, which helps prevent cholesterol buildup.
- **Triglycerides**, the blood fats released into the bloodstream after a meal.

## What Is a Healthy Cholesterol Reading?

Total cholesterol is the sum of all the cholesterol in your blood. Less than 200 mg/dL total cholesterol is ideal, and 200–239 mg/dL is borderline-high. Total cholesterol above 240 mg/dL is high and doubles your risk of heart disease. However, total cholesterol is not the only crucial number you should know. Because LDL increases your risk for heart disease, you always should find out your LDL level. Even if your total cholesterol is higher than 200, you may not be at high risk for a heart attack. Some people—such as women before menopause and young, active men who have no other risk factors—may have high HDL cholesterol and desirable LDL levels. Ask your doctor to interpret your results so you both know

your numbers and understand what they mean. (See Table 15.2.)

HDL, good cholesterol, also is important, particularly in women. Federal guidelines define an HDL reading of less than 40 mg/dL as a major risk factor for developing heart disease. HDL levels of 60 mg/dL or more are protective and lower the risk of heart disease.

Triglycerides, the free-floating molecules that transport fats in the bloodstream, ideally should be below 150 mg/dL. Individuals with readings of 150 to 199 mg/dL, considered borderline, as well as those with higher readings, may benefit from weight control, physical activity, and, if necessary, medication.

## Lowering Cholesterol

According to federal guidelines, about one in five Americans may require treatment to lower his or her cholesterol level.[32] However, nearly half of people who need cholesterol treatment, which can reduce the risk of heart disease by 30 percent over five years, don't get it. The National Cholesterol Education Program (NCEP) estimates that some 36 million Americans should be watching their diet and exercising more. Another 65 million should be taking cholesterol-lowering drugs. Depending on your lipoprotein profile and an assessment of other risk factors, your physician may recommend that you take steps to lower your LDL cholesterol.

*Lifestyle Changes* Some individuals with elevated cholesterol can improve their lipoprotein profile with lifestyle changes:

- **Dietary changes.** In the past, dietary changes produced relatively modest improvements compared to the effects of medications, which can cut cholesterol by as much as 35 percent. However, a diet consisting of cholesterol-lowering foods, including nuts, soy, oats, and plant sterols (in margarine and green leafy vegetables), reduced LDL cholesterol by about 30 percent. An added benefit: a reduction in C-reactive protein, discussed later in this chapter. Researchers are recommending this diet as an effective first treatment for individuals with high cholesterol levels, particularly when coupled with exercise and weight loss.

## How to Get an Accurate Lipoprotein Profile

- Go to your primary health-care provider to get a lipoprotein profile. Although cholesterol tests at shopping malls or health fairs can help identify people at risk, the analyzers are often not certified technicians, and the readings may be inaccurate.

- Ask about accuracy. Find out if the lab is using the National Institutes of Health standards, and ask about the lab's margin for error (which should be less than 5 percent).

- Fast beforehand. Cholesterol tests are most accurate after a 9- to 14-hour fast. Women may not want to get tested at the end of their menstrual cycles, when minor elevations in cholesterol levels occur because of lower estrogen levels. Cholesterol levels can also rise 5 to 10 percent during periods of stress. Reschedule the test if you come down with an intestinal flu because the viral infection could interfere with the absorption of food and thus with cholesterol levels. Let your doctor know if you're taking any drugs. Common medications, including birth control pills and hypertension drugs, can affect cholesterol levels.

- Sit down before allowing blood to be drawn or your finger to be pricked. Don't let a technician squeeze blood from your finger, which forces fluid from cells, diluting the blood sample and possibly leading to a falsely low reading.

Table 15.2 **How to Interpret Your Lipoprotein Profile**

| Total Cholesterol Level | Category |
|---|---|
| **Less than 200 mg/dL** | **Desirable level that puts you at lower risk for coronary heart disease. A cholesterol level of 200 mg/dL or higher raises your risk.** |
| **200 to 239 mg/dL** | **Borderline high** |
| **240 mg/dL and above** | **High blood cholesterol. A person with this level has more than twice the risk of coronary heart disease as someone whose cholesterol is below 200 mg/dL.** |
| HDL Cholesterol Level | Category |
| **Less than 40 mg/dL (for men)** | |
| **Less than 50 mg/dL (for women)** | **Low HDL cholesterol. A major risk factor for heart disease.** |
| **60 mg/dL and above** | **High HDL cholesterol. An HDL of 60 mg/dL and above is considered protective against heart disease.** |
| LDL Cholesterol Level | Category |
| **Less than 100 mg/dL** | **Optimal** |
| **100 to 129 mg/dL** | **Near or above optimal** |
| **130 to 159 mg/dL** | **Borderline high** |
| **160 to 189 mg/dL** | **High** |
| **190 mg/dL and above** | **Very high** |

**Your LDL cholesterol goal depends on how many other risk factors you have.**

- If you don't have coronary heart disease or diabetes and have one or no risk factors, your LDL goal is less than 160 mg/dL.

- If you don't have coronary heart disease or diabetes and have two or more risk factors, your LDL goal is less than 130 mg/dL.

- If you do have coronary heart disease or diabetes, your LDL goal is less than 100 mg/dL.

| Triglyceride Level | Category |
|---|---|
| **Less than 150 mg/dL** | **Normal** |
| **150-199 mg/dL** | **Borderline high** |
| **200-499 mg/dL** | **High** |
| **500 mg/dL or above** | **Very high** |

Source: National Cholesterol Education Program (NCEP) and American Heart Association. Adapted from http://www.americanheart.org/presenter.jhtml?identifier54500.

- **Weight management.** For individuals who are overweight, losing weight can help lower LDL. This is especially true for those with high triglyceride levels and/or low HDL levels and those who have a large waist measurement (more than 40 inches for a man and more than 35 inches for a woman).

- **Physical activity.** Regular activity can help lower LDL, lower blood pressure, reduce triglycerides, and particularly important, raise HDL. Again, these benefits are especially important for those with high triglyceride levels or large waist measurements.

Lifestyle changes can lower harmful LDL levels by 5 to 10 percent. However, a greater reduction of 30 to 40 percent requires either intensive lifestyle changes, including an extremely low-fat diet, or the addition of cholesterol-lowering medication.

*Medications*  Drugs called statins—better known by brand names such as Lipitor, Mevacor, Pravachol, and Zocor—can cut the risk of dying of a heart attack by as much as 40 percent. Initially tested in men, statins have proved equally beneficial for women, including those whose cholesterol levels rise after menopause.

Statins also protect patients who have not had a heart attack but are at high risk for developing cardiovascular disease because of high cholesterol or other risk factors. Large-scale studies indicate that statins protect against heart attacks and strokes even in older adults without known cardiovascular disease or diabetes and with low cholesterol—if these patients also have high levels of CRP or C-reactive protein (discussed on p. 508).

Statins work in the liver to block production of cholesterol. When the liver can't make cholesterol, it draws LDL cholesterol from the blood to use as raw material. This means that less LDL is available to trigger or promote the artery-clogging process known as atherosclerosis. Statins also appear to stabilize cholesterol-filled deposits in artery walls and to cool down inflammation. Long-term therapy with statins reduces the risk for death, heart attack, and stroke among people with heart disease, even when LDL levels are not elevated. The lower the LDL, the lower the risk.

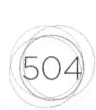

**atrium (plural atria)** Either of the two upper chambers of the heart, which receive blood from the veins.

**ventricle** Either of the two lower chambers of the heart, which pump blood out of the heart and into the arteries.

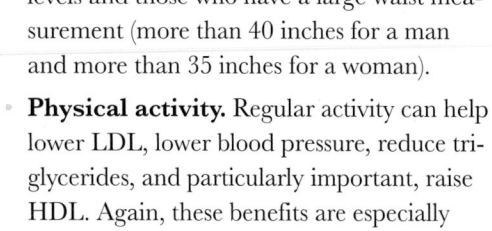

# Cardiovascular (Heart) Disease

In the United States, death rates from cardiovascular disease have dropped by 60 percent since 1950, one of the major U.S. health achievements of the twentieth century. The medical advances described in this chapter have contributed to this decline, but much of the credit goes to lifestyle changes, such as quitting smoking and making dietary changes that lower blood pressure and cholesterol levels.

Yet we still have a long way to go to keep the hearts of all Americans healthy. Only one of nearly 2,000 middle-aged Americans meets the criteria for ideal heart health as defined by the American Heart Association.[33] These criteria are:

- Never smoked or quit more than a year ago.
- Body Mass Index (BMI) less than 25.
- Physical exercise—at least 150 minutes of moderate intensity or 75 minutes of vigorous intensity a week.
- At least four components of a healthful diet, such as fewer calories and more fruits and vegetables (see Chapter 5).
- Total cholesterol lower than 200.
- Blood pressure below 120/80.
- Fasting blood sugar below 100.

Nearly 2,600 Americans die of heart disease every day—that's one every 34 seconds. More than 64 million Americans have heart disease. Each year an estimated 1 million Americans suffer a heart attack; nearly half of them die. The costs of treating heart disease and stroke are expected to triple in the next 20 years to an estimated $818 billion, according to the American Heart Association.[34]

## How the Heart Works

The heart is a hollow, muscular organ with four chambers that serve as two pumps (see Figure 15.5). It is about the size of a clenched fist. Each pump consists of a pair of chambers formed of muscles. The upper two—each called an **atrium**—receive blood, which then flows through valves into the lower two chambers, the **ventricles**, which contract to pump blood out into the arteries through a second set of valves. A thick wall divides the right side of the heart from the left side; even though the two sides are separated, they contract at almost the same time. Contraction of the ventricles is called **systole**; the period of relaxation between contractions is called **diastole**. The heart valves, located at the entrance and exit of the ventricular chambers, have flaps that open and close to allow blood to flow through the chambers of the heart.

The *myocardium* (heart muscle) consists of branching fibers that enable the heart to contract, or beat, between 60 and 80 times per minute, or about 100,000 times a day. With each beat, the heart pumps about 2 ounces of blood. This may not sound like much, but it adds up to nearly 5 quarts of blood pumped by the heart in one minute, or about 75 gallons per hour.

The heart is surrounded by the *pericardium*, which consists of two layers of a tough membrane. The space between the two contains a lubricating fluid that allows the heart muscle to move freely. The *endocardium* is a smooth membrane lining the inside of the heart and its valves.

Blood circulates through the body by means of the pumping action of the heart, as shown in Figure 15.6. The right ventricle (on your own right side) pumps blood, via the *pulmonary arteries*, to the lungs, where it picks up oxygen (a gas essential to the body's cells) and gives off carbon dioxide (a waste product of metabolism). The blood returns from the lungs via the *pulmonary veins* to the left side of the heart, which pumps it, via the **aorta**, to the arteries in the rest of the body.

The arteries divide into smaller and smaller branches and finally into **capillaries**, the smallest blood vessels of all (only slightly larger in diameter than a single red blood cell). The blood within the capillaries supplies oxygen and nutrients to the cells of the tissues and takes up various waste products. Blood returns to the heart via the veins: The blood from the upper body (except the lungs) drains into the heart through the *superior vena cava*, while blood from the lower body returns via the *inferior vena cava*.

The workings of this remarkable pump affect your entire body. If the flow of blood to or through the heart or to the rest of the body is reduced, or if a disturbance occurs in the small bundle of highly specialized cells in the heart

## Figure 15.5 The Healthy Heart

The heart muscle is nourished by blood from the coronary arteries, which arise from the aorta. (b) The cross section shows the four chambers and the myocardium, the muscle that does the heart's work. The pericardium is the outer covering of the heart.

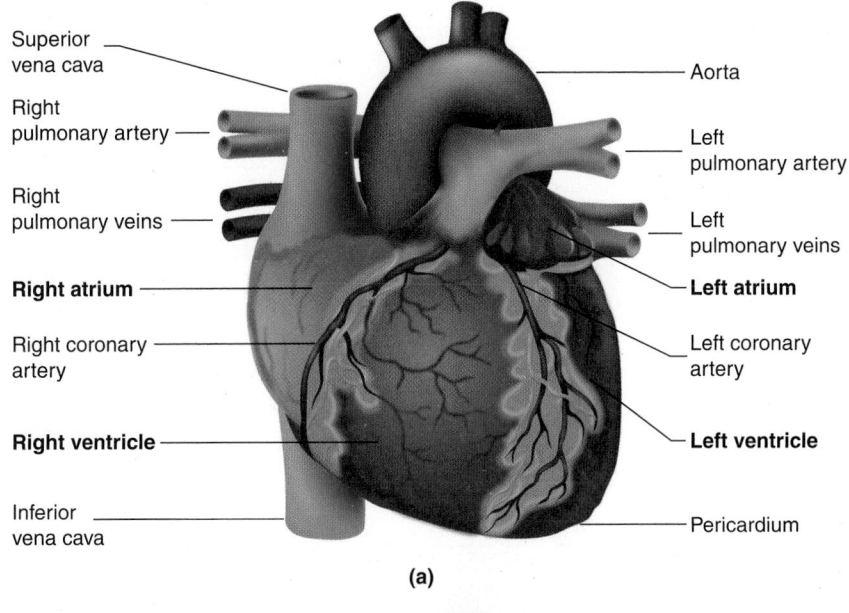

(a)

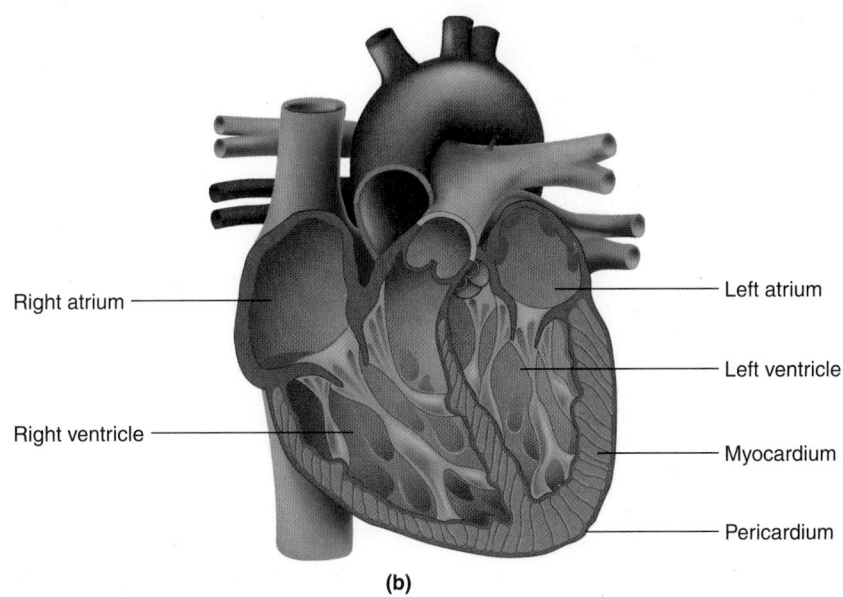

(b)

that generate electrical impulses to control heartbeats, the result may at first be too subtle to notice. However, without diagnosis and treatment, these changes could develop into a life-threatening problem.

Perhaps the biggest breakthrough in the field of cardiology has been not a test or a treatment but a realization: Heart disease is not inevitable. We can keep our hearts healthy for as long as we live, but the process of doing so must start early and continue throughout life.

**systole** The contraction phase of the cardiac cycle.

**diastole** The period between contractions in the cardiac cycle, during which the heart relaxes and dilates as it fills with blood.

**aorta** The main artery of the body, arising from the left ventricle of the heart.

**capillary** A minute blood vessel that connects an artery to a vein.

## Figure 15.6 The Path of Blood Flow

Blood is pumped from the right ventricle into the pulmonary arteries, which lead to the lungs, where gas exchange (oxygen for carbon dioxide) occurs. Oxygenated blood returning from the lungs drains into the left atrium and is then pumped into the left ventricle, which sends the blood into the aorta and its branches. The oxygenated blood flows through the arteries, which extend to all parts of the body. Again, gas exchange occurs in the body tissues; this time oxygen is "dropped off" and carbon dioxide "picked up."

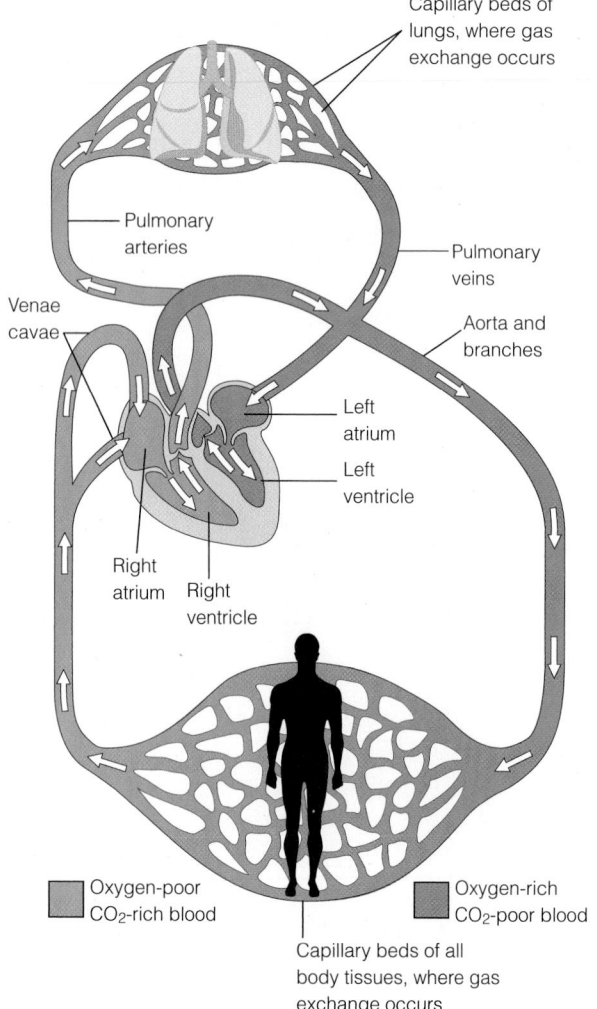

Capillary beds of lungs, where gas exchange occurs

Pulmonary arteries

Pulmonary veins

Venae cavae

Aorta and branches

Left atrium

Left ventricle

Right atrium   Right ventricle

Oxygen-poor CO$_2$-rich blood

Oxygen-rich CO$_2$-poor blood

Capillary beds of all body tissues, where gas exchange occurs

## Heart Risks on Campus

 Many people, including college students and other young adults, are unaware of habits and conditions that put their hearts at risk. Many undergraduates view heart disease as mainly a problem for white men and underestimate the risks for women and ethnic groups. Students rate their own knowledge of heart disease as lower than that of sexually transmitted infections and psychological disorders. Yet heart disease is the third-leading cause of death among adults age 25 to 44. Diabetes, family history, and other risk factors increase their likelihood of heart disease.

Young athletes face special risks. Each year seemingly healthy teens or young adults die suddenly on playing fields and courts. The culprit in one of every three cases of sudden cardiac death in young athletes is a silent condition called hypertrophic cardiomyopathy (HCM), an excessive thickness of the heart muscle. Because of HCM, the heart is more prone to dangerous heart irregularities.

In research studies, cardiac screening with an electrocardiogram has revealed abnormalities in 21 to 37 percent of student athletes. Most were mild, but approximately 1 percent of the students had significant electrical problems in the heart that would have been missed without electrocardiography. Some medical groups have recommended routine electrocardiograms to reduce risk of sudden cardiac death in competitive collegiate sports; others believe that a simpler physical exam-based screening is sufficient.

## Hearts and Minds: Psychosocial Risk Factors

As discussed in Chapter 2, our psychological and social health affects not just our minds but our bodies, including the heart. While problems such as depression and stress may increase cardiovascular risk, happiness may help keep our hearts healthy. In a study that followed men and women for ten years, those who showed more "positive" emotions—such as enthusiasm, joy, and contentment—were less likely to develop heart disease than less happy individuals. The happier people were, the lower their risk of heart disease became.[35]

Other factors also may protect the heart. In a study of adults in 52 nations, education—but not family income, occupation, or material possessions—lowered the risk of having a heart attack. Even with lifestyle, age, and income taken into consideration, people with low education levels (grade school or less) were significantly more likely to suffer a heart attack than those whose education extended beyond high school.[36]

How you respond to everyday sources of stress can affect your heart as well as your overall health. While you may not be able to control the sources of stress, you can change how you habitually respond to it.

Researchers classify psychological risk factors for heart disease into three categories: chronic, episodic, and acute. Chronic factors, such as job strain or lack of social support, play an important role in the buildup of artery-clogging plaque and may increase blood pressure. Even feeling that life has treated you unfairly boosts a person's chance of having a heart attack.

Episodic factors, such as depression, can last from several weeks to two years and may lead to the creation of "unstable" plaque, which is more likely to break off and block a blood vessel within the heart. Short-term or acute psychological risk factors, such as an angry outburst, can directly trigger a heart attack in people with underlying heart disease.

These factors may act alone or combine and exert different effects at different ages and stages of life. They may influence behaviors such as smoking, diet, alcohol consumption, and physical activity, as well as directly cause changes in physiology.

*Depression*  Depression and heart disease often occur together. People with heart disease are more likely to be depressed, and some seemingly healthy people with depression are at greater risk of heart problems. Depressed women younger than age 60 are more likely to suffer a heart attack than those who do not suffer from depression. After a heart attack, depression is common in both men and women, but physicians are less likely to recognize and treat depression in women.

Patients who suffer heart attacks and develop clinical depression have higher rates of complications and an increased risk of dying from another heart attack or other heart problems. People who are physically healthy with no risk factors for heart disease but who are prone to anger, hostility, and mild depression have higher levels of C-reactive protein, a substance linked to increased risk of heart disease.

*Anger and Hostility*  Anger and hostility have both short- and long-term consequences for the heart, particularly for men. In general the angriest men are three times more likely to develop heart disease than the most placid ones. Hostility more than doubles the risk of

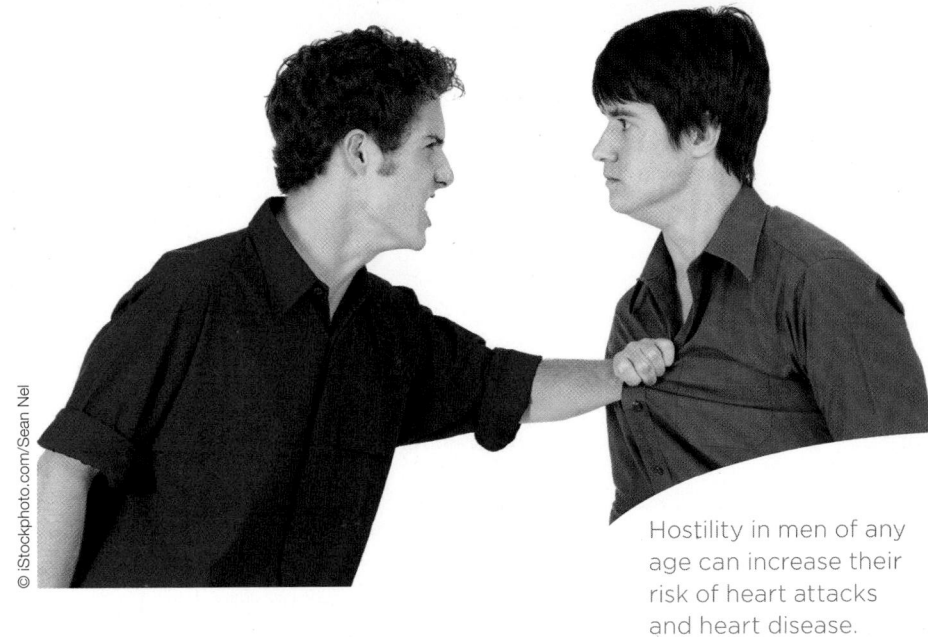

Hostility in men of any age can increase their risk of heart attacks and heart disease.

recurrent heart attacks in men (but not women). Research has linked hostility to increased cardiac risk factors, to decreased survival in men with coronary artery disease below the age of 61, to an increased risk of heart attack in men with metabolic syndrome, and to an increased risk of abnormal heart rhythms. Adults whose spouses rate them high in "antagonism"—a tendency to be argumentative, competitive, or cold—are more likely to have calcium buildup in their heart arteries.

Angry young men may be putting their future heart health in jeopardy. In a study that tracked more than 1,000 physicians for 36 years and took into account other physical and psychological risk factors, the angriest young men were six times more likely to suffer heart attacks by 55 and three times more likely to develop any form of cardiovascular disease. (See Health in Action: "Taming a Toxic Temper.")

How does hostility harm the heart? Anger triggers a surge in stress hormones that can provoke abnormal and potentially lethal heart rhythms and activates platelets, the tiny blood cells that trigger blood clotting. High levels of anger can also trigger a spasm in a coronary artery, which results in the additional narrowing of a partially blocked blood vessel.

In women, anger and hostility do not always lead to heart troubles. However, women who outwardly express anger may be at increased risk if they also have other risk factors for heart disease, such as diabetes or unhealthy levels of lipoproteins.

**Personality Types** In addition to stress, anger, and depression, other psychological traits can increase the risk of heart disease. Based on more than a decade of research, Dutch scientists have identified a "Type D" (for distressed) personality type. Type D people tend to be anxious, self-conscious, irritable, insecure, and negative, and go to great lengths not to say or do anything that others might not like. In the Dutch study, almost four times as many Type D individuals as others in cardiac rehabilitation programs died within an eight-year period.

In the past, other personality types have been linked to disease, for example, hard-charging, hostile Type As to heart disease and conflict-avoiding, emotion-suppressing Type Cs to cancer. However, these traits have not proved to be significant risk factors for these illnesses.

## Other Risk Factors

Researchers have identified other potential threats to heart health.

**Inflammation and C-Reactive Protein** Inflammation—the process by which the body responds to fever, injury, or infection—plays an essential role in healing and recovering from infection. However, chronic low-grade inflammation may contribute to atherosclerosis and set the stage for heart attacks, strokes, and other forms of cardiovascular disease. The most common triggers of inflammation are smoking, lack of exercise, high-fat and high-calorie meals, and highly processed foods.

C-reactive protein (CRP), produced in the liver, rises whenever the body responds to inflammation. Individuals with the highest CRP levels are more likely to develop heart disease than those with the lowest levels. High concentrations of CRP also may predict greater risk of sudden death.

**Homocysteine** High levels of *homocysteine*—an amino acid in the blood—have been linked to a greater risk of heart disease and stroke. Homocysteine may have an effect on atherosclerosis by damaging the inner lining of arteries and promoting blood clots. Several clinical trials are under way to test whether lowering homocysteine will reduce the risk of heart disease.

**Illegal Drugs** Illegal drugs pose many dangers—one of the most serious is their potentially deadly impact on the cardiovascular system. Ecstasy, amphetamines, and cocaine can cause a sudden rise in blood pressure, heart rate, and contractions of the left ventricle (the pumping chamber) of the heart, which can increase the risk of a heart attack.

The hallucinogens lysergic acid diethylamide (LSD) and psilocybin (psychoactive mushrooms) also have the potential for triggering irregular heartbeats and heart attacks, although less serious cardiac complications, such as a temporary rise in blood pressure, are more common. Morphine and heroin, which account for almost half of drug-related deaths, can lower blood pressure and affect the heart rate. Inhalants can produce fatal heartbeat irregularities. Marijuana, the most widely used illegal drug among young adults, can affect blood pressure and heart rate, but it is not known whether it can trigger a heart attack.

**Bacterial Infection** Certain bacteria may indeed put the heart at risk. *Streptococcus sanguis*, the bacterium found in dental plaque, has been implicated in the buildup of atherosclerotic plaque. Individuals with periodontal disease are at increased risk of heart disease and stroke. Regular brushing, flossing, and dental visits can reduce this danger.

Another common bacterium, *Chlamydia pneumoniae*, long linked to respiratory infections, also may threaten the heart. Individuals with high levels of antibodies to this bacteria are more likely to suffer a heart-related problem. Researchers have reported that antibiotics, taken to treat common infections, may protect against first-time heart attacks. A national clinical trial to determine whether antibiotics can reduce the risk of heart attack and stroke is under way.

## The Heart of a Woman

Many people still think of heart disease as a "guy problem." Men do have a higher incidence of cardiovascular problems than women before age 45. Although women develop heart problems later in life, by about age 65, their risk is about the same as men's. Heart disease, which now kills one in four women in the United States, is the largest single cause of death of women worldwide. Death rates from heart disease are rising among American women ages 35 to 54. American women are four to six times more likely to die of heart disease than of breast cancer.

Doctors no longer classify women as "low risk" or "intermediate risk" but consider them either to have ideal cardiovascular health or to be at risk of cardiovascular "events," such as a heart attack or stroke.

According to revised guidelines to prevent cardiovascular disease, women should strive for the following:

- BMI of less than 25
- Abstinence from smoking
- 150 minutes of moderate or 75 minutes of vigorous exercise every week (for additional benefits, 300 minutes of moderate or 150 minutes of vigorous exercise weekly)
- Diet high in fruits and vegetables, fiber, and whole grains and low in saturated fat, cholesterol, sugar, and sodium
- Non-HDL cholesterol level of less than 230 mg/dL
- Blood pressure of 120/80 mm Hg
- Fasting blood glucose of less than 100 mg/dL

The guidelines also encourage omega-3 fatty acids (discussed in Chapter 6) in fish or capsule form for women who have high cholesterol or triglycerides and advise all women to avoid therapies with risks that outweigh potential benefits, including postmenopausal hormone therapy, antioxidant vitamin supplements, folic acid supplements except during childbearing years to prevent birth defects, and routine use of aspirin if under age 65.[37]

According to the American Heart Association, all women with at least one major cardiometabolic risk factor are at risk for heart disease. Nine in ten women may meet this standard. Many women don't get a proper diagnosis because they have a form of heart disease that doesn't show up on the usual diagnostic tests. In women with *vascular dysfunction*, the blood vessels—both the large coronary arteries and the small microvessels—supplying the heart do not expand properly to accommodate increased blood flow. Standard diagnostic procedures, including stress tests and coronary angiograms, do not reveal this condition. However, newer tests, including ultrasound of the blood vessels,

# Health in Action

## Taming a Toxic Temper

Are you a hothead? Do you lose it, blow up, explode, go ballistic, have a fit? The terms we use for getting angry reveal its dangers. Anger is a bomb, and if you have a short fuse, you and everyone around you are in harm's way. In the long run, chronic rage puts your life at risk—especially if you're an angry young male. In a study that tracked more than 1,000 physicians for 36 years, the angriest young men were six times more likely to suffer heart attacks by 55 and three times more likely to develop any form of cardiovascular disease. Anger and hostility also threaten the hearts of women with other cardiac risk factors.

"Taming a Toxic Temper" in *Labs for IPC* shows you how to recognize the earliest signs of anger and analyze the situations that trigger your anger—so you can handle them, change the ways in which you respond, and keep in mind the consequences of an angry outburst. It is important that you, not your temper, be in control of your life. Here's a preview.

Begin by asking yourself these questions:

- Do people describe you as hotheaded?
- Do you get so annoyed when someone tries to get ahead of you in a line that you confront the person?
- Do you get so angry you forget what you're thinking?
- Did you ever become so angry with someone that you felt as if you would explode?

After reviewing your answers, you rate your temper on a scale of 1 (tranquil) to 10 (red-hot). You also review your anger history by describing the five worst rage explosions of your life

and listing all of the negative consequences of your anger and outbursts.

The next step involves setting aside time to practice anger-reduction exercises you learn and writing journal entries.

Taming your temper is a six-step process. You learn one step each week, and each week add a new one. Here's a sampling of the first one:

**WEEK 1. Tune into your cues.** To control your anger, you must be mindful and sensitive to subtle cues that you are becoming angry as *early as possible*. What is the earliest sign of anger you experience in your body . . . ?

- Do you clench your fists?
- Do you tighten your jaw?
- Do you feel heat?

Whenever you feel the first sensation, look for something subtle that comes before it—a thought, perhaps, or a perception of something about another person that does not set right with you. The earlier you sense that something is beginning to make you angry, the greater the opportunity . . . The other five steps are:

- Identify your triggers.
- Talk yourself down.
- Rely on anger-reducers.
- Develop better coping tools.
- Take it to the street.

In the final stage you continue to monitor your anger levels, triggers, and cues daily and continue to rehearse in real life, by deliberately putting yourself in circumstances that used to set off angry outbursts. Let someone take the last bagel even though you were obviously reaching for it. Stand next to the student talking loudly on her cell phone. . . .

can reveal heart problems that angiograms fail to pick up.

Women are less likely to survive heart attacks than men, perhaps because they don't seek or receive treatment as soon as men. That's why women need to know the early signs and symptoms of female heart disease:

- Tiredness, even after getting adequate sleep.
- Trouble breathing.
- Trouble sleeping.
- Feeling sick to the stomach.
- Feeling scared or nervous.
- New or worse headaches.
- An ache in the chest.
- Feeling "heavy" or "tight" in the chest.
- A burning feeling in the chest.
- Pain in the back, between the shoulders.
- Pain or tightness in the chest that spreads to the jaw, neck, shoulders, ear, or the inside of the arms.
- Pain in the belly, above the belly button.

Researchers long believed that postmenopausal hormone therapy (HT) protected women from heart disease. However, more recent large-scale studies have shown little, if any, benefit. In fact, in older women HT increases the risk of cardiovascular problems and blood clots. However, women in their 50s who take estrogen therapy have lower levels of dangerous calcium deposits in their arteries, suggesting that supplemental estrogen for younger women with menopausal symptoms may benefit their hearts.

In light of these inconclusive and contradictory results, the AHA guidelines recommend against use of hormone therapy simply to prevent heart disease. They also recommend not using antioxidant supplements or folic acid, which have proven ineffective.

## Aspirin and the Heart

Daily low-dose aspirin has been recommended as a preventive step for men at high risk of cardiovascular disease because it reduces the stickiness of platelets (cells that cause blood clotting). This lowers the risk of blood clots, which can block a blood vessel and trigger a heart attack or stroke. Several research studies have demonstrated an association between aspirin use and reductions in heart attacks in men. However, while aspirin lowers the likelihood of heart attack, it may slightly increase stroke risk.

According to new recommendations from the U.S. Preventive Services Task Force, people should consider various factors including age, gender, diabetes, blood pressure, cholesterol levels, smoking, and risk of gastrointestinal bleeding before deciding to use aspirin. The more risk factors they have, the more likely they are to benefit from aspirin.

The Task Force recommends that men between the ages of 45 and 79 should use aspirin to reduce their risk for heart attacks when the benefits outweigh the harm from potential gastrointestinal bleeding. Women between ages 55 and 70 should use aspirin to reduce their risk for ischemic stroke when the benefits outweigh the risk from gastrointestinal bleeding. The Task Force recommends against aspirin use in men under age 45 or women under age 55 because heart attacks and strokes are less likely in these age groups.[38]

Small doses of aspirin can lower the risk of heart attack in men who have never had heart disease, but the drug does not cut the chances of dying from the disease. A U.S. Preventative Services Task Force has recommended low-dose aspirin for men between ages 45 and 79 to stave off heart attacks and for women over 65 to prevent strokes.[39]

Aspirin can produce side effects, including gastrointestinal bleeding, allergic reactions, and peptic ulcers. However, the very low doses recommended for heart disease prevention generally do not cause serious problems. Aspirin is not advised for people taking anticlotting medication, who have stomach ulcers, or who have kidney or liver disease. Some individuals are aspirin-resistant and do not benefit from its protective effects.

Researchers are testing a "polypill," a single pill that contains a statin, three blood pressure medications, and aspirin to see if this combination might best reduce the risk of heart attack, stroke, and other cardiovascular problems.[40]

# Crises of the Heart

**Coronary Artery Disease** The general term for any impairment of blood flow through the blood vessels, often referred to as "hardening of the arteries," is **arteriosclerosis**. The most common form is **atherosclerosis**, a disease of the lining of the arteries in which **plaque**—deposits of fat, fibrin (a clotting material), cholesterol, other cell parts, and calcium—narrows the artery channels. Twenty-first-century research has revealed that inflammation also plays a crucial role.

**Atherosclerosis** This process begins when LDL cholesterol penetrates the wall of an artery. Ideally, HDL cholesterol carries the cholesterol out of the artery wall to the liver for disposal. However, if LDL accumulates, the artery responds by releasing chemical messengers called cytokines, which trigger active inflammation in the artery wall. T-lymphocytes and macrophages, specialized white blood cells that are part of the body's defensive immune system, move from the bloodstream into the artery and engulf the LDL. As they ingest the LDL, the macrophages enlarge and become foam cells, which rupture, releasing cholesterol into the artery wall, where the cycle of damage begins again. In response, the smooth muscle cells in the artery wall create a fibrous cap over the inflamed area (Figure 15.7).

These hard-capped plaques are dangerous: They narrow arteries, reduce the flow of blood, and produce angina (chest pain). However, the usual culprits in heart attacks are smaller, softer plaques that can rupture. As the body responds with clotting factors, platelets, and blood cells, a blood clot, or thrombus, forms on the disrupted plaque's surface. The clot ultimately blocks the artery and kills heart muscle cells. Similar clots can block blood flow to the brain and lead to other complications, including kidney failure and circulation problems in the legs and feet.

**Unclogging the Arteries** Reversing the buildup of plaque inside the arteries is possible with cholesterol-lowering drugs and a low-fat diet. A strict program of dietary and lifestyle change without any medication, developed by Dean Ornish, M.D., of the University of California, San Francisco, also has proved effective in reversing coronary artery disease. The following are the key elements of this approach:

- **A very low-fat, vegetarian diet,** including nonfat dairy products and egg whites, keeping fat intake to below 8 percent of total calories consumed. Ornish's recommended diet allows no meat, poultry, fish, butter, cheese, ice cream, or any form of oil.

- **Moderate exercise,** consisting of an hour of aerobic activity three times a week. Walking is recommended because more rigorous exercise might be dangerous for heart patients, who may develop increased risk of blood clots, irregular heartbeats, or coronary artery spasms during exertion.

**arteriosclerosis** Any of a number of chronic diseases characterized by degeneration of the arteries and hardening and thickening of arterial walls.

**atherosclerosis** A form of arteriosclerosis in which fatty substances (plaque) are deposited on the inner walls of arteries.

**plaque** The sludgelike substance that builds up on the inner walls of arteries.

Figure 15.7 **How Atherosclerosis Happens**
LDL cholesterol penetrates an artery wall, and the accumulation of LDL cholesterol triggers an inflammation. Macrophages engulf the LDL and become foam cells. The artery wall creates a fibrous cap over this plaque, and the artery is narrowed. If the plaque ruptures, blood clots can block blood flow to the heart or to the brain.

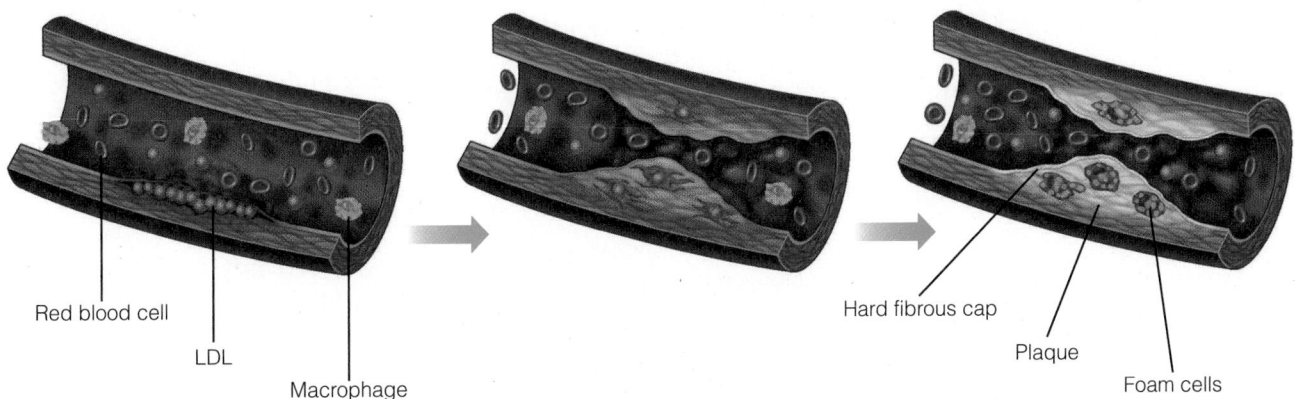

Red blood cell

LDL

Macrophage

Hard fibrous cap

Plaque

Foam cells

- **Stress counseling.** Ornish's patients learn how the body's stress response can cause a rapid heartbeat and narrowing of the arteries, and how stress reduction can reduce cholesterol levels.

- **An hour a day of yoga, meditation, breathing, and progressive relaxation.** Some patients use visualization, for instance, imagining their arteries being cleared by a tunneling machine.

*Angina Pectoris*   A temporary drop in the supply of oxygen to the heart tissue causes feelings of pain or discomfort in the chest known as **angina pectoris**. Some people suffer angina only when the demands on their hearts increase, such as during exercise or when under stress. Many people have angina for years and yet never suffer a heart attack; in some, the angina even disappears. However, angina should be considered a warning of danger if it becomes more severe or more frequent, occurs with less activity or exertion, begins to waken a person from a sound sleep at night, persists for more than 10 to 15 minutes, or causes unusual perspiration.

*Heart Attack (Myocardial Infarction)* Each year, about 1.5 million Americans suffer a heart attack. About 500,000 die. Half of the deaths occur within an hour of the start of symptoms and before the person reaches the hospital. The medical name for a heart attack, or coronary, is **myocardial infarction (MI)**. The *myocardium* is the cardiac muscle layer of the wall of the heart. It receives its blood supply, and thus its oxygen and other nutrients, from the coronary arteries. If an artery is blocked by a clot or plaque, or by a spasm, the myocardial cells do not get sufficient oxygen, and the portion of the myocardium deprived of its blood supply begins to die.

Although such an attack may seem sudden, usually it has been building up for years, particularly if the person has ignored risk factors and early warning signs. According to research, 80 to 90 percent of those who develop heart disease and 95 percent of those who suffer a fatal heart attack have at least one major risk factor.

*Is It a Heart Attack?*   If they experience the following symptoms, individuals should seek immediate medical care and take an aspirin (325 milligrams) to keep the blood clot in a coronary artery from getting any bigger:

- A tight ache, heavy, squeezing pain, or discomfort in the center of the chest, which may last for 30 minutes or more and is not relieved by rest.
- Chest pain that radiates to the shoulder, arm, neck, back, or jaw.
- Anxiety.
- Sweating or cold, clammy skin.
- Nausea and vomiting.
- Shortness of breath.
- Dizziness, fainting, or loss of consciousness.

As noted on page 508, women often experience heart attacks differently than men. In the month before an attack, many report unusual fatigue and disturbed sleep. Far fewer women than men experience chest pain. More common symptoms are shortness of breath, weakness and fatigue, a clammy sweat, dizziness, and nausea.

Many everyday activities—eating, drinking coffee, having sex, even breathing—can spur a heart attack. In a recent major analysis of heart attack triggers, air pollution from traffic posed the greatest risk, causing about 7 percent of heart attacks. Coffee was linked to 5 percent of heart attacks, and alcohol to another 5 percent. Physical exertion may trigger 6 percent of heart attacks, eating a heavy meal, 3 percent. And having sex, 2 percent.[41]

If you're with someone who's exhibiting the classic signs of heart attack, and if they last for two minutes or more, act at once. Expect the person to deny the possibility of anything as serious as a heart attack, but insist on taking prompt action.

Time is of the essence when a heart attack occurs. If you develop symptoms or if you're with someone who does, call 911 immediately. The sooner emergency personnel get to a heart attack victim and administer cardiac life support, the greater the odds of survival. Yet according to the American Heart Association, most patients wait three hours after the initial symptoms begin before seeking help. By that time, half of the affected heart muscle may already be lost.

*Cardiac Arrest*   Cardiac arrest occurs when the heart stops beating. If circulation isn't restored within four or five minutes, the brain shuts down completely, and the person dies.

**angina pectoris** A severe, suffocating chest pain caused by a brief lack of oxygen to the heart.

**myocardial infarction (MI)** A condition characterized by the dying of tissue areas in the myocardium, caused by interruption of the blood supply to those areas; the medical name for a heart attack.

**Cardiopulmonary resuscitation (CPR)** is an emergency procedure for a person whose heart has stopped or who is no longer breathing. CPR can maintain circulation and breathing until emergency medical help arrives.

The combination of mouth-to-mouth "rescue" breathing and chest compressions performed by individuals trained in CPR is the most effective method. However, according to the most recent research, chest compressions or "hands-only" CPR, which does not require extensive training, also can keep blood circulating until emergency help arrives. (For video instructions on hands-on CPR, go to: http://handsonlycpr.eisenberginc .com/)

Automated external defibrillators (AEDs), portable computerized devices, can actually restart a heart with a lethal rhythm (ventricular fibrillation) or that is not beating at all. The machines, widely available on airplanes and in public places like stadiums and terminals, also can be purchased by individuals. Written and voice instructions allow lay people as well as trained professionals to use them in case of emergency. A combination of CPR and defibrillation boosts the survival rate much higher than from CPR alone.

*Saving Hearts* State-of-the-art treatments for heart attacks include clot-dissolving drugs, early administration of medications to thin the blood, intravenous nitroglycerin, and in some cases, a beta-blocker (which blocks many of the effects of adrenaline in the body, particularly its stimulating impact on the heart).

*Percutaneous transluminal coronary angioplasty (PTCA)*, also called balloon angioplasty, is the most often performed heart operation. Less costly and less risky than bypass surgery, PTCA opens blood vessels in the heart that are narrowed but not completely blocked. PTCA involves a precise, time-consuming technique called *cardiac catheterization*—the threading of a narrow tube or catheter through an artery to the heart. An X-ray taken with a special dye injected into the arteries reveals the location and extent of a blockage. By inflating a tiny balloon at the tip of the catheter, physicians can break up the clog and widen the narrowed artery. When they deflate the balloon, circulation is restored. Stents can help prevent balloon-opened arteries from clogging again.

A *coronary bypass* is a procedure in which an artery from the patient's leg or chest wall is grafted onto a coronary artery to detour blood around the blocked area. Each year hundreds of thousands of coronary bypasses are performed in the United States; about 1 to 5 percent of these patients die as a result of surgical complications. Surgery or angioplasty to improve blood flow in patients with moderate to severe levels of blood flow restriction to the heart reduces the risk of cardiac death more than drugs alone.

# Stroke

When the blood supply to a portion of the brain is blocked, a cerebrovascular accident, or **stroke**, occurs. The proportion of strokes among young adults between ages 20 and 45 has been rising, probably as a consequence of the higher incidence of obesity, hypertension, and diabetes.[42] About two-thirds of the almost 800,000 strokes that occur every year in the United States strike women. However, before age 85, men experience more strokes. Nonetheless, women of every age fare worse than men in the prevention, diagnosis, treatment, and outcome of stroke. An estimated 20 percent of stroke victims die within three months; 50 to 60 percent are disabled. About half of those who have a stroke are partially paralyzed on one side of their body; between a quarter and a half are partially or completely dependent on others for daily living; a third become depressed; a fifth cannot walk. Quick treatment with a clot-busting drug at a hospital can reduce the chance of disability after a stroke, but few people recognize the signs of a stroke and seek medical care within three hours of the first symptoms.[43]

Strokes rank third, after heart disease and cancer, as a cause of death in this country. Worldwide, stroke is second only to heart disease as a cause of death. After decades of steady decline, the number of strokes per year has begun to rise. The main reasons seem to be that more people in the United States are living longer, advanced medical care is allowing more people to survive heart disease, and doctors are better able to diagnose and detect strokes. Yet 80 percent of strokes are preventable, primarily through lifestyle modification. The most important steps are treating hypertension, not

**cardiopulmonary resuscitation (CPR)** A method of artificial stimulation of the heart and lungs; a combination of mouth-to-mouth breathing and chest compression.

**stroke** A cerebrovascular event in which the blood supply to a portion of the brain is blocked.

smoking, managing diabetes, lowering cholesterol, and taking aspirin, which reduces stroke risk in women, but not men.[44]

## Risk Factors

Risk factors for stroke, like those for heart disease, include some that can't be changed (such as gender, race, and age) and some that can be controlled:

- **Gender.** Men have a greater risk of stroke than women. However, women are at increased risk at times of marked hormonal changes, particularly pregnancy and childbirth. Past studies have shown an association between oral contraceptive use and stroke, particularly in women over age 35 who smoke. The newer low-dose oral contraceptives have not shown an increased stroke risk among women ages 18 to 44. Early menopause (before age 42) may double a woman's stroke risk.

- 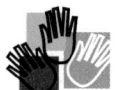 **Race.** The incidence of strokes is two to three times greater in blacks than whites in the same communities. Hispanics also are more likely to develop hemorrhagic strokes than whites.

- **Age.** A person's risk of stroke more than doubles every decade after age 55.

- **Obesity.** According to a recent longitudinal study of middle-aged Americans, the more overweight individuals are, the more likely they are to have a stroke. Obesity may increase stroke risk by contributing to high blood pressure and diabetes.

- **Hypertension.** Detection and treatment of high blood pressure are the best means of stroke prevention.

- **High red blood cell count.** A moderate to marked increase in the number of a person's red blood cells increases the risk of stroke.

- **Heart disease.** Heart problems can interfere with the flow of blood to the brain; clots that form in the heart can travel to the brain, where they may clog an artery.

- **Blood fats.** Although the standard advice from cardiologists is to lower harmful LDL levels, what may be more important to lower stroke risk is an increase in the levels of protective HDL.

- **Diabetes mellitus.** Diabetics have a higher incidence of stroke than nondiabetics.

- **Estrogen therapy.** In the Women's Health Initiative—a series of clinical trials of hormone therapy for postmenopausal women—estrogen-only therapy significantly increased the risk of stroke.

- **A diet high in fat and sodium.** Individuals consuming the largest amounts of fatty foods and sodium are at much greater risk then those eating low-fat, low-salt diets.

## Causes of Stroke

There are two types of stroke: *ischemic stroke*, which is the result of a blockage that disrupts blood flow to the brain, and *hemorrhagic stroke*, which occurs when blood vessels rupture. One of the most common causes of ischemic stroke is the blockage of a brain artery by a thrombus, or blood clot—a *cerebral thrombosis*. Clots generally form around deposits sticking out from the arterial wall. Sometimes a wandering blood clot (embolus), carried in the bloodstream, becomes wedged in one of the cerebral arteries. This is called a *cerebral embolism*, and it can completely plug up a cerebral artery.

In hemorrhagic stroke, a diseased artery in the brain floods the surrounding tissue with blood. The cells nourished by the artery are deprived of blood and can't function, and the blood from the artery forms a clot that may interfere with brain function. This is most likely to occur if the patient suffers from a combination of hypertension and atherosclerosis. Hemorrhage (bleeding) may also be caused by a head injury or by the bursting of an aneurysm, a blood-filled pouch that balloons out from a weak spot in the wall of an artery.

Brain tissue, like heart muscle, begins to die if deprived of oxygen, which may then cause difficulty speaking and walking, and loss of memory. (See Figure 15.8.) These effects may be slight or severe, temporary or permanent, depending on how widespread the damage and whether other areas of the brain can take over the function of

Figure 15.8  **The Effects of Stroke on the Brain**

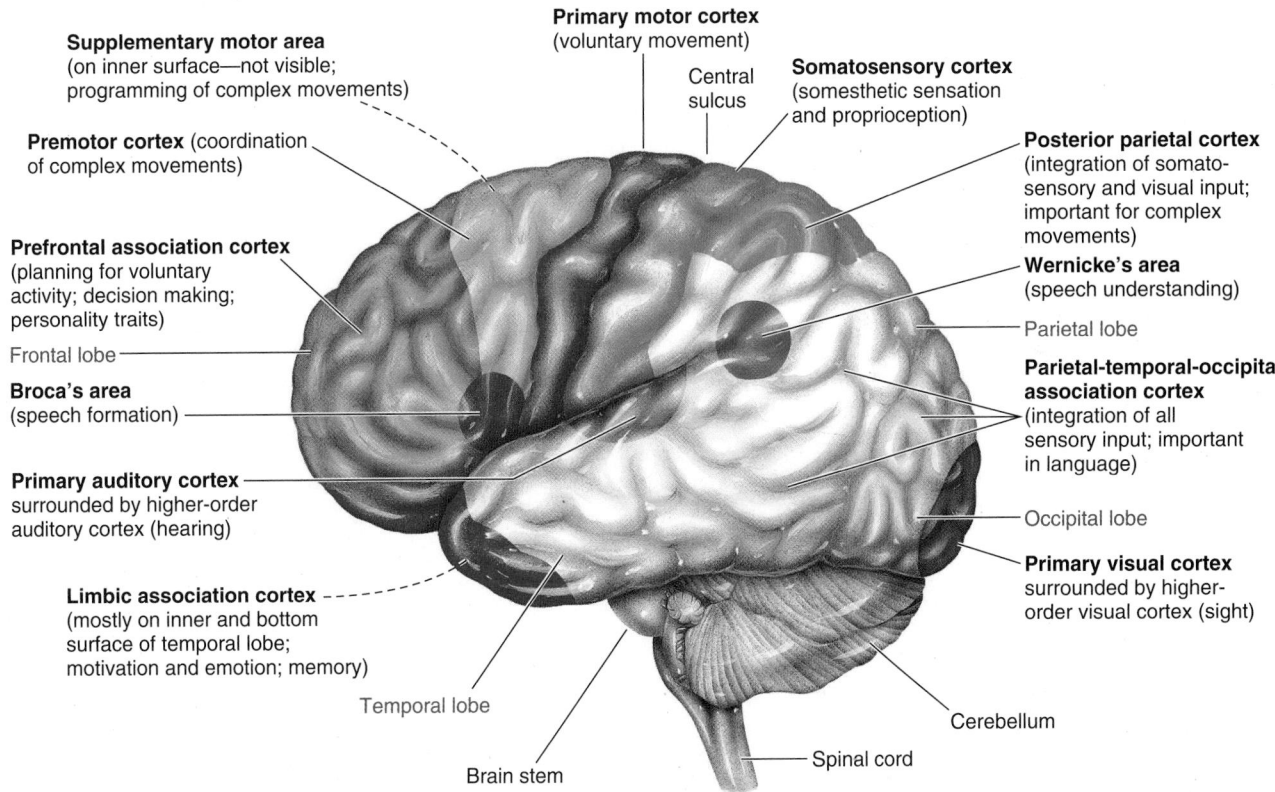

**(a)** Regions of the cerebral cortex responsible for various functions

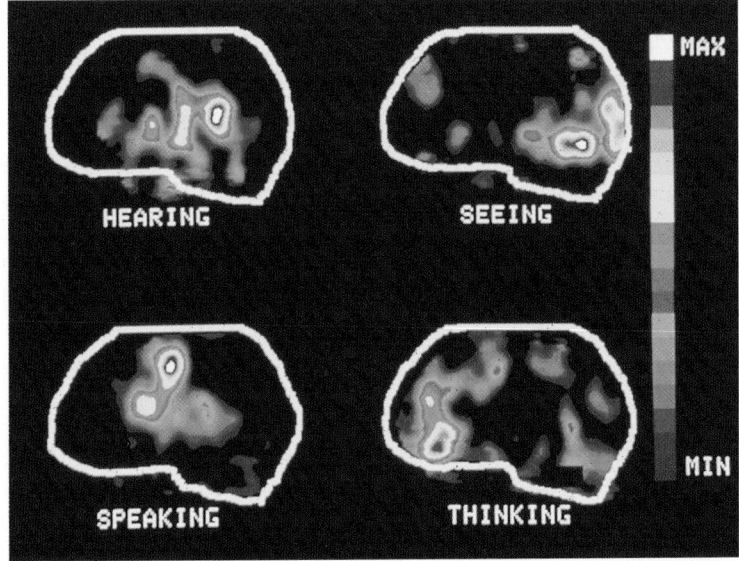

**(b)** Regions of increased blood flow during different tasks

the damaged area. About 30 percent of stroke survivors develop dementia, a disorder that robs a person of memory and other intellectual abilities.

## Silent Strokes

As many as one in ten middle-aged adults may suffer a "silent" stroke, known as a "silent cerebral infarct," that does not produce clear symptoms but causes damage within the brain. According to new research, silent strokes may be at least five times more common than full-blown strokes in people under age 65 and are not uncommon in those younger than 50. The parts of the brain affected by the stroke may not involve motion or speech, but silent strokes can affect mood or memory.

Doctors note that mild strokes are not really silent but "whisper," causing very subtle symptoms that people might ignore. However, on tests of mental and physical functioning, individuals who've had very mild strokes suffer clear impairments. Even if they do not cause symptoms, brain imaging techniques such as MRIs can detect their effects. The best medical advice: know the warning signs of a stroke and seek immediate treatment.

## Transient Ischemic Attacks (TIAs)

Sometimes a person will suffer **transient ischemic attacks (TIAs)**, "little strokes" that cause minimal damage but serve as warning signs of a potentially more severe stroke. A TIA doubles the risk for a heart attack.[45] One of three people who suffer TIAs will have a stroke during the following five years if they don't get treatment. The two major types of TIAs are:

- **Transient monocular blindness.** Blurring, a blackout or whiteout of vision, a sense of a shade coming down, or another visual disturbance in one eye.

- **Transient hemispheral attack.** Diminished blood flow to one side of the brain, causing numbness or weakness of one arm, leg, or side of the face, or problems speaking or thinking.

Many TIAs are caused by a narrowing of blood vessels in the neck (carotid arteries) because of a buildup of plaque. Specialists can diagnose this problem by feeling and listening to the arteries, by ultrasound, by measuring the pressure or circulation rate from the carotid arteries to the eyes, or by arterial angiography (injection of a dye into the arteries as X-rays are taken), a procedure that can be either dangerous, even deadly, or lifesaving.

Surgery to widen the carotid arteries may be recommended for individuals with significant narrowing (50 to 80 percent or more). For other patients, aspirin and other drugs that make platelets less sticky and interfere with clotting may be effective.

## Treatments for Strokes

Extremely rapid beating of the heart's upper chambers causes blood clots to form; they may enter the bloodstream and travel to the brain, where they can get stuck and choke off the blood supply. In the past, the only way to prevent such strokes was regular use of a medication called warfarin, which inhibits blood clotting and therefore increases the risk of severe bleeding. However, aspirin proved as effective as warfarin—without that dangerous side effect. Daily low-dose aspirin can cut in half the risk of strokes caused by abnormal heartbeats, which strike 75,000 Americans each year.

For patients who suffer a thrombotic stroke, thrombolytic drugs such as tissue-type plasminogen activator (tPa) can restore brain blood flow and save blood cells. Other medications called heparinoids can reduce the blood's tendency to clot. For thrombolytic drugs to be effective, they must be administered within three hours after the stroke; heparinoids must be given within 24 hours. People who get to a hospital within an hour of having the first symptoms of a stroke are twice as likely to receive tPa. However, the average person does not seek help for 22 hours or longer.

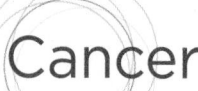

# Cancer

The rate of new cancers in the United States has dropped by almost 1 percent a year, and the rate of death from new cancers has fallen 1.6 percent a year. For the first time, lung cancer deaths have decreased in women as well as men—a drop attributed to a decline in smoking.[46]

**transient ischemic attack (TIA)** A cerebrovascular event in which the blood supply to a portion of the brain is blocked temporarily; repeated attacks are predictors of more severe strokes.

According to a recent study by the American Cancer Society, the majority of the world's new cancer cases (7.1 million) and deaths (4.8 million) now occur in developing countries. These numbers are expected to double by 2030 as the world's population grows and ages.[47]

Healthier lifestyles could prevent some 340,000 cancers a year.[48] A third of cancers are related to smoking; another third, to obesity, poor diet, and lack of exercise.

The number of survivors living with cancer in the United States has risen to an all-time high of 11.7 million, including 7 million age 65 or older.[49] In addition to improvements due to early detection and advances in treatment, psychosocial support has proven effective in extending survival in patients with melanoma, leukemia, and cancer of the breast, lung, and gastrointestinal tract.[50] (See "Self-Survey," p. 529.)

## Understanding Cancer

The uncontrolled growth and spread of abnormal cells causes cancer. Normal cells follow the code of instructions embedded in DNA (the body's genetic material); cancer cells do not. Think of the DNA within the nucleus of a cell as a computer program that controls the cell's functioning, including its ability to grow and reproduce itself. If this program or its operation is altered, the cell goes out of control. The nucleus no longer regulates growth. The abnormal cell divides to create other abnormal cells, which again divide, eventually forming *neoplasms* (new formations), or tumors.

Tumors can be either benign (slightly abnormal, not considered life-threatening) or malignant (cancerous). The only way to determine whether a tumor is benign is by microscopic examination of its cells. Cancer cells have larger nuclei than the cells in benign tumors; they vary more in shape and size; and they divide more often. In general, one billion cancer cells need to have formed before a cancer can be detected. This is the number of cells in a tumor that measures one centimeter (about a third of an inch.)

At one time cancer was thought to be a single disease that attacked different parts of the body. Now scientists believe that cancer comes in countless forms, each with a genetically determined molecular "fingerprint" that indicates how deadly it is. With this understanding, doctors can identify how aggressively a tumor should be treated.

Without treatment, cancer cells continue to grow, crowding out and replacing healthy cells. This process is called **infiltration**, or invasion. Cancer cells may also **metastasize**, or spread to other parts of the body via the bloodstream or lymphatic system (Figure 15.9). For many cancers, as many as 60 percent of patients may

**infiltration** A gradual penetration or invasion.

**metastasize** To spread to other parts of the body via the bloodstream or lymphatic system.

Figure 15.9 **Metastasis, or Spread of Cancer**
Cancer cells can travel through the blood vessels to spread to other organs or through the lymphatic system to form secondary tumors.

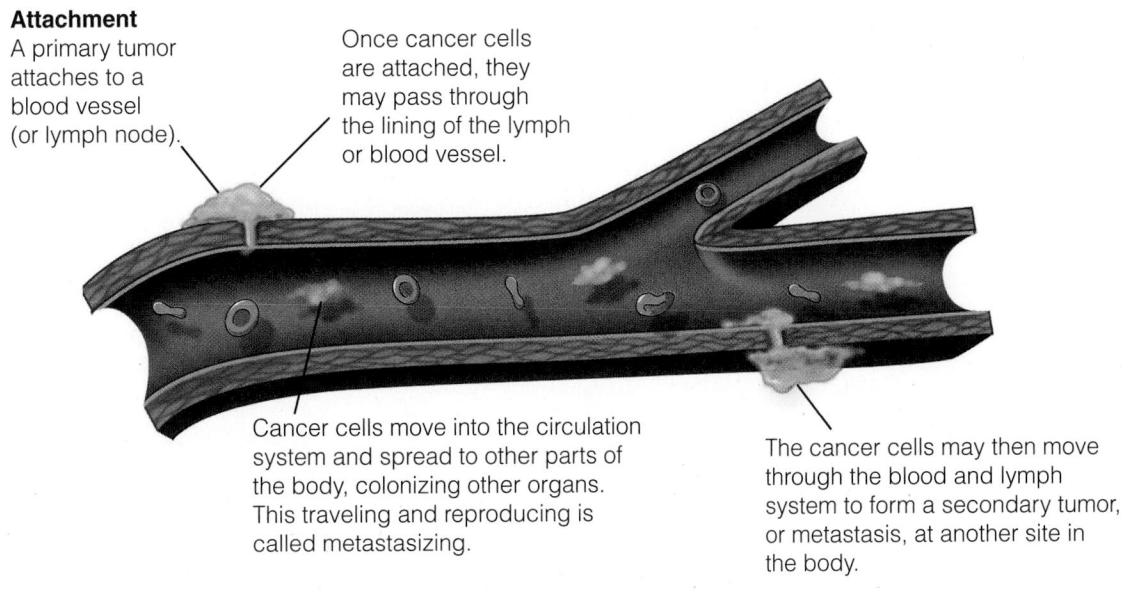

**Attachment**
A primary tumor attaches to a blood vessel (or lymph node).

Once cancer cells are attached, they may pass through the lining of the lymph or blood vessel.

Cancer cells move into the circulation system and spread to other parts of the body, colonizing other organs. This traveling and reproducing is called metastasizing.

The cancer cells may then move through the blood and lymph system to form a secondary tumor, or metastasis, at another site in the body.

have metastases (which may be too small to be felt or seen without a microscope) at the time of diagnosis. Early detection and treatment result in the highest rate of cure.

## Risk Factors for Cancer

According to the American Cancer Society, almost 1.5 million individuals are diagnosed with cancer each year; about 563,000 die of it. The five-year survival rate for all cancer is 66 percent, up from 50 percent three decades ago.[51]

Cancer strikes individuals at all social, economic, and educational levels. However, not everyone receives a prompt diagnosis and equal high-quality care. Those who lack health insurance or whose policies do not cover all the costs of treatments often face delays in detecting a cancer and in beginning treatment.

Since the occurrence of cancer increases over time, most cases affect adults who are middle-aged or older. In the United States, men have a one in two lifetime risk of developing cancer; for women, the risk is one in three (see Figure 15.10).

The term **relative risk** compares the risk of developing cancer in people with a certain exposure or trait to the risk in those who do not have this exposure or trait. Smokers, for instance, have a ten-times-greater relative risk of developing lung cancer than nonsmokers. Most relative risks are smaller. For example, women who have a first-degree (mother, sister, or daughter) family history of breast cancer have about a twofold increased risk of developing breast cancer compared with women who do not have a family history of the disease. This means that they are about twice as likely to develop breast cancer.

**relative risk** The risk of developing cancer in persons with a certain exposure or trait compared to the risk in persons who do not have the same exposure or trait.

**Figure 15.10 Sex Differences in Cancer Rates and Deaths**

| Estimated New Cases* | | Estimated Deaths | |
|---|---|---|---|
| **Male** | **Female** | **Male** | **Female** |
| Prostate 218,890 (29%) | Breast 178,480 (26%) | Lung & bronchus 89,510 (31%) | Lung & bronchus 70,880 (26%) |
| Lung & bronchus 114,760 (15%) | Lung & bronchus 98,620 (15%) | Prostate 27,050 (9%) | Breast 40,460 (15%) |
| Colon & rectum 79,130 (10%) | Colon & rectum 74,630 (11%) | Colon & rectum 26,000 (9%) | Colon & rectum 26,180 (10%) |
| Urinary bladder 50,040 (7%) | Uterine corpus 39,080 (6%) | Pancreas 16,840 (6%) | Pancreas 16,530 (6%) |
| Non-Hodgkins lymphoma 34,200 (4%) | Non-Hodgkins lymphoma 28,990 (4%) | Leukemia 12,320 (4%) | Ovary 15,280 (6%) |
| Melanoma of the skin 33,910 (4%) | Melanoma of the skin 26,030 (4%) | Liver & intrahepatic bile duct 11,280 (4%) | Leukemia 9,470 (4%) |
| Kidney and renal pelvis 31,590 (4%) | Thyroid 25,480 (4%) | Esophagus 10,900 (4%) | Non-Hodgkins lymphoma 9,060 (3%) |
| Leukemia 24,800 (3%) | Ovary 22,430 (3%) | Urinary bladder 9,630 (3%) | Uterine corpus 7,400 (3%) |
| Oral cavity & pharynx 24,180 (3%) | Kidney and renal pelvis 19,600 (3%) | Non-Hodgkins lymphoma 9,600 (3%) | Brain & other nervous system 5,590 (2%) |
| Pancreas 18,830 (2%) | Leukemia 19,440 (3%) | Kidney & renal pelvis 8,080 (3%) | Liver and intrahepatic bile duct 5,500 (2%) |
| All Sites 766,860 (100%) | All sites 678,060 (100%) | All sites 289,550 (100%) | All sites 270,100 (100%) |

* Excludes basal and squamous cell skin cancers and in situ carcinoma except urinary bladder.

Medical experts recommend that cancer survivors exercise regularly, eat at least five servings of fruits and vegetables daily, and not smoke. However, only a small minority—5 percent in one study—are following all three recommendations.

*Heredity* An estimated 13 to 14 million Americans may be at risk of a hereditary cancer. In hereditary cancers, such as retinoblastoma (an eye cancer that strikes young children) or certain colon cancers, a specific cancer-causing gene is passed down from generation to generation. The odds of any child with one affected parent inheriting this gene and developing the cancer are 50–50.

Other people are born with genes that make them susceptible to having certain cells grow and divide uncontrollably, which may contribute to cancer development. The most well-known are mutations of the BRCA gene, linked with increased risk of breast, colon, and ovarian cancer.

Genetic tests can identify some individuals who are born with an increased susceptibility to cancer. By spotting a mutated gene in an individual, doctors can sometimes detect cancer years earlier through increased cancer screening. The most likely sites for inherited cancers to develop are the breast, brain, blood, muscles, bones, and adrenal glands.

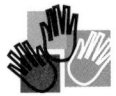 **Racial and Ethnic Groups** Although overall cancer death rates have fallen in the United States, black Americans still bear the biggest brunt of fatal cancers. The death rate from cancer among black men is 32 percent higher than that of white men while the cancer death rate among black women is about 16 percent above that of white women.[52]

African American women have the highest incidence of colorectal and lung cancers of any ethnic group, while black men have the highest rates of prostate, colorectal, and lung cancer. African Americans also have higher rates of incidence and deaths from other cancers, including those of the mouth, throat, esophagus, stomach, pancreas, and larynx.

Cancer rates also vary in other racial and ethnic groups. Hispanics have a six times lower risk of developing melanoma than Caucasians, yet tend to have a worse prognosis than Caucasians when they do develop this skin cancer. The incidence of female breast cancer is highest among white women and lowest among Native American women. Cervical cancer is most common in Hispanic women.

Asian Americans, both those born in the United States and immigrants, generally have lower cancer rates than other ethnic groups. Vietnamese men have much higher rates of liver cancer than whites, while Korean men and women are much more likely to develop stomach cancer. Compared with other Asian Americans, Chinese and Vietnamese women have higher rates of lung cancer. Asian Americans who have lived in the United States the longest are likely to develop the cancers that are most common here, such as breast and colon cancer, although at lower rates than whites.

*Obesity* Long recognized as threats to cardiovascular health, overweight and obesity may play a role in an estimated 90,000 cancer deaths each year. According to American Cancer Society researchers who examined the relationship between body mass index (BMI) and risk of dying from cancer, 14 percent of cancer deaths in men and 20 percent of cancer deaths in women may stem from excess weight.

The higher an individual's BMI, the greater the likelihood of dying of cancer. An unhealthy body weight increases the risk of many types of cancer, including breast (in postmenopausal women), colon and rectum, kidney, cervix, ovary, uterus, esophagus, gallbladder, stomach (in men), liver, pancreas, prostate, non-Hodgkin's lymphoma, and multiple myeloma.

The degree to which extra pounds affect cancer risk varies by site. Obesity elevates the risk of esophageal cancer fivefold; increases the risk of breast or uterine cancer by two to four times; and boosts the risk for colon cancer by 35 percent to twofold.

*Infectious Agents* Worldwide, an estimated 17 percent of cancers can be attributed to infection. In economically developing countries, infections cause or contribute to 26 percent of cancers. In developed countries, they play a role in 7 percent of new cases of cancer.

Among the cancers that have been linked with infectious agents are human papillomavirus

(HPV) with cervical cancer and *Helicobacter pylori* with stomach cancer. Viruses have been implicated in certain leukemias (cancers of the blood system) and lymphomas (cancers of the lymphatic system), cancers of the nose and pharynx, liver cancer, and cervical cancer. (See Chapter 10 for details on the human papillomavirus.) Human immunodeficiency virus (HIV) can lead to certain lymphomas and leukemias and to a type of cancer called Kaposi's sarcoma.

Generally, the presence of a bacterium or a virus per se is not enough to cause cancer. A predisposing environment and other cofactors—most still unknown—are needed for cancer development and growth.

## Common Types of Cancer

Cancer refers to a group of more than a hundred diseases characterized by abnormal cell growth. Although all cancers have similar characteristics, each is distinct. Some cancers are relatively simple to cure, whereas others are more threatening and mysterious. The earlier any cancer is found, the easier it is to treat and the better the patient's chances of survival.

Cancers are classified according to the type of cell and the organ in which they originate, such as the following:

- **Carcinoma**, the most common kind, which starts in the epithelium, the layers of cells that cover the body's surface or line internal organs and glands.
- **Sarcoma**, which forms in the supporting, or connective, tissues of the body: bones, muscles, blood vessels.
- **Leukemia**, which begins in the blood-forming tissues: bone marrow, lymph nodes, and the spleen.
- **Lymphoma**, which arises in the cells of the lymph system, the network that filters out impurities.

If you note any of the following seven warning signs, immediately schedule an appointment with your doctor:

- Change in bowel or bladder habits.
- A sore that doesn't heal.
- Unusual bleeding or discharge.
- Thickening or lump in the breast, testis, or elsewhere.
- Indigestion or difficulty swallowing.
- Obvious change in a wart or mole.
- Nagging cough or hoarseness.

***Skin Cancer*** One of every five Americans can expect to develop skin cancer in their lifetimes. Once scientists thought exposure to the B range of ultraviolet light (UVB), the wavelength of light responsible for sunburn, posed the greatest danger. However, longer-wavelength UVA, which penetrates deeper into the skin, also plays a major role in skin cancers. An estimated 80 percent of total lifetime sun exposure occurs during childhood, so sun protection is especially important in youngsters. Tanning salons and sunlamps also increase the risk of skin cancer because they produce ultraviolet radiation. A half-hour dose of radiation from a sunlamp can be equivalent to the amount you'd get from an entire day in the sun. Often skin damage is invisible to the naked eye but shows up under special diagnostic lights.

 Young adults spend the most time in the sun and also frequent tanning salons. Even when they perceive the seriousness of skin cancer, college students—particularly women—describe suntanned skin as attractive, healthy, and athletic-looking and view the benefits of getting a suntan as outweighing the risks of skin cancer or premature aging. Some students actually become addicted to tanning. (See Consumer Alert, p. 522.) However, a CDC report concluded that indoor tanning is "simply not safe" and causes sunburn, infection, eye damage, and increased risk of skin cancer.

The most common skin cancers are *basal cell* (involving the base of the epidermis, the top level of the skin) and *squamous cell* (involving cells in the epidermis). Their incidence is increasing among men and women under the age of 40. Long-term exposure to the sun is the biggest risk factor for these cancers.

Every year more than 5 million Americans develop skin lesions known as actinic keratoses (AKs), rough red or brown scaly patches that develop in the upper layer of the skin, usually on the face, lower lip, bald scalp, neck, back of the hands, and forearms. Forty percent of squamous cell carcinomas, the second leading cause of skin cancer deaths, begin as AKs. Treatments include surgical removal, cryosurgery (freezing the skin), electrodesiccation (heat generated by an electric current), topical chemotherapy, and removal with lasers, chemical peels, or dermabrasion.

Malignant *melanoma*, the deadliest type of skin cancer, causes 1 to 2 percent of all cancer deaths. Melanoma has become the most common cancer among young adults between ages 25 and 29 and the second most common cancer among 15- to 24-year-olds.[53] During the 1930s, the lifetime risk of melanoma was about 1 in 1,500. Today it is 1 in 75. This increase in risk is due mostly to overexposure to UV radiation. The use of a tanning bed ten times or more a year doubles the risk for individuals over age 30.

Both the amount and the intensity of lifetime sun exposure play key roles in determining risk for melanoma. People living in areas where the sun's ultraviolet rays reach Earth with extra intensity, such as tropical or high-altitude regions, are at increased risk. Although melanoma occurs more often among people over 40, it is increasing in younger people, particularly those who had severe sunburns in childhood. The rate of increase in melanoma also has risen more in men (4.6 percent a year) than in women (3.2 percent). Men are more likely than women to be diagnosed with melanoma after age 40.

Individuals with any of the following characteristics are at increased risk:

- Fair skin, light eyes, or fair hair.
- A tendency to develop freckles and to burn instead of tan.
- A history of childhood sunburn or intermittent, intense sun exposure.
- A personal or family history of melanoma.
- A large number of nevi, or moles (200 or more, or 50 or more if under age 20), or dysplastic (atypical) moles.

**Detection**  The most common predictor for melanoma is a change in an existing mole or development of a new and changing pigmented mole. The most important early indicators are change in color, an increase in diameter, and changes in the borders of a mole (Figure 15.11). An increase in height signals a corresponding growth in depth under the skin. Itching in a new or long-standing mole also should not be ignored.

## Save Your Skin

- **Once a month, stand in front of a full-length mirror to examine your front and back, and your left and right sides with your arms raised.** Check the backs of your legs, the tops and soles of your feet, and the surfaces between your toes. Use a hand mirror to check the back of your neck, behind your ears, and your scalp.

- **Watch for changes in the size, color, number, and thickness of moles.** Suspicious moles are likely to be asymmetrical (one half doesn't match the other), with ragged, notched, or blurred edges. Also look for any signs of darkly pigmented growth, oozing, scaliness, bleeding, or a change in sensation, itchiness, tenderness, or pain.

- **Don't put too much faith in sunscreens.** Wearing sunscreen (with a sun protection factor, or SPF, of at least 15) is good, but protective clothing is better—and staying in the shade is best. Check your shadow. One simple guideline for reducing the risk of skin cancer is avoiding the sun anytime your shadow is shorter than you are. According to the National Cancer Institute (NCI), this shadow method—based on the principle that the closer the sun comes to being directly overhead, the stronger its ultraviolet rays—works for any location and at any time of year.

- **Check for photosensitivity.** If you are taking any drugs, ask your doctor or pharmacist to see if the medication could make you more sensitive to sun damage. Be especially cautious about sun exposure if you have been using a synthetic preparation derived from vitamin A (Retin A) as an acne or anti-wrinkle treatment; it can increase your susceptibility.

- **Use extra caution near water, snow, and sand since they reflect the damaging rays of the sun and increase the risk of sunburn.** Wear protective clothing, such as a wide-brimmed cap or hat, whenever possible.

## Figure 15.11 ABCD: The Warning Signs of Melanoma

An estimated 95 percent of cases of melanoma arise from an existing mole. A normal mole is usually round or oval, less than 6 millimeters (about ¼ inch) in diameter, and evenly colored (black, brown, or tan). Seek prompt evaluation of any moles that change in ways shown in the photo.

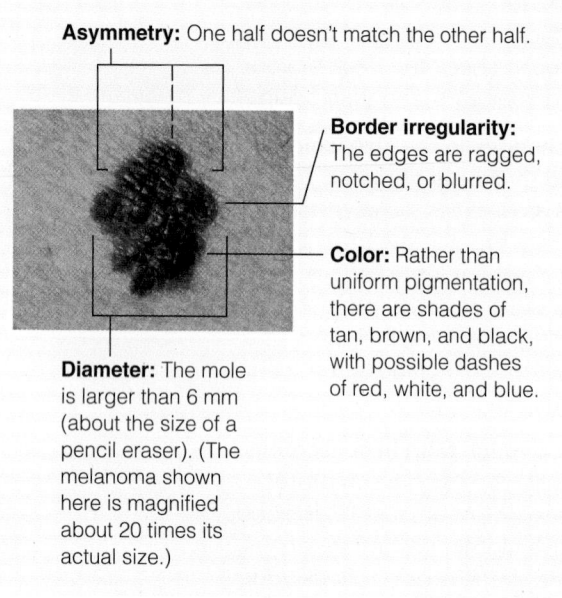

**Asymmetry:** One half doesn't match the other half.

**Border irregularity:** The edges are ragged, notched, or blurred.

**Color:** Rather than uniform pigmentation, there are shades of tan, brown, and black, with possible dashes of red, white, and blue.

**Diameter:** The mole is larger than 6 mm (about the size of a pencil eraser). (The melanoma shown here is magnified about 20 times its actual size.)

Courtesy of the Skin Cancer Foundation

## CONSUMER ALERT

### Are You Addicted to Tanning?

You know that exposure to ultraviolet rays increases your risk of developing skin cancer, but maybe you still can't stay out of the sun or a tanning booth. Why?

**Facts to Know**

- Researchers theorize that repetitive tanning behavior may be the result of a kind of addiction.

- Texas beachgoers, asked questions about their tanning habits, gave replies similar to those who gamble or drink compulsively.

**Steps to Take**

- Test your risk of "ultraviolet light (UVL) dependency" by taking the CAGE screening testing for addictive behavior.

- Ask yourself the following questions;

  - **C**ut: Ever felt you ought to cut down on your behavior?

  - **A**nnoyed: Have people annoyed you by criticizing your behavior?

  - **G**uilt: Ever felt bad or guilty about your behavior?

  - **E**ye Opener: Ever engaged in your behavior to steady your nerves in the morning?

Answering yes to two of the CAGE questions is a strong indication for an addictive behavior; answering yes to three confirms it.

---

**Treatment** If caught early, melanoma is highly curable, usually with surgery alone. Once it has spread, chemotherapy with a single drug or a combination can temporarily shrink tumors in some people. However, the five-year survival rate for metastatic melanoma is only 14 percent.

*Breast Cancer* Every 3 minutes, a woman in the United States learns that she has breast cancer. Every 12 minutes, a woman dies of breast cancer. Many women misjudge their own likelihood of developing breast cancer, either overestimating or underestimating their susceptibility. In a national poll, one in every ten surveyed considered herself at no risk at all. This is never the case. Every woman is at risk for breast cancer simply because she's female.

The most common risk factors include the following:

- **Age.** As shown in Table 15.3, at 25, a woman's chance of developing breast cancer is 1 in 19,608; by age 45, it has increased to 1 in 93; by 65, it is 1 in 17. The mean age at which women are diagnosed is 63.

### Table 15.3 A Woman's Risk of Developing Breast Cancer

| | |
|---|---|
| By age 25 | 1 in 19,608 |
| By age 30 | 1 in 2,525 |
| By age 35 | 1 in 622 |
| By age 40 | 1 in 217 |
| By age 45 | 1 in 93 |
| By age 50 | 1 in 50 |
| By age 55 | 1 in 33 |
| By age 60 | 1 in 24 |
| By age 65 | 1 in 17 |
| By age 70 | 1 in 14 |
| By age 75 | 1 in 11 |
| By age 80 | 1 in 10 |
| By age 85 | 1 in 9 |
| Ever | 1 in 8 |

- **Family history.** The overwhelming majority of breast cancers—90 to 95 percent—are not due to strong genetic factors. However, having a first-degree relative—mother, sister, or daughter—with breast cancer does increase risk, and if the relative developed breast cancer before menopause, the cancer is more likely to be hereditary.

- **Long menstrual history.** Women who had their first period before age 12 are at greater risk than women who began menstruating later. The reason is that the more menstrual cycles a woman has, the longer her exposure to estrogen, a hormone known to increase breast cancer danger. For similar reasons, childless women, who menstruate continuously for several decades, are also at greater risk. Neither miscarriage nor induced abortion increases the risk of breast cancer.

- **Age at birth of first child.** An early pregnancy—in a woman's teens or 20s—changes the actual maturation of breast cells and decreases risk. But if a woman has her first child in her 40s, precancerous cells may actually flourish with the high hormone levels of the pregnancy.

- **Breast biopsies.** Even if laboratory analysis finds no precancerous abnormalities, women who require such tests are more likely to develop breast cancer. Fibrocystic breast disease, a term often used for "lumpy" breasts, is not a risk factor.

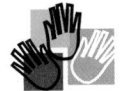 **Race and ethnicity.** Breast cancer rates are lower in Hispanic and Asian American populations than in whites and in African American women. Caucasian women over 40 have the highest incidence rate for breast cancer in this country, but African American women at every age have a greater likelihood of dying from breast cancer.

BRCA1 mutations indicate a higher risk of aggressive forms of breast cancer and of ovarian cancer. Hispanic women, particularly those of Mexican descent, are more likely than white or black women to have hereditary forms of cancer.

- **Occupation.** Based on two decades of following more than a million women, Swedish researchers have developed a list of jobs linked with a high risk of breast cancer. These include pharmacists, certain types of teachers, schoolmasters, systems analysts and programmers, telephone operators, telegraph and radio operators, metal platers and coaters, and beauticians.

- **Alcohol.** Women's risk of breast cancer increases with the amount of alcohol they drink. Those who take two or more drinks per day are 40 percent more likely to develop breast cancer than women who don't drink at all. For a nondrinking woman, the lifetime risk of breast cancer by age 80 is 1 in 11. For heavy drinkers it's about 1 in 7, regardless of race, education, family history, use of hormone therapy, or other risk factors.

- **Hormone therapy (HT).** Several studies confirm an increased risk with a combination of estrogen and progestin, particularly in women who use combination HT for five years or longer. With the decreasing use of hormone therapy, breast cancer rates have declined, especially among affluent women over 50.[54]

- **Obesity.** Excess weight, particularly after menopause, increases the risk of getting breast cancer. Overweight women, both pre- and postmenopausal, with breast cancer are more likely to die of their disease.

- **Sedentary lifestyle.** According to the World Health Organization, regular physical activity may cut the risk of developing breast cancer by 20 to 40 percent, regardless of a woman's menopausal status or the type or intensity of the activity. The reason may be that exercise lowers levels of circulating ovarian hormones.

**Detection** Doctors have long advised women to perform monthly breast self-exams (BSEs) after their periods (Figure 15.12). In its newest guidelines, the American Cancer Society now describes BSE as "an option" for women starting in their twenties and urges all women to report any breast changes promptly. It recommends a breast exam by a trained practitioner every three years for women in their twenties and thirties and every year for women 40 and over and a yearly mammogram for all women, starting at age 40.

The best tool for early detection is the diagnostic X-ray exam called **mammography**. Women whose breast cancer is detected by screening mammography have a significantly better prognosis than those whose cancer is found another way—even if the cancer has already spread to their lymph nodes. A likely reason is that mammography can detect tumors that are both slower growing and less biologically lethal than others.

Mammography has proven effective in detecting breast cancer at an early stage, when treatment is more effective and a cure more likely. The American College of Obstetricians and Gynecologists now recommends annual mammography for women who are 40 and older. Previous guidelines had suggested mammograms every one or two years after age 40.[55]

**mammography** A diagnostic X-ray exam used to detect breast cancer.

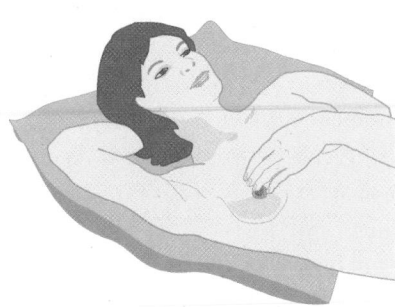

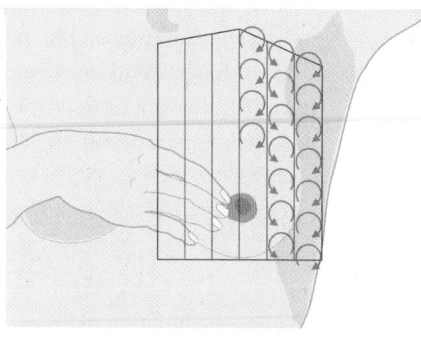

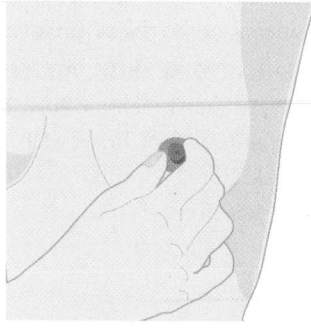

1. Lie flat on your back. Place a pillow or towel under one shoulder, and raise that arm over your head. With the opposite hand, you'll feel with the pads, not the fingertips, of the three middle fingers, for lumps or any change in the texture of the breast or skin.

2. The area you'll examine is from your collarbone to your bra line and from your breastbone to the center of your armpit. Imagine the area divided into vertical strips. Using small circular motions (the size of a dime), move your fingers up and down the strips. Apply light, medium, and deep pressure to examine each spot. Repeat this same process for your other breast.

3. Gently squeeze the nipple of each breast between your thumb and index finger. Any discharge, clear or bloody, should be reported to your doctor immediately.

Women who were diagnosed in their 40s and died of breast cancer account for at least one-third of all potential years of life lost to this disease.[56] Of the 40,000 women who die of breast cancer every year, 18 percent are diagnosed in their 40s.[57]

Magnetic Resonance Imaging may be more accurate than mammography for detecting early forms of breast cancer before they progress to more aggressive forms. The American Cancer Society now recommends MRI screening for women with a strong family history of breast or ovarian cancer and those who have been treated for Hodgkin's disease. Women who've had cancer in one breast or those with extremely dense breasts may also benefit.

**Treatment** Breast cancer can be treated with surgery, radiation, and drugs (chemotherapy and hormonal therapy). Doctors may use one of these options or a combination, depending on the type and location of the cancer and whether the disease has spread.

Most women undergo some type of surgery. **Lumpectomy**, or breast-conserving surgery, removes only the cancerous tissue and a surrounding margin of normal tissue. A modified radical **mastectomy** includes the entire breast and some of the underarm lymph nodes. Removing underarm lymph nodes is important to determine if the cancer has spread, but a technique called sentinel node biopsy allows

physicians to pinpoint the first lymph node into which a tumor drains (the sentinel node) and remove only the nodes most likely to contain cancer cells.

Radiation therapy is treatment with high-energy rays or particles to destroy cancer. In almost all cases, lumpectomy is followed by six to seven weeks of radiation. Chemotherapy is used to reach cancer cells that may have spread beyond the breast—in many cases even if no cancer is detected in the lymph nodes after surgery.

The use of drugs such as tamoxifen and aromatase inhibitors, in addition to standard chemotherapy, can significantly lower the risk of recurrence.

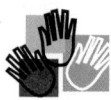 *Cervical Cancer* Cervical cancer, the second most common cancer in women worldwide, claims 250,000 lives every year. Approximately 85 percent of these deaths occur in developing countries where women do not have access to effective cervical cancer screening. An estimated 11,000 cases of invasive cervical cancer are diagnosed in the United States every year. The highest incidence rate occurs among Vietnamese women; Alaska Native, Korean, and Hispanic women also have higher rates than the national average.

Women are at higher risk for cervical cancer if they engaged in sexual activity before the age of

**lumpectomy** The surgical removal of a breast tumor and its surrounding tissue.

**mastectomy** The surgical removal of an entire breast.

16 or have had multiple sexual partners (more than five in a lifetime). Genital herpes, smoking, and secondhand smoke increase the danger. However, as numerous studies have conclusively demonstrated in the last two decades, human papillomavirus (HPV) infection is the primary risk factor for cervical cancer.

HPV infection is very common in young women. In some studies one in five sexually active women under age 30 has HPV. However, only about 13 of the hundred-plus types of HPV cause dysplasia, or precancerous changes in cervical cells. Women should be tested for HPV if they have an abnormal or unclear PAP smear result (Table 15.4).

For a more detailed discussion of HPV, see Chapter 10.

*Ovarian Cancer* Ovarian cancer is the leading cause of death from gynecological cancers. Risk factors include a family history of ovarian cancer; personal history of breast cancer; obesity; infertility (because the abnormality that interferes with conception may also play a role in cancer development); and low levels of transferase, an enzyme involved in the metabolism of dairy foods. Ovarian cancer may be diagnosed by pelvic examination, ultrasound, MRI, computed tomography, or PET (positron emission tomography) scan. Women with ovarian cancer are more likely to report abdominal pain, feeling full quickly after eating, and urinary urgency, but these symptoms are so common that they are often overlooked or dismissed.[58]

*Testicular Cancer* In the last 20 years the incidence of testicular cancer has risen 51 percent in the United States—from 3.61 to 5.44 per 100,000. It is not clear why testicular cancer is on the rise, although researchers speculate that changing environmental or socioeconomic risk factors could have a role. Chronic use of marijuana increases the risk of an especially aggressive form of testicular cancer. Testicular cancer occurs mostly among young men between the ages of 18 and 35, who are not normally at risk of cancer. At highest risk are men with an undescended testicle (a condition that is almost always corrected in childhood to prevent this danger). To detect possibly cancerous growths, men should perform monthly testicular self-exams, as shown in Figure 15.13.

Table 15.4 **What Your Pap Test Results Mean**

A Pap test may come back as "normal," "unclear," or "abnormal."

| | | |
|---|---|---|
| **Normal** | 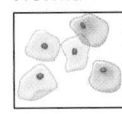 | A normal (or "negative") result means that no cell changes were found on the cervix. |
| **Unclear** | 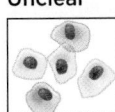 | It is common for test results to come back unclear. Doctors may use other words to describe this result such as inconclusive, or ASC-US. These all mean the same thing: that some cervical cells could be abnormal, perhaps because of an infection. An HPV test will indicate if the changes are related to HPV. |
| **Abnormal** | 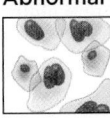 | An abnormal result means that cell changes were found on the cervix. This usually does not indicate cervical cancer. Abnormal changes on your cervix are likely caused by HPV. The changes may be minor (low-grade) or serious (high-grade). Most of the time, minor changes go back to normal on their own. But more serious changes can turn into cancer if the cells are not removed. The more serious changes are often called "pre-cancer" because they are not yet cancer but could turn into cancer over time. |

Figure 15.13 **Testicular Self-Exam**
The best time to examine your testicles is after a hot bath or shower, when the scrotum is most relaxed. Place your index and middle fingers under each testicle and the thumb on top, and roll the testicle between the thumb and fingers. If you feel a small, hard, usually painless lump or swelling, or anything unusual, consult a urologist.

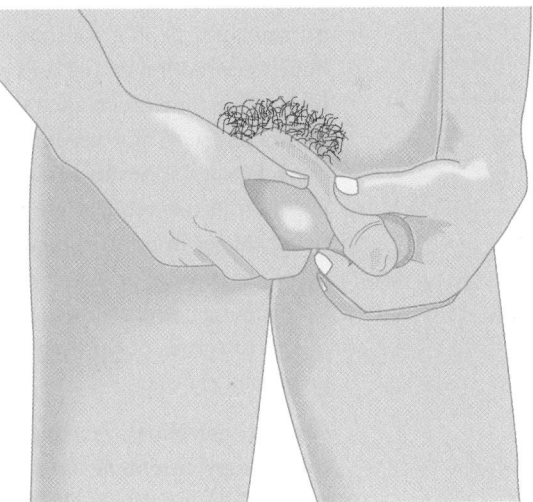

Often the first sign of this cancer is a slight enlargement of one testicle. There also may be a change in the way it feels when touched. Sometimes men with testicular cancer report a dull ache in the lower abdomen or groin, along with a sense of heaviness or sluggishness. Lumps on the testicles also may indicate cancer.

A man who notices any abnormality should consult a physician. If a lump is indeed present, a surgical biopsy is necessary to find out if it is cancerous. If the biopsy is positive, a series of tests generally is needed to determine whether the disease has spread.

Treatment for testicular cancer generally involves surgical removal of the diseased testis, sometimes along with radiation therapy, chemotherapy, and the removal of nearby lymph nodes. The remaining testicle is capable of maintaining a man's sexual potency and fertility. Only in rare cases is removal of both testicles necessary. Testosterone injections following such surgery can maintain potency. The chance for a cure is very high if testicular cancer is spotted early.

*Colon and Rectal Cancer*   Colon and rectal, or colorectal, cancer is the third most common cancer and accounts for 10 percent of cancer deaths. Most cases occur after age 50. Both age and gender influence the risk of colon cancer. Older individuals and men are more likely to develop polyps (nonmalignant growths that may turn cancerous at some point) and tumors in the colon than young people and women.

Risk factors include age (over 50), personal or family history of colon and rectal cancer, polyps in the colon or rectum, ulcerative colitis, smoking, alcohol consumption, prolonged high consumption of red and processed meat, high-fat or low-fiber diet, and inadequate intake of fruits and vegetables. In the landmark Women's Health Initiative trials, a low-fat diet did not reduce the risk of colon and rectal cancer in postmenopausal women. Low doses of aspirin or other nonsteroidal anti-inflammatory drugs appear to reduce the risk of precancerous polyps that can lead to colon and rectal cancer.

Current guidelines recommend a screening colonoscopy beginning at age 50, earlier for those at higher risk based on personal, family, or medical history. The initial screening is crucial because it detects the largest, most dangerous polyps, which can then be removed.

Early signs of colorectal cancer are bleeding from the rectum, blood in the stool, or a change in bowel habits. Treatment may involve surgery, radiation therapy, and/or chemotherapy.

*Prostate Cancer*   After skin cancer, prostate cancer is the most common form of cancer in American men. The risk of prostate cancer is 1 in 6; the risk of death due to metastatic prostate cancer is 1 in 30. More than a quarter of men diagnosed with cancer have prostate cancer. The disease strikes African American men more often than white; Asian and American Indian men are affected less often.

The risk of prostate cancer increases with age, family history, exposure to the heavy metal cadmium, high number of sexual partners, and history of frequent sexually transmitted infections. A diet high in saturated fat may be a risk factor. An inherited predisposition may account for 5 to 10 percent of cases. A purported link between vasectomy and prostate cancer has been disproved. Statin drugs, commonly prescribed to lower cholesterol, also may lower the risk of prostate cancer.

The development of a simple annual screening test that measures levels of a protein called prostate-specific antigen (PSA) in the blood has revolutionized the diagnosis of prostate cancer. PSA testing is recommended for men at high risk (African Americans and men with close relatives with prostate cancer) starting at age 45 and for all men at age 50. It remains controversial, however. Some claim that PSA testing saves lives; others, that it leads to unnecessary and potentially harmful treatments. Annual screening has not reduced deaths from the disease in older men, and new guidelines recommend against screening for men age 75 or older. There is insufficient evidence to assess the balance of benefits and risks in younger men.[59]

Treatment may include hormones, chemotherapy, a low-fat diet, and radiation. About 60,000 men undergo radical prostate surgery in the United States every year. The five-year survival rate has increased from 67 percent to 99 percent over the past 20 years.

# Other Major Illnesses

Other noninfectious diseases have a debilitating effect on many people. But most of the diseases discussed in this section can be controlled, if not cured.

## Epilepsy and Seizure Disorders

About 10 percent of all Americans will have at least one seizure at some time. Between 0.5 and 1 percent of all Americans have recurrent seizures. Derived from the Greek word for seizure, **epilepsy** is the term used to refer to a variety of neurological disorders characterized by sudden attacks (seizures) of violent muscle contractions and unconsciousness. Epilepsy is rarely fatal; the primary danger to life is to suffer an attack while driving or swimming.

Seizures can be major, referred to as *grand mal*; minor, referred to as *petit mal*; or psychomotor. In a grand-mal seizure, the person loses consciousness, falls to the ground, and experiences convulsive body movements. Petit-mal seizures are brief, characterized by a loss of consciousness for 10 to 30 seconds, by eye or muscle flutterings, and occasionally by a loss of muscle tone. About 90 percent of all epileptics have grand-mal seizures; 40 percent suffer both petit-mal and grand-mal seizures. The frequency of attacks defines the severity of the epilepsy. Diagnosis is based on a history of recurring attacks and a study of the brain's electrical activity, called an electroencephalogram (EEG).

About half of all cases of epilepsy have no known cause and are therefore classified as *idiopathic*. Others stem from conditions that affect the brain, such as trauma, tumors, congenital malformations, or inflammation of the membranes covering the brain. Idiopathic epilepsy usually begins between the ages of 2 and 14. Seizures before age 2 are usually related to developmental defects, birth injuries, or a metabolic disease affecting the brain. (Fever-induced convulsions are not related to epilepsy.) Seizures after age 14 are generally symptoms of brain disease or injury.

Seizure disorders don't reflect or affect intellectual or psychological soundness; people who suffer from them have normal intelligence. Therapy with anticonvulsant drugs can control seizures in most people, and once seizures are under control, epileptics can live full, normal lives by continuing to take their medications.

If you're with a person who suffers a grand-mal seizure, make sure he or she isn't injured during the attack. Don't try to restrain the person or interfere with his or her movements, and don't try to force anything into the person's mouth.

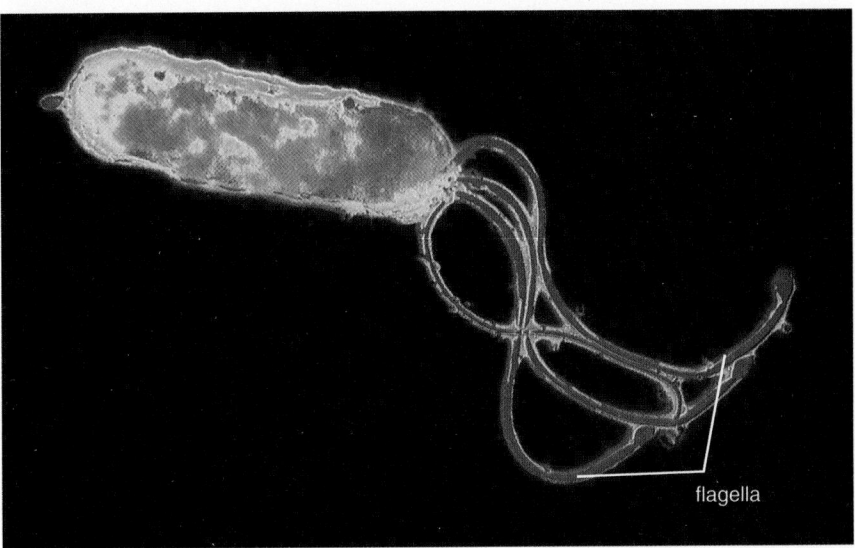

flagella

The bacterium *Helicobacter pylori* has flagella that enable it to tunnel beneath the protective layer coating the stomach lining.

## Asthma

**Asthma** is a disease characterized by constriction of the breathing passages. As with allergy, asthma rates have skyrocketed in the last two decades. Approximately 20 million Americans have asthma. Asthma-related problems account for more than half a million hospital stays each year and 14 deaths each day in the United States, according to the Asthma and Allergy Foundation of America.

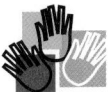 Asthma is more common among inner-city residents and blacks. The disease disproportionately affects African Americans. A black man in New York City is 11 times more likely to die from asthma than other men in the city.

While asthma is not always linked to allergy, the two are related. Among people with asthma, 90 percent of the children, 70 percent of young adults, and 50 percent of older adults also have allergies. According to epidemiologic research, 23 percent of youngsters diagnosed with allergies by age 1 develop asthma by age 6. Of those diagnosed after age 1, 13 percent eventually become asthmatic. Symptoms include wheezing, coughing, shortness of breath, and chest tightness. If the symptoms are untreated or undertreated, they can worsen and damage the lungs. Oral contraceptives increase the risk in some women.[60]

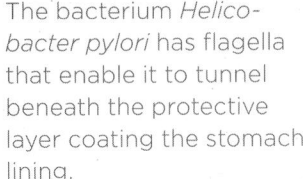

**epilepsy** A variety of neurological disorders characterized by sudden attacks (seizures) of violent muscle contractions and unconsciousness.

**asthma** A disease or allergic response characterized by bronchial spasms and difficult breathing.

The number of people with asthma continues to increase into adulthood. However, as shown by a study that followed college students for 23 years, most report that their symptoms improve or disappear.

Over the last decade advances in asthma medications and tools have significantly improved management of this disease. Inhaled corticosteroids, long-acting bronchodilators (such as Advair), and leukotriene receptor antagonists (such as Singulair) have proven particularly helpful in controlling symptoms and preventing serious attacks that would require treatment with oral steroids.[61]

If you have asthma, here are some steps you should take:

- **Get away from the asthma trigger** (cigarette smoke, cat, pollen, etc.).

- **Assess the severity of the attack.** The most precise way to do so is with a peak flow meter. If your peak flow is less than half your best value, the attack is severe.

- **Use a quick reliever.** The fastest way to relieve an asthma attack is to use a quick-acting bronchodilator such as albuterol.

- **Suppress inflammation.** Quick-relief bronchodilators treat only the constricted muscles surrounding the bronchial tubes. Treating the overproduction of mucus requires an anti-inflammatory medication, typically a corticosteroid, such as prednisone.

- **Know when to call for help.** Severe asthma attacks can be dangerous. If you don't feel improvement, get help immediately from your doctor or an urgent care or emergency health care center, or call 911.

**ulcer** A lesion in, or an erosion of, the mucous membrane of an organ.

## Ulcers

Open sores, often more than an inch wide, that develop in the lining of the stomach or the duodenum (the first part of the small intestine) are called **ulcers.** They are caused by excessive acidic digestive juices. The major symptom is a burning pain felt throughout the upper abdomen. The pain may come and go, lasting up to three hours. It may begin either right after eating or several hours later.

One in five men and one in ten women get ulcers of the stomach or duodenum, but the number of ulcers is declining. Risk factors include heavy use of cigarettes, alcohol, or caffeine; the ingestion of large amounts of painkillers that contain aspirin or ibuprofen; and advanced age. Bleeding is not common but may be dangerous, even life-threatening. An untreated stomach ulcer can lead to serious weight loss and anemia.

Researchers have identified a bacterium, *Helicobacter pylori*, that may infect the digestive system and set the stage for ulcers. According to various studies, most ulcer patients carry this organism. One theory is that infection leads to an inflammation of the stomach lining called gastritis, which increases vulnerability to other stressors, such as smoking, alcohol, or anxiety. Treatment with antibiotics leads to improvement in most patients.

Conventional therapy for ulcers includes self-help measures, such as avoiding aspirin; eating small, frequent meals; taking antacids; and not smoking or drinking alcohol or caffeine. Drugs such as cimetidine, ranitidine, and sucralfate can reduce the amount of acid produced by the stomach and relieve ulcer symptoms.

# Preventing Serious Illness

You may not be able to control every risk factor in your life or environment, but you can protect yourself from the obvious ones.

_____ **Not smoking.** There's no bigger favor you can do for your heart or your lungs—your entire body.

_____ **Cutting down on saturated fats and cholesterol.** This can help prevent high blood cholesterol levels, obesity, and heart disease.

_____ **Watching your weight.** Even relatively modest gains can have a big effect on your risk of heart disease. Overweight and obesity are associated with increased risks for cancers at several sites: breast (among postmenopausal women), colon, endometrium, esophagus (adenocarcinoma), and kidney.

_____ **Moving more.** Regular exercise can help lower your blood pressure, lower LDL, and reduce triglycerides.

_____ **Lowering your stress levels.** If too much stress is a problem in your life, try the relaxation techniques described in Chapter 3.

_____ **Getting your blood pressure checked regularly.** Knowing your numbers can alert you to a potential problem long before you develop any symptoms.

_____ **Avoiding excessive exposure to ultraviolet light.** If you spend a lot of time outside, protect your skin by using sunscreen and wearing long-sleeve shirts and a hat. Also, wear sunglasses to protect your eyes. Don't purposely put yourself at risk by binge-sunbathing or by using sunlamps.

_____ **Controlling your alcohol intake.** The risk of cancers of the mouth, pharynx, larynx, esophagus, liver, and breast increases substantially with intake of more than two drinks per day for men or one drink for women.

_____ **Being alert to changes in your body.** You know your body's rhythms and appearance better than anyone else, and only you will know if certain things aren't right. Changes in bowel habits, skin changes, unusual lumps or discharges—anything out of the ordinary—may be clues that require further medical investigation.

# Are You at Risk of Cancer?

Answer the following questions:

1. Do you protect your skin from overexposure to the sun? _____

2. Do you abstain from smoking or using tobacco in any form? _____

3. If you're over 40 or if family members have had colon cancer, do you get routine digital rectal exams? _____

4. Do you eat a balanced diet that includes the recommended daily value for vitamins A, B, and C? _____

5. If you're a woman, do you have regular Pap tests and pelvic exams? _____

6. If you're a man over 40, do you get regular prostate exams? _____

7. If you have burn scars or a history of chronic skin infections, do you get regular checkups? _____

8. Do you avoid smoked, salted, pickled, and high-nitrite foods? _____

9. If your job exposes you to asbestos, radiation, cadmium, or other environmental hazards, do you get regular checkups? _____

10. Do you limit your consumption of alcohol? _____

11. Do you avoid using tanning salons or home sunlamps? _____

12. If you're a woman, do you examine your breasts every month for lumps? _____

13. Do you eat plenty of vegetables and other sources of fiber? _____

14. If you're a man, do you perform regular testicular self-exams? _____

15. Do you wear protective sunglasses in sunlight? _____

16. Do you follow a low-fat diet? _____

17. Do you know the cancer warning signs? _____

_Scoring_

_If you answered no to any of the questions, your risk for developing various kinds of cancer may be increased._

# Making Change Happen

## Detecting Cancer

| Site | Recommendation |
|---|---|
| **Breast** | • Yearly mammograms are recommended starting at age 40. The age at which screening should be stopped should be individualized by considering the potential risks and benefits of screening in the context of overall health status and longevity.<br>• Clinical breast exam should be part of a periodic health exam, about every 3 years for women in their 20s and 30s, and every year for women 40 and older.<br>• Women should know how their breasts normally feel and report any breast change promptly to their health care providers. Breast self-exam is an option for women starting in their 20s.<br>• Women at increased risk (e.g., family history, genetic tendency, past breast cancer) should talk with their doctors about the benefits and limitations of starting mammography screening earlier, having additional tests (i.e., breast ultrasound and MRI), or having more frequent exams. |
| **Colon and Rectum** | Beginning at age 50, men and women should begin screening with one of the examination schedules that follow:<br>• A fecal occult blood test (FOBT) or fecal immunochemical test (FIT) every year.<br>• A flexible sigmoidoscopy (FSIG) every 5 years.<br>• Annual FOBT or FIT and flexible sigmoidoscopy every 5 years.*<br>• A double-contrast barium enema every 5 years.<br>• A colonoscopy every 10 years. |
| **Prostate** | The PSA test and the digital rectal examination should be offered annually, beginning at age 50, to men who have a life expectancy of at least 10 years. Men at high risk (African American men and men with a strong family history of one or more first-degree relatives diagnosed with prostate cancer at an early age) should begin testing at age 45. For both men at average risk and high risk, information should be provided about what is known and what is uncertain about the benefits and limitations of early detection and treatment of prostate cancer so that they can make an informed decision about testing. |
| **Uterus** | **Cervix:** Screening should begin approximately 3 years after a woman begins having vaginal intercourse, but no later than 21 years of age. Screening should be done every year with regular Pap tests or every 2 years using liquid-based tests. At or after age 30, women who have had three normal test results in a row may get screened every 2 to 3 years. Alternatively, cervical cancer screening with human papillomavirus (HPV) DNA testing and conventional or liquid-based cytology could be performed every 3 years. However, doctors may suggest that a woman get screened more often if she has certain risk factors, such as HIV infection or a weak immune system. Women 70 years and older who have had three or more consecutive normal Pap tests in the last 10 years may choose to stop cervical cancer screening. Screening after total hysterectomy (with removal of the cervix) is not necessary unless the surgery was done as a treatment for cervical cancer.<br><br>**Endometrium:** The American Cancer Society recommends that at the time of menopause all women should be informed about the risks and symptoms of endometrial cancer, and strongly encouraged to report any unexpected bleeding or spotting to their physicians. Annual screening for endometrial cancer with endometrial biopsy beginning at age 35 should be offered to women with or at risk for hereditary nonpolyposis colon cancer (HNPCC). |
| **Cancer-Related Checkup** | For individuals undergoing periodic health examinations, a cancer-related checkup should include health counseling, and, depending on a person's age and gender, might include examinations for cancers of the thyroid, oral cavity, skin, lymph nodes, testes, and ovaries, as well as for some nonmalignant diseases. |

*Combined testing is preferred over either annual FOBT or FIT, or FSIG every 5 years, alone. People who are at moderate or high risk for colorectal cancer should talk with a doctor about a different testing schedule. If you want to write your own goals for lowering your risk for major diseases, access the Behavior Change Planner in CengageNOW at www.cengagebrain.com.

Source: Adapted from American Cancer Society, *Cancer Facts and Figures—2007*. Copyright © 2007 American Cancer Society, Inc. www.cancer.org

# Making This Chapter Work for You

## Review Questions

1. The heart
   a. has four chambers, which are responsible for pumping blood into the veins for circulation through the body.
   b. pumps blood first to the lungs where it picks up oxygen and discards carbon dioxide.
   c. beats about 10,000 times and pumps about 75 gallons of blood per day.
   d. has specialized cells that generate electrical signals to control the amount of blood that circulates through the body.

2. A heart attack
   a. occurs when the myocardium receives an excessive amount of blood from the coronary arteries.
   b. is typically suffered by individuals who have irregular episodes of atherosclerosis.
   c. can be treated successfully up to four hours after the event.
   d. occurs when the myocardial cells are deprived of oxygen-carrying blood, causing them to die.

3. You can protect yourself from certain types of cancer by
   a. not smoking.
   b. avoiding people who have had cancer.
   c. wearing sunscreen with an SPF of less than 15.
   d. using condoms during sexual intercourse.

4. Which of the following statements about skin cancer is true?
   a. Individuals with a large number of moles are at decreased risk for melanoma.
   b. The most serious type of skin cancer is squamous cell carcinoma.
   c. The safest way to get a tan and avoid skin cancer is to use tanning salons and sunlamps instead of sunbathing in direct sunlight.
   d. Individuals with a history of childhood sunburn are at increased risk for melanoma.

5. A woman's risk of developing breast cancer increases if
   a. she is Caucasian over the age of 40.
   b. she had her first child when in her teens or 20s.
   c. her husband's mother had breast cancer.
   d. she began menstruating when she was 15 or 16.

6. Prostate cancer
   a. occurs mostly among men between the ages of 18 and 35.
   b. is usually more aggressive in white men.
   c. has a low survival rate.
   d. can be detected through a screening test that measures the levels of prostate-specific antigen in the blood.

7. You can control all of these cardiometabolic risk factors *except*
   a. lipoprotein levels.
   b. high blood glucose.
   c. family history.
   d. overweight.

8. Which of the following statements about diabetes mellitus is *false*?
   a. Individuals with type 2 diabetes can often control the disease without taking insulin.
   b. The incidence of diabetes has decreased in the last decade, especially among African Americans, Native Americans, and Latinos.
   c. Individuals with diabetes must measure the levels of glucose in their blood to ensure that it does not rise to unsafe levels.
   d. Untreated or uncontrolled diabetes can lead to coma and eventual death.

9. Hypertension
   a. is diagnosed when blood pressure is consistently lower than 130/85 mm Hg.
   b. may be treated with dietary changes, which include eating low-fat foods and avoiding sodium.
   c. can cause fatty deposits to collect on the artery walls.
   d. usually does not respond to medication, especially in severe cases.

10. In your lipoprotein profile, having a high level of this blood element is a good thing.
    a. HDL cholesterol
    b. LDL cholesterol
    c. C-reactive protein
    d. triglyceride

*Answers to these questions can be found on page 672.*

## Critical Thinking

1. Have you had your blood pressure checked lately? If your reading was high, what steps are you now taking to help reduce your blood pressure?

2. Have you had a lipoprotein profile lately? Do you think it's necessary for you to obtain one? If your reading was/is borderline or high, what lifestyle changes can you make to help control your cholesterol level?

3. Do you have family members who have had cancer? Were these individuals at risk for cancer because of specific environmental factors, such as long-term exposure to tobacco smoke? If no particular cause was identified, what other factors could have triggered their diseases?

Are you concerned that you might have inherited a genetic predisposition to any particular type of cancer because of your family history?

4. A friend of yours, Karen, discovered a small lump in her breast during a routine self-examination. When she mentions it, you ask if she has seen a doctor. She tells you that she hasn't had time to schedule an appointment; besides, she says, she's not sure it's really the kind of lump one has to worry about. It's clear to you that Karen is in denial and procrastinating about seeing a doctor. What advice would you give her?

## Media Menu

Visit www.cengagebrain.com to access course materials and companion resources for this text that will:

- Help you evaluate your knowledge of the material.

- Allow you to prepare for exams with interactive quizzing.

- Use the CengageNOW product to develop a Personalized Learning Plan targeting resources that address areas you should study.

- Coach you through identifying target goals for behavioral change and creating and monitoring your personal change plan throughout the semester using the Behavior Change Planner available in the CengageNOW resource.

## Internet Connections

**www.diabetes.org**
Here you will find the latest information on both type 1 and type 2 diabetes mellitus, including suggestions regarding diet and exercise. The online bookstore features meal planning guides, cookbooks, and self-care guides. Type in your zip code to find community resources.

**www.americanheart.org**
This comprehensive site features a searchable database of all major cardiovascular diseases, plus information on healthy lifestyles, current research, CPR, cardiac warning signs, risk awareness, low-cholesterol diets, and family health. The interactive Heart Profilers® provides personalized information about treatment options for common cardiovascular conditions such as hypertension, heart failure, and cholesterol.

**www.fi.edu/biosci/heart.html**
This interesting site, developed by the Franklin Institute of Science, provides an interactive multimedia tour of the heart, as well as statistics, resources, links, and information on how to monitor your heart's health by becoming aware of your vital signs.

**www.cdc.gov/cancer**
This site, sponsored by the Centers for Disease Control and Prevention (CDC), features current information on cancer of the breast, cervix, prostate, skin, and colon. The site also provides monthly spotlights on specific cancers, as well as links to the National Comprehensive Cancer Control Program and the National Program of Cancer Registries.

## Key Terms

The terms listed are used on the page indicated. Definitions of the terms are in the Glossary at the end of the book.

angina pectoris   512

aorta   505

arteriosclerosis   511

asthma   527

atherosclerosis   511

atrium   504

capillary   505

cardiometabolic   488

cardiopulmonary
   resuscitation (CPR)   513

cholesterol   490

diabetes mellitus   494

diastole   505

diastolic blood pressure   490

epilepsy   527

hypertension   490

infiltration   517

lipoprotein   491

lumpectomy   524

mammography   523

mastectomy   524

metabolic syndrome   492

metastasize   517

myocardial infarction (MI)   512

plaque   511

prehypertension   500

relative risk   518

stroke   513

systole   505

systolic blood pressure   490

transient ischemic attack (TIA)   516

triglyceride   491

ulcer   528

ventricle   504

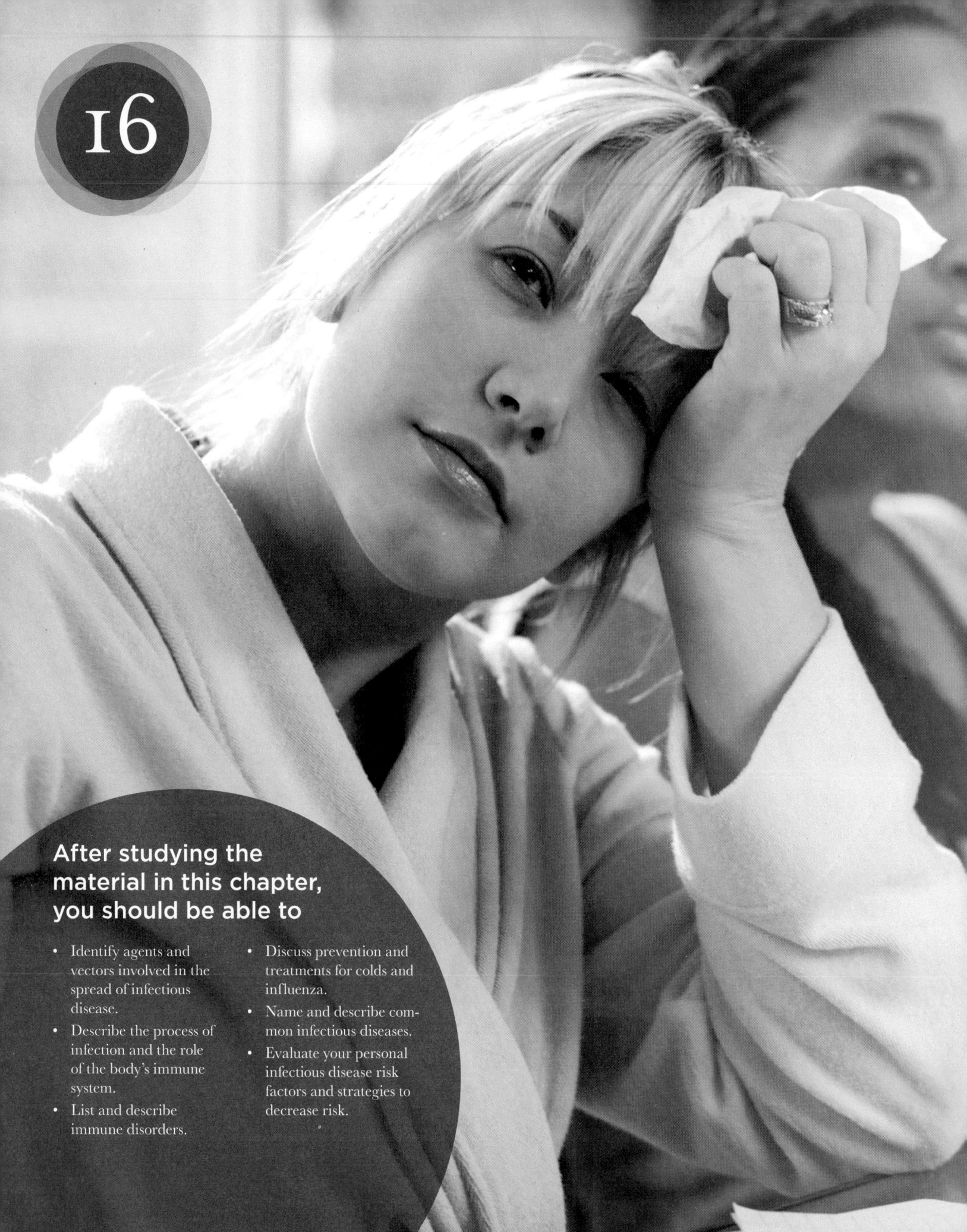

# 16

## After studying the material in this chapter, you should be able to

- Identify agents and vectors involved in the spread of infectious disease.
- Describe the process of infection and the role of the body's immune system.
- List and describe immune disorders.

- Discuss prevention and treatments for colds and influenza.
- Name and describe common infectious diseases.
- Evaluate your personal infectious disease risk factors and strategies to decrease risk.

*Zach shrugged off the headache and sore throat he woke up with and rushed to class. During the lecture he started shivering. When he got up to leave, his legs felt shaky, and it hurt to walk. His entire body seemed stiff. Back in his dorm, Zach collapsed onto his bed. He felt feverish. His head throbbed. He started vomiting. Dark blotches broke out on his forehead, arms, and legs.*

# Infectious Illnesses

That evening his resident advisor drove Zach to the emergency room. The pain in his legs was excruciating, but his blood pressure was so low that the doctors couldn't give him pain medication. A spinal tap revealed that Zach had bacterial meningitis, a potentially deadly infection that causes swelling in the brain and spinal cord. Intensive treatment saved Zach's life, although he suffered hearing loss and severe nerve damage that required months of rehabilitation. Zach considers himself lucky. Bacterial meningitis can strike so unexpectedly and worsen so quickly that it can kill a healthy young person within days.

Throughout history, infectious diseases have claimed more lives than any military conflict or natural disaster. Although modern medicine has won many victories against the agents of infection, we remain vulnerable to a host of infectious illnesses. Drug-resistant strains of tuberculosis and Staphylococcus bacteria challenge current therapies. New infectious diseases such as H1N1 flu are emerging and traveling around the world. Agents of infection also can be used as weapons of war and terrorism.

This chapter is a lesson in self-defense against all forms of infection. The information it provides can help you boost your defenses, recognize and avoid enemies, shield yourself from infections, and realize when to seek help.

## Understanding Infection

We live in a sea of microbes. Most of them don't threaten our health or survival; some, such as the bacteria that inhabit our intestines, are actually beneficial. Yet in the course of history, disease-causing microorganisms have claimed millions of lives. The twentieth century brought the conquest of infectious killers such as cholera and scarlet fever. Although modern science has won many victories against the agents of infection, infectious illnesses remain a serious health threat. (See "Health in the Headlines," p. 537.)

Infection is a complex process, triggered by various **pathogens** (disease-causing organisms) and countered by the body's own defenders. Physicians explain infection in terms of a

**pathogen** A microorganism that produces disease.

Visit www.cengagebrain.com to access course materials for this text, including the Behavior Change Planner, interactive quizzes, tutorials, and more. See the preface on page xv for details.

© iStockphoto.com/Rubberball

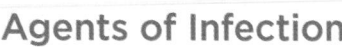

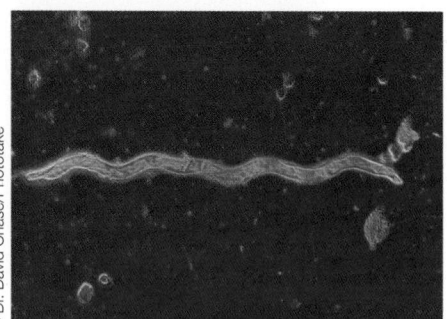

host (either a person or a population) that contacts one or more agents in an environment. A **vector**—a biological or physical vehicle that carries the agent to the host—provides the means of transmission.

## Agents of Infection

The types of microbes that can cause infection are viruses, bacteria, fungi, protozoa, and helminths (parasitic worms).

*Viruses* The tiniest pathogens—**viruses**—are also the toughest; they consist of a bit of nucleic acid (DNA or RNA, but never both) within a protein coat. Unable to reproduce on its own, a virus takes over a body cell's reproductive machinery and instructs it to produce new viral particles, which are then released to enter other cells. The common cold, the flu, herpes, hepatitis, and AIDS are viral diseases.

The most common viruses are these types:

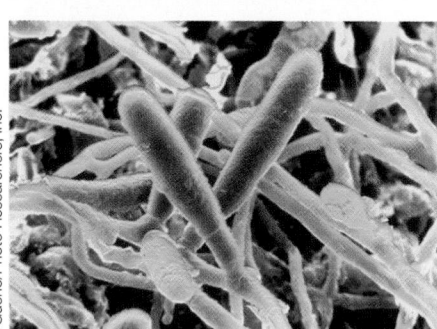

- **Rhinoviruses and adenoviruses**, which get into the mucous membranes and cause upper respiratory tract infections and colds.

- **Coronaviruses**, named for their corona, or halo-like appearance, are second only to rhinoviruses in causing the common cold and other respiratory infections. A coronavirus is the cause of severe acute respiratory syndrome (SARS).

- **Influenza viruses**, which can change their outer protein coats so dramatically that individuals

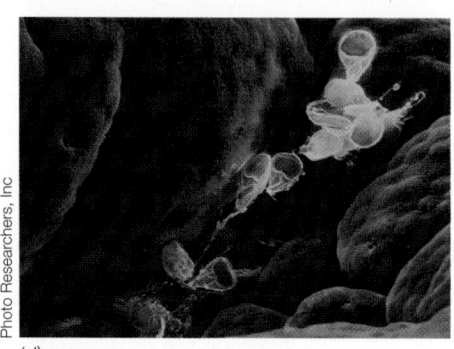

resistant to one strain cannot fight off a new one. (See page 548 for a discussion of the H1N1 virus.)

- **Herpes viruses**, which take up permanent residence in the cells and periodically flare up.

- **Papilloma viruses**, which cause few symptoms in women and almost none in men but may be responsible, at least in part, for a rise in the incidence of cervical cancer among younger women.

- **Hepatitis viruses**, which cause several forms of liver infection, ranging from mild to life-threatening.

- **Slow viruses**, which give no early indication of their presence but can produce fatal illnesses within a few years.

- **Retroviruses**, which are named for their backward (retro) sequence of genetic replication compared to other viruses. One retrovirus, human immunodeficiency virus (HIV), causes acquired immune deficiency syndrome (AIDS).

- **Filoviruses**, which resemble threads and are extremely lethal.

The problem in fighting viruses is that it's difficult to find drugs that harm the virus and not the cell it has commandeered. **Antibiotics** (drugs that inhibit or kill bacteria) have no effect on viruses. **Antiviral drugs** don't completely eradicate a viral infection, although they can decrease its severity and duration. Because viruses multiply very quickly, antiviral drugs are most effective when taken before an infection develops or in its early stages.

*Bacteria* Simple one-celled organisms, **bacteria** are the most plentiful microorganisms as well as the most pathogenic. Most kinds of bacteria don't cause disease; some, like certain strains of *Escherichia coli* that aid in digestion, play important roles within our bodies. Even friendly bacteria, however, can get out of hand and cause acne, urinary tract infections, vaginal infections, and other problems.

Bacteria harm the body by releasing either enzymes that digest body cells or toxins that produce the specific effects of such diseases as diphtheria or toxic shock syndrome. In self-defense, the body produces specific proteins (called *antibodies*) that attack and inactivate the invaders. Tuberculosis, tetanus, gonorrhea, scarlet

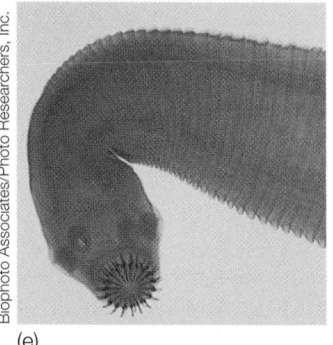

Examples of the major categories of organisms that cause disease in humans. Except for the helminths (parasitic worms), pathogens are microorganisms that can be seen only with the aid of a microscope. (a) Viruses: common cold, (b) Bacteria: syphilis, (c) Fungi: athlete's foot fungus, (d) Protozoa: Giardia lamblia, (e) Helminths: tapeworm.

fever, and diphtheria are examples of bacterial diseases.

Because bacteria are sufficiently different from the cells that make up our bodies, antibiotics can kill them without harming our cells. Antibiotics work only against specific types of bacteria. If your doctor thinks you have a bacterial infection, tests of your blood, pus, sputum, urine, or stool can identify the particular bacterial strain.

*Fungi* Single-celled or multicelled organisms, **fungi** consist of threadlike fibers and reproductive spores. Fungi lack chlorophyll and must obtain their food from organic material, which may include human tissue. Fungi release enzymes that digest cells and are most likely to attack hair-covered areas of the body, including the scalp, beard, groin, and external ear canals. They also cause athlete's foot. Treatment consists of antifungal drugs.

*Protozoa* These single-celled, microscopic animals release enzymes and toxins that destroy cells or interfere with their function. Diseases caused by **protozoa** are not a major health problem in this country, primarily because of public health measures. Around the world, however, some 2.24 billion people (more than 40 percent of the world's population) are at risk for acquiring malaria—a protozoan-caused disease. Up to 3 million die from this disease annually. Many more come down with amoebic dysentery. Treatment for protozoa-caused diseases consists of general medical care to relieve the symptoms, replacement of lost blood or fluids, and drugs that kill the specific protozoan.

The most common disease caused by protozoa in the United States is *giardiasis,* an intestinal infection caused by microorganisms in human and animal feces. It has become a threat at day-care centers, as well as among campers and hikers who drink contaminated water. Symptoms include nausea, lack of appetite, gas, diarrhea, fatigue, abdominal cramps, and bloating. Many people recover in a month or two without treatment. However, in some cases the microbe causes recurring attacks over many years. Giardiasis can be life-threatening in small children and the elderly, who are especially prone to severe dehydration from diarrhea. Treatment usually consists of antibiotics.

*Helminths (Parasitic Worms)* Small parasitic worms that attack specific tissues or organs and compete with the host for nutrients are called **helminths**. One major worldwide health problem is *schistosomiasis,* a disease caused by a parasitic worm, the fluke, that burrows through the skin and enters the circulatory system. Infection with another helminth, the tapeworm, may be contracted from eating undercooked beef, pork, or fish containing larval forms of the tapeworm. Helminthic diseases are treated with appropriate medications.

## How Infections Spread

The major *vectors,* or means of transmission, for infectious disease are animals and insects, people, food, and water.

*Animals and Insects* Disease can be transmitted by house pets, livestock, birds, and wild animals. Insects also spread a variety of diseases. The housefly may spread dysentery, diarrhea, typhoid fever, or trachoma (an eye disease rare in the United States but common in other parts of the world). Other insects, including mosquitoes, ticks, mites, fleas, and lice, can transmit such diseases as malaria, yellow fever, encephalitis, dengue fever (a growing threat in Mexico), and Lyme disease.

New threats in the United States include West Nile virus (WNV), which can be spread to humans by mosquitoes that bite infected birds, and monkeypox virus, carried by various animals, including prairie dogs. Concern has grown about avian influenza, or bird flu, which has spread to wild and domestic birds around the world. H1N1 (swine) flu, which can be transmitted between humans and pigs, caused a global pandemic in 2009. (These illnesses are discussed later in this chapter.)

*People* The people you're closest to can transmit pathogens through the air, through touch, or through sexual contact. To avoid infection, stay out of range of anyone who's coughing, sniffling, or sneezing, and don't share food or dishes. Carefully wash your dishes, utensils, and hands, and abstain from sex or make self-protective decisions about sexual partners.

*Food* Every year foodborne illnesses strike millions of Americans, sometimes with fatal consequences. Bacteria account for two-thirds of foodborne infections, and thousands of suspected cases of infection with *Escherichia*

## Health in the Headlines

### Infection Update

Up-to-date, accurate information is one of your best defenses against the dangers of infection. After accessing Global Health Watch, click on "Diseases" and then on "Infectious Diseases." Scan the list of major infectious diseases and choose one, such as "Common Cold" or "Meningitis." When you click on this topic, you'll find a list of headlines under "Latest news." Read through the latest research reports, and summarize in your online journal.

**host** A person or population that contracts one or more pathogenic agents in an environment.

**vector** A biological or physical vehicle that carries the agent of infection to the host.

**virus** A submicroscopic infectious agent; the most primitive form of life.

**antibiotics** Substances produced by microorganisms, or synthetic agents, that are toxic to bacteria.

**antiviral drug** A substance that decreases the severity and duration of a viral infection if taken prior to or soon after onset of the infection.

**bacteria** (singular, bacterium) One-celled microscopic organisms; the most plentiful pathogens.

**fungi** (singular, fungus) Organisms that reproduce by means of spores.

**protozoa** Microscopic animals made up of one cell or a group of similar cells.

**helminth** A parasitic roundworm or flatworm.

*coli* bacteria in undercooked or inadequately washed food have been reported. (See Chapter 6 for more on *E. coli* outbreaks.)

Every year as many as 4 million Americans have a bout with *Salmonella* bacteria, which have been found in about a third of all poultry sold in the United States. These infections can be serious enough to require hospitalization and can lead to arthritis, neurological problems, and even death. Consumers can greatly reduce the number of salmonella infections by proper handling, cooking, and refrigeration of poultry (see Chapter 6).

*Water* Waterborne diseases, such as typhoid fever and cholera, are still widespread in less developed areas of the world. They have been rare in the United States, although outbreaks caused by inadequate water purification have occurred.

## The Process of Infection

If someone infected with the flu sits next to you on a bus and coughs or sneezes, tiny viral particles may travel into your nose and mouth. Immediately, the virus finds or creates an opening in the wall of a cell, and the process of infection begins. During the **incubation period**, the time between invasion and the first symptom, you're unaware of the pathogen multiplying inside you. In some diseases, incubation may go on for months, even years; for most, it lasts several days or weeks.

The early stage of the battle between your body and the invaders is called the *prodromal period*. As infected cells die, they release chemicals that help block the invasion. Other chemicals, such as *histamines*, cause blood vessels to dilate, thus allowing more blood to reach the battleground. During all of this, you feel mild, generalized symptoms, such as headache, irritability, and discomfort. You're also highly contagious. At the height of the battle—the typical illness period—you cough, sneeze, sniffle, ache, feel feverish, and lose your appetite.

Recovery begins when the body's forces gain the advantage. With time, the body destroys the last of the invaders and heals itself. However, the body is not able to develop long-lasting immunity to certain viruses, such as colds, flu, or HIV.

## Who Is at Highest Risk?

Like human bullies, the viruses responsible for the most common infectious illnesses tend to pick on those least capable of fighting back. Among the most vulnerable are the following groups:

- **Children and their families.** Youngsters get up to a dozen colds annually; adults average two a year. When a flu epidemic hits a community, about 40 percent of school-age boys and girls get sick, compared with only 5 to 10 percent of adults. But parents get up to six times as many colds as other adults.

- **The elderly.** Statistically, fewer older men and women are likely to catch a cold or flu, yet when they do, they face greater danger than the rest of the population. People over 65 who get the flu have a one in ten chance of being hospitalized for pneumonia or other respiratory problems, and a one in fifty chance of dying from the disease.

- **The chronically ill.** Lifelong diseases, such as diabetes, kidney disease, or sickle-cell anemia, decrease an individual's ability to fend off infections. Individuals taking medications that suppress the immune system, such as steroids, are more vulnerable to infections, as are those with medical conditions that impair immunity, such as infection with HIV.

- **Smokers and those with respiratory problems.** Smokers are a high-risk group for respiratory infections and serious complications, such as pneumonia. Chronic breathing disorders, such as asthma and emphysema, also greatly increase the risk of respiratory infections.

- **Those who live or work in close contact with someone sick.** Health-care workers who treat high-risk patients, nursing home residents, and others living in close quarters—such as students in dormitories—face greater odds of catching others' colds and flus.

- **Residents or workers in poorly ventilated buildings.** Building technology has helped spread certain airborne illnesses, such as tuberculosis, via recirculated air. Indoor air quality can be closely linked with disease transmission in winter, when people spend a great deal of time in tightly sealed rooms.

**incubation period** The time between a pathogen's entrance into the body and the first symptom.

Figure 16.1 **The Human Lymphatic System and Its Functions**

The lymphatic system helps filter impurities from the body.

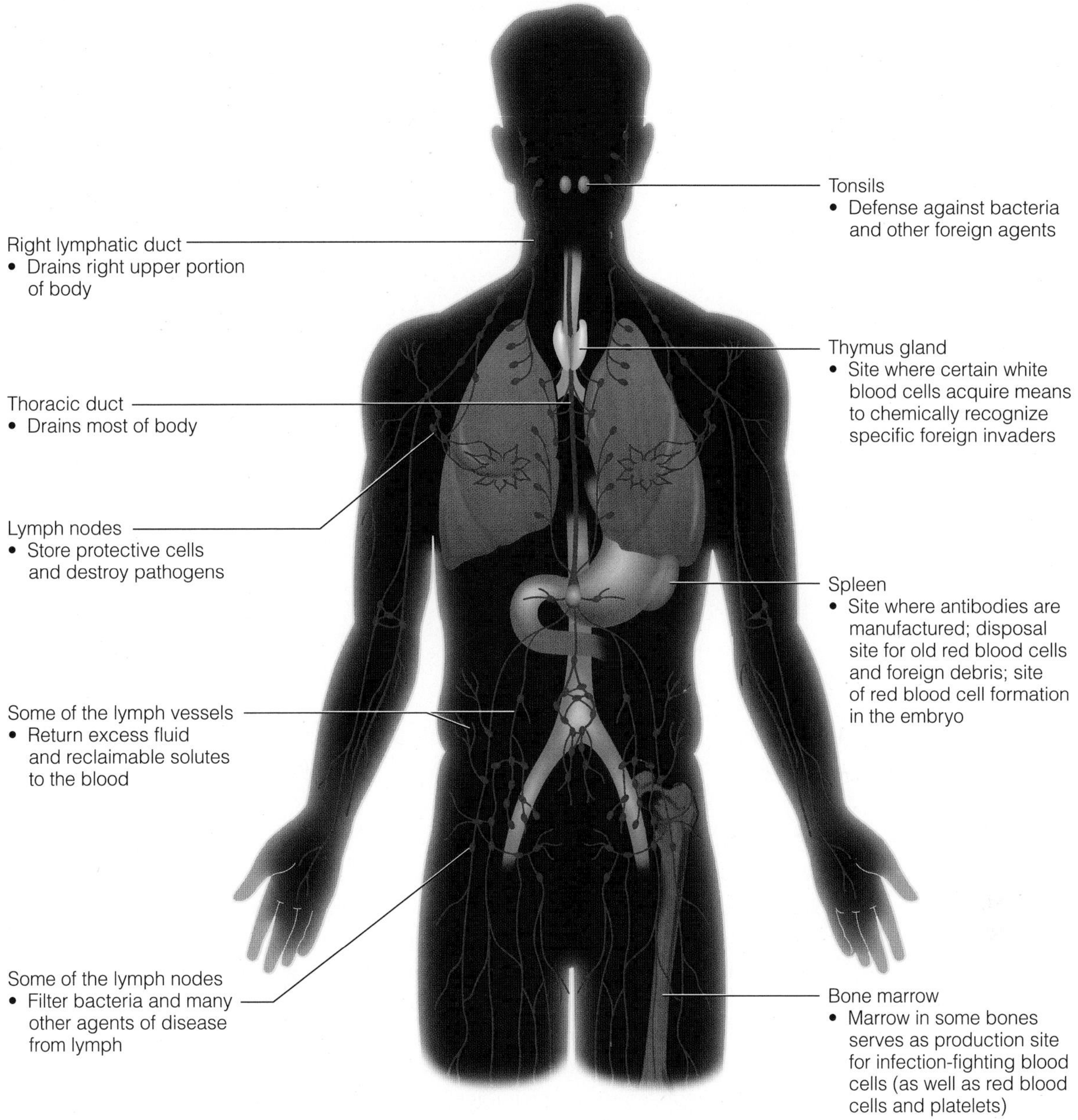

Tonsils
• Defense against bacteria and other foreign agents
Right lymphatic duct
• Drains right upper portion of body
Thymus gland
• Site where certain white blood cells acquire means to chemically recognize specific foreign invaders
Thoracic duct
• Drains most of body
Lymph nodes
• Store protective cells and destroy pathogens
Spleen
• Site where antibodies are manufactured; disposal site for old red blood cells and foreign debris; site of red blood cell formation in the embryo
Some of the lymph vessels
• Return excess fluid and reclaimable solutes to the blood
Some of the lymph nodes
• Filter bacteria and many other agents of disease from lymph
Bone marrow
• Marrow in some bones serves as production site for infection-fighting blood cells (as well as red blood cells and platelets)


# How Your Body Protects Itself

Various parts of your body safeguard you against infectious diseases by providing **immunity**, or protection, from these health threats. Your skin, when unbroken, keeps out most potential invaders. Your tears, sweat, skin oils, saliva, and mucus contain chemicals that can kill bacteria. Cilia, the tiny hairs lining your respiratory passages, move mucus, which traps inhaled bacteria, viruses, dust, and foreign matter, to the back of the throat, where it is swallowed; the digestive system then destroys the invaders.

When these protective mechanisms can't keep you infection-free, your body's immune system, which is on constant alert for foreign substances that might threaten the body, swings into action. (See "Health in Action: Infection Protection.") The immune system includes structures of the lymphatic system—the spleen, thymus gland, lymph nodes, and lymph vessels—that help filter impurities from the body (Figure 16.1). The **lymph nodes**, or glands, are small tissue masses in which some protective cells are stored.

**immunity** Protection from infectious diseases.

**lymph nodes** Small tissue masses in which some immune cells are stored.

Figure 16.2  **The Immune Response**

Some T cells can kill infected body cells. B cells churn out antibodies to tag pathogens for destruction by macrophages and other white blood cells.

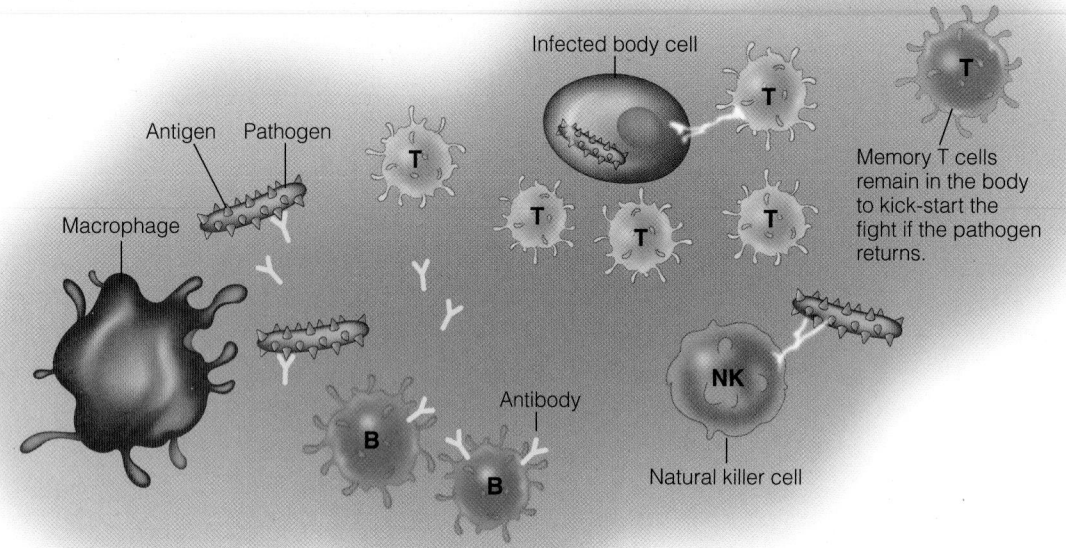

If pathogens invade your body, many of them are carried to the lymph nodes to be destroyed. This is why your lymph nodes often feel swollen when you have a cold or the flu.

More than a dozen different types of white blood cells (lymphocytes) are concentrated in the organs of the lymphatic system or patrol the entire body by way of the blood and lymph vessels. Some of these white blood cells are generalists and some are specialists. The generalists include *macrophages*, which are large scavenger cells with insatiable appetites for foreign cells, diseased and run-down red blood cells, and other biological debris (Figure 16.2). The specialists are the *B cells* and *T cells*, which respond to specific invaders.

An *antigen* is any substance the white blood cells recognize as foreign. B cells create antibodies, which are proteins that bind to antigens and mark them for destruction by other white blood cells. Antigens are specific to the pathogen, and the antibody to a particular antigen binds only to that antigen (Figure 16.2). Once the human body produces antibodies against a specific antigen—the mumps virus, for instance— you're protected against that antigen for life. If you're again exposed to mumps, the antibodies

previously produced prevent another episode of the disease.

But you don't have to suffer through an illness to acquire immunity. Inoculation with a vaccine containing synthetic or weakened antigens can give you the same protection. The type of long-lasting immunity in which the body makes its own antibodies to a pathogen is called *active immunity*. Immunity produced by the injection of **gamma globulin**, the antibody-containing part of the blood from another person or animal that has developed antibodies to a disease, is called *passive immunity*.

## Immune Response

Attacked by pathogens, the body musters its forces and fights. Sometimes the invasion is handled like a minor border skirmish; other times a full-scale battle is waged throughout the body. Together, the immune cells work like an internal police force. When an antigen enters the body, the T cells aided by macrophages engage in combat with the invader. Certain T cells (cytotoxic T cells) can destroy infected body cells or tumor cells by "touch-killing." Meanwhile, the B cells churn out antibodies, which rush to the

**gamma globulin** The antibody-containing portion of the blood fluid (plasma).

scene and join in the fray. Also busy at surveillance are natural killer cells that, like the elite forces of a SWAT team, seek out and destroy viruses and cancer cells (Figure 16.2).

If the microbes establish a foothold, the blood supply to the area increases, bringing oxygen and nutrients to the fighting cells. Tissue fluids, as well as antibacterial and antitoxic proteins, accumulate. You may develop redness, swelling, local warmth, and pain—the signs of **inflammation**.

Chronic low-grade inflammation increases by twofold to fourfold the levels of cytokines, substances secreted by certain immune cells, in the bloodstream. These elevated levels serve as inflammatory markers that have emerged as major players in the development of several major diseases, including atherosclerosis, hypertension, and other cardiovascular disorders, insulin resistance, metabolic syndrome, type 2 diabetes, and cancer. Recent research has linked chronic inflammation with depression in college students as well.

 Medical scientists are continuing to investigate the role of inflammatory markers and to identify ways to reduce elevated levels. In a number of studies, vigorous exercise, including cycling, running, swimming, and resistance training, did reduce markers of inflammation. The impact of these markers on disease risk and progression is not yet clear.

As more tissue is destroyed, a cavity, or **abscess**, forms and fills with fluid, battling cells, and dead white blood cells (pus). If the invaders aren't killed or inactivated, the pathogens are able to spread into the bloodstream and cause what is known as **systemic disease**.

Some people have an **immune deficiency**—either inborn or acquired. A very few children are born without an effective immune system; their lives can be endangered by any infection. Although still experimental, therapy to implant a missing or healthy gene may offer new hope for a normal life.

## Immunity and Stress

Whenever we confront a crisis, large or small, our bodies produce powerful hormones that provide extra energy. However, this stress response dampens immunity, reducing the number of some key immune cells and the responsiveness of others.

 As discussed in Chapter 4, stressful experiences in childhood can have a long-term effect on health. Students' stress and mental health affects their susceptibility to infections. In an analysis of ACHA data on more than 47,000 undergraduates, those who did not report depression, anxiety, or exhaustion were least likely to develop an acute infectious illness (bronchitis, ear infection, sinus infection, or strep throat). The more exhausted students said they were, the greater their probability of coming down with an infection.[1]

Stress affects the body's immune system in different ways, depending on two factors: the controllability or uncontrollability of the stressor and the mental effort required to cope with the stress. An uncontrollable stressor that lasts longer than 15 minutes may interfere with cytokine interleukin-6, which plays an essential role in activating the immune defenses. Uncontrollable stressors also produce high levels of the hormone cortisol, which suppresses immune system functioning. The mental efforts required to cope with high-level stressors produce only brief immune changes that appear to have little consequence for health. However, stress has been shown to slow pro-inflammatory cytokine production, which is essential for healing.

## Immunity and Gender

When the flu hits a household, the last one left standing is likely to be Mom. The female immune system responds more vigorously to common infections, offering extra protection against viruses, bacteria, and parasites.

The genders also differ in their vulnerability to allergies and autoimmune disorders. Although both men and women frequently develop allergies, allergic women are twice as likely to experience potentially fatal anaphylactic shock. A woman's robust immune system also is more likely to overreact and turn on her own organs and tissues. On average, three of four people with autoimmune disorders, such as multiple sclerosis, Hashimoto's thyroiditis, and scleroderma, are women.

**inflammation** A localized response by the body to tissue injury, characterized by swelling and the dilation of the blood vessels.

**abscess** A localized accumulation of pus and disintegrating tissue.

**systemic disease** A pathologic condition that spreads throughout the body.

**immune deficiency** Partial or complete inability of the immune system to respond to pathogens.

# Health in Action

## Infection Protection

Some day medical science may develop vaccines or other means of providing total protection against infectious diseases. Until then your best defense is to take commonsense steps to promote well-being and reduce the risks of infection. Here are some basic principles of self-defense:

- **Eat a balanced diet** to be sure you get essential vitamins and minerals. Severe deficiencies in vitamins B6, B12, and folic acid impair immunity. Keep up your iron and zinc intake. Iron influences the number and vigor of certain immune cells, whereas zinc is crucial for cell repair. Too little vitamin C also may increase susceptibility to infectious diseases.

- **Avoid fatty foods.** A low-fat diet can increase the activity of immune cells that hunt down and knock out cells infected with viruses.

- **Get enough sleep.** Without adequate rest, your immune system cannot maintain and renew itself.

- **Exercise regularly.** Aerobic exercise stimulates the production of an immune-system booster called interleukin-2.

- **Don't smoke.** Smoking decreases the levels of some immune cells and increases susceptibility to respiratory infections.

- **Control your alcohol intake.** Heavy drinking interferes with normal immune responses and lowers the number of defender cells.

- **Wash your hands frequently with hot water and soap.** In a public restroom, use a paper towel to turn off the faucet after you wash your hands, and avoid touching the doorknob. Wash objects used by someone with a cold.

- **Don't share food, drinks, silverware, glasses,** and other objects that may carry infectious microbes.

- **Spend as little time as possible in crowds during cold and flu season,** especially closed places, such as elevators and airplanes. When out, keep your distance from sneezers and coughers.

- **Don't touch your eyes, mouth, and nose,** especially after being with someone who has cold symptoms.

- **Use tissues** rather than cloth handkerchiefs, which may harbor viruses for hours or days.

- **Avoid irritating air pollutants** whenever possible.

In your online journal, write your own goals and top strategies for preventing infection.

**allergy** A hypersensitivity to a particular substance in one's environment or diet.

Why are there such large gender differences in susceptibility? Scientists believe that the sex hormones have a great impact on immunity. Through a woman's childbearing years, estrogen, which protects heart, bone, brain, and blood vessels, also bolsters the immune system's response to certain infectious agents. Women produce greater numbers of antibodies when exposed to an antigen.

In contrast, testosterone may suppress this response—possibly to prevent attacks on sperm cells, which might otherwise be mistaken as alien invaders. When the testes are removed from mice and guinea pigs, their immune systems become more active.

# Immune Disorders

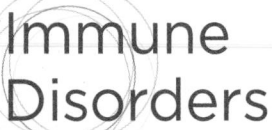

Sometimes our immune system overreacts to certain substances, mistakes the body's own tissues for enemies, or doesn't react adequately. The result is immune disorders such as allergies and autoimmune disorders.

## Allergies

An **allergy** represents a hypersensitivity to a substance in the environment or diet that does not bother most other people. Allergies are the sixth leading cause of chronic disease. More than half of Americans between ages 6 and 59 are sensitive to one or more allergens. Allergies consistently rate as one of the top health problems among college students. In one study, almost half of college students reported a problem with allergies in the previous year.

Among the substances that trigger allergic reactions are:

- Pollen.
- Dust mites.
- Mold spores.
- Pet dander.
- Food (discussed in Chapter 6).
- Insect stings.
- Medicine.

In an allergic reaction, the immune system reacts as if it were defending the body against germs such as bacteria and viruses. When an allergic person first comes into contact with an allergen, the immune system generates large amounts of a type of antibody called immunoglobulin E or IgE. Each IgE antibody is specific for one particular substance, such as a particular pollen. The next time the allergen encounters its specific IgE, it attaches to it like a key fitting into a lock. This signals the cell to produce or release powerful chemicals like histamine that cause inflammation and the symptoms of allergy. The most common are:

- Runny or clogged nose.
- Sneezing.
- Coughing.
- Itching eyes, nose, and throat.
- Eye irritation.

Allergy sufferers run annual tabs of up to $2 billion in doctor visits, diagnostic tests, prescriptions, and decreased productivity. Every year allergies account for more than 10 million workdays missed; every day they keep 10,000 children out of school.

Thanks to treatment breakthroughs, allergy sufferers no longer have to choose between feeling better or feeling alert. Treatment options include nonsedating oral medications, nasal sprays, and **immunotherapy**, which consists of a series of injections of small but increasing doses of an allergen. Allergy shots are not necessarily more costly or time-consuming than taking medicine to relieve symptoms and may, over time, reduce health care costs.[2]

*Autoimmune Disorders*  Sometimes the body's defenses go awry, and the immune system declares war on the cells, tissues, or organs it normally protects. **Autoimmune disorders** rank among the top ten killers and disablers of American adults, particularly women. They strike about three times as many women as men, possibly because of the effects of female hormones on the immune system. Women are most vulnerable in the prime of life, during their reproductive years. (See Table 16.2.)

Some autoimmune disorders directly damage a single organ, as happens with Addison's disease, which targets the adrenal glands, or Crohn's disease, which affects the gastrointestinal tract. Other autoimmune disorders attack multiple organs. Systemic lupus erythematosus, for instance, can affect the skin, joints, kidneys, heart, brain, and red blood cells.

For many people with autoimmune disorders, the biggest challenge is finding out what's wrong. Early symptoms, such as low-grade fever or achiness, often wax and wane and are dismissed or misdiagnosed by doctors. New blood tests for lupus and multiple sclerosis are promising faster, more accurate diagnoses, but for many autoimmune disorders, there are no conclusive laboratory tests.

**Table 16.1 Vaccines Recommended for College Students**

| Tetanus-Diphtheria-Pertussis (Tdap) vaccine |
| Meningococcal vaccine* |
| HPV vaccine series |
| Hepatitis A vaccine series |
| Hepatitis B vaccine series |
| Polio vaccine series |
| Measles-Mumps-Rubella (MMR) vaccine series |
| Varicella (chicken pox) vaccine series |
| Influenza vaccine |
| Pneumococcal polysaccharide (PPV) vaccine |

*Recommended for previously unvaccinated college freshmen living in dormitories.

© Capifrutta/Shutterstock.com

Patients should keep a detailed record of when symptoms start, recur, flare, or subside, and seek a specialist—a rheumatologist, dermatologist, immunologist, or gastroenterologist, depending on symptoms—who has expertise in autoimmune disorders. New treatments are revolutionizing treatments for many autoimmune disorders, including rheumatoid arthritis.

# Immunization for Adults

One of the great success stories of modern medicine has been the development of vaccines that provide protection against many infectious diseases. Immunization has reduced cases of measles, mumps, tetanus, whooping cough, and other life-threatening illnesses by more than 95 percent. Nonetheless some parents remain reluctant to vaccinate their children.

Although many people associate vaccination with children's health, the vast majority of vaccine-preventable deaths occur among adults. An estimated 40,000 to 50,000 American adults die every year from diseases that vaccines could have prevented. Only slightly more than a third of adults get an annual flu shot; many seniors have not gotten a pneumonia vaccination, a one-time shot recommended for everyone over age 65. Table 16.1 lists the vaccines recommended for college students and Figure 16.3 shows the recommended adult immunization

**immunotherapy** A series of injections of small but increasing doses of an allergen, used to treat allergies.

**autoimmune disorder** Resulting from the attack on body tissue by an immune system that fails to recognize the tissue as self.

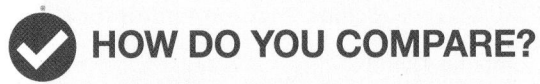

## HOW DO YOU COMPARE?

# VACCINATIONS ON CAMPUS

| Vaccinated against | Percentage of students | Vaccinated against | Percentage of students |
|---|---|---|---|
| Hepatitis B | 73 | Varicella (chicken pox) | 43.4 |
| Measles, Mumps, Rubella | 70.9 | Influenza (within last | |
| Meningococcal Meningitis | 54.7 | 12 months) | 39.9 |

## HOW DO YOU COMPARE?

Vaccinations are your first line of defense against potentially serious infectious diseases. Do you know your vaccination history? Do you keep track of recommendations for new or booster shots? Do you get a flu vaccination every year? Jot down what you see as the pros and cons of up-to-date vaccinations in your online journal.

Source: American College Health Association, *American College Health Association-National College Health Assessment II: Reference Group Executive Summary Spring 2010* (Linthicum, MD: American College Health Association, 2010).

Figure 16.3 **Recommended Adult Immunization Schedule, by Vaccine and Age Group—United States, 2011**

| Vaccine | 19–26 years | 27–49 years | 50–59 years | 60–64 years | ≥ 65 years |
|---|---|---|---|---|---|
| Tetanus, diphtheria, pertussis [Td/Tdap]* | Substitute 1-time dose of Tdap for Td booster; then boost with TD every 10 yrs | | | | Td booster every 10 yrs |
| Human papillomavirus (HPV)* | 3 doses (females) | | | | |
| Measles, mumps, rubella (MMR)* | 1 or 2 doses | | 1 dose | | |
| Varicella (chicken pox)* | 2 doses | | | | |
| Influenza* | 1 dose annually | | | | |
| Pneumococcal (polysaccharide) | 1–2 doses | | | | 1 dose |
| Hepatitis A* | 2 doses | | | | |
| Hepatitis B* | 3 doses | | | | |
| Meningococcal* | 1 or more doses | | | | |
| Zoster | | | | 1 dose | |

\* Covered by the Vaccine Injury Compensation Program

For all persons in this category who meet the age requirements and who lack evidence of immunity (e.g., lack documentation of vaccination or have no evidence of previous infection)

Recommended if some other risk factor is present (e.g., based on medical, occupational, lifestyle, or other indications)

No recommendation

schedule.[3] The percentage of students vaccinated against different diseases varies greatly. How do you compare? (See How Do You Compare? page 544.)

# Common Cold

There are more than 200 distinct cold viruses. Although in a single season you may develop a temporary immunity to one or two, you may then be hit by a third. Americans come down with 1 billion colds annually.

Every year, about 25 million cold sufferers in the United States visit their family doctors with uncomplicated upper respiratory infections. The common cold results in about 20 million days of absence from work and 22 million days of absence from school.

 College and university students are at increased risk for colds and influenza-like illnesses. In one study that followed more than 3,000 students from fall to spring, nine in ten had at least one cold or flu-like illness. Colds can strike in any season, but different cold viruses are more common at different times of years. Rhinoviruses cause most spring, summer, and early fall colds and tend to cause more symptoms above the neck (stuffy nose, headache, runny eyes). Adenoviruses, para-influenza viruses, coronaviruses, influenza viruses, and others that strike in the winter are more likely to get into the trachea and bronchi (the breathing passages) and cause more fever and bronchitis.

Cold viruses spread by coughs, sneezes, and touch. Cold sufferers who sneeze and then touch a doorknob or countertop leave a trail of highly contagious viruses behind them. The best preventive tactics are frequent hand washing, replacing toothbrushes regularly, exercising regularly, and avoiding stress overload.

A lack of sleep can increase your odds of getting a cold. People who get less than seven hours of sleep a night are three times more likely to catch a cold. Those who sleep poorly are five times more susceptible.

High levels of stress increase the risk of becoming infected by respiratory viruses and

## Caring for Your Cold

Fortunately, the most effective treatments for a cold are inexpensive—or even free:

- **Drink plenty of fluids, particularly warm ones.** Warmth is important because the aptly named "cold" viruses replicate at lower temperatures. Hot soups and drinks (particularly those with a touch of something pungent, like lemon or ginger) raise body temperature and help clear the nose. Tea may enhance the immune system.

- **Get plenty of rest.** Taking it easy reduces demands on the body, which helps speed recovery.

- **Do not take antibiotics.** They are ineffective against colds and flu.

- **Do not take aspirin or acetaminophen (Tylenol), which may suppress the antibodies the body produces to fight cold viruses and increase symptoms such as stuffiness.** Children, teenagers, and young adults should never take aspirin for a cold or flu because of the danger of Reye's syndrome, a potentially deadly disorder that can cause convulsions, coma, swelling of the brain, and kidney damage. A better alternative for achiness is ibuprofen (brand names include Motrin, Advil, and Nuprin), which doesn't seem to affect immune response.

- **Choose the right medicines for your symptoms.**

| If you want to: | Choose medicine with: |
|---|---|
| Unclog a stuffy nose | Nasal decongestant |
| Quiet a cough | Cough suppressant |
| Loosen mucus so that you can cough it up | Expectorant |
| Stop runny nose and sneezing | Antihistamine |
| Ease fever, headaches, minor aches and pains | Pain reliever (analgesic) |

- **Know when to call your doctor.** You usually do not have to call a doctor right away if you have signs of a cold or flu. But be sure to call in these situations:
  - Your symptoms get worse.
  - Your symptoms last a long time.
  - After feeling a little better, you show signs of a more serious problem. Some of these signs are a sick-to-your-stomach feeling, vomiting, high fever, shaking, chills, chest pain, or coughing with thick, yellow-green mucus.

developing cold symptoms. People who feel unable to deal with everyday stresses have an exaggerated immune reaction that may intensify cold or flu symptoms once they've contracted a virus. Those with a positive emotional outlook are less vulnerable.

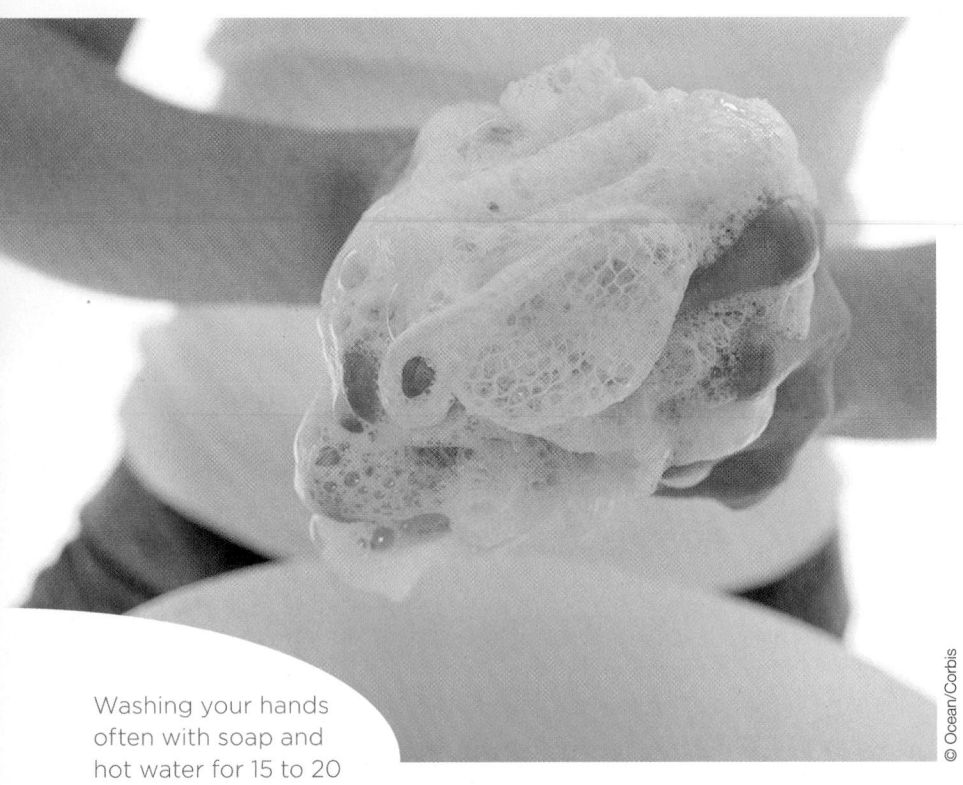
© Ocean/Corbis

Washing your hands often with soap and hot water for 15 to 20 seconds will help protect you from germs. When soap and water are not available, you can use alcohol-based disposable hand wipes or gel sanitizers. If using gel, rub your hands until the gel is dry; the alcohol in the gel kills the germs.

Although colds and sore throats—a frequent cold symptom—are caused by viruses, many people seek treatment with antibiotics, which are effective only against bacteria. Unless you're coughing up green or foul yellow mucus (signs of a secondary bacterial infection), antibiotics won't help. They have no effect against viruses and may make your body more resistant to such medications when you develop a bacterial infection in the future. An estimated 5 to 17 percent of sore throats in adults are caused by bacteria (*Group A streptococci*). For effective treatments, see Health on a Budget at right.

Excess prescribing for antibiotics accounts for more than half of all prescriptions and costs more than $700 million a year. In addition to their costs, antibiotics may increase risks to users and their contacts. An increasing number of studies show that antibiotics foster the growth of one or more strains of antibiotic-resistant bacteria for at least two to six months inside the person taking the pills—who can pass on this drug-resistant bug to family, roommates, and others.

According to a recent review of 30 published studies, taking vitamin C every day does not ward off the common cold or shorten its length or severity. However, some people might

indeed benefit—those exposed to short bouts of extreme physical exercise or cold temperatures. Tests of high-dose vitamin C after the onset of cold symptoms showed no consistent effect on either the length of a cold or the severity of its symptoms.

The latest findings on *Echinacea* are also mixed. In previous studies, the herbal supplement cut the chances of catching a cold by more than half and shortened the duration of a cold by an average of 1.4 days. However, a more recent report found no significant impact on the length or severity of a cold.[4]

In a recent review, lozenges or syrup containing zinc, a mineral that inhibits rhinoviral replication, did help reduce the duration and severity of the common cold in healthy people, when taken within 24 hours of onset of symptoms. The use of zinc supplements for at least five months also reduced the incidence of colds and school absenteeism. Individuals taking zinc lozenges (not syrup or tablet form) were more likely to complain of bad taste or nausea.[5] (See "Health on a Budget: Caring for Your Cold," p. 545.)

To avoid getting a cold:

- Avoid people with colds when possible.

- Sneeze or cough into a tissue and then throw the tissue away.

- Clean surfaces you touch with a germ-killing disinfectant.

- Don't touch your nose, eyes, or mouth. Germs can enter your body easily by these paths.

- Wash your hands often. Use hot water and lather up, covering the back of your hands as well as your fingers and palms. Scrub for at least 15 seconds—about the time it takes to sing one chorus of "Happy Birthday to You."

- Don't switch to alcohol-based hand sanitizers. While they are handy when you can't get to a sink, they must come into contact with all surfaces of your hands in order to be effective. Even then, they cleanse no better than plain soap and water.

- Dry your hands thoroughly. Wet hands are more likely to spread germs than dry ones.

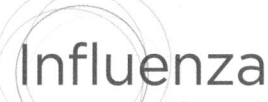

# Influenza

Although similar to a cold, **influenza**—or the flu—causes more severe symptoms that last longer.

## Seasonal Influenza

Every year 10 to 20 percent of Americans develop seasonal influenza, more than 200,000 are hospitalized, and 36,000 die.

Flu viruses, transmitted by coughs, sneezes, laughs, and even normal conversation, are extraordinarily contagious, particularly in the first three days of the disease. The usual incubation period is two days, but symptoms can hit hard and fast. Two varieties of viruses—influenza A and influenza B—cause most flus.

The CDC now recommends an annual flu shot for everyone over the age of six months, except for those with certain medical conditions. Vaccination with the live, nasal-spray flu vaccine (FluMist) is an option for healthy people ages 5 to 49 years who are not pregnant. The spray represents a particular advantage for children since more than 30 percent of youngsters get the flu, but most don't receive a flu shot. However, its recipients are likely to have more health-care visits related to flu and pneumonia than those given standard flu shots.

For those who don't get vaccinated, antiviral drugs, which must be taken within 36 to 48 hours of the first flu symptom, have provided the next best line of defense. Two of the oldest of these medications, amantadine and rimantadine, which work only against the type A flu virus, are no longer effective, possibly because the flu virus has mutated and become resistant. Two newer agents, Tamiflu (oseltamivir) and Relenza (zanamivir), fight both type A and type B influenza.

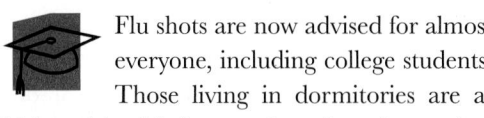
Flu shots are now advised for almost everyone, including college students. Those living in dormitories are at higher risk of influenza than those in nondormitory settings. The specific aspects of dormitory life that increase the risk of flu symptoms include the number of roommates and the presence/absence of carpeting. Students living in "triples," with three beds to a room; those sleeping in the same room with a roommate in a

## How to Protect Yourself and Others from Influenza

### If You Are Well

- **Get vaccinated.**

- **Do not share cups, glasses, bottles, dishes, or silverware.**

- **Wash your hands frequently, especially after close contact with other people (on buses, in stores, at the gym, etc.)** with soap and water. Alcohol-based hand sanitizers are also effective.

- **Avoid touching your eyes, nose, or mouth.**

- **Try to avoid close contact with sick people.**

- **Reduce time in crowded settings.**

- **Stay in good general health: get plenty of sleep, be physically active, manage daily stress, drink plenty of fluids, eat nutritious food.**

- **Follow public health advice regarding school closures, avoiding crowds, and other social distancing measures.**

- **Improve airflow in your living space by opening windows as much as possible.**

- **There is no evidence that wearing a face mask in open areas (as opposed to enclosed spaces while in close contact with a person with flu-like symptoms) reduces the risk.** If you do choose to wear one, place it carefully so it covers the mouth and nose with minimal gaps between the face and mask. Once it's on, avoid touching the mask. Wash your hands immediately after removing it. Replace a mask with a new clean, dry one as soon as it becomes damp. Do not reuse single-use masks.

### If You Have Symptoms

- **Cover your nose and mouth with a tissue when you cough or sneeze.** Throw the tissue in the trash after you use it.

- **Wash your hands often with soap and water, especially after you cough or sneeze.**

- **Be prepared to stay home, in your room, or in a designated quarantined area for a week or until you have been fever-free for at least a day.** Get a supply of over-the-counter medicines, alcohol-based hand rubs, tissues, and other related items to avoid the need to go out in public while you are sick and contagious.

- **To prevent the spread of influenza virus among family members or roommates, keep surfaces (especially bedside tables, bathroom sinks, kitchen counters) clean by wiping them down with a household disinfectant.** Wash linens, eating utensils, and dishes before sharing them.

**influenza** Any type of fairly common, highly contagious viral diseases.

double; and those with uncarpeted floors have higher rates of flu symptoms, such as fever, sore throat, and fatigue.

# H1N1 Influenza (Swine Flu)

The H1N1 virus is an influenza type A virus that was detected in people in the United States in April 2009, following infections in Mexico and other countries. It was originally referred to as "swine flu" because many of its genes were similar to influenza viruses that normally occur in pigs in North America. However, further study has shown that H1N1 is distinctive, with two genes from flu viruses that normally circulate in pigs in Europe and Asia plus avian genes and human genes. Scientists call this a "quadruple reassortant" virus.

The symptoms of H1N1 flu are similar to the symptoms of regular flu: fever, cough, sore throat, body aches, headache, chills, fatigue. A significant number of people infected with H1N1 also have reported diarrhea and vomiting. As with seasonal flu, severe illness and death have occurred as a result of infection with this virus.

Federal health officials estimate that the H1N1 pandemic of 2009 sickened some 57 to 84 million people, causing 378,000 hospitalizations and 17,160 deaths (lower than that in prior flu seasons). H1N1 did not prove as infectious among young adults as was first feared. However, pregnant women (particularly those with asthma, obesity, or diabetes), school-age children, and the morbidly obese were much more likely to become seriously ill or die.

A vaccine specifically targeting H1N1 proved highly effective. Annual flu shots now provide protection against both seasonal and H1N1 flu.[6]

# The Threat of a Pandemic

Public health officials differentiate between an outbreak, an epidemic, and a pandemic:

- An outbreak is a sudden rise in the incidence of a disease.
- An epidemic affects an atypically large number of individuals within a population, community, or region at the same time.
- A pandemic occurs over a wide geographic area and affects an exceptionally high proportion of the population. Influenza pandemics tend to occur when disease-causing organisms that typically affect only animals adapt and infect humans, then further adapt so they can pass easily from human to human. The flu pandemic of 1918–1919 claimed half a million lives.

Among the challenges health professionals face in a pandemic are inadequate supplies of vaccines or antiviral drugs; a shortage of medical supplies and facilities; and difficult decisions as to who should receive antiviral drugs and vaccines. A pandemic also has a significant economic and social impact as communities cancel events, businesses and schools close, and travel is restricted.

In case of a pandemic, here are some ways you can protect yourself:

- **Stay informed**. Check reliable sources of information, such as the federal website www.pandemicflu.gov.
- **Get an annual flu shot**, which now contains a vaccine against H1N1 as well as seasonal influenza.
- **See your doctor** within two days of developing flu symptoms.
- **Think carefully about travel in flu season.** Viruses are easily transmitted in confined spaces such as airplanes, trains, and buses. If possible, don't travel to places with outbreaks of potentially deadly viruses.

# Meningitis

**Meningitis**, or invasive meningococcal disease, attacks the membranes around the brain and spinal cord and can result in hearing loss, kidney failure, and permanent brain damage. One of the most common types is caused by the bacterium *Neisseria meningitis*. Viral meningitis is typically less severe.

**meningitis** An extremely serious, potentially fatal illness that attacks the membranes around the brain and spinal cord; caused by the bacterium *Neisseria meningitis*.

Most common in the first year of life, the incidence of bacterial meningitis rises in young people between ages 15 and 24. Adolescents and young adults account for nearly 30 percent of all cases of meningitis in the United States. If not treated early, meningitis can lead to death or permanent disabilities. One in five of those who survive suffers from long-term side effects, such as brain damage, hearing loss, seizures, or limb amputation. Fatality rates are five times higher among 15- to 24-year-olds.

Each year 100 to 125 cases of meningitis occur on college campuses. An estimated 5 to 15 students die as a result. One in five survivors suffers long-term side effects. Individuals living in crowded living situations, such as dormitories, sleep-away camps, and barracks, are at increased risk.

Meningitis spreads through the exchange of respiratory droplets, which can come from sharing a drink, cigarette, or silverware; kissing; coughing; or sneezing. Even inhaling second-hand smoke can infect you with the disease.

## Preventing Meningitis

Vaccination protects against four of the five most common types of meningococcal bacteria. These four strains cause more than 80 percent of cases in adolescents and young adults. As with other immunizations, minor reactions may occur. These include pain and swelling at the injection site, headache, fatigue, or a vague sense of discomfort. The incidence of life-threatening meningitis has declined substantially since the vaccine was developed.

The CDC and other major health organizations, such as the American College Health Association, recommend routine vaccination with a new type of meningococcal vaccine, which provides longer-lasting protection than the previous type, and booster shots at age 16 for those previously vaccinated.[7]

## Recognizing Meningitis

The early symptoms of meningitis may be mild and resemble symptoms of flu or other less severe infections. Bacterial meningitis symptoms may develop within hours; viral meningitis symptoms may develop quickly or over several days. Fever, headache, and neck stiffness are the hallmark symptoms of meningitis. Not all symptoms may appear, but they can progress very quickly, killing an otherwise healthy person in 48 hours or less, so it is critical to seek medical attention quickly.

The most common symptoms of meningitis are:

- Sudden high fever.
- Severe, persistent headache.
- Neck stiffness and pain that makes it difficult to touch the chin to the chest.
- Nausea and vomiting, sometimes along with diarrhea.
- Confusion and disorientation (acting "goofy").
- Drowsiness or sluggishness.
- Eye pain or sensitivity to bright light.
- Pain or weakness in the muscles or joints.

Other possible signs and symptoms include:

- Abnormal skin color.
- Stomach cramps.
- Ice-cold hands and feet.
- Dizziness.
- Reddish or brownish skin rash or purple spots.
- Numbness and tingling.
- Seizures.

## When to Seek Medical Care

If two or more of the symptoms of meningitis appear at the same time or if the symptoms are very severe or appear suddenly, seek medical care right away. If a red rash appears along with fever, see if the rash disappears when a glass is pressed against it. If it does not, this could be a sign of blood infection, which is a medical emergency. Call 911 without delay. Other symptoms that might require emergency treatment include loss of consciousness, seizures, muscle weakness, or sudden severe dementia.

A new rapid test can determine the presence of viral meningitis in just 2.5 hours. Because it can help quickly distinguish between viral and bacterial meningitis, the test could help reduce the unnecessary use of antibiotics. About one in ten people who get meningitis dies from it. Of those who survive, another 11 to 19 percent lose fingers, arms, or legs, become deaf, have problems

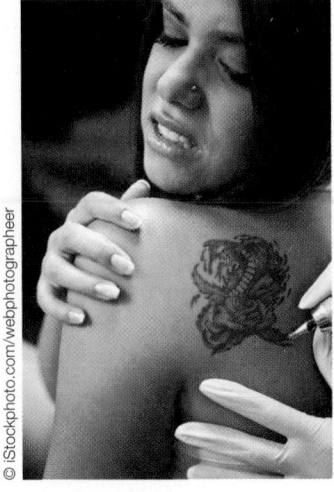

Getting a tattoo or a piercing can pose health risks, including bacterial infection and hepatitis.

with their nervous systems, or suffer seizures, strokes, or brain damage. Thus it is critical to seek medical care for this infection. A new concern is the emergence of the first U.S. cases of bacterial meningitis resistant to a widely used antibiotic.

Who should be vaccinated:

- All children when they turn 11 or 12 or when they enter high school, if they have not been previously vaccinated.
- College freshmen living in dorms.
- Military recruits.
- People who may have been exposed to meningitis during an outbreak.

Who should not get vaccinated for meningitis or should wait:

- Anyone who has had a severe, life-threatening reaction or allergy to any vaccine component.
- Anyone who is moderately or severely ill at the time of the scheduled immunization.
- Anyone who has ever had Guillain-Barre syndrome (a neurological disorder).
- Pregnant women.

# Hepatitis

An estimated 500,000 Americans contract hepatitis each year. At least five different viruses, referred to as **hepatitis** A, B, C, Delta, and E, can cause this inflammation of the liver. Newly identified viruses also may be responsible for some cases of what is called "non-A, non-B" hepatitis. Thanks largely to effective vaccines, rates of hepatitis A and hepatitis B infections have declined to their lowest rates in decades. Although there is no vaccine for hepatitis C, its incidence also has declined significantly.

All forms of hepatitis target the liver, the body's largest internal organ. Symptoms include headaches, fever, fatigue, stiff or aching joints, nausea, vomiting, and diarrhea. The liver becomes enlarged and tender to the touch; sometimes the yellowish tinge of jaundice develops. Treatment consists of rest, a high-protein diet, and the avoidance of alcohol and drugs that may stress the liver. Alpha interferon, a protein that boosts

**hepatitis** An inflammation and/or infection of the liver caused by a virus, often accompanied by jaundice.

immunity and prevents viruses from replicating, may be used for some forms.

Most people begin to feel better after two or three weeks of rest, although fatigue and other symptoms can linger. As many as 10 percent of those infected with hepatitis B and up to two-thirds of those with hepatitis C become carriers of the virus for several years or even life. Some have persistent inflammation of the liver, which may cause mild or severe symptoms and increase the risk of liver cancer.

## Hepatitis A

Hepatitis A, a less serious form, is generally transmitted by poor sanitation, primarily fecal contamination of food or water, and is less common in industrialized nations than in developing countries. As many as 30 percent of individuals in the United States show evidence of past infection with the virus. Among those at highest risk in the United States are children and staff at day-care centers, residents of institutions for the mentally handicapped, sanitation workers, and workers who handle primates such as monkeys. Gamma globulin can provide short-term immunity; vaccines against hepatitis A have been approved by the FDA. The CDC recommends routine immunization against hepatitis A in states with high rates, as well as for travelers to countries where hepatitis A is common, men who have sex with men, and persons who use illegal drugs.

## Hepatitis B

Hepatitis B, a potentially fatal disease transmitted through the blood and other bodily fluids, infects an estimated 300 million people around the world.[8] Once spread mainly by contaminated tattoo needles, needles shared by drug users, or transfusions of contaminated blood, hepatitis B is now transmitted mostly through sexual contact. Many cases resolve on their own, but hepatitis B can cause chronic liver infection, cirrhosis, and liver cancer. Medications for hepatitis B often must be taken long-term, or the disease comes back even stronger.

Hepatitis B is a particular threat to young people; 75 percent of new cases are diagnosed in those between ages 15 and 39. They usually contract hepatitis B through high-risk behaviors such as multiple sex partners and use of injected drugs. Athletes in contact sports, such as wrestling and football, may transmit the hepatitis B virus in sweat. With the discovery that HBV is more common in athletes than had been suspected, health experts are calling for mandatory HBV testing and vaccination against hepatitis B for all athletes.

Individuals who have tattoos or body piercing may also be at risk if procedures are not done under regulated conditions. (See "Consumer Alert.") At highest risk are male homosexuals, heterosexuals with multiple sex partners, health-care workers with frequent contact with blood, injection drug users, and infants born to infected mothers. Vaccination can prevent hepatitis B and is recommended for all newborns and, if not already vaccinated, for travelers to certain regions, health-care workers, dialysis patients, and anyone engaging in unprotected sexual activity (homosexual or heterosexual).[9]

## Hepatitis C

Hepatitis C virus (HCV) is four times as widespread as HIV, infecting about 2 percent of Americans. However, rates have fallen dramatically since the early 1980s—to about 7 per million Americans.[10] A simple blood test can show if you are infected with HCV. However, few of the estimated 3 to 4 million carriers in the United States realize they are infected. Of those infected with HCV, 80 percent have no symptoms.

The risk factors for HCV infection are blood transfusion or organ transplant before 1992, exposure to infected blood, illegal drug use, tattoos, or body piercing. If you choose to have a body piercing, avoid piercing guns, and make certain that the piercing equipment has been sterilized. Hepatitis C virus is not spread by casual contact, such as hugging, kissing, or sharing food utensils. There is controversy over whether HCV can be transmitted sexually.

About three-quarters of those infected with HCV develop chronic or long-term hepatitis. About one-quarter develop progressive, irreversible liver damage, with scar tissue (cirrhosis) gradually replacing healthy liver tissue. Hepatitis C also increases the risk of a rare form of liver cancer. If the liver no longer functions adequately, a patient may require liver transplantation. Hepatitis C infection also increases

the risk of non-Hodgkin's lymphoma by up to 30 percent.

The most common treatment for hepatitis C is a combination of interferon, which stops the virus from making copies of itself, and ribavirin, an antiviral medication. The treatment lasts for 6 to 12 months and can be extremely difficult to endure.

## ❗ CONSUMER ALERT

### The Perils of Piercing

"Body art"—tattoos and piercings—has become increasingly widespread. In a national sampling of 500 men and women between ages 18 and 50, 24 percent had tattoos. In surveys of college students, higher percentages have reported permanent tattoos or body piercing. As many as one in five individuals with body piercing may suffer medical complications. In a British study, almost half of tongue piercings resulted in infections and other problems.

#### Facts to Know

- With no state or federal regulations of "body artists," unsafe tattooing and piercing practices can put consumers in danger. In one survey of "skin-penetration operators," only half said that they followed governmental guidelines for infection control.

- Epidemiologists have identified tattooing as a strong, independent risk factor for testing positive for hepatitis C virus (HCV) but not for development of acute hepatitis. In other words, individuals for tattoos may acquire HCV but may not develop symptoms themselves.

- Even so-called temporary tattooing with henna is not without risk. Dermatologists have reported an increasing number of skin reactions. Piercings of the tongue, lips, or cheeks present different dangers, including recessed gums; loose, chipped, or fractured teeth; pain; infection; inflammation; nerve damage; and tooth loss.

- You may think you're safe if you go to a licensed tattoo or piercing salon. However, there are no formal schools, no certification requirements, and no diplomas for these practitioners. In many states it is possible to get a license without the benefit of any kind of training.

#### Steps to Take

- **Ask to see certification that the autoclave—a high-temperature pressure cooker used for medical instruments—has been sterilized.**

- **Make sure the artist is wearing standard medical latex gloves.**

- **Find out if the artist is vaccinated for hepatitis B.** Can he or she show you proof, such as a doctor's record, of vaccination?

- **Make sure the artist uses only new sterile needles.**

- **Make sure the artist doesn't "double-dip."** The ink should be new, used on only one client—you.

- **If you require prophylactic antibiotics for dental cleanings or other procedures, do not get a tattoo.** Consumers with rheumatic heart disease and other conditions that increase their risk of infections have died as a result of bacterial infection contracted from a tattoo.

# Epstein-Barr Virus and Infectious Mononucleosis

Epstein-Barr virus (EBV), a member of the herpes virus family, infects most people at some time in their lives. As many as 95 percent of American adults between ages 35 and 45 have been infected. When infected in childhood, boys and girls usually show no or very mild symptoms. However, when infection with EBV occurs during adolescence or young adulthood, it causes infectious mononucleosis 35 to 50 percent of the time.[11]

You can get **mononucleosis** through kissing—or any other form of close contact. "Mono" is a viral disease that targets people 15 to 24 years old. Its symptoms include a sore throat, headache, fever, nausea, and prolonged weakness. The spleen is swollen and the lymph nodes are enlarged. You may also develop jaundice or a skin rash similar to rubella (German measles).

The major symptoms usually disappear within two to three weeks, but weakness, fatigue, and often depression may linger for at least two more weeks. The greatest danger is from physical activity that might rupture the spleen, resulting in internal bleeding. The liver may also become inflamed. A blood test can determine whether you have mono. However, there's no specific treatment other than rest.

# Chronic Fatigue Syndrome (CFS)

More than a million Americans have the array of symptoms known as **chronic fatigue syndrome (CFS)**. CFS is a complex disorder characterized by profound fatigue that does not improve with bed rest and that may get worse with physical or mental activity. Other symptoms include weakness, muscle pain, impaired memory or concentration, insomnia, and postexertion fatigue that lasts for more than

24 hours. Symptoms can persist for years. CFS affects four times as many women as men.

Diagnosis of CFS remains difficult, although numerous studies have found significant immune abnormalities, such as high levels of certain immune cells (B lymphocytes and cytokines) that act as if they were constantly battling a viral infection. There is no known cure, but a combination of therapies can help relieve symptoms.

# Herpes Gladiatorum (Mat Herpes, Wrestler's Herpes, Mat Pox)

*Herpes gladiatorum* is a skin infection caused by the herpes simplex type 1 virus and spread by direct skin-to-skin contact. It most commonly occurs among wrestlers, judo players, or other athletes who have with very close skin contact with each other.

Within a few days of infection, some people develop a sore throat, swollen lymph nodes, fever, or tingling on the skin. *Herpes gladiatorum* lesions appear as a cluster of blisters on the face, extremities, or trunk. Generally, lesions appear within eight days after exposure to an infected person, but they may take longer to emerge. All wrestlers with skin sores or lesions should see a physician for evaluation and should not participate in practice or competition until their lesions have healed (usually four to five days).

*Herpes gladiatorum* infections can recur. The virus can "hide out" in the nerves and reactivate later, causing another infection. Generally, recurrent infections are less severe and don't last as long. However, a recurring infection is just as contagious as the original infection, so the same precautions are needed to prevent infecting others.

You can reduce your risk of mat herpes by taking the following precautions:

- Shower at school immediately after practice, using soap and water. Bring your own plastic bottle of liquid soap.

**mononucleosis** An infectious viral disease characterized by an excess of white blood cells in the blood, fever, bodily discomfort, a sore throat, and kidney and liver complications.

**chronic fatigue syndrome (CFS)** A cluster of symptoms whose cause is not yet known; a primary symptom is debilitating fatigue.

- Use your own towel, and don't share your towel with anyone else. Wash your towel after each use, using hot water with detergent (and bleach if possible), and dry on high-heat setting.

- Change your practice and competition gear every day.

- Clean your headgear daily with the same soap you use for showering.

- Clean the soles of your shoes before stepping on the mat. Use a towel soaked in a disinfectant solution.

# Group A and Group B Strep Infection

Sore throats are common winter complaints, but those caused by group A streptococcus bacteria—*strep throats*—are more than a trivial threat. If not treated promptly with antibiotics, strep bacteria can travel to the kidneys, the liver, or the heart, where they can cause rheumatic fever—an inflammation of the heart that can cause weakness, shortness of breath, joint pain, and an abnormal heartbeat. In recent years clusters of rheumatic fever have sprung up in several major cities. The best way to prevent further increases in rheumatic fever and heart disease is accurate diagnosis and thorough treatment of strep throat.[12] Rapid new diagnostic tests can identify strep within minutes. If the test is positive, treatment with penicillin or a similar antibiotic is indicated. Brief treatment (five days) with Omnicef, a newer antibiotic, has proved as effective as ten days of oral penicillin.

Toxic streptococcal shock syndrome, or toxic strep, is an invasive form of the disease in which strep gains access to the blood and causes a drop in blood pressure, a very high fever, and the production of exotoxins (substances that can attack various organs, such as the kidneys, heart, or in rare cases, flesh). Toxic strep is rather rare and usually doesn't occur with strep throats. Prompt treatment is critical.

Group B streptococcus (GBS), the leading cause of life-threatening perinatal infections in the United States, is primarily a threat to newborns.

Because some 15 to 40 percent of pregnant women carry GBS but have no symptoms, the American Academy of Pediatrics has called for universal screening of expectant mothers. Each year 12,000 newborns are infected, most of them during childbirth; more than 1,600 die; and another 1,600 suffer permanent brain damage from meningitis. Women at high risk of infecting their newborns with GBS are those who have premature labor, early rupture of their amniotic membranes, fever, and a high group B strep count before or during pregnancy, or who have previously borne an infant infected with GBS. Also at risk are diabetics, low-income women, and those under age 20.

# Toxic Shock Syndrome

As discussed in Chapter 9, toxic shock syndrome (TSS) is a potentially deadly disease associated with the use of tampons, particularly high-absorbency types. It is caused by *Staphylococcus aureus* and group A *Streptococcus pyogenes* bacteria that release toxins (poisonous waste products) into the bloodstream. Symptoms include a high fever; a rash that leads to peeling of the skin on the fingers, toes, palms, and soles; dizziness; dangerously low blood pressure; and abnormalities in several organ systems (the digestive tract and the kidneys) and in the muscles and blood.

In addition to women who use high-absorbency tampons, or leave their tampons in too long, those who have given birth within the preceding six to eight weeks are at greater risk. Children (including newborns), men, and postmenopausal women also have developed TSS, which usually has been traced to bacteria in skin abscesses, boils, cuts, or postsurgical wounds.

Without prompt treatment, TSS can cause severe and permanent damage, including muscle weakness, partial paralysis, amnesia, disorientation, an inability to concentrate, and impaired lung and kidney function. Sometimes toxic shock weakens the blood vessels, increasing the risk of heart problems. Victims can enter the life-threatening crisis called shock, in which blood flow throughout the body is inadequate to sustain life. Treatment usually consists of

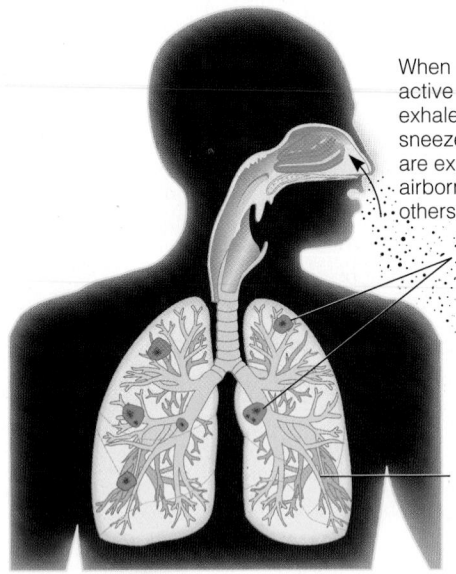

When someone with active tuberculosis exhales, coughs, or sneezes, TB bacteria are expelled in tiny airborne droplets that others may inhale.

The TB bacteria lodge mainly in the lungs, where they slowly multiply, creating patches, then cavities.

Other parts of the lung are affected, including the bronchi and the lining of the lung.

If untreated, TB can eventually spread to and damage the brain, bone, eyes, liver and kidneys, spine, and skin.

immediate hospitalization, intravenous administration of fluids, medications to raise blood pressure, and powerful antibiotics; intravenous administration of immunoglobins that attack the toxins produced by these bacteria may also be beneficial.

# Tuberculosis

A bacterial infection of the lungs that was once the nation's leading killer, **tuberculosis (TB)** still claims the lives of more people than any acute infectious disease other than pneumonia (Figure 16.4). About 30 percent of the world's population is infected with the TB organism, although not all develop active disease. In the United States, rates have fallen to an all-time low.[13] Immigration from countries where TB is common, poverty, homelessness, alcoholism and drug abuse, the HIV/AIDS epidemic, and the emergence of resistant strains of TB account for most new cases.

Although TB is most prevalent among high-risk groups, the overall danger increases as more people develop active disease because TB is highly contagious. TB outbreaks have occurred throughout the country in hospitals,

**tuberculosis (TB)** A highly infectious bacterial disease that primarily affects the lungs and is often fatal.

nursing homes, prisons, and office buildings, where inadequate ventilation increases the risk of infection.

# The "Superbug" Threat: MRSA

For decades most strains of the bacterium *Staphylococcus aureus* responded to treatment with penicillin. When the bacterium became resistant to penicillin, physicians switched to a newer antibiotic, methicillin. Within a year the first case of methicillin-resistant *S. aureus* (MRSA) was detected. This "superbug," which fights off traditional antibiotics, has become a major health threat.

One in three healthy people carry *S. aureus* bacteria on their skin. Of these as many as 1 in 100 may be carrying MRSA. In medical terms, these individuals are "colonized" but not infected. For infection to occur, MRSA must enter the body through an accidental injury such as a scrape or burn or via a deliberate break in the skin such as a surgical incision.

The rate of MRSA infections is highest in hospitals and health-care facilities, but MRSA also can develop among sports teams, child-care attendees, and prison inmates.

MRSA spreads by touch. In health-care settings, it can spread from patient to patient through contact with doctors and nurses with unwashed hands or contaminated gloves or contact with unsterile medical equipment.

## Preventing MRSA

Health advocates are calling for increased screening of patients for MRSA, isolating and treating MRSA carriers, more conscientious hand washing, and more diligent use of gowns, gloves, and masks to prevent transmission of MRSA.

Outside hospitals, community-associated MRSA (CA-MRSA) can occur in people without any established risks, including college students, who often live in close quarters and participate in contact sports such as football, wrestling, and fencing. According to a recent study, the risk of infection in a community gym is low, and commonsense health precautions can lower your risk.[14]

According to CDC estimates, some 94,000 American get serious MRSA infections each year, and nearly 19,000 die. A post-surgical infection with MRSA causes such serious complications that it can cost $60,000 to treat.[15] The number of these infections has decreased significantly in hospital intensive care units since 2001.[16] Among the simple steps responsible for this decline are closer monitoring of hand washing, better means of disinfecting rooms, and improved tracking of patients as they transfer from one hospital or room to another.

Enhanced cleaning of hospital intensive care units has proven effective in reducing patients' risk of MRSA infections.[17] However, the single most effective protective step is hand-washing, along with steps such as screening of incoming patients for MRSA and use of clean gloves and gowns by health professionals.[18]

## Who Is at Highest Risk?

People at high risk of becoming infected with MRSA are those in close contact with carriers, as hospital patients are. MRSA poses the greatest danger to individuals who have:

- A weakened immune system.
- A preexisting infection.
- Open wounds, cuts, or burns.

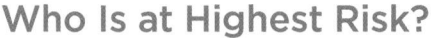

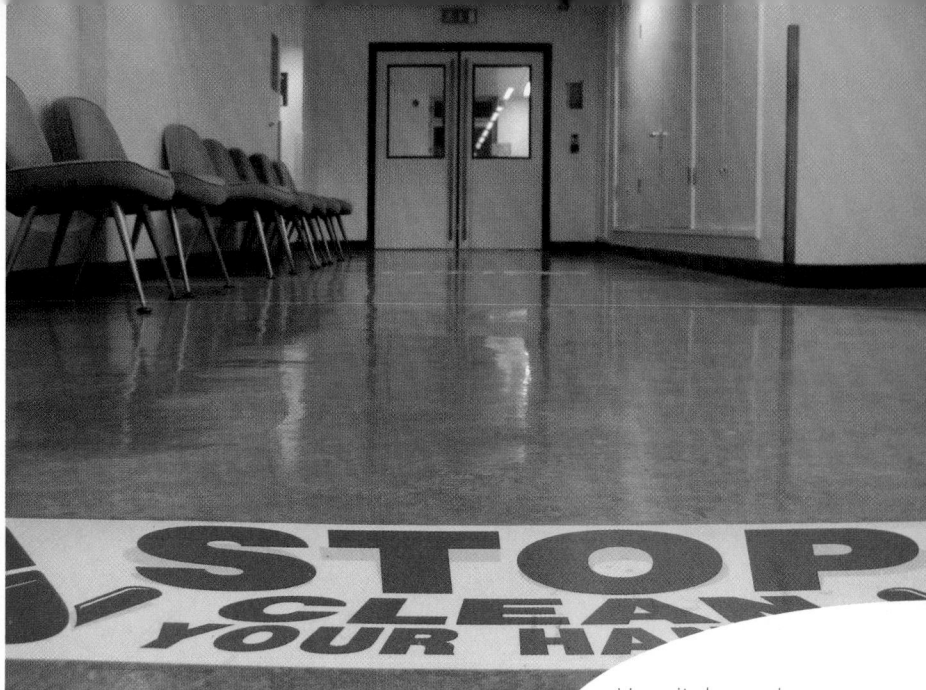

Hospitals can be dangerous places. MRSA spreads from patient to patient when hand washing is inadequate or when gloves or equipment are contaminated.

- Other types of wounds, such as skin breaks from an intravenous drug line.
- Undergone surgery.
- Taken antibiotics recently or for a long period.

Also at great risk are:

- Athletes in contact sports.
- Elderly individuals
- Premature or newborn babies.

*Your Strategies for Prevention*

## How to Avoid MRSA

- **Wash hands thoroughly and frequently.**
- **Ask health-care professionals if they've washed their hands before examining or treating you.**
- **Keep cuts and scrapes clean.** Cover them with a Band-Aid.
- **Avoid touching other people's cuts, incisions, or dressings.**
- **Don't share personal items such as towels or razors.**
- **If you go to a gym, wipe the equipment before working out.** Use a clean towel to prevent your skin from coming into direct contact with the machines. Shower after each workout.

# Insect- and Animal-Borne Infections

Common insects and animals, including ticks and mosquitoes, can transmit dangerous infections, among them Lyme disease and West Nile virus. Of all emerging infections, 75 percent originate in animals; of these, 61 percent can be transmitted to humans.[19]

## Lyme Disease

**Lyme disease**, a bacterial infection, is spread by ixodid ticks that carry a particular bacterium—the spirochete *Borrelia burgdorferi*. An

**Lyme disease** A disease caused by a bacterium carried by a tick; it may cause heart arrhythmias, neurological problems, and arthritis symptoms.

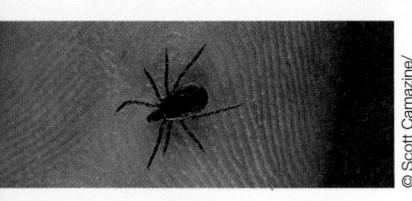

Ticks are responsible for the spread of Lyme disease. If you spot a tick, remove it as soon as possible with tweezers or small forceps. Put it in a plastic bag or sealed bottle and save it. If you develop a rash or other symptoms, take it with you to the doctor.

infected person may have various symptoms, including joint inflammation, heart arrhythmias, blinding headaches, and memory lapses. The disease can also cause miscarriages and birth defects. Lyme disease is by far the most commonly reported vector-borne infectious disease in the United States.

The primary culprit in most cases of Lyme disease is the deer tick, although other ticks, including the western black-legged tick and the Lone Star tick, also may transmit the bacterium that causes Lyme disease. Dog ticks are not usually a threat.

You are not likely to get Lyme disease if a tick is attached to your skin for less than 48 hours. About 70 to 80 percent of infected individuals develop a red rash at the site of the tick bite. Over a period of days to weeks, the rash grows larger. A ring of skin just beyond the bite site may fade, creating a ring or "bull's-eye" appearance. Rarely, the rash may burn or itch. Once diagnosed, Lyme disease is treated with antibiotics. Nonsteroidal anti-inflammatory drugs, such as aspirin or ibuprofen, can relieve fever and pain.

About 60 percent of untreated individuals develop arthritis, and their joints become swollen and painful. If Lyme disease spreads to the nervous system, it can cause neurological symptoms, including memory loss, inability to concentrate, muscle weakness with tingling and numbness in the arms and legs, and Bell's palsy, a facial droop caused by muscle paralysis.

## West Nile Virus

West Nile virus (WNV) is transmitted by a mosquito that feeds on an infected bird and then bites a human. The first cases in the United States occurred in 1999. Experts now see WNV as a seasonal epidemic that flares up in the summer and continues into the fall in cities and the areas around them. WNV also can be spread through blood transfusions, organ transplants, breast-feeding, and from mother to fetus during pregnancy.

WNV interferes with normal central nervous system functioning and causes inflammation of brain tissue. The risk of catching WNV is low. Relatively few mosquitoes carry WNV, and fewer than 1 percent of people who are bitten by mosquitoes experience any symptoms. Repellents that contain DEET, picaridin, and oil of lemon eucalyptus can protect against these mosquitoes.

There is no specific treatment for WNV infection. People with more severe cases usually require hospitalization and supportive treatment, including intravenous fluids and help with breathing. An antiviral drug, interferon, which might lessen the symptoms and duration of the illness in infected patients, is undergoing testing.

## Avian Influenza

Avian influenza, or bird flu, is caused by viruses that occur naturally among wild birds. Most strains of bird flu virus cannot infect humans, but a few can, usually with great difficulty. Influenza viruses jumped from birds to humans three times in the twentieth century. In each case a mutation in the genes of the virus allowed it to infect humans. Then a further change allowed the virus to pass easily from one human to another, rapidly spreading around the world in a deadly pandemic.

A virus called H5N1, previously found only in birds, spread to domestic poultry and infected people who had worked closely with sick birds in Hong Kong in 1997. The H5N1 virus has spread to wild migratory birds, which have carried it to other countries and continents.

# Emerging Infectious Diseases

The twenty-first century has ushered in new agents of infection and new apprehension about the potential use of infectious diseases as instruments of terror and mass destruction.

## SARS

Severe acute respiratory syndrome (SARS) became a new global health threat in 2003, with major outbreaks in several Asian countries, including China and Hong Kong, and in Toronto.

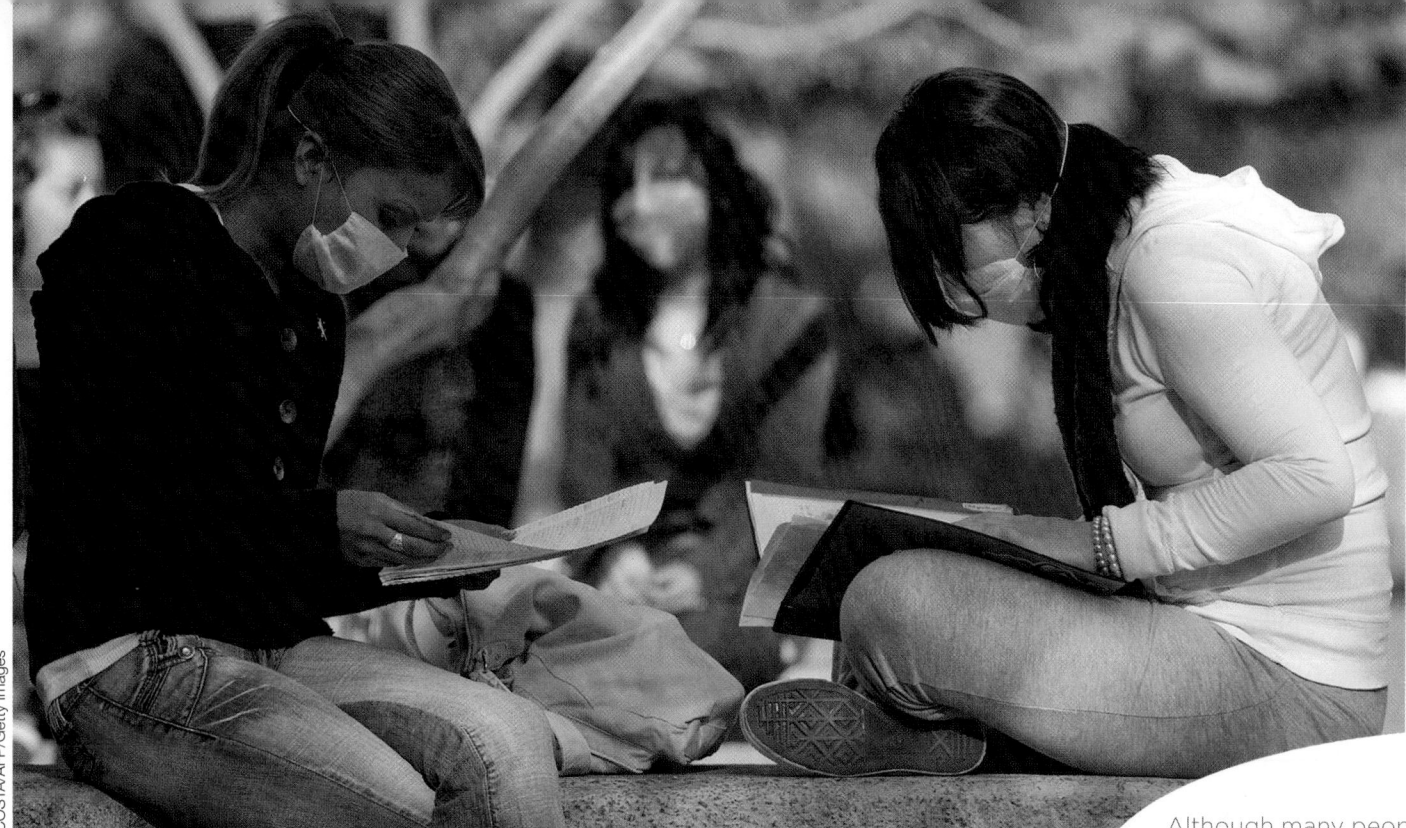

Although many people try to protect themselves by wearing face masks, there is no evidence that masks lower the risk of infection in open spaces.

Another outbreak occurred in China in 2004. SARS-associated coronavirus (SARS-CoV) spreads by close face-to-face contact, most often by droplets expelled into the air when an infected person coughs or sneezes. The virus is believed capable of living outside the body for at least 24 hours. A few persons may be especially infectious and are more likely to spread the SARS virus to others in the same airplane, household, school, workplace, or hospital. Doctors do not know how long a person remains contagious.

The average incubation period for SARS is six to ten days. Symptoms include high fever, coughing, headache, chills, muscle aches, and shortness of breath. Most of those infected develop pneumonia. There are no specific treatments for SARS. Patients receive supportive care, such as fluids to prevent dehydration and ventilators to aid breathing. Scientists are developing possible vaccines and antiviral agents.

## Bioterror Threats

Americans have learned firsthand that certain infectious agents can be used as weapons of terrorism and war. Bioterror agents, such as anthrax and, potentially, smallpox, botulism, and tularemia, have been added to the ranks of emerging infectious diseases.

*Anthrax*   Anthrax, which is found naturally in wild and farm animals, can also be produced in a laboratory. The disease is spread through exposure to anthrax spores, not through exposure to an infected person.

*Smallpox*   Smallpox is a serious, contagious, and sometimes fatal infectious disease. Smallpox was eradicated decades ago after a successful worldwide vaccination program. The last case of smallpox in the United States was in 1949. The last naturally occurring case in the world was in Somalia in 1977. There is no treatment, and up to 30 percent of those infected with smallpox die.

Because of fear that terrorists might use smallpox as a biological weapon, the U.S. government has stockpiled enough vaccine to inoculate everyone in the event of an emergency. Most individuals vaccinated before 1972, when mandated smallpox immunization ended in the United States, retain some immunity for many years, some for up to 75 years. However, half of all Americans have never received the smallpox vaccine, and many scientists believe protection wanes over time for those who did. Those vaccinated in the past can safely be revaccinated for optimum protection. An Institute of Medicine committee has recommended against vaccinating the entire population at this time.

*Botulism*  Botulism is a muscle-paralyzing disease caused by a toxin made by the bacterium *Clostridium botulinum*. Botulinum toxin is among the most lethal substances known, and it can kill within 24 hours. Botulism causes muscle weakness and eventual paralysis that starts at the top of the body and works its way down. The disease kills by paralyzing muscles used to breathe. The CDC and some state health departments keep an antidote to botulinum toxin in storage. Treatment includes taking the antidote and possibly using a ventilator for breathing until the toxin works its way out of the system.

*Tularemia*  Tularemia is an illness that normally infects wild animals, such as rabbits and squirrels. Humans can acquire the illness by coming in contact with the blood or body fluids of infected animals, from the bite of a fly or tick that carries blood from an infected animal, or from contaminated food or water. As a biological weapon, tularemia-causing bacteria could be dispersed through the air to be inhaled.

# Reproductive and Urinary Tract Infections

Reproductive and urinary tract infections are very common. Many are not spread exclusively by sexual contact, so they are not classified as sexually transmitted diseases.

## Vaginal Infections

Vaginal complaints account for approximately 10 million medical office visits a year. The most common are trichomoniasis, candidiasis, and bacterial vaginosis (Table 16.2).

Protozoa (*Trichomonas vaginalis*) that live in the vagina can multiply rapidly, causing itching, burning, and discharge—all symptoms of

**trichomoniasis**. Male carriers usually have no symptoms, although some may develop urethritis or an inflammation of the prostate and seminal vesicles. Anyone with this infection should be screened for syphilis, gonorrhea, chlamydia, and HIV. Sexual partners must be treated with oral medication (metronidazole, trade name Flagyl), even if they have no symptoms, to prevent reinfection.

Populations of a yeast called *Candida albicans*—normal inhabitants of the mouth, digestive tract, and vagina—are usually held in check. Under certain conditions, however (such as poor nutrition, stress, or antibiotic use), the microbes multiply, causing burning, itching, and a whitish discharge, and producing what is commonly known as a yeast infection. Common sites for **candidiasis**, which is also called *moniliasis*, are the vagina, vulva, penis, and mouth.

The women most likely to test positive for candidiasis have never been pregnant, use condoms for birth control, have sexual intercourse more than four times a month, and have taken antibiotics in the previous 15 to 30 days. Vaginal medications, such as GyneLotrimin and Monistat, are nonprescription drugs that provide effective treatment. Women should keep the genital area dry and wear cotton underwear.

Male sexual partners may be advised to wear condoms during outbreaks of candidiasis.

**Bacterial vaginosis** is characterized by alterations in the microorganisms that live in the vagina, including depletion of certain bacteria and overgrowth of others. It typically causes a white or gray vaginal discharge with a distinctive fishy odor similar to that of trichomoniasis. Its underlying cause is unknown, although it occurs most frequently in women with multiple sex partners. Long-term dangers include pelvic inflammatory disease and pregnancy complications. Metronidazole, either in the form of a pill or a vaginal gel, is the primary treatment. According to CDC guidelines, treatment for male sex partners appears to be of little benefit, but some health practitioners recommend treatment for both partners in cases of recurrent infections. Antibiotic therapy may help prevent an infected woman from acquiring an STI.

**trichomoniasis** An infection of the protozoan Trichomonas vaginalis; females experience vaginal burning, itching, and discharge, but male carriers may be asymptomatic.

**candidiasis** An infection of the yeast Candida albicans, commonly occurring in the vagina, vulva, penis, and mouth and causing burning, itching, and a whitish discharge.

**bacterial vaginosis** A vaginal infection caused by overgrowth and depletion of various microorganisms living in the vagina, resulting in a malodorous white or gray vaginal discharge.

Table 16.2 **Common Reproductive Tract Infections**

| Infection | Transmission | Symptoms | Treatment |
|---|---|---|---|
| **Bacterial vaginosis** | Most common causative agent, *Gardnerella vaginalis bacterium*, sometimes transmitted through coitus | Women: Fishy- or musty-smelling thin discharge, like flour paste in consistency and usually gray<br>Men: Mostly asymptomatic | Metronidazole (Flagyl) by mouth or intravaginal applications of topical metronidazole gel or clindamycin cream |
| **Candidiasis (yeast infection)** | *Candida albicans* fungus may accelerate growth when the chemical balance of the vagina is disturbed; also transmitted through sexual interaction | Women: White, "cheesy" discharge; irritation of vaginal and vulval tissues | Vaginal suppositories or topical cream, such as clotrimazol (GyneLotrimin) and miconazole (Monistat), or oral fluconazole |
| **Trichomoniasis** | Protozoan parasite *Trichomonas vaginalis*, usually passed through genital sexual contact | Women: White or yellow vaginal discharge with an unpleasant odor; sore and irritated vulva<br>Men: No symptoms | Metronidazol (Flagyl) for both women and men |

# Urinary Tract Infections

A urinary tract infection (UTI) can be present in any of the three parts of the urinary tract: the urethra, the bladder, or the kidneys. An infection involving the urethra is known as **urethritis**. If the bladder is also infected, it's called **cystitis**. If it reaches the kidneys, it's called *pyelonephritis*.

An estimated 40 percent of women report having had a UTI at some point in their lives. Three times as many women as men develop UTIs, probably for anatomical reasons. A woman's urethra is only 1.5 inches long; a man's is 6 inches. Therefore, bacteria, the major cause of UTIs, have a shorter distance to travel to infect a woman's bladder and kidneys. About one-fourth to one-third of all women between ages 20 and 40 develop UTIs, and 80 percent of those who experience one infection develop recurrences.

Conditions that can set the stage for UTIs include irritation and swelling of the urethra or bladder as a result of pregnancy, bike riding, irritants (such as bubble bath, douches, or a diaphragm), urinary stones, enlargement of the prostate gland in men, vaginitis, and stress. Early diagnosis is critical because infection can spread to the kidneys and, if unchecked, result in kidney failure. Symptoms include frequent, burning, or painful urination; chills; fever; fatigue; and blood in the urine.

Recurrent UTIs, a frequent problem among young women, have been linked with a genetic predisposition, sexual intercourse, and the use of diaphragms. Women often attribute urinary tract infections to lifestyle habits, poor hygiene, negligence, or even "a penalty of growing old."

**urethritis** Infection of the urethra.

**cystitis** Infection of the urinary bladder.

# Protecting Yourself

As with other aspects of your well-being, your choices and behaviors affect your risk of acquiring infectious diseases. Which of the following steps have you taken?

_____ **Getting your "shots."** Keep track of the vaccinations you've received and the dates you received them. Check with your doctor about any booster shots you may require. Get a tetanus booster every five years (an easy way not to forget: get one every time you celebrate a birthday ending in a 5 or 0, such as 25 and 30). Get your flu shot or spray. If you're a woman and have not been vaccinated against human papillomavirus (HPV), talk to your doctor about the potential benefits for you.

_____ **Practicing good health habits.** Take this chapter's Self Survey in Your *Personal Wellness Guide* to check your infection protection IQ. Identify the areas where you may need to boost your defenses, and follow the guidelines in Your Health Action Plan.

_____ **Making sexual health a priority.** Whether you are having sex or not, both men and women need regular checkups to make sure they are sexually healthy.

_____ **Talking first.** Get to know your partner. Before having sex, establish a committed relationship that allows trust and open communication. You should be able to discuss past sexual histories and any previous STIs or IV drug use. You should not feel cajoled, coerced, or forced into having sex.

_____ **Staying sober.** Alcohol and drugs impair your judgment, make it harder to communicate clearly, and can lead to forgetting or failing to use condoms properly.

_____ **Being honest.** If you have an STI, like HPV or herpes, advise any prospective sexual partner. Allow him or her to decide what to do. If you mutually agree on engaging in sexual activity, use latex condoms and other protective measures.

_____ **Being prepared for a sex emergency.** Consider carrying two condoms with you just in case one breaks or tears. Both men and women are equally responsible for preventing STIs, and both should carry condoms.

# What's Your Infection IQ?

Check the items that apply to you.

_____ I wash my hands with soap and water after I use the restroom.

_____ I wash my hands with soap and water before I eat.

_____ Before and after using exercise equipment, I wipe the handles.

_____ I wash my hands with soap and water after working out with weights or exercise equipment at a gym.

_____ I avoid contact with people who are coughing and sneezing.

_____ I wash my hands with soap and water more often during the cold and flu season.

_____ All of my vaccinations are current.

_____ I eat at least 3 balanced meals a day.

_____ I get 6 to 8 hours of sleep at night.

_____ I use relaxation techniques to lower my stress level.

_____ I do not smoke.

_____ I do not drink or I keep alcohol consumption to a minimum.

_____ I do not use drugs of any kind, including steroids.

_____ I throw leftovers out after 3 days.

_____ I wash fruits and vegetables before eating.

_____ I check expiration dates on food items.

_____ I apply insect spray (containing DEET) when I am outdoors.

_____ I wear long-sleeved clothing and long pants when hiking.

_____ I check myself for ticks after a hike.

Add up your checkmarks, and look for patterns in your protective behaviors. Are you conscientious about exercise and sleep, but careless about washing your hands or wiping down gym equipment? Do you protect yourself against food infections (discussed in Chapter 6) but not against sexually transmitted infections (discussed in Chapter 11)? Identify the aspects of infection protection that need the most work, and start practicing the defensive behaviors that will lower your risk.

# *Making Change Happen*

## Sleep Power

Sleep, as decades of research have shown, has the power to keep you well. Without adequate sleep, your immune system weakens, your heart becomes more vulnerable, and your risk of diabetes, obesity, and other illnesses increases. Unfortunately, college students can be notoriously poor sleepers. Many keep irregular schedules, bolt high-caffeine energy drinks, and pull all-nighters. However, if you want to tap into the power of sleep instead of searching for shortcuts or substitutes, "Sleep Power" in *Labs for IPC* can help. Here's a preview.

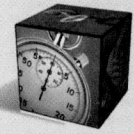

### Get Real

In this stage, you test your rest by completing a sleep log for a week and recording information such as how much sleep you got and how sleepy you were morning, afternoon, and evening. You also assess your "sleep smarts" by indicating which of ten statements apply to you, including the following:

• I get up at the same time most weekdays. _____

• I never drink caffeinated beverages after 6:00 p.m. _____

• I don't take long naps, especially in the evening. _____

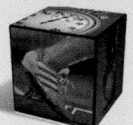

### Get Ready

As part of your preparation, you assess your sleep environment by answering questions such as:

• Where do you sleep? In a dorm room with one or more roommates? In your room at your parents' house? In an apartment?

• What is the state of your bed? The mattress may be old, but do you have a comfortable pillow? Are the sheets clean?

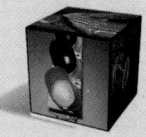

### Get Going

In this stage you find eight strategies for better sleeping and greater energy. Here is our favorite:

• **Power Nap.** A short nap of about 15 to 20 minutes can boost mood, motivation, and performance, and lower stress as well as improve memory and learning. As researchers have demonstrated, you can train yourself to take efficient daytime naps. Here are some basic guidelines:

• Try a nap in the late morning or just after lunch.

• In the hour or two before your nap, avoid caffeine or foods that are heavy in fat and sugar.

If you don't have time or can't find a place for a power nap, try the following:

• **A mini-nap.** Just 5 to 15 minutes of sleep can increase alertness and stamina.

• **A micro-nap.** Rather than struggling to keep your eyes open, give yourself 2 to 5 minutes of rest, which has proven effective in overcoming sleepiness.

• **A nano-nap.** Just 10 to 20 seconds of releasing all thoughts and tension from your body provides a breather for your brain.

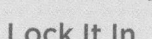

### Lock It In

You audit your sleep and sleepiness and use the information to make the most of your "down time."

# Making This Chapter Work for You

## Review Questions

1. Which of the following statements about the common cold and influenza is *true*?
   a. Influenza is just a more severe form of the common cold.
   b. Aspirin should be avoided by children and young adults who have a cold or influenza.
   c. The flu vaccine is also effective against most of the viruses that cause the common cold.
   d. Antibiotics are appropriate treatments for colds but not for influenza.

2. The meningitis vaccination
   a. is recommended for all college freshmen.
   b. protects against four of the five most common types of meningococcal bacteria.
   c. also protects against gonorrhea.
   d. may cause minor reactions such as fever or hives.

3. Hepatitis B
   a. is spread mainly through contaminated needles.
   b. infects mostly middle-aged people.
   c. does not have a preventive vaccine.
   d. can be spread in the sweat of athletes.

4. Which statement about methicillin-resistant *Staphylococcus* aureus (MRSA) is *false*?
   a. MRSA can be spread by doctors in a hospital.
   b. MRSA can be spread by athletes playing contact sports.
   c. MRSA is carried on the skin of as many as 1 in 100 people.
   d. MRSA can cause lung infections.

5. Which of the following statements is *true*?
   a. Lyme disease is a bacterial infection transmitted by ticks.
   b. West Nile virus is transmitted to humans by birds.
   c. West Nile virus is the most commonly reported vector-borne infectious disease in the United States.
   d. Avian flu has been transmitted from human to human.

6. Which statement about reproductive and urinary tract infections is *false*?
   a. Yeast infections can be treated with nonprescription drugs.
   b. Symptoms of UTIs include burning urination, chills, fever, and blood in the urine

   c. Three times as many women as men develop UTIs.
   d. Bacterial vaginosis usually causes a vaginal discharge with a rotten-egg odor.

7. Public health officials define a pandemic as
   a. a sudden rise in the incidence of a particular disease.
   b. an atypically large number of people in a region suffering from the same disease.
   c. a high proportion of the population over a wide geographic area suffering from the same disease.
   d. more than 25 percent the world's population suffering from the same disease.

8. Which of the following statements is *true*?
   a. The Lyme disease vaccine stimulates the immune system to produce antibodies against the bacterium *Borrelia burgdorferi*.
   b. West Nile virus is transmitted to humans by birds.
   c. The West Nile virus is the most commonly reported vector-borne infectious disease in the United States.
   d. Avian flu has been transmitted from human to human.

9. Which of the following statements about specific infectious diseases is *false*?
   a. Symptoms of SARS include high fever, coughing, headache, and chills.
   b. Anthrax can be found in wild and farm animals.
   c. Hepatitis A is usually transmitted through contaminated needles, transfusions, and sexual contact.
   d. College freshmen are at higher risk for contracting meningitis than the general population of young people between the ages of 18 and 23.

10. Which statement about reproductive and urinary tract infections is *false*?
    a. Yeast infections can be treated with nonprescription drugs.
    b. Symptoms of UTIs include burning urination, chills, fever, and blood in the urine.
    c. Three times as many women as men develop UTIs.
    d. Bacterial vaginosis usually causes a vaginal discharge with a rotten-egg odor.

*Answers to these questions can be found on page 672.*

## Critical Thinking

1. Prior to reading this chapter, describe what you did to avoid contracting infectious disease. Now that you have read the chapter, will you be making any changes in your practices? Briefly explain the convenience, advantages, and disadvantages of each practice that you have and/or will be using to prevent infection.

2. At the pharmacy, the shelves are full of medications for cold and flu. How do you sort through them? Do you get recommendations from family and friends? Do you study the labels? Do you keep track of what works for you?

3. Did you get vaccinated for meningitis? Why or why not? Where did you get your information on the disease and the vaccine, and how did you make your decision?

## Media Menu

Visit www.cengagebrain.com to access course materials and companion resources for this text that will:

- Help you evaluate your knowledge of the material.

- Allow you to prepare for exams with interactive quizzing.

- Use the CengageNOW product to develop a Personalized Learning Plan targeting resources that address areas you should study.

- Coach you through identifying target goals for behavioral change and creating and monitoring your personal change plan throughout the semester using the Behavior Change Planner available in the CengageNOW resource.

## Internet Connections

**www.immunize.org**
This site features comprehensive vaccination information for children, adolescents, and adults.

**www3.niaid.nih.gov**
The National Institute of Allergy and Infectious Diseases is part of the National Institutes of Health. Its website provides information about current research and includes fact sheets about all manner of topics related to allergies and infectious diseases.

**www.cdc.gov/ncidod**
This comprehensive site, sponsored by the Centers for Disease Control and Prevention (CDC), features an infectious disease index, news on emerging infectious diseases, and a section for travelers.

## Key Terms

The terms listed are used on the page indicated. Definitions of the terms are in the Glossary at the end of the book.

| | | |
|---|---|---|
| abscess 541 | gamma globulin 540 | lymph nodes 539 |
| allergy 542 | helminth 537 | meningitis 548 |
| antibiotics 536 | hepatitis 550 | mononucleosis 552 |
| antiviral drug 536 | host 536 | pathogen 535 |
| autoimmune disorder 543 | immune deficiency 541 | protozoa 537 |
| bacteria 536 | immunity 539 | systemic disease 541 |
| bacterial vaginosis 558 | immunotherapy 543 | trichomoniasis 558 |
| candidiasis 559 | incubation period 538 | tuberculosis (TB) 554 |
| chronic fatigue syndrome (CFS) 552 | inflammation 541 | urethritis 559 |
| cystitis 558 | influenza 547 | vector 536 |
| fungi 537 | Lyme disease 555 | virus 536 |

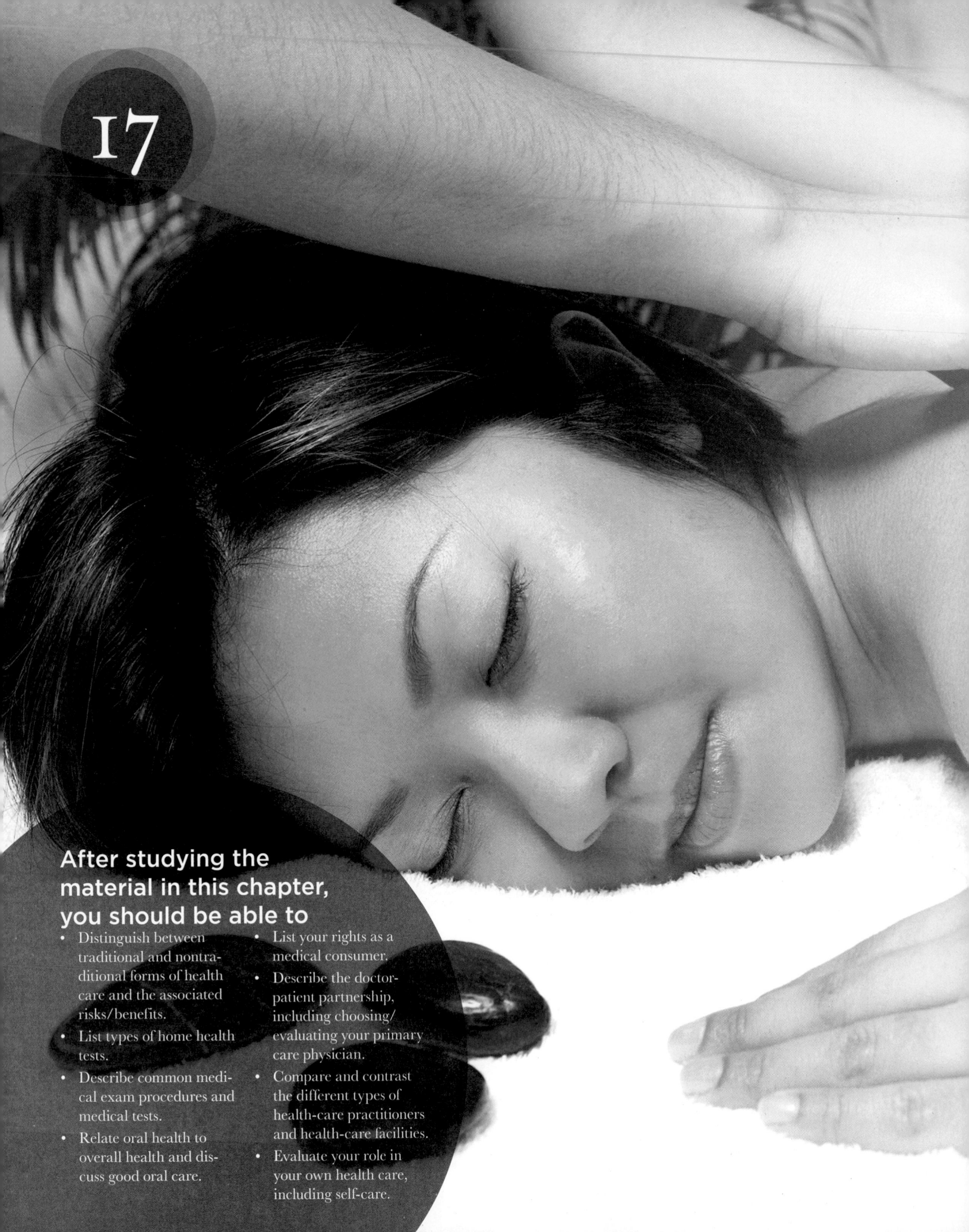

# 17

## After studying the material in this chapter, you should be able to

- Distinguish between traditional and nontraditional forms of health care and the associated risks/benefits.

- List types of home health tests.

- Describe common medical exam procedures and medical tests.

- Relate oral health to overall health and discuss good oral care.

- List your rights as a medical consumer.

- Describe the doctor-patient partnership, including choosing/evaluating your primary care physician.

- Compare and contrast the different types of health-care practitioners and health-care facilities.

- Evaluate your role in your own health care, including self-care.

Long after she immigrated to the United States from India, Tapu's grandmother refused to go to Western doctors. She preferred practitioners who used the herbs and techniques she had relied on in her homeland. Tapu's father, an American-trained physician, would argue with his mother-in-law about what he considered her old-fashioned views. As a doctor's daughter, Tapu grew up believing in the superiority of Western medicine.

# Traditional and Nontraditional Health Care

In her sophomore year at college, Tapu found out that she needed oral surgery. To her surprise, the oral surgeon suggested an alternative method of controlling postoperative pain: acupuncture. "My dad's never going to approve," she said. "And he's the one who's still paying my medical bills." The doctor referred Tapu—and her father—to recent studies conducted by National Institute of Health researchers on acupuncture's efficacy in relieving postsurgical pain. After doing more research online, Tapu agreed to try acupuncture following her operation.

Like Tapu, millions of Americans are turning to complementary and alternative medicine (CAM), a term that includes a broad range of healing philosophies, approaches, and therapies not traditionally taught in medical schools or provided in hospitals. But consumers are learning that they have to be just as savvy—and skeptical—about these therapies and practitioners as they are with any other form of health care.

By describing most of today's many health-care choices, this chapter, particularly "Health Assurance" in Making Change Happen and *Labs for IPC*, will help you take greater responsibility for your personal well-being. Whether you are monitoring your blood pressure, taking medication, or deciding whether to try an alternative therapy, you need to gather information, ask questions, weigh advantages and disadvantages, and take charge of your health. The reason: No one cares more about your health than you and no one will do more to promote your well-being.

## Quality Health Care

Quality matters in health care perhaps more than anywhere because your life may depend on it. Yet the quality of health care varies greatly in this country. Some physicians, some hospitals,

Visit www.cengagebrain.com to access course materials for this text, including the Behavior Change Planner, interactive quizzes, tutorials, and more. See the preface on page xv for details.

# Personalizing Your Health Care

Thanks to advances in genomics (the study of the entire set of human genes), physicians are tailoring tests and treatments to individual patients. "Personalized" medicine can alert your doctor to potential threats that might be prevented, delayed, or detected at an earlier, more treatable stage and, if you do develop a disease, pinpoint the mediations that will do the most good and cause the least harm.

But "personalizing" health care is also a personal responsibility. You can take charge of your own health by compiling a family health history and informing yourself about risks related to your gender, race, and ethnicity.

You can learn about your future health risks by asking your parents, grandparents, uncles, and aunts about any medical conditions they may have.

© Pixland/Jupiterimages

some health-care plans do a better job of helping people stay healthy or get better if they become ill. At one time, patients simply put their faith in physicians and assumed that they knew best and would make the correct medical decisions. Today health care has become far more complex and impersonal. Increasingly, doctors as well as consumer advocates insist that patients need to take responsibility for their own care. Rather than assuming that health-care providers will do whatever is necessary and appropriate, you must take the initiative to ensure that you get quality care.[1]

Quality begins with you. (See Self-Survey.) By learning how to maintain your health, evaluate medical information, and spot early signs of a problem, you're more likely to get the best possible care—and to keep down your medical bills. Self-care means head-to-toe maintenance, including good oral care, appropriate screening tests, knowing your medical rights, and understanding the health-care system.

Chances are that you've tried—or will try—alternative therapies. Many use a "whole-person" approach that addresses all the dimensions of health. You need to be just as savvy a consumer when considering a complementary or alternative treatment as you would with a more mainstream one. You also need to continue your best healthy practices throughout your life so you can function at your best for as long as possible. But your future begins with the healthy choices you make today and every day.

## Your Family Health History

Someday a DNA scan from a single drop of blood may tell you the diseases you're most likely to develop. A family history can do the same—now.

Mapping your family medical history can help identify health risks you may face in the future. One way of charting your health history is to draw a medical family "tree" that includes your parents and siblings (who share half your genes), as well as grandparents, uncles, aunts, and cousins. Depending on how much information you're able to obtain for each relative, your medical family tree can include health issues each family member has faced, including illnesses with a hereditary component, such as high blood pressure, diabetes, some cancers, and certain psychiatric disorders. Although having a relative with a certain disease may increase your risk, your likelihood of ending up with the same condition also depends on your health habits, such as diet and exercise. Knowing now that you're at risk can motivate you to change any unhealthy behaviors. Realizing that you have a relative with, say, colon cancer could mean that you should start screening tests ten years before others because you're at risk of developing a tumor at an earlier age.

For guidance on creating a family history, check these websites: **www.mayoclinic.com** or **www.ashg.org/genetics/ashg/educ/007.shtml**.

## Men and Women as Health-Care Consumers

The genders differ significantly in the way they use health-care services in the United States. Women see doctors more often than men, take more prescription drugs, are hospitalized more, and control the spending of three of every four health-care dollars. In a national telephone poll, 76 percent of American women—but only 60 percent of men—said they had had a health exam in the last 12 months.

Many experts believe that the need for birth control and reproductive health services gets women into the habit of making regular visits to health-care professionals, primarily gyne-cologists. There are no comparable specialists for men, who tend to visit urologists, specialists in male reproductive organs, only when they develop problems. Men also are conditioned to take a stoic, tough-it-out attitude to early symptoms of a disease.

Men feel they are not allowed to manifest illness unless it's overt, says family practitioner Martin Miner, M.D., who has conducted research on men and health care. One reason men die earlier than women is because of the length of time they wait to go for treatment.

The genders also differ in the symptoms and syndromes they develop. For instance, men are more prone to back problems, muscle sprains and strains, allergies, insomnia, and digestive problems. Men develop heart disease about a decade earlier in life than women. More men develop ulcers and hernias; women are more likely to get gallbladder disease and irritable bowel syndrome. An estimated 3 to 6 percent of men suffer from migraines, compared with 15 to 17 percent of women. Yet women and men spend similar proportions of their lifetimes—about 81 percent—free of disability. For men, whose lifespans are shorter, this translates into an average of 58.8 years; for women, 63.9 years.

## Self-Care

Most people do treat themselves. You probably prescribe aspirin for a headache, chicken soup or orange juice for a cold, or a weekend trip to unwind from stress. At the very least, you should know what your **vital signs** are and how they compare against normal readings (Figure 17.1).

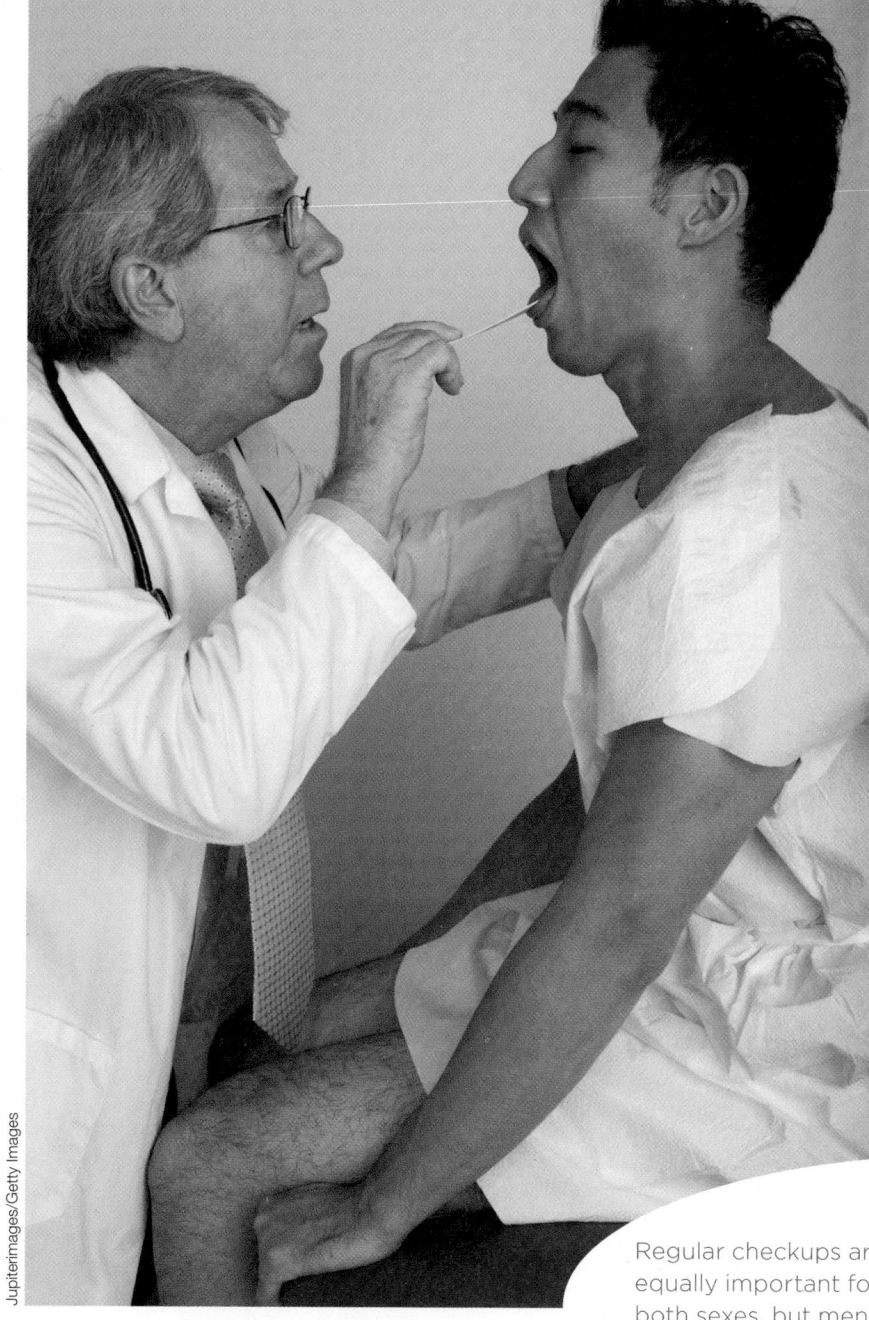

Jupiterimages/Getty Images

Regular checkups are equally important for both sexes, but men often put off seeing a physician until symptoms become too serious to ignore.

Once a thermometer was the only self-testing equipment found in most American homes. Now hundreds of home tests are available to help consumers monitor everything from fertility to blood pressure to cholesterol levels (Table 17.1). More convenient and less expensive than a visit to a clinic or doctor's office, the new tests are generally as accurate as those administered by a professional.

Self-care also can mean getting involved in the self-help movement, which has grown into a major national trend. An estimated 20 million

**vital signs** Measurements of physiological functioning; specifically, temperature, blood pressure, pulse rate, and respiration rate.

Figure 17.1 **Take Your Own Vital Signs**

| Vital Sign | Normal Values |
|---|---|
| Temperature | 98.9° F in the morning or 99.9° F later in the day is upper limit of the normal oral temperature for people 40 years old or younger.<br><br>• Women's temperatures are slightly higher than men's.<br>• African Americans' temperatures are slightly higher than European Americans'.<br><br>Measure your temperature with a mercury or digital thermometer. |
| Blood pressure | Below 120 (systolic) and below 80 (diastolic). You can measure your own blood pressure if you want to invest in blood pressure equipment. Check your local drugstore to purchase a blood pressure cuff or digital blood pressure monitor. |
| Pulse | 72 beats per minute. Take your pulse rate at your wrist or at the carotid artery in your neck. |
| Respiration rate | 15–20 breaths per minute. |

Table 17.1 **Home Health Tests: A Consumer's Guide**

| Type of Test | What It Does |
|---|---|
| Pregnancy | Determines if a woman is pregnant by detecting the presence of human chorionic gonodatropin in urine. Considered 99 percent accurate. |
| Fertility | Measures levels of luteinizing hormone (LH), which rise 24 to 36 hours before a woman conceives. Can help women increase their odds of conceiving. |
| Blood pressure | Measures blood pressure by means of an automatically inflating armband or a cuff for the finger or wrist; helps people taking hypertension medication or suffering from high blood pressure to monitor their condition. |
| Cholesterol | Checks cholesterol in blood from a finger prick; good for anyone concerned about cholesterol. |
| Colon cancer | Screening test to detect hidden blood in stool; recommended for anyone over 40 or concerned about colorectal disease. |
| Urinary tract infection | Diagnoses infection by screening for certain white blood cells in urine; advised for women who get frequent UTIs and whose doctors will prescribe antibiotics without a visit. |
| HIV infection | Detects antibodies to HIV in a blood sample sent anonymously to a lab. Controversial because no face-to-face counseling is available for those who test positive. |

© bilderlounge/Jupiterimages

people participate in self-help support groups. Millions of others join virtual support communities online.

## Oral Health

Oral health involves more than healthy teeth—it refers to the entire mouth, including all the structures that allow us to talk, bite, chew, taste, swallow, smile, scream, or scowl. Oral health is a critical part of overall health. Research has revealed links between chronic oral infection and heart and lung diseases, stroke, low birthweight, premature births, and diabetes.

Poor oral health can lead to a variety of health problems. People with gum disease are at higher risk for developing heart disease, stroke, uncontrolled diabetes, preterm births, and respiratory disease. One recent study found an increased risk of pancreatic cancer in individuals who had experienced tooth loss.

Thanks to fluoridated water and toothpaste and improved dental care, Americans' oral health is better than in the past. However, without good self-care, you probably will lose some teeth to decay and gum disease. The best way to prevent such problems is through proper and regular brushing and flossing.

**Gum**, or periodontal, **disease** is an inflammation that attacks the gum and bone that hold your teeth in place. The culprit is **plaque**, the sticky film of bacteria that forms on teeth. More than 300 species of bacteria live under the gum line, and about half a dozen have been linked to serious gum problems. The early stage of gum disease is called **gingivitis**. If untreated, it develops into a more serious form known as **periodontitis**, in which plaque moves down the tooth to the roots, which then become infected. In advanced periodontitis, the infection destroys the bone and fibers that hold teeth in place.

Symptoms of gum disease include bleeding during brushing or flossing, redness and puffiness of gums, tenderness or pain, persistent bad breath or a bad taste in the mouth, receding gums, shifted or loosened teeth, and changes in the way your teeth fit together when you bite. New treatments, which offer an alternative to traditional gum surgery, include a single antibiotic injection or the implant of a small

## How to Take Care of Your Mouth

- **Brush your teeth every morning and every night.** Oral bacteria reach their highest count during sleep because fluids in the mouth accumulate. Nighttime cleaning reduces the bacterial population; morning cleaning lets you reduce the buildup.

- **Use a toothpaste that has the American Dental Association (ADA) seal of acceptance and a toothbrush with soft, rounded bristles.** Replace your toothbrush every three months.

- **Hold the brush at a 45-degree angle from your gums.** Pay particular attention to the space between your teeth and gums, especially on the inside, toward your tongue. Brush for two to five minutes. Don't brush too vigorously. If you scrub as hard as you can, you may damage your teeth and gums. Abrasion—a problem for more than half of American adults—erodes tooth surfaces, weakens teeth, and increases sensitivity to hot and cold foods. There is some evidence that powered toothbrushes are better at removing plaque and reducing the risk of gum disease than are ordinary manual toothbrushes.

- **Because brushing can't reach plaque and food trapped between teeth, daily flossing is essential.** Using waxed or unwaxed floss, start behind the upper and lower molars at one side of your mouth and work toward the other side.

- **See your dentist twice a year for routine cleaning and examination.** Your dentist should take a complete medical history from you and update it every six months, examine your mouth for signs of cancer, and thoroughly outline all treatment options.

- **Make sure that everyone who works on the inside of your mouth wears a mask and rubber gloves** to reduce the risk of disease transmission (that is, bacterial and viral infections, such as hepatitis, herpes, and HIV).

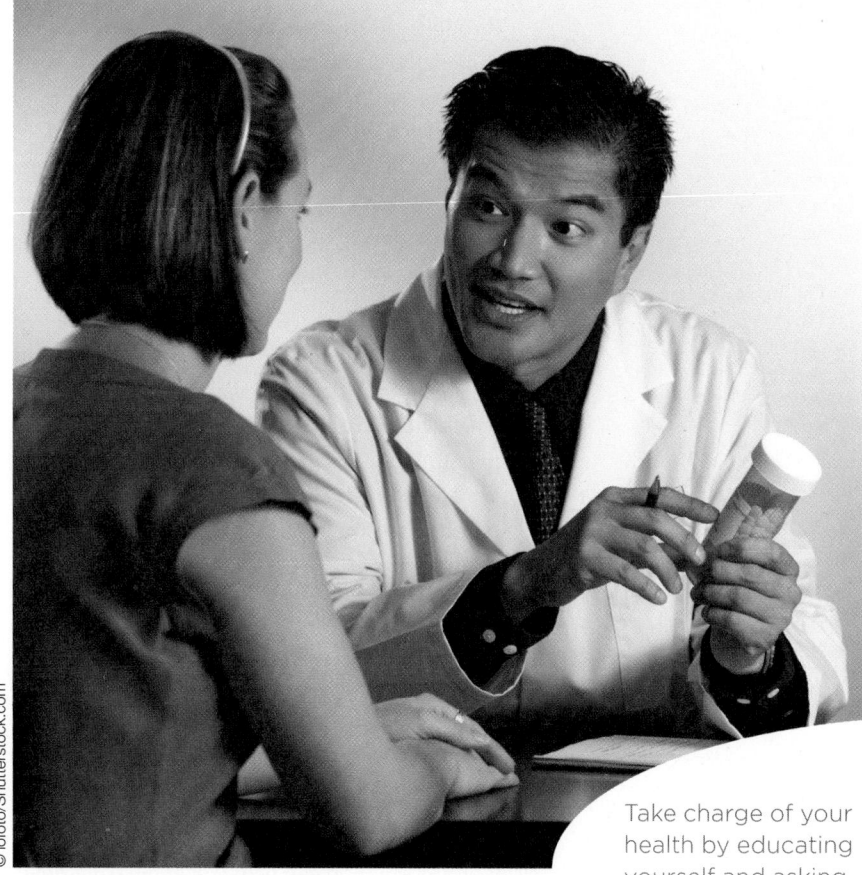

© iofoto/Shutterstock.com

Take charge of your health by educating yourself and asking your doctor questions about your health and treatments.

antibiotic chip in the periodontal pockets to promote healing.

Taking care of your mouth isn't important only for dental health: It may affect how long you live. Gingivitis and periodontitis trigger an inflammatory response that causes the arteries to swell, which leads to a constriction of blood flow that can increase the incidence of cardiovascular disease. Periodontal disease also leads to a higher white blood cell count, an indicator that the immune system is under increased stress. The good news: You can prevent these problems by flossing daily and brushing your teeth and your tongue (to get rid of bacteria that can cause gum disease and bad breath).

## The Doctor-Patient Partnership

Once the family doctor was indeed part of the family. The family doctor brought babies into the world, shepherded them through childhood, comforted and counseled them, stood by their bedside in their darkest hours. Patients entrusted the doctor with their cares, their

**gum disease** Inflammation of the gum and bones that hold teeth in place.

**plaque** The sticky film of bacteria that forms on teeth.

**gingivitis** Inflammation of the gums.

**periodontitis** Severe gum disease in which the tooth root becomes infected.

confidences, their very lives. Dramatic break-throughs in diagnosing and treating illness shifted the focus in medicine from the family physician to the specialist, from basic caring to high-tech medical care. Patients today are more likely to be cured of a vast array of illnesses than were patients a century ago. However, they often complain of insensitive, uncaring physicians who focus on their diseases rather than on them as individuals.

As more physicians have joined managed-care organizations (discussed later in this chapter), which emphasize efficiency, they sometimes feel pressure to see more patients a day, to spend less time with each, and to discourage expensive tests and treatments.

Because physicians have less time and less autonomy, patients today must do more. Your first step should be learning more about your body, any medical conditions or problems you develop, and your options for treatment. You can find a great deal of information via computer online services, patient advocacy and support organizations, and libraries.

This information can help you know what questions to ask and how to evaluate what your doctor says. But you have to be willing to speak up. Busy doctors give patients less than a minute on average during a routine visit to say what's bothering them before they interrupt. This doesn't mean your doctor isn't interested, but it does mean that you have to develop good communication skills so you can tell physicians what they need to know to help you.

# Choosing a Primary Care Physician

Why does a healthy young adult need a doctor? To stay healthy as long as possible. At some point in early adulthood, you should establish a relationship with a physician who will do basic screening tests (Table 17.2), record your family history, and help you prevent problems down the road. The primary care physicians who are playing increasingly important roles in

American health care include family practitioners, general internists, and pediatricians.

Obstetrician-gynecologists serve as the primary providers of health care for more than half of all women. If you're a woman and your gynecologist is the only physician you see, make sure that he or she performs other tests—such as measuring your blood pressure—in addition to a pelvic and breast exam. If you develop other symptoms or health concerns, ask for an appropriate referral.

 At college health centers, clinics, and some health-care organizations, consumers may be assigned to a primary physician or restricted to certain doctors. Even if your choices are limited, don't suspend your critical judgment. If your assigned physician does not listen to your concerns or is not providing adequate care, you can—and should—request another physician. Your rapport with your primary physician and the feelings of mutual trust and respect that develop between you can have as much of an impact on your well-being as your doctor's technical expertise.

One key to making the health-care system work for you lies in choosing a good physician. After seeing your primary care physician, ask yourself the following questions to evaluate the quality of care you are getting.

- Did your physician take a comprehensive history? Was the physical examination thorough?

- Did your physician explain what he or she was doing during the exam?

- Did he or she spend enough time with you?

- Did you feel free to ask questions? Did your physician give you straight answers? Did he or she reassure you when you were worried?

- Does your physician seem willing to admit that he or she doesn't know the answers to some questions?

- Does your physician hesitate to refer you to a specialist even when you have a complex problem that warrants such care?

Look back at your answers. If they make you feel uneasy, have a talk with your physician. Or find a physician or a health plan that provides better service.

Here are some guidelines for talking with your doctor:

- **Prepare in advance.** Write down your questions, organize them in a logical fashion, and select the top ten queries you want answered. Make a copy of all your questions to review and leave with your doctor.

- **Ask about a "question hour."** Many health-care practitioners set aside a specific time of day for patients with call-in questions. Find out if your college health center offers this service. Does a nurse field all calls? Can you get specific advice?

- **Go online.** Many doctors' offices answer queries by e-mail. Ask your doctor if you can e-mail follow-up questions or progress reports on how you're feeling.

- **Interrupt the interrupter.** If you're having difficulty explaining what's wrong, say so. If your doctor tries to put words in your mouth, say, "Please just listen so I can tell you the whole story without getting sidetracked."

## Your Medical Exam

Although analysts have not found evidence that an annual screening physical is warranted for healthy adults, primary care physicians feel differently. In a recent survey about two-thirds agreed that an annual physical examination is necessary. The benefits, as doctors see them, include time to counsel patients about preventive health services, detection of underlying illnesses before symptoms develop, and improved patient-physician relationships.

Your physician will want a past **medical history**, including major illnesses, surgery, and treatments. Report any allergies you have, particularly to drugs, and the medications you take, including aspirin, antacids, sleeping pills, oral contraceptives, and recreational drugs, even if illegal. Your physician may also want to know about topics you consider private, such as sexually transmitted infections. Remember that he or she needs all this information to provide you with comprehensive treatment. Note, too, that a physician must report certain information—for example, certain sexually transmitted diseases—to health authorities.

### Table 17.2 **Screening Tests and Recommendations**

**Anemia**
Beginning in adolescence, all nonpregnant women should be screened every five to ten years until menopause.

**Clinical Breast Exam/Mammogram**
Women ages 20 to 39 should receive a clinical breast exam every three years. Women age 40 and older should receive an annual clinical breast exam and a mammogram.

**Cervical Cancer Screening (Pap Smear)**
Three years after first sexual intercourse or by age 21, whichever comes first, until age 30, women should receive an annual Pap smear. After age 30, the screening rate may decrease. See "Making Change Happen: Detecting Cancer" in Chapter 15, page 530.

**Cholesterol and Lipids**
Adults over age 20 should have a lipoprotein panel test every five years.

**Colorectal Cancer Screening**
Adults age 50 and older should receive an annual fecal occult blood test and colonoscopy every ten years.

**Type 2 Diabetes**
Beginning at age 45, adults should have a fasting blood glucose test every three years.

**Hypertension Screening**
Adults age 18 and older should have an annual blood pressure (BP) check. If the BP is less than 130/85, it should be checked every two years. If the blood pressure is between 130–139/85–89, it should be checked annually. After age 60, blood pressure should be checked annually.

**Osteoporosis**
Women age 65 and older should have a baseline bone mineral density test. To reduce the risk of fractures, women should increase dietary calcium and vitamin D, perform weight-bearing exercise, stop smoking, and moderate alcohol intake.

**Prostate Cancer Screening**
Men age 50 and older should discuss potential benefits and known harms of screening with PSA and digital rectal exam.

**Skin Cancer Screening**
Adults should receive an annual skin exam.

**Visual Exam**
Adults ages 18 to 40 should have a complete visual examination every two to three years; ages 41 to 60, every two years; and age 61 and older, every year.

After the physician has asked you questions about your complaints, medical history, and lifestyle, he or she will probably perform the standard tests described below. During the examination, point out any pains, lumps, or skin growths you've noticed. If you feel pain when the physician palpates (feels) any part of your body, say so.

- **Head.** Using a flashlightlike instrument called an *ophthalmoscope*, the physician will look at the lens, retina, and blood vessels of your eyes. He or she also will examine your ears, mouth, tongue, teeth, and gums.

**medical history** The health-related information collected during the interview of a client by a health-care professional.

- **Neck.** Feeling around your neck, the physician will check for enlarged lymph glands (a sign of infection), for lumps in the thyroid gland, and for warning signs of stroke in the neck arteries.

- **Chest.** With a *stethoscope*, the physician will listen to the sounds made by your heart, to detect heart murmurs and irregular contractions, and by your lungs, to detect asthma or emphysema. By tapping on your chest and back with his or her fingers, the physician can tell the size and shape of your heart, which may reveal some forms of heart disease, and whether any fluid has collected in your lungs. The physician will also check for abnormal lumps in a woman's breasts.

- **Abdomen.** Here the physician uses his or her fingers to probe for tender spots and malformations of the liver and other organs, which may reveal signs of alcoholism, hepatitis, or hernias.

- **Rectum and genitals.** With a gloved hand, the physician can feel in the rectum for growths and hemorrhoids. A rectal examination can also reveal enlargement of the male's prostate gland. The physician will check male testicles and spermatic cords for abnormalities.

- **Pelvic examination.** During a pelvic examination, a woman lies on her back, with her heels in stirrups at the end of the examining table and her legs spread out to the sides. The physician inspects the labia, clitoris, and vaginal opening. Using two gloved, lubricated fingers, the physician will check for abnormalities in the vagina, uterus, fallopian tubes, and ovaries. Many physicians will also perform a rectal or rectovaginal (one finger in the rectum and one in the vagina) examination. A nurse or other health-care worker should be present throughout the exam.

  The *speculum* is a medical instrument that spreads the walls of the vagina so that the inside can be seen. As discussed in Chapters 11 and 16, doctors are using HPV tests as well as the conventional **Pap smear** to screen for cervical cancer.

- **Extremities.** The physician may check your knees and other joints for reflexes, which can indicate nerve disorders, and look for tremors in outstretched hands or in the face. The color, elasticity, and wetness or dryness of your skin can alert him or her to nutritional problems, or can indicate diabetes or skin cancer. Hair and nails can give indications of internal health, such as blood disorders. Swelling of the ankles can be an indication of heart, kidney, or liver disease.

- **Pulse and blood pressure.** Your physician may check your pulse in various places, looking for signs of poor circulation. The rhythm and speed of the heart may also signal diseases of the heart or thyroid gland. High blood pressure can be an early warning sign of possible heart attack, stroke, or kidney damage.

## Medical Tests

Besides the diagnostic tests just listed, the physician may order some laboratory and other tests, including the following:

- **Chest X-ray.** A chest X-ray can reveal abnormalities of the heart and lungs; if you're a smoker, the physician may insist on one.

- **Electrocardiogram.** The *electrocardiogram*, performed while you're at rest, records the electrical activity of your heart. It can show irregularities in heart rhythm or muscle damage, as well as hardening of the arteries.

- **Urinalysis.** Your urine may be analyzed by a medical laboratory. If sugar (glucose) is found in your urine, your physician may order a separate blood test to check for diabetes. The presence of blood cells may indicate infection of the bladder or kidneys. Abnormal amounts of albumin (protein) in the urine may also suggest kidney disease.

- **Blood tests.** The physician or laboratory technician may draw blood to do a blood cell count. An excess of white blood cells may indicate an infection or, occasionally, leukemia. A deficiency of red blood cells may indicate anemia. Your blood also may be analyzed to measure the levels of its various components. High levels of glucose can indicate diabetes, and high levels of uric acid may mean gout or kidney stones. Your lipoprotein profile may indicate cardiac risk (see Chapter 15).

**Pap smear** A test in which cells removed from the cervix are examined under a microscope for signs of cancer; also called a Pap test.

See the Hales Health Almanac found on the companion website for a comprehensive guide to medical tests.

## Preventing Medical Errors

More people die from medical errors than from motor vehicle accidents, breast cancer, or AIDS. Medical errors occur when a planned part of medical care doesn't work properly or when the wrong plan was used in the first place. They can happen anywhere in the health-care system, from doctors' offices to pharmacies to hospitals to patients' homes. They may involve medications, diagnoses, tests, lab equipment, surgery, or infection. They are most likely to occur when doctors and patients have problems communicating.

Your best defense against medical errors is information. Your questions about your treatments can keep you safe and ensure you get quality health care. (See Health on a Budget.)

# Your Medical Rights

As a consumer, you have basic rights that help ensure that you know about any potential dangers, receive competent diagnosis and treatment, and retain control and dignity in your interactions with health-care professionals. Many hospitals publish a patient's bill of rights, including your rights to know whether a procedure is experimental; to refuse to undergo a specific treatment; to designate someone else to make decisions about your care if and when you cannot; and to leave the hospital, even against your physician's advice.

You have the right to be treated with respect and dignity, including being called "Mr." or "Ms." or whatever you wish, rather than by your first name. Make clear your preferences. If you feel that health-care professionals are being condescending or inconsiderate, say so—in the same tone and manner that you would like others to use with you. If you're hospitalized, find out if there's a patient advocate or representative at your hospital. These individuals can help you communicate with physicians, make any special arrangements, and get answers to questions or complaints.

## Your Right to Information

By law, a patient must give consent for hospitalization, surgery, and other major treatments. **Informed consent** is a right, not a privilege. Use this right to its fullest. Ask questions. Seek other opinions. Make sure that your expectations are realistic and that you understand the potential risks, as well as the possible benefits, of a prospective treatment.

## Your Right to Privacy and Access to Medical Records

Your medical records are your property. You have the right to see them whenever you choose and to limit who else can see them. Federal standards protecting the privacy of patients' medical information guarantee patients access to their medical records, give them more control over how personal health information is disclosed, and limit the ways that health plans, pharmacies, and hospitals can use personal medical information.

**informed consent** Permission (to undergo or receive a medical procedure or treatment) given voluntarily, with full knowledge and understanding of the procedure—or treatment and its possible consequences.

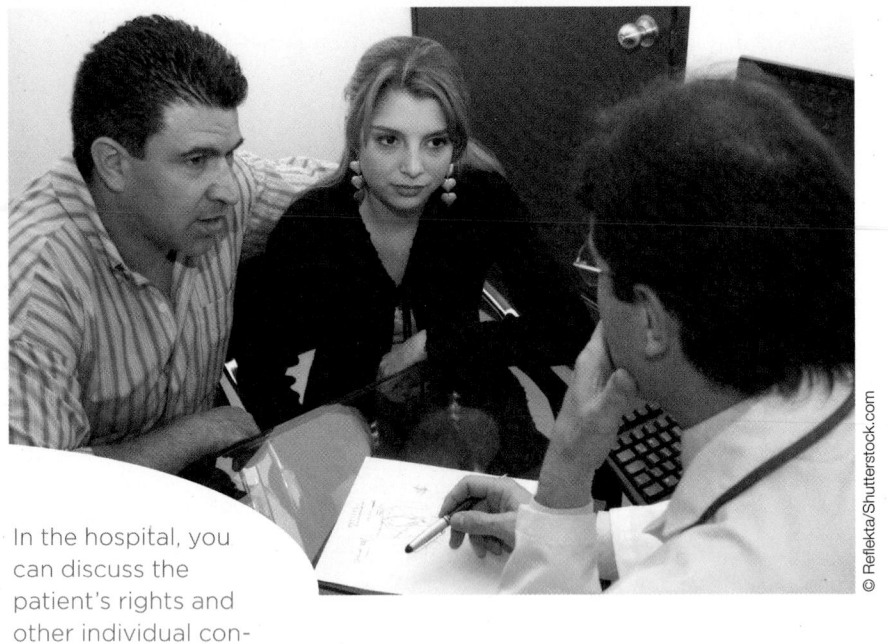

In the hospital, you can discuss the patient's rights and other individual concerns with a patient advocate.

Key provisions include:

- **Access to medical records.** As a patient, you should be able to see and obtain copies of your medical records and request corrections if there are errors. Health-care providers must provide these within 30 days; they may charge for the cost of copying and mailing records.
- **Notice of privacy practices.** Your providers must inform you of how they use personal medical information. Doctors, nurses, and other providers may not disclose information for purposes not related to your health care.
- **Prohibition on marketing.** Pharmacies, health plans, and others must obtain specific authorization before disclosing patient information for marketing.
- **Confidentiality.** Patients can request that doctors take reasonable steps to ensure confidential communications, such as calling a cell phone rather than home or office.

## Your Right to Quality Health Care

The essence of a *malpractice* suit is the claim that the physician failed to meet the standard of quality care required of a reasonably skilled and careful medical doctor. Although physicians don't have to guarantee good results to their patients and aren't held liable for unavoidable errors, they are required to use the same care

and judgment in treatment that other physicians in the same specialty would use under similar circumstances. To protect themselves financially, physicians, particularly those in surgical specialties who are most likely to be sued, pay tens of thousands of dollars a year in malpractice insurance premiums. Some of this cost is passed on to patients.

Most lawsuits are based on negligence and assert that a physician failed to render diagnosis and treatment with appropriate professional knowledge and skill. Other cases are brought for failure to provide information, obtain consent, or respect a patient's confidentiality. However, analysis of malpractice cases has shown that, in 70 to 80 percent, a doctor's attitude and inability to communicate effectively—by devaluing patients' views, delivering information poorly, failing to understand patients' perspectives, or displaying an air of superiority—also played a role.

# Elective Treatments

As medical technology has developed new options, millions of Americans are trying elective procedures and products that are not medically necessary but that promise to enhance health or appearance. Some are new alternatives for correcting common problems, such as poor vision, while others offer the promise of looking younger or more attractive. In some cases, the procedures are scams or hoaxes. (See Consumer Alert.)

## Vision Surgery

Millions of people in the United States have undergone laser surgery to correct their vision. In LASIK (laser-assisted in situ keratomileusis), the most common technique, a surgeon uses a razorlike instrument to lift a flap of the cornea—the clear stiff outer layer over the colored iris—and then reshapes the exposed area using a laser. The surgery alters the way the eye focuses light, correcting nearsightedness, farsightedness, and some astigmatism. Laser surgery cannot make an aging eye's lens flexible again to improve close-up vision in middle-aged adults. Numbing eye drops make the treatment painless, although burning and scratchiness are normal for a couple of hours afterward. An estimated 10 to 30 percent of patients require additional surgery, or "enhancements," to sharpen their vision. Other complications include glare, sensitivity to bright lights, and poor night vision.

Prices have fallen, but ophthalmologists have warned consumers that some laser surgery centers have cut corners to cut prices, such as hiring inexperienced surgeons or using optometrists or technicians rather than MDs for pre- and post-operative checkups. A qualified eye surgeon should have a record of 100 or more LASIK procedures and at least 25 enhancements—but no more than 20 percent of his or her patients should require enhancements. Ideally, the surgeon should also be the one doing your pre- and postprocedure checks.

*When Is LASIK Not for You?* You are probably NOT a good candidate for refractive surgery[2] if:

- **You are not a risk taker.** Certain complications are unavoidable in a percentage of patients, and there are no long-term data available for current procedures.

- **Cost is an issue.** Most medical insurance will not pay for refractive surgery. Although the cost is coming down, it is still significant.

- **You required a change in your contact lens or glasses prescription in the past year.** This is called refractive instability. Patients who are in their early 20s or younger, whose hormones are fluctuating due to disease such as diabetes, who are pregnant or breast-feeding, or who are taking medications that may cause fluctuations in vision are more likely to have refractive instability and should discuss the possible additional risks with their doctor.

- **You have a disease or are on medications that may affect wound healing.** Certain conditions, such as autoimmune diseases and diabetes, and some medications may prevent proper healing after a refractive procedure.

- **You actively participate in contact sports.** If you participate in boxing, wrestling, martial arts, or other activities in which blows to the face and eyes are a normal occurrence, LASIK is probably not right for you.

- **You are under 18.** Currently, no lasers are approved for LASIK on persons under the age of 18.

- **It will jeopardize your career.** Some jobs, including certain military assignments, prohibit refractive procedures.

## Cosmetic Surgery

Approximately 11 million cosmetic treatments are performed every year.[3] About a quarter of those undergoing plastic surgery are between the ages of 18 and 29. The number of teenagers opting for cosmetic procedures—primarily liposuction, nose reshaping, and breast augmentation—is increasing. Nonsurgical cosmetic procedures such as injections of synthetic collagen and botulinum toxin (Botox®) also have become more popular. Health insurance rarely covers cosmetic procedures, which can run into the tens of thousands of dollars.

The most common cosmetic operation is liposuction, the removal of fatty tissue by means of a vacuum device. It can be performed on many areas of the body, from sagging jowls to midsection "love handles" or "muffin tops." The doctor first flushes the target area with a solution of lidocaine (a local anesthetic with a numbing effect), saline, and epinephrine (a drug that reduces bleeding by constricting blood vessels). Inserting a hollow, wandlike cannula under the skin, the doctor breaks up fatty deposits and suctions them, along with other body fluids, with a vacuum device.

Risks and complications include infection, numbness, bleeding, discoloration, lumpiness, and, if too much tissue is removed without proper cautions, potentially fatal complications. The American Society of Plastic and Reconstructive Surgeons estimates the mortality rate is one in 5,000 liposuction patients. Several states are considering legislation to tighten restrictions on training and credentialing doctors who perform liposuction.

Breast augmentation is another cosmetic procedure. The Institute of Medicine, after reviewing all available evidence, has reported that there appears to be no link between breast implants and autoimmune disease, connective tissue disorders, or cancer. However, today's surgeons use implants filled with a saltwater solution. Patients still face possible complications,

## Health Hoaxes

Every year millions of Americans go searching for medical miracles that never happen. In all, they spend more than $10 billion on medical **quackery**, unproven health products and services. Those who lose only money are the lucky ones. Many also waste precious time, during which their conditions worsen. Some suffer needless pain, along with crushed expectations.

### Facts to Know

Promoters of fraudulent health products often use similar claims and practices to trick consumers into buying their products. Be suspicious when you see:

- Claims that a product is a "scientific breakthrough," "miraculous cure," "secret ingredient," or "ancient remedy."

- Claims that the product is an effective cure for a wide range of ailments. No product can cure multiple conditions or diseases.

- Claims that use impressive-sounding medical terms. They're often covering up a lack of good science.

- Undocumented case histories of people who've had amazing results. It's too easy to make them up. And even if true, they can't be generalized to the entire population. Anecdotes are not a substitute for valid science.

- Claims that the product is available from only one source and payment is required in advance.

- Claims of a "money-back" guarantee.

- Websites that fail to list the company's name, physical address, phone number, or other contact information.

### Steps to Take

To keep from risking your life on false hope, follow these guidelines:

- Arm yourself with up-to-date information about your condition or disease from appropriate organizations, such as the American Cancer Society or the Arthritis Foundation, which keep track of unproven and ineffective methods of treatment.

- Ask for a written explanation of what a treatment does and why it works, evidence supporting all claims (not just testimonials), and published reports of the studies, including specifics on numbers treated, doses, and side effects. Be skeptical of self-styled "holistic practitioners," treatments supported by crusading groups, and endorsements from self-proclaimed experts or authorities.

- Don't part with your money quickly. Insurance companies won't reimburse for unproven therapies.

- Don't discontinue your current treatment without your physician's approval. Many physicians encourage supportive therapies—such as relaxation exercises, meditation, or visualization—as a supplement to standard treatments.

Source: Federal Trade Commission, www.ftc.gov/bcp/consumer.shtm.

**quackery** Medical fakery; unproven practices claiming to cure diseases or solve health problems.

including rupture, scarring, infection, and leaking or hardening of their implants.

# Nontraditional Health Care

**Complementary and alternative medicine (CAM)** refers to various medical and health care systems, practices, and products that are not considered part of conventional medicine because there is not yet sufficient proof of their safety and effectiveness. CAM's varied healing philosophies, approaches, and therapies include preventive techniques designed to delay or prevent serious health problems before they start and **holistic** methods that focus on the whole person and the physical, mental, emotional, and spiritual aspects of well-being. Some approaches are based on the same physiological principles as traditional Western methods; others, such as acupuncture, are based on different healing systems. The most commonly used are nonvitamin, nonmineral, natural products (such as fish or omega 3 oil and echinacea) and deep breathing exercises. (See Table 17.3.)

Most people who choose CAM want to improve their overall health and well-being or to relieve the symptoms associated with chronic or terminal illnesses or the side effects of conventional treatments for such diseases. Some are seeking a transformational experience that changes their worldview or want greater control over their health. The overwhelming majority of patients use CAM as a complement to rather than a substitute for conventional care.

The list of available CAM treatment changes constantly as treatments that are proven safe and effective become adopted into conventional health care and as new approaches to health care emerge. Informed consent remains an issue because there are no widespread standards for disclosing risks, discussing alternatives, and assessing potential benefits.

About 25 percent of the scientific reviews of various CAM approaches that have been done in recent years have found sufficient evidence to conclude that certain therapies are effective for certain conditions. For instance, acupuncture

Table 17.3 **10 Most Common CAM Therapies among Adults**

Source: NIH MedlinePlus Magazine, www.n/m.nih.gov/medlineplus/magazine/.

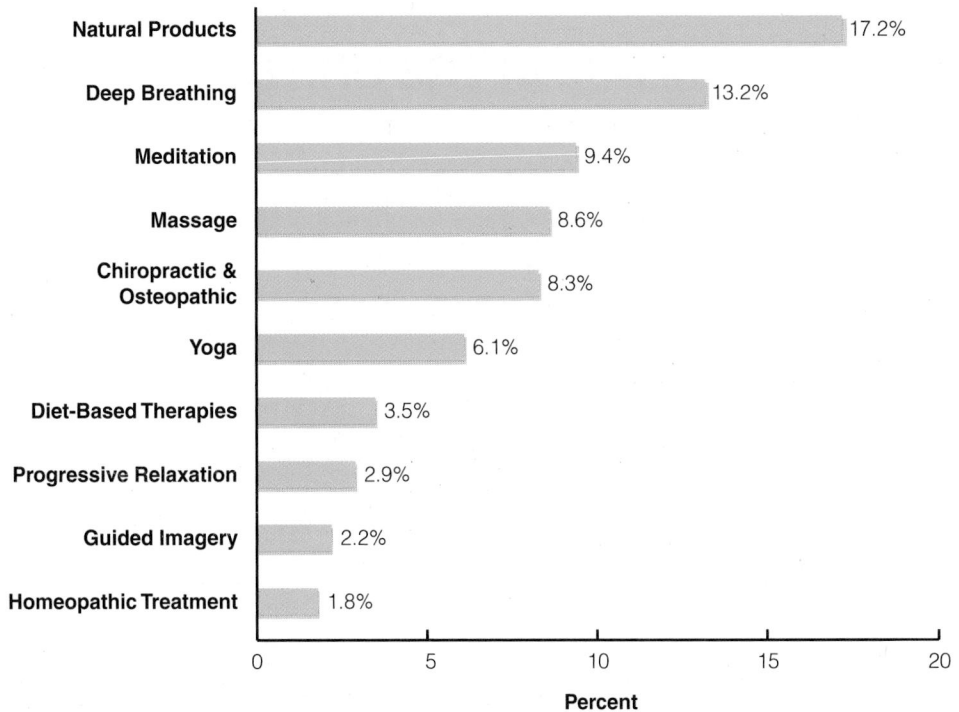

## Who Uses CAM

According to recent surveys, 38 percent of adults in the United States report use of CAM therapy in the previous 12 months. The most frequent reasons are back pain or other problems, head or chest colds, neck pain or problems, joint pain or stiffness, and anxiety or depression. Individuals with cancer, cardiovascular diseases, and lung disorders also are likely to try CAM. Not all CAM users have health problems. About one-fifth of adults with no health conditions and a quarter of those who had not visited a doctor in the past 12 months used CAM therapies. (See Health in Action.)

About one in nine children has used CAM, including natural products, chiropractic or osteopathic manipulation, deep breathing exercises, yoga, and homeopathic remedies. Youngsters whose parents use CAM are much more likely to receive CAM treatments than those whose parents do not. For both adults and

and, to a lesser extent, massage therapy are now included among the recommended therapies for treating back pain in guidelines released by the American College of Physicians and the American Pain Society.

children, individuals worried about costs were more likely to delay conventional care and try CAM.

The populations most likely to use CAM are:

- Women.
- Adults between ages 30 and 69.
- Cancer survivors.[4]
- Adults with higher levels of education.
- Individuals who are physically active during their leisure time.
- People who have existing medical conditions or made frequent medical visits in the prior year.
- Residents of Western states.
- Former smokers.
- People with private health insurance (for those under age 65).

CAM is more widely used in many other countries. In Germany, for instance, 82 percent of patients use CAM treatments, with acupuncture, massage, and relaxation techniques the most widely used.

Some states have mandated health insurance coverage for CAM therapies, which also

**complementary and alternative medicine (CAM)** A term used to apply to all health-care approaches, practices, and treatments not widely taught in medical schools, not generally used in hospitals, and not usually reimbursed by medical insurance companies.

**holistic** An approach to medicine that takes into account body, mind, emotions, and spirit.

## ✔ HOW DO YOU COMPARE?

# CAM USE IN THE UNITED STATES

| Ethnic/Racial Group | Percentage Who Have Used CAM |
|---|---|
| American Indian/Alaska Native | 50 |
| White | 43 |
| Asian | 40 |
| African American | 26 |
| All Americans | 38 |

## HOW DO YOU COMPARE?

Ethnicity is only one factor that influences the use of complementary and alternative medicine. Have you tried a CAM therapy? If so, do you think that your racial or ethnic background played any role in this decision? What other factors have shaped your health-care choices? Record your observations in your online journal.

Source: National Center for Complementary and Alternative Medicine, http://nccam.nih.

**integrative medicine** An approach that combines traditional medicine with alternative/complementary therapies.

**acupuncture** A Chinese medical practice of puncturing the body with needles inserted at specific points to relieve pain or cure disease.

are becoming more common in Canada and Europe. Many medical schools now include training in CAM in their curricula. **Integrative medicine**, which combines selected elements of both conventional and alternative medicine in a comprehensive approach to diagnosis and treatment, has gained greater acceptance within the medical community.

## Types of CAM

The National Center for Complementary and Alternative Medicine (NCCAM) has classified CAM therapies into five categories (Figure 17.2).

- **Alternative medical systems.**
- **Mind-body medicine.**
- **Biologically based therapies.**
- **Manipulative and body-based methods.**
- **Energy therapies.**

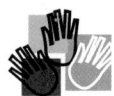 *Alternative Medical Systems* Systems of theory and practice other than traditional Western medicine are included in this group. They include acupuncture, Eastern medicine, t'ai chi, external and internal qi, Ayurvedic medicine, naturopathy, and unconventional Western systems, such as homeopathy and orthomolecular medicine. (See "Health in the Headlines.")

**Acupuncture** is an ancient Chinese form of medicine, based on the philosophy that a cycle of energy circulating through the body controls health. Pain and disease are the result of a disturbance in the energy flow, which can be corrected by inserting long, thin needles at specific points along longitudinal lines, or *meridians*, throughout the body. Each point controls a

Figure 17.2 **The Five Categories of CAM**

Source: NCCAM, http://nccam.nih.gov.

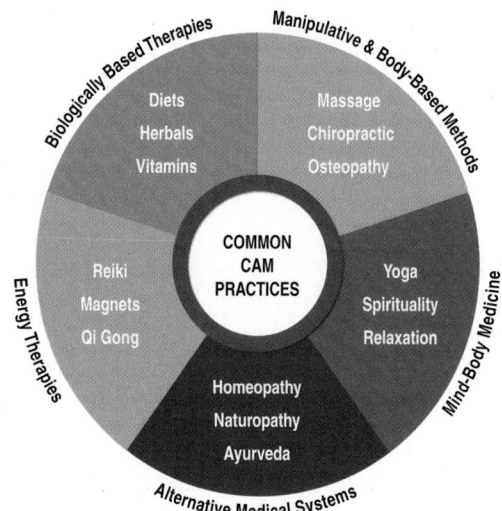

different corresponding part of the body. Once inserted, the needles are rotated gently back and forth or charged with a small electric current for a short time. Western scientists aren't sure exactly how acupuncture works, but some believe that the needles alter the functioning of the nervous system.

Since the 1990s, studies have looked at acupuncture's effect on specific health conditions and how it affects the brain and nervous system; the neurological properties of meridians and acupuncture points; and methods for improving the quality of acupuncture research.[5]

High-quality, randomized, controlled trials have shown that various forms of acupuncture, including so-called sham acupuncture during which no needles actually penetrate the skin, are equally effective for low-back pain—and more beneficial than standard care. However, even sham acupuncture can produce adverse effects, including infection and trauma.[6]

Recent studies have found that acupuncture:

- Helps alleviate nausea in cancer patients undergoing chemotherapy.
- Relieves pain and improves function for some people with osteoarthritis of the knee.
- Helps in treating chronic lower back pain.
- May or may not be of value for many other conditions, including irritable bowel syndrome and some neurologic disorders.[7]

Considered alternative in this country, **Ayurveda** is a traditional form of medical treatment in India, where it has evolved over thousands of years. Its basic premise is that illness stems from incorrect mental attitudes, diet, and posture. Practitioners use a discipline of exercise, meditation, herbal medication, and proper nutrition to cope with such stress-induced conditions as hypertension, the desire to smoke, and obesity.

**Homeopathy** is based on three fundamental principles: like cures like; treatment must always be individualized; and less is more—the idea that increasing dilution (and lowering the dosage) can increase efficacy. By administering doses of animal, vegetable, or mineral substances to a large number of healthy people to see if they all develop the same symptoms, homeopaths determine which substances may be given, in small

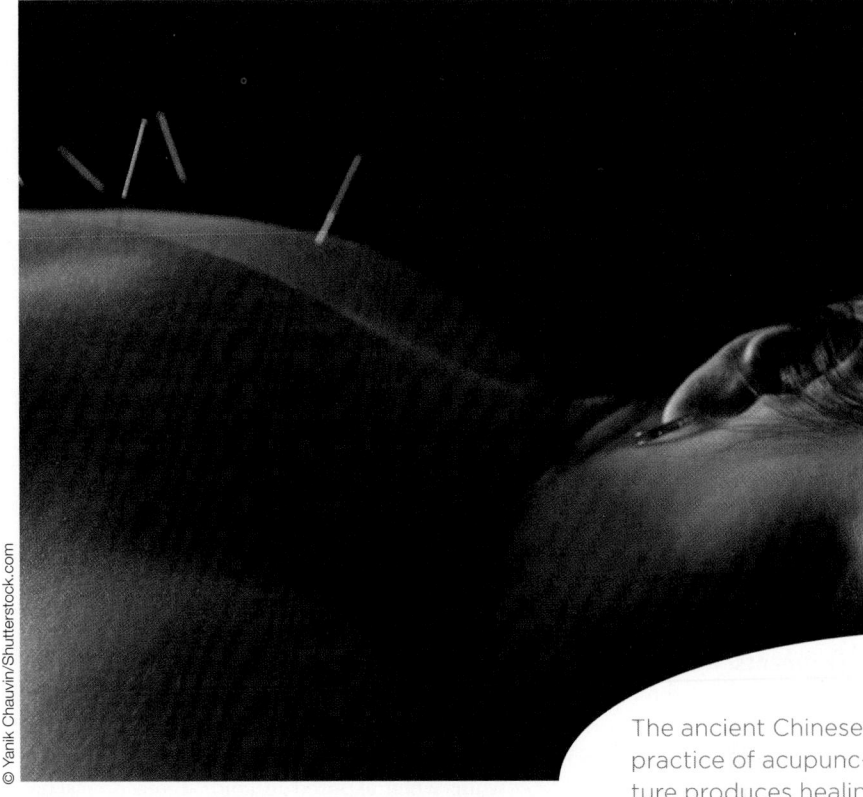

© Yanik Chauvin/Shutterstock.com

quantities, to alleviate the symptoms. Some of these substances are the same as those used in conventional medicine: nitroglycerin for certain heart conditions, for example, although the dose is minuscule.

**Naturopathy** emphasizes natural remedies, such as sun, water, heat, and air, as the best treatments for disease. Therapies might include dietary changes (such as more vegetables and no salt or stimulants), steam baths, and exercise. Some naturopathic physicians (who are not MDs) work closely with medical doctors in helping patients.

*Mind-Body Medicine* Mind-body medicine uses techniques designed to enhance the mind's capacity to affect bodily function and symptoms. Some techniques that were considered alternative in the past have become mainstream (for example, patient support groups and cognitive-behavioral therapy). Other mind-body approaches are still considered CAM, including meditation, prayer (see Chapter 2), yoga, t'ai chi, visual imagery, mental healing, and therapies that use creative outlets such as art, music, or dance. About 30 percent of Americans report using relaxation techniques and imagery, biofeedback, and hypnosis; 50 percent use prayer.

**Ayurveda** A traditional Indian medical treatment involving meditation, exercise, herbal medications, and nutrition.

**homeopathy** A system of medical practice that treats a disease by administering dosages of substances that would in healthy persons produce symptoms similar to those of the disease.

**naturopathy** An alternative system of treatment of disease that emphasizes the use of natural remedies such as sun, water, heat, and air. Therapies may include dietary changes, steam baths, and exercise.

# Health in Action

The physical and emotional risks of using mind-body interventions are minimal. Although we need much more research on how these approaches work and when to apply them most effectively, there is considerable evidence that mind-body interventions have positive effects on psychological functioning and quality of life and may be particularly helpful for patients coping with chronic illnesses.

Mind-body approaches definitely have won some acceptance in modern medical care. Techniques such as hypnosis have proved helpful in reducing discomfort and complications during and after various surgical procedures and in relieving hot flashes in breast cancer survivors. With *biofeedback*, people can learn to control usually involuntary functions, such as circulation to the hands and feet, tension in the jaws, and heartbeat rates. Biofeedback has been used to treat dozens of ailments, including asthma, epilepsy, pain, and Raynaud's disease (a condition in which the fingers become painful and white when exposed to cold). Biofeedback has become accepted as a mainstream therapy,[8] and many health insurers now cover biofeedback treatments.

Creative *visualization* (also discussed in Chapter 4) helps patients heal, including some diagnosed as terminally ill with cancer. Other patients use visualization to create a clear idea of what they want to achieve, whether the goal is weight loss or relaxation.

*Biologically Based Therapies* Biologically based CAM therapies use substances such as herbs, foods, and vitamins. They include **herbal medicine** (botanical medicine or phytotherapy), the use of individual herbs or combinations; special diet therapies, such as macrobiotics, Ornish, Atkins, and high fiber; orthomolecular medicine (use of nutritional and food supplements for preventive or therapeutic purposes); and use of other products (such as shark cartilage) and procedures applied in an unconventional manner.

In the last ten years, sales of herbal supplements have skyrocketed by 100 percent, but most people don't consider evidence-based indications before trying them. According to recent research, two-thirds of people who use herbs do not do so in accordance with scientific guidelines. Although more than 1,500 different preparations are on the U.S. market, just a few single-herb preparations account for about half the sales in the United States: echinacea, garlic, ginkgo biloba, ginseng, kava, St. John's wort, and valerian. Unlike medications, herbal products are exempt from the FDA's regulatory scrutiny. The ingredients and the potency of active ingredients can vary from batch to batch.

Rigorous research studies are producing the first scientific evidence on the safety and efficacy of herbal supplements. Their benefits generally have proved modest (Table 17.4). Acai berry products, for example, have been widely marketed for weight-loss and anti-aging purposes, but there is no definitive scientific evidence to support the claims for this so-called superfood. The Federal Trade Commission has asked federal courts to temporarily suspend a series of fake news websites that have been marketing acai berry weight-loss products. People who are using or are considering using natural products, including acai, should discuss this decision with their health-care provider.[9]

Most of the herbs tested have proved generally safe, although side effects such as headache and nausea can occur. However, some herbs can cause serious, even fatal dangers. Echinacea may cause liver damage if taken in combination with anabolic steroids. Several widely used herbs, including ginger, garlic, and ginkgo biloba, are dangerous if taken prior to surgery.

The FDA has prohibited the sale of dietary supplements containing ephedra, which was linked with dozens of deaths and more than 1,000 adverse reactions. It has issued warnings on other potentially dangerous herbs, including chaparral, comfrey, yohimbe, lobelia, germander, willow bark, jin bu huan, and products containing magnolia or stephania.

*Manipulative and Body-Based Methods* CAM therapies based on manipulation and/or movement of the body are divided into three subcategories:

- **Chiropractic medicine.**

- **Massage therapy and body work** (including osteopathic manipulation, Swedish massage, Alexander technique, reflexology, Pilates, acupressure, and rolfing).

**Table 17.4 Evidence-Based Evaluations of Herbal Supplements**

| Herb | Evidence |
|------|----------|
| Saw palmetto | Reduces an enlarged prostate, but the effect is small compared with prescription medication |
| Ginseng | Improves energy of cancer patients |
| Echinacea and vitamin C | Mixed results warding off colds |
| Kava | May reduce anxiety, but can cause liver damage |
| Ginkgo biloba | No improvement in memory or thinking in the healthy elderly, but a small benefit for patients with dementia |
| Garlic | Not effective in lowering cholesterol |
| Black cohosh | No more effective than placebo for hot flashes; long-term effects unknown |

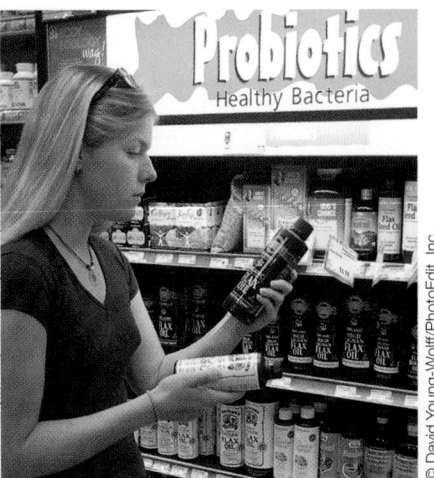
© David Young-Wolff/PhotoEdit, Inc.

- **Unconventional physical therapies** (including colonics, hydrotherapy, and light and color therapies).

**Chiropractic** is a treatment method based on the theory that many human diseases are caused by misalignment of the spine (subluxation). Chiropractors are licensed in all 50 states, but chiropractic is considered a mainstream therapy by some and a form of CAM by others. Significant research in the last ten years has demonstrated its efficacy for acute lower-back pain. NIH is funding research on other potential benefits, including headaches, asthma, middle ear inflammation, menstrual cramps, and arthritis.

Chiropractors, who emphasize wellness and healing without drugs or surgery, may use X-rays and magnetic resonance imaging (MRI) as well as orthopedic, neurological, and manual examinations in making diagnoses. However, chiropractic treatment consists solely of the manipulation of misaligned discs that may be putting pressure on nerve tissue and affecting other parts of the body. Many HMOs offer chiropractic services, which are the most widely used alternative treatment among managed care patients.

*Energy Therapies* Various approaches focus on energy fields believed to exist in and around the body. Some use external energy sources, such as electromagnetic fields. Magnets are marketed to relieve pain, but there is little scientific evidence of their efficacy. Others, such as therapeutic touch, use a therapist's healing energy to repair imbalances in an individual's biofield.

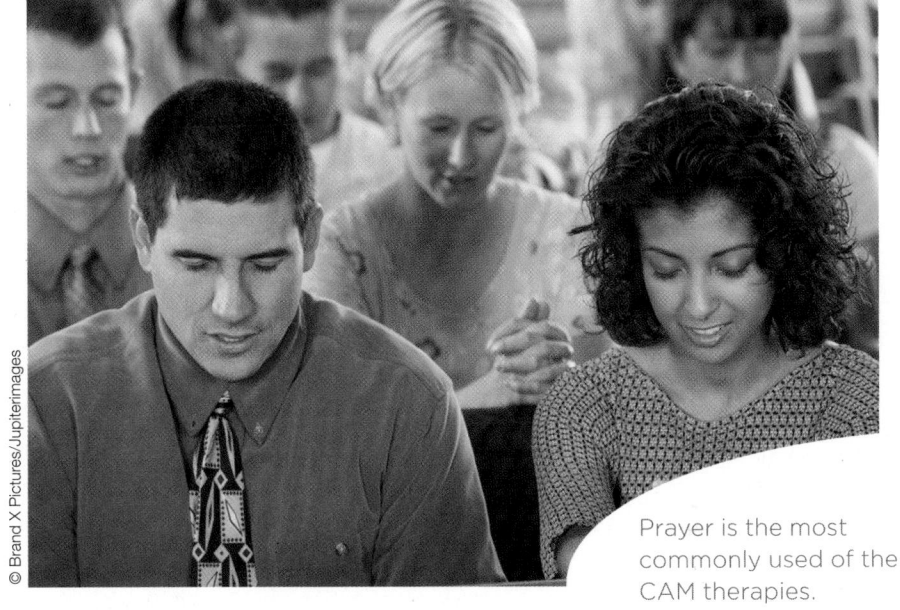
© Brand X Pictures/Jupiterimages

Prayer is the most commonly used of the CAM therapies.

## The Health-Care System

As a college student, you can turn to the student health service if you get sick. There, a nurse, nurse practitioner, physician's assistant, or medical doctor may evaluate your symptoms and provide basic care. However, you may rely on a primary care physician in your hometown to perform regular checkups or manage a chronic condition like asthma. If you're injured in an accident, you probably will be treated at the nearest emergency room. If you become seriously ill and

**herbal medicine** An ancient form of medical treatment using substances derived from trees, flowers, ferns, seaweeds, and lichens to treat disease.

**chiropractic** A method of treating disease, primarily through manipulating the bones and joints to restore normal nerve function.

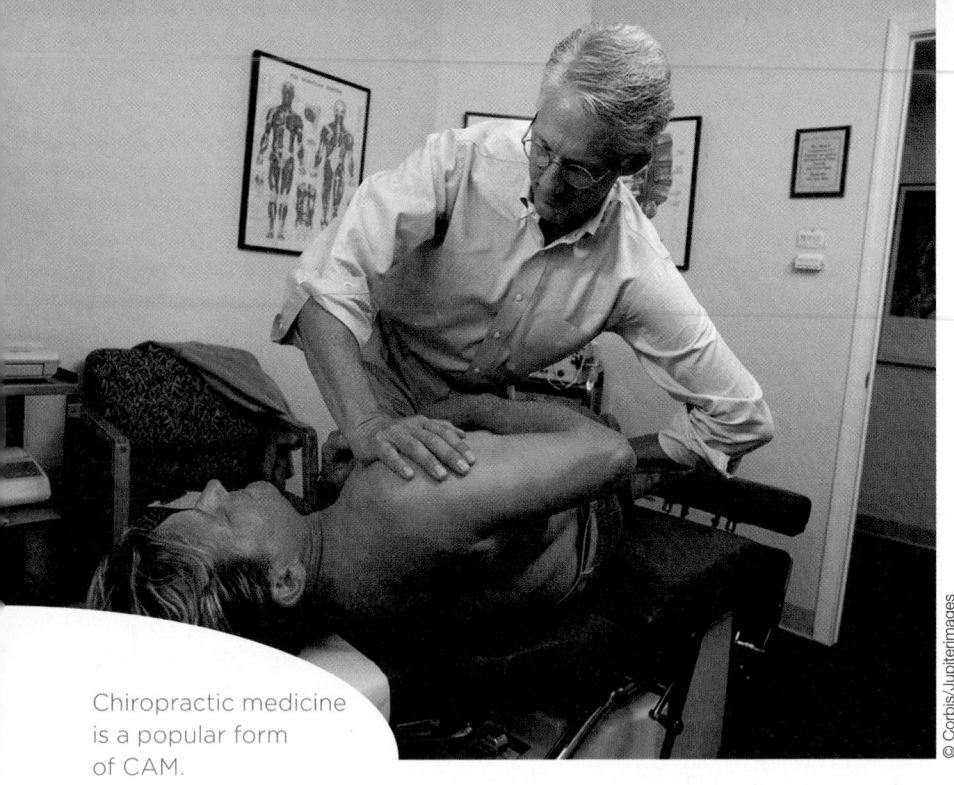

Chiropractic medicine is a popular form of CAM.

## Alternative Medicine

In recent years rigorous scientific studies have confirmed the effectiveness of some forms of CAM and refuted the claimed benefits of others. To get the latest evidence on a particular approach, access Global Health Watch and click on "Alternative Medicine." Scan the list of therapies and choose one, such as "Acupuncture" or "Meditation." Once you've selected your topic, read through the headlines under "Latest news" and summarize one article in your online journal.

require highly specialized care, you may have to go to a university-affiliated medical center to receive state-of-the-art treatment.

Students can often continue their health-care coverage under their parents' policy until the age of 26. However, if a parent belongs to an HMO with a local network of providers, the student may not be covered for anything outside the plan's service area except emergency care. A more open plan, like a preferred provider organization, may allow students to see doctors near school, but the costs may be high.

Most colleges offer some type of health insurance plan, with the student health center acting as the primary care provider. Many schools require enrollment if the student is not covered under any other plan. Check the plan carefully. Physicals, gynecological visits, and other preventive care may not be covered. College plans also may not cover preexisting conditions, such as asthma.

## Health-Care Practitioners

Fewer than 10 percent of health-care practitioners are physicians; other types of health professionals are assuming more important roles in delivering primary, or basic, health services. As a consumer, you should be aware of the range and special skills of the most common types of health-care providers.

*Physicians* A medical doctor (M.D.) trained in American medical schools usually takes at least three years of premedical college courses (with an emphasis on biology, chemistry, and physics) and then completes four (but sometimes three or five) years of medical school. The first two years of medical school are devoted to the study of human anatomy, embryology, pharmacology, and similar basic subjects. During the last two years, students work directly with physicians in hospitals. Medical students who pass a series of national board examinations then enter a one-year internship in a hospital, followed by another two to five years of residency (depending on their specialty), which leads to certification in a particular field, or specialty.

About 500,000 of the nation's 700,000 physicians are specialists or subspecialists, who focus on a specific part of the body, organ system, type of disease, or type of treatment. Traditionally, they have had greater status and earned much larger incomes than primary care physicians—family practitioners, pediatricians, and internists—who provide preventive care, regular checkups, and routine treatments of uncomplicated medical conditions. However, changes in health policy (such as increases in Medicare payments to primary care physicians) and in the delivery of services have given a more prominent role to primary care physicians. They now often function as "gatekeepers" who decide whether a patient needs to see a medical specialist.

*Nurses* A registered nurse (RN) graduates from a school of nursing approved by a state board and passes a state board examination. RNs may have a bachelor's or an associate degree and may specialize in certain areas, such as intensive care or nurse-midwifery. Nurse practitioners, RNs with advanced training and experience, may run community clinics or provide screening and preventive care at group medical practices. Some have independent practices.

Licensed practical nurses (LPNs), also called licensed vocational nurses, are licensed by the state. After graduating from state-approved schools of practical nursing, they must take a board exam. They work under the supervision of RNs or physicians. Certified nursing assistants (CNAs), nursing aides, and orderlies assist registered and practical nurses in providing services directly related to the comfort and well-being of hospitalized patients.

***Specialized and Allied-Health Practitioners*** More than 60 types of health practitioners work with physicians and nurses in providing medical services. Some, such as *occupational therapists*, have at least a bachelor's degree. Allied-health professionals may specialize in a variety of fields. *Clinical psychologists* have graduate degrees and provide a wide range of mental health services but don't prescribe medications—as do *psychiatrists. Optometrists*, trained in special schools of optometry, diagnose visual abnormalities and prescribe lenses or visual aids; however, they don't prescribe drugs, diagnose or treat eye diseases, or perform surgery—functions performed by *ophthalmologists. Podiatrists* are specially trained, licensed health-care professionals who specialize in problems of the feet.

***Dentists*** Most dental students earn a bachelor's degree and then complete two more years of training in the basic sciences and two years of clinical work before graduating with a degree of D.D.S. or D.M.D. (Doctor of Dental Surgery or Doctor of Medical Dentistry). To qualify for a license, graduates must pass both a written and a clinical examination. Dentists may work in general practice or choose a specialty, such as orthodontics (straightening teeth).

***Chiropractors*** Chiropractors hold the degree of Doctor of Chiropractic (D.C.), which signifies that they have had two years of college-level training, plus four years in a health-care school specializing in chiropractic, described earlier in this chapter.

## Health-Care Facilities

As a prospective patient, you can choose from various options: a physician's office, a clinic, an emergency room, or a hospital. Most **primary care**—also referred to as ambulatory or outpatient care—is provided by a physician in an office, emergency room, or clinic. *Secondary care* usually is provided by specialists or subspecialists in either an outpatient or inpatient (hospital) setting. *Tertiary care*, available at university-affiliated hospitals and regional referral centers, includes special procedures such as kidney dialysis, open-heart surgery, and organ transplants.

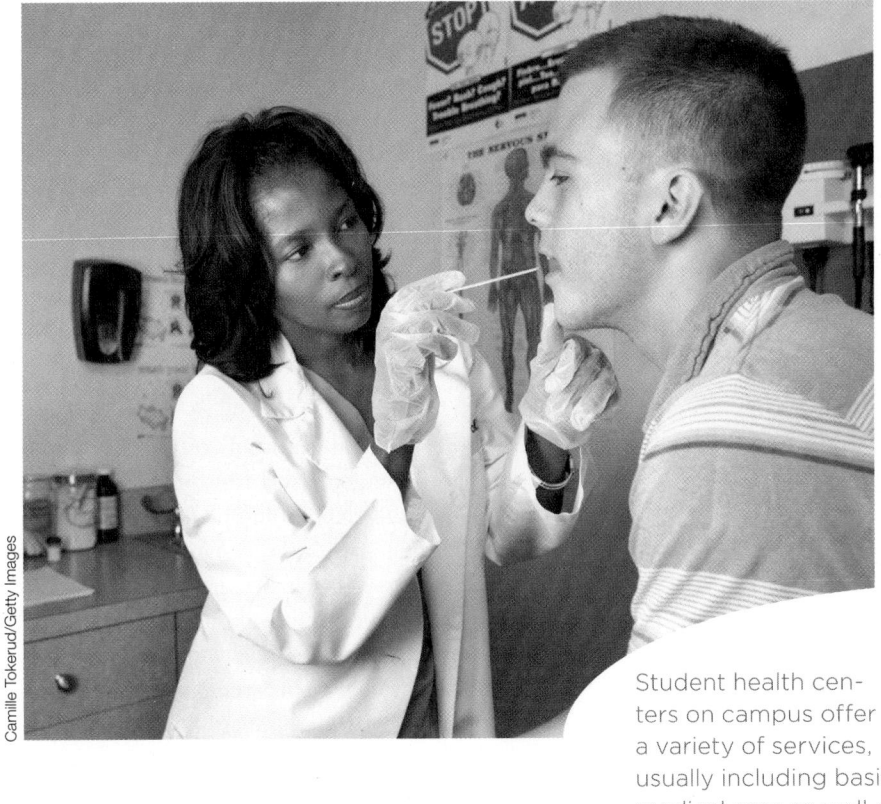

Camille Tokerud/Getty Images

Student health centers on campus offer a variety of services, usually including basic medical care as well as counseling on health-related issues.

 ***College Health Centers*** The American College Health Association estimates that 1,500 institutions of higher learning provide direct health services. Student health centers, initially developed by departments of physical education and hygiene, range in size from small dispensaries staffed by nurses to large-scale, multispecialty clinics that provide both inpatient and outpatient care and are fully accredited by the Joint Commission on Accreditation of Healthcare Organizations. Some serve only students; others provide services for faculty, staff, and family members.

On some campuses, health educators work with the student health centers to provide counseling on such topics as nutrition; tobacco, drug, and alcohol abuse; exercise and fitness; sexuality; and contraception. Some college health centers provide psychological counseling, as well as dental, pharmacy, and optometric services. Some campuses also provide sports-medicine services for student athletes. Services are paid for by various combinations of prepaid health fees, general university funds, fee-for-service charges, and health-insurance reimbursements.

**primary care** Ambulatory or outpatient care provided by a physician in an office, emergency room, or clinic.

***Outpatient Treatment Centers*** Increasingly, procedures that once required hospitalization, such as simple surgery, are being performed at outpatient centers, which may be freestanding or affiliated with a medical center. Patients have any necessary tests performed beforehand, undergo surgery or receive treatment, and return home after a few hours to recuperate. Outpatient centers can handle many common surgical procedures, including cataract removal, tonsillectomy, breast biopsy, dilation and curettage (D and C), vasectomy, and face-lifts.

Without the high overhead costs of a hospital, outpatient surgery costs run only about 30 to 50 percent of standard hospital fees. Today, 70 percent of hospitals do outpatient, or "in-and-out," surgery. To cut health-care costs, insurance companies are encouraging, or in some cases requiring, their policyholders to choose outpatient surgery. However, operations requiring prolonged general anesthesia or extensive postoperative care still must be performed on an inpatient basis.

Freestanding emergency or urgent-care centers (those not part of a hospital) claim that they deliver high-quality medical treatment with maximum convenience in minimal time. Rather than going to crowded hospital emergency rooms when they slice a finger in the kitchen, patients can go to a freestanding emergency center and receive prompt attention.

***Hospitals and Medical Centers*** Different types of hospitals offer different types of care. The most common type of hospital is the *private*, or *community*, *hospital*, which may be run on a profit or a nonprofit basis, generally contains 50 to 400 beds, and provides more personalized care than public hospitals do. The quality of care individual patients receive depends mostly on the physicians themselves. *Public hospitals* include city, county, public health service, military, and Veterans Administration hospitals. The quality of patient care depends on the overall quality of the institution.

Of the more than 6,500 hospitals nationwide, about 300 are major *academic medical centers* or *teaching hospitals*. Affiliated with medical schools, they generally provide the most up-to-date and experienced care, because staff physicians must stay current in order to teach their students. These centers, with the best equipment, researchers, and resources, offer high-technology care—at a price. The cost of treatment at all teaching hospitals averages approximately 20 percent higher than at nonteaching hospitals. At major teaching hospitals with large graduate training programs for physicians and other health providers, the costs are as much as 45 percent higher than those at nonteaching hospitals.

The Joint Commission on the Accreditation of Healthcare Organizations (JCAH) reviews all hospitals every three years. Eighty percent of hospitals qualify for JCAH accreditation. If you have to enter a hospital and your health insurance or plan allows a choice, try to find out as much as you can about the alternatives available to you:

- Talk to your physician about a hospital and why he or she recommends it.

- As a cost-cutting strategy, many hospitals have cut back on the use of registered nurses. Check with the local nursing association about the ratio of patients to nurses, and the ratio of RNs to LPNs.

- Find out room rates and charges for ancillary services, including tests, lab work, X-rays, and medications. Check with your health plan to see whether you need preapproval for any of these costs and ask what you will be expected to pay.

- Ask how many times in the past year the hospital has performed the procedure recommended for you, and what the success and complication rates have been. Ask about the hospital's nosocomial (hospital-caused) infection rate and accident rate. You also have the right to information on the number and types of malpractice claims filed against a hospital.

- If possible, go on a tour of the hospital. Does the setting seem comfortable? Is the staff courteous? Does the hospital seem clean and efficiently run?

***Emergency Services*** Hospital emergency rooms should be used only in a true emergency. Most are overwhelmed, understaffed, and underfinanced—particularly in big cities. Patients usually see a different physician each time; he or she deals with the main complaints but doesn't have time for a full examination. Extensive tests and procedures are difficult to arrange in an emergency room, and patients who don't have truly urgent problems may have to wait for a long time. Emergency-room fees are higher than those for standard office visits and are not always covered by medical insurance.

*Inpatient Care* Inpatient hospital care remains the most expensive form of health care. Health-insurance companies and health-care plans (described on pages 586–587) often demand a second opinion or make their own evaluation before approving coverage of an elective, or nonemergency, hospital admission. As another means of controlling costs, health insurers (including Medicare) may limit hospital stays or pay for hospital care on the basis of diagnostic-related groups, or DRGs. Under this system, hospitals are paid according to a patient's diagnosis—for example, a set number of dollars for every appendectomy. If the hospital can treat and discharge patients more quickly than the national average for that DRG, it makes money. On the other hand, if a patient develops unexpected complications or is slow to recover, the hospital loses money.

Because hospital stays are shorter than in the past, patients often leave "quicker and sicker"—after a shorter stay and not as far along in their recovery. Nevertheless, the benefits of shorter hospital stays, including reduced risk of infection and more rapid resumption of normal life activities, may outweigh the slightly increased risks associated with early discharge.

*Home Health Care* With hospitals discharging patients sooner, **home health care**—the provision of equipment and services to patients in the home to restore or maintain comfort, function, and health—has become a major industry. Advances in technology have made it possible for treatments once administered only in hospitals—such as kidney dialysis, chemotherapy, and traction—to be performed at home at 10 to 40 percent of the cost. The physician's house call, once considered an anachronism, has also come back in fashion. According to various surveys, the majority of primary care physicians will see patients in their homes.

Hospital discharge planners usually arrange home health care for patients who've been hospitalized. Families can also contact health aides, nurses, and other needed professionals on their own. According to the Health Insurance

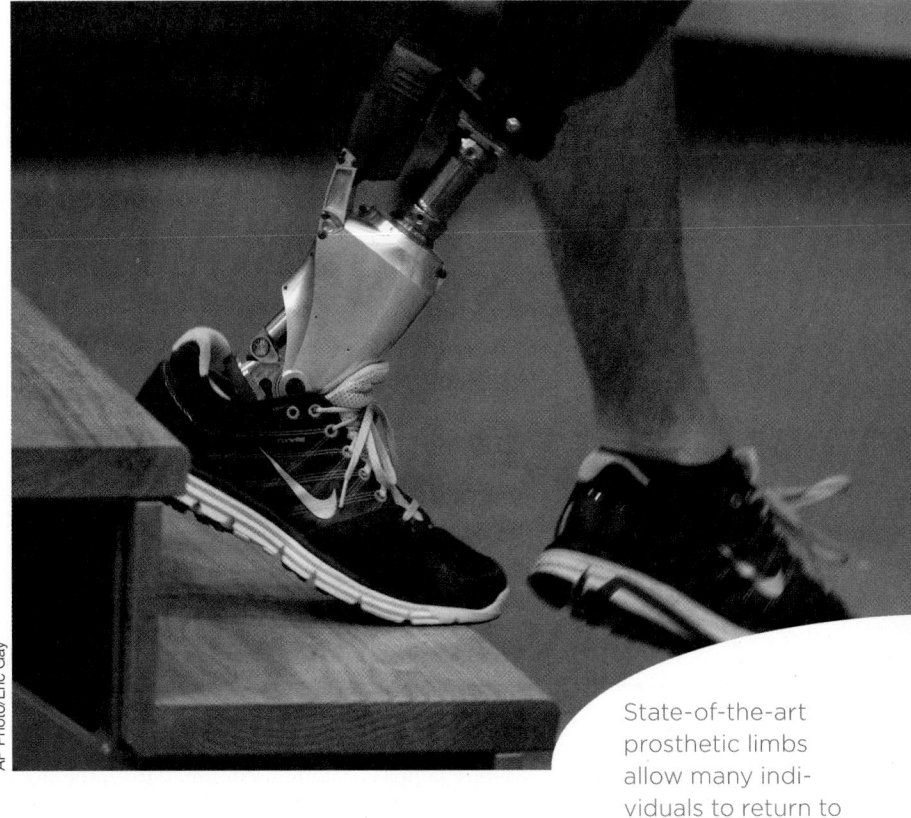

AP Photo/Eric Gay

State-of-the-art prosthetic limbs allow many individuals to return to full, active lives.

Association of America, most private insurance policies offer some coverage for these home health-care costs.

## Health-Care Financing

Health-care spending in the United States has soared to $2.2 trillion—$7,421 per man, woman, and child. Although the rate of growth in health-care spending has been declining in the last few years, it still remains higher than overall inflation.

Your health plan affects many things, including:

- **Who** will care for you (doctors and other health-care providers), and how much choice you will have.
- **What** kind of care you will receive (for example, which preventive services are covered).
- **Where** you will receive your care (which hospitals, for example).
- **When** you will receive your care (will you receive it when you need it).
- **How** you will be cared for (the quality of care you receive).
- **How much** you will pay.

**home health care** Provision of medical services and equipment to patients in the home to restore or maintain comfort, function, and health.

### Managed Care

**Managed care** has become the predominant form of health care in the United States. Managed-care organizations, which take various forms, deliver care through a network of physicians, hospitals, and other health-care professionals who agree to provide their services at fixed or discounted rates. Nine in ten physicians in the United States have contracted with managed-care companies.

Consumers in a managed-care group must follow certain procedures in advance of seeking care (for example, getting prior approval for a test or treatment) and must abide by a limit on reimbursement for certain services. Some procedures may be deemed unnecessary and not be covered at all. Patients who choose to see a physician who is not a participating member of the medical-insurance coverage group may have to pay the entire fee themselves.

Managed-care plans have been criticized for pressuring providers to "undertreat" patients—for example, sending them home from the hospital too soon or denying them costly tests or treatments. Members have complained of long waits, the need to switch primary physicians if their doctor leaves the plan, difficulty getting approval for needed services, and a sense that providers pay more attention to the bottom line than to the health needs of their patients.

As dissatisfaction with managed care has grown, consumers have demanded more choice of physicians, direct access to specialists, and the ability to go "out of network." In response to patients' complaints, many states have approved "patient protection acts" or "comprehensive consumer bills of rights."

According to the National Committee for Quality Assurance, managed-care plans have shown improvement in the delivery of care, but health-care costs continue to rise. As a result, employers are cutting back coverage and asking employees to shoulder more of the burden of their health care in the belief that consumers will seek more efficient care when they are required to pay more out of pocket.

### Health Maintenance Organizations

**Health maintenance organizations**, or **HMOs**, are managed-care plans that emphasize routine care and prevention by providing complete medical services in exchange for a predetermined monthly payment. In a *group-model HMO*, physicians provide care in offices at a clinic run by the HMO. In an *individual practice association (IPA)*, or network HMO, independent physicians provide services in their own offices. HMOs generally pay a fixed amount per patient to a physician or hospital, regardless of the type and number of services actually provided. This is called *capitation*.

Members of HMOs pay a regular, pre-set fee that usually includes diagnostic tests, routine physical exams, and vaccinations as well as treatment of illnesses. HMOs usually do not require a deductible, and copayments for medications or services are small. The primary drawback of standard HMOs is that the consumer is limited to a particular health-care facility and staff.

### Preferred Provider Organizations

In a **preferred provider organization (PPO)**, a third party—a union, an insurance company, or a self-insured business—contracts with a group of physicians and hospitals to treat members at a discount. PPO members may choose any physician within the network, and usually pay a 10 percent copayment for care within the system and a higher percentage (20 to 30 percent) for care elsewhere. PPOs generally require prior approval for expensive tests or major procedures.

A *point-of-service* (POS) plan is a PPO that permits patients to use physicians outside the network. Consumers pay the difference between the preferred provider's discounted fee and the outside physician's fee. A *gatekeeper* plan requires members to choose a primary physician, as in an HMO, who must approve all referrals to specialists.

When deciding on an HMO or PPO, use these questions as a guide:

- How many doctors can I choose from?
- Is the network made up of private or group practice physicians?
- Which doctors are accepting new patients?
- Can I change my primary care physician?
- What is the procedure for referrals to specialists?
- How easy is it to get an appointment?
- How far in advance must routine visits be scheduled?

**managed care** Health-care services and reimbursement predetermined by third-party insurers.

**health maintenance organization (HMO)** An organization that provides health services on a fixed-contract basis.

**preferred provider organization (PPO)** A group of physicians contracted to provide health care to members at a discounted price.

- What arrangements are there for handling emergency care?
- What health-care services are offered?
- Are there limits on medical tests, surgery, or other services?
- What if I want or need a special service that is not covered?
- Which hospitals are used?
- What happens if I'm out of town and need medical attention?
- What is the yearly total for monthly premiums?
- Are there any copayments? For which services and how much?

*Medicare/Medicaid*   The government, through programs like Medicare and Medicaid, funds 45 percent of total U.S. health spending. Under Medicare, the federal government pays 80 percent of most medical bills, after a deductible fee, for people over age 65. Medicare also offers options for coverage of prescription medications.

Medicaid, a federal and state insurance plan that protects people with very low or no incomes, is the chief source of coverage for the unemployed. However, many unemployed Americans don't qualify because their family incomes are above the poverty line. Publicly insured patients are more likely than those with private insurance to receive inadequate care and to experience adverse health outcomes.

*Health-Care Reform*   On March 23, 2010, President Obama signed into law comprehensive health reform legislation, the Patient Protection and Affordable Care Act, which will eventually provide insurance coverage for 32 million uninsured Americans. In the long term, the legislation will require most Americans to obtain health insurance, offer federal subsidies to lower premiums, and significantly expand eligibility for Medicaid. Because of these changes, 94 percent of legal residents not covered by Medicare will have health insurance, up from 83 percent in 2010.

If you are under 26, the law mandates that you can be covered by your parents' health policy. Some plans already extend coverage to adult dependents as long as they are full-time students. If you buy coverage on your own, you will pay less than those who are older.

Other changes include significant new restrictions on the insurance industry, new protections for consumers who already have health insurance, lower prices for certain medications, and coverage for people who have lost health insurance and can't qualify for an individual policy. Insurance companies no longer can rescind a policy once someone gets sick, nor can they impose lifetime limits on coverage.[10] Although no one yet knows the full impact the controversial legislation will have on the costs of health care, the Congressional Budget Office has said that by 2016 the new law will result in little, if any, increase in premiums for people with employer-sponsored plans.

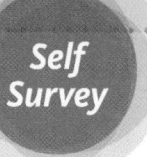

# Safeguarding Your Health

You can do more to safeguard and enhance your well-being than any health-care provider. Here are some recommendations to keep in mind. Check the ones you have used or plan to use in the future; then survey your health-care savvy in *Your Personal Wellness Guide.*

\_\_\_\_\_ **Trusting your instincts.** You know your body better than anyone else. If something is bothering you, it deserves medical attention. Don't let your health-care provider—or your health plan administrator—dismiss it without a thorough evaluation.

\_\_\_\_\_ **Doing your homework.** Go to the library or online and find authoritative articles that describe what you're experiencing. The more you know about possible causes of your symptoms, the more likely you are to be taken seriously.

\_\_\_\_\_ **Finding a good primary care physician who listens carefully and responds to your concerns.** Look for a family doctor or general internist who takes a careful history, performs a thorough exam, and listens and responds to your concerns.

\_\_\_\_\_ **Seeing your doctor regularly.** If you're in your 20s or 30s, you may not need an annual exam, but it's important to get checkups at least every two or three years so you and your doctor can get to know each other and develop a trusting, mutually respectful relationship.

\_\_\_\_\_ **Getting a second opinion.** If you are uncertain of whether to undergo treatment or which therapy is best, see another physician and listen carefully for any doubts or hesitation about what you're considering.

\_\_\_\_\_ **Seeking support.** Patient support and advocacy groups can offer emotional support, information on many common problems, and referral to knowledgeable physicians.

\_\_\_\_\_ **If your doctor cannot or will not respond to your concerns, getting another one.** Regardless of your health coverage, you have the right to replace a physician who is not meeting your health-care needs.

\_\_\_\_\_ **Speaking up.** If you don't understand, ask. If you feel that you're not being taken seriously or being treated with respect, say so. Sometimes the only difference between being a patient or becoming a victim is making sure your needs and rights are not forgotten or overlooked.

\_\_\_\_\_ **Bringing your own advocate.** If you become intimidated or anxious talking to physicians, ask a friend to accompany you, to ask questions on your behalf and to take notes.

# Are You a Savvy Health-Care Consumer?

1. You want a second opinion, but your doctor dismisses your request for other physicians' names as unnecessary. What do you do?

   a. Assume that he or she is right and you would merely be wasting time.

   b. Suspect that your physician has something to hide and immediately switch doctors.

   c. Contact your health plan and request a second opinion.

2. As soon as you enter your doctor's office, you get tongue-tied. When you try to find the words to describe what's wrong, your physician keeps interrupting. When giving advice, your doctor uses such technical language that you can't understand what it means. What do you do?

   a. Prepare better for your next appointment.

   b. Pretend that you understand what your doctor is talking about.

   c. Decide you'd be better off with someone who specializes in complementary/alternative therapies and seems less intimidating.

3. You feel like you're running on empty, tired all the time, worn to the bone. A friend suggests some herbal supplements that promise to boost energy and restore vitality. What do you do?

   a. Immediately start taking them.

   b. Say that you think herbs are for cooking.

   c. Find out as much as you can about the herbal compounds and ask your doctor if they're safe and effective.

4. Your hometown physician's office won't give you a copy of your medical records to take with you to college. What do you do?

   a. Hope you won't need them and head off without your records.

   b. Threaten to sue.

   c. Politely ask the office administrator to tell you the particular law or statute that bars you from your records.

5. Your doctor has been treating you for an infection for three weeks, and you don't seem to be getting any better. What do you do?

   a. Talk to your doctor, by phone or in person, and say, "This doesn't seem to be working. Is there anything else we can try?"

   b. Stop taking the antibiotic.

   c. Try an herbal remedy that your roommate recommends.

6. Your doctor suggests a cutting-edge treatment for your condition, but your health plan or HMO refuses to pay for it. What do you do?

   a. Try to get a loan to cover the costs.

   b. Settle for whatever treatment options are covered.

   c. Challenge your health plan.

7. You call for an appointment with your doctor and are told nothing is available for four months. What do you do?

   a. Take whatever time you can get whenever you can get it.

   b. Explain your condition to the nurse or receptionist, detailing any symptoms and pain you're experiencing.

   c. Give up and decide you don't need to see a doctor at all.

8. Even though you've been doing sit-ups faithfully, your waist still looks flabby. When you see an ad for waist-whittling liposuction, what do you do?

   a. Call for an appointment.

   b. Talk to a health-care professional about a total fitness program that may help you lose excess pounds.

   c. Carefully research the risks and costs of the procedure.

9. You have a condition that you do not want anyone to know about, including your health insurer and any potential employer. What do you do?

   a. Use a false name.

   b. Give your physician a written request for confidentiality about this condition.

   c. Seek help outside the health-care system.

10. Your doctor suggests a biopsy of a funny-looking mole that's sprouted on your nose. Rather than using a laboratory that specializes in skin analysis, your HMO requires that all samples be sent to a general lab, where results may not be as precise. What do you do?

    a. Ask your doctor to request that a specialty pathologist at the general lab perform the analysis.

    b. Hope that in your case, the general lab will do a good-enough job.

    c. Threaten to change HMOs.

*Answers*

1: c; 2: a; 3: c; 4: c; 5: a; 6: c; 7: b; 8: b and c; 9: b; 10: a

# *Making Change Happen*

## Health Assurance

You—your resources, your common sense, your choices, your feelings of self-efficacy and self-worth—determine how long and how well you live. Nothing and no one else has a greater impact on your health than you. Knowledge about health and health care is indeed power, but information alone isn't enough. Action is the key. The habits you form now, the decisions you make while in college, will affect you for decades to come. "Health Assurance" in *Labs for IPC* can equip you with the basic skills and tools you need to ensure and assure yourself of a healthy future. Here's a preview.

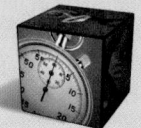

### Get Real

In this stage you evaluate your sense of self-efficacy (discussed in Chapter 1) for your health by answering True or False to ten questions, including the following:

- I can avoid getting sick by taking care of myself. _____

- Most people do not realize how much circumstances contribute to their illnesses. _____

- The only way to protect my health is to do what my doctor tells me to do. _____

You also evaluate how well you are taking care of yourself by answering 16 questions, including the following:

- Have you had your blood glucose checked? (This is a test for prediabetes and diabetes.)

- Do you check your entire body for changes in moles and other early signs of skin cancer at least once a year?

- Do you wear a helmet when you ride a bicycle or motorcycle?

Based on your answers, you rate your conscientiousness in taking care of your health on a scale of 1 (whatever happens happens) to 10 (ever vigilant).

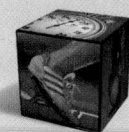

### Get Ready

You get ready for the exercises in this lab by gathering information on your health and family history and scheduling medical appointments.

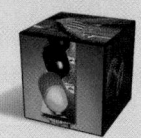

### Get Going

You create your personal health record as both an electronic file and a hard-copy file that includes basic information such as:

- Dates and results of tests and screenings.

- Major illnesses and surgeries, with dates.

- A list of your medicines, dosages, and how long you've taken them.

You also assemble your family history, including all major illnesses and tendencies toward conditions such as allergies or migraines.

Every week you select a personally relevant topic, such as high blood pressure or diabetes, based on your personal or family medical history, and research it. You also prepare for your next doctor's visit by following directions for what to ask; what to tell; what to do if you get a diagnosis; what to do if you need a lab test, an X-ray, or another kind of test; what to do if you receive a prescription for a new medicine; and how to follow up.

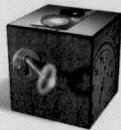

### Lock It In

To maintain your health, you give yourself a checkup every week, recording any new health problems.

You also keep up with health news, particularly any conditions that affect you or your family.

# Making This Chapter Work for You

## Review Questions

1. Periodontal disease
   a. results from poor eating habits.
   b. can lead to cardiovascular problems.
   c. in its early stage can be prevented by brushing alone.
   d. is caused by a variety of bacteria and viruses.

2. During a medical exam, your doctor will
   a. check your cardiovascular system by listening to your heart and feeling your neck arteries.
   b. check your lungs by probing for tender spots and malformations.
   c. look into your eyes to see if you have vision problems that require glasses or contact lenses.
   d. evaluate your joints by tapping on the knees and elbows.

3. Informed consent means that
   a. the patient has informed the doctor of his or her symptoms and has consented to treatment.
   b. the physician has informed the patient about the treatment to be given and has consented to administer the treatment.
   c. the patient has informed the doctor of his or her symptoms, and the doctor has consented to administer treatment.
   d. the physician has informed the patient about the treatment to be given, and the patient has consented to the treatment.

4. Patients have all the following *rights* except the right
   a. to access their medical records.
   b. to medical care that meets accepted standards of quality.
   c. to donate a body part for compensation.
   d. to leave the hospital against their physician's advice.

5. People use complementary and alternative therapies
   a. to spend less money on health care.
   b. to take an active role in their own treatment.
   c. to show their disdain for the medical establishment.
   d. to take more prescription drugs.

6. Which statement is *false*?
   a. Acupuncture has been shown to control nausea in patients after surgery.
   b. Chiropractic has been shown to relieve acute lower-back pain.
   c. People can learn to control involuntary functions through biofeedback.
   d. Naturopathy is based on the premise that like cures like.

7. Which of the following statements about the health-care system is *true*?
   a. Primary care is usually provided by specialists in a hospital.
   b. Nurses can perform some surgical procedures once they are board certified.
   c. Most hospitals in the United States are teaching hospitals and affiliated with medical schools.
   d. The length of hospital stays may be determined by a patient's diagnosis rather than the person's pace of recovery.

8. Managed care features all of the following *except*
   a. health maintenance organizations.
   b. a fee-for-service system of insurance.
   c. preferred provider organizations.
   d. limitations on reimbursement for certain health services.

9. Personalizing health care—tailoring medical care to individual patients—may include all the following *except*
   a. DNA testing.
   b. mapping a family medical history.
   c. taking into account gender and ethnic background.
   d. taking into account economic status.

10. Which of the following is *not* a common form of CAM therapy?
    a. taking multivitamins
    b. meditation
    c. massage
    d. using guided imagery

*Answers to these questions can be found on page 672.*

## Critical Thinking

1. Think about an experience you've had with a traditional medical practitioner. How did you feel during the physical examination? Did you trust the practitioner? Were you comfortable with the level of communication? Evaluate your experience and give your opinion of the value of the checkup.

2. Have you used any complementary or alternative approaches to health care? If so, were you satisfied with the results? How did your experience with the CAM therapist compare with your most recent experience with a traditional medical practitioner? Do you feel confident that you know the difference between alternative care and quackery?

3. Jocelyn has been experiencing a great deal of fatigue and frequent headaches for the past couple of months. She doesn't have health insurance and doesn't want to spend money on a doctor visit. So she did some research on the Internet about ways to relieve her symptoms and was considering taking a couple of herbal supplements that were touted as potential treatments. If she asked you for your advice, what would you tell her? Do you think that self-care is appropriate in this situation?

## Media Menu

Visit www.cengagebrain.com to access course materials and companion resources for this text that will:

- Help you evaluate your knowledge of the material.

- Allow you to prepare for exams with interactive quizzing.

- Use the CengageNOW product to develop a Personalized Learning Plan targeting resources that address areas you should study.

- Coach you through identifying target goals for behavioral change and creating and monitoring your personal change plan throughout the semester using the Behavior Change Planner available in the CengageNOW resource.

## Internet Connections

**www.health.gov/nhic/**
This excellent site, sponsored by the National Health Information Center (NHIC) of the U.S. Office of Disease Prevention and Health Promotion, is a health information referral service providing health professionals and consumers with a database of various health organizations. The site provides a searchable database, publications, and a list of toll-free numbers for health information.

**http://nccam.nih.gov**
This National Institutes of Health site features a variety of fact sheets on alternative therapies and dietary supplements, research, current news, and databases for the public as well as for practitioners.

**www.medicinenet.com**
This comprehensive site is written for the consumer by board-certified physicians and contains medical news, a

directory of procedures, a medical dictionary, a pharmacy, and first aid information. You can use the information at MedicineNet.com to prepare for a doctor visit, learn about a diagnosis, or understand a prescribed treatment or procedure.

**www.fda.gov**
In addition to providing information on regulation and legislation relating to food and drugs, the FDA website offers information on strategies for evaluating health products and services.

**www.odsw.od.nih.gov/Health_Information/Health_ Information.aspx**
Health information on dietary supplements, including vitamins and minerals.

## Key Terms

The terms listed are used on the page indicated. Definitions of the terms are in the Glossary at the end of the book.

acupuncture  578

Ayurveda  579

chiropractic  581

complementary and alternative medicine (CAM)  577

gingivitis  568

gum disease  568

health maintenance organization (HMO)  586

herbal medicine  580

holistic  577

home health care  585

homeopathy  579

informed consent  573

integrative medicine  578

managed care  586

medical history  571

naturopathy  579

Pap smear  572

periodontitis  568

plaque  568

preferred provider organization (PPO)  586

primary care  583

quackery  576

vital signs  567

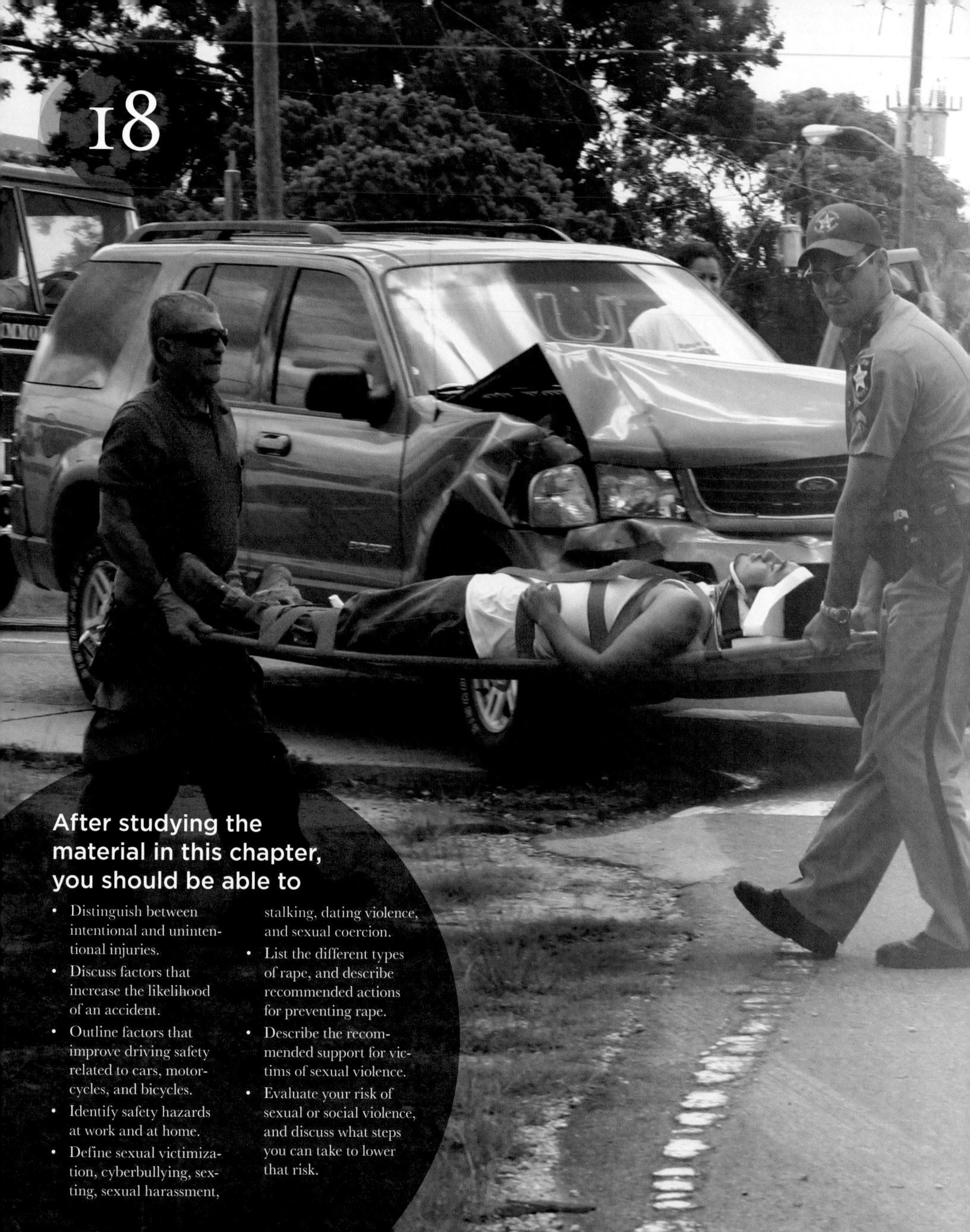

# 18

## After studying the material in this chapter, you should be able to

- Distinguish between intentional and unintentional injuries.
- Discuss factors that increase the likelihood of an accident.
- Outline factors that improve driving safety related to cars, motorcycles, and bicycles.
- Identify safety hazards at work and at home.
- Define sexual victimization, cyberbullying, sexting, sexual harassment,

stalking, dating violence, and sexual coercion.
- List the different types of rape, and describe recommended actions for preventing rape.
- Describe the recommended support for victims of sexual violence.
- Evaluate your risk of sexual or social violence, and discuss what steps you can take to lower that risk.

"This can't be happening to me!" This was the phrase that first ran through Parker's mind when the car swerved out of control. He kept repeating it to himself as he heard the sickening sound of metal hitting metal and felt a terrible crushing pain shoot up through his legs. Later at the hospital, when he woke up after surgery, it was his first thought. And all through the long months of rehabilitation, on the days when he thought life would never go back to normal, he'd try to tell himself that this too couldn't be happening to him.

# Personal Safety

Most young people think the same way. Accidents, injuries, assaults, crimes—all seem like things that happen only to other people, only in other places. But no one, regardless of how young, healthy, or strong, is immune from danger. The risks to college students include alcohol-associated injuries and illnesses, traffic accidents, and physical and sexual assaults.

Recognizing the threat of intentional and unintentional injury is the first step to ensuring your personal safety. You may think that the risk of something bad happening is simply a matter of chance, of being in the wrong place at the wrong time. That's not the case. Certain behaviors, such as using alcohol or drugs or not buckling your seat belt, greatly increase the risk of harm.

Ultimately, you have more control over your safety than anyone or anything else in your life. This chapter is a primer in self-protection that could help safeguard—perhaps even save—your

life. Included are recommendations for commonsense safety on the road, at home, and at work. This chapter also explores other serious threats to personal safety in our society: violence and sexual victimization.

## Unintentional Injury

The major threat to the lives of college students isn't illness but injury. Almost 75 percent of deaths among Americans 15 to 24 years old are caused by "unintentional injuries" (a term public health officials prefer), suicides, and homicides. Accidents, especially motor vehicle crashes, kill more college-age men and women than all other causes combined; the greatest number of lives lost to accidents is among those 25 years of age.[1]

Visit www.cengagebrain.com to access course materials for this text, including the Behavior Change Planner, interactive quizzes, tutorials, and more. See the preface on page xv for details.

Life can never be risk-free, but you can do more than anyone else to avoid unnecessary hazards and to maximize your ability to cope with potentially dangerous situations. According to research on survivors of various types of disasters, those who respond well in a crisis tend to have three underlying psychological attributes:

- They believe that they can influence events. (Refer to the discussion of self-efficacy in Chapter 1.)
- They are able to find meaningful purpose in turmoil and trauma. (See the discussion on spirituality in Chapter 2.)
- They know that they can learn from both positive and negative experiences. (See Chapter 3, "The School of Life," in *IPC*.)[2]

## Why Accidents Happen

Some of the many factors that influence an individual's risk of accident or injury are these:

- **Age.** Injury is the leading cause of death during the first four decades of life in the United States. Every day more than 2,000 children and teenagers die from an injury that could have been prevented. The five most common causes of unintentional injury are road traffic injuries, drowning, burns, falls, and poisoning. Most victims of fatal accidents are males. Feeling full of life and energy, they may take dangerous risks because they think they're invulnerable.
- **Alcohol.** An estimated 40 percent of Americans are involved in an alcohol-related accident sometime during their lives. Alcohol plays a role in about a quarter of fatal motor vehicle accidents and half of fatal motorcycle crashes.
- **Stress.** When we're tense and anxious, we all pay less attention to what we're doing. One common result is an increase in accidents. If you find yourself having a series of small mishaps or near-misses, do something to lower your stress level, rather than wait for something more harmful to happen (see Chapter 4). When facing danger, take deep, controlled, regular breaths—a technique first-responders learn in their training.
- **Situational Factors.** Some situations—such as driving on a curvy, wet road in a car

## What to Do in an Emergency

Life-threatening situations rarely happen more than once or twice in any person's life. When they do, you must think and act quickly to prevent disastrous consequences.

- **Stop, look, and listen.** Your immediate response to an emergency may be overwhelming fear and anxiety. Take several deep breaths. Start by assessing the circumstances. Look for any possible dangers to you or the victim, such as a live electrical wire or a fire. Listen for sounds, such as a cry for help or a siren. Don't attempt rescue techniques, such as cardiopulmonary resuscitation (CPR), unless you're trained.

- **Don't wait for symptoms to go away or get worse.** If you suspect that someone is having a heart attack or stroke, or has ingested something poisonous, *phone for help immediately*. A delay could jeopardize the person's life.

- **Don't move a victim.** The person may have a broken neck or back, and attempting to move him or her could cause extensive damage or even death.

- **Don't drive.** Even if the hospital is just ten minutes away, you're better off waiting for a well-equipped ambulance with trained paramedics who can deliver emergency care on the spot.

- **Don't do too much.** Often well-intentioned good Samaritans make injuries worse by trying to tie tourniquets, wash cuts, or splint broken limbs. Also, don't give an injured person anything to eat or drink.

- **At home, keep a supply of basic first-aid items in a convenient place.** Beyond the emergency number 911, make sure that telephone numbers for your doctor and neighbors are handy.

with worn tires—are so inherently dangerous that they greatly increase the odds of an accident. But even when there's greater risk, you can lower the danger: For instance, you can make sure your tires and brakes are in good condition.

- **Thrill Seeking.** To some people, activities that others might find terrifying—such as skydiving or parachute jumping—are stimulating. These thrill seekers may have lower than normal levels of the brain chemicals that regulate excitement. Because the stress of potentially hazardous sports may increase the levels of these chemicals, they feel pleasantly aroused rather than scared.

Accidents can happen to anyone at any time, so it's important that you be prepared.

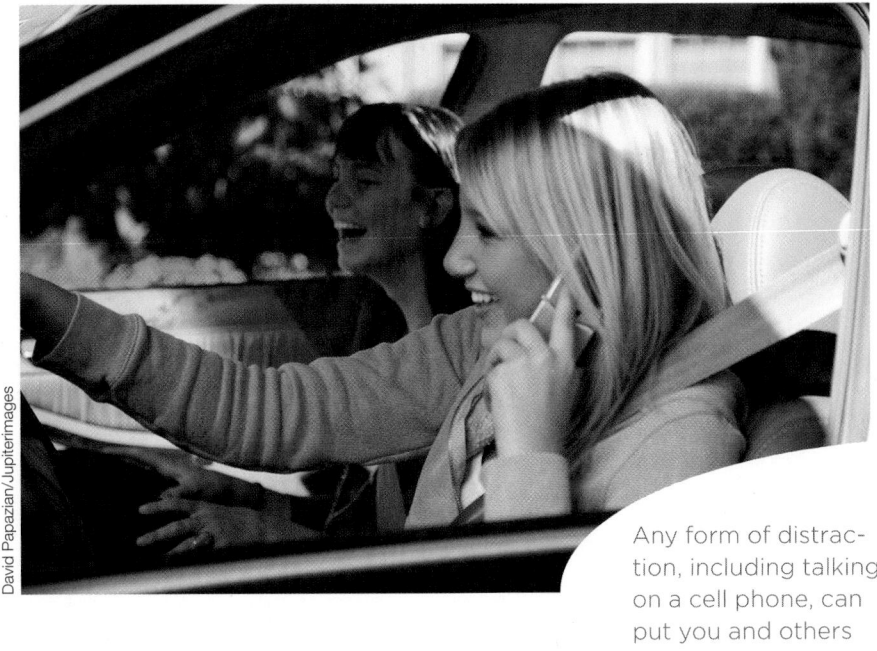

Any form of distraction, including talking on a cell phone, can put you and others at risk.

# Safety on the Road

The annual number of traffic fatalities has fallen in recent years. This decline, according to the National Highway Traffic Safety Administration, is due to several factors, including increased vehicle safety and rigorous campaigns to curtail drunk driving and encourage seat belt use.[3] Yet drivers feel less safe on the road than they did five years ago. In a recent national study by the AAA Foundation for Traffic Safety, these wary drivers blamed distractions as the biggest reasons why.[4]

An average of 117 people die every day in motor vehicle crashes—approximately one every twelve minutes. Alcohol use is a factor in about 40 percent of these crashes; speeding, in about one-third. Rollovers caused by drivers who lose control of their vehicles kill about 25 people daily. Crashes involving teen drivers result in about 25 fatalities each day.

According to a new study, most accidents involving young drivers are due to three all-too-common driving errors: failure to "scan" the environment by looking ahead and to the left and the right while driving, going too fast for road conditions (even if under the speed limit), and being distracted by something inside or outside the vehicle.[5]

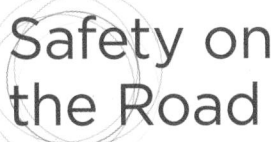 College students aren't necessarily safer drivers than others their age. According to national data, full-time college students drink and drive more often than part-time students and other young adults, but they also are more likely to wear seat belts while driving and riding in cars. How can you increase your odds of staying safe on the road? Some key factors are staying sober and alert, using your seat belt, making sure your vehicle has working air bags, and controlling road rage. The number one culprit in car crashes is distraction—whether by chatting on the phone, fiddling with a CD player, or eating.

## Avoid Distracted Driving

Distracted driving refers to any nondriving activity a person engages in that has the potential to distract him or her from the primary task of driving and increase the risk of crashing. Common distractions include talking on a cell phone; texting; eating; drinking; talking to passengers; using a navigation device; grooming; changing the radio station, CD, or mp3 player; and watching a video.

The three types of distraction are:

- Visual—taking your eyes off the road
- Manual—taking your hands off the wheel
- Cognitive—taking your mind off what you're doing

Although all distractions can endanger drivers' safety, texting is the most alarming because it involves all three types of distraction.

Distracted driving may be responsible for 20 percent of injury crashes, more than 5,000 deaths, and almost 450,000 injuries.[6] Young drivers under age 20 are most likely to become distracted, but drivers of all ages who use hand-held devices are four times as likely to get into crashes serious enough to injure themselves.

## Don't Text or Talk

Even if the cell phone is a hands-free model, using it while driving is as dangerous as driving drunk. The reason is that talking or texting while driving distracts the brain as well as the eyes—much more so than talking to another person in the vehicle.

Conversation on any type of phone disrupts a driver's attention to the visual environment, leading to what researchers call "inattention blindness," the inability to recognize objects encountered in the driver's visual field. This form of cognitive impairment may distract drivers for up to two minutes after the phone conversation has ended. Phone conversations have proven more distracting than those between drivers and passengers, who tend to slow down or stop speaking as driving conditions change and often alert drivers to potential dangers.

Using a cell phone while driving, whether it's a handheld or hands-free, delays a driver's reactions as much as having a blood alcohol concentration at the legal limit of .08 percent.[7] Many states have passed laws banning use of a cell phone to text or talk while driving. You can check the laws in your state at http://distraction.gov/state-laws/index.html.

Drivers talking on cell phones are more likely to hit, injure, and kill pedestrians.

The U.S. Department of Transportation offers these suggestions to avoid distractions while driving:

- Never text or talk on your cell phone while you're behind the wheel.

- Turn off the ringer on your phone, and set it out of reach while you're driving.

- Never eat, drink, primp, use a GPS device, read, or surf through radio stations or CD tracks while you drive.

- If you happen to call someone who is driving, suggest that the driver call you back upon arrival.[8]

## Stay Sober and Alert

The number of fatalities caused by drunk driving, particularly among young people, has dropped. The National Highway Traffic Safety Administration (NHTSA) attributes this decline to increases in the drinking age, to educational programs aimed at reducing nighttime driving by teens, to the formation of Students Against Destructive Decisions (SADD, originally called Students Against Drunk Driving) and similar groups, and to changes in state laws that lowered the legal blood-alcohol concentration level for drivers under age 21 (some states have zero tolerance blood-alcohol level [BAC] for drivers under 21). Although most drunk drivers are men, more young women are driving drunk and getting into fatal car accidents than ever before.

Falling asleep at the wheel is second only to alcohol as a cause of serious motor vehicle accidents. About half of drivers in the United States drive while drowsy. Nearly 14 million have fallen asleep at the wheel in the past year, according to the National Sleep Foundation. Men and young adults between the ages of 18 and 29 are at the highest risk for driving while drowsy or falling asleep at the wheel.

## Buckle Up

Seat belt use has reached an all-time high, with three in four Americans buckling up. States with seat belt laws have even higher rates of use: 80 percent. However, young people are less likely to use seat belts. Men between ages 19 and 29 are least likely to wear seat belts while driving or riding in a car. By official estimates, two-thirds of 15- to 20-year-olds killed in motor vehicle accidents were not wearing seat belts. Most college students buckle up in cars, but are less likely to wear helmets on bicycles, motorcycles, and skates.[9] (See Table 18.1).

Seat belts save an estimated 9,500 lives in the United States each year. When lap-shoulder belts are used properly, they reduce the risk of fatal injury to front-seat passengers by 45 percent and the risk of moderate to critical injury by 50 percent. Because an unrestrained passenger can injure others during a crash, the risk of death is lowest when all occupants wear seat belts, according to federal analysts. Seat belt use by everyone in a car may prevent about one in six deaths that might otherwise occur in a crash.

## Check for Air Bags

An air bag, either with or without a seat belt, has proved the most effective means of preventing adult death, somewhat more so for women than for men. The combination of airbags and seat belts affords the best protection against spine fractures; an airbag alone decreases this risk but to a lesser extent.

Because there is controversy over the potential hazard air bags pose to children, the American Academy of Pediatrics recommends that children be placed in the backseat, whether or not the car is equipped with a passenger air bag.

## Rein in Road Rage

The emotional outbursts known as road rage are a factor in as many as two-thirds of all fatal car crashes and one-third of nonfatal accidents, according to the NHTSA. Psychologist Arnold Nerenberg of Whittier, California, a specialist in motorway mayhem, estimates 1.78 billion episodes of road rage occur each year, resulting in more than 28,000 deaths and 1 million injuries.[10]

Some strategies for reducing road rage include the following:

* **Lower the stress in your life.** Take a few moments to breathe deeply and relax your shoulders before putting the key in the ignition.
* **Consciously decide not to let other drivers get to you.** Decide that whatever happens, it's not going to make your blood pressure go up.
* **Slow down.** If you're going five or ten miles over the speed limit, you won't have the time you need to react to anything that happens.
* **Modify bad driving habits one at a time.** If you tend to tailgate slow drivers,

Table 18.1 **Student Safety Strategies**

| | Percent (%) | | |
|---|---|---|---|
| | Never | Rarely or sometimes | Mostly or always |
| Wear a seat belt when you ride in a car | 0.4 | 3.7 | 95.8 |
| Wear a helmet when you ride a bicycle | 42.2 | 23.5 | 34.4 |
| Wear a helmet when you ride a motorcycle | 7.8 | 6.4 | 85.8 |
| Wear a helmet when you are inline skating | 55.1 | 15.2 | 29.7 |

Source: American College Health Association, *American College Health Association-National College Health Health Assessment II: Reference Group Executive Summary Spring 2010* (Linthicum, MD: American College Health Association, 2010).

spend a week driving at twice your usual following distance. If you're a habitual horn honker, silence yourself.

* **Be courteous—even if other drivers aren't.** Don't dawdle in the passing lane. Never tailgate or switch lanes without signaling. Don't use your horn or high beams unless absolutely necessary.
* **Never retaliate.** Whatever another driver does, keep your cool. Count to ten. Take a deep breath. If you yell or gesture at someone who's upset with you, the conflict may well escalate.
* **If you do something stupid, show that you're sorry.** On its website, the AAA Foundation for Traffic Safety solicited suggestions for automotive apologies. The most popular: slapping yourself on your forehead or the top of your head to indicate that you know you goofed. Such gestures can soothe a miffed motorist—and make the roads a slightly safer place for all of us.

## Cycle Safely

Per vehicle mile, motorcyclists are 35 times more likely to die in a crash than passenger car occupants. The most common motorcycle injury is head trauma, which can lead to physical disability, including paralysis and general weakness, as well as problems reading and thinking. It can also cause personality changes and psychiatric problems, such as depression, anxiety, uncontrollable mood swings, and anger. Complete recovery from head trauma can take four to six years, and the costs can be staggering. Head injury can also result in permanent disability, coma, and death.

After years of steady increases, motorcycle deaths have begun to fall.[11] Much of the credit goes to helmets, which are required in most states and dramatically reduce the risk not just of death but of head injury and spinal trauma that could otherwise lead to paralysis.[12]

More than 80 million people ride bicycles, about half for basic transportation rather than recreation. Each year, bicycle crashes kill about 700 of these individuals and send 450,000 to 587,000 to emergency rooms. Men are more likely to suffer cycling injuries. Head injury is the cause of 75 percent of bicycle crash deaths.

Only about half of cyclists wear helmets. On college campuses, even fewer students—12 to 25 percent—opt for helmets. Yet in a study of students requiring emergency care for a bicycle-related head injury, only 4 percent were wearing helmets. Among the reasons college students give for not wearing helmets are physical discomfort, cost, biking only a short distance, inconvenience, vanity, concerns about ridicule, and vision impairment associated with wearing a helmet. In a recent study, the primary determinant of whether students wear helmets is the influence of friends and family. Encouraging someone you care about to wear a helmet can make a difference.[13] (See Consumer Alert.)

# Safety at Work

The workplace is second only to the home as the most frequent site of accidents. The industries with the highest fatality rates are mining; transportation, communication, and public utilities; construction; and agriculture, forestry, and fishing. Whatever your job, find out about potential hazards and learn the proper safety regulations. (Chapter 19 discusses some potential environmental hazards at work, including noise and toxic substances.)

According to a report by the National Research Council and Institute of Medicine, annually about one million workers suffer musculoskeletal disorders of the lower back and upper extremities as a result of their "particular jobs

and working conditions—including heavy lifting, repetitive and forceful motions, and stressful working conditions." Many can be prevented.

## Computers and Your Health

As computers have become part of daily life for everyone from preschoolers to seniors, health professionals have learned a great deal about potential health problems, including repetitive motion injuries and vision-related difficulties.

**Repetitive Motion Injuries** **Repetitive motion injuries (RMIs)** have surpassed back and neck injuries as the number one claim for workers compensation injuries. Repeated motions—such as the hand and arm movements made while using a computer keyboard—all day, every day, can result in muscle and tendon strain and inflammation. About 20 percent of people with pain, tingling, or numbness in the hands may have carpal tunnel syndrome, an overuse injury caused by repetitive motions in the hands and wrists. Symptoms include pain, swelling, and numbness and weakness in the hands or the arms. If these problems are identified early, permanent damage can generally be avoided by altering the work environment and allowing for more breaks during the day.

The slope and height of a computer keyboard can affect the likelihood of repetitive motion injuries. If you work at a computer, good posture and correct positioning of the computer screen and keyboard can help prevent repetitive motion injuries, eyestrain, and back strain (Figure 18.1). Here are some additional tips:

- Place the keyboard so that your elbows are bent at a 90-degree angle and you don't have to bend your wrists to type.

- Use a chair that provides ample back support. Keep your thighs parallel to the floor and your feet on the floor. If your feet don't reach the floor, use a footrest.

- If you experience neck strain, place a document holder next to your screen so that you can view the materials more easily.

- Every 15 minutes take a 30-second break, stretch your arms, and walk around the office. Take a 15-minute break at least once every two hours.

**Vision Problems** **Computer vision syndrome** is a condition marked by tired and sore eyes, blurred vision, headaches, and neck, shoulder, and back pain. The American Optometric Association estimates that it afflicts nearly 90 percent of workers who use computers and also is common among children and students of all ages. The symptoms result from repeatedly stressing some aspect of the visual system, but they often disappear as soon as the person stops working at the computer.

Figure 18.1 **Safe Computing**
By paying attention to your posture and your computer's position, you can help protect yourself from repetitive motion injury, back strain, and eyestrain.

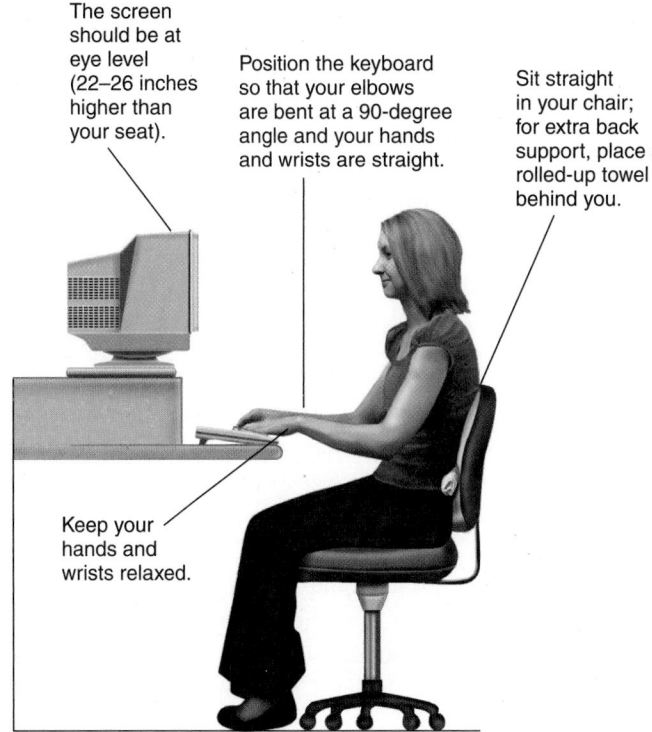

The screen should be at eye level (22–26 inches higher than your seat).

Position the keyboard so that your elbows are bent at a 90-degree angle and your hands and wrists are straight.

Sit straight in your chair; for extra back support, place a rolled-up towel behind you.

Keep your hands and wrists relaxed.

The eye focuses on a computer image differently from the way it focuses on a printed one. The pixels that appear on a computer screen, unlike printed characters, are bright in the center and gradually fade away into the background color. This makes it difficult for the eye to sustain focus. Optometrists have developed a specific method, called a **PRIO** examination, that simulates how the eye responds to pixels on a computer screen. It can determine the need and proper prescription for computer-only eyeglasses.

# Safety at Home

Every year home accidents cause nearly 25 million injuries. Over 30 percent of fatal injuries to adolescents occur in the home. According to a recent study of home safety, households tend to be safe in some ways but not in others. For instance, some homes have smoke detectors but also have exposed electrical cords. Poison poses the greatest threat, causing about 30,000 deaths every year; 93 percent are the result of

**repetitive motion injury (RMI)** Inflammation of or damage to a part of the body due to repetition of the same movements.

**computer vision syndrome** A condition caused by computer use marked by tired and sore eyes, blurred vision, headaches, and neck, shoulder, and back pain.

drug overdose, mostly from opioid pain medications.[14] Half a million children swallow poisonous materials each year. Adults may also be poisoned by mistakenly taking someone else's prescription drugs or taking medicines in the dark and swallowing the wrong one. In case of poisoning, call 911 or 1-800-222-1222 for help 24 hours every day.

Falls of all kinds are the second leading cause of death from unintentional injury in the United States. High heels or worn footgear, poor lighting, slippery or uneven walkways, broken stairs and handrails, loose or worn rugs, and objects left where people walk all increase the likelihood of a slip.

You can prevent fires by making sure that the three ingredients of fire—fuel, a heat source, and oxygen—don't get a chance to mix. Almost anything can act as fuel for fire, including paper, wood, and flammable liquids such as oils, gasoline, and some paints. A heat source can be a spark from a lighted match, a pilot light, or an electrical wire. Oxygen is necessary for the chemical reaction between the fuel and heat source that causes combustion.

If a fire starts and it's small, you may be able to put it out with a portable fire extinguisher before it spreads. However, if the fire does get out of control, you might have only two to five minutes to get out of the house or building alive. A fire-escape plan can save time and lives. Sketch a plan of your house, apartment building, dormitory, or fraternity or sorority house. Identify two ways out of each room or apartment. Make sure everyone is familiar with these escape routes. Designate an area outside where all family members or dorm residents should meet after escaping from a fire.

 In a national survey, the majority of colleges had at least one dorm without a sprinkler system. If a fire breaks out in your dorm room, get out as quickly as possible, but don't run. Before opening a room door, place your hand on it. If it's hot, don't open it. If the door feels cool, open it slightly to check for smoke; if there's none, leave by your planned escape route. If you're on an upper floor and your escape routes are blocked, open a window (top and bottom, if possible) and wait or signal from the window for help. Never try to use an elevator in a fire.

# Which Gender Is at Greater Risk?

Just like illness, injury doesn't discriminate against either gender. Both men and women can find themselves in harm's way—but for different reasons. Here are some gender differences in vulnerability:

- Men are ten times more likely to die of an occupational injury than women.

- Males are most often the victims and the perpetrators of homicides in the United States. In about 68 percent of cases reported by the Bureau of Justice Statistics, both the offender and the victim were male.

- Overall, men are 3.6 times more likely than women to be murdered and 9 times more likely to commit murder. Both men and women are more likely to kill or attempt to kill male victims than female victims.

- Men are more likely than women to be assaulted as adults.

- The genders also differ in their fear of crime. In a recent study, women—but not men—tended to become less apprehensive and to feel less vulnerable as they became older. Increased income correlated with higher levels of fear for men but lower levels for women.[15]

# Living in a Dangerous World

The World Health Organization (WHO) defines violence as "the intentional use of physical force or power, threatened or actual, against oneself, another person, or a group or community, that either results in, or has a high likelihood of resulting in, injury, death, psychological harm, maldevelopment, or deprivation." A simpler way of putting it is that "violence is anything you wouldn't want someone to do to you." Although anyone is capable of violent crime, being aware of certain behaviors in a person may keep you safer.

After more than a decade of declining rates, violent crime in the United States seems to be increasing. Guns are the second-leading cause of injury-related death in the United States after car accidents. About 260 Americans are injured by firearms every day; one-third die from their wounds. Gun violence annually takes the lives of nearly 30,000 Americans. The cost of hospital treatment for the victims of violence (including attempted suicide and murder, fights, rapes, and assaults) exceeds $2.3 billion a year.[16]

Although men commit nine times more violent crimes than women, the rates are getting closer. Individuals with mental illness are somewhat more likely to become violent and to be the victims of violent crimes.

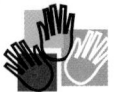 There are ethnic and racial differences in patterns of violence. African Americans are at greater risk of victimization by violent crime than whites or persons of other racial groupings. Hispanics are at greater risk of violent victimization than non-Hispanics. There is little difference between white women and nonwhite women in rape, physical assault, or stalking. Native American and Alaska Native women are significantly more likely than white women or African American women to report being raped. Mixed-race women also have a significantly higher incidence of rape than white women. Native American and Alaska Native men report significantly more physical assaults than Asian and Pacific Islander men.

# Crime and Violence on Campus

 Most college students feel safe on campus, especially in the day, but less so at night and in the community surrounding their school.[17] (See How Do You Compare?) According to the Bureau of Justice, college students are victims of almost half a million violent crimes a year, including assault, robbery, sexual assault, and rape. While this number may seem high, the overall violent crime rate has dropped from 88 to 41 victimizations per 1,000 students in the last decade. You can take steps to lower your risk—at little or no financial cost. (See Health on a Budget, p. 604.)

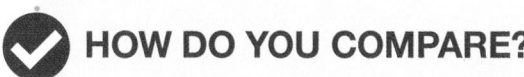
College students ages 18 to 24 are less likely to be victims of violent crime, including robbery and assault, than nonstudents of the same age. More than half (58 percent) of crimes against students are committed by strangers. More than nine in ten occur off campus, most often in an open area or street, on public transportation, in a place of business, or at a private home. In about two-thirds of the crimes, no weapon is involved. Most off-campus crimes occur at night, while on-campus crimes are more frequent in the day.

Male college students are twice as likely to be victims of overall violence as female students. White undergraduates have higher rates of violent victimization than students of other races. Simple assault accounts for two-thirds of violent crimes against students; sexual assault or rape accounts for around 6 percent.

Substance use increases the risk of sexual and physical victimization of college students. College women are more likely to report sexual violence associated with most forms of substance use, while college men are more likely to be victims of physical violence.

About three in four campus crimes are never reported to the police. The main reasons

# A Do-It-Yourself Security Program

These simple, no-cost steps can provide greater protection than an elaborate alarm system. The key is to employ them every day and never let your guard down.

- **Avoid walking alone in the evening or night.** Take advantage of campus shuttle or escort services. If none are available, stick to well-lit routes.

- **Train yourself to be aware of your surroundings and the people around you.** Visualize potential exit routes in case of an emergency.

- **Always carry your cell phone and enough money so that you can take a taxi home if you find yourself in a dicey situation.**

- **Program the campus security number into your cell phone's speed dial numbers so you can access it with a single key stroke.**

- **Always lock your doors and any first- and second-floor windows at night.** Don't compromise your safety for a roommate or friend who asks you to leave the door unlocked.

- **Never leave your ID, wallet, checkbook, jewelry, cameras, and other valuables in open view.**

- **Be careful what information and which photographs you post online on social networking sites.** You never know who will see them.

- **Never drive when you're drowsy or under the influence of alcohol or drugs.** Always wear a seat belt. Never give a ride to hitchhikers or anyone you don't know.

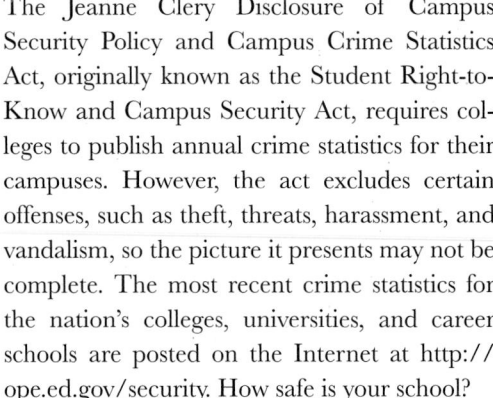

The Jeanne Clery Disclosure of Campus Security Policy and Campus Crime Statistics Act, originally known as the Student Right-to-Know and Campus Security Act, requires colleges to publish annual crime statistics for their campuses. However, the act excludes certain offenses, such as theft, threats, harassment, and vandalism, so the picture it presents may not be complete. The most recent crime statistics for the nation's colleges, universities, and career schools are posted on the Internet at http://ope.ed.gov/security. How safe is your school?

Campuses have implemented dozens of programs to halt violence, and many have proven effective. One school used a poster campaign to raise awareness of dating violence. Others have designed sexual violence prevention programs for members of fraternities, sororities, and intercollegiate athletic teams. Many have established codes of conduct barring the use of alcohol and drugs, fighting, and sexual harassment, and have instituted policies requiring suspension or expulsion for students who violate this code.[18] Some schools are experimenting with social media messages to increase awareness of and prevent problems such as violence against women.[19]

## Hazing

**Hazing** refers to any activity that humiliates, degrades, or poses a risk of emotional or physical harm for the sake of joining a group or maintaining full status in that group. This behavior may occur in fraternities and sororities, athletic teams, or other campus organizations. Its forms include verbal ridicule and abuse, forced consumption of alcohol or ingestion of vile substances, sexual violation, sleep deprivation, paddling, beating, burning, or branding.

## Hate or Bias Crimes

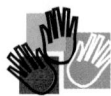

Recent years have seen the emergence of violent crimes motivated by hatred of a particular person's (or group of persons') race, ethnicity, religion, sexual orientation, or political values.

More than half of hate or bias crimes on campus are motivated by race. Twenty percent of students, faculty, and staff surveyed fear for their physical safety because of their sexual

students give for not reporting crimes are that they are too minor or private or they are not certain that the action was a crime. Individuals also may be too ashamed or emotionally overwhelmed to contact authorities.

According to researchers, only 2 percent of victimized college women report crimes to the police. The most frequent reason for not reporting sexual and physical incidents is that they didn't seem serious enough. However, women who were sexually victimized also felt ashamed, feared that they would be held responsible, or didn't want anyone to know what happened. Nonwhite women were significantly more likely than white women to say that they did not report an incident to the police because they thought they would be blamed or because they did not want the police involved.

**hazing** Any activity that humiliates, degrades, or poses a risk of emotional or physical harm for the sake of joining a group or maintaining full status in that group.

orientation or gender identity. These crimes can take the form of graffiti; verbal slurs; bombings; threatening notes, e-mails, or phone calls; and physical attacks. They often generate fear and intimidation in large groups of students, undermining health, academic work, and the basic security of a campus.

## Shootings, Murders, and Assaults

Shootings of students and faculty have occurred at several campuses in recent years. However, like murder and manslaughter, they remain uncommon. There are about 3,000 aggravated assaults—an attack with a weapon or one that causes serious injury—each year. Weapons were involved in about a third of violent college crimes. Firearms were used in 9 percent of all violent crimes and 8 percent of assaults.

Campus shootings have a psychological impact on students on other campuses as well. In a study of students at a school in the same geographical area, the most common reaction was greater caution in social settings.

The American College Health Association has recommended various strategies to keep campuses safe, including:

- Enforcing codes of conduct.
- Tougher sanctions, including expulsion, for serious misconduct.
- Zero-tolerance policies for campus violence.
- Building a sense of community.
- Screening out students who pose a real threat.
- Warning students about criminal activity at orientation, through the campus newspaper, in residence halls, and through campus Internet communications devices.

## Consequences of Campus Violence

The toll of crime and violence at colleges and universities is high. Violence can cripple as well as claim lives. Moreover, the victims of violent crime often suffer lasting psychological and emotional effects. Some victims take a leave of absence or transfer to another school. Those who remain in school may have problems

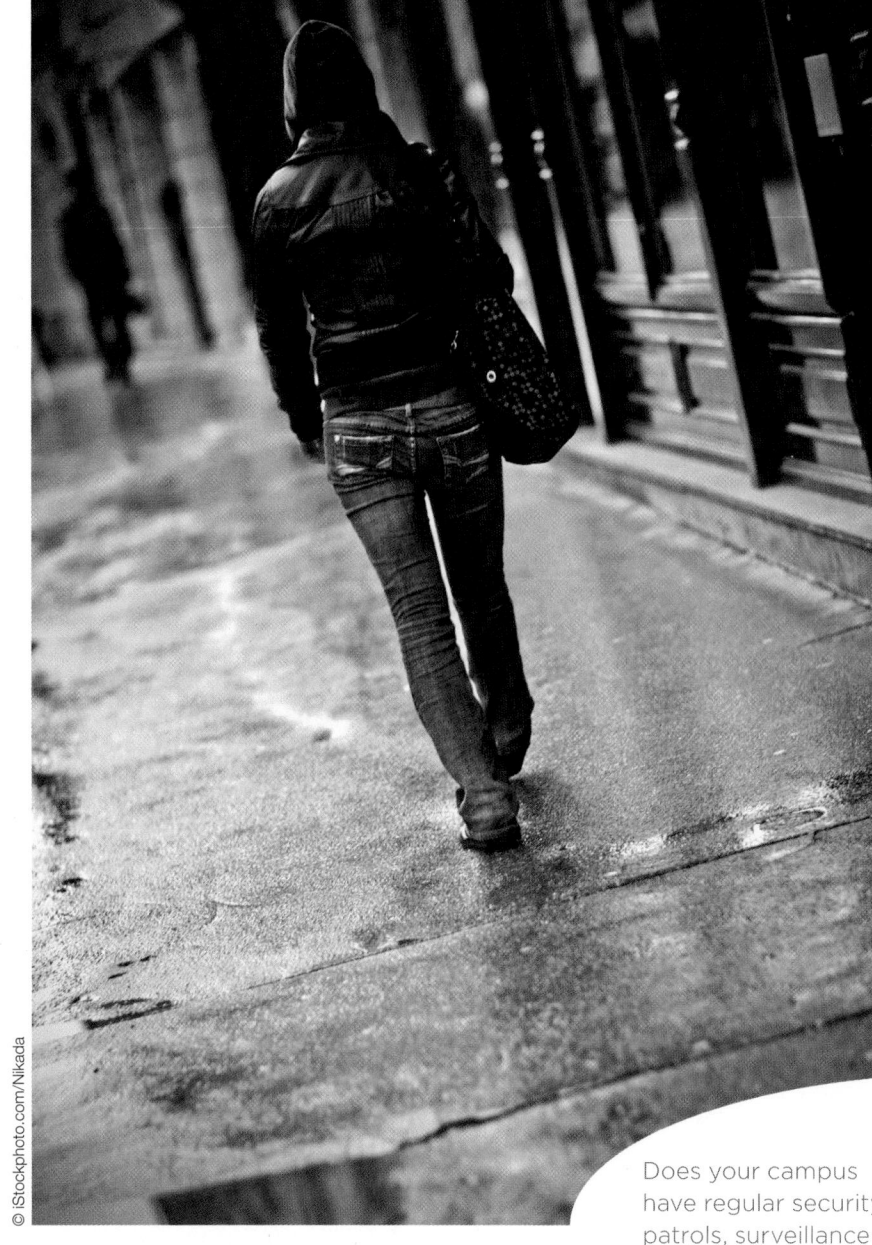

© iStockphoto.com/Nikada

Does your campus have regular security patrols, surveillance cameras, or late-night escorts? Have you taken advantage of these services?

concentrating, studying, and attending classes, and may avoid academic and social activities. Some develop clinical symptoms that affect their mental and physical health (see Chapter 2).

# Sexual Victimization and Violence

Sexual victimization refers to any situation in which a person is deprived of free choice and

## Campus Violence

Violence can intrude in our world, including colleges and universities. After accessing Global Health Watch, click on "Preventing Injury and Violence" and then on "Campus Violence." Scan the headlines and select a recent report either on a problem related to violence in a school setting or on the steps being taken to prevent such occurrences. Write a summary in your online journal.

**sexual harassment** Uninvited and unwanted sexual attention.

forced to comply with sexual acts. This is not only a woman's issue; in fact, men also are victimized. In recent years, researchers have come to view acts of sexual victimization along a continuum, ranging from street hassling, stalking, and obscene telephone calls to rape, battering, and incest. Sexual violence has its roots in social attitudes and beliefs that demean women and condone aggression. According to international research, much sexual violence takes place within families, marriage, and dating relationships. In many settings, rape is a culturally approved strategy to control and discipline women. In these places, laws and policies to improve women's status are critical to ending sexual coercion.

## Cyberbullying and Sexting

The Internet, which brought friends and fans together to share common interests, also has given rise to new forms of victimization. One is cyberbullying, defined as "an aggressive, intentional act carried out by a group or individual using electronic forms of contact repeatedly and over time against a victim who cannot easily defend him- or herself."[20] In some studies as many as 20 percent of adolescents and young adults have reported being cybervictims or cyberbullies; some describe themselves as both.

Both cyberbullies and their victims are likely to experience psychiatric and psychosomatic problems, according to a study of more than 2,000 adolescents. One in four of those who had been victimized reported fearing for his or her safety.[21]

In focus groups on one university campus, male and female undergraduates agreed that cyberbullying is easier than face-to-face bullying because it is less personal and more indirect. Many students minimized it as a problem and argued that simply using technology—signing up for Facebook, for instance—qualifies as consent. However, the students also acknowledged that cyberbullying can have serious consequences.[22]

Many teens engage in "sexting," the sending of nude or partially nude photos and sexually explicit messages via cell phones. A photo that may be sent as a joke or intended for only one person can quickly make its way to countless viewers. As discussed in Chapter 5, such violations of privacy can be emotionally devastating.

In some states they also are illegal, and tough new laws are cracking down on cyberbullying and the transmission of sexual materials.

## Sexual Harassment

All forms of **sexual harassment** or unwanted sexual attention—from the display of pornographic photos to the use of sexual obscenities to a demand for sex by anyone in a position of power or authority—are illegal.

 Nearly two-thirds of students experience sexual harassment at some point during college, including nearly one-third of first-year students. Nearly one-third of students say they have experienced physical harassment, such as being touched, grabbed, or pinched in a sexual way. Sexual comments and jokes are the most common form of harassment. More than half of female students and nearly half of male students say they have experienced this type of harassment. Lesbian, gay, bisexual, and transgender (LGBT) students, as well as those with physical disabilities such as deafness, are more likely than other students to be sexually harassed.[23]

Sexual harassment takes an especially heavy toll on female students, who often feel upset, self-conscious, embarrassed, or angry. Men are much less likely to admit to being very or somewhat upset. A third of harassed college women say they felt afraid; one-fifth say they were disappointed in their college experience as a result of sexual harassment.

 About half of college men and a third of women admit that they have sexually harassed someone on campus. Private college students are more likely than their public college peers to have ever done so. Students at large schools (population of 10,000 or more) are more likely than students at small schools with fewer than 5,000 students to say they have experienced sexual harassment. The most common rationale for harassment is "I thought it was funny." Harassment occurs in dorms or student housing as well as outside on campus grounds and in classrooms or lecture halls.

If you encounter sexual harassment as a student, report it to the department chair or dean. If you don't receive an adequate response to your complaint, talk with the campus representatives who handle matters involving affirmative action or civil rights. Federal guidelines prevent any discrimination against you in terms of grades or the loss of a job or scholarship if you report harassment. Schools that do not take measures to remedy harassment could lose federal funds.

## Stalking

The "willful, repeated, and malicious following, harassing, or threatening of another person," as **stalking** is defined, is common on college campuses—perhaps more so than in the general population. Most college women know their stalkers. About half are acquaintances; a high percentage of these are classmates, boyfriends, or ex-boyfriends. In one study, about half of the women said they had not sought help from anyone. Those who did seek assistance turned to friends, parents, residence hall advisors, or police.[24]

 College students may be targeted for several reasons. Simply because they are young and still learning how to manage complex social relationships, some individuals may not recognize their behavior as stalking or even as disturbing. In addition, college students tend to live close to each other and to have flexible schedules and large amounts of unsupervised time.

Stalking is not a benign behavior and can result in emotional or psychological distress, physical harm, or sexual assault. By some estimates, 10 percent of stalking incidents result in forced or attempted sexual contact. The most common consequence is psychological, with victims reporting emotional or psychological distress.

## Dating Violence

Actual or threatened physical or sexual violence or psychological and emotional abuse of a current or former dating partner is a form of violence. It can occur between heterosexual, homosexual, or bisexual partners.

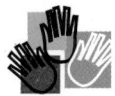  Violence in dating relationships is common on campuses around the world. In the International Dating Violence study, which surveyed 15,927 college students in 22 locations, 30 percent had physically assaulted a dating partner in the previous 12 months. The proportion of students who reported being the victims of a physical assault ranged from 14 to 39 percent. India, Korea, New Zealand, Germany, Greece, Russia, the United Kingdom, the United States, and Canada had consistently high rates of assault, injury, and sexual coercion, while Israel, Australia, Belgium, Sweden, and Switzerland had lower rates.[25]

In the United States, one in seven college student couples reported at least one episode of male-to-female violence in the preceding 12 months. In dating relationships, 39 percent of college women and 33 percent of men reported being a victim of violence from their dating partners. Young women ages 15 to 24 are at greater risk if they report that a partner tried to "control" them, for instance, by preventing them from seeing friends.[26]

In research on students at American universities, a larger percentage of women than men assault a dating partner by, for example, throwing something that could hurt at a partner, pushing, shoving, grabbing, or slapping. However, the rates of perpetrating an assault resulting in an injury, as well as being a victim of an assault that resulted in an injury, are overwhelmingly higher for males.

 About 20 percent of students say they coerced a partner into sex in the previous 12 months, while 24 percent of students report being victims of sexual coercion. Rates of sexual coercion—for example, making a partner have sex without a condom or insisting on sex when a partner did not want to—were higher for men than women.

In addition to physical injury, victims of violence in their intimate relationships—male as well as female—are at increased risk of posttraumatic stress disorder (PTSD), depression, and suicidal thoughts.[27] Women exposed to acute or previous domestic violence are more likely than other women to have made suicide attempts. In general, suicide attempt rates among battered women are high, ranging from 20 to 26 percent.

## Nonvolitional Sex and Sexual Coercion

**Nonvolitional sex** is sexual behavior that violates a person's right to choose when and with whom to have sex and what sexual behaviors

**stalking** The willful, repeated, and malicious following of another person.

**nonvolitional sex** Sexual behavior that violates a person's right to choose when and with whom to have sex and what sexual behaviors to engage in.

to engage in. The more extreme forms of this behavior include sexual coercion or forced sex, rape, childhood sexual abuse, and violence against people with nonconventional sexual identities. Other forms, such as engaging in sex to keep one's partner or to pass as heterosexual, are so common that many think of them as normal. In a recent study, 32 percent of students reported being victims of sexual coercion, and 78 percent reported having verbally aggressive partners.[28]

**Sexual coercion** can take many forms, including exerting peer pressure, taking advantage of one's desire for popularity, threatening an end to a relationship, getting someone intoxicated, stimulating a partner against his or her wishes, or insinuating an obligation based on the time or money one has expended. Men may feel that they need to live up to the sexual stereotype of taking advantage of every opportunity for sex. Women are far more likely than men to encounter physical force. Alcohol use increases a woman's risk.[29]

 Many schools are alerting incoming female students about what researchers call "the red zone," a period of time early in one's first undergraduate year when women are at particularly high risk for unwanted sexual experiences. One university defines the red zone more precisely as "the time period between freshman move-in and fall break wherein there is a particularly high risk of victimization." Unwanted touching and attempted intercourse are the most common behaviors reported, although researchers also have documented sexual assaults and rapes. Women who had a nonconsensual sexual experience while drinking prior to college are at higher risk.[30]

## Rape

**Rape** refers to sexual intercourse with an unconsenting partner under actual or threatened force. Sexual intercourse between a male over the age of 16 and a female under the age of consent (which ranges from 12 to 21 in different states) is called *statutory rape*. In *acquaintance rape*, or *date rape*, the victim knows the rapist. In *stranger rape*, the rapist is an unknown assailant. Both acquaintance and stranger rapes are serious crimes that can have a devastating impact on their victims.

All states now recognize as rape the assault of a victim who is incapable of giving consent because of alcohol or other substances. However, many women who experience a sexual encounter that meets this legal definition do not label it as a rape or even as sexual victimization. Compared with stranger rapes, these assaults are typically less violent and involve less force by the assailant, less resistance by the victim, and less injury to her. Yet women who do not acknowledge an unwanted sexual experience as rape nonetheless suffer psychological consequences, including distress and other trauma symptoms.[31]

 Over the course of five years (the national average for a college career), including summers and vacations, one of every four or five female students is raped. In a single academic year, 3 percent of coeds are raped—35 rapes for every 1,000 women. According to the U.S. Department of Justice, a campus with 6,000 coeds averages one rape a day every day for the entire school year.[32]

In nine surveys of male university students, between 3 and 6 percent had been raped by other men; up to 25 percent had been sexually assaulted. Like female rape victims, male victims suffer long-term psychological problems and physical injuries, and are at risk of contracting a sexually transmitted infection.

For many years, the victims of rape were blamed for doing something to bring on the attack. However, researchers have shown that women are raped because they encounter sexually aggressive men, not because they look or act a certain way. Although no woman is immune to attack, many rape victims are children or adolescents.

Women who successfully escape rape attempts do so by resisting verbally and physically, usually by yelling and fleeing. Women who use forceful verbal or physical resistance (screaming, hitting, kicking, biting, and running) are more likely to avoid rape than women who try pleading, crying, or offering no resistance.

***Types of Rape*** Although rape has long been viewed as an act of violence and domination, recent studies indicate that not all rapes fit into a single pattern. Within the broad category of rape are specific, but not mutually exclusive, subcategories of the crime, including anger

**sexual coercion** Sexual activity forced upon a person by the exertion of psychological pressure by another person.

**rape** Sexual penetration of a female or a male by means of intimidation, force, or fraud.

rape, power rape, sadistic rape, gang rape, and sexual gratification rape.

*Anger* rape, usually on a total stranger, is motivated by hatred and a desire for revenge for the rejection the rapist feels he's suffered from women. Anger rapists often harbor long-standing hostility toward women, use far more physical violence than is needed for submission, and usually don't find the rape sexually gratifying.

*Power* rape is a generally premeditated attack motivated by a desire to dominate and control another person. Power rapists, unable to deal with stress and their sense of failure, may rape to regain a sense of power. They use only as much force as needed to make their victims submit and may find the rape sexually gratifying, even though that's not their primary motive.

*Sadistic* rape is a premeditated assault that often involves bondage, torture, or sexual abuse. Sadistic rapists find power and anger sexually arousing and may subject victims to rituals of humiliation or torture. They're often preoccupied with violent pornography; their motives are more complex and difficult to understand than those of other types of rapists.

*Gang* rape involves three or more rapists. Men in close groups that drink and party together—such as fraternities or athletic teams—are more likely to participate in such assaults. The reasons may go beyond aggression and sexual gratification to the excitement and camaraderie the men feel while sharing the experience.

*Sexual gratification* rape is usually an impulsive attack by someone willing to use physical coercion for the sake of sex. These rapists generally use no more force than needed to get a partner to submit and may stop the attack if it becomes clear they'll have to use extreme violence to overcome resistance. Many acquaintance rapes fit into this category.

**Acquaintance, or Date, Rape** According to data from the U.S. Bureau of Justice, nine in ten reported rapes and sexual assaults in the United States involve a single offender with whom the victim had a prior relationship.

Both women and men report having been forced into sexual activity by someone they know. Many college students are in the age group most likely to face this threat: women ages 16 to 25 and men under 25. Women are most vulnerable

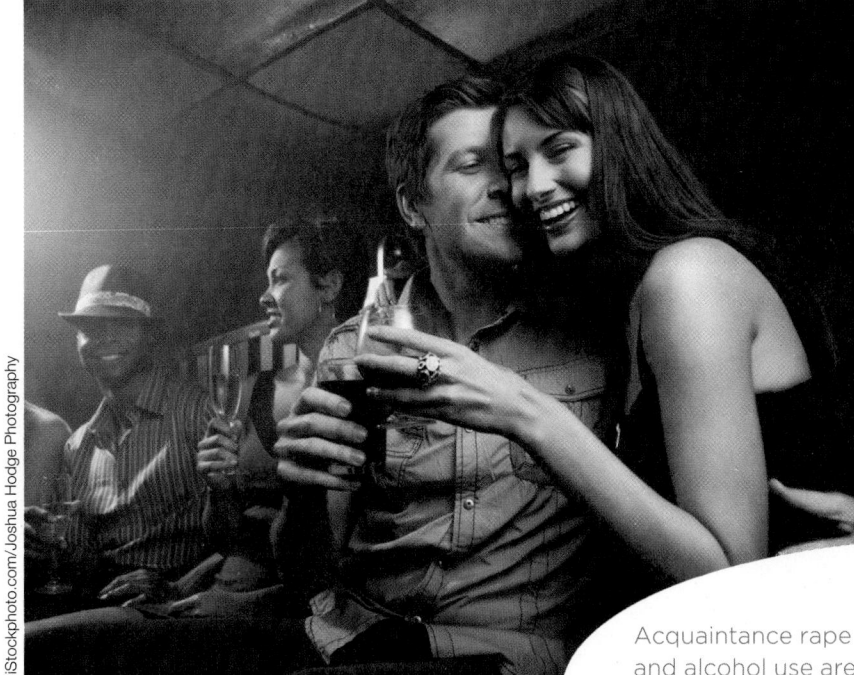

© iStockphoto.com/Joshua Hodge Photography

Acquaintance rape and alcohol use are very closely linked. Both men and women may find their judgment impaired or their communications unclear as a result of drinking.

and men are most likely to commit assaults during their senior year of high school and their first year of college.

Women who describe incidents of sexual coercion that meet the legal definition of rape often don't label it as such. They may have a preconceived notion that true rape consists of a blitz-like attack by a stranger. Or they may blame themselves for getting into a situation in which they couldn't escape. They may feel some genuine concern for others who would be devastated if they knew the truth (for example, if the rapist was the brother of a good friend or the son of a neighbor).

The same factors that lead to other forms of sexual victimization can set the stage for date rape. Socialization into an aggressive role, acceptance of rape myths, and a view that force is justified in certain situations increase the likelihood of a man's committing date rape. (See "Health in Action: How to Avoid Date Rape.") Other factors can also play a role, including the following:

- **Personality and early sexual experiences.** Certain factors may predispose individuals to sexual aggression, including first sexual experience at a very young age, earlier and more frequent than usual childhood sexual experiences (both forced and voluntary), hostility toward women, irresponsibility, lack of social consciousness, and a need for dominance over sexual partners.

- **Situational variables (what happens during the date).** Men who initiate a date, pay all expenses, and provide transportation are more likely to be sexually aggressive, perhaps because they feel they can call all the shots.

- **Rape myths.** As several studies have confirmed, college men hold more rape-tolerant attitudes than do college women. For example, college men are significantly more likely than college women to agree with statements such as, "Some women ask to be raped and may enjoy it" and "If a woman says 'no' to having sex, she means 'maybe' or even 'yes.'"[33]

  Some social groups, such as fraternities and athletic teams, may encourage the use of alcohol; reinforce stereotypes about masculinity; and emphasize violence, force, and competition. The group's shared values, including an acceptance of sexual coercion, may keep individuals from questioning their behavior. They also may keep bystanders from intervening to prevent a potential rape.[34]

- **Drinking.** Alcohol use is one of the strongest predictors of acquaintance rape. Men who've been drinking may not react to subtle signals, may misinterpret a woman's behavior as a come-on, and may feel more sexually aroused. At the same time, drinking may impair a woman's ability to effectively communicate her wishes and to cope with a man's aggressiveness.[35]

- **Date rape drugs.** Drugs such as Rohypnol (flunitrazepam) and GHB (gamma hydroxybutyrate) have been implicated in cases of acquaintance, or date, rape. Since both drugs are odorless and tasteless, victims have no way of knowing their drink has been tampered with. The subsequent loss of memory leaves victims with no explanation for where they've been or what's happened.

  Rohypnol—which can cause impaired motor skills and judgment, lack of inhibitions, dizziness, confusion, lethargy, very low blood pressure, coma, and death—has been outlawed in the United States. Deaths also have been attributed to GHB overdoses.

 College women often aren't aware of the possibility that their drinks may be tampered with or that they may have been given a date-rape drug. In one study, female undergraduates did not perceive any risk in leaving their drinks unattended. Even if they started feeling ill at a party, many did not suspect that a date-rape drug could be the cause. The victims of prior assaults were slower at picking up on and responding to potentially dangerous dating situations, possibly because they feel that personal risks are unavoidable and beyond their control.

- **Gender differences in interpreting sexual cues.** In research comparing college men and women, the men typically overestimated the woman's sexual availability and interest, seeing friendliness, revealing clothing, and attractiveness as deliberately seductive. In one study of date rape, the men reported feeling "led on," in part because their female partners seemed to be dressed more suggestively than usual.

*Stranger Rape*  Rape prevention consists primarily of making it as difficult as possible for a rapist to make you his victim:

- **Don't advertise that you're a woman living alone.** Use initials on your mailbox. Install and use secure locks on doors and windows, changing door locks after losing keys or moving into a new residence.

- **Don't open your door to strangers.** If a repairman or public official is at your door, ask him to identify himself and call his office to verify that he is a reputable person on legitimate business.

- **Lock your car when it is parked, and drive with locked car doors.** Should your car break down, attach a white cloth to the antenna and lock yourself in. If someone other than a uniformed officer stops to offer help, ask this person to call the police or a garage but do not open your locked car door.

- **Avoid dark and deserted areas,** and be aware of the surroundings where you're walking. Should a driver ask for directions when you're a pedestrian, avoid approaching his car. Instead, call out your reply from a safe distance.

- **Have house or car keys in hand as you approach the door.** Check the back seat before getting into your car.
- **Carry a device for making a loud noise,** like a whistle or, even better, a pint-sized compressed air horn available in many sporting goods and boat supply stores. Sound the noise alarm at the first sign of danger.

### Male Nonconsensual Sex and Rape

No one knows how common male rape is because men are less likely to report such assaults than women. Researchers estimate that the victims in about 10 percent of acquaintance rape cases are men. These hidden victims often keep silent because of embarrassment, shame, or humiliation, as well as their own feelings and fears about homosexuality and conforming to conventional sex roles.

Although many people think men who rape other men are always homosexuals, most male rapists consider themselves to be heterosexual. Young boys aren't the only victims. The average age of male rape victims is 24. Rape is a serious problem in prison, where men may experience brutal assaults by men who usually resume sexual relations with women once they're released.

**Impact of Rape** Rape-related injuries include unexplained vaginal discharge, bleeding, infections, multiple bruises, and fractured ribs. Victims of sexual violence often develop chronic symptoms, such as headaches, backaches, high blood pressure, sleep disorders, pelvic pain, and sexual fertility problems. But sexual violence has both a physical and a psychological impact. The psychological scars of a sexual assault take a long time to heal. Therapists have linked sexual victimization with hopelessness, low self-esteem, high levels of self-criticism, and self-defeating relationships. An estimated 30 to 50 percent of women develop posttraumatic stress disorder (see Chapter 3) following a rape. Many do not seek counseling until a year or more after an attack, when their symptoms have intensified or become chronic.

Acquaintance rape may cause fewer physical injuries but greater psychological torment. Often too ashamed to tell anyone what happened, victims may suffer alone, without skilled therapists or sympathetic friends to reassure them. Women raped by acquaintances blame themselves more, see themselves less positively,

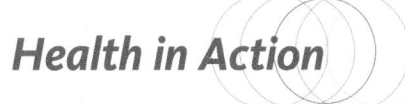

# Health in Action

### How to Avoid Date Rape

Here are strategies that can lower your risk of being involved in a date rape:

#### For Men:
- Remember that it's okay not to "score" on a date.
- Don't assume that a sexy dress or casual flirting is an invitation to sex.
- Be aware of your partner's actions. If she pulls away or tries to get up, understand that she's sending you a message—one you should acknowledge and respect.
- Restrict drinking, drug use, or other behaviors (such as hanging out with a group known to be sexually aggressive in certain situations) that could affect your judgment and ability to act responsibly.
- Think of the way you'd want your sister or a close female friend to be treated by her date. Behave in the same manner.

#### For Women:
- If the man pays for all expenses, he may think he's justified in using force to get "what he paid for." If you cover some of the costs, he may be less aggressive.
- Back away from a man who pressures you into other activities you don't want to engage in on a date, such as chugging beer or drag racing with his friends.
- Avoid misleading messages and avoid behavior that may be interpreted as sexual teasing. Don't tell him to stop touching you, talk for a few minutes, and then resume petting.
- Despite your clearly stated intentions, if your date behaves in a sexually coercive manner, use a strategy of escalating forcefulness—direct refusal, vehement verbal refusal, and, if necessary, physical force.
- Avoid using alcohol or other drugs when you definitely do not wish to be sexually intimate with your date.

Reflect on your experiences in social situations that became sexually uncomfortable or aggressive. Write a brief description of how you will prevent or handle such situations in the future in your online journal.

question their judgment, have greater difficulty trusting others, and have higher levels of psychological distress. Nightmares, anxiety, and flashbacks are common. The women may avoid others, become less capable of protecting themselves, and continue to be haunted by sexual violence for years. A therapist can help these victims begin the slow process of healing.

 **What to Do in Case of Rape**
Fewer than 5 percent of college rapes are reported. Women who are raped should call a friend or a rape crisis center. A rape victim should not bathe or change her clothes before calling. Semen, hair, and material under her fingernails or on her apparel all may be useful in identifying the man who raped her.

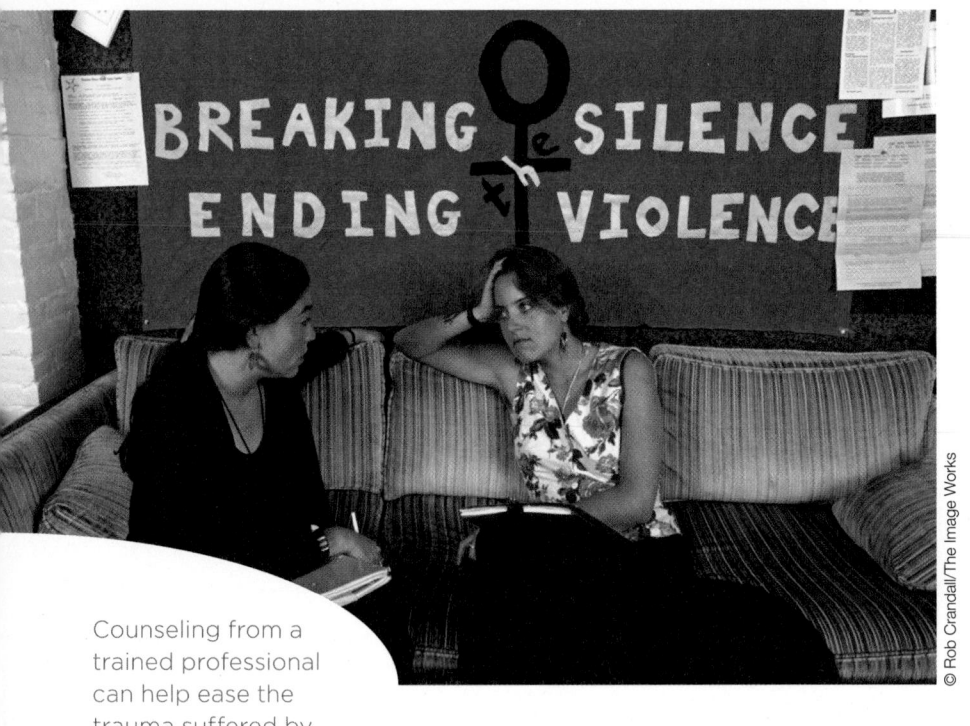

Counseling from a trained professional can help ease the trauma suffered by a rape victim.

© Rob Crandall/The Image Works

physical and psychological treatment and a haven where women can begin to rebuild their shattered self-esteem, as well as their daily lives. Rape counseling and crisis centers on college campuses and in the community provide various forms of assistance to victims of rape. In many cities, the telephone directory lists hot lines and resources. More than 400 victims' advocacy groups have been set up across the country to advise those hurt by crime. Support organizations help many survivors deal with the emotional aftermath of their experiences.

Sometimes well-intentioned friends and relatives add to the stress felt by the victims of violence. Here's how to offer comfort without implying criticism:

- **Don't try to deny that it happened.** Although it may be hard to talk about—or even listen to—what happened, the reality of the event must not be ignored. Denial makes victims doubt their own experience and question themselves at a time when they crave reassurance.

- **Don't pressure the victim to talk—or not to talk.** Some individuals need to go over every detail of what happened, again and again, until they work out their feelings of outrage and become ready to get on with their lives. Others find going into details too humiliating. Let the victim set the tone and limits for disclosure. Don't pry or prod.

- **Don't blame the victim.** Even when no one doubts that the victim is completely innocent, individuals may be plagued by regrets and self-accusation: Why didn't I lock the windows? Why did I park on that dark street? Any second-guessing or implied criticism adds to this burden of blame and shame.

- **Don't try to rush the victim to leave the past behind and get on with his or her life.** Recovery from any traumatic event takes time, and only the victim knows the appropriate pace. If, however, months pass without any lessening of symptoms or improvement in day-to-day functioning, family members and friends shouldn't hesitate to recommend that their loved one see a mental health professional.

A rape victim who chooses to go to a doctor or hospital should remember that she may not necessarily have to talk to police. However, a doctor can collect the necessary evidence, which will then be available if she later decides to report the rape to police. All rape victims should talk with a doctor or health-care worker about testing and treatment for sexually transmitted infections and postintercourse conception.

Even an unsuccessful rape attempt should be reported because the information a woman may provide about the attack—the assaulter's physical characteristics, voice, clothes, car, even an unusual smell—may prevent another woman from being raped.

## Helping the Victims of Violence

As their numbers have grown and their anguish has been recognized, the victims of violence have received greater attention. Hundreds of shelters for battered wives and their children have been set up across the country. They offer

# Staying Safe on Campus

Like other aspects of your health, safety is your personal responsibility. Are you as safe as you can be? Review the following list and check the precautions you've already taken. Make a to-do list of those you will implement in the future.

## Fundamentals

____ Freshmen should "respectfully decline" to have photo and personal information published for distribution to the campus community. Fraternities and upperclassmen have abused this type of publication to "target" naive freshmen.

____ Study the campus and neighborhood with respect to routes between your residence and class/activities schedule. Know where emergency phones are located if you do not have a cell phone.

____ Share your class/activities schedule with parents and a network of close friends, effectively creating a type of "buddy" system. Give network telephone numbers to your parents, advisors, and friends.

____ Survey the campus, academic buildings, residence halls, and other facilities while classes are in session and after dark to see that buildings, walkways, quadrangles, and parking lots are adequately secured, lit, and patrolled. Are emergency phones, escorts, and shuttle services adequate?

____ To gauge the social scene, drive down fraternity row on weekend nights and stroll through the student hangouts. Are people behaving responsibly, or does the situation seem reckless and potentially dangerous? Remember, alcohol and/or drug abuse is involved in about 90 percent of campus crime. Carefully evaluate off-campus student apartment complexes and fraternity houses if you plan to live off-campus.

## Residence

____ Doors and windows to your residence hall should be equipped with quality locking mechanisms. Room doors should be equipped with peep holes and deadbolts. Always lock them when you are absent. Do not loan out your key. Rekey locks when a key is lost or stolen.

____ Card access systems are far superior to standard metal key and lock systems. Card access enables immediate lock changes when keys are lost, stolen, or when housing arrangements change. Most hotels and hospitals have changed to card access systems for safety reasons. Higher education institutions need to adopt similar safety features.

____ Dormitories should have a central entrance/exit lobby where nighttime access is monitored, as well as an outside telephone which visitors must use to gain access.

____ Dormitory residents should insist that residential assistants and security patrols routinely check for propped doors—day and night.

____ Know your neighbors and don't be reluctant to report illegal activities and suspicious loitering.

## Off-Campus Residents

Off-campus residents should contact their student legal aid representative to draft leases that stipulate minimum standards of security and responsibility. Students and parents should also consult any Neighborhood Watch association active in the community or the municipal police regarding local crime rates.

Source: Reprinted with permission by Security on Campus, Inc., http://www .securityoncampus.org. Security on Campus assists victims of campus crime.

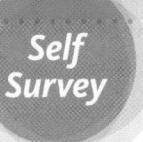

# How Safe Is Your School?

### Residence Hall Security

| YES | NO | |
|---|---|---|
| ____ | ____ | Single-sex residence halls |
| ____ | ____ | Coed residence halls |
| ____ | ____ | Freshman residence halls |
| ____ | ____ | Substance-free residence halls |
| ____ | ____ | Senior residence halls |
| ____ | ____ | Alcohol prohibited |
| ____ | ____ | Drugs prohibited |
| ____ | ____ | Propped door alarms |
| ____ | ____ | Coed bathrooms |
| ____ | ____ | Card swipe—like hotels—for exterior and interior residence hall rooms |
| ____ | ____ | Patented keys |
| ____ | ____ | Standard keys |
| ____ | ____ | Automatic locked doors |
| ____ | ____ | Propped doors |
| ____ | ____ | Doors locked at night |

YES NO

___ ___ Doors never locked
___ ___ Doors always locked
___ ___ Guards on duty 24 hours/day
___ ___ Guards on duty at night
___ ___ Apartments on campus
___ ___ Fire sprinklers
___ ___ Peep hole in room door
___ ___ Dead bolt on room door
___ ___ Safety chain on room door
___ ___ Bath in room
___ ___ Bathrooms down hallway
___ ___ Single-sex bathrooms kept locked
___ ___ Floors locked—all floors
___ ___ Secure windows—all floors
___ ___ Peer education programming
___ ___ Safety education programming
___ ___ Alcohol and other drug programming
___ ___ Support groups—depression, eating disorders, etc.
___ ___ Wellness center
___ ___ Women's center
___ ___ Panic alarms in rooms

## Campus Security

YES NO

**Campus Security Force**
___ ___ Sworn police
___ ___ Unsworn security
___ ___ Security guards
___ ___ Trained volunteer students
___ ___ Arrest power
___ ___ Patrolling day
___ ___ Patrolling night
___ ___ Carry firearms
___ ___ Bicycle patrols
___ ___ Surveillance cameras
___ ___ Emergency phones in working condition
___ ___ Escort services—24 hours
___ ___ Shuttle services
___ ___ Personal alarm devices

## Parental Notification

YES NO

___ ___ For suicide attempts
___ ___ For depression
___ ___ For alcohol poisoning
___ ___ For DUI
___ ___ For stalking
___ ___ For acts of violence
___ ___ For illegal drug use
___ ___ For underage drinkers
___ ___ For public drunkenness
___ ___ For housing firearms
___ ___ For sexual assault
___ ___ For hate crimes or speech

## Visitors

YES NO

___ ___ Phone/intercom at entrance
___ ___ Leave ID with guard
___ ___ Guest passes with guard
___ ___ Sign in guests with guard

## Security Patrols in Residence Halls

YES NO

___ ___ By police nightly
___ ___ By security nightly
___ ___ By students—RA or equivalent
___ ___ By no one

## Roommate Conflicts

YES NO

**Offending Roommate Quickly Transferred:**
___ ___ For using illegal drugs
___ ___ For having sex while roommate present
___ ___ For binge/underage drinking
___ ___ For noisy parties
___ ___ For hate speech
___ ___ For physical abuse or violence
___ ___ For vandalism

## Health Services

YES NO

___ ___ Rape crisis center
___ ___ Alcohol–drug counselors
___ ___ Student AA meetings on campus
___ ___ For academic probation
___ ___ For disciplinary probation
___ ___ For residence hall violations
___ ___ For off-campus citations

## Campus Judicial System

YES NO

___ ___ Releases results in hearings involving crimes of violence
___ ___ Open campus judicial hearings
___ ___ Reveals names of campus sex offenders

*Get campus crime statistics from* **www.ope.ed/gov/security** *or from your admissions office.*

## Criminal Offenses

Murder ___
Forcible sex offenses ___
Nonforcible sex offenses ___
Robbery ___
Aggravated assault ___
Burglary ___
Arson ___
Motor vehicle theft ___
Hate crimes ___
**Total criminal offenses** ___
**Per student crime ratio** ___

Liquor law violations      _____

Drug law violations        _____

Weapons violations         _____

**Total Campus Arrests**   _____

Calculate campus crimes per thousand students and compare them with other schools. Also, attempt a balanced evaluation by combining your subjective impressions with any calculations.

Source: Security on Campus, Inc., www.securityoncampus.org.

# Making Change Happen

## Become Your Own Guardian Angel

In a world full of many potential dangers, we all need someone to watch over us and keep us safe from harm. Whether or not you believe in guardian angels, there is always someone who—better than any other—can look out for you. That person is you.

"Your Guardian Angel" in *Labs for IPC* provides a comprehensive personal security program, based on the Stages of Change, discussed in Chapter 1 of this text and in *IPC*. By systematically working through this lab, you will come to value yourself so much that you avoid unwise risks, and you will consistently take the necessary measures to safeguard your physical and psychological well-being. Here's a preview.

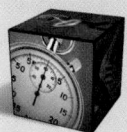

### Get Real

In this stage, you assess your values by ranking the importance of seven dimensions of safety on a scale of 0 to 100. Try these two examples:

- physical safety, protection of life and limbs from accidents and injury _____

- safety in intimate situations _____

You then do a self-appraisal of your risk awareness by assigning a numerical score to 15 behaviors, including these:

- If someone behaves strangely, I move away and keep my distance. _____

- I do not let people "guilt" me into situations that I do not want to be in. _____

- I am careful to observe people long and well before allowing them an intimate position in my life. _____

You also rate your accident prevention skills on the road, at home, out and about, and on a date. Here are just three of the 42 skills covered in the lab:

- Do you always wear a seat belt? _____

- Do you never lend your keys or ID to anyone? _____

- Do you never leave a party, concert, or bar with someone you just met or don't know well? _____

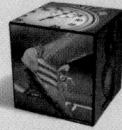

### Get Ready

The next stage includes five steps to prepare for change. Here is the first:

- Decide in which areas of your life you are going to put special focus on being a better guardian angel to yourself. Choose at least three, but do not limit yourself to these.

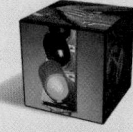

### Get Going

This is the stage where you start taking action with concrete steps that you incorporate into your daily life. Here is one example:

- **Become more mindful.** For the first four weeks of this lab, once a week survey the risk factors in a familiar or unfamiliar environment. For example, if you have heard about a new club or bar, take someone along with you and scope out the place. Or go to a campus event and see what risks might formerly have escaped your attention . . .

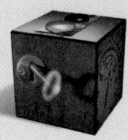

### Lock It In

You never outgrow your need for a guardian angel. That's why it's important to know how to steer clear of danger by taking steps such as the following:

- **Watch over yourself.** At the end of each week, identify any circumstances under which you might have put yourself in harm's way—consciously or not. In your *IPC Journal*, write about how you perceived the possible risks to yourself at the time and how you see them now . . .

## Review Questions

1. Signs of a potentially violent person include
   a. crying jags.
   b. heightened focus on schoolwork.
   c. frequent loss of temper.
   d. increased social activity.

2. Which of the following is *not* a safe-driving tip?
   a. Avoid driving at night for the first year after getting a license.
   b. Make sure your car has snow tires or chains before driving in hazardous snowy conditions.
   c. If riding with an intoxicated driver, keep talking to him so that he doesn't fall asleep at the wheel.
   d. Don't let packages or people obstruct the rear or side windows.

3. Which of the following statements about home safety is *true*?
   a. Falls pose the greatest threat of injury in the home, followed by poison.
   b. The three ingredients of fire are fuel, a heat source, and oxygen.
   c. The risk of falls is lowest in the elderly.
   d. If you're on the top floor of the dorm when a fire breaks out, get to the elevator quickly.

4. Which statement about violence on college campuses is *false*?
   a. Campus hazing often involves activities that would be called torture if perpetrated elsewhere.
   b. Most crimes against students occur on campus.
   c. Many campuses have codes of conduct on alcohol, drugs, and fighting.
   d. Crime statistics for colleges and universities are posted on the Internet.

5. Sexual victimization
   a. includes sexual harassment, sexual coercion, and rape.
   b. is gender-specific, affecting women who are violated emotionally or physically by men.
   c. is rare in academic environments such as college campuses.
   d. most commonly takes the form of physical assault and stalking.

6. You can avoid computer health hazards by
   a. positioning the monitor so that you are looking up at it.
   b. positioning the keyboard so that you don't have to bend your wrists to use it.
   c. sustaining focus on the screen with the PRIO method.
   d. taking a 15-minute break every 30 minutes.

7. Which of the following statements about rape is *true*?
   a. When a person is sexually attacked by a stranger, it is referred to as *rape*. When a person is sexually attacked by an acquaintance, it is referred to as *sexual coercion*.
   b. Statutory rape is defined as sexual intercourse initiated by a woman under the age of consent.
   c. Men who rape other men usually consider themselves heterosexuals.
   d. Women who flirt and dress provocatively are typically more willing to participate in aggressive sex than women who dress conservatively and do not flirt.

8. Seat belt use
   a. is optional if your car has air bags.
   b. is higher in teenage men than women.
   c. reduces the risk of serious injury by about 50 percent.
   d. is declining in the United States.

9. Ways to protect or prevent rape include which of the following?
   a. Use alcohol and drugs only in familiar surroundings.
   b. Take a self-defense class.
   c. To avoid angering a sexually aggressive person, become passive and quiet.
   d. Do not discuss your sexual limits on a first or second date because just talking about sex will encourage your date to think you are interested in a sexual relationship.

10. Which of the following factors affects an individual's risk of accident or injury?
    a. hunger level
    b. stress level
    c. amount of automobile insurance coverage
    d. knowledge of CPR

*Answers to these questions can be found on page 672.*

## Critical Thinking

1. Can you name two risk factors in your daily life that might increase the likelihood of accidental injury? What actions have you taken to keep yourself safe? Are there other risk factors you could minimize or eliminate? What might you do about them?

2. A friend of yours, Eric, frequently makes crude or derogatory comments about women. When you finally call him on this, his response is, "I didn't say anything wrong. I like women." What might you say to him?

## Media Menu

Visit www.cengagebrain.com to access course materials and companion resources for this text that will:

- Help you evaluate your knowledge of the material.

- Allow you to prepare for exams with interactive quizzing.

- Use the CengageNOW product to develop a Personalized Learning Plan targeting resources that address areas you should study.

- Coach you through identifying target goals for behavioral change and creating and monitoring your personal change plan throughout the semester using the Behavior Change Planner available in the CengageNOW resource.

## Internet Connections

**www.rainn.org**
This site provides great information from an organization fighting against rape, assault, and incest.

**www.rapecrisis.com**
This private nonprofit organization provides support to victims of sexual violence and their families, including a 24/7 crisis hotline and several advocacy programs.

**www.nsc.org**
The mission of the NSC is to educate and influence society to adopt safety, health, and environmental policies,

practices, and procedures that prevent human suffering and economic losses arising from preventable causes.

**www.safeyouth.org**
This site is a gateway to resources for professionals, parents, youth, and individuals working to prevent and end violence committed by and against young people.

## Key Terms

The terms listed are used on the page indicated. Definitions of the terms are in the Glossary at the end of the book.

| | | |
|---|---|---|
| computer vision syndrome 601 | rape 608 | sexual harassment 606 |
| hazing 604 | repetitive motion injury (RMI) 601 | stalking 608 |
| nonvolitional sex 607 | sexual coercion 608 | |

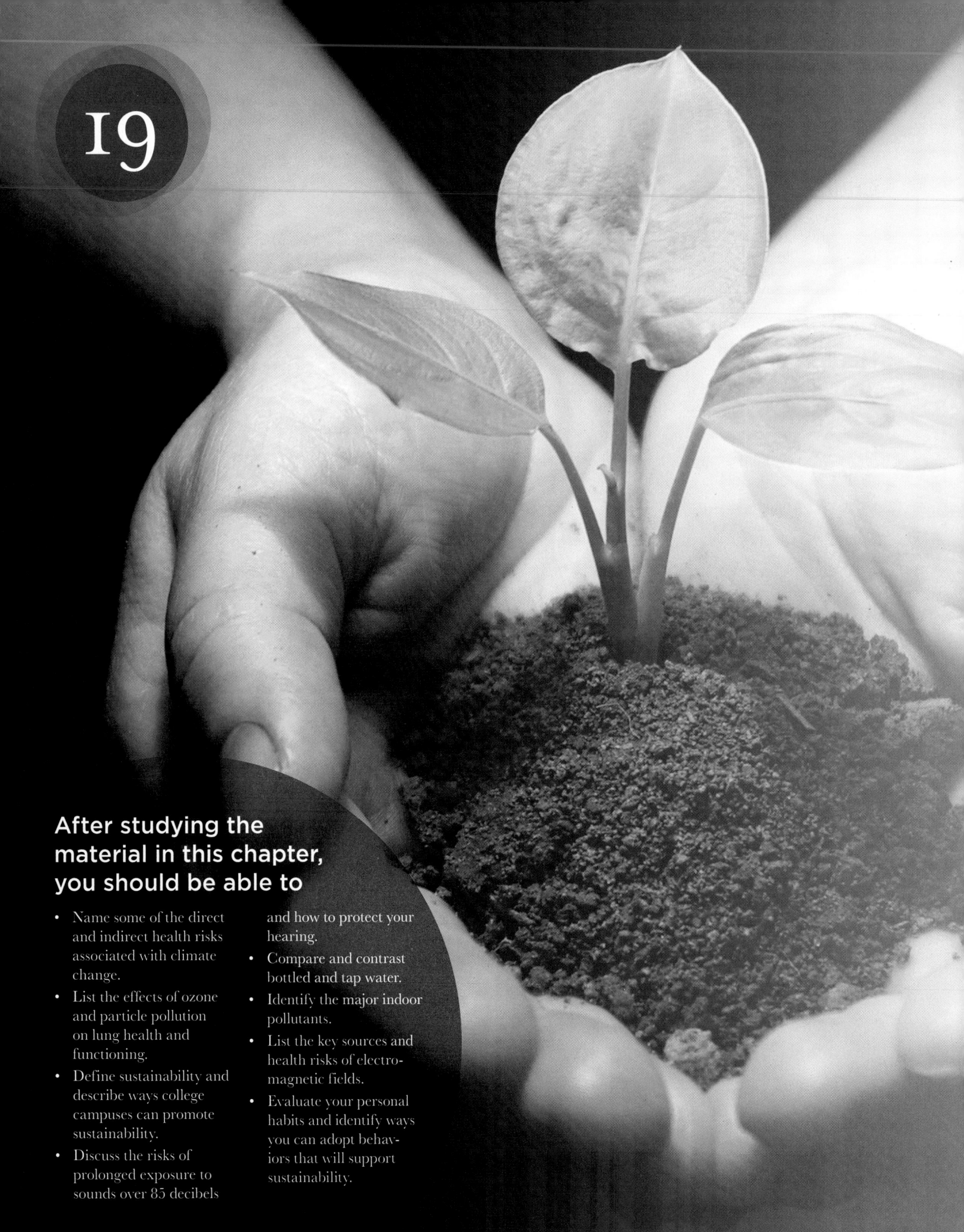

# 19

## After studying the material in this chapter, you should be able to

- Name some of the direct and indirect health risks associated with climate change.
- List the effects of ozone and particle pollution on lung health and functioning.
- Define sustainability and describe ways college campuses can promote sustainability.
- Discuss the risks of prolonged exposure to sounds over 85 decibels and how to protect your hearing.
- Compare and contrast bottled and tap water.
- Identify the major indoor pollutants.
- List the key sources and health risks of electro-magnetic fields.
- Evaluate your personal habits and identify ways you can adopt behaviors that will support sustainability.

Until college Neri's commitment to the environment consisted of carrying the recyclables out to the curb every week. She opted to live in a "green" residence hall on campus because she liked the light, airy architecture, the plantings everywhere, and the opportunity to join a community of individuals committed to a shared cause. But as Neri learned more about energy sources and usage, living green became a way of life. She stopped

# A Healthier Environment

buying plastic bottles of water, relied on natural light whenever possible, and switched to energy-efficient lightbulbs. Like a growing number of students, she joined an environmental action group whose activities include planting trees, setting up recycling centers, and launching energy-conservation makeovers on campus. (See "How Do You Compare?")

Some describe the campaign to create a healthier environment and combat climate change as this generation's equivalent of the civil rights movement. Without doubt these issues cannot be ignored. Although environmental concerns may seem so enormous that nothing any individual can do will have an effect, this is not the case. All of us, as citizens of the world, can help find solutions to the challenges confronting our planet. The first step is realizing that you have a personal responsibility for safeguarding the health of your environment and, thereby, your own well-being.

This chapter explores the complex interrelationships between your world and your well-being. It discusses major threats to the

environment, including climate changes; atmospheric changes; air, water, and noise pollution; chemical risks; and radiation.

## The Environment and Your Health

Ours is a planet in peril. Glaciers are melting. Sea levels are rising. Forests are being destroyed. Droughts have become more frequent and more intense. Heat waves have killed tens of thousands of people. Hurricanes and floods have ravaged cities. Millions have died from the effects of air pollution and contaminated water.

The planet Earth—once taken for granted as a ball of rock and water that existed for our use for all time—is a single, fragile **ecosystem** (a community of organisms that share a physical and chemical environment). Our environment is a closed ecosystem, powered by the sun. The materials needed for the survival of this planet must be recycled over and over again.

**ecosystem** A community of organisms sharing a physical and chemical environment and interacting with each other.

Visit www.cengagebrain.com to access course materials for this text, including the Behavior Change Planner, interactive quizzes, tutorials, and more. See the preface on page xv for details.

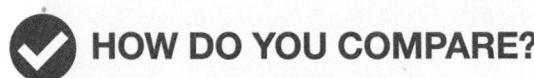

# DO STUDENTS CARE ABOUT THE ENVIRONMENT?

| Incoming freshmen who consider it very important to | | Percent |
|---|---|---|
| *become involved in programs to clean up the environment | | 27.3 |
| | Men | 24.5 |
| | Women | 29.7 |
| *adopt "green" practices to protect the environment | | 42.3 |
| | Men | 37.0 |
| | Women | 46.6 |

## HOW DO YOU COMPARE?

How would you describe your commitment to a healthier environment? Have you participated in any environmental cleanups? Have you adopted "green" practices in your life? Describe what you've done or what you are ready to commit to doing for the environment's sake in your online journal.

Source: J. H. Pryor, S. Hurtado, L. DeAngelo, L. Palucki Blake, and S. Tran, *The American Freshman: National Norms Fall 2010* (Los Angeles: Higher Education Research Institute, UCLA, 2010).

Increasingly, we're realizing just how important the health of this ecosystem is to our own well-being and survival. (See Health in Action.)

The World Health Organization (WHO) has identified the three major environmental threats to health: unsafe water, sanitation, and hygiene; indoor air pollution from solid fuel use; and outdoor air pollution. Improving water, sanitation, hygiene, and indoor and outdoor air could prevent an estimated 4 million deaths a year and greatly reduce child mortality in the world's lowest-income countries.[1]

For good or for ill, we cannot separate our individual health from that of the environment in which we live. However, efforts to clean up the environment are paying off. According to the American Lung Association, air quality in many cities, particularly in the Northeast and Midwest, has improved in the last decade. In addition to air quality, the water we drink and the chemicals we use also have an impact on the quality of our lives. At the same time, the lifestyle choices we make, the products we use, the efforts we undertake to clean up a beach or save wetlands affect the quality of our environment. For some ideas on what you can do, see Health on a Budget.

## Climate Change

The International Panel on Climate Change of the United Nations, made up of leading scientists from around the world, has reported with absolute certainty that the world's climate is changing in significant ways and will continue to do so in the foreseeable future. These experts predict an increase in extreme weather events (such as hurricanes and heat waves), greater weather variability, and rising water temperatures. The American Association for the Advancement of Science (AAAS) and other prestigious institutions around the world have issued warnings on the growing dangers of global climate change.

## Global Warming

Earth's average temperature increased about 1 degree in the 20th century to approximately 59 degrees, but the rate of warming in the last three decades has been three times the average rate since 1900. Seas have risen about six to eight feet globally over the last century and are rising at a higher rate.

Why is our planet getting warmer? Figure 19.1 shows the normal greenhouse effect: Certain

## Figure 19.1 The Greenhouse Effect

The normal greenhouse effect warms Earth to a hospitable temperature. An increase in greenhouse gases intensifies the greenhouse effect, trapping more heat and raising Earth's temperature.

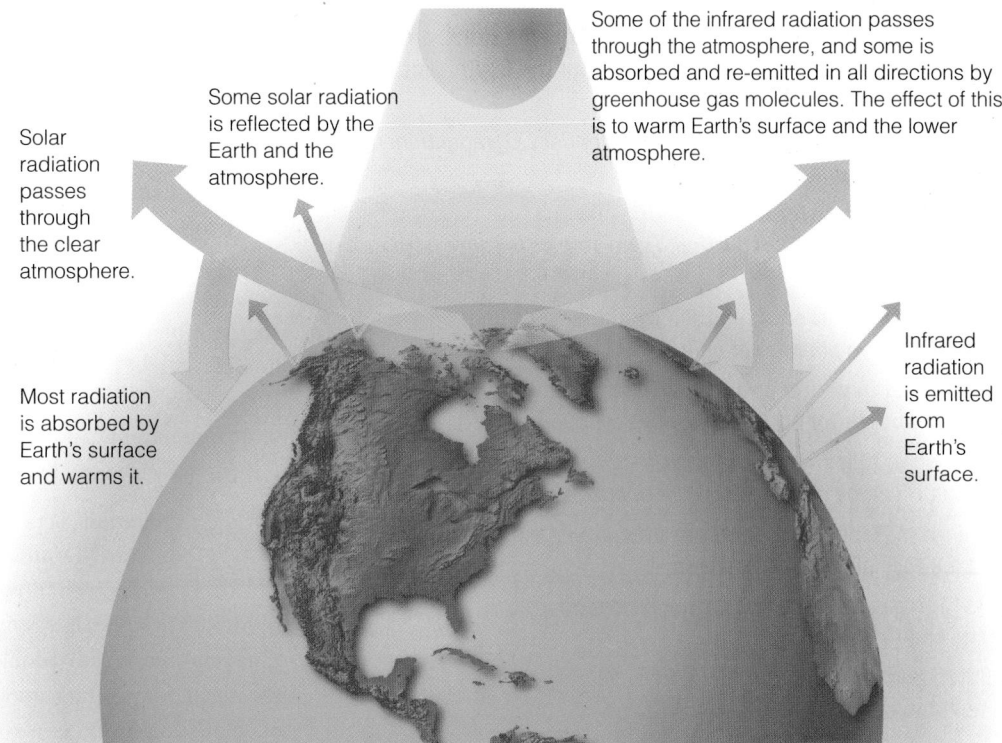

Some of the infrared radiation passes through the atmosphere, and some is absorbed and re-emitted in all directions by greenhouse gas molecules. The effect of this is to warm Earth's surface and the lower atmosphere.

Some solar radiation is reflected by the Earth and the atmosphere.

Solar radiation passes through the clear atmosphere.

Most radiation is absorbed by Earth's surface and warms it.

Infrared radiation is emitted from Earth's surface.

gases in Earth's atmosphere trap energy from the sun and retain heat somewhat like the glass panels of a greenhouse. These "greenhouse" gases include carbon dioxide, methane, and nitrous oxide. Human activities, scientists now say with 90 percent certainty, have increased the greenhouse gases in our atmosphere. We burn fossil fuels (oil, natural gas, coal) and wood products, which release carbon dioxide into the atmosphere. We produce coal, natural gas, and oil, which emit methane. Livestock and the decomposition of organic wastes also produce methane. Agricultural and industrial processes emit nitrous oxide. These emissions enhance the normal greenhouse effect, trapping more heat and raising the temperature of the atmosphere and Earth's surface.

After years of doubt and debate, most leading experts agree that the buildup of greenhouse gases is changing natural climate and weather patterns in new and potentially dangerous ways. Carbon dioxide levels are higher now than at any time in the past 800,000 years and, according to the AAAS, are "heading for levels not experienced for millions of years."[2]

## The Health Risks

No individual is immune to the effects of climate change. WHO estimates that climate change is already causing at least 150,000 excess deaths a year and that this number will climb to at least 300,000 annually by 2030.[3]

Climate change can imperil health directly—for example, as the result of floods or heat waves—and indirectly—by changing the patterns of infectious diseases, supplies of fresh water, and food availability. For example, as the planet continues to warm, infectious diseases—particularly mosquito-borne illnesses such as malaria, dengue fever, yellow fever, and encephalitis—may spread to more regions. Already in the United States, mosquitoes and other insects that carry diseases such as West Nile virus, Rocky Mountain spotted fever, and Lyme disease are spreading to areas once considered too cold for these insects to survive. The rise in global temperatures has already led to a greater pollen load and more allergies among more people.[4]

# Health in Action

## Protecting the Planet

Simple steps can help save energy, lower carbon dioxide ($CO_2$) emissions, and cut down on energy costs. Here are some recommendations from the Environmental Defense and World Wildlife Fund:

- Wash laundry in warm or cold water, not hot. *Average annual $CO_2$ reduction: up to 500 pounds for two loads of laundry a week.*

- Buy products sold in the simplest possible packaging. Carry a tote bag or recycle shopping bags. *Average annual $CO_2$ reduction: 1,000 pounds because garbage is reduced 25 percent.*

- Switch from standard lightbulbs to energy-efficient fluorescent ones. *Average annual $CO_2$ reduction: about 500 pounds per bulb.*

- Set room thermostats lower in winter and higher in summer. *Average annual $CO_2$ reduction: about 500 pounds for each two-degree reduction.*

- Run dishwashers only when full, and choose the energy-saving mode rather than the regular setting. *Average annual $CO_2$ reduction: 200 pounds.*

- Bike, carpool, or take mass transit whenever possible. *Average annual $CO_2$ reduction: 20 pounds for each gallon of gasoline saved.*

- Drive a car that gets high gas mileage and produces low emissions. Keep your speed at or below the speed limit.

- Keep your tires inflated and your engine tuned. Recycle old batteries and tires. (Most stores that sell new ones will take back old ones.)

- Turn off your engine if you're going to be stopped for more than a minute.

- Collect all fluids that you drain from your car (motor oil, antifreeze) and recycle or properly dispose of them.

If you want to write your own goals for working toward a healthy environment, access the Behavior Change Planner in CengageNOW at **www.cengagebrain.com**.

## The Impact of Pollution

Any change in the air, water, or soil that could reduce its ability to support life is a form of *pollution*. Natural events, such as smoke from fires triggered by lightning, can cause pollution. However, most sources of pollution are man-made. There are now about ten times as many cars around the world as there were 50 years ago. The number of people living in cities has increased by more than a factor of four, and global energy consumption by nearly a factor of five.

The effects of pollution depend on the concentration (amount per unit of air, water, or soil) of the **pollutant**, how long it remains in the environment, and its chemical nature. An *acute effect* is a severe, immediate reaction, usually after a single, large exposure. For example, pesticide poisoning can cause nausea and dizziness, even

**pollutant** A substance or agent in the environment, usually the by-product of human industry or activity, that is injurious to human, animal, or plant life.

**mutagen** An agent that causes alterations in the genetic material of living cells.

**carcinogen** A substance or agent that causes cancer.

death. A *chronic effect* may take years to develop or may be a recurrent or continuous reaction, usually after repeated exposure. Years of exposure to traffic pollution, for instance, has been linked to an increase in blood pressure.

Environmental agents that trigger changes, or *mutations*, in the genetic material (the DNA) of living cells are called **mutagens**. The changes that result can lead to the development of cancer. A substance or agent that causes cancer is a **carcinogen**: All carcinogens are mutagens; most mutagens are carcinogens. Furthermore, when a mutagen affects an egg or a sperm cell, its effects can be passed on to future generations. Mutagens that can cross the placenta of a pregnant woman and cause a spontaneous abortion or birth defects in the fetus are called *teratogens*.

 Pollution is a hazard to all who breathe. Deaths caused by air pollution exceed those from motor vehicle injuries. Those with respiratory illnesses and other chronic health problems are at greatest risk during days when smog or allergen counts are high. However, as a recent study showed, even healthy college students suffer impairments in their heart and circulatory systems as a result of urban air pollution. The effects of carbon monoxide are much worse in smokers, who already have higher levels of the gas in their blood.

As carbon dioxide levels in the air rise due to the greenhouse effect, air quality will worsen. Gases found in polluted air—such as ozone, sulfur dioxide, and nitrogen dioxide—contribute to heart disease and worsen the health of individuals who already have heart conditions. Poor air quality also contributes to breathing difficulties and may be responsible for the dramatic increase in asthma in recent decades. Elevated carbon dioxide levels can trigger asthma attacks and allergies by increasing ragweed pollen. Greater carbon dioxide in the air also stimulates the growth of poison ivy and other nuisance plants.

Toxic substances in polluted air can enter the human body in three ways: through the skin, through the digestive system, and through the lungs. The combined interaction of two or more hazards can produce an effect greater than that of either one alone. Pollutants can affect an organ or organ system directly or indirectly.

Among the health problems that have been linked with pollution are the following:

- Headaches and dizziness.
- Eye irritation and impaired vision.
- Nasal discharge.
- Cough, shortness of breath, and sore throat.
- Constricted airways.
- Constriction of blood vessels and increased risk of heart disease.
- Chest pains and aggravation of the symptoms of colds, pneumonia, bronchial asthma, emphysema, chronic bronchitis, lung cancer, and other respiratory problems.
- Birth defects and reproductive problems including lower success with in-vitro fertilization.
- Nausea, vomiting, and stomach cancer.
- Allergy and asthma from diesel fumes in polluted air.
- Higher mortality from strokes.

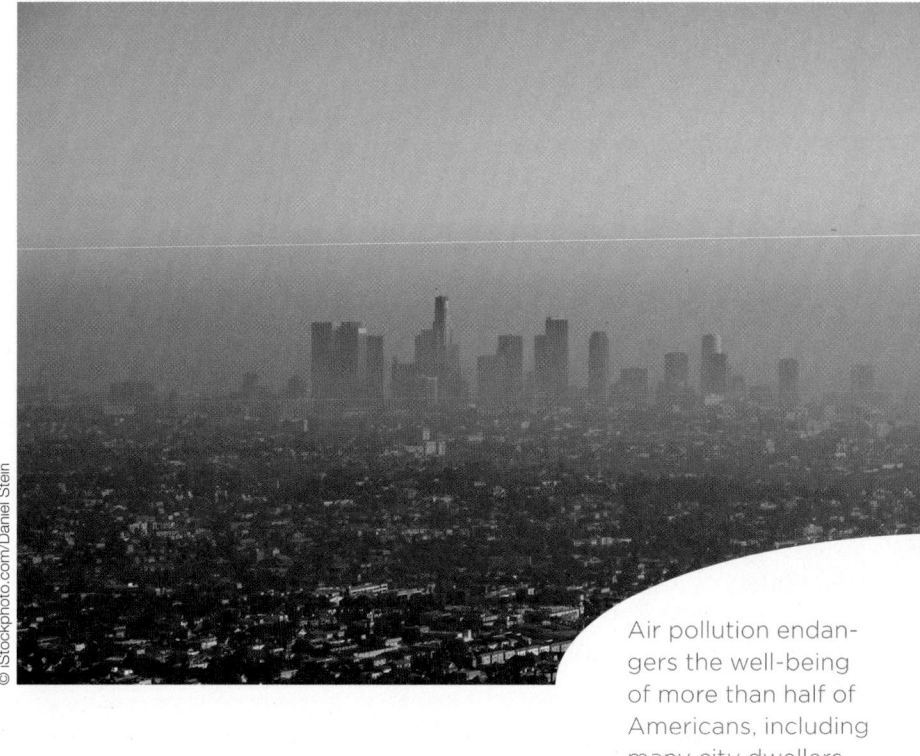

© iStockphoto.com/Daniel Stein

Air pollution endangers the well-being of more than half of Americans, including many city dwellers.

## The Air You Breathe

Remember the last time you stood at a busy intersection as a bus or truck spewed brownish fumes in your face? Maybe your eyes stung, or your throat burned. But breathing polluted air can do more than irritate: It can take months or even years off your life.

An estimated 154.5 million people—more than half the nation's population—live in areas with dangerous levels of air pollution. As pollutants destroy the hairlike cilia that remove irritants from the lungs, individuals may suffer chronic bronchitis, characterized by excessive mucus flow and continuous coughing. Emphysema may develop or worsen, as pollutants constrict the bronchial tubes and destroy the air sacs in the lungs, making breathing more difficult.

When air pollution levels are high, heart attacks, strokes, heart failure flare-ups, and lung troubles increase. Air contamination also has enduring effects on heart health and increases atherosclerosis and deaths due to heart disease. For the elderly and people with asthma or heart disease, polluted air can be life-threatening. In children,

it can impair lung development.[5] Even healthy individuals can be affected, particularly if they exercise outdoors during high-pollution periods or spend long periods in dirty air. Breathing air pollution while stuck in traffic may trigger 7.4 percent of heart attacks.[6]

### Ozone

**Ozone**, the primary ingredient of smog air pollution, can impair the body's immune system and cause long-term lung damage. (Ozone in the upper atmosphere protects us by repelling harmful ultraviolet radiation from the sun, but ozone in the lower atmosphere is a harmful component of air pollution.) Automobiles also produce carbon monoxide, a colorless and odorless gas that diminishes the ability of red blood cells to carry oxygen. The resulting oxygen deficiency can affect breathing, hearing, and vision in humans and stunt the growth of plants and trees.

Several large investigations have confirmed that ozone at levels currently found in the United States can shorten lives. Even on days when ozone levels are below the national standard, the risk of premature death is greater in areas with higher levels. The individuals most vulnerable to the effects of ozone are children, senior citizens, people who work or exercise outdoors, those with a respiratory disease such as asthma,

**ozone** A form of oxygen that is a harmful component of air pollution.

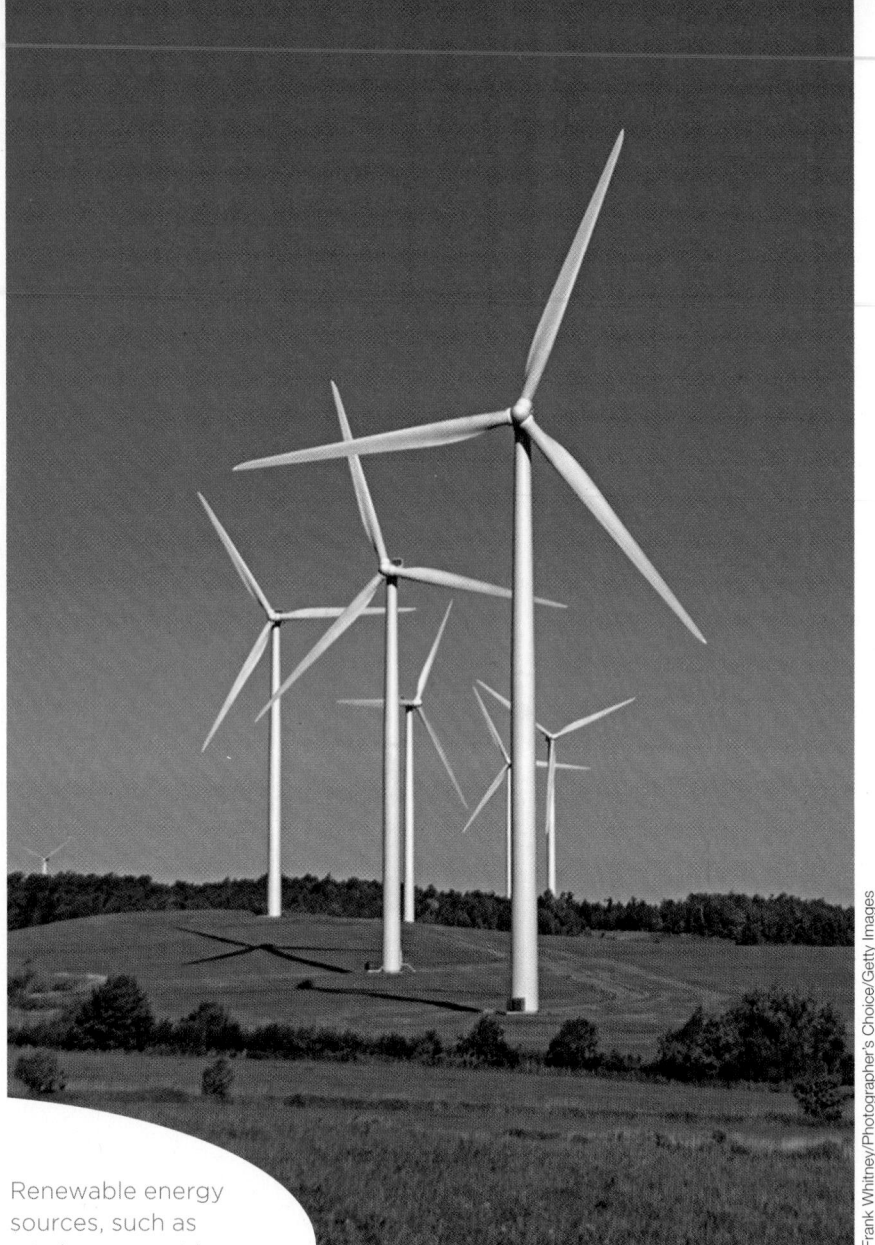

Renewable energy sources, such as wind, can provide more environmentally friendly alternatives. However, individual choices and behaviors also have an impact on the state of our world.

**sustainability** A method of using a resource so that the resource is not depleted or permanently damaged.

## Particle Pollution

Scientists refer to the mix of very tiny solid and liquid particles in the air as *particle pollution*. The particles themselves can range in size from microscopic to one-tenth the diameter of a strand of hair. Our natural defenses help us to cough or sneeze large particles out of our bodies, but they don't keep out smaller particles, which get trapped in the lungs. The smallest ones pass through the lungs into the bloodstream.

Particle pollution damages the body in ways similar to cigarette smoking. Even short-term exposure can be deadly because particle pollution increases the risk of heart attacks and strokes, especially among the elderly and those with heart conditions. It also diminishes lung function, causes inflammation of lung tissue in young, healthy adults, increases the number and severity of asthma attacks, and increases mortality in infants and young children.

Living near highways or spending time in heavy traffic, whether driving or taking public transportation, may be especially dangerous. Several studies have found an increased risk of premature death in those who live, work, drive, or ride in high-traffic areas. Air pollution may permanently impair the capacity of the lungs of 10- to 18-year-olds who live within about a third of a mile of a freeway, limiting their ability to breathe for the rest of their lives and increasing their risk of serious lung diseases.[8]

Particle pollution—considered the most dangerous because it can be an immediate as well as a long-term threat to life—has increased in the eastern part of the United States but decreased in the West. Cities that have reduced particle pollution—such as Pittsburgh, Buffalo, Los Angeles, Indianapolis, and St. Louis—have reported gains in life expectancy.[9]

and "responders" who are otherwise healthy but respond intensely to ozone.

Ozone's other ill effects include shortness of breath, chest pain when inhaling deeply, wheezing, coughing, and increased susceptibility to respiratory infections. Studies of college freshmen who were lifelong residents of Los Angeles or the San Francisco Bay Area found that long exposure to elevated ozone levels had reduced their "lung function," that is, their lungs' ability to work efficiently. Although ozone levels have declined, Los Angeles, Bakersfield, and Visalia, all in California, remain the most ozone-polluted cities in the United States.[7]

## Working toward Sustainability

More universities are developing programs to achieve **sustainability**, the use of as little as possible of resources that cannot be renewed. Innovative programs include "green" dorms and campaigns to reduce energy waste. Not all undergraduates share this concern, but higher numbers express commitment to environmental action than in the past.

Three important paths to sustainability are precycling, recycling, and compositing. **Precycling** refers to buying products packaged in recycled materials. According to the consumer group Earthworks, packaging makes up a third of what people in the United States throw away. When you precycle, you consider how you're going to dispose of a product and the packaging materials before purchasing it. For example, you might choose eggs in recyclable cardboard packages, rather than in foam cartons, and look for juice and milk in refillable bottles.

**Recycling**—collecting, reprocessing, marketing, and reusing materials once considered trash—serves several important functions, including:

- **Preserving natural resources.** Reprocessing used materials to make new products and packaging reduces the consumption of natural resources. Recycling steel saves iron ore, coal, and limestone. Recycling newsprint, office paper, and mixed paper saves trees.

- **Saving energy.** Recycling used aluminum cans, for instance, requires only about 5 percent of the energy needed to produce aluminum. Recycling just one can save enough electricity to light a 100-watt bulb for $3\frac{1}{2}$ hours.

- **Reducing greenhouse gas emissions.** Recycling cuts these gases by decreasing the amount of energy used to produce and transport new products.

- **Decreasing the need for landfill storage or incineration**. Both are more costly and can contribute to air pollution.

Different communities take different approaches to recycling. Many provide regular curbside pickup of recyclables, and others have drop-off centers. Buyback centers pay for recyclables. In some places, reverse vending machines accept returned beverage containers and provide deposit refunds.

Discarded computers, other electronic devices, and printer cartridges also should be recycled, by donating them to schools or charitable organizations. "Tech trash" buried in landfills is creating a new hazard because trace amounts of

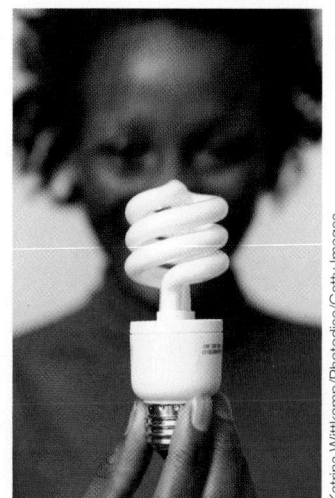

Katrina Wittkamp/Photodisc/Getty Images

potentially hazardous agents, such as lead and mercury, can leak into the ground and water. Find out if your campus has a program to recycle electronic devices.

With *composting*—which some people describe as nature's way of recycling—the benefits can be

**precycling** The use of products that are packaged in recycled or recyclable material.

**recycling** The processing or reuse of manufactured materials to reduce consumption of raw materials.

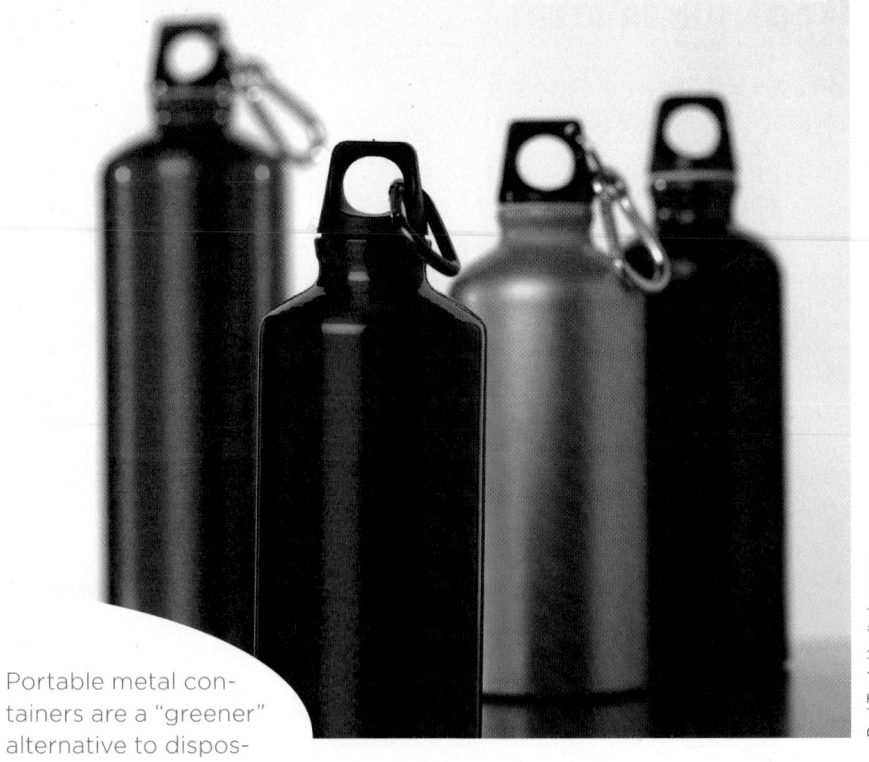

Portable metal containers are a "greener" alternative to disposable plastic water bottles.

Paul Tearle/Jupiterimages

Each year the CDC reports an average of 7,400 cases of illness related to the water people drink. The most common culprits include parasites, bacteria, viruses, chemicals, and lead. Traces of prescription drugs also have been found in the water of some communities. Home filters can block certain pathogens that can cause diarrhea and other gastrointestinal problems, but they do not seem to remove most chemical contaminants. If you decide to use a filter, clean it regularly to prevent a buildup of bacteria.

## Is Bottled Better?

Consumers seem convinced that bottled water is purer than tap. The market for bottled water in the United States has been growing by 10 percent per year, making it second only to soft drinks as America's favorite beverage. On average we drink about 25 gallons of bottled water every year, compared to 51.5 gallons of soft drinks and 21 gallons of beer.[10]

However, medical researchers have not found a scientific reason to recommend bottled water over tap water. This conclusion held true even after very low levels of radioactive iodine were detected in surface water and rain water in the United States following the damage to nuclear reactors in Japan caused by the tsunami of Spring 2011.[11]

Dentists report an increase in cavities among children and teenagers who drink bottled water rather than fluoridated tap water. An estimated 25 to 30 percent of bottled water sold in this country is, in fact, tap water, sometimes further treated and sometimes not. Despite images of mountain streams and glacier peaks on the labels, most comes from an urban water supply.

## Portable Water Bottles

The simplest, safest, most ecofriendly water container is a glass. If you want to carry water with you, you have plenty of alternatives, but some portable drinking containers may pose risks to you or to the environment.

Most disposable water bottles are made with lightweight polyethylene terephthalate (PET). Reusing these bottles may pose some health dangers, although there is little scientific agreement on how serious these risks may be. Your mouth leaves a residue of bacteria when you drink from

seen as close as your backyard. Organic products, such as leftover food and vegetable peels, are mixed with straw or other dry material and kept damp. Bacteria eat the organic material and turn it into a rich soil. Some people keep a compost pile (which should be stirred every few days) in their backyard; others take their organic garbage (including mowed grass and dead leaves) to community gardens or municipal composting sites.

# The Water You Drink

Fears about the public water supply have led many Americans to turn off their taps. About two-thirds take steps to drink purer water, either by using filtration and distillation methods or by drinking bottled water. However, Consumers Union, a nonprofit advocacy group, maintains that the United States has the safest water supply in the world. The Environmental Protection Agency has set standards for some 80 contaminants. These include many toxic chemicals and heavy metals—including lead, mercury, cadmium, and chromium—that can cause kidney and nervous system damage and birth defects.

a bottle, and these bacteria may accumulate with repeated use. Disposable bottles also pose a risk to the environment. The manufacture of the estimated 30 billion PET water bottles sold annually in the United States requires about 17 million barrels of oil. About 86 percent of these bottles become waste, which may take as long as 400 to 1,000 years to degrade.

Many consumers have switched to harder bottles made with polycarbonate plastic (known by the brand name Nalgene). Portable metal containers are another option. One popular brand is aluminum with a nontoxic liner; a second is simply made of stainless steel.

# Indoor Pollutants: The Inside Story

You may think of pollution as primarily a threat when you're outdoors, but people in industrialized societies spend more than 90 percent of their time inside buildings. Think of how much time you spend in your dorm, apartment, or home and in classrooms, dining halls, movie theaters, offices, stores, and shops. The quality of the air you breathe inside these places can have an even greater impact on your well-being than outdoor pollution. (See Health in the Headlines.)

Some sources—such as building materials and household products such as air fresheners—release pollutants more or less continuously. Other sources—such as tobacco smoke, solvents in cleaning products, and pesticides—can produce high levels of pollutants that remain in the air for long periods after their use.

## Environmental Tobacco Smoke (ETS)

The mixture of smoke from the burning end of a cigarette, pipe, or cigar and a smoker's exhalations contains over 4,000 compounds, more than 40 of which are known to cause cancer in humans or animals. More than half of U.S. states have enacted smoking bans in private worksites, restaurants, bars, airports, schools, hospitals, and many other locations. However, some states, mainly in the South and parts of

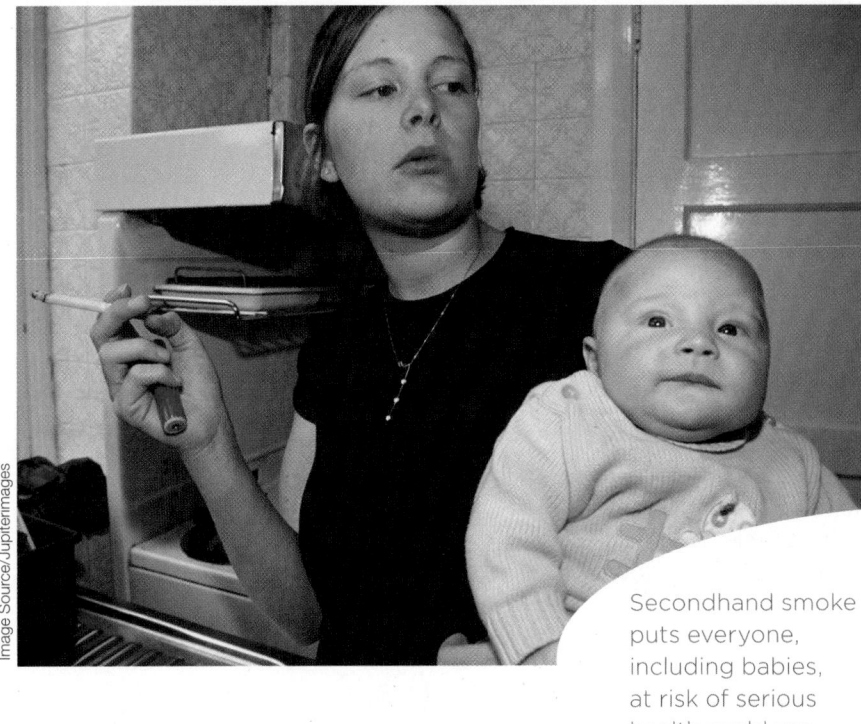

Image Source/Jupiterimages

Secondhand smoke puts everyone, including babies, at risk of serious health problems.

the West, have resisted comprehensive bans. As a result, about 88 million nonsmokers in the United States are still exposed to environmental tobacco smoke.[12]

***Secondhand Smoke*** At greatest risk for the dangers of "passive smoking" or "secondhand smoke" are infants and young children and youngsters with asthma or other respiratory problems. Children exposed to secondhand smoke face a much higher likelihood of high blood pressure and other risks for heart disease by age 13 than other children.[13] (See Chapter 14 for a further discussion of the health risks of environmental tobacco smoke.)

Health effects of secondhand smoke include eye, nose, and throat irritation; headaches; lung cancer; and possible contribution to heart disease. In children, the health effects include increased risk of lower respiratory tract infections, such as bronchitis and pneumonia, and ear infections; buildup of fluid in the middle ear; increased severity and frequency of asthma episodes; and decreased lung function. Pregnant women who live or work with smokers may be at higher risk of having a stillbirth.[14]

***Thirdhand Smoke*** Tobacco smoke creates more than an odor in a room. According to a recent study, tobacco residue—dubbed "thirdhand smoke"—contains cancer-causing toxins that stick to a variety of surfaces, where they can

## Environmental Threats

A wide host of agents in the air we breathe and the water we drink can affect our well-being. To get the most recent findings on environmental health threats, access Global Health Watch and search for one of the topics covered in this chapter, such as "radon" or "electromagnetic fields." Scan the headlines and select a relevant article. Write a summary in your online journal.

get into the dust and be picked up on the fingers. Babies and young children are most likely to be exposed to these harmful chemicals.

## Radon

Created by the breakdown of uranium in rocks, soil, and water, radon is the second-leading cause of lung cancer. Colorless and odorless, this radioactive gas enters homes through dirt floors, cracks in concrete walls and floors, floor drains, and sumps. When radon becomes trapped in buildings and concentrations build up indoors, exposure to the gas becomes a concern.

- **Sources:** Earth and rock beneath home; well water; building materials. Houses in the Northeast and Midwest tend to have higher radon levels than those elsewhere in the United States.[15]

- **Health Effects:** No immediate symptoms. Exposure to high levels of radon increases the risk of lung cancer. Smokers are at higher risk of developing radon-induced lung cancer.

- **Steps to Reduce Exposure**:

  - If you have any reason to suspect a radon problem in your home, you can buy inexpensive, do-it-yourself radon test kits online and in hardware stores. Look for ones that are state-certified or have met the requirements of a national radon proficiency program.

  - If testing reveals unsafe levels, contractors trained to fix radon problems can make changes to reduce the risk.

  - For more information on radon, contact your state radon office, or call 800-SOS-RADON.

## Molds and Other Biological Contaminants

Bacteria, mildew, viruses, animal dander, cat saliva, house dust mites, cockroaches, and pollen can all pose a threat to health. One of the oldest and most widespread substances on Earth, mold—a type of fungus that decomposes organic matter and provides plants with nutrients—has emerged as a major health concern. Common molds include *Aspergillus*, *Penicillium*, and *Stachybotrys*, a slimy, dark green mold that

has been blamed for infant deaths and various illnesses, from Alzheimer's disease to cancer, in adults that breathe in its spores. Faulty ventilation systems and airtight buildings have been implicated as contributing to the increased mold problem.

- **Sources:** Wet or moist walls, ceilings, carpets, and furniture; poorly maintained humidifiers, dehumidifiers, and air conditioners; bedding; household pets.

- **Health Effects:** Eye, nose, and throat irritation; shortness of breath; dizziness; lethargy; fever; digestive problems. Diseases like humidifier fever are associated with exposure to toxins that can grow in ventilation systems of large buildings. However, these diseases can also be traced to microorganisms in home heating and cooling systems and humidifiers. Children, the elderly, and people with breathing problems, allergies, and lung diseases are particularly susceptible to disease-causing biological agents in the indoor air.

- **Steps to Reduce Exposure**:

  - Use fans vented to outdoors in kitchens and bathrooms.

  - Clean cool-mist and ultrasonic humidifiers in accordance with manufacturer's instructions and refill with clean water daily.

  - Empty water trays in air conditioners, dehumidifiers, and refrigerators frequently.

  - Keep your personal living space clean. No, your mother may not be checking on you, but regular cleaning reduces house dust mites, pollens, animal dander, and other allergy-causing agents.

## Household Products

The liquids, foams, gels, and other materials you use to clean, disinfect, degrease, polish, wax, and preserve contain powerful chemicals that can pollute indoor air during and for long periods after their use. EPA researchers have found levels of about a dozen common organic pollutants to be two to five times higher inside homes than outside, regardless of whether the homes were located in rural or highly industrial areas.

- **Sources:** Paints, paint strippers, and other solvents; wood preservatives; aerosol sprays;

cleansers and disinfectants; moth repellents and air fresheners; stored fuels and automotive products; hobby supplies; dry-cleaned clothing.

- **Health Effects:** Eye, nose, and throat irritation; headaches, loss of coordination, nausea; damage to liver, kidney, and central nervous system. They also may lower estrogen and lead to earlier menopause.[16] Some organics can cause cancer in animals; some are suspected or known to cause cancer in humans.

- **Steps to Reduce Exposure**:
  - Follow instructions carefully. If the label says to use the product in a well-ventilated area, go outdoors or open windows to provide the maximum amount of outdoor air possible.
  - Use one household care product at a time. Mixing can create dangerous chemical reactions.[17]
  - Throw away partially full containers of old or unneeded chemicals, which can leak gases even when closed. Do not simply toss them in the garbage can. Find out if your local government or any organization in your community sponsors special days for the collection of toxic household wastes. If no such collection days are available, think about organizing one.
  - Buy limited quantities. Purchase only as much as you will use right away.
  - Keep to a minimum any exposure to emissions from products containing methylene chloride, such a paint strippers, adhesive removers, and aerosol spray paints. Methylene chloride is converted to carbon monoxide in the body and can cause symptoms associated with exposure to carbon monoxide.

## Formaldehyde

Some indoor pollutants come from the very materials that buildings are made of and from the appliances inside them. Formaldehyde is commonly used in building materials, carpet backing, furniture, foam insulation, plywood, and particle board. This chemical can cause nausea, dizziness, headaches, heart palpitations, stinging eyes, and burning lungs. Formaldehyde

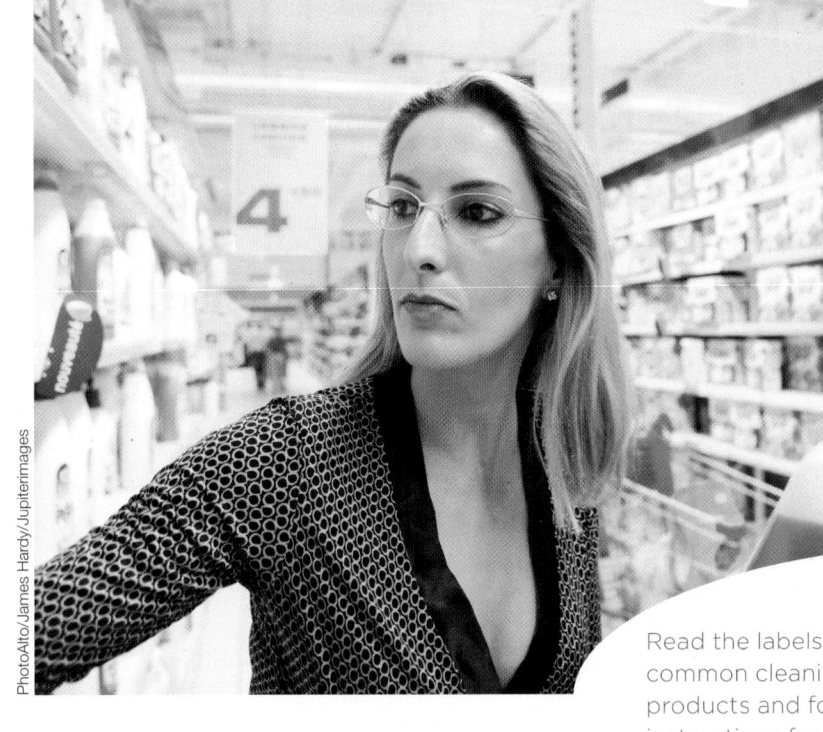

PhotoAlto/James Hardy/Jupiterimages

Read the labels on common cleaning products and follow instructions for use and storage to avoid possible health risks.

gas, which is colorless and odorless, has been shown to cause cancer in animals. Most manufacturers have voluntarily quit using it, but many homes already contain materials made with urea-formaldehyde, which can seep into the air.

The rate at which products like pressed wood or textiles release formaldehyde can change. Formaldehyde emissions will generally decrease as products age. When the products are new, high indoor temperatures or humidity can cause increased release of formaldehyde from these products.

- **Sources:** Pressed wood products (hardwood plywood wall paneling, particle board, fiberboard) and furniture made with these pressed wood products; urea-formaldehyde foam insulation (UFFI); combustion sources and environmental tobacco smoke; durable press drapes, other textiles, and glues.

- **Health Effects:** Watery eyes, burning sensations in the eyes and throat, nausea, and difficulty in breathing. High concentrations may trigger attacks in people with asthma. Has been shown to cause cancer in animals and may cause cancer in humans.

- **Steps to Reduce Exposure**:
  - Use "exterior-grade" pressed wood products (lower-emitting because they contain phenol resins, not urea resins).

# No- and Low-Cost Ways to "Green" Your Space

Whether you live in a dorm, apartment, or house, you can take simple, inexpensive steps to create a greener personal environment. Here are some ways to get started. (See Figure 19.2 for more ideas.)

- Buy furniture and household items secondhand, or recycle your parents' things. If you can't find everything you need in the attic or basement, try a website such as **www.freecycle.com**, where you can barter your way to greener furnishings.

- Choose recycled notebooks and printer paper and ecofriendly shampoos, conditioners, and lotions.

- Rather than relying on air-conditioning or central heat, use a space heater or fan, depending on the season, to regulate the temperature around you.

- Buy a stainless steel or coated aluminum water bottle instead of using disposable bottles.

- Use green cleaning products like vinegar and baking soda instead of expensive and potentially harmful chemicals.

- Tote books and groceries in canvas bags rather than paper or plastic ones.

- Chip in with roommates or friends so you can buy in bulk, which saves money and requires less packaging.

- Don't throw anything out before asking yourself if it can be recycled, donated, or simply used in another way.

termites (termiticides), rodents (rodenticides), fungi (fungicides), and microbes (disinfectants). They are sold as sprays, liquids, sticks, powders, crystals, balls, and foggers.

The EPA requires manufacturers to put information on the label about when and how to use a pesticide. Remember that the "-cide" in pesticides means "to kill." Pesticides are also made up of ingredients that are used to carry the active agent. These carrier agents are called "inerts" because they are not toxic to the targeted pest; nevertheless, some inerts are capable of causing health problems.

- **Sources:** Products used to kill household pests or on lawns and gardens (if the product drifts or is tracked inside the house).

- **Health Effects:** High levels of certain pesticides can produce various symptoms, including headaches, dizziness, muscle twitching, weakness, tingling sensations, and nausea. They also might cause long-term damage to the liver and the central nervous system, as well as an increased risk of cancer.

- **Steps to Reduce Exposure:**

  - Follow instructions. It is illegal to use any pesticide in any manner inconsistent with the directions on its label.

  - Use only the pesticides approved for use by the general public and then only in recommended amounts; increasing the amount does not offer more protection. Ventilate the area well after pesticide use.

  - If possible, take plants and pets outside when applying pesticides to them.

  - Dispose of unwanted pesticides according to the directions on the label or on special household hazardous waste collection days.

  - Use nonchemical methods of pest control where possible.

  - Keep indoor spaces clean, dry, and well ventilated to avoid pest and odor problems.

  - Minimize exposure to moth repellents, which contain paradichlorobenzene, a chemical known to cause cancer in animals. If using mothballs, place them and the items to be protected in trunks or other containers that can be stored in areas such as attics and detached garages.

- Use air conditioning and dehumidifiers to maintain moderate temperature and reduce humidity levels.

- Increase ventilation, particularly after bringing new sources of formaldehyde into the home.

- Always ask about the formaldehyde content of pressed wood products, including building materials, cabinetry, and furniture before you purchase them.

## Pesticides

According to a recent survey, 75 percent of U.S. households used at least one pesticide product indoors during the past year. Products used most often are insecticides and disinfectants. Pesticides used in and around the home include products to control insects (insecticides),

Figure 19.2 **Greening Your Space**

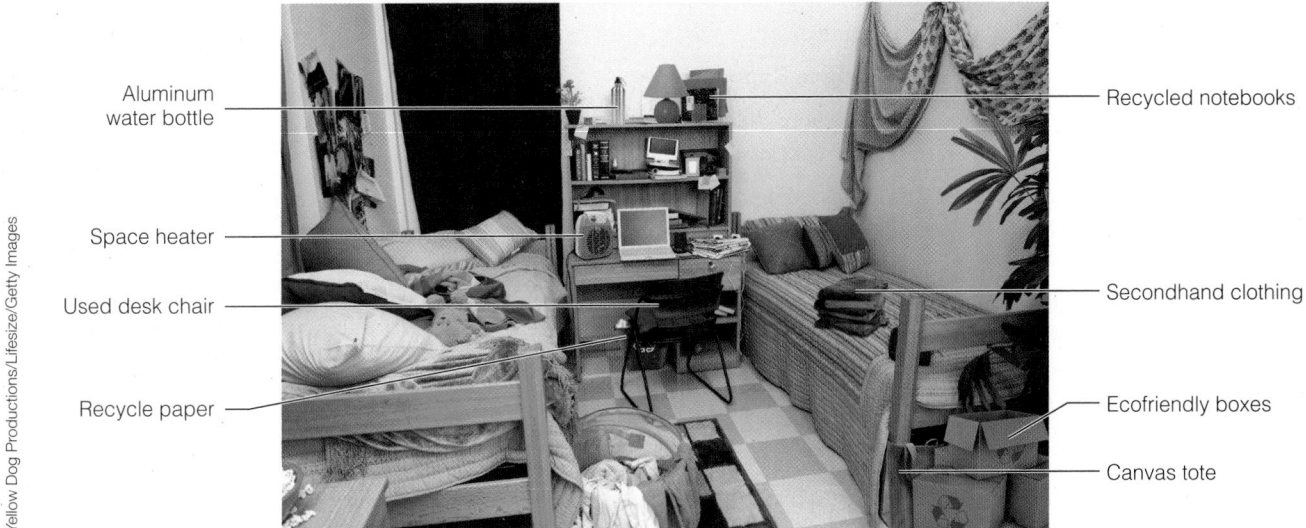

Aluminum water bottle

Space heater

Used desk chair

Recycle paper

Recycled notebooks

Secondhand clothing

Ecofriendly boxes

Canvas tote

Yellow Dog Productions/Lifesize/Getty Images

Do not buy air fresheners that contain paradichlorobenzene.

## Asbestos

This mineral fiber has been used commonly in a variety of building construction materials for insulation and as a fire-retardant. The government has banned several asbestos products, and manufacturers have also voluntarily limited use of asbestos. Today asbestos is most commonly found in older homes, pipe and furnace insulation materials, asbestos shingles, millboard, textured paints, and floor tiles.

- **Sources:** Deteriorating, damage, or disturbed insulation, fireproofing, acoustical materials, and floor tiles.

- **Health Effects:** Too small to be visible, the most dangerous asbestos fibers accumulate in the lungs and can cause lung cancer, mesothelioma (a cancer of the chest and abdominal linings), and asbestosis (irreversible lung scarring that can be fatal). Symptoms of these diseases do not show up until many years after exposure began. Smokers are at higher risk of developing asbestos-induced lung cancer.

- **Steps to Reduce Exposure**:
  - Leave undamaged asbestos material alone if it is not likely to be disturbed.

- Use trained and qualified contractors for control measures that may disturb asbestos and for cleanup.

- Follow proper procedures in replacing woodstove door gaskets that may contain asbestos.

## Lead

People are exposed to lead, a long-recognized health threat, through air, drinking water, food, contaminated soil, deteriorating paint, and dust. Airborne lead enters the body when an individual breathes or swallows lead particles or dust. Before its risks were known, lead was used in paint, gasoline, water pipes, and many other products.

- **Sources:** Lead-based paint; contaminated soil, dust, and drinking water.

- **Health Effects:** Lead affects practically all systems within the body. Lead at high levels can cause convulsions, coma, and even death. Lower levels of lead can cause adverse health effects on the central nervous system, kidney, and blood cells. In pregnant women, even small amounts can significantly increase blood pressure.[18] Infants and children are more vulnerable to lead exposure than adults—lead is more easily absorbed into growing bodies and the tissues of small children are more sensitive to the damaging effects of lead. Children may have higher exposures since they are more likely to get lead dust on their hands and then put their fingers or other lead-contaminated objects into their mouths.

- **Steps to Reduce Exposure**:

  - Keep areas where children play as dust-free and clean as possible.

  - Leave lead-based paint undisturbed if it is in good condition; do not sand or burn off paint that may contain lead.

  - Do not remove lead paint yourself.

  - Do not bring lead dust into the home.

  - If your work or hobby involves lead, change clothes and use doormats before entering your home.

  - Eat a balanced diet, rich in calcium, iron, and vitamin C. High levels of ascorbic acid (vitamin C) have been associated with a lower rate of elevated blood lead levels.

## Carbon Monoxide and Nitrogen Dioxide

Carbon monoxide (CO) gas—which is tasteless, odorless, colorless, and nonirritating—can be deadly. Produced by the incomplete combustion of fuel in space heaters, furnaces, water heaters, and engines, CO reduces the delivery of oxygen in the blood. Every year an estimated 10,000 Americans seek treatment for CO inhalation; at least 250 die because of this silent killer. Those most at risk are the chronically ill, the elderly, pregnant women, and infants.

- **Sources**: Unvented kerosene and gas space heaters; leaking chimneys and furnaces; back-drafting from furnaces, gas water heaters, woodstoves, and fireplaces; gas stoves; automobile exhaust from attached garages.

- **Health Effects:** At low concentrations, fatigue in healthy people and chest pain in people with heart disease. At higher concentrations, impaired vision and coordination; headaches; dizziness; confusion; nausea. Can cause flu-like symptoms that clear up after leaving home. Fatal at very high concentrations.

Another dangerous gas, nitrogen dioxide ($NO_2$), can reach very high levels if you use a natural gas or propane stove in a poorly ventilated kitchen. This gas may lead to respiratory illnesses. Pilot

lights are a steady source of nitrogen dioxide; to reduce exposure, switch to spark ignition.

- **Sources:** Kerosene heaters, unvented gas stoves and heaters.

- **Health Effects:** Eye, nose, and throat irritation. May cause impaired lung function and increased respiratory infections in young children.

- **Steps to Reduce Exposure of Both CO and $NO_2$:**

  - Keep appliances properly adjusted.

  - Open flues when fireplaces are in use.

  - Do not idle a car inside the garage.

# Chemical Risks

Various chemicals, including benzene, asbestos, and arsenic, have been shown to cause cancer in humans. Probable carcinogens include DDT and PCB. Risks can be greatly increased with simultaneous exposures to more than one carcinogen, for example, tobacco smoke and asbestos.[19]

According to the CDC, the levels of potentially harmful chemicals, including pesticides and lead, in Americans' blood have declined. Still, an estimated 50,000 to 70,000 U.S. workers die each year of chronic diseases related to past exposure to toxic substances, including lung cancer, bladder cancer, leukemia, lymphoma, chronic bronchitis, and disorders of the nervous system. **Endocrine disruptors**, chemicals that act as or interfere with human hormones, particularly estrogen, may pose a different threat. Scientists are investigating their impact on fertility, falling sperm counts, and cancers of the reproductive organs. Exposure to toxic chemicals causes about 3 percent of developmental defects.

## Agricultural Pesticides

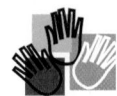 High quantities of toxic chemical waste from unused or obsolete pesticides are posing a continuing and worsening threat to people and the environment in Eastern Europe, Africa, Asia, the Middle East, and Latin America. In the United States, the FDA estimates that 33 to 39 percent of our food supply contains residues of pesticides that

**endocrine disruptors** Synthetic chemicals that interfere with the ways that hormones work in humans and wildlife.

may pose a long-term danger to our health. Scientists have detected traces of pesticides in groundwater in both urban and rural areas. Exposure to pesticides may pose a risk to pregnant women and their unborn children. Men whose jobs routinely expose them to pesticides may be at increased risk of prostate cancer. Parental exposure does not increase the likelihood of childhood brain cancer.

**Chlorinated hydrocarbons** include several high-risk substances—such as DDT, kepone, and chlordane—that have been restricted or banned because they may cause cancer, birth defects, neurological disorders, and damage to wildlife and the environment. They are extremely resistant to breakdown.

**Organophosphates**, including chemicals such as malathion, break down more rapidly than the chlorinated hydrocarbons. Most are highly toxic, causing cramps, confusion, diarrhea, vomiting, headaches, and breathing difficulties. Higher levels in the blood can lead to convulsions, paralysis, coma, and death.

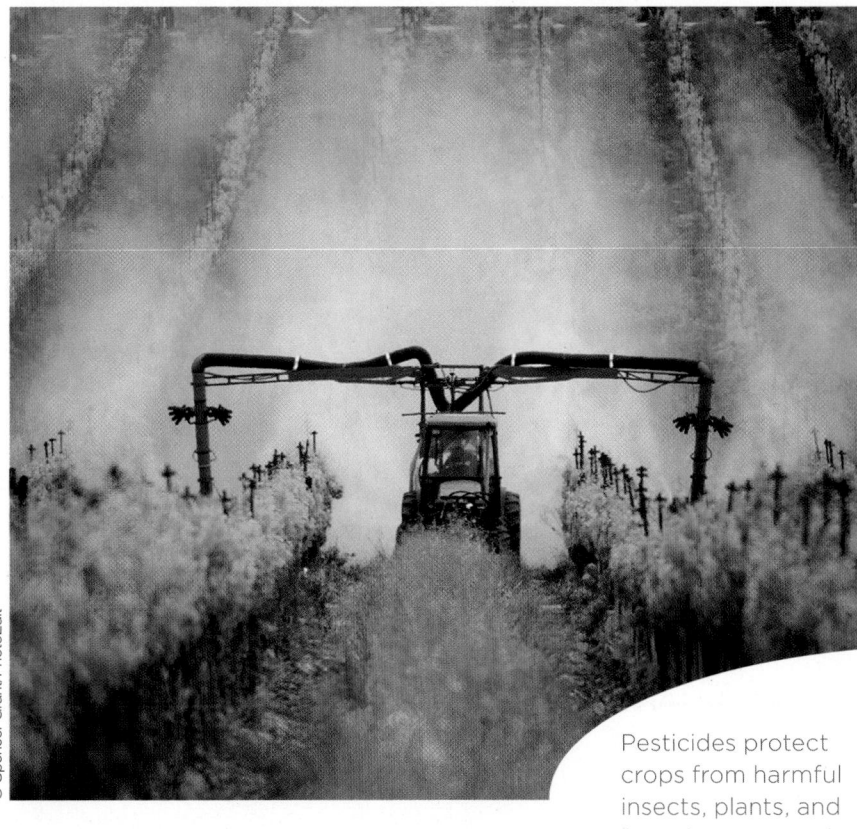

© Spencer Grant/PhotoEdit

Pesticides protect crops from harmful insects, plants, and fungi but may endanger human health.

## Chemical Weapons

Terrorist threats include the possibility of the use of chemical weapons. Possible bioterror agents include poison gases, herbicides, and other types of chemical substances that can kill, maim, or temporarily incapacitate. Chemical agents can be dispersed as liquids, vapors, gases, and aerosols that attack nerves, blood, skin, or lungs. In contrast to biological weapons, chemical weapons can kill rapidly, often within hours or minutes, and sometimes with just a small drop. Possible protection against chemical weapons includes gas masks, shelters, and sealed suits and vehicles. Treatment and antidotes can sometimes help after exposure. If contaminated, you need to flush your eyes and skin immediately for at least five to ten minutes while awaiting emergency help.

## Multiple Chemical Sensitivity

The proliferation of chemicals in modern society has led to an entirely new disease, **multiple chemical sensitivity (MCS)**, also called environmentally triggered illness, universal allergy, or chemical AIDS. MCS was first described almost a half century ago when a Chicago allergist treated a number of patients who reported becoming ill after being exposed to various petrochemicals. Since that time, many more cases of MCS have been reported, yet there is no agreed-upon definition of the condition, no medical test that can diagnose it, and no proven treatment.

According to medical theory, people become chemically sensitive in a two-step process: First, they experience a major exposure to a chemical, such as a pesticide, a solvent, or a combustion product. The sensitized person then begins to react to low-level chemical exposures from ordinary substances, such as perfumes and tobacco smoke. Symptoms include a runny nose, breathing difficulties, memory problems, chest pain, depression, dizziness, fatigue, headache, inability to concentrate, nausea, aches and pains in muscles and joints, and heart palpitations.

# Invisible Threats

Among the unseen threats to health are various forms of *radiation*, energy radiated in the form of waves or particles.

**chlorinated hydrocarbons** Highly toxic pesticides, such as DDT and chlordane, that are extremely resistant to breakdown; may cause cancer, birth defects, neurological disorders, and damage to wildlife and the environment.

**organophosphates** Toxic pesticides that may cause cancer, birth defects, neurological disorders, and damage to wildlife and the environment.

**multiple chemical sensitivity (MCS)** A sensitivity to low-level chemical exposures from ordinary substances, such as perfumes and tobacco smoke, that results in physiological responses such as chest pain, depression, dizziness, fatigue, and nausea. Also known as environmentally triggered illness.

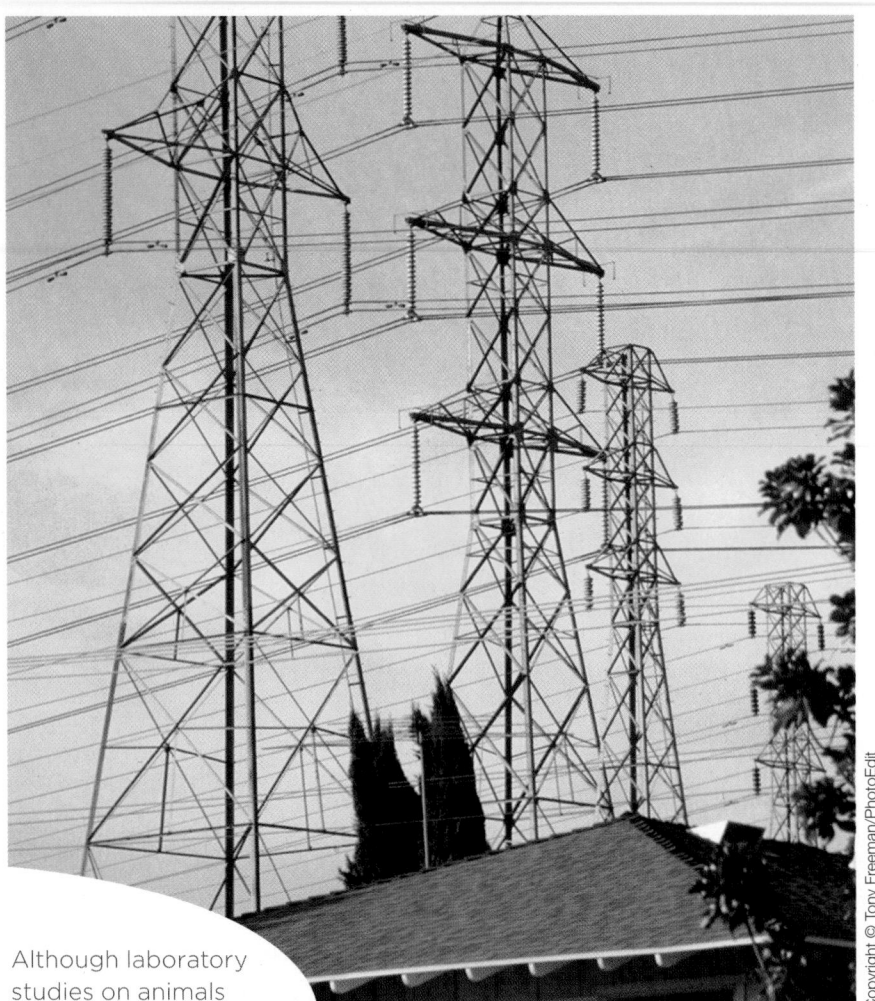
Copyright © Tony Freeman/PhotoEdit

Although laboratory studies on animals indicate that EMFs affect human cell membranes, research on humans has found only a weak connection between EMFs and disease.

**electromagnetic fields (EMFs)**
The invisible electric and magnetic fields generated by an electrically charged conductor.

## Electromagnetic Fields

Any electrically charged conductor generates two kinds of invisible fields: electric and magnetic. Together they're called **electromagnetic fields** (**EMFs**). For years, these fields, produced by household appliances, home wiring, lighting fixtures, electric blankets, and overhead power lines, were considered harmless. However, epidemiological studies have revealed a link between exposure to high-voltage lines and cancer (especially leukemia, a blood cancer) in electrical workers and children.

Laboratory studies on animals have shown that alternating current, which changes strength and direction 60 times a second (and electrifies most of North America), emits EMFs that may interfere with the normal functioning of human cell membranes, which have their own electromagnetic fields. The result may be mood disorders,

changes in circadian rhythms (our inner sense of time), miscarriage, developmental problems, or cancer. Researchers have documented increases in breast cancer deaths in women who worked as electrical engineers, electricians, or in other high-exposure jobs, and a link between EMF exposure and increased risk of leukemia and possibly brain cancer.

The National Institute of Environmental Health Sciences concluded that the evidence of a risk of cancer and other human disease from the electric and magnetic fields around power lines is "weak." This finding applies to the extremely low frequency electric and magnetic fields surrounding both the big power lines that distribute power and the smaller but closer electric lines in homes and appliances. However, the researchers also noted that EMF exposure "cannot be recognized as entirely safe."

## Cell Phones

Since cellular phone service was introduced in the United States in 1984, mobile and handheld phones have become ubiquitous, and concern has grown about their possible health risks. The federal government sets upper exposure limits to electromagnetic energy from cell phones known as the specific absorption rate, or SAR. A phone emits the most radiation during a call, but it also emits small amounts periodically whenever it's turned on.

Can exposure to low levels of electromagnetic energy that the body absorbs from a cell phone be harmful? Researchers have found that a one-hour cell phone conversation stimulates the areas of the brain closest to the phone's antenna, but they do not know if these effects pose any long-term risk.[20] More than 70 research papers on the potentially harmful effects of cell phone use have raised concerns about cancer, neurological disorders, sleep problems, or headaches; others have shown no association or were inconclusive. A recent British study found no significant increase in the incidence of brain tumors in men and women in the decade after cell phones became widespread.[21]

The Food and Drug Administration (FDA) and Federal Communications Commission (FCC) have stated that "the available scientific evidence does not show that any health problems are associated with using wireless phones. There is no proof, however, that wireless phones are absolutely safe." Additional studies are under way.

Researchers have documented an increase in ear canal temperature with cell phone use, protein changes in human cells exposed to cell phone radiation, and an increased rate of benign brain tumors. Other research found no impact on the daily patterns of hormones secreted by the gonads, pituitary, or adrenal glands in men.[22] Some health experts have discouraged children from using cell phones largely because of concerns that their developing nervous systems may be especially vulnerable.

As discussed in Chapter 18, cell phones do pose one serious health risk. Drivers distracted by cell phones are more likely to get into accidents and to hit—and kill—pedestrians.[23]

## Microwaves

**Microwaves** (extremely high frequency electromagnetic waves) increase the rate at which molecules vibrate; this vibration generates heat. There's no evidence that existing levels of microwave radiation encountered in the environment pose a health risk to people, and all home microwave ovens must meet safety standards for leakage.

A concern about the safety of microwave ovens stems from the chemicals in plastic wrapping and plastic containers used in microwave ovens. Chemicals may leak into food. In high concentrations, some of the chemicals (such as DEHA, which makes plastic more pliable) can cause cancer in mice. Consumers should be cautious about using clingy plastic wrap when reheating leftovers, and plastic-encased metal "heat susceptors" included in convenience foods such as popcorn and pizza. Although these materials seem safe when tested in conventional ovens at temperatures of 300° to 350° Fahrenheit, microwave ovens can boost temperatures to 500° Fahrenheit.

## Ionizing Radiation

Radiation that possesses enough energy to separate electrons from their atoms, leaving charged ions, is called **ionizing radiation**. Its effects on health depend on many factors, including the amount, length of exposure, type, part of the body exposed, and the health and age of the individual.

We're surrounded by low-level ionizing radiation every day. Most comes from cosmic rays and radioactive minerals, which vary according to geography. (Denver has more than Atlanta, for instance, because of its altitude.) Man-made sources, including medical and dental X-rays, account for approximately 18 percent of the average person's lifetime exposure.

Radiation exposure in humans is measured in units called rads and rems. A rad (radiation absorbed dose) is a measure of the energy deposited by ionizing radiation when it's absorbed by an object. A rem (roentgen equivalent man) is a measure of the biological effect of ionizing radiation. Different types of radiation cause different amounts of damage. The rem measurement takes this into account. For X-rays, rads and rems are equivalent. A quantity of 1 rad or 1 rem is a substantial dose of radiation. Smaller doses are measured in millirads (thousandths of a rad) or millirems (thousandths of a rem). The average annual radiation exposure for a person in the United States is about one-tenth of a rem.

## Diagnostic X-Rays

The EPA estimates that 30 to 50 percent of the 700 million X-rays taken every year in the United States are unnecessary. However, doctors sometimes prescribe X-rays or newer imaging techniques involving radiation, such as CT scans, to protect themselves from malpractice suits, and hospitals benefit financially from the heavy use of X-ray equipment.

Dental X-rays involve little radiation, but many people receive so many so often that they're second only to chest examinations in frequency. New technology has significantly reduced radiation exposure.

# Your Hearing Health

Hearing loss is the third-most common chronic health problem, after high blood pressure and arthritis, among older Americans.

**microwaves** Extremely high frequency electromagnetic waves that increase the rate at which molecules vibrate, thereby generating heat.

**ionizing radiation** A form of energy emitted from atoms as they undergo internal change.

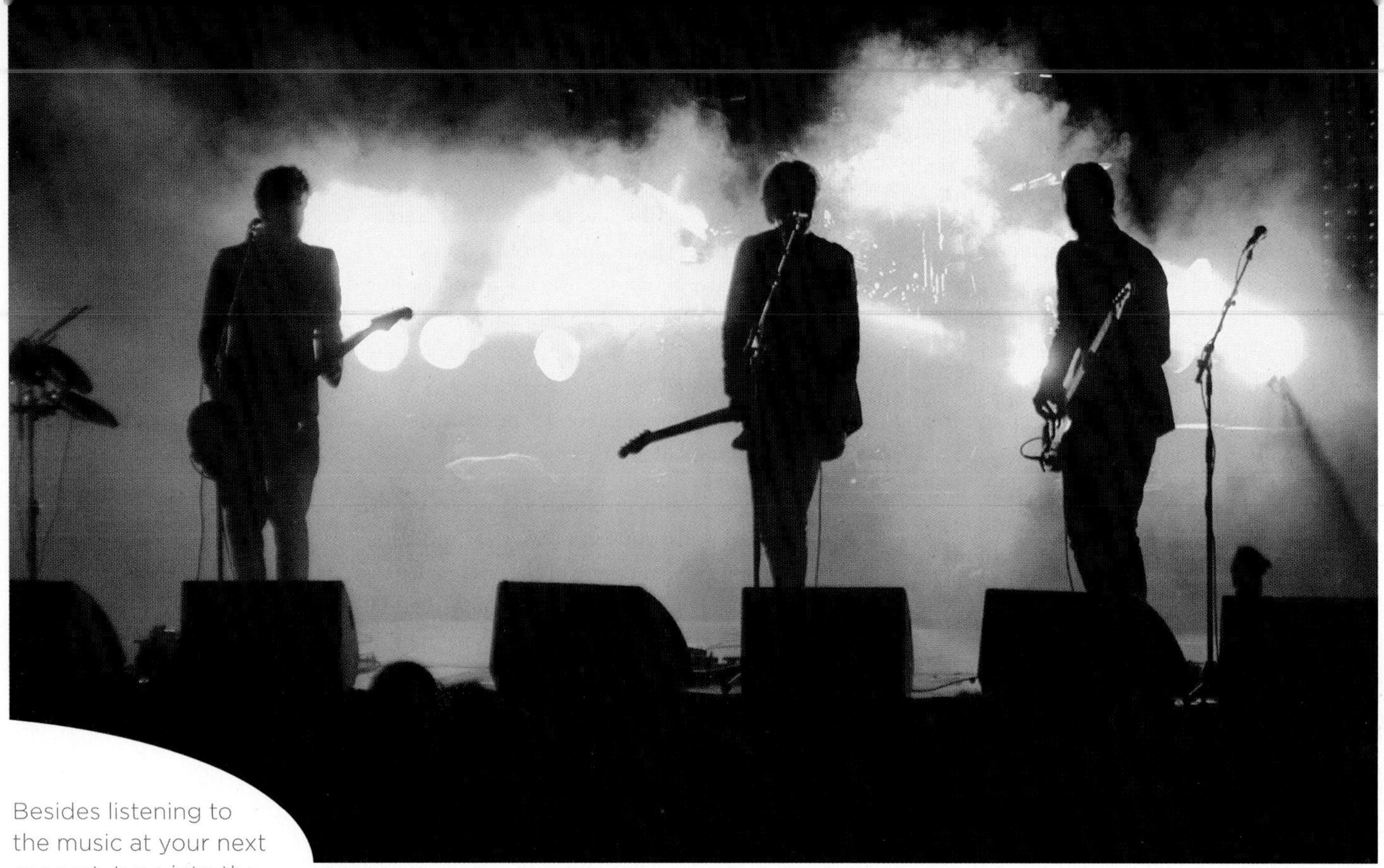

Besides listening to the music at your next concert, tune into the noise level and how your ears are feeling.

Noise-induced hearing loss is the most frequent preventable disability. Nearly 22 million Americans between ages 20 and 69 have irreversibly damaged hearing because of excessive noise exposure. Regular use of over-the-counter pain-killers also can lead to hearing loss, especially in younger men.[24]

## How Loud Is That Noise?

Loudness, or the intensity of a sound, is measured in **decibels** (**dB**). A whisper is 20 decibels; a conversation in a living room is about 50 decibels. On this scale, 50 isn't two and a half times louder than 20, but 1,000 times louder: Each 10-dB rise in the scale represents a tenfold increase in the intensity of the sound. Very loud but short bursts of sounds (such as gunshots and fireworks) and quieter but longer-lasting sounds (such as power tools) can induce hearing loss.

Sounds under 75 dB don't seem harmful. However, prolonged exposure to any sound over 85 dB (the equivalent of a power mower or food blender) or brief exposure to louder sounds can harm hearing. The noise level at rock concerts can reach 110 to 140 dB, about as loud as an air raid siren.

## Effects of Noise

Noise-induced hearing loss is 100 percent preventable—and irreversible. Hearing aids are the only treatment, but they do not correct the problem; they just amplify sound to compensate for hearing loss.

The healthy human ear can hear sounds within a wide range of frequencies (measured in hertz), from the low-frequency rumble of thunder at 50 hertz to the high-frequency overtones of a piccolo at nearly 20,000 hertz. High-frequency noise damages the delicate hair cells that serve as sound receptors in the inner ear. Damage first begins as a diminished sensitivity to frequencies around 4,000 hertz, the highest notes of a piano.

Early symptoms of hearing loss include difficulty understanding speech and *tinnitus* (ringing in the ears). Brief, very loud sounds, such as an explosion or gunfire, can produce immediate, severe, and permanent hearing loss. Longer exposure to less intense but still hazardous sounds, such

**decibel (dB)** A unit for measuring the intensity of sounds.

as those common at work or in public places, can gradually impair hearing, often without the individual's awareness.

Conductive hearing loss, often caused by ear infections, cuts down on perception of low-pitched sounds. Sensorineural loss involves damage or destruction of the sensory cells in the inner ear that convert sound waves to nerve signals.

Noise can harm more than our ears: High-volume sound has been linked to high blood pressure and other stress-related problems that can lead to heart disease, insomnia, anxiety, headaches, colitis, and ulcers. Noise frays the nerves; people tend to be more anxious, irritable, and angry when their ears are constantly barraged with sound.

## Are Earbuds Hazardous to Hearing?

Although there is limited research, audiologists (who specialize in hearing problems) report seeing greater noise-induced hearing loss in young people. One probable culprit is extended use of earbuds, tiny earphones used with portable music players that deliver sound extremely close to the eardrum. Hearing loss can be temporary or permanent.

The dangers to your hearing depend on how loud the music is and how long you listen. Because personal music players have long-lasting rechargeable batteries, people—especially young ones—both listen for long periods and turn up the volume because they feel "low personal vulnerability" to hearing loss. As long as the sound level is within safety levels (see Figure 19.3), you can listen as long as you'd like. If you listen to music so loud that someone else can hear it two or three feet away, it's too loud.

For safe listening, limit listening to a portable music player with earphones or earbuds at 60 percent of its potential volume to one hour a day. At the very least, take a five-minute break after an hour of listening and keep the volume low.

Ask yourself the following questions to determine if you should have your hearing checked:

- Do you frequently have to ask people to repeat themselves?

Figure 19.3 **Louder and Louder**

The human ear perceives a 10-decibel increase as a doubling of loudness. Thus, the 100 decibels of a subway train sound much more than twice as loud as the 50 decibels of a rushing stream.

*Note: The maximum exposure allowed on the job by federal law, in hours per day: 90 decibels, 8 hours; 100 decibels, 2 hours; 110 decibels, ½ hour.

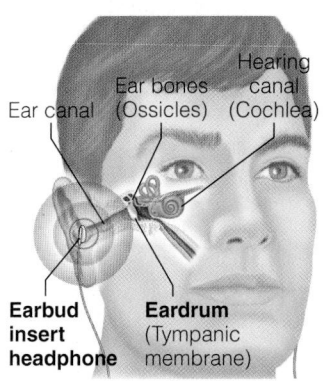

| Decibels | Example | Zone |
|---|---|---|
| 0 | The softest sound a typical ear can hear | Safe |
| 10 dB | Just audible | |
| 20 dB | Watch ticking; leaves rustling | |
| 30 dB | Soft whisper at 16 feet | |
| 40 dB | Quiet office; suburban street (no traffic) | |
| 50 dB | Interior of typical urban home; rushing stream | 1,000 times louder than 20 dB |
| 60 dB | Normal conversation; busy office | |
| 70 dB | Vacuum cleaner at 10 feet; hair dryer | |
| 80 dB | Alarm clock at 2 feet; loud music; average daily traffic | 1,000 times louder than 50 dB |
| 90 dB* | Motorcycle at 25 feet; jet 4 miles after takeoff | Risk of injury |
| 100 dB* | Video arcade; loud factory; subway train | |
| 110 dB* | Car horn at 3 feet; symphony orchestra; chain saw | 1,000 times louder than 80 dB |
| 120 dB | Jackhammer at 3 feet; boom box; nearby thunderclap | Injury |
| 130 dB | Rock concert; jet engine at 100 feet | |
| 140 dB | Jet engine nearby; amplified car stereo; firearms | 1,000 times louder than 110 dB |

## How to Protect Your Ears

- **If you must live or work in a noisy area, wear hearing protectors to prevent exposure to blasts of very loud noise.** Don't think cotton or facial tissue stuck in your ears can protect you; foam or soft plastic earplugs are more effective. Wear them when operating lawn mowers, weed trimmers, or power tools.

- **Give your ears some quiet time.** Rather than turning up the volume on your personal music player to blot out noise, look for truly quiet environments, such as the library, where you can rest your ears and focus your mind.

- **Soundproof your home by using draperies, carpets, and bulky furniture.** Put rubber mats under washing machines, blenders, and other noisy appliances. Seal cracks around windows and doors.

- **Beware of large doses of aspirin.** Researchers have found that eight aspirin tablets a day can aggravate the damage caused by loud noise; twelve a day can cause ringing in the ears (tinnitus).

- **Don't drink in noisy environments.** Alcohol intensifies the impact of noise and increases the risk of lifelong hearing damage.

- **When you hear a sudden loud noise, press your fingers against your ears.** Limit your exposure to loud noise. Several brief periods of noise seem less damaging than one long exposure.

- Do you have difficulty hearing when someone speaks in a whisper?

- Do people complain that you turn up the volume too much when watching television or listening to music?

- Do you have difficulty following conversation in a noisy environment?

- Do you avoid groups of people because of hearing difficulty?

- Have your friends or family suggested you might have hearing loss?

## Hearing Loss

 In a recent study, as many as one-quarter of college students suffered mild hearing loss, including some who believed their hearing was normal. This loss could be the result of use of personal music devices such as mp3 players.[25]

Hearing loss generally increases with age, affecting an estimated 21 percent of Americans ages 48 to 59 and 90 percent of those over age 80.[26] Yet only one in five Americans older than age 70 uses hearing aids, even though a much greater number have difficulty hearing and following conversations.[27]

# Taking Care of Mother Earth

Environmental problems can seem so complex that you may think there's little you can do about them. That's not the case. This world can be made better instead of worse. The job isn't easy, and all of us have to do our part. Just as many diseases of the previous century have been eradicated, so in time we may be able to remove or reduce many environmental threats. Your future—and our planet's future—may depend on it.

_____ **Plant a tree.** Even a single tree helps absorb carbon dioxide and produces cooling that can reduce the need for air conditioning.

_____ **Limit your driving.** If you usually drive to campus, check out alternatives, such as carpooling and public or campus transportation.

_____ **Precycle.** Surf the web for sites that sell products made from recycled materials. Click on **http://www.ecomall.com/** for listings.

_____ **Save the juice.** Plug your appliances and e-gadgets, which drain electricity even when turned off, into a power strip. Whenever you leave, flicking off the switch effectively unplugs them.

_____ **Integrate a new "green" habit into your life every week.** Turn the thermostat down in winter and up in summer. Spend a few minutes less in the shower. Use both sides of printer paper. Once a week declare a "spare the air" day and don't drive.

_____ **Avoid disposables.** Use a mug instead of a paper or foam cup, a sponge instead of a paper towel, a cloth napkin instead of a paper one.

_____ **Recycle.** Buy products made from recycled materials. Shop for used furniture or clothing. Don't throw away anything someone else may be able to use.

_____ **Be water wise.** Turn off the tap while you shave or brush your teeth. Install water-efficient faucets, toilets, and shower heads. Wash clothes in cold water. Drink tap rather than bottled water.

_____ **Spare the seas.** If you live near the coast or are picnicking or hiking near the ocean, don't use plastic bags (which are often blown into the water) or plastic six-pack holders (which can get caught around the necks of sea birds).

**Self Survey**

# Are You Doing Your Part for the Planet?

You may think that there is little you can do, as an individual, to save Earth. But everyday acts can add up and make a difference in helping or harming the planet on which we live.

|  | Almost Never | Sometimes | Always |
|---|---|---|---|
| 1. Do you walk, cycle, carpool, or use public transportation as much as possible to get around? | _____ | _____ | _____ |
| 2. Do you recycle? | _____ | _____ | _____ |
| 3. Do you reuse plastic and paper bags? | _____ | _____ | _____ |
| 4. Do you try to conserve water by not running the tap as you shampoo or brush your teeth? | _____ | _____ | _____ |
| 5. Do you use products made of recycled materials? | _____ | _____ | _____ |
| 6. Do you drive a car that gets good fuel mileage and has up-to-date emission control equipment? | _____ | _____ | _____ |

|  | Almost Never | Sometimes | Always |
|---|---|---|---|
| 7. Do you turn off lights, televisions, and appliances when you're not using them? | _____ | _____ | _____ |
| 8. Do you avoid buying products that are elaborately packaged? | _____ | _____ | _____ |
| 9. Do you use glass jars and waxed paper rather than plastic wrap for storing food? | _____ | _____ | _____ |
| 10. Do you take brief showers rather than baths? | _____ | _____ | _____ |
| 11. Do you use cloth towels and napkins rather than paper products? | _____ | _____ | _____ |
| 12. When listening to music, do you keep the volume low? | _____ | _____ | _____ |
| 13. Do you try to avoid any potential carcinogens, such as asbestos, mercury, or benzene? | _____ | _____ | _____ |
| 14. Are you careful to dispose of hazardous materials (such as automobile oil or antifreeze) at appropriate sites? | _____ | _____ | _____ |
| 15. Do you follow environmental issues in your community and write your state or federal representatives to support "green" legislation? | _____ | _____ | _____ |

Count the number of items you've checked in each column. If you've circled 10 or more in the "always" column, you're definitely helping to make a difference. If you've mainly circled "sometimes," you're moving in the right direction, but you need to be more consistent and more conscientious. If you've circled 10 or more in the "never" column, carefully read this chapter and "Your Health Action Plan for Protecting the Planet" to find out what you can do.

## Making Change Happen

## Going Green

Environmental concerns may seem so enormous that you may think that nothing you do will have an effect. This is not the case. The world can be made better instead of worse. You have the power to make choices and changes that will protect the environment we all share.

The lab "OurSpace" in *Labs for IPC* provides a systematic approach to living a "greener" life. Based on the Stages of Change discussed in Chapter 1 of this text and in *IPC*, the lab provides a blueprint that will guide you as you make changes that will benefit you and your environment. Here's a preview:

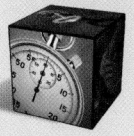

### Get Real

Before you know where you're going, you need to understand where you are. In this stage, you evaluate your environmental values by rating how important (on a scale of 0 to 100) each of 11 goals is to you, including:

- Slowing or stopping global warming. _____

- Improving air quality. _____

You record a second number for how involved you are with each item, with 0 representing not involved and 100 as involved in taking action as humanly possible.

You also assess how green your lifestyle is by checking which of 19 things you do regularly. These behaviors include:

- I buy products packaged simply in recycled or recyclable materials. _____

- I limit use of disposables such as paper napkins and plastic utensils. _____

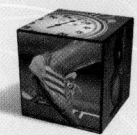

### Get Ready

Your next step is to prepare for change by following recommendations such as the following:

- **Check out campus resources.** Look for a local chapter of groups such as the Campus Climate Challenge, Student Environmental Action Coalition, or the Sierra Club. These organizations launch energy-conservation campaigns for their campuses, sponsor conferences, and so on. Download their calendars of scheduled activities for the term and get involved.

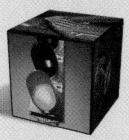

### Get Going

This is the stage where you start taking action with concrete steps that you incorporate into your daily life. Here is an excerpt from the comprehensive six-week green makeover included in the lab.

- **Adopt a space.** Take personal responsibility for a piece of the planet. This could be part of a path you walk every day to class, the stairs outside your dorm or apartment building, a neglected flower bed on the quad, your bus stop, whatever. Check on it regularly, and . . .

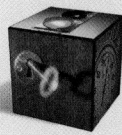

### Lock It In

Your planet is going to need your help for the rest of your life. That's why it's important to make your new environmentally friendly habits permanent. Here is an excerpt from one suggestion of how to do so:

- **Keep informed of environmental issues.** Americans are paying more attention to global warming and other environmental threats. Follow political discussions. Become familiar with the environmental positions of political candidates. Note which businesses are taking the initiative in fostering innovative, energy-saving programs. Be aware of . . .

# Making This Chapter Work for You

## Review Questions

1. Which of the following statements about climate change is *true*?
   a. Increasing carbon dioxide production will slow the progress of global warming.
   b. Most experts say that the buildup of greenhouse gases is changing natural climate and weather patterns.
   c. Climate change poses no health risks for humans in the next 20 years.
   d. Increasing tree cover and agricultural lands will contribute to global warming.

2. An example of the concept of sustainability is
   a. getting enough to eat at every meal.
   b. lowering the price of gas to 1990 levels.
   c. using wind power to generate electricity.
   d. maintaining our current levels of energy usage.

3. Mutagens
   a. are caused by birth defects.
   b. result in changes to the DNA of body cells.
   c. are agents that trigger changes in the DNA of body cells.
   d. are caused by repeated exposure to pollutants.

4. Drinking water safety
   a. may be compromised if your water comes from a well.
   b. is low in the United States because of chemical treatment.
   c. can be guaranteed by using bottled water, which is completely free of chemical contaminants.
   d. is measured by the cases of illness reported each year.

5. Threats to the environment include
   a. an open ecosystem.
   b. depletion of the oxygen layer.
   c. ecological processes.
   d. global warming.

6. Pesticide risks to health include
   a. reduced male fertility.
   b. higher incidence of childhood brain cancer if parents have been exposed.
   c. higher incidence of cancer and birth defects from chlorinated hydrocarbons such as DDT.
   d. higher incidence of diabetes.

7. One of the most important things you can do to help protect the environment is
   a. use as much water as possible to help lower the ocean water levels.
   b. recycle paper, bottles, cans, and unwanted food.
   c. avoid energy-depleting fluorescent bulbs.
   d. use plastic storage containers and plastic wrap to save trees from being cut down.

8. Precycling is
   a. planning ahead about recycling.
   b. buying products packaged in recycled material.
   c. removing excess packaging and leaving it in the store where an item was purchased.
   d. preparing to recycle.

9. You can protect your hearing by
   a. avoiding prolonged exposure to sounds under 75 decibels.
   b. using foam earplugs when operating noisy tools or attending rock concerts.
   c. limiting noise exposure to short bursts of loud sounds such as fireworks.
   d. drinking alcohol in noisy environments to mute the sounds.

10. Which of the following statements about air pollution is *false*?
    a. More than 80 percent of the people in the United States live in counties with unhealthy levels of ozone or particle pollution.
    b. Ozone in the upper atmosphere protects us from harmful ultraviolet radiation from the sun, but in the lower atmosphere, it is a harmful air pollutant.
    c. Air pollution can cause the same types of respiratory health problems as smoking.
    d. Particle pollution diminishes lung function and increases the severity of asthma attacks.

*Answers to these questions can be found on page 672.*

## Critical Thinking

1. How do you contribute to environmental pollution? How might you change your habits to protect the environment?

2. An excerpt from a recent newspaper article stated, "Children living in a public housing project near a local refinery suffer from a high rate of asthma and allergies, and an environmental group says the plant may be to blame." The refinery has met all the local air quality standards, employs hundreds in the community, and pays substantial city taxes, which support police, fire, and social services. If you were a city council member, how would you balance health and environmental concerns with the need for industry in your community? What actions would you recommend in this particular situation?

3. In one Harris poll, 84 percent of Americans said that, given a choice between a high standard of living (but with hazardous air and water pollution and the depletion of natural resources) and a lower standard of living (but with clean air and drinking water), they would prefer clean air and drinking water and a lower standard of living. What about you? What exactly would you be willing to give up: air conditioning, convenience packaging and products, driving your own car rather than using public transportation? Do you think most people are willing to change their lifestyles to preserve the environment?

## Media Menu

Visit www.cengagebrain.com to access course materials and companion resources for this text that will:

- Help you evaluate your knowledge of the material.

- Allow you to prepare for exams with interactive quizzing.

- Use the CengageNOW product to develop a Personalized Learning Plan targeting resources that address areas you should study.

- Coach you through identifying target goals for behavioral change and creating and monitoring your personal change plan throughout the semester using the Behavior Change Planner available in the CengageNOW resource.

## Internet Connections

**www.envirolink.org**
Envirolink is a nonprofit organization that brings together individuals and groups concerned about the environment and provides access to a wealth of online environmental resources.

**www.seac.org**
Since 1988, the Student Environmental Action Coalition has been empowering students and youth to fight for environmental and social justice in our schools and communities.

**www.campusclimatechallenge.org**
The Challenge leverages the power of young people to organize on college campuses and high schools across

Canada and the United States to win 100% Clean Energy policies at their schools.

**www.stopglobalwarming.org**
This site is a nonpartisan effort to bring citizens together to declare that global warming is here now and that it is time to demand solutions.

**www.cdc.gov/nceh/**
This site, sponsored by the U.S. Centers for Disease Control and Prevention, features a searchable database as well as fact sheets and brochures on a variety of environmental topics, from emergency preparedness and public health tracking to environmental hazards and lead poisoning prevention.

## Key Terms

The terms listed are used on the page indicated. Definitions of the terms are in the Glossary at the end of the book.

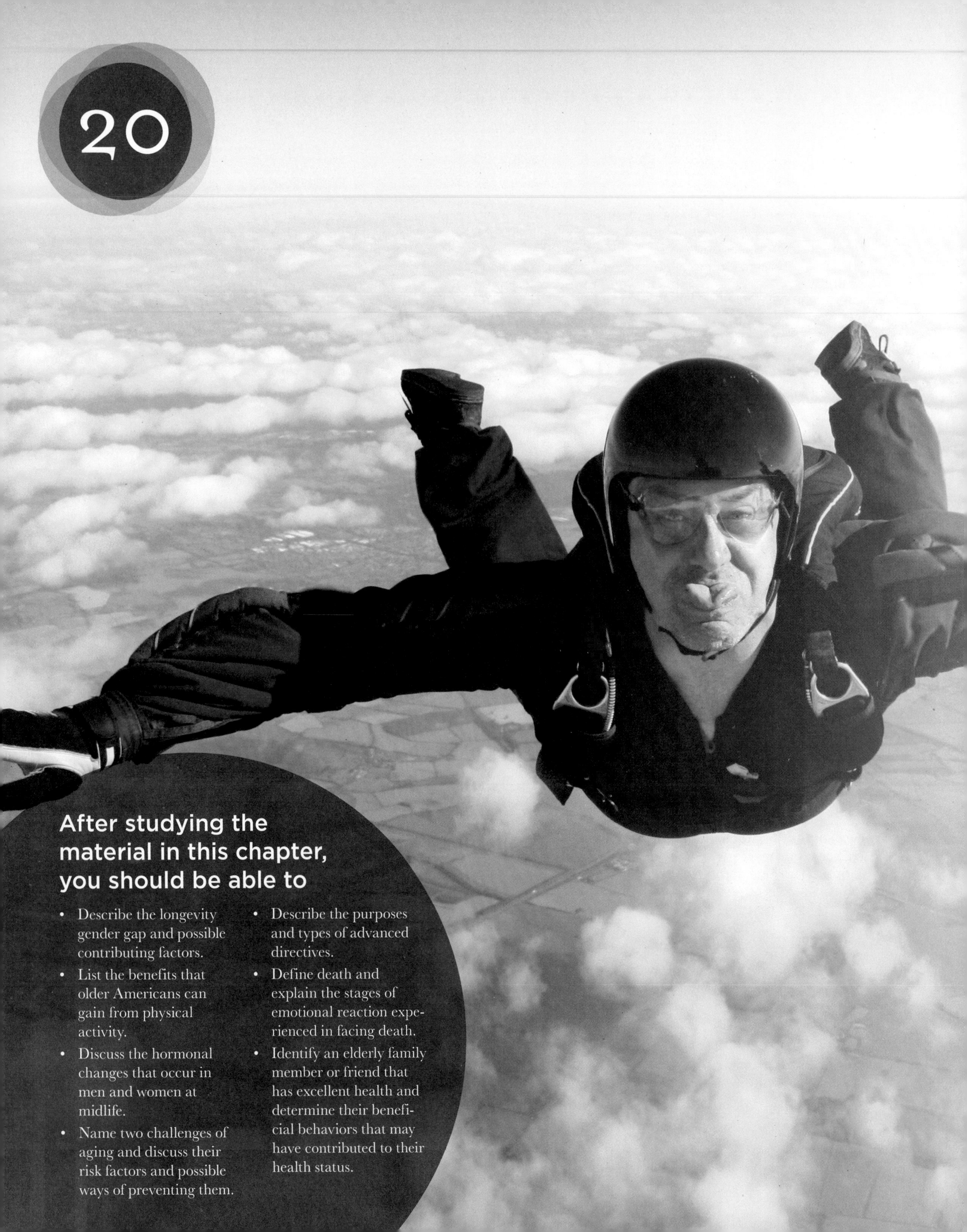

**20**

## After studying the material in this chapter, you should be able to

- Describe the longevity gender gap and possible contributing factors.
- List the benefits that older Americans can gain from physical activity.
- Discuss the hormonal changes that occur in men and women at midlife.
- Name two challenges of aging and discuss their risk factors and possible ways of preventing them.

- Describe the purposes and types of advanced directives.
- Define death and explain the stages of emotional reaction experienced in facing death.
- Identify an elderly family member or friend that has excellent health and determine their beneficial behaviors that may have contributed to their health status.

Frank didn't feel old until he enrolled in a college personal health course. Formal at first, the other students—young enough to be his children—started calling him "Pop." When the professor announced that the next week's topic would be aging, Frank beamed, "I'll be the expert!"

# A Lifetime of Health

More of us can expect to say the same. In the United States, the number of people over age 65 is expected to increase from 12 to nearly 20 percent of the population—an estimated 71.5 million in 2030.

Although **aging**—the characteristic pattern of normal life changes that occurs as humans, plants, and animals grow older—remains inevitable, you can do a great deal to influence the impact that the passage of time has on you. Whether you're in your teens, 20s, 30s, or older, now is the time to take the steps that will add healthy, active, productive years to your life.

This chapter provides a preview of the changes age brings, the steps you can take to age healthfully, and the ways you can make the most of all the years of your life.

Invariably, though, no one gets out of this life alive. Death is the natural completion of things, as much a part of the real world as life itself. In time we all lose people we cherish: grandparents, aunts and uncles, parents, friends, neighbors, coworkers, siblings. With each loss, part of us may seem to die, yet each loss also reaffirms how precious life is.

This chapter explores the meaning of death, describes the process of dying, provides infor-

mation on end-of-life issues, and offers advice on comforting the dying and helping their survivors.

## The Aging of America

About one in eight Americans—approximately 12 percent of the population—is over age 65. With millions of baby boomers reaching retirement age, one in every five Americans will be older than 65 by the year 2030. (See Figure 20.1.)

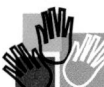 Older Americans are as diverse as other segments of our population. About one in five (19 percent) comes from a minority group. The largest percentage of these are African American (9 percent) or Hispanic (6 percent). Asians or Pacific Islanders make up about 3 percent of older Americans.

About three in four older Americans describe their health as good or better. Older African Americans, American Indians/Alaska Natives, and Hispanics are less likely to say they are in top health than are whites. Most older people have at least one chronic condition; many have several health problems. Women report more arthritis; men, more heart disease and cancer.

**aging** The characteristic pattern of normal life changes that occur as living things grow older.

Visit www.cengagebrain.com to access course materials for this text, including the Behavior Change Planner, interactive quizzes, tutorials, and more. See the preface on page xv for details.

Figure 20.1  **The Age Boom**

The baby boomers (those born between 1946 and 1964) started turning 65 in 2011, and the number of older people will increase dramatically. The older population in 2030 is projected to be twice as large as in 2000.

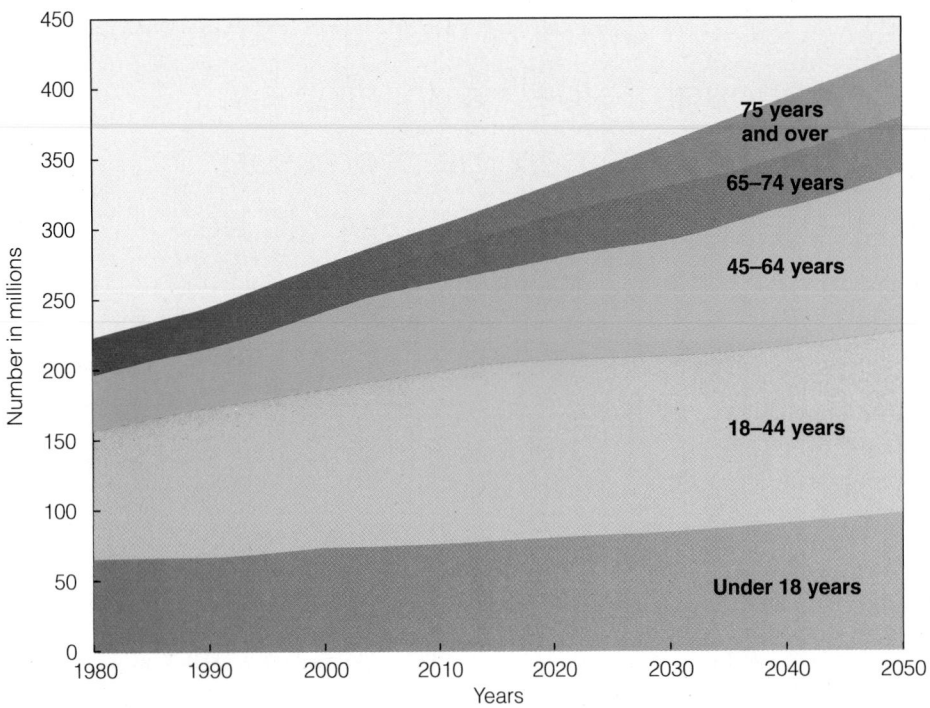

## How Long Can You Expect to Live?

The answer depends on you. Statistically, you're likely to live longer than your parents or grandparents. Life expectancy has been increasing steadily over the last century and now is 78.2 years. According to the National Center for Health Statistics, life expectancy for American women now stands at 80.6 years; for men, it is a record high of 75.7 years.[1]

Medical advances, including new medications, are driving down the rates of major killers such as heart disease, cancer, and stroke and are contributing to longer life expectancies. Death rates have fallen for men, women, whites, blacks, and Hispanics.[2] However, behavioral or lifestyle choices also make a big difference.

According to a recent study, Americans who smoke, have high blood pressure, have high blood sugar, and are overweight may be shortening their life expectancy by an average of four years. The patterns of smoking, high blood pressure, high blood glucose, and overweight/obesity account for almost 75 percent of differences in cardiovascular deaths and up to 50 percent of differences in cancer deaths in various areas of the United States.

Here is the difference in life expectancy each of these health hazards can make:

- **High blood pressure:** 1.5 years for men, 1.6 years for women.
- **Obesity:** 1.3 years for men, 1.3 years for women.
- **High blood sugar:** .5 years for men, .3 years for women.
- **Smoking:** 2.5 years for men, 1.8 years for women.[3]

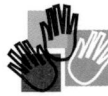 The causes of death vary with age (see "How Do You Compare?"). In the teen and young adult years, males are more likely to die than females, typically from accidents, suicides, and homicides, and older teens are more likely to die than younger ones.[4] Teenage black males are 20 times more likely to die from homicide than are white males. Teenage black and Hispanic females are also more likely to die from homicide than are American Indian, white, and Asian teen girls.[5] As a person reaches 45, the top risk of death is

from cancer, followed by heart disease. At around age 65, the risks swap: a person is most likely to die from heart disease, followed by cancer.[6]

## The Longevity Gender Gap

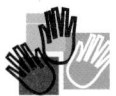 Women's lifespans average 5 to 10 percent longer than men's. No one knows exactly why. This longevity gender gap has been shrinking since 1990 and now stands at 4.9 years.[7] Women in other developed nations—Australia, Canada, France, Greece, Italy, Japan, the Netherlands, Norway, Spain, Sweden, Switzerland—live up to two years longer than those in the United States and about seven years longer than men. In the former Soviet Union, life expectancy for females is 13 years longer than for males.

Why do men die sooner? The female edge may begin at conception with the extra X chromosome, which provides a backup for defects on the X gene and a double dose of the genetic factors that regulate the immune system. In addition, the female hormone estrogen bolsters immunity and protects heart, bone, brain, and blood vessels.

In some cancers, estrogen may somehow protect against distant metastases. In contrast, testosterone may dampen the immune response in males—possibly to prevent attacks on sperm cells that might otherwise be mistaken as alien invaders. When the testes are removed from mice and guinea pigs, their immune systems become more active. In men, lessened immunity may lower resistance to cancer as well as infectious disease.

Testosterone also has been implicated in men's risk of heart disease and stroke. Originally designed to equip men with an instantaneous burst of power—essential for survival in Stone Age times—this potent male hormone may surge so intensely that it wreaks havoc throughout the cardiovascular system.

Males also die more often as a result of intentional and nonintentional injury. Overall, men are three times more likely than women to die in accidents, mainly in cars and on the job. Men also are four times more likely to die violently. Nine in ten murderers and eight in ten murder victims are men.

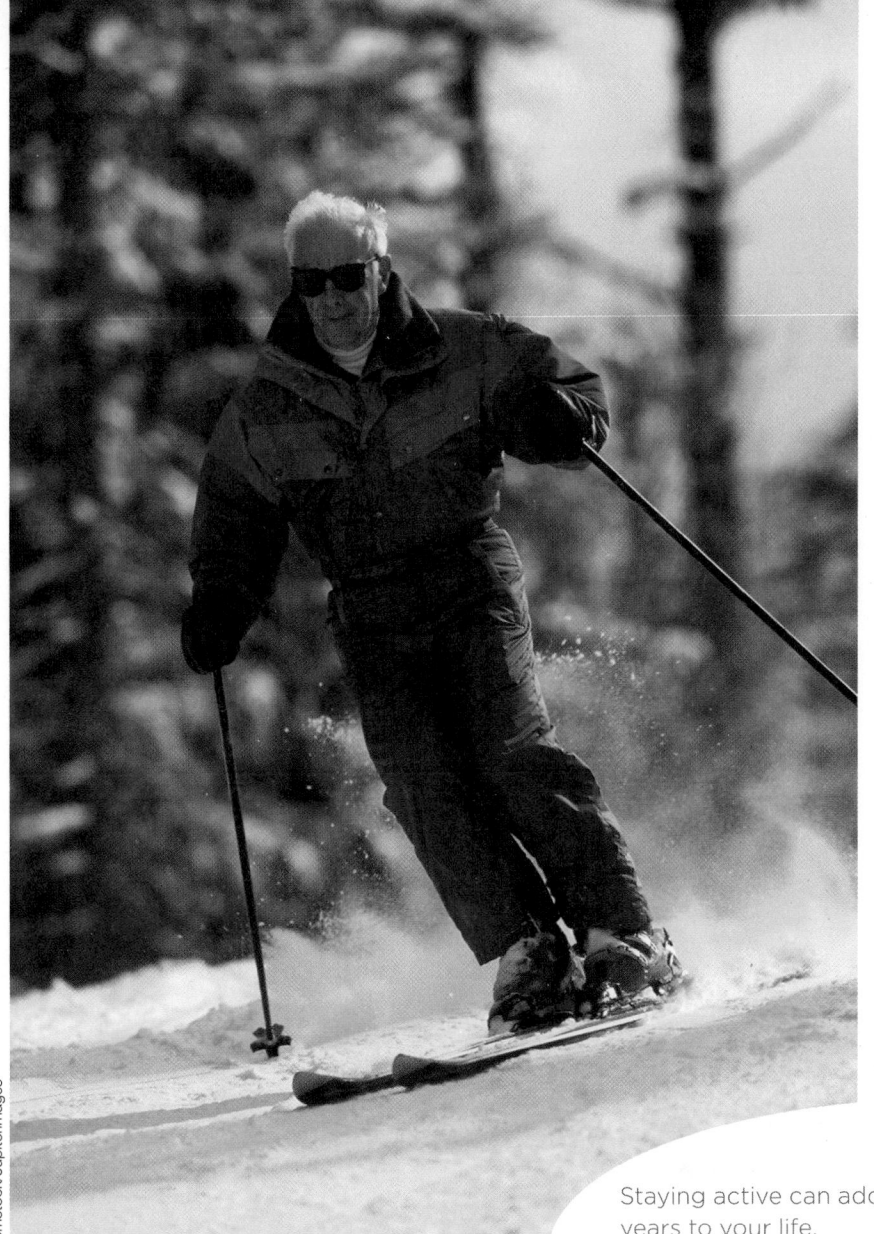

Comstock/Jupiterimages

Staying active can add years to your life.

## Successful Aging

Although Americans are living longer than ever, many may not reach old age in prime condition. According to a recent survey, physical disabilities that limit mobility are increasing among middle-aged Americans. In a recent survey, more than 40 percent of those between ages 50 and 64 reported problems such as difficulty standing for two hours, stooping, walking a quarter mile, or climbing ten steps without resting.[8] Middle-aged women who are not fit show increasing rates of physical frailty throughout life.[9]

According to research on "exceptional longevity" (survival to at least age 90), the key factors

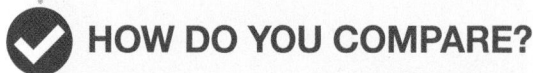
to living long and well are maintaining a healthy lifestyle (including regular exercise, weight management, and no smoking) and avoiding or delaying chronic illnesses. Among the growing number of "centenarians" who live past their hundredth birthday, two-thirds did not develop age-related conditions such as diabetes, dementia, heart disease, osteoporosis, Parkinson's disease, or stroke until age 85 or older. Men who make it to the century mark have significantly better mental and physical functioning than women their age.

When surveyed, about half of Americans ages 65 to 69 say, "These are the best years of my life." Many people in their 70s and 80s agree. When asked about the keys to a meaningful and vital life, older adults rate having family and friends and taking care of their health as most important, followed by spiritual life.

## Physical Activity: It's Never Too Late

The effects of ongoing activity are so profound that gerontologists sometimes refer to exercise as "the closest thing to an antiaging pill." Exercise slows many changes associated with advancing age, such as loss of lean muscle tissue, increase in body fat, and decreased work capacity. Consistent lifelong exercise preserves heart muscle

in the elderly to levels that match or even exceed those of healthy young sedentary individuals.[10]

The benefits of exercise extend to both men and women. In one study of healthy older men, regular exercise was associated with a nearly 30 percent lower mortality rate. In a study of overweight, postmenopausal women, exercise improved physical and mental well-being—and the more the women exercised, the greater the improvements in their quality of life. In other research on Canadian women older than 65, those who took part in regular aerobic activity had higher scores of cognitive function than their sedentary peers. The bottom line: What you *don't* do may matter more than what you do.

No one is ever too old to get in shape. The American College of Sports Medicine encourages seniors to engage in the full range of physical activities, including aerobic conditioning. With regular conditioning, 60-year-olds can regain the fitness they had at age 40 to 45. Adults over the age of 72 who exercise more and smoke less than their peers are most likely to enjoy long, healthy, and happy lives, according to a study that followed 1,000 seniors for nine years.

Exercise lowers the risk of diabetes, heart disease, and stroke in the elderly—and greatly improves general health. Male and female runners over age 50 have much lower rates of disability and much lower health-care expenses than less active seniors. Even less-intense activities, such as gardening, dancing, and brisk walking, can delay chronic physical disability and cognitive decline.

According to the U.S. surgeon general, physical activity offers older Americans additional benefits, including the following:

• Greater ability to live independently.

• Reduced risk of falling and fracturing bones.

• Lower risk of dying from coronary heart disease and of developing high blood pressure, colon cancer, and diabetes.

• Reduced blood pressure in some people with hypertension.

• Fewer symptoms of anxiety and depression.

• Improvements in mood and feelings of well-being.

Despite these potential benefits, many seniors are not active. By age 75, about one in three men and one in two women engage in no physical activity. Yet even sedentary individuals in their 80s and 90s can participate in an exercise program—and gain significant benefits.

At any age, staying fit doesn't have to be expensive. (See Health on a Budget, p. 650.) Older adults who take part in low-cost fitness programs offered by YMCAs or senior centers have shown significant improvement in their daily functioning and lower risk of becoming disabled.

The American College of Sports Medicine and American Heart Association recommend developing a fitness plan with a health professional to manage risks and take health conditions into account. Its basics should consist of:

• Moderately intense aerobic exercise 30 minutes a day, five days a week

    or

• Vigorously intense aerobic exercise 20 minutes a day, three days a week

    and

• 8 to 10 strength-training exercises, with 10 to 15 repetitions of each exercise, two or three times a week

    and

• balance exercises.

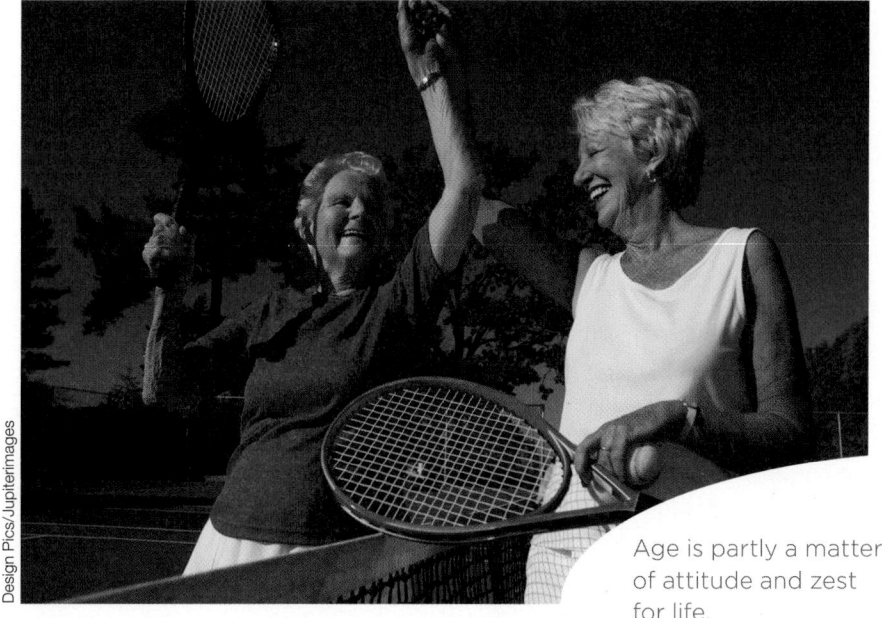

Design Pics/Jupiterimages

Age is partly a matter of attitude and zest for life.

## Nutrition and Obesity

The most common nutritional disorder in older persons is obesity. Overweight men and women over age 65 face higher risk of diabetes, heart disease, stroke, and other health problems, including arthritis.

Many elderly people who live independently do not get adequate amounts of one or more essential nutrients. The reasons are many: limited income, difficulty getting to stores, chronic illness, medications that interfere with the metabolism of nutrients, problems chewing or digesting, poor appetite, inactivity, illness, depression. Nutritionists urge the elderly, like other Americans, to concentrate on eating healthful foods; many also recommend daily nutritional supplements, which may provide the added benefit of improving cognitive function in healthy people over 65.

## The Aging Brain

Scientists used to think that the aging brain, once worn out, could never be fixed. Now they know that the brain can and does repair itself. When neurons (brain cells) die, the surrounding cells develop "fingers" to fill the gaps and establish new connections, or synapses, between surviving neurons. Although self-repair occurs more quickly in young brains, the process continues in older brains. Even victims of Alzheimer's disease, the most devastating form of senility,

# "Buy" Yourself a Longer Life

You don't need money for the only anti-aging program that has been proven to add years to life expectancy. All you have to do is follow four basic steps:

- **Keep your arteries young.**
  If your arteries are clear and healthy, you're more likely to have a healthy heart and a sharper brain and less likely to develop high blood pressure, high cholesterol, kidney problems, and memory impairment. For your arteries' sake, exercise regularly, avoid high-fat foods, watch your weight, and find ways to manage daily stress (see Chapter 4).

- **Avoid illness.** Most individuals who live to celebrate their hundredth birthday don't suffer from chronic diseases. Defend yourself by eating a healthy diet, not smoking, avoiding

weight gain in middle age, recognizing and treating conditions like high blood pressure and elevated cholesterol, and keeping up with immunizations.

- **Stay strong.** As landmark studies with frail nursing home residents in their 80s and 90s have shown, strength training at any age builds muscle and bone, speeds up metabolic rate, improves sleep and mobility, boosts the spirit, and enhances self-confidence.

- **Maintain your zest for living.** Just as with muscles, the best advice to keep your brain strong is "use it or lose it." Keep challenging yourself, asking questions, and pursuing new passions. Individuals who are optimistic, sociable, and happy generally outlive their more pessimistic, grumpier peers.

---

have enough healthy cells in the diseased brain to regrow synapses. Scientists hope to develop drugs that someday may help the brain repair itself.

Mental ability does not decline along with physical vigor. In fact, we do indeed get wiser as we get older. Older adults are better equipped than younger ones to see multiple points of view, to search for compromise, and to solve social conflicts. However, they may find it more difficult to multitask and split their focus between two tasks.[11]

Researchers have been able to reverse the supposedly normal intellectual declines of 60- to 80-year-olds by tutoring them in problem solving. Reaction time, intellectual speed and efficiency, nonverbal intelligence, and maximum work rate for short periods may diminish by age 75. However, understanding, vocabulary, ability to remember key information, and verbal intelligence remain about the same.

**menopause** The complete cessation of ovulation and menstruation for 12 consecutive months.

Aspirin, even at low doses, appears to prevent declines in key areas of the brain, according to brain-imaging studies. However, long-term use of low-dose aspirin did not lead to improved thinking, memory, and other cognitive skills in women over age 65 participating in the landmark Women's Health Study. In other research, nonsteroidal anti-inflammatory drugs (NSAIDs) failed to prevent Alzheimer's disease in older men and women with a family history of the disorder. The herbal supplement ginkgo biloba also has no clear-cut benefit in preventing memory problems.

*Memory*   According to data from a National Institute of Aging survey, memory loss and cognitive problems are becoming less common among older Americans. The reasons may be that today's seniors have more formal education, higher economic status, and better health care for problems such as high blood pressure and high cholesterol that can jeopardize brain function.

Higher education does not prevent cognitive decline over time, according to recent research, but schooling does yield an advantage. Individuals with more education continue to have a higher level of cognitive functioning into old age so they remain independent for a longer period. There is growing evidence that using your brain as you age—by reading, playing games, solving crossword puzzles, and doing crafts such as pottery or quilting—greatly decreases the risk of memory loss.

## Women at Midlife

In the next two decades some 40 million American women will end their reproductive years. "The primary misconception is that this is a terrible time when all women suffer horrible symptoms," says Sherry Sherman, M.D., project officer for the National Institute of Aging's Study of Women Across the Nation, which has followed 3,300 women through midlife since 1996. "When you look at healthy women in the community in terms of what actually affects their lives, their periods stop. That's it."[12]

*Perimenopause*   While the average age of **menopause**—defined as the complete cessation of menstrual periods for 12 consecutive months—is 51.5, a woman's reproductive system begins changing more than a decade earlier.

"The change of life starts in our thirties with irregular menstrual cycles and then heats up in our forties with hot flashes and night sweats," says psychiatrist Marsha Speller, M.D., author of *The Menopause Answer Book*.[13]

For many women, **perimenopause**—the four-to-ten-year span before a woman's last period—is more baffling and bothersome than the years after. During this time the egg cells, or oocytes, in a woman's ovaries start to senesce, or die off, at a faster rate. Eventually, the number of egg cells drops to a tiny fraction of the estimated 2 million packed into her ovaries at birth. Trying to coax some of the remaining oocytes to ripen, the pituitary gland churns out extra follicle-stimulating hormone (FSH). This surge is the earliest harbinger of menopause, occurring six to ten years before a woman's final periods. Eventually, the other menstrual messenger, luteinizing hormone (LH), also increases, but at a slower rate.

These hormonal shifts can trigger an array of symptoms. The most common is night sweats (a *subdromal hot flash*, in medical terms), which can be intense enough to disrupt sleep. The drop in estrogen levels also may cause hot flashes (bursts of perspiration that last from a few seconds to 15 minutes). Women who have night sweats and hot flashes at the start of menopause may be less likely to have a heart attack. Those who develop these symptoms later in menopause may have higher heart disease risks.[14]

A woman's habits and health history also have an impact. Women with a lifelong history of depression are more likely to experience early perimenopause. The fluctuating hormones of perimenopause may increase depressive symptoms even in women who have never had previous depressions. Smokers experience more symptoms at an earlier age than nonsmokers. Heavier women also have more severe symptoms.

*Menopause* About 10 to 15 percent of women breeze through this transition with only trivial symptoms. Another 10 to 15 percent are virtually disabled. The majority fall somewhere in between these extremes. Women who undergo surgical or medical menopause (the result of removal of their ovaries or chemotherapy) often experience abrupt symptoms, including flushing, sweating, sleeplessness, early morning awakenings, involuntary urination,

changes in libido, mood swings, perception of memory loss, and changes in cognitive function.

 Race and ethnicity profoundly affect women's experience. African American women report more hot flashes and night sweats but have more positive attitudes toward menopause. Japanese and Chinese women experience more muscle stiffness and fewer hot flashes but view menopause more negatively. Hispanic women reach menopause a year or two earlier than Caucasian women; Asian women, a year or two later.

Dwindling levels of estrogen subtly affect many aspects of a woman's health, from her mouth (where dryness, unusual tastes, burning, and gum problems can develop) to her skin (which may become drier, itchier, and overly sensitive to touch). With less estrogen to block them, a woman's androgens, or male hormones, may have a greater impact, causing acne, hair loss, and according to some anecdotal reports, surges in sexual appetite. (Other women, however, report a drop in sexual desire.)

At the same time, a woman's clitoris, vulva, and vaginal lining begin to shrivel, sometimes resulting in pain or bleeding during intercourse. Since the thinner genital tissues are less effective in keeping out bacteria and other pathogens, urinary tract infections may become more common. Some women develop breast or ovarian cysts, which usually go away on their own. Eventually, a woman's ovaries don't respond at all to her pituitary hormones. After the last ovulatory cycle, progesterone is no longer secreted, and estrogen levels decrease rapidly. A woman's testosterone level also falls.

In the United States, the average woman who reaches menopause has a life expectancy of about 30 more years. However, she faces risks of various diseases, including an increased risk of obesity, metabolic syndrome, heart disease, stroke, and breast cancer. Women can reduce these risks by exercise, good nutrition, and weight control both before and after menopause.

"Exercise is the best thing a woman can do for herself at midlife," says JoAnn Pinkerton, M.D., of the National Women's Health Resource Center. "It improves your heart function so you have less chance of heart disease. It improves your cognition so you think better. It decreases your risk of breast cancer. It helps your mood. It

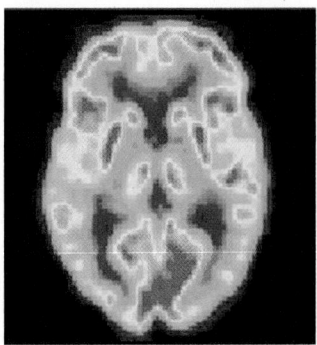
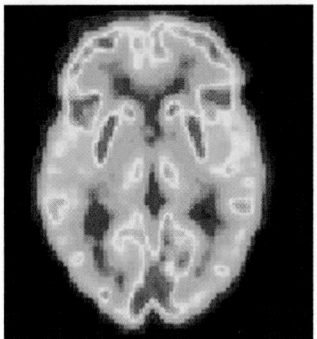

In these PET scans, the red and yellow show greater neuron activity in the young adult. The brain of the older person shows less activity and more dark areas, indicating that the fluid-filled ventricles have grown larger. Recent research shows, however, that older brains do repair themselves.

**perimenopause** The period from a woman's first irregular cycles to her last menstruation.

lessens the likelihood of depression. It increases energy and protects your bones."[15] In a recent study, walking proved effective in easing anxiety, boosting mood, and improving the quality of life of women during menopause.

*Hormone Therapy* **Hormone therapy (HT)** was long believed to prevent heart disease and strokes and help women live longer. But medical thinking on HT, particularly a combination of estrogen and progestin, has changed completely in recent years. HT is no longer recommended for reasons other than short-term relief of symptoms such as hot flashes and night sweats.

The Women's Health Initiative (WHI)—a series of clinical trials begun in 1991 on postmenopausal women—halted its study of combination estrogen/progestin therapy in July 2002 and its study of estrogen-only therapy in 2004 because of safety concerns. As various studies have confirmed, combination therapy increases the risk of breast cancer, heart disease, blood clots, and stroke. In the latest analysis of the WHI data, the risks to women who took estrogen-only therapy faded after they stopped their treatment.[16] Thus, women and their doctors are opting for treatments that are safer, can be taken at lower doses, can be administered via different routes (such as sprays), and do not include progesterone.

Hormonal therapy does reduce the risk of postmenopausal osteoporosis, but its risks and benefits need to be weighed against those of other available treatments. Women who stop hormonal therapy have about a 50 percent chance that their menopausal symptoms will recur, regardless of their age or how long they used HT. In controlled trials, black cohosh, the most popular herbal treatment, either alone or with other herbs, proved no more effective than placebo in relieving hot flashes and other menopause symptoms. In a controlled trial, acupuncture also failed to provide reliable relief of menopausal hot flashes. Among other promising approaches are soy (although it is less effective than hormone therapy)[17] and classes in mindfulness (discussed in Chapter 4) and stretching.[18]

## Men at Midlife

Although men don't experience the dramatic hormonal upheaval that women do, they do experience a decline by as much as 30 to 40 percent in their primary sex hormone, testosterone, between the ages of 48 and 70. This change, sometimes called *andropause*, may cause a range of symptoms, including decreased muscle mass, greater body fat, loss of bone density, flagging energy, lowered fertility, and impaired virility. Some researchers are experimenting with testosterone supplements now available in various forms, including under-the-skin implants, transdermal patches, and gel. In tests with young men, testosterone has increased lean body mass and decreased body fat—at least temporarily. However, other researchers warn that, particularly in older men, excess testosterone might raise the risk of prostate cancer and heart disease.

After age 40, the prostate gland, which surrounds the urethra at the base of the bladder, enlarges. This condition, called *benign prostatic hypertrophy*, occurs in every man. By age 50, half of all men have some enlargement of the gland; after 70, three-quarters do. As it expands, the prostate tends to pinch the urethra, decreasing urinary flow and creating a sense of urinary urgency, particularly at night. Other warning signs of prostate problems include difficult urination, blood in the urine, painful ejaculation, or constant lower-back pain.

Medical treatments for benign prostate hypertrophy include drugs that improve urine flow and reduce obstruction of the bladder outlet as well as medications that partially shrink the enlarged prostate by lowering the level of the major male hormone inside the prostate. In some cases, surgical treatment is necessary.

## Sexuality and Aging

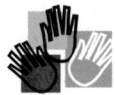 Health and sexuality interact in various ways as we age. When they are healthy and have a willing partner, a substantial number of older men remain sexually active. The fittest men and women report more frequent sexual activity. Better health translates into a better sex life. Healthy people are more likely to express an interest in sex, engage in sex, and enjoy sex.

In a recent analysis, researchers calculated the "sexual life expectancy" of men and women. According to their data, on average 55-year-old men can expect to remain sexually active for another 15 years while women the same

**hormone therapy (HT)** The use of supplemental hormones during and after menopause.

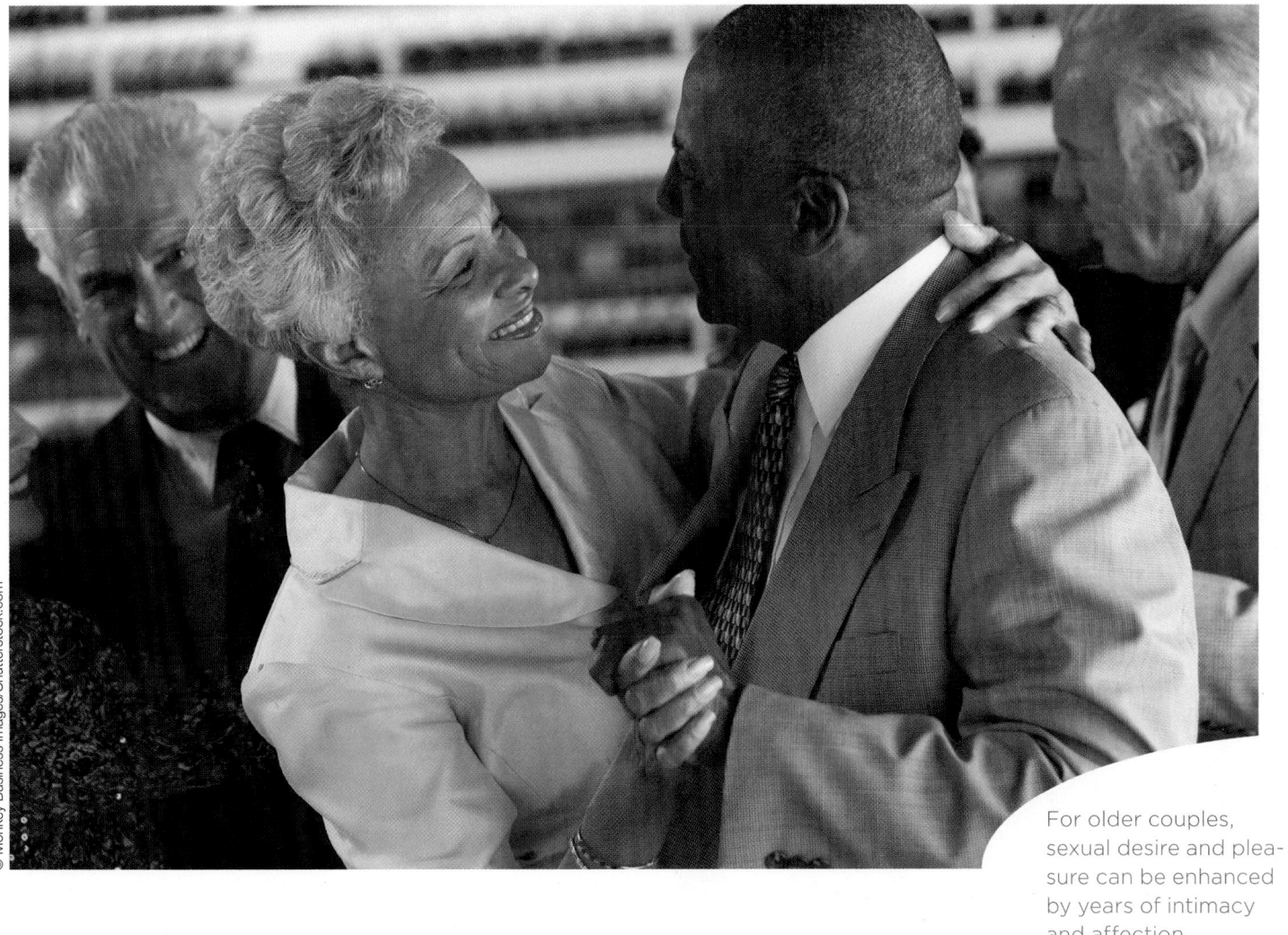

For older couples, sexual desire and pleasure can be enhanced by years of intimacy and affection.

age could expect about 11 more sexually active years. Women with partners remain sexually active longer. Men in good health gain an additional five to seven years of sexual life expectancy.[19]

Other research has found a relationship between sex and longevity. A Swedish study found that men, but not women, who had discontinued intercourse had higher death rates. A study of the entire male population of a small Welsh town found that the sexually active men had half the mortality of the inactive group. In a Duke University study, longevity in women correlated with enjoyment of sexual intercourse, rather than with its frequency.

Aging does cause some changes in sexual response: Women produce less vaginal lubrication. An older man needs more time to achieve an erection or orgasm and to attain another erection after ejaculating. Both men and women experience fewer contractions during orgasm. However, none of these changes reduces sexual pleasure or desire.

# The Challenges of Age

No matter how well we eat, exercise, and take care of ourselves, some physical changes are inevitable as we age. (See Consumer Alert, p. 656.) Figure 20.2 shows some of these changes, but most of them are not debilitating, and people can remain active and vital into extreme old age. Aging brains and bodies do become vulnerable to diseases like Alzheimer's and osteoporosis. Other common life problems, such as depression, substance misuse, and safe driving, become more challenging as we age.

Figure 20.2   **The Effects of Aging on the Body**

## Alzheimer's

Alzheimer's disease is the most common form of dementia in those aged 65 or older. Although this memory disorder is still incurable, researchers are developing new insights and approaches to treatment. To get the most recent information, access Global Health Watch and go to "Diseases." Scroll down, and click on "Alzheimer's Disease." Scan the headlines under "Latest news," and select a relevant article. Write a summary in your online journal.

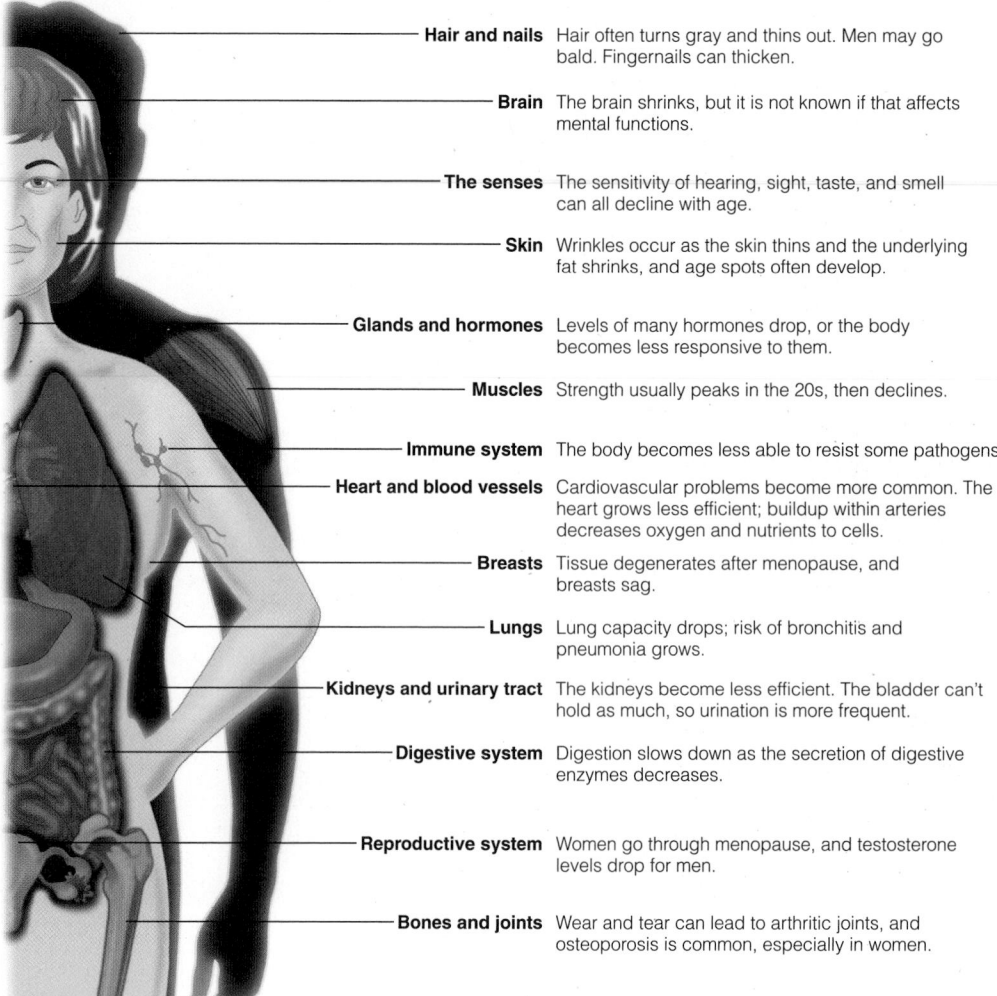

**Hair and nails**   Hair often turns gray and thins out. Men may go bald. Fingernails can thicken.

**Brain**   The brain shrinks, but it is not known if that affects mental functions.

**The senses**   The sensitivity of hearing, sight, taste, and smell can all decline with age.

**Skin**   Wrinkles occur as the skin thins and the underlying fat shrinks, and age spots often develop.

**Glands and hormones**   Levels of many hormones drop, or the body becomes less responsive to them.

**Muscles**   Strength usually peaks in the 20s, then declines.

**Immune system**   The body becomes less able to resist some pathogens.

**Heart and blood vessels**   Cardiovascular problems become more common. The heart grows less efficient; buildup within arteries decreases oxygen and nutrients to cells.

**Breasts**   Tissue degenerates after menopause, and breasts sag.

**Lungs**   Lung capacity drops; risk of bronchitis and pneumonia grows.

**Kidneys and urinary tract**   The kidneys become less efficient. The bladder can't hold as much, so urination is more frequent.

**Digestive system**   Digestion slows down as the secretion of digestive enzymes decreases.

**Reproductive system**   Women go through menopause, and testosterone levels drop for men.

**Bones and joints**   Wear and tear can lead to arthritic joints, and osteoporosis is common, especially in women.

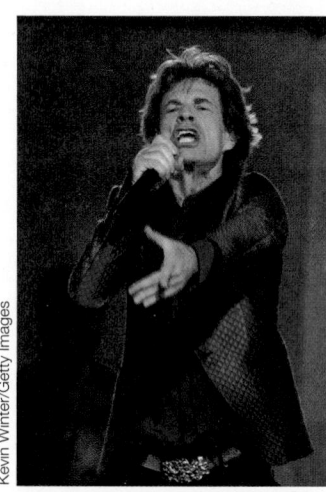

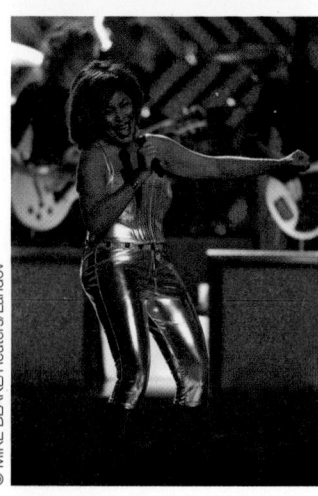

What life after 60 can look like.

## Alzheimer's Disease

About 15 percent of older Americans lose previous mental capabilities, a brain disorder called **dementia**. Sixty percent of these—an estimated 2.4 to 4.5 million—suffer from the type of dementia called **Alzheimer's disease**, a progressive deterioration of brain cells and mental capacity.

Age is the top risk factor for Alzheimer's, but cognitive decline may begin up to six years before it is evident.[20] Someone in America develops Alzheimer's every 72 seconds; by 2050 the rate will increase to every 33 seconds. The percentage of people with Alzheimer's doubles for every five-year age group beyond 65. By age 85, nearly half of men and women have Alzheimer's. A person with the disease typically lives eight years after the onset of symptoms,

but some live as long as 20 years. Some 7.7 million older Americans will develop Alzheimer's by 2030. The greatest increase will be among people age 85 and older.

People whose parents have been diagnosed with Alzheimer's disease or dementia may be more likely to experience memory loss themselves in middle age. Scientists have identified multiple genes that make people more likely to develop Alzheimer's.[21]

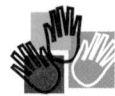 Women are more likely to develop Alzheimer's than men, and women with Alzheimer's perform significantly worse than men in various visual, spatial, and memory tests. Black Americans are about two times more likely to develop Alzheimer's than whites; Hispanics face about 1.5 times the risk.[22]

Various factors, such as regular exercise and weight management, may lower the likelihood of Alzheimer's. A healthful diet—rich in nuts, fish, tomatoes, poultry, and dark and green leafy vegetables and low in high-fat foods, red meat, and butter—may help protect the brain. Individuals who say their lives have a purpose also are less likely to develop Alzheimer's or other forms of cognitive impairment than those who scored lower on "purpose in life" evaluations.

However, an independent NIH-sponsored panel has determined that there still is not sufficient evidence to prove that any preventive strategy—from dietary supplements to mental stimulation or exercise—can prevent Alzheimer's.

The early signs of dementia—insomnia, irritability, increased sensitivity to alcohol and other drugs, and decreased energy and tolerance of frustration—are usually subtle and insidious. Diagnosis requires a comprehensive assessment of an individual's medical history, physical health, and mental status, often involving brain scans and a variety of other tests.

Cholesterol-lowering statin drugs, discussed in Chapter 15, may reduce the risk of Alzheimer's, regardless of the medication used or the person's genetic risk for the disease. Vitamin C or vitamin E, once touted as possible memory preservers, have not proven to lower the risk of dementia or Alzheimer's in older adults.

Even though medical science cannot restore a brain that is in the process of being destroyed by an organic brain disease like Alzheimer's, medications can control difficult behavioral symptoms and enhance or partially restore cognitive ability. Often physicians find other medical or psychiatric problems, such as depression, in these patients; recognizing and treating these conditions can have a dramatic impact.

The FDA has approved several prescription drugs for people with mild to moderate dementia, including Aricept, Exelon, Reminyl, and Mamenda. None has proven superior to the others.

## Osteoporosis

Another age-related disease is *osteoporosis*, a condition in which losses in bone density become so severe that a bone will break with even slight trauma or injury. A chronic disease, osteoporosis

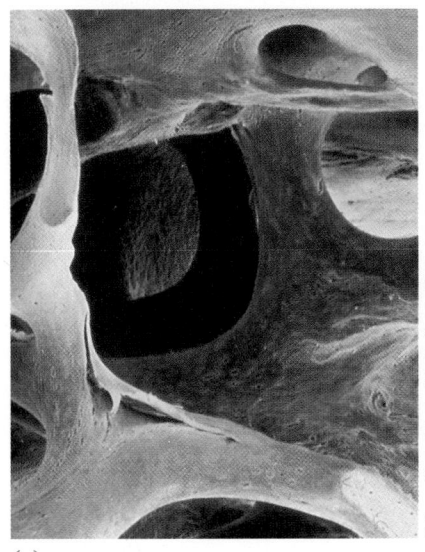
(a)
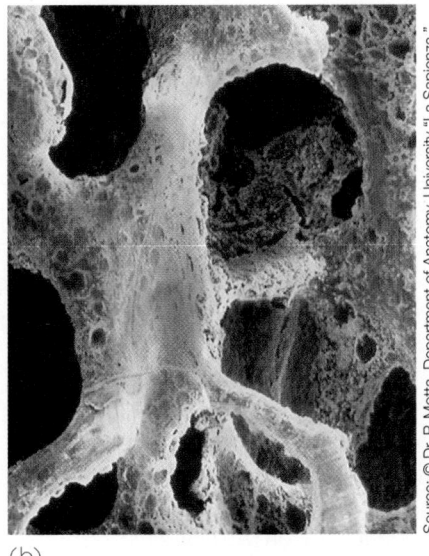
(b)

Source: © Dr. P. Motta, Department of Anatomy, University "La Sapienza," Rome/SciencePhoto Library/Photo Researchers, Inc.
SciencePhoto Library/Photo Researchers, Inc.

The effect of osteoporosis on bone density. (a) Normal bone tissue. (b) After the onset of osteoporosis, bones lose density and become hollow and brittle.

is silent for years or decades before a fracture occurs. Each year more than a third of Americans ages 65 and older experience a fall, and nearly 16,000 die as a result of their injuries. Even a low-trauma fracture increases the risk of dying during the subsequent five years, while a hip fracture heightens this risk for ten years.

Women, who have smaller skeletons, are more vulnerable than men; in extreme cases, their spines may become so fragile that just bending causes severe pain. But although commonly seen as an illness of women, osteoporosis occurs frequently in men. One in every two women and one in four men over 50 will have an osteoporosis-related fracture in their lifetimes.

Regardless of your age and gender, you can prevent future bone problems by taking some protective steps now. The most important guidelines are as follows:

- **Get adequate calcium.** Increased calcium intake, particularly during childhood and the growth spurt of adolescence, can produce a heavier, denser skeleton and reduce the risk of the complications of bone loss later in life. College-age women also can strengthen their bones and reduce their risk of osteoporosis by increasing their calcium intake and physical activity.

- If you do not get enough calcium in your diet, **take daily supplements.**

- **Drink alcohol only moderately.** More than two or three alcoholic beverages a day impairs intestinal calcium absorption.

**dementia** Deterioration of mental capability.

**Alzheimer's disease** A progressive deterioration of intellectual powers due to physiological changes within the brain; symptoms include diminishing ability to concentrate and reason, disorientation, depression, apathy, and paranoia.

- **Don't smoke.** Smokers tend to be thin and enter menopause earlier, thus extending the period of jeopardy from estrogen loss.

- **Let the sunshine in (but don't forget your sunscreen).** Vitamin D, a vitamin produced in the skin in reaction to sunlight, boosts calcium absorption.

- **Exercise regularly.** Both aerobic exercise and weight training can help preserve bone density.

**advance directives** Documents that specify an individual's preferences regarding treatment in a medical crisis.

# Preparing for Medical Crises and the End of Life

Throughout this book, we have stressed the ways in which you can determine how well and how long you live. You can also make decisions about the end of your life. When facing a serious, potentially life-threatening illness, people typically have practical, realistic goals, such as maintaining their quality of life, remaining independent, being comfortable, and providing for their families. (See "Health in Action.")

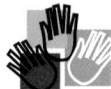 Various racial and ethnic groups have different preferences for their end-of-life wishes. Many Arab Americans prefer not to go to nursing homes as they near the end of their lives, while many African Americans are comfortable with nursing homes and hospitals. Hispanic individuals express strong concerns about dying with dignity. Many white people don't want their families to take care of them, although they—like members of most other racial and ethnic groups—want their families nearby as they live out their last days.

## Advance Directives

All states and the District of Columbia have laws authorizing the use of **advance directives** to specify the kind of medical treatment individuals want in case of a medical crisis. These documents are important because, without clear indications of a person's preferences, hospitals and other institutions often make decisions on an individual's behalf, particularly if family members are not available or disagree among themselves.

The two most common advance directives are health-care proxies and living wills. Each state has different legal requirements for these forms. You can find state-specific forms at **www.caring info.org**. Once the forms are completed, make copies of your advance directives and give them to anyone who might have input in decisions on your behalf. Also give copies to your physician or health-care organization and ask that they be made part of your medical record.

*Health-Care Proxy* A *health-care proxy* is an advance directive that gives someone else the power to make health decisions on your behalf. This advance directive is also called Medical Power of Attorney or Health-Care Power of Attorney. People typically name a relative or close friend as their agent. Let family and friends know that you have completed a health-care proxy. Tell your primary physician, but you should not designate your doctor as your agent. Many states prohibit this. Even when allowed, it is not a good idea because your doctor's primary responsibility is to administer care.

*Living Will* Individuals can use a **living will** (also called health-care directive or physician's directive) to indicate whether they want or don't want all possible medical treatments and technology used to prolong their lives. Living wills are most effective when they focus on priorities and goals, not so much on how to achieve them.

Most states recognize living wills as legally binding, and a growing number of health-care professionals and facilities offer patients help in drafting living wills. Figure 20.3 shows a physician's directive for Texas and notes where state laws may differ.

*The Five Wishes* An innovative document called "Five Wishes" helps the aged, the seriously ill, their loved ones, and caregivers prepare for medical crises. Written with the help of the American Bar Association's Commission on the Legal Problems of the Elderly, the Five Wishes document has a health-care proxy, a health-care directive, and three other "wishes." Persons using this document can specify:

- Which person they want to make health-care decisions for them when they are no longer able to do so.

- Which kinds of medical treatments they do or don't want.

- How comfortable they want to be made.

- How they want people to treat them.

- What they want loved ones to know.

The Five Wishes document (at **www.aging withdignity.org**) is legally valid in 38 states. Churches, synagogues, hospices, hospitals, physicians, social service agencies, and employers

## Preparing for a Medical Crisis in an Aging Relative

"Medical crises are more common and more likely to lead to serious complications after age 60," says Kenneth Brummel-Smith, M.D., former president of the American Geriatrics Society. As your parents, grandparents, and other relatives get older, here is what you can do in advance:

- **Watch for warning signals.** If your relative begins stumbling or having near-misses on the highway, make sure he or she sees a doctor before a serious fall or accident occurs. There may be a cure or, if not a cure, a way to improve functioning.

- **Suggest a surrogate.** Even if a couple has been married for 40 years, neither has the legal right to make medical decisions for a spouse. The same is true for children and other relatives. The only way to get that right is to fill out a form, usually called an advance directive or medical power of attorney.

- **Talk to loved ones.** "Waiting for something bad to happen doesn't make it any easier to talk about," says Dr. Brummel-Smith, who suggests sitting down for a formal discussion at some point after a relative reaches age 65 "but definitely before age 75."

- **Focus on values.** "You don't have to discuss every possible drug or surgery or intervention," says Dr. Brummel-Smith. "What's important is that you understand the older person's values. What are fates worse than death? Independence may be more important then living a longer life." Many families use the "Five Wishes" form (available online at **www.agingwithdignity.org**) to discuss preferences for medical, personal, emotional, and spiritual care.

- **Involve the person's primary physician.** Often it's not a question of what doctors can do medically in a crisis, but of what they should do, which is the patient's decision. Encourage loved ones to discuss "what ifs" with their doctors and make their desires clear. For instance, a primary physician should know which treatments patients want (such as resuscitation during surgery) as well as those they don't want (such as remaining on a ventilator if unable to breathe on their own).

- **Investigate alternative living options.** Aging parents should visit retirement communities or nursing homes while they're still healthy, not with the idea of moving into them, but of knowing what's available. They also should find out if their health plan provides services for seniors after a medical crisis.

- **Make sure you know where to find key documents.** An easily accessible folder with copies of the latest lab reports, consultations, and advance directives helps to avoid unnecessary tests and get faster treatment when a crisis does occur.

also are distributing the document to help people plan for their own care or that of aging parents.

*DNR Order* You can also sign an advance directive specifying that you want to be allowed to die naturally—you do not want to be resuscitated in case your heart stops beating. **Do-not-resuscitate (DNR)** orders apply mainly to hospitalized, terminally ill patients and must be signed by a physician. However, in some states, it is possible to complete a *nonhospital DNR* form that specifies an individual's wish not to be

**living will** An advance directive providing instructions for the use of life-sustaining procedures in the event of terminal illness or injury.

**do-not-resuscitate (DNR)** An advance directive expressing an individual's preference that resuscitation efforts not be made during a medical crisis.

Figure 20.3  **Preparing a Physician's Directive**

Source: *A Guide to the Living Will,* Hippocrates (May/June, 1988).

Directives are effective until they're revoked. Still, it's considered a good idea to initial and date your directive every few years to show that it still expresses your wishes.

In some states the directive is valid for pregnant women. Others exclude women during all or part of their pregnancy, although that has been challenged on the grounds that a woman's right to privacy doesn't end when she becomes pregnant.

You can revoke or amend your directive at any time simply by making a statement to a physician, nurse, or other health-care worker.

---

### DIRECTIVE TO PHYSICIANS
#### For Persons 18 Years of Age and Over

I, _____, recognize that the best health care is based upon a partnership of trust and communication with my physician. My physician and I will make health care decisions together as long as I am of sound mind and able to make my wishes known. If there comes a time that I am unable to make medical decisions about myself because of illness or injury, I direct that the following treatment preferences be honored:

If, in the judgment of my physician, I am suffering with a terminal condition from which I am expected to die within six months, even with available life-sustaining treatment provided in accordance with prevailing standards of medical care:

____ I request that all treatments other than those needed to keep me comfortable be discontinued or withheld and my physician allow me to die as gently as possible; OR

____ I request that I be kept alive in this terminal condition using available life-sustaining treatment (THIS SELECTION DOES NOT APPLY TO HOSPICE CARE).

If, in the judgment of my physician, I am suffering with an irreversible condition so that I cannot care for myself or make decisions for myself and am expected to die without life-sustaining treatment provided in accordance with prevailing standards of care:

____ I request that all treatments other than those needed to keep me comfortable be discontinued or withheld and my physician allow me to die as gently as possible; OR

____ I request that I be kept alive in this irreversible condition using available life-sustaining treatment (THIS SELECTION DOES NOT APPLY TO HOSPICE CARE).

Additional requests: (After discussion with your physician, you may wish to consider listing particular treatments in this space that you do or do not want in specific circumstances, such as artificial nutrition and fluids, intravenous antibiotics, etc. Be sure to state whether you do or do not want the particular treatment).

After signing this DIRECTIVE, if my representative or I elect hospice care, I understand and agree that only those treatments needed to keep me comfortable would be provided and I would not be given available life-sustaining treatments.

If I do not have a Medical Power of Attorney and I am unable to make my wishes known, I designate the following person(s) to make treatment decisions with my physician compatible with my personal values.

Name _____

Address _____

Name _____

Address _____

(If a Medical Power of Attorney has been executed, then an agent already has been named and you should not list additional names in this document.)

If the above persons are not available, or if I have not designated a spokesperson, I understand that a spokesperson will be chosen for me following standards specified in the laws of Texas. If, in the judgment of my physician, my death is imminent within minutes to hours, even with the use of all available medical treatment provided within the prevailing standard of care, I acknowledge that all treatments may be withheld or removed except those needed to maintain my comfort.

I understand that under Texas law this Directive has no effect if I have been diagnosed as pregnant. This DIRECTIVE will remain in effect until I revoke it. No other person may do so. I understand that I may revoke this DIRECTIVE at any time.

I understand the full import of this DIRECTIVE and I am emotionally and mentally competent to make this DIRECTIVE.

Signed _____

City, County, and State of Residence _____

Date _____

Two competent witnesses must sign below, acknowledging your signature. The witness designated as "Witness 1" may not be a person designated to make a treatment decision for the patient and may not be related to the patient by blood or marriage. The witness may not be entitled to any part of the estate and may not have a claim against the estate of the patient. The witness may not be the attending physician or an employee of the attending physician. If this witness is an employee of the health care facility in which the patient is being cared for, this witness may not be involved in providing direct patient care to the patient. This witness may not be an officer, director, partner, or business office employee of the health care facility in which the patient is being cared for or of any parent organization of the health care facility.

Witness 1 _____

Witness 2 _____

TEXAS LAW DOES NOT REQUIRE THIS DIRECTIVE TO BE NOTARIZED.

---

In most states, directives will have a space to specify treatment you do or don't want. Ask your physician what to include here. You can:

• Ask for or prohibit use of artificial feeding tubes, cardiopulmonary resuscitation, antibiotics, dialysis, and respirators.

• Ask for pain medication to keep you comfortable.

• State whether you would prefer to die in the hospital or at home.

• Designate a proxy— someone to make decisions about your treatment when you're unable.

• Donate organs or other body parts.

In some states your signature must be notarized. Elsewhere, the signature of the witnesses is adequate, although if you're in a hospital or nursing home, in some states you may need as an additional witness the chief of staff or medical director.

resuscitated at home. Patients in the final stages of advanced cancer or AIDS may choose to use such forms to protect their rights in case paramedics are called to their home.

*Holographic Wills*   Perhaps you think that only wealthy or older people need to write wills. However, if you're married, have children, or own property, you should either hire a lawyer to draw up a will or at least write a **holographic will** yourself, specifying who should inherit your possessions. If you die *intestate* (without a will), the state will make these decisions for you. Even a modest estate can be tied up in court for a long period of time, depriving family members of money when they need it most.

A holographic will is a handwritten (not typed) statement that some states will recognize. You can:

- **Name a family member or friend** as the executor, the person who sees that your wishes are carried out.
- **List the things you own** and to whom you want them to go; include addresses and telephone numbers, if possible.
- **Select a guardian for your children** (if any), presumably someone whose ideas about raising children are similar to your own. Be sure that any named guardians are willing and able to accept this responsibility before writing them into your will.
- **Specify any funeral arrangements.**

Be sure to keep the will in a safe place, where your executor, family members, or closest beneficiary can find it quickly and easily; tell them where it is.

## Ethical Dilemmas

Modern medicine can do more to delay or defy death than was once thought possible. However, the ability to sustain life in patients with no hope of recovery has created wrenching medical and moral dilemmas. Increasingly, lawyers, ethicists, and consumer advocates are arguing that health-care providers must recognize a fundamental right of patients: the right to die.

Health economists, noting that more than half of U.S. health-care dollars are spent in the last year of life, have questioned "heroic" measures to prolong the life of chronically ill elderly patients or those with fatal diseases. Policies on such aggressive measures vary from hospital to hospital and state to state; often medical staff are not aware of patients' wishes.

Some health-care facilities require that staff members try to resuscitate any patient whose heart stops unless a do-not-resuscitate (DNR) order has been written, usually with the family's permission.

Families may demand aggressive medical care near the end of life on the basis of religious grounds, such as a conviction that every moment of life is a gift from God worth preserving at any cost. However, doctors are not obliged to provide a treatment they consider medically inappropriate or inhumane simply because of the family's religious beliefs. Ideally, doctors and family members, perhaps with the aid of a chaplain, work together to reach a consensus on the appropriate limits to life-sustaining treatment.

Another major ethical concern is the fate of an estimated 5,000 to 10,000 unconscious Americans who are being kept alive by artificial means. Some are in a **coma**, a state of total unconsciousness. They may have no sense of where they are, no memory, and no experience of pain. Others are in a **persistent vegetative state**, in which they're awake and yet unaware. They open their eyes; their brain waves show the characteristic patterns of waking and sleep. They can usually breathe on their own after a few weeks on artificial respiration; they can cough; the pupils of their eyes respond to light; but they do not respond to pain.

## The Gift of Life

If you're at least 18 years old, you can fill out a donor card (Figure 20.4), agreeing to designate, in the event of your death, any organs or tissues needed for transplantation. Corneas may help a blind person see, for example. Kidneys, or even a heart, may be transplanted. The donation takes effect upon your death and is a generous way of giving others the possibilities for life that you have had yourself. The card should be filled out and signed; some must be signed in the presence of two witnesses. Attach the donor card to the back of your driver's license or I.D. card. (Whole-body donations may require other arrangements.)

**holographic will** A will wholly in the handwriting of its author.

**coma** A state of total unconsciousness.

**persistent vegetative state** A state of being awake and capable of reacting to physical stimuli, such as light, while being unaware of pain or other environmental stimuli.

Figure 20.4 **Example of a Uniform Donor Card**

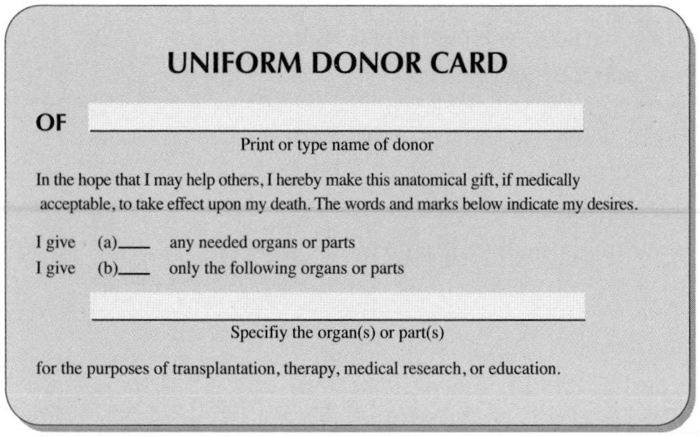

---

**UNIFORM DONOR CARD**

OF _____
Print or type name of donor

In the hope that I may help others, I hereby make this anatomical gift, if medically
acceptable, to take effect upon my death. The words and marks below indicate my desires.

I give    (a)_____    any needed organs or parts
I give    (b)_____    only the following organs or parts

_____
Specifiy the organ(s) or part(s)

for the purposes of transplantation, therapy, medical research, or education.

---

The reasons for becoming an organ donor or agreeing to donate a loved one's organs are complex. Older men and women generally have higher donation rates. Families often base their decision on a loved one's explicit desire either to donate organs or not. Concerns about disfigurement and feelings of emotional exhaustion also play a role.

# Death and Dying

Some 2.4 million people die in the United States each year. Although most are older, death occurs in all age groups. The causes of death vary with both age and gender. Among those under age 35, intentional and nonintentional injury are the primary causes of death. Among older Americans, cancer and heart disease are the top killers. In fact, cancer, heart disease, and stroke continue to claim the most lives around the world. Men typically die at a younger age than women. College-age individuals are most likely to die as a result of accidents or assaults.

## Defining Death

In our society, death isn't a part of everyday life, as it once was. Because machines can now keep alive people who, in the past, would have died, the definition of death has become more complex. Death has been broken down into the following categories:

- **Functional death.** The end of all vital functions, such as heartbeat and respiration.

- **Cellular death.** The gradual death of body cells after the heart stops beating. If placed

in a tissue culture or, as is the case with various organs, transplanted to another body, some cells can remain alive indefinitely.

- **Death.** The moment when the heart stops beating.

- **Brain death.** The end of all brain activity, indicated by an absence of electrical activity (confirmed by an electroencephalogram, or EEG) and a lack of reflexes. The notion of brain death is bound up with what we consider to be the actual person, or self. The destruction of a person's brain means that his or her personality no longer exists; the lower brain centers controlling respiration and circulation no longer function.

- **Spiritual death.** The moment when the soul, as defined by many religions, leaves the body.

When does a person actually die? The traditional legal definition of death is failure of the lungs or heart to function. However, because respiration and circulation can be maintained by artificial means, most states have declared that an individual is considered dead only when the brain, including the brain stem, completely stops functioning. Brain-death laws prohibit a medical staff from "pulling the plug" if there is any hope of sustaining life.

## Denying Death

Most of us don't quite believe that we're going to die. A reasonable amount of denial helps us focus on the day-to-day realities of living. However, excessive denial can be life-threatening. Some drivers, for instance, refuse to buckle their seat belts because they refuse to acknowledge that a drunk driver might collide with them. Similarly, cigarette smokers deny that lung cancer will ever strike them, and people who eat high-fat meals deny that they'll ever suffer a heart attack.

One important factor in denial is the nature of the threat. It's easy to believe that death is at hand when someone's pointing a gun at you; it's much harder to think that cigarette smoking might cause your death 20 or 30 years down the road. The late Elisabeth Kübler-Ross, a psychiatrist who extensively studied the process of dying, described the downside of denying death in *Death: The Final Stage of Growth*:

It is the denial of death that is partially responsible for people living empty, purposeless lives; for when you live as if you'll live forever, it becomes too easy to postpone the things you know that you must do. You live your life in preparation for tomorrow or in the remembrance of yesterday—and meanwhile, each today is lost. In contrast, when you fully understand that each day you awaken could be the last you have, you take the time that day to grow, to become more of who you really are, to reach out to other human beings.[23]

## Emotional Responses to Dying

Kübler-Ross identified five typical stages of reaction that a person goes through when facing death (Figure 20.5).

1. **Denial ("No, not me")**. At first knowledge that death is coming, a terminally ill patient rejects the news. The denial overcomes the initial shock and allows the person to begin to gather together his or her resources. Denial, at this point, is a healthy defense mechanism. It can become distressful, however, if it's reinforced by the relatives and friends of the dying patient.

2. **Anger ("Why me?")**. In the second stage, the dying person begins to feel resentment and rage regarding imminent death. The anger may be directed at God or at the patient's family and caregivers, who can do little but try to endure any expressions of anger, provide comfort, and help the patient on to the next stage.

3. **Bargaining ("Yes, me, but . . .")**. In this stage, a patient may try to bargain, usually with God, for a way to reverse or at least postpone dying. The patient may promise, in exchange for recovery, to do good works or to see family members more often. Alternatively, the patient may say, "Let me live long enough to see my grandchild born" or "to see the spring again."

4. **Depression ("Yes, it's me")**. In the fourth stage, the patient gradually realizes the full consequences of his or her condition. This may begin as grieving for health that has been lost and then become

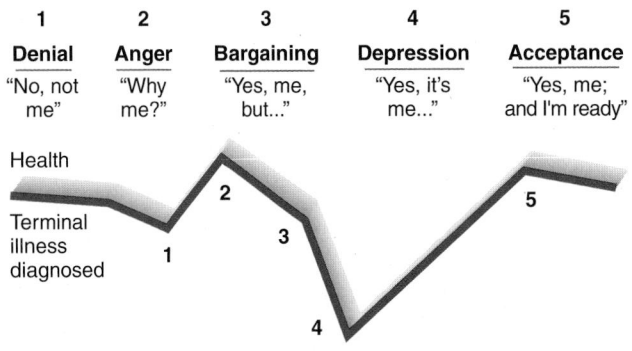

Figure 20.5  **Kübler-Ross's Five Stages of Adjustment to Facing Death**

anticipatory grieving for the loss that is to come of friends, loved ones, and life itself. This stage is perhaps the most difficult: The dying person should not be left alone during this period. Neither should loved ones try to cheer up the patient, who must be allowed to grieve.

5. **Acceptance ("Yes, me; and I'm ready")**. In this last stage, the person has accepted the reality of death: The moment looms as neither frightening nor painful, neither sad nor happy—only inevitable. The person who waits for the end of life may ask to see fewer visitors, to separate from other people, or perhaps to turn to just one person for support.

Several stages may occur at the same time and some may happen out of sequence. Each stage may take days or only hours or minutes. Throughout, denial may come back to assert itself unexpectedly, and hope for a medical breakthrough or a miraculous recovery is forever present.

Some experts dispute Kübler-Ross's basic five-stage theory as too simplistic and argue that not all people go through such well-defined stages in the dying process. The way a person faces death is often a mirror of the way he or she has faced other major stresses in life: Those who have had the most trouble adjusting to other crises will have the most trouble adjusting to the news of their impending death.

An individual's will to live can postpone death for a while. In a study of elderly Chinese women, researchers found that their death rate decreased before and during a holiday during which the senior women in a household play a central role; it increased after the celebration. A similar temporary drop occurs among Jews at the time of Passover. However, different events may have different effects. The prospect of an upcoming birthday postpones death in women but hastens it in men. The will to live typically fluctuates in terminal patients, varying along with depression, anxiety, shortness of breath, and a sense of well-being.

The family of a dying person experiences a spectrum of often wrenching emotions. Family members, too, may deny the verdict of death, rage at the doctors and nurses who can't do more to save their loved one, bargain with God to give up their own health if necessary, sink into helplessness and depression, and finally accept the reality of their anticipated loss. Dying can be seen from different perspectives. The Renz model, for example, views it as a process of maturation consisting of pretransition, transition, and posttransition. The initial response is an upsurge of emotions, including anger, grief, feelings of personal emptiness, and despair. These may emerge again and again.

However, as patients confront reality, they eventually can "let go and let be." As one researcher observed, "There is happiness and well-being in the midst of illness. In the course of the dying process spiritual experiences of such intensity often happen more than just once. After a shorter or longer struggle, patients reach a new mental state, a gift of grace beyond human endeavor and power."

# How We Die

Life can end in very different ways. Sudden death, by accident or murder, for instance, brings an abrupt end to life in individuals who may have been in optimal health. A terminal illness, such as an aggressive and fatal cancer, can lead to a steep drop in functioning prior to death. When organs such as the kidneys fail, a patient's well-being tends to plummet and then recover but in a downward pattern. The frailty of old age leads to a gradual decline to ever lower levels of functioning and eventual death.

Most people who have a fatal or **terminal illness** prefer to know the truth about their health and chances for recovery. Even when they're not officially informed by a doctor or relative, most fatally ill people know or strongly suspect that they're dying. Dying people usually make it clear whether they want to talk about death and to what extent. The most frequent concern is how much time is left. Usually physicians can give only a rough estimate, such as "several weeks or months."

## A "Good" Death

As life expectancy has increased and high-technology interventions have multiplied, many health-care professionals as well as citizens and social organizations have begun to demand a better way of caring for those who are dying. The Center to Improve Care of the Dying, in Washington, D.C., has set goals for reintegrating dying within living, thus enhancing the prospect for growth at the end of life. These experts talk of "dying well," "living while dying," and "physician-assisted living." They aim to change our way of thinking about dying so that we view the end of life as a time of love and reconciliation, and transcendence of suffering.

Physicians who care for the dying are being urged to do all that they can to eliminate pain. They are encouraged not to withhold opioid drugs, such as morphine, simply out of fear of addiction. More efforts are being made for patients to be taken care of at home, with appropriate support and well-informed guidance.

Various psychological factors can affect those at risk of dying. Elderly people who lack hope in the future are much more likely to die within the next few years. Researchers speculate that hopelessness may lead to biochemical and nervous system abnormalities or that hopeless individuals may not eat well, take medications as prescribed, or follow a doctor's recommendations.

Spirituality plays a major role. In various surveys, many patients say they want their doctors and nurses to address their spiritual concerns. In one survey, even 45 percent of nonreligious patients thought physicians should inquire politely about patients' spiritual needs. However, some worry that such queries may be inappropriate or detract from a doctor's primary mission.

## Caregiving

When someone becomes terminally ill, a woman—usually the patient's wife, daughter, or sister—is most likely to provide day-to-day care,

**terminal illness** An illness in which death is inevitable.

often for periods longer than a year. Caregiving takes a different toll on men and women. In one study of adult daughters and husbands caring for terminally ill breast cancer patients, the daughters experienced more symptoms of anxiety and depression and greater family strain.

The impact of caregiving continues even after the death of an ill spouse. In one study, the health of older caregivers who had experienced strain prior to a spouse's death did not deteriorate. They showed no increase in depressive symptoms or use of antidepressant drugs and did not lose weight. Those who had not been caregivers were more likely to experience depression and weight loss.

## Hospice: Caring When Curing Isn't Possible

A **hospice** is a homelike health-care facility or program that helps dying men and women who can afford such care to live their final days to the fullest, as free as possible from disabling pain and mental anguish.

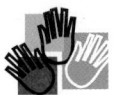 Race and ethnicity affect the use of hospice. In a study of patients over age 65 (and all covered by Medicare) with terminal cancer, Asian American and black patients were less likely to enroll in a hospice program than whites and Hispanics. They also were more likely to be hospitalized in an intensive care unit at least twice during their last month of life.[24]

Hospice workers generally work in teams, usually consisting of a nurse, physician, social worker, chaplain, and trained volunteers. Other professionals, such as a physical therapist, may join the team when needed. These workers provide the comfort, support, and care dying patients need until they do die.

Hospice programs offer a combination of medical and emotional care that involves not only the patient but also the family members or others concerned with caring for the patient. Most hospice patients have life expectancies of six months or less and are no longer receiving treatments aimed at curing their diseases. When someone is available to provide care, patients remain in their own homes. Hospice nurses regularly visit all home patients and are available around the clock.

For patients requiring care that the family cannot provide, round-the-clock care is available at the hospice facility. Unlike a traditional hospital, where the focus is on diagnosis, cure, and treatment, a hospice works to make what is left of life pain-free and comfortable. Visiting hours for relatives and friends are flexible, with no restrictions on visits by children and grandchildren. Hospice services are covered, in full or in part, by most major insurance companies.

## Near-Death Experiences

Reports of near-death experiences have grown, thanks largely to advances in emergency medical care. Most are remarkably similar, whether they occur in children or adults, whether they're the result of accidents or illnesses, even whether the individuals actually are near death or only think they are. Some individuals who have survived a close brush with death report **autoscopy** (watching, from several feet in the air, resuscitation attempts on their own bodies) or **transcendence** (the sense of passing into a foreign region or dimension). Some see light, often at the end of a tunnel. Their vision seems clearer; their hearing, sharper. Some recall scenes from their lives or feel the presence of loved ones who have died. Many report profound feelings of joy, calm, and peace. Fewer than 1 percent of those who've reported near-death experiences described them as frightening or distressing, although a larger number recall transitory feelings of fear or confusion.

Many near-death experiences occur in individuals who've been sedated or given other medications; however, many others do not. Several studies have shown that individuals who received medication or anesthesia were actually less likely to remember near-death experiences than those who hadn't had any drugs. Some scientists have speculated that lack of oxygen, changes in blood gases, altered brain functioning, or the release of neurotransmitters (messenger chemicals in the brain) may play a role in near-death experiences. However, there's little solid evidence that physiological events are responsible. There's also no proof that wishful thinking, cultural conditioning, posttraumatic stress, or other psychological mechanisms may be at work. For now, the most that scientists can say for sure about this medical mystery is that it needs further study.

**hospice** A homelike health-care facility or program committed to supportive care for terminally ill people.

**autoscopy** The sensation of one's self being outside its body, often experienced by individuals in near-death medical crises.

**transcendence** The sense of passing into a foreign region or dimension, often experienced by a person near death.

# Suicide

Suicide increases with age and is most common in persons age 65 and older. This age group accounts for 18 percent of all suicides in the United States. For every completed suicide, there are 10 to 40 unsuccessful attempts. (Chapter 5 presents a detailed discussion of the risk factors and warning signs of suicide.)

One of the main factors leading to suicide is illness, especially terminal illness. A great deal of debate centers on quality of life, yet there is no reliable or consistent way to measure this. Patients who are dying may feel some quality of life, even when others do not recognize it, or their evaluations of the quality of their lives may fluctuate. Dying patients who say their lives are not worth living may be suffering from depression; hopelessness is one of its characteristic symptoms.

## "Rational" Suicide

An elderly widow suffering from advanced cancer takes a lethal overdose of sleeping pills. A young man with several AIDS-related illnesses shoots himself. A woman in her 50s, diagnosed as having Alzheimer's disease, asks a doctor to help her end her life. Are these suicides "rational" because these individuals used logical reasoning in deciding to end their lives?

The question is intensely controversial. Advocates of the right to "self-deliverance" argue that individuals in great pain or faced with the prospect of a debilitating, hopeless battle against an incurable disease can and should be able to decide to end their lives. As legislatures and the legal system tackle the thorny questions of an individual's right to die, mental health professionals worry that, even in those with fatal diseases, suicidal wishes often stem from undiagnosed depression.

Because depression may indeed warp the ability to make a rational decision about suicide, mental health professionals urge physicians and family members to make sure individuals with chronic or fatal illnesses are evaluated for depression and given medication, psychotherapy, or both. It is also important for everyone to allow enough time—an average of three to eight weeks—to see if treatment for depression will make a difference in their desire to keep living.

## Physician-Assisted Suicide

According to U.S. surveys, there is greater support for physician-assisted suicide and euthanasia among patients and the general public than among physicians. More Caucasians support these practices than members of ethnic minority groups.

Oregon is the first state to legalize physician-assisted suicide for terminally ill patients. The Supreme Court has upheld the state's Death with Dignity Act, which bars suicide assistance for anyone whose judgment may be impaired by a mental disorder.

If patients have a right to die, should doctors help them end their lives? Physicians could stop any extraordinary efforts to sustain life (for example, by withholding oxygen or ending intravenous feedings); such actions are referred to as passive *euthanasia*, or *dyathanasia*. Euthanasia, the active form of so-called mercy killing, has generally been viewed as illegal and unethical. Euthanasia is tolerated and legally pardoned in the Netherlands but remains illegal in all European countries. The demand for physician-assisted death in the Netherlands has not risen; and patients and physicians have become more reluctant to ask for or offer this option over the past few years.

Some medical groups, such as the American Medical Association, oppose as unethical any physician's involvement in euthanasia. Others argue that individuals have the right to end their own lives and that physicians who provide prescriptions for lethal doses of certain drugs are acting out of compassion and respect for patients' wishes.

# The Practicalities of Death

At a time of great emotional pain, grieving family members must cope with medical, legal, and practical concerns, including obtaining a medical certificate of the cause of death, registering the death, and making funeral arrangements.

They also may want to arrange for organ donations and, in some circumstances, an autopsy.

## Funeral Arrangements

A body can be either buried or cremated. Burial requires the purchase of a cemetery plot, which many families do decades before death. A burial is typically the third most expensive purchase of a lifetime, behind the cost of a house and car. The average national costs range as high as $6,000, although they vary considerably. Memorial societies are voluntary groups that help people plan in advance for death. They obtain services at moderate cost, keep the arrangements simple and dignified, and—most important, perhaps—ease the emotional and financial burden on the rest of the family when death finally does come.

If the body is to be cremated, you must comply with some additional formalities, with which the funeral director can help you. After a *cremation* (incineration of the remains), you can either collect the ashes to keep, bury, or scatter yourself, or ask the crematorium to dispose of them.

The tradition of a funeral may help survivors come to terms with the death, enabling them to mourn their loss and to celebrate the dead person's life. Funerals are usually held two to four days after the death. Many have two parts: a religious ceremony at a church or funeral home, and a burial ceremony at the grave site.

Alternatively, the body may be disposed of immediately, through burial, cremation, or bequeathal to a medical school, and a memorial service held later. In a memorial service, the body is not present, which may change the focus of the service from the person's death to his or her life.

## Autopsies

An autopsy is a detailed examination of a body after death, also called a postmortem exam. There are two types:

- **Medicolegal.** This type of autopsy is performed to establish the cause of death and to gather information about the death for use as evidence in any legal proceedings. It is done to detect any crimes and to help identify the proper person for prosecution, to investigate

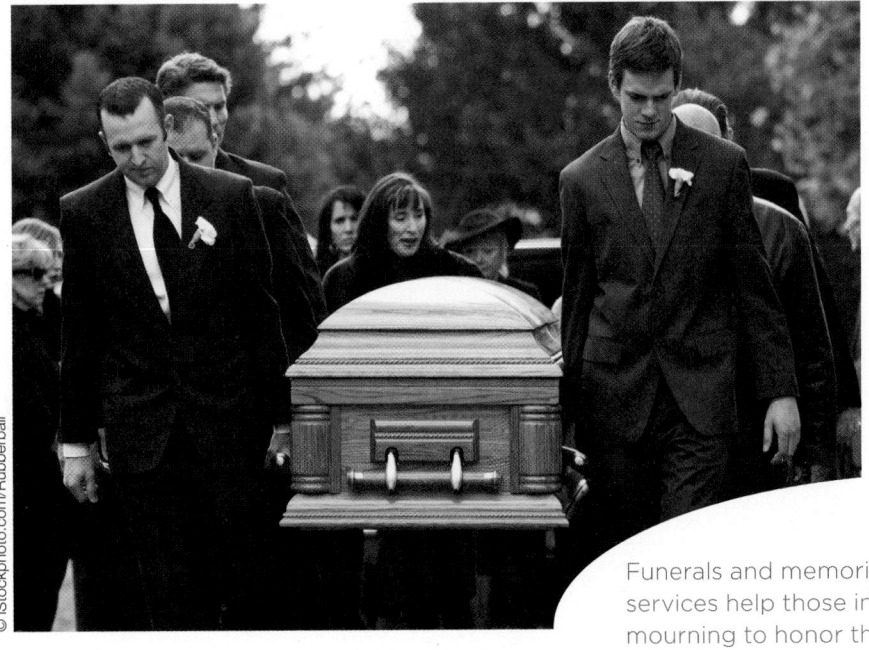

possible industrial hazards or contagious diseases that may endanger the public health, or to establish the cause of death for insurance purposes.

- **Medical/educational.** This type of autopsy is performed, usually in the hospital where the person died, to increase medical knowledge and to determine a more exact cause of death. It may be requested by the attending physician or the family, but it cannot be performed without the family's permission.

Autopsies can be extremely valuable in establishing an accurate cause of death, revealing a different diagnosis that might have led to a change in therapy and prolonged survival in about 10 percent of cases. Thirty years ago about 50 percent of patients who died in hospitals were autopsied. However, the autopsy rate in the United States has been steadily declining, and today about 10 to 20 percent of deaths in teaching hospitals are autopsied.

## Grief

An estimated 8 million Americans lose a member of their immediate family each year. Each death leaves an average of five people bereaved. Such loss may be the single most upsetting and feared event in a person's life. It produces a

Funerals and memorial services help those in mourning to honor the deceased and to come to terms with their loss.

wide range of reactions, including anxiety, guilt, anger, and financial concern. Many may see the death of an old person as less tragic than the death of a child or young person. A sudden death is more of a shock than one following a long illness. A suicide can be particularly devastating, because family members may wonder whether they could have done anything to prevent it. The cause of death also can affect the reactions of friends and acquaintances. Some people express less sympathy and support when individuals are murdered or take their own lives.

According to the stage theory of grief, individuals respond to the loss of a loved one by progressing through several steps, just like people facing death. These consist of shock-numbness, yearning-searching, disorganization-despair, and reorganization. All these reactions can occur simultaneously, although most peak within six months. Acceptance continues to increase over time. The most common and one of the most painful experiences is the death of a parent. When both parents die, even adult individuals may feel like orphaned children. They mourn not just for the father and mother who are gone, but also for their lost role of being someone's child.

Bereavement is not a rare occurrence on college campuses, but it is largely an ignored problem. Counselors have called upon universities to help students who have lost a loved one through initiatives such as training nonbereaved students to provide peer support and raising consciousness about bereavement.

## Grief's Effects on Health

Men and women who lose partners, parents, or children endure so much stress that they're at increased risk of serious physical and mental illness, and even of premature death. Studies of the health effects of grief have found the following:

- Grief produces changes in the respiratory, hormonal, and central nervous systems and may affect functions of the heart, blood, and immune systems.

- Grieving adults may experience mood swings between sadness and anger, guilt and anxiety.

- Grievers may feel physically sick, lose their appetite, sleep poorly, or fear that they're

## How to Cope with Grief

- **Accept your feelings—sorrow, fear, emptiness, whatever—as normal.** Don't try to deny emotions such as anger, guilt, despair, or relief.

- **Let others help you—by bringing you food, taking care of daily necessities, providing companionship and comfort.** (It will make them feel better, too.)

- **Face each day as it comes.** Let yourself live in the here-and-now until you're ready to face the future. Give yourself time—perhaps more than you ever imagined—for the pain to ebb, the scars to heal, and your life to move on.

- **Don't think there's a right or wrong way to grieve.** Mourning takes many forms, and there's no set timetable for working through the various stages of grief.

- **Seek professional counseling if you remain intensely distressed for more than six months or your grief does not ease over time.** Therapy can help prevent potentially serious physical and psychological problems.

going crazy because they "see" the deceased person in different places.

- Friendships and remarriage offer the greatest protection against health problems.

- Some widows may have increased rates of depression, suicide, and death from cirrhosis of the liver. The greatest risk factors are poor previous mental and physical health and a lack of social support.

- Grieving parents, partners, and adult children are at increased risk of serious physical and mental illness, suicide, and premature death.

Sometimes grief progresses from an emotionally painful but normal experience to a more persistent problem, called *complicated grief*. Individuals who experience very long-lasting or severe symptoms, including inability to accept a loved one's death, persistent thoughts about the death, and preoccupation with the lost loved one, can benefit from professional treatment.

# Living Long and Well

"Every man desires to live long," wrote Jonathan Swift, "but no man would be old." We all wish for long lives, yet we want to avoid the disease and disability that can tarnish our golden years. Which of the following steps will you take to ensure a lifetime of health?

_____ **Exercise regularly.** By improving blood flow, staving off depression, warding off heart disease, and enhancing well-being, regular workouts help keep mind and body in top form.

_____ **Don't smoke.** Every cigarette you puff can snuff out seven minutes of your life, according to the Centers for Disease Control and Prevention.

_____ **Watch your weight and blood pressure.** Increases in these vital statistics can increase your risk of hypertension, cardiovascular disease, and other health problems.

_____ **Eat more fruits and vegetables.** These foods, rich in vitamins and protective antioxidants, can reduce your risk of cancer and damage from destructive free radicals.

_____ **Cut down on fat.** Fatty foods can clog the arteries and contribute to various cancers.

_____ **Limit drinking.** Alcohol can undermine physical health and sabotage mental acuity.

_____ **Cultivate stimulating interests.** Elderly individuals with complex and interesting lifestyles are most likely to retain sharp minds and memories beyond age 70.

_____ **Don't worry; be happy.** At any age, emotional turmoil can undermine well-being. Relaxation techniques, such as meditation, help by reducing stress.

_____ **Reach out.** Try to keep in contact with other people of all ages and experiences. Make the effort to invite them to your home or go out with them. On a regular basis, do something to help another person.

_____ **Make the most of your time.** Greet each day with a specific goal—to take a walk, write letters, visit a friend.

# What Is Your Aging IQ?

*Answer True or False*

T  F  1. Everyone becomes "senile" sooner or later, if he or she lives long enough.

T  F  2. American families have by and large abandoned their older members.

T  F  3. Depression is a serious problem for older people.

T  F  4. The numbers of older people are growing.

T  F  5. The vast majority of older people are self-sufficient.

T  F  6. Mental confusion is an inevitable, incurable consequence of old age.

T  F  7. Intelligence declines with age.

T  F  8. Sexual urges and activity normally cease around ages 55 to 60.

T  F  9. If a person has been smoking for 30 or 40 years, it does no good to quit.

T  F  10. Older people should stop exercising and rest.

T  F  11. As you grow older, you need more vitamins and minerals to stay healthy.

T  F  12. Only children need to be concerned about calcium for strong bones and teeth.

T  F  13. Extremes of heat and cold can be particularly dangerous to old people.

T  F  14. Many older people are hurt in accidents that could have been prevented.

T  F  15. More men than women survive to old age.

T  F  16. Deaths from stroke and heart disease are declining.

T  F  17. Older people on the average take more medications than younger people.

T  F  18. Snake oil salesmen are as common today as they were on the frontier.

T  F  19. Personality changes with age, just like hair color and skin texture.

T  F  20. Sight declines with age.

## Scoring

1. False. Even among those who live to be 80 or older, only 20 to 25 percent develop Alzheimer's disease or some other incurable form of brain disease. "Senility" is a meaningless term that should be discarded.

2. False. The American family is still the number one caretaker of older Americans. Most older people live close to their children and see them often; many live with their spouses. In all, eight out of ten men and six out of ten women live in family settings.

3. True. Depression, loss of self-esteem, loneliness, and anxiety can become more common as older people face retirement, along with the deaths of relatives and friends, and other such crises—often at the same time. Fortunately, depression is treatable.

4. True. By the year 2030, one in four people will be over 65 years of age.

5. True. Only a small percentage of the older population live in nursing homes. The rest live independently or with relatives or caregivers.

6. False. Mental confusion and serious forgetfulness in old age can be caused by Alzheimer's disease or other conditions that cause incurable damage to the brain, but some 100 other problems can cause the same symptoms. A minor head injury, a high fever, poor nutrition, adverse drug reactions, and depression can all be treated and the confusion will be cured.

7. False. Intelligence per se does not decline without reason. Most people maintain their intellect or improve as they grow older.

8. False. Most older people can lead an active, satisfying sex life.

9. False. Stopping smoking at any age not only reduces the risk of cancer and heart disease, it also leads to healthier lungs.

10. False. Many older people enjoy—and benefit from—exercises such as walking, swimming, and bicycle riding. Exercise at any age can help strengthen the heart and lungs, and lower blood pressure. See your physician before beginning a new exercise program.

11. False. Although certain requirements, such as that for "sunshine" vitamin D, may increase slightly with age, older people need the same amounts of most vitamins and minerals as younger people. Older people in particular should eat nutritious food and cut down on sweets, salty snack foods, high-calorie drinks, and alcohol.

12. False. Older people require fewer calories, but adequate intake of calcium for strong bones can become more important as you grow older. This is particularly true for women, whose risk of osteoporosis increases after menopause. Milk and cheese are rich in calcium as are cooked dried beans, collards, and broccoli. Some people need calcium supplements as well.

13. True. The body's thermostat tends to function less efficiently with age, and the older person's body may be less able to adapt to heat or cold.

14. True. Falls are the most common cause of injuries among the elderly. Good safety habits, including proper lighting, nonskid carpets, and keeping living areas free of obstacles, can help prevent serious accidents.

15. False. Women tend to live 5 to 10 percent longer than men.

16. True. Fewer men and women are dying of stroke or heart disease.

17. True. The elderly consume 25 percent of all medications and, as a result, have many more problems with adverse drug reactions.

18. True. Medical quackery is a $10 billion business in the United States. People of all ages are commonly duped into "quick cures" for aging, arthritis, and cancer.

19. False. Personality doesn't change with age. Therefore, all old people can't be described as rigid and cantankerous. You are what you are for as long as you live. But you can change what you do to help yourself to good health.

20. False. Although changes in vision become more common with age, any change in vision, regardless of age, is related to a specific disease. If you are having problems with your vision, see your doctor.

*Source: National Institute on Aging, www.counselingnotes.com/seniors/age/age_iq.htm.*

## Making Change Happen

## Finding Life's Meaning

If you're in your teens, 20s, or 30s, aging and death seem remote, even unimaginable. That's normal. But whatever your age, coming to terms with the stark reality that life is not infinite—that it must end—can give greater meaning to your days.

The lab "Finity" in *Labs for IPC*, based on the Stages of Change discussed in Chapter 1 of this text and in *IPC*, celebrates living as fully, as richly, as joyfully as possible. By making smart choices every day, you can do a great deal to ensure that you live longer. By making conscious, creative choices, you also can ensure that your life is more enjoyable, meaningful, and fulfilling.

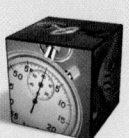

### Get Real

In this section, you take a comprehensive inventory of your life so far. You begin with the Satisfaction with Life Scale, a reliable indicator of how individuals perceive their personal happiness. Using a scale of 7 (strongly agree) to 1 (strongly disagree), you respond to five statements, including:

- In most ways my life is close to my ideal.
- If I could live my life over, I would change almost nothing.

You also answer yes or no to 23 questions about the last 24 hours of your life, including:

- Did you look at the sky?
- Did you taste something absolutely yummy?
- Did you make someone smile?

Social psychology has identified the key components of a fulfilling, happy, high-quality life. You can see how yours compares by assessing:

- Your close relationships.
- Your sense of spirituality or a higher purpose.
- Your positive qualities.
- Your engagement with a passionate pursuit—for family, work, sport, or other experiences—that adds great satisfaction to your life.

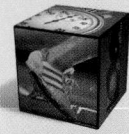

### Get Ready

In this section you block out time for the experiential exercises this lab requires in the action stage.

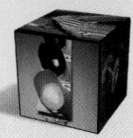

### Get Going

You review a list of 25 adjectives, including descriptives such as:

- Cheerful
- Mean-spirited
- Hard-working
- Whiny

You pick one adjective that you want to describe you (or one that you want to erase from any description of you), and weave appropriate behaviors into your actions that day. You work with a "signature behavior" that you'd like to have associated with you.

- You make up a life list of the things you want to do before you die and do a series of imaginative and creative activities with goals you'd like to accomplish, experiences you'd like to have, things you don't want to regret . . .
- In your *IPC Journal* you develop an outline for your life— past, present, and future—with . . .

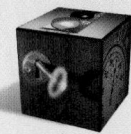

### Lock It In

Living a life fully requires paying attention each and every day. In this section, you develop and deepen simple practices to ensure that you do so, such as:

- **Make your day.** Record in your *IPC Journal* the nicest thing that happened. It might be as small as a bus driver's hearty hello or a "Well done!" on an assignment, or as big as making a team, acing a final exam, or hearing a longed-for "I love you."

# Making This Chapter Work for You

## Review Questions

1. Steps for protecting against bone loss include
   a. having at least two drinks per day.
   b. getting moderate exposure to sunlight.
   c. avoiding heavy exercise.
   d. having a diet low in calcium.

2. When should concern change to intervention?
   a. Uncle Charlie is 85 and continues to drive himself to the grocery store and to the senior center during the daytime.
   b. Nana takes pills at breakfast, lunch, and dinner but sometimes mixes them up.
   c. Mom's hot flashes have become a family joke.
   d. Your older brother can never remember where he put his car keys.

3. You can best help a friend who is bereaved by
   a. encouraging him to have a few drinks to forget his pain.
   b. simply spending time with her.
   c. avoiding talking about his loss because it is awkward.
   d. reminding her about all she still has in her life.

4. Physically fit people over age 60
   a. have lower risk of dying from chronic heart disease.
   b. can regain the fitness level of a 25-year-old.
   c. show no difference in levels of anxiety and depression.
   d. have higher health-care expenses.

5. Which statement about aging is *false*?
   a. The most common nutritional disorder in the elderly is obesity.
   b. In men, sexual activity and longevity are linked.
   c. Hormone therapy reduces the risk of heart disease in menopausal women.
   d. Seniors who take up new hobbies late in life may slow aging within the brain.

6. The gender gap related to longevity
   a. is due to deficiencies in the Y chromosome.
   b. results from the presence of a mutant gene.
   c. may be due to the X chromosome and its hormonal influences on the immune system.
   d. is about 13 years in the United States.

7. Which of the following is a change associated with aging that is slowed by exercise?
   a. loss of connective tissue in skin
   b. decrease in certain hormone levels
   c. loss of lean muscle tissue
   d. decreased interest in food

8. Factors that contribute to staying healthy longer include all of the following *except*
   a. avoiding illness.
   b. moderate smoking.
   c. regular exercise.
   d. lifelong learning.

9. Which statement about the aging brain is *false*?
   a. When brain cells die, surrounding cells can fill the gaps to maintain cognitive function.
   b. Remembering names and recalling information may take longer.
   c. "Use it or lose it."
   d. Mental ability and physical ability both decline with age.

10. An advance directive
    a. indicates who should have your property in the event you die.
    b. may authorize which individuals may not participate in your health care if you are unable to care for yourself.
    c. can specify your desires related to the use of medical treatments and technology to prolong your life.
    d. should specify which physician you designate to be your health-care proxy.

*Answers to these questions can be found on page 672.*

## Critical Thinking

1. How are your parents or other mentors staying fit and alert as they age? Do you think you might use similar strategies?

2. Do you think that coming to terms with mortality allows an individual to live each day to its fullest, rather than putting off what he or she would like to do until tomorrow? How does this concept affect your own life? Explain. Do you believe in a next life? How does this affect your view of life and death?

3. Have your living parents and grandparents written advanced directives or a living will? Have you discussed with them their preferences regarding treatment in the event of a medical crisis? If you haven't had this discussion with your family, how can you begin the process of helping your parents or grandparents communicate their wishes?

4. As many as 10,000 people in this country are chronically unconscious, kept alive by artificial respirators and

feeding tubes. If you were in an accident that left you in a vegetative state, would you want doctors to do everything possible to fight for your life? Would you want to spend months or even years totally unaware of your surroundings? Should health-care professionals have the right to declare that anyone is too old, too ill, or too frail to try to save? Should they have the right to insist that someone live on even if that person isn't experiencing much of a life?

## Media Menu

Visit www.cengagebrain.com to access course materials and companion resources for this text that will:

- Help you evaluate your knowledge of the material.

- Allow you to prepare for exams with interactive quizzing.

- Use the CengageNOW product to develop a Personalized Learning Plan targeting resources that address areas you should study.

- Coach you through identifying target goals for behavioral change and creating and monitoring your personal change plan throughout the semester using the Behavior Change Planner available in the CengageNOW resource.

## Internet Connections

### www.nia.nih.gov
This government site features a comprehensive array of resources on aging, including publications on a variety of geriatric health topics, current news events, and a resource directory for older people.

### www.realage.com
This site features diet and exercise assessment tools—such as a BMI calculator, exercise estimator, and RealAge assessment quizzes on a variety of health topics—to help you determine your risk of disease and what you can do to reduce this risk. The main feature is an interactive, online personal lifestyle assessment that also gives you options for "growing younger."

### http://aoa.gov
This site, part of the Department of Health and Human Services, has information for seniors and their families on promoting healthy lifestyles and general aging topics.

### www.npr.org/programs/death/
This site, sponsored by National Public Radio, contains transcripts and resources from an *All Things Considered* series focusing on how Americans deal with death and dying. Features include personal stories, a place where you can tell your own story, and a comprehensive list of organizations that can help families who are coping with death, dying, and the diseases of old age.

## Key Terms

The terms listed are used on the page indicated. Definitions of the terms are in the Glossary at the end of the book.

advance directives  656

aging  645

Alzheimer's disease  654

autoscopy  663

coma  659

dementia  654

do-not-resuscitate (DNR)  657

holographic will  659

hormone therapy (HT)  652

hospice  663

living will  657

menopause  650

perimenopause  651

persistent vegetative state  659

terminal illness  662

transcendence  663

# Making This Chapter Work for You

**Answers to Review Questions**

**Chapter 1**
1. b; 2. c; 3. c; 4. c; 5. b; 6. b; 7. c; 8. d; 9. c; 10. c

**Chapter 2**
1. b; 2. b; 3. d; 4. b; 5. a; 6. b; 7. c; 8. c; 9. c; 10. a

**Chapter 3**
1. d; 2. a; 3. a; 4. b; 5. a; 6. b; 7. b; 8. c; 9. d; 10. d

**Chapter 4**
1. b; 2. c; 3. a; 4. d; 5. d; 6. d; 7. b; 8. a; 9. c; 10. a

**Chapter 5**
1. b; 2. b; 3. d; 4. d; 5. d; 6. d; 7. c; 8. c; 9. a; 10. a

**Chapter 6**
1. d; 2. c; 3. b; 4. c; 5. a; 6. d; 7. a; 8. a; 9. b; 10. d

**Chapter 7**
1. c; 2. a; 3. a; 4. a; 5. d; 6. b; 7. c; 8. d; 9. c; 10. b

**Chapter 8**
1. c; 2. d; 3. c; 4. b; 5. b; 6. b; 7. b; 8. c; 9. b; 10. a

**Chapter 9**
1. d; 2. d; 3. c; 4. b; 5. a; 6. d; 7. d; 8. b; 9. a; 10. c

**Chapter 10**
1. c; 2. d; 3. c; 4. b; 5. d; 6. b; 7. a; 8. c; 9. c; 10. a

**Chapter 11**
1. c; 2. d; 3. b; 4. c; 5. a; 6. d; 7. b; 8. b; 9. a; 10. c

**Chapter 12**
1. b; 2. a; 3. c; 4. a; 5. b; 6. d; 7. c; 8. d; 9. c; 10. d

**Chapter 13**
1. b; 2. b; 3. a; 4. d; 5. b; 6. d; 7. a; 8. d; 9. b; 10. c

**Chapter 14**
1. d; 2. c; 3. d; 4. b; 5. d; 6. c; 7. a; 8. b; 9. a; 10. c

**Chapter 15**
1. b; 2. d; 3. a; 4. d; 5. a; 6. d; 7. c; 8. b; 9. b; 10. a

**Chapter 16**
1. b; 2. b; 3. d; 4. c; 5. a; 6. d; 7. c; 8. a; 9. c; 10. a

**Chapter 17**
1. b; 2. a; 3. d; 4. c; 5. b; 6. d; 7. d; 8. b; 9. d; 10. a

**Chapter 18**
1. c; 2. c; 3. a; 4. b; 5. a; 6. b; 7. c; 8. c; 9. b; 10. b

**Chapter 19**
1. b; 2. c; 3. c; 4. a; 5. d; 6. c; 7. b; 8. b; 9. b; 10. a

**Chapter 20**
1. b; 2. b; 3. b; 4. a; 5. c; 6. c; 7. c; 8. b; 9. d; 10. c

# Glossary

**abscess** A localized accumulation of pus and disintegrating tissue.

**absorption** The passage of substances into or across membranes or tissues.

**abstinence** Voluntary refrainment from sexual intercourse.

**acculturation** The process of psychosocial change by which an ethnic minority changes as a consequence of contact with the ethnic majority.

**acquired immune deficiency syndrome (AIDS)** The final stages of HIV infection, characterized by a variety of severe illnesses and decreased levels of certain immune cells.

**active stretching** A technique that involves stretching a muscle by contracting the opposing muscle.

**acupuncture** A Chinese medical practice of puncturing the body with needles inserted at specific points to relieve pain or cure disease.

**acute injuries** Physical injuries, such as sprains, bruises, and pulled muscles, which result from sudden traumas, such as falls or collisions.

**adaptive response** The body's attempt to reestablish homeostasis or stability.

**addiction** A behavioral pattern characterized by compulsion, loss of control, and continued repetition of a behavior or activity in spite of adverse consequences.

**additive** Characterized by a combined effect that is equal to the sum of the individual effects.

**adoption** The legal process for becoming the parent to a child of other biological parents.

**advance directives** Documents that specify an individual's preferences regarding treatment in a medical crisis.

**aerobic exercise** Physical activity in which sufficient or excess oxygen is continually supplied to the body.

**aging** The characteristic pattern of normal life changes that occur as living things grow older.

**alcohol abuse** Continued use of alcohol despite awareness of social, occupational, psychological, or physical problems related to its use, or use of alcohol in dangerous ways or situations, such as before driving.

**alcohol dependence** Development of a strong craving for alcohol due to the pleasurable feelings or relief of stress or anxiety produced by drinking.

**alcoholism** A chronic, progressive, potentially fatal disease characterized by impaired control of drinking; a preoccupation with alcohol; continued use of alcohol despite adverse consequences; and distorted thinking, most notably denial.

**allergy** A hypersensitivity to a particular substance in one's environment or diet.

**altruism** Acts of helping or giving to others without thought of self-benefit.

**Alzheimer's disease** A progressive deterioration of intellectual powers due to physiological changes within the brain; symptoms include diminishing ability to concentrate and reason, disorientation, depression, apathy, and paranoia.

**amenorrhea** The absence or suppression of menstruation.

**amino acids** Organic compounds containing nitrogen, carbon, hydro—gen, and oxygen; the essential building blocks of proteins.

**amnion** The innermost membrane of the sac enclosing the embryo or fetus.

**amphetamine** Any of a class of stimulants that trigger the release of epinephrine, which stimulates the central nervous system; users experience a state of hyperalertness and energy, followed by a crash as the drug wears off.

**anaerobic exercise** Physical activity in which the body develops an oxygen deficit.

**androgyny** The expression of both masculine and feminine traits.

**angina pectoris** A severe, suffocating chest pain caused by a brief lack of oxygen to the heart.

**anorexia nervosa** A psychological disorder in which refusal to eat and/or an extreme loss of appetite leads to malnutrition, severe weight loss, and possibly death.

**antagonistic** Opposing or counteracting.

**antibiotics** Substances produced by microorganisms, or synthetic agents, that are toxic to bacteria.

**antidepressant** A drug used primarily to treat symptoms of depression.

**antioxidants** Substances that prevent the damaging effects of oxidation in cells.

**antiviral drug** A substance that decreases the severity and duration of a viral infection if taken prior to or soon after onset of the infection.

**anxiety disorders** A group of psychological disorders involving episodes of apprehension, tension, or uneasiness, stemming from the anticipation of danger and sometimes accompanied by physical symptoms, which cause significant distress and impairment to an individual.

**aorta** The main artery of the body, arising from the left ventricle of the heart.

**appetite** A desire for food, stimulated by anticipated hunger, physiological changes within the brain and body, the availability of food, and other environmental and psychological factors.

**arteriosclerosis** Any of a number of chronic diseases characterized by degeneration of the arteries and hardening and thickening of arterial walls.

**artificial insemination** The introduction of viable sperm into the vagina by artificial means for the purpose of inducing conception.

**Asperger syndrome** is a high-functioning form of autism characterized by difficulty interacting socially, repetitive behaviors, clumsiness, and delays in motor development.

**asthma** A disease or allergic response characterized by bronchial spasms and difficult breathing.

**atherosclerosis** A form of arteriosclerosis in which fatty substances (plaque) are deposited on the inner walls of arteries.

**atrium (plural atria)** Either of the two upper chambers of the heart, which receive blood from the veins.

**attention-deficit/hyperactivity disorder (ADHD)** A spectrum of difficulties in controlling motion and sustaining attention, including hyperactivity, impulsivity, and distractibility.

**autoimmune disorder** Resulting from the attack on body tissue by an immune system that fails to recognize the tissue as self.

**autonomy** The ability to draw on internal resources; independence from familial and societal influences.

**autoscopy** The sensation of one's self being outside its body, often experienced by individuals in near-death medical crises.

**aversion therapy** A treatment that attempts to help a person overcome a dependence or bad habit by making the person feel disgusted or repulsed by that habit.

**axon terminal** The ending of an axon, from which impulses are transmitted to a dendrite of another neuron.

**axon** The long fiber that conducts impulses from the neuron's nucleus to its dendrites.

**Ayurveda** A traditional Indian medical treatment involving meditation, exercise, herbal medications, and nutrition.

**bacteria** (singular, bacterium) One-celled microscopic organisms; the most plentiful pathogens.

**bacterial vaginosis** A vaginal infection caused by overgrowth and depletion of various microorganisms living in the vagina, resulting in a malodorous white or gray vaginal discharge.

**ballistic stretching** Rapid bouncing movements.

**barbiturates** Antianxiety drugs that depress the central nervous system, reduce activity, and induce relaxation, drowsiness, or sleep; often prescribed to relieve tension and treat epileptic seizures or as a general anesthetic.

**barrier contraceptives** Birth control devices that block the meeting of egg and sperm, either by physical barriers, such as condoms, diaphragms, or cervical caps, or by chemical barriers, such as spermicide, or both.

**basal metabolic rate (BMR)** The number of calories required to sustain the body at rest.

**behavioral therapy** A technique that emphasizes application of the principles of learning to substitute desirable responses and behavior patterns for undesirable ones.

**benzodiazepines** Antianxiety drugs that depress the central nervous system, reduce activity, and induce relaxation, drowsiness, or sleep; often prescribed to relieve tension, muscular strain, sleep problems, anxiety, and panic attacks; also used as an anesthetic and in the treatment of alcohol withdrawal.

**bidis** Skinny, sweet-flavored cigarettes.

**binge eating** The rapid consumption of an abnormally large amount of food in a relatively short time.

**binge** For a man, having five or more alcoholic drinks at a single sitting; for a woman, having four drinks or more at a single sitting.

**biofeedback** A technique of becoming aware, with the aid of external monitoring devices, of internal physiological activities in order to develop the capability of altering them.

**bipolar disorder** Severe depression alternating with periods of manic activity and elation.

**bisexual** Sexually oriented toward both sexes.

**blastocyst** In embryonic development, a ball of cells with a surface layer and an inner cell mass.

**blended family** A family formed when one or both of the partners bring children from a previous union to the new marriage.

**blood-alcohol concentration (BAC)** The amount of alcohol in the blood, expressed as a percentage.

**body composition** The relative amounts of fat and lean tissue (bone, muscle, organs, water) in the body.

**body mass index (BMI)** A mathematical formula that correlates with body fat; the ratio of weight to height squared.

**bulimia nervosa** Episodic binge eating, often followed by forced vomiting or laxative abuse, and accompanied by a persistent preoccupation with body shape and weight.

**burnout** A state of physical, emotional, and mental exhaustion resulting from constant or repeated emotional pressure.

**caesarean delivery** The surgical procedure in which an infant is delivered through an incision made in the abdominal wall and uterus.

**calorie balance** The relationship between calories consumed from foods and beverages and calories expended in normal body functions and through physical activity. If the calories consumed equals calories expended, you have calorie balance.

**calorie** The amount of energy required to raise the temperature of 1 gram of water by 1 degree Celsius. In everyday usage related

to the energy content of foods and the energy expended in activities, a calorie is actually the equivalent of a thousand such calories, or a kilocalorie.

**candidiasis** An infection of the yeast Candida albicans, commonly occurring in the vagina, vulva, penis, and mouth and causing burning, itching, and a whitish discharge.

**capillary** A minute blood vessel that connects an artery to a vein.

**carbohydrates** Organic compounds, such as starches, sugars, and glycogen, that are composed of carbon, hydrogen, and oxygen, and are sources of bodily energy.

**carbon monoxide** A colorless, odorless gas produced by the burning of gasoline or tobacco; displaces oxygen in the hemoglobin molecules of red blood cells.

**carcinogen** A substance or agent that causes cancer.

**cardiometabolic** Referring to the heart and to the biochemical processes involved in the body's functioning.

**cardiopulmonary resuscitation (CPR)** A method of artificial stimulation of the heart and lungs; a combination of mouth-to-mouth breathing and chest compression.

**cardiorespiratory fitness** The ability of the heart and blood vessels to circulate blood through the body efficiently.

**celibacy** Abstention from sexual activity; can be partial or complete, permanent or temporary.

**certified social worker or licensed clinical social worker (LCSW)** A person who has completed a two-year graduate program in counseling people with mental problems.

**cervical cap** A thimble-size rubber or plastic cap that is inserted into the vagina to fit over the cervix and prevent the passage of sperm into the uterus during sexual intercourse; used with a spermicidal foam or jelly, it serves as both a chemical and a physical barrier to sperm.

**cervix** The narrow, lower end of the uterus that opens into the vagina.

**chancroid** A soft, painful sore or localized infection usually acquired through sexual contact.

**chiropractic** A method of treating disease, primarily through manipulating the bones and joints to restore normal nerve function.

**chlamydia** A sexually transmitted infection caused by the bacterium *Chlamydia trachomatis*, often asymptomatic in women, but sometimes characterized by urinary pain; if undetected and untreated, may result in pelvic inflammatory disease (PID).

**chlorinated hydrocarbons** Highly toxic pesticides, such as DDT and chlordane, that are extremely resistant to breakdown; may cause cancer, birth defects, neurological disorders, and damage to wildlife and the environment.

**cholesterol** An organic substance found in animal fats; linked to cardiovascular disease, particularly atherosclerosis.

**chronic fatigue syndrome (CFS)** A cluster of symptoms whose cause is not yet known; a primary symptom is debilitating fatigue.

**circumcision** The surgical removal of the foreskin of the penis.

**clitoris** A small erectile structure on the female, corresponding to the penis on the male.

**club drugs** Illegally manufactured psychoactive drugs that have dangerous physical and psychological effects.

**cocaine** A white crystalline powder extracted from the leaves of the coca plant that stimulates the central nervous system and produces a brief period of euphoria followed by a depression.

**codependency** An emotional and psychological behavioral pattern in which the spouses, partners, parents, children, and friends of individuals with addictive behaviors allow or enable their loved ones to continue their self-destructive habits.

**cognitive therapy** A technique used to identify an individual's beliefs and attitudes, recognize negative thought patterns, and educate in alternative ways of thinking.

**cohabitation** Two people living together as a couple, without official ties such as marriage.

**coitus interruptus** The removal of the penis from the vagina before ejaculation.

**coma** A state of total unconsciousness.

**complementary and alternative medicine (CAM)** A term used to apply to all health-care approaches, practices, and treatments not widely taught in medical schools, not generally used in hospitals, and not usually reimbursed by medical insurance companies.

**complementary proteins** Incomplete proteins that, when combined, provide all the amino acids essential for protein synthesis.

**complete proteins** Proteins that contain all the amino acids needed by the body for growth and maintenance.

**complex carbohydrates** Starches, including cereals, fruits, and vegetables.

**computer vision syndrome** A condition caused by computer use marked by tired and sore eyes, blurred vision, headaches, and neck, shoulder, and back pain.

**conception** The merging of a sperm and an ovum.

**condom** A latex sheath worn over the penis during sexual acts to prevent conception and/or the transmission of disease; the female condom lines the walls of the vagina.

**contraception** The prevention of conception; birth control.

**corpus luteum** A yellowish mass of tissue that is formed, immediately after ovulation, from the remaining cells of the follicle; it secretes estrogen and progesterone for the remainder of the menstrual cycle.

**Cowper's glands** Two small glands that discharge into the male urethra; also called bulbourethral glands.

**culture** The set of shared attitudes, values, goals, and practices of a group that are internalized by an individual within the group.

**cunnilingus** Sexual stimulation of a woman's genitals by means of oral manipulation.

**cystitis** Infection of the urinary bladder.

**decibel (dB)** A unit for measuring the intensity of sounds.

**defense mechanism** A psychological process that alleviates anxiety and eliminates mental conflict; includes denial, displacement, projection, rationalization, reaction formation, and repression.

**delirium tremens (DTs)** The delusions, hallucinations, and agitated behavior following withdrawal from long-term chronic alcohol abuse.

**dementia** Deterioration of mental capability.

**dendrites** Branching fibers of a neuron that receive impulses from axon terminals of other neurons and conduct these impulses toward the nucleus.

**detoxification** The supervised removal of a poisonous or harmful substance (such as a drug) from the body; a therapy for alcoholics in which they are denied alcohol in a controlled environment.

**diabetes mellitus** A disease in which the inadequate production of insulin leads to failure of the body tissues to break down carbohydrates at a normal rate.

**diaphragm** A bowl-like rubber cup with a flexible rim that is inserted into the vagina to cover the cervix and prevent the passage of sperm into the uterus during sexual intercourse; used with a spermicidal foam or jelly, it serves as both a chemical and a physical barrier to sperm.

**diastole** The period between contractions in the cardiac cycle, during which the heart relaxes and dilates as it fills with blood.

**diastolic blood pressure** Lowest blood pressure between contractions of the heart.

**diathesis stress model** A psychological theory that explains behavior as a result of both nature and nurture.

**dietary fiber** The nondigestible form of carbohydrates found in plant foods, such as leaves, stems, skins, seeds, and hulls.

**dilation and evacuation (D and E)** A medical procedure in which the contents of the uterus are removed through the use of instruments.

**distress** A negative stress that may result in illness.

**do-not-resuscitate (DNR)** An advance directive expressing an individual's preference that resuscitation efforts not be made during a medical crisis.

**dopamine** A brain chemical associated with feelings of satisfaction and euphoria.

**drug abuse** The excessive use of a drug in a manner inconsistent with accepted medical practice.

**drug** Any substance, other than food, that affects bodily functions and structures when taken into the body.

**drug dependence** Continued substance use even when its use causes cognitive, behavioral, and physical symptoms.

**drug diversion** The transfer of a drug from the person for whom it was prescribed to another individual.

**drug misuse** The use of a drug for a purpose (or person) other than that for which it was medically intended.

**dynamic flexibility** The ability to move a joint quickly and fluidly through its entire range of motion with little resistance.

**dysfunctional** Characterized by negative and destructive patterns of behavior between partners or between parents and children.

**dysmenorrhea** Painful menstruation.

**dyspareunia** A sexual difficulty in which a woman experiences pain during sexual intercourse.

**dysthymia** Frequent, prolonged mild depression.

**eating disorders** Bizarre, often dangerous patterns of food consumption, including anorexia nervosa and bulimia nervosa.

**ecosystem** A community of organisms sharing a physical and chemical environment and interacting with each other.

**Ecstasy (MDMA)** A synthetic compound, also known as methylenedioxymethamphetamine, that is similar in structure to methamphetamine and has both stimulant and hallucinogenic effects.

**ectopic pregnancy** A pregnancy in which the fertilized egg has implanted itself outside the uterine cavity, usually in the fallopian tube.

**ejaculation** The expulsion of semen from the penis.

**ejaculatory duct** The canal connecting the seminal vesicles and vas deferens.

**electromagnetic fields (EMFs)** The invisible electric and magnetic fields generated by an electrically charged conductor.

**embryo** An organism in its early stage of development; in humans, the embryonic period lasts from the second to the eighth week of pregnancy.

**emergency contraception (EC)** Types of oral contraceptive pills, usually taken within 72 hours after intercourse, that can prevent pregnancy.

**emotional health** The ability to express and acknowledge one's feelings and moods and exhibit adaptability and compassion for others.

**emotional intelligence** A term used by some psychologists to evaluate the capacity of people to understand themselves and relate well with others.

**enabling factors** The skills, resources, and physical and mental capabilities that shape our behavior.

**enabling** Unwittingly contributing to a person's addictive or abusive behavior. Components of enabling include shielding or covering up for an abuser/addict; controlling him or her; taking over responsibilities; rationalizing addictive behavior; or cooperating with him or her.

**endocrine disruptors** Synthetic chemicals that interfere with the ways that hormones work in humans and wildlife.

**endocrine system** The group of ductless glands that produce hormones and secrete them directly into the blood for transport to target organs.

**endometrium** The mucous membrane lining the uterus.

**endorphins** Mood-elevating, pain-killing chemicals produced by the brain.

**environmental tobacco smoke** Secondhand cigarette smoke; the third-leading preventable cause of death.

**epididymis** That portion of the male duct system in which sperm mature.

**epilepsy** A variety of neurological disorders characterized by sudden attacks (seizures) of violent muscle contractions and unconsciousness.

**erectile dysfunction (ED)** The consistent inability to maintain a penile erection sufficient for adequate sexual relations.

**erogenous** Sexually sensitive.

**essential nutrients** Nutrients that the body cannot manufacture for itself and must obtain from food.

**estrogen** The female sex hormone that stimulates female secondary sex characteristics.

**ethyl alcohol** The intoxicating agent in alcoholic beverages; also called ethanol.

**eustress** Positive stress, which stimulates a person to function properly.

**evidence-based medicine** The choice of a medical treatment on the basis of large randomized controlled research trials and large prospective studies.

**failure rate** The number of pregnancies that occur per year for every 100 women using a particular method of birth control.

**fallopian tubes** The pair of channels that transport ova from the ovaries to the uterus; the usual site of fertilization.

**family** A group of people united by marriage, blood, or adoption; residing in the same household; maintaining a common culture; and interacting with one another on the basis of their roles within the group.

**fellatio** Sexual stimulation of a man's genitals by means of oral manipulation.

**fertilization** The fusion of sperm and egg nucleus.

**fetal alcohol effects (FAE)** Milder forms of FAS, including low birth weight, irritability as newborns, and permanent mental impairment as a result of the mother's alcohol consumption during pregnancy.

**fetal alcohol syndrome (FAS)** A cluster of physical and mental defects in the newborn, including low birth weight, smaller-than-normal head circumference, intrauterine growth retardation, and permanent mental impairment caused by the mother's alcohol consumption during pregnancy.

**fetus** The human organism developing in the uterus from the ninth week until birth.

**FITT** A formula that describes the frequency, intensity, type, and length of time for physical activity.

**flexibility** The range of motion allowed by one's joints; determined by the length of muscles, tendons, and ligaments attached to the joints.

**folic acid** A form of folate used in vitamin supplements and fortified foods.

**functional fiber** Isolated, nondigestible carbohydrates with beneficial effects in humans.

**functional fitness** The ability to perform real-life activities, such as lifting a heavy suitcase.

**fungi** (singular, fungus) Organisms that reproduce by means of spores.

**gamma globulin** The antibody-containing portion of the blood fluid (plasma).

**GBL (gamma butyrolactone)** The main ingredient in gamma hydroxybutyrate (GHB); once ingested, GBL converts to GHB and can cause the ingestor to lose consciousness.

**gender** Maleness or femaleness, as determined by a combination of anatomical and physiological factors, psychological factors, and learned behaviors.

**general adaptation syndrome (GAS)** An anxiety disorder characterized as chronic distress.

**generalized anxiety disorder (GAD)** An anxiety disorder characterized as chronic distress.

**generic** A consumer product with no brand name or registered trademark.

**GHB (gamma hydroxybutyrate)** A brain messenger chemical that stimulates the release of human growth hormone; commonly abused for its high and its alleged ability to trim fat and build muscles. Also known as "blue nitro" or the "date rape drug."

**gingivitis** Inflammation of the gums.

**glia** Support cells for neurons in the brain and spinal cord that separate the brain from the bloodstream, assist in the growth of neurons, speed transmission of nerve impulses, and eliminate damaged neurons.

**gonadotropins** Gonad-stimulating hormones produced by the pituitary gland.

**gonorrhea** A sexually transmitted infection caused by the bacterium *Neisseria gonorrhoeae*; symptoms include discharge from the penis; women are generally asymptomatic.

**gum disease** Inflammation of the gum and bones that hold teeth in place.

**hallucinogen** A drug that causes hallucinations.

**hashish** A concentrated form of a drug, derived from the cannabis plant, containing the psychoactive ingredient THC, which causes a sense of euphoria when inhaled or eaten.

**hazing** Any activity that humiliates, degrades, or poses a risk of emotional or physical harm for the sake of joining a group or maintaining full status in that group.

**health** A state of complete well-being, including physical, psychological, spiritual, social, intellectual, and environmental dimensions.

**health belief model (HBM)** A model of behavioral change that focuses on the individual's attitudes and beliefs.

**health literacy** Ability to understand health information and use it to make good decisions about health and medical care.

**health maintenance organization (HMO)** An organization that provides health services on a fixed-contract basis.

**health promotion** Any planned combination of educational, political, regulatory, and organizational supports for actions and conditions of living conducive to the health of individuals, groups, or communities.

**helminth** A parasitic roundworm or flatworm.

**hepatitis** An inflammation and/or infection of the liver caused by a virus, often accompanied by jaundice.

**herbal medicine** An ancient form of medical treatment using substances derived from trees, flowers, ferns, seaweeds, and lichens to treat disease.

**herpes simplex** A condition caused by one of the herpes viruses and characterized by lesions of the skin or mucous membranes; herpes simplex virus 2 is sexually transmitted and causes genital blisters or sores.

**heterosexual** Primary sexual orientation toward members of the other sex.

**holistic** An approach to medicine that takes into account body, mind, emotions, and spirit.

**holographic will** A will wholly in the handwriting of its author.

**homeopathy** A system of medical practice that treats a disease by administering dosages of substances that would in healthy persons produce symptoms similar to those of the disease.

**homeostasis** The body's natural state of balance or stability.

**homosexual** Primary sexual orientation toward members of the same sex.

**hormone** Substance released in the blood that regulates specific bodily functions.

**hormone therapy (HT)** The use of supplemental hormones during and after menopause.

**hospice** A homelike health-care facility or program committed to supportive care for terminally ill people.

**host** A person or population that contracts one or more pathogenic agents in an environment.

**human immunodeficiency virus (HIV)** A type of virus that causes a spectrum of health problems, ranging from a symptomless infection to changes in the immune system, to the development of life-threatening diseases because of impaired immunity.

**human papillomavirus (HPV)** A pathogen that causes genital warts and increases the risk of cervical cancer.

**hunger** The physiological drive to consume food.

**hypertension** High blood pressure occurring when the blood exerts excessive pressure against the arterial walls.

**hypothermia** An abnormally low body temperature; if not treated appropriately, coma or death could result.

**immune deficiency** Partial or complete inability of the immune system to respond to pathogens.

**immunity** Protection from infectious diseases.

**immunotherapy** A series of injections of small but increasing doses of an allergen, used to treat allergies.

**implantation** The embedding of the fertilized ovum in the uterine lining.

**incomplete proteins** Proteins that lack one or more of the amino acids essential for protein synthesis.

**incubation period** The time between a pathogen's entrance into the body and the first symptom.

**infertility** The inability to conceive a child.

**infiltration** A gradual penetration or invasion.

**inflammation** A localized response by the body to tissue injury, characterized by swelling and the dilation of the blood vessels.

**influenza** Any type of fairly common, highly contagious viral diseases.

**informed consent** Permission (to undergo or receive a medical procedure or treatment) given voluntarily, with full knowledge and understanding of the procedure—or treatment and its possible consequences.

**inhalants** Substances that produce vapors having psychoactive effects when sniffed.

**integrative medicine** An approach that combines traditional medicine with alternative/complementary therapies.

**intercourse** Sexual stimulation by means of entry of the penis into the vagina; coitus.

**interpersonal therapy (IPT)** A technique used to develop communication skills and relationships.

**intimacy** A state of closeness between two people, characterized by the desire and ability to share one's innermost thoughts and feelings with each other either verbally or nonverbally.

**intoxication** Maladaptive behavioral, psychological, and physiologic changes that occur as a result of substance abuse.

**intramuscular** Into or within a muscle.

**intrauterine device (IUD)** A device inserted into the uterus through the cervix to prevent pregnancy by interfering with implantation.

**intravenous** Into a vein.

**ionizing radiation** A form of energy emitted from atoms as they undergo internal change.

**isokinetic** Having the same force; exercise with specialized equipment that provides resistance equal to the force applied by the user throughout the entire range of motion.

**isometric** Of the same length; exercise in which muscles increase their tension without shortening in length, such as when pushing an immovable object.

**isotonic** Having the same tension or tone; exercise requiring the repetition of an action that creates tension, such as weight lifting or calisthenics.

**labia majora** The fleshy outer folds that border the female genital area.

**labia minora** The fleshy inner folds that border the female genital area.

**labor** The process leading up to birth: effacement and dilation of the cervix; the movement of the baby into and through the birth canal, accompanied by strong contractions; and contraction of the uterus and expulsion of the placenta after the birth.

**lacto-vegetarians** People who eat dairy products as well as fruits and vegetables (but not meat, poultry, or fish).

**Lamaze method** A method of childbirth preparation taught to expectant parents to help the woman cope with the discomfort of labor; combines breathing and psychological techniques.

**laparoscopy** A surgical sterilization procedure in which the fallopian tubes are observed with a laparoscope inserted through a small incision, and then cut or blocked.

**lipoprotein** A compound in blood that is made up of proteins and fat; a high-density lipoprotein (HDL) picks up excess cholesterol in the blood; a low-density lipoprotein (LDL) carries more cholesterol and deposits it on the walls of arteries.

**living will** An advance directive providing instructions for the use of life-sustaining procedures in the event of terminal illness or injury.

**locus of control** An individual's belief about the sources of power and influence over his or her life.

**LSD (lysergic acid diethylamide)** A synthetic psychoactive substance originally developed to explore mental illness.

**lumpectomy** The surgical removal of a breast tumor and its surrounding tissue.

**Lyme disease** A disease caused by a bacterium carried by a tick; it may cause heart arrhythmias, neurological problems, and arthritis symptoms.

**lymph nodes** Small tissue masses in which some immune cells are stored.

**macronutrients** Nutrients required by the human body in the greatest amounts, including water, carbohydrates, proteins, and fats.

**mainstream smoke** The smoke inhaled directly by smoking a cigarette.

**major depression** Sadness that does not end; ongoing feelings of utter helplessness.

**mammography** A diagnostic X-ray exam used to detect breast cancer.

**managed care** Health-care services and reimbursement predetermined by third-party insurers.

**marijuana** The drug derived from the cannabis plant, containing the psychoactive ingredient THC, which causes a mild sense of euphoria when inhaled or eaten.

**marriage and family therapist** A psychiatrist, psychologist, or social worker who specializes in marriage and family counseling.

**mastectomy** The surgical removal of an entire breast.

**masturbation** Manual (or nonmanual) self-stimulation of the genitals, often resulting in orgasm.

**medical abortion** Method of ending a pregnancy within nine weeks of conception using hormonal medications that cause expulsion of the fertilized egg.

**medical history** The health-related information collected during the interview of a client by a health-care professional.

**meditation** A group of approaches that use quiet sitting, breathing techniques, and/or chanting to relax, improve concentration, and become attuned to one's inner self.

**menarche** The onset of menstruation at puberty.

**meningitis** An extremely serious, potentially fatal illness that attacks the membranes around the brain and spinal cord; caused by the bacterium *Neisseria meningitis*.

**menopause** The complete cessation of ovulation and menstruation for 12 consecutive months.

**menstruation** Discharge of blood from the vagina as a result of the shedding of the uterine lining at the end of the menstrual cycle.

**mental disorder** Behavioral or psychological syndrome associated with distress or disability or with a significantly increased risk of suffering death, pain, disability, or loss of freedom.

**mental health** The ability to perceive reality as it is, respond to its challenges, and develop rational strategies for living.

**MET (metabolic equivalent of task)** The amount of energy a person uses at rest.

**metabolic syndrome** A cluster of disorders of the body's metabolism that make diabetes, heart disease, or stroke more likely.

**metastasize** To spread to other parts of the body via the bloodstream or lymphatic system.

**micronutrients** Vitamins and minerals needed by the body in very small amounts.

**microwaves** Extremely high frequency electromagnetic waves that increase the rate at which molecules vibrate, thereby generating heat.

**mindfulness** A method of stress reduction that involves experiencing the physical and mental sensations of the present moment.

**minerals** Naturally occurring inorganic substances, small amounts of some being essential in metabolism and nutrition.

**minipill, progestin-only pill** An oral contraceptive containing a small amount of progestin and no estrogen, which prevents contraception by making the mucus in the cervix so thick that sperm cannot enter the uterus.

**miscarriage** A pregnancy that terminates before the twentieth week of gestation; also called spontaneous abortion.

**mononucleosis** An infectious viral disease characterized by an excess of white blood cells in the blood, fever, bodily discomfort, a sore throat, and kidney and liver complications.

**monophasic pill** An oral contraceptive that releases synthetic estrogen and progestin at constant levels throughout the menstrual cycle.

**mons pubis** The rounded, fleshy area over the junction of the female pubic bones.

**mood** A sustained emotional state that colors one's view of the world for hours or days.

**multiphasic pill** An oral contraceptive that releases different levels of estrogen and progestin to mimic the hormonal fluctuations of the natural menstrual cycle.

**multiple chemical sensitivity (MCS)** A sensitivity to low-level chemical exposures from ordinary substances, such as perfumes and tobacco smoke, that results in physiological responses such as chest pain, depression, dizziness, fatigue, and nausea. Also known as environmentally triggered illness.

**muscular endurance** The ability to withstand the stress of continued physical exertion.

**muscular strength** Physical power; the maximum weight one can lift, push, or press in one effort.

**mutagen** An agent that causes alterations in the genetic material of living cells.

**myocardial infarction (MI)** A condition characterized by the dying of tissue areas in the myocardium, caused by interruption of the blood supply to those areas; the medical name for a heart attack.

**naturopathy** An alternative system of treatment of disease that emphasizes the use of natural remedies such as sun, water, heat, and air. Therapies may include dietary changes, steam baths, and exercise.

**NEAT (nonexercise activity thermogenesis)** Nonvolitional movement that can be an effective way of burning calories.

**neuron** A nerve cell; the basic working unit of the brain, which transmits information from the senses to the brain and from the brain to specific body parts; each neuron consists of a cell body, an axon terminal, and dendrites.

**neuropsychiatry** The study of the brain and mind.

**neurotransmitters** Chemicals released by neurons that stimulate or inhibit the action of other neurons.

**nicotine** The addictive substance in tobacco; one of the most toxic of all poisons.

**nocturnal emissions** Ejaculations while dreaming; wet dreams.

**nongonococcal urethritis (NGU)** Inflammation of the urethra caused by organisms other than the *Gonococcus* bacterium.

**nonvolitional sex** Sexual behavior that violates a person's right to choose when and with whom to have sex and what sexual behaviors to engage in.

**nucleus** The central part of a cell, contained in the cell body of a neuron.

**nutrition** The science devoted to the study of dietary needs for food and the effects of food on organisms.

**obesity** The excessive accumulation of fat in the body; class 1 obesity is defined by a BMI between 30.0 and 34.9; class 2 obesity by a BMI between 35.0 and 39.9; class 3, or severe obesity, is a BMI of 40 or higher.

**obsessive-compulsive disorder (OCD)** An anxiety disorder characterized by obsessions and/or compulsions that impair one's ability to function and form relationships.

**opioids** Drugs that have sleep-inducing and pain-relieving properties, including opium and its derivatives and nonopioid, synthetic drugs.

**optimism** The tendency to seek out, remember, and expect pleasurable experiences.

**oral contraceptives** Preparations of synthetic hormones that inhibit ovulation; also referred to as birth control pills or simply the pill.

**organic** Term designating food produced with, or production based on the use of, fertilizers originating from plants or animals, without the use of pesticides or chemically formulated fertilizers.

**organophosphates** Toxic pesticides that may cause cancer, birth defects, neurological disorders, and damage to wildlife and the environment.

**orgasm** A series of contractions of the pelvic muscles occurring at the peak of sexual arousal.

**osteoporosis** A condition in which the bones become increasingly soft and porous, making them susceptible to injury.

**outcomes** The ultimate impacts of particular treatments or absence of treatment.

**ovary** The female sex organ that produces egg cells, estrogen, and progesterone.

**over-the-counter (OTC) drugs** Medications that can be obtained legally without a prescription from a medical professional.

**overload principle** Providing a greater stress or demand on the body than it is normally accustomed to handling.

**overloading** Method of physical training involving increasing the number of repetitions or the amount of resistance gradually to work the muscle to temporary fatigue.

**overtrain** Working muscles too intensely or too frequently, resulting in persistent muscle soreness, injuries, unintended weight loss, nervousness, and an inability to relax.

**overuse injuries** Physical injuries to joints or muscles, such as strains, fractures, and tendonitis, which result from overdoing a repetitive activity.

**overweight** A condition of having a BMI between 25.0 and 29.9.

**ovo-lacto-vegetarians** People who eat eggs, dairy products, and fruits and vegetables (but not meat, poultry, or fish).

**ovulation** The release of a mature ovum from an ovary approximately 14 days prior to the onset of menstruation.

**ovum** (plural, ova) The female gamete (egg cell).

**ozone** A form of oxygen that is a harmful component of air pollution.

**panic attack** A short episode characterized by physical sensations of light-headedness, dizziness, hyperventilation, and numbness of extremities, accompanied by an inexplicable terror, usually of a physical disaster such as death.

**panic disorder** An anxiety disorder in which the apprehension or experience of recurring panic attacks is so intense that normal functioning is impaired.

**passive stretching** A stretching technique in which an external force or resistance (your body, a partner, gravity, or a weight) helps the joints move through their range of motion.

**pathogen** A microorganism that produces disease.

**PCP (phencyclidine)** A synthetic psychoactive substance that produces effects similar to other psychoactive drugs when swallowed, smoked, sniffed, or injected, but also may trigger unpredictable behavioral changes.

**pelvic inflammatory disease (PID)** An inflammation of the internal female genital tract, characterized by abdominal pain, fever, and tenderness of the cervix.

**penis** The male organ of sex and urination.

**perimenopause** The period from a woman's first irregular cycles to her last menstruation.

**perineum** The area between the anus and vagina in the female and between the anus and scrotum in the male.

**periodontitis** Severe gum disease in which the tooth root becomes infected.

**persistent vegetative state** A state of being awake and capable of reacting to physical stimuli, such as light, while being unaware of pain or other environmental stimuli.

**phobia** An anxiety disorder marked by an inordinate fear of an object, a class of objects, or a situation, resulting in extreme avoidance behaviors.

**physical dependence** The physiological attachment to, and need for, a drug.

**physical fitness** The ability to respond to routine physical demands, with enough reserve energy to cope with a sudden challenge.

**phytochemicals** Chemicals such as indoles, coumarins, and capsaicin, which exist naturally in plants and have disease-fighting properties.

**placenta** An organ that develops after implantation and to which the embryo attaches, via the umbilical cord, for nourishment and waste removal.

**plaque** The sludgelike substance that builds up on the inner walls of arteries.

**plaque** The sticky film of bacteria that forms on teeth.

**pollutant** A substance or agent in the environment, usually the by-product of human industry or activity, that is injurious to human, animal, or plant life.

**polyabuse** The misuse or abuse of more than one drug.

**posttraumatic stress disorder (PTSD)** The repeated reliving of a trauma through nightmares or recollection.

**potentiating** Making more effective or powerful.

**practice guidelines** Recommendations for diagnosis and treatment of various health problems based on evidence from scientific research.

**preconception care** Health care to prepare for pregnancy.

**precycling** The use of products that are packaged in recycled or recyclable material.

**predisposing factors** The beliefs, values, attitudes, knowledge, and perceptions that influence our behavior.

**predrinking** Consuming alcoholic beverages, usually with friends, before going out to bars or parties; also called pre-gaming, pre-loading, or front-loading.

**preferred provider organization (PPO)** A group of physicians contracted to provide health care to members at a discounted price.

**prehypertension** A condition of slightly elevated blood pressure, which is likely to worsen in time.

**premature ejaculation** A sexual difficulty in which a man ejaculates so rapidly that his partner's satisfaction is impaired.

**premature labor** Labor that occurs after the twentieth week but before the thirty-seventh week of pregnancy.

**premenstrual dysphoric disorder (PMDD)** A disorder that causes symptoms of psychological depression during the last week of the menstrual cycle.

**premenstrual syndrome (PMS)** A disorder that causes physical discomfort and psychological distress prior to a woman's menstrual period.

**prevention** Information and support offered to help healthy people identify their health risks, reduce stressors, prevent potential medical problems, and enhance their well-being.

**primary care** Ambulatory or outpatient care provided by a physician in an office, emergency room, or clinic.

**progesterone** The female sex hormone that stimulates the uterus, preparing it for the arrival of a fertilized egg.

**progressive overloading** Gradually increasing physical challenges once the body adapts to the stress placed upon it to produce maximum benefits.

**progressive relaxation** A method of reducing muscle tension by contracting, then relaxing, certain areas of the body.

**proof** The alcoholic strength of a distilled spirit, expressed as twice the percentage of alcohol present.

**prostate gland** A structure surrounding the male urethra that produces a secretion that helps liquefy the semen from the testes.

**protection** Measures that an individual can take when participating in risky behavior to prevent injury or unwanted risks.

**proteins** Organic compounds composed of amino acids; one of the essential nutrients.

**protozoa** Microscopic animals made up of one cell or a group of similar cells.

**psychiatric drugs** Medications that regulate a person's mental, emotional, and physical functions to facilitate normal functioning.

**psychiatric nurse** A nurse with special training and experience in mental health care.

**psychiatrist** Licensed medical doctor with additional training in psychotherapy, psychopharmacology, and treatment of mental disorders.

**psychoative** Mind-affecting.

**psychodynamic** Interpreting behaviors in terms of early experiences and unconscious influences.

**psychological dependence** The emotional or mental attachment to the use of a drug.

**psychologist** Mental health care professional who has completed doctoral or graduate program in psychology and is trained in psychotherapeutic techniques, but who is not medically trained and does not prescribe medications.

**psychotherapy** Treatment designed to produce a response by psychological rather than physical means, such as suggestion, persuasion, reassurance, and support.

**quackery** Medical fakery; unproven practices claiming to cure diseases or solve health problems.

**range of motion** The fullest extent of possible movement in a particular joint.

**rape** Sexual penetration of a female or a male by means of intimidation, force, or fraud.

**rapid eye movement (REM) sleep** Regularly occurring periods of sleep during which the most active dreaming takes place.

**Rating of Perceived Exertion (RPE)** A self-assessment scale that rates symptoms of breathlessness and fatigue.

**receptors** Molecules on the surface of neurons on which neurotransmitters bind after their release from other neurons.

**recycling** The processing or reuse of manufactured materials to reduce consumption of raw materials.

**refractory period** The period of time following orgasm during which the male cannot experience another orgasm.

**reinforcing factors** Rewards, encouragement, and recognition that influence our behavior in the short run.

**relapse prevention** An alcohol recovery treatment method that focuses on social skills training to develop ways of preventing or minimizing a relapse.

**relative risk** The risk of developing cancer in persons with a certain exposure or trait compared to the risk in persons who do not have the same exposure or trait.

**rep (or repetition)** In weight training, a single performance of a movement or exercise.

**repetitive motion injury (RMI)** Inflammation of or damage to a part of the body due to repetition of the same movements.

**resting heart rate** The number of heartbeats per minute during inactivity.

**reuptake** Reabsorption by the originating cell of neurotransmitters that have not connected with receptors and have been left in synapses.

**reversibility principle** The physical benefits of exercise are lost through disuse or inactivity.

**rhythm method** A birth control method in which sexual intercourse is avoided during those days of the menstrual cycle in which fertilization is most likely to occur.

**rubella** An infectious disease that may cause birth defects if contracted by a pregnant woman; also called German measles.

**salvia** An herb with hallucinogenic properties when smoked or inhaled.

**same-sex marriage** Governmentally, socially, or religiously recognized marriage in which two people of the same sex live together as a family.

**satiety** A feeling of fullness after eating.

**saturated fats** A chemical term indicating that a fat molecule contains as many hydrogen atoms as its carbon skeleton can hold. These fats are normally solid at room temperature.

**schizophrenia** A general term for a group of mental disorders with characteristic psychotic symptoms, such as delusions, hallucinations, and disordered thought patterns during the active phase of the illness, and a duration of at least six months.

**scrotum** The external sac or pouch that holds the testes.

**secondary sex characteristics** Physical changes associated with maleness or femaleness, induced by the sex hormones.

**self-actualization** A state of wellness and fulfillment that can be achieved once certain human needs are satisfied; living to one's full potential.

**self-compassion** A healthy form of self-acceptance in the face of perceived inadequacy or failure.

**self-disclosure** Sharing personal information and experiences with another that he or she would not otherwise discover; self-disclosure involves risk and vulnerability.

**self-efficacy** Belief in one's ability to accomplish a goal or change a behavior.

**self-esteem** Confidence and satisfaction in oneself.

**semen** The viscous whitish fluid that is the complete male ejaculate; a combination of sperm and secretions from the prostate gland, seminal vesicles, and other glands.

**seminal vesicles** Glands in the male reproductive system that produce the major portion of the fluid of semen.

**set** In weight training, the number of repetitions of the same movement or exercise.

**sex** Maleness or femaleness, resulting from genetic, structural, and functional factors.

**sexual coercion** Sexual activity forced upon a person by the exertion of psychological pressure by another person.

**sexual dysfunction** The inability to react emotionally and/or physically to sexual stimulation in a way expected of the average healthy person or according to one's own standards.

**sexual harassment** Uninvited and unwanted sexual attention.

**sexual health** The integration of the physical, emotional, intellectual, social, and spiritual aspects of sexual being in ways that are positively enriching and that enhance personality, communication, and love.

**sexual orientation** The direction of an individual's sexual interest, either to members of the opposite sex or to members of the same sex.

**sexuality** The behaviors, instincts, and attitudes associated with being sexual.

**sexually transmitted disease (STD)** A disease that is caused by a sexually transmitted infection that produces symptoms.

**sexually transmitted infection (STI)** The presence in the human body of an infectious agent that can be passed from one sexual partner to another.

**sidestream smoke** The smoke emitted by a burning cigarette and breathed by everyone in a closed room, including the smoker; contains more tar and nicotine than mainstream smoke.

**simple carbohydrates** Sugars; like all carbohydrates, they provide the body with glucose.

**social norm** A behavior or attitude that a particular group expects, values, and enforces.

**social phobia** A severe form of social anxiety marked by extreme fears and avoidance of social situations.

**specificity principle** Each part of the body adapts to a particular type and amount of stress placed upon it.

**sperm** The male gamete produced by the testes and transported outside the body through ejaculation.

**spermatogenesis** The process by which sperm cells are produced.

**spiritual health** The ability to identify one's basic purpose in life and to achieve one's full potential.

**spiritual intelligence** The capacity to sense, understand, and tap into ourselves, others, and the world around us.

**spirituality** A belief in someone or something that transcends the boundaries of self.

**stalking** The willful, repeated, and malicious following of another person.

**static flexibility** The ability to assume and maintain an extended position at one end point in a joint's range of motion.

**static stretching** A gradual stretch held for a short time of 10 to 30 seconds.

**sterilization** A surgical procedure to end a person's reproductive capability.

**stimulant** An agent, such as a drug, that temporarily relieves drowsiness, helps in the performance of repetitive tasks, and improves capacity for work.

**stress** The nonspecific response of the body to any demands made upon it; may be characterized by muscle tension and acute anxiety, or may be a positive force for action.

**stressors** Specific or nonspecific agents or situations that cause the stress response in a body.

**stroke** A cerebrovascular event in which the blood supply to a portion of the brain is blocked.

**subcutaneous** Under the skin.

**suction curettage** A procedure in which the contents of the uterus are removed by means of suction and scraping.

**sustainability** A method of using a resource so that the resource is not depleted or permanently damaged.

**synapse** A specialized site at which electrical impulses are transmitted from the axon terminal of one neuron to a dendrite of another.

**synergistic** Characterized by a combined effect that is greater than the sum of the individual effects.

**syphilis** A sexually transmitted infection caused by the bacterium *Treponema pallidum* and characterized by early sores, a latent period, and a final period of life-threatening symptoms, including brain damage and heart failure.

**systemic disease** A pathologic condition that spreads throughout the body.

**systole** The contraction phase of the cardiac cycle.

**systolic blood pressure** Highest blood pressure when the heart contracts.

**tar** A thick, sticky dark fluid produced by the burning of tobacco, made up of several hundred different chemicals, many of them poisonous, some of them carcinogenic.

**target heart rate** Sixty to 85 percent of the maximum heart rate; the heart rate at which one derives maximum cardiovascular benefit from aerobic exercise.

**terminal illness** An illness in which death is inevitable.

**testes** (singular, testis) The male sex organs that produce sperm and testosterone.

**testosterone** The male sex hormone that stimulates male secondary sex characteristics.

**toxic shock syndrome (TSS)** A disease characterized by fever, vomiting, diarrhea, and often shock, caused by a bacterium that releases toxic waste products into the bloodstream.

**toxicity** Poisonousness; the dosage level at which a drug becomes poisonous to the body, causing either temporary or permanent damage.

**trans fat** Fat formed when liquid vegetable oils are processed to make table spreads or cooking fats; also found in dairy and beef products; considered to be especially dangerous dietary fats.

**transcendence** The sense of passing into a foreign region or dimension, often experienced by a person near death.

**transgender** Having a gender identity opposite one's biological sex.

**transient ischemic attack (TIA)** A cerebrovascular event in which the blood supply to a portion of the brain is blocked temporarily; repeated attacks are predictors of more severe strokes.

**transtheoretical model** A model of behavioral change that focuses on the individual's decision making; it states that an individual progresses through a sequence of six stages as he or she makes a change in behavior.

**trichomoniasis** An infection of the protozoan Trichomonas vaginalis; females experience vaginal burning, itching, and discharge, but male carriers may be asymptomatic.

**triglyceride** A fat that flows through the blood after meals and is linked to increased risk of coronary artery disease.

**tubal ligation** The suturing or tying shut of the fallopian tubes to prevent pregnancy.

**tubal occlusion** The blocking of the fallopian tubes to prevent pregnancy.

**tuberculosis (TB)** A highly infectious bacterial disease that primarily affects the lungs and is often fatal.

**12-step programs** Self-help group programs based on the principles of Alcoholics Anonymous.

**ulcer** A lesion in, or an erosion of, the mucous membrane of an organ.

**unsaturated fats** A chemical term indicating that a fat molecule contains fewer hydrogen atoms than its carbon skeleton can hold. These fats are normally liquid at room temperature.

**urethra** The canal through which urine from the bladder leaves the body; in the male, also serves as the channel for seminal fluid.

**urethral opening** The outer opening of the thin tube that carries urine from the bladder.

**urethritis** Infection of the urethra.

**uterus** The female organ that houses the developing fetus until birth.

**vagina** The canal leading from the exterior opening in the female genital area to the uterus.

**vaginal contraceptive film (VCF)** A small dissolvable sheet saturated with spermicide that can be inserted into the vagina and placed over the cervix.

**vaginal spermicide** A substance that kills or neutralizes sperm, inserted into the vagina in the form of a foam, cream, jelly, suppository, or film.

**vaginismus** A sexual difficulty in which a woman experiences painful spasms of the vagina during sexual intercourse.

**values** The criteria by which one makes choices about one's thoughts, actions, goals, and ideals.

**vas deferens** Two tubes that carry sperm from the epididymis into the urethra.

**vasectomy** A surgical sterilization procedure in which each vas deferens is cut and tied shut to stop the passage of sperm to the urethra for ejaculation.

**vector** A biological or physical vehicle that carries the agent of infection to the host.

**vegans** People who eat only plant foods.

**ventricle** Either of the two lower chambers of the heart, which pump blood out of the heart and into the arteries.

**virus** A submicroscopic infectious agent; the most primitive form of life.

**visualization, or guided imagery** An approach to stress control, self-healing, or motivating life changes by means of seeing oneself in the state of calmness, wellness, or change.

**vital signs** Measurements of physiological functioning; specifically, temperature, blood pressure, pulse rate, and respiration rate.

**vitamins** Organic substances that are needed in very small amounts by the body and carry out a variety of functions in metabolism and nutrition.

**waist-to-hip-ratio (WHR)** The proportion of one's waist circumference to one's hip circumference.

**wellness** A deliberate lifestyle choice characterized by personal responsibility and optimal enhancement of physical, mental, and spiritual health.

**withdrawal** Development of symptoms that cause significant psychological and physical distress when an individual reduces or stops drug use.

**zygote** A fertilized egg.

# References

## Chapter 1

1. Preamble to the Constitution of the World Health Organization as adopted by the International Health Conference, New York, 19–22 June, 1946; signed on 22 July 1946 by the representatives of 61 States (Official Records of the World Health Organization, no. 2, p. 100) and entered into force on 7 April 1948amended since 1948.
2. Morozink, J.A., et al. "Socioeconomic and Psychological Predictors of Interleukin-6 in the MIDUS National Sample." *Health Psychology*, Vol. 29, No. 6, November 2010, pp. 626–635.
3. Crimmins, E. M., et al. "Explaining Divergent Levels of Longevity in High-Income Countries." *International*, January 31, 2011 (e-pub), http://www.nap.edu/openbook.php?record_id=13089&page=1.
4. McCullough, M. L., et al. "Following Cancer Prevention Guidelines Reduces Risk of Cancer, Cardiovascular Disease and All-Cause Mortality." *Cancer Biomarkers, Epidemiology, and Prevention*, April 5, 2011 (e-pub).
5. "Health, United States, 2010: With Special Feature on Death and Dying." National Center for Health Statistics, February 2011, www.cdc.gov/nchs/hus.htm.
6. "Healthy People 2020—Improving the Health of Americans." U.S. Department of Health and Human Services, http://www.healthypeople.gov/2020.
7. Ibid.
8. "Health, United States, 2010."
9. Bloom, B., and R. A. Cohen. "Young Adults Seeking Medical Care: Do Race and Ethnicity Matter?" *NCHS Data Brief*, Vol. 55, January 2011, http://www.cdc.gov/nchs/data/databriefs/db55.pdf.
10. "Healthy People 2020."
11. American College Health Association. *American College Health Association-National College Health Assessment II: Reference Group Executive Summary Spring 2010*, www.acha-ncha.org/.../ACHA-NCHA-II_ReferenceGroup_ExecutiveSummary_Spring2010.pdf.
12. Ibid.
13. Ibid.
14. Sacco, R. "Young Adults' Beliefs about Their Health Clash with Risky Behaviors." American Heart Association and American Stroke Association, May 2, 2011 (e-pub).
15. Ibid.
16. Schappert, S. M., and E. A. Rechtsteiner. "Ambulatory Medical Care Utilization Estimates for 2007." *Vital and Health Statistics Series*, Vol. 13, No. 169, May 2011, http://www.cdc.gov/nchs/data/series/sr_13/sr13_169.pdf.
17. American College Health Association. *American College Health Association-National College Health Assessment II: Reference Group Executive Summary Spring 2010*.
18. "Health Literacy: Statistics At-a-Glance." Partnership for Clear Health Communication at the National Patient Safety Foundation, http://www.npsf.org/askme3/pdfs/STATS_GLANCE_EN.pdf.
19. Peterson, P. N., et al. "Health Literacy and Outcomes among Patients with Heart Failure." *Journal of the American Medical Association*, Vol. 305, No. 16, April 2011, pp. 1695–1701.
20. Khaw, K. T., et al. "Combined Impact of Health Behaviours and Mortality in Men and Women: The EPIC-Norfolk Prospective Population Study." *Public Library of Science Medicine*, Vol. 5, No. 1, e1t2 doi:10.1371/journal.pmed.0050012.
21. Hales, Dianne, and Kenneth W. Christian. *An Invitation to Personal Change*. Belmont, CA: Cengage Publishing, 2009.
22. Robinson, L. M., et al. "An Integrative Review of Adolescent Smoking Cessation Using the Transtheoretical Model of Change." *Journal of Pediatric Health Care*, February 28, 2011 (e-pub).
23. Hart, I. E. "Transtheoretical Model Mediators of Fruit and Vegetable Intakes in the 5+YourWay® Study." Thesis. University of Otago, 2011, http://otago.ourarchive.ac.nz/handle/10523/1657.

## Chapter 2

1. Pronk, N. P., et al. "Adherence to Optimal Lifestyle Behaviors Is Related to Emotional Health Indicators among Employees." *Population Health Management*, November 19, 2010, (e-pub ahead of print).
2. Wood, A. M., and N. Tarrier. "Positive Clinical Psychology: A New Vision and Strategy for Integrated Research and Practice." *Clinical Psychology Review*, Vol. 30, No. 7, November 2010, pp. 819–829.
3. Antonuccio, David, and Robert Jackson. "The Science of Forgiveness." *"Positive Psychology in Practice." Harvard Mental Health Letter*, Vol. 24, No. 11, May 28, pp. 1–3.
4. Wood, "Positive Clinical Psychology."
5. Quoidbach, J., et al. "Positive Emotion Regulation and Well-Being: Comparing the Impact of Eight Savoring and Dampening Strategies." *Personality and Individual Differences*, Vol. 49, No. 5, October 2010, pp. 368–373.
6. Neely, M. E., et al. "Self-Kindness When Facing Stress: The Role of Self-Compassion, Goal Regulation, and Support in College Students' Well-Being." *Motiv Emot*, Vol. 33, 2009, pp. 88–97.
7. Martins, A., et al. "A Comprehensive Meta-Analysis of the Relationship between Emotional Intelligence and Health." *Personality and Individual Differences*, Vol. 49, No. 6, October 2010, pp. 554–564.
8. Raynor, Douglas, and Heidi Levein. "Association between the Five-Factor Model of Personality and Health Behaviors among College Students." *Journal of American College Health*, Vol. 58, No. 1, July–August 2009, pp. 73–81.
9. Ibid.
10. Seligman, Martin. Personal interview.
11. Flora, Carla. "The Pursuit of Happiness." *Psychology Today*, Vol. 42, No. 1, February 2009, pp. 61–69.
12. Falkenstern, M., et al. "Mood over Matter: Can Happiness Be Your Undoing?" *Journal of Positive Psychology*, Vol. 4, No. 5, September 2009, pp. 365–371.
13. "Experiences Bring More Joy Than Possessions Do." *HealthDay*, February 9, 2009, www.medlineplus.gov.
14. Lyubomirsky, Sonja. Personal interview.
15. Kim, J., and R. L. Jong-Eun. "The Facebook Paths to Happiness: Effects of the Number of Facebook Friends and Self-Presentation on Subjective Well-Being." *Cyberpsychology, Behavior, and Social Networking*, November 2010 (e-pub ahead of print).
16. Carver, C. S., et al. "Optimism." *Clinical Psychology Review*, Vol. 30, No. 7, November 2010, pp. 879–889.
17. Ibid.
18. Larsen, Randy. Personal interview.
19. Bhugra, D. "Commentary: Religion, Religious Attitudes and Suicide." *International Journal of Epidemiology*, Vol. 39, No. 6, October 2010, pp. 1496–1498.
20. Lawler-Row, K. A., and J. Elliott. "The Role of Religious Activity and Spirituality in the Health and Well-Being of Older Adults." *Journal of Health Psychology*, Vol. 14, No. 1, 2009, pp. 43–52.
21. Chida, Yoichi, et al. "Religiosity/Spirituality and Mortality: A Systematic Quantitative Review." *Psychotherapy and Psychosomatics*, Vol. 78, No. 2, January 2009, pp. 81–90.
22. Newberg, Andrew, and Mark Robert Waldman. *How God Changes Your Brain: Breakthrough Findings from a Leading Neuroscientist*. New York: Ballantine Books, 2009.
23. Edwards, Paul. Personal interview.
24. Krageloh, C. U., et al. "How Religious Coping Is Used Relative to Other Coping Strategies Depends on the Individual's Level of Religiosity and Spirituality." *Journal of Religion and Health*, November 2010 (e-pub ahead of print).
25. Koenig, Harold. Personal interview.
26. Wood, Alex M. "Gratitude Predicts Psychological Well-Being above the Big Five Facets." *Personality and Individual Differences*, Vol. 46, 2009, pp. 443–447.
27. Lambert, N. M., et al. "Can Prayer Increase Gratitude?" *Psychology of Religion and Spirituality*, Vol. 1, No. 3, 2009, pp. 139–149.
28. Kashdan, T. B., et al. "Gender Differences in Gratitude: Examining Appraisals, Narratives, the Willingness to Express Emotions, and Changes in Psychological Needs." *Journal of Personality*, Vol. 77, No. 3, June 2009.
29. Ibid.
30. Wood, A. M., et al. "Gratitude and Well-Being: A Review and Theoretical Integration." *Clinical Psychology Review*, Vol. 30, No. 7, November 2010, pp. 890–905.
31. Ibid.
32. Grant, A. M., and F. Gino. "A Little Thanks Goes a Long Way: Explaining Why Gratitude Expressions Motivate Prosocial Behavior." *Journal of Personality and Social Psychology*, Vol. 98, No. 6, June 2010, pp. 946–955.
33. Fincham, Frank. "Forgiveness: Integral to a Science of Close Relationships?" *Prosocial Motives, Emotions, and Behavior: The Better Angels of Our Nature*. Mario Mikulincer and Phillip R. Shaver (eds.), Washington, DC: American Psychological Association, 2010, pp. 347–365.
34. Karremans, J. C., et al. "The Malleability of Forgiveness." *Prosocial Motives, Emotions, and Behavior: The Better Angels of Our Nature*. Mario Mikulincer and Phillip R. Shaver (eds.), Washington, DC: American Psychological Association, 2010, pp. 285–301.
35. "Perceived Insufficient Rest or Sleep Among Adults—United States, 2008." *MMWR*, Vol. 58, No. 42, October 30, 2009, pp. 1175–1179.
36. Smolensky, M. H., et al. "Sleep Disorders, Medical Conditions, and Road Accident Risk." *Accident Analysis and Prevention*, Vol. 43, No. 2, March 2011, pp. 533–548.
37. Taylor, D. J., and A. D. Bramoweth. "Patterns and Consequences of Inadequate Sleep in College Students: Substance Use and Motor Vehicle Accidents." *Journal of Adolescent Health*, Vol. 46, No. 6, June 2010, pp. 610–612.
38. Miller, N. L., et al. "Longitudinal Study of Sleep Patterns of United States Military Academy Cadets." *Sleep*, Vol. 33, No. 12, December 2010, pp. 1623–1631.
39. Gaultney, J. F. "The Prevalence of Sleep Disorders in College Students: Impact on Academic Performance." *Journal of American College Health*, Vol. 59, No. 2, October 2010, pp. 91–97.
40. Ibid.
41. Ibid.
42. Taylor and Bramoweth, "Patterns and Consequences of Inadequate Sleep in College Students."
43. "Sleep: Snooze or Lose." University of Michigan Health Services, www.uhs.umich.edu/wellness/other/sleep.html.

44. Vail-Smith, Karen, et al. "Relationship between Sleep Quality and Health Risk Behaviors in Undergraduate College Students." *College Student Journal*, Vol. 43, No. 3, 2009.

45. Ratner, David. "Sleep and Academic Performance." Dissertation Abstracts International: Section B: The Sciences and Engineering, Vol. 69(8-B), 2009, p. 5097.

46. Paunio, T., et al. "Longitudinal Study on Poor Sleep and Life Dissatisfaction in a Nationwide Cohort of Twins." *American Journal of Epidemiology*, Vol. 169, No. 2, January 15, 2009.

47. Cohen, S., et al. "Sleep Habits and Susceptibility to the Common Cold." *Archives of Internal Medicine*, Vol. 169, No. 1, 2009, pp. 62–67.

48. "The Importance of Sleep and Health: Six Reasons Not to Scrimp on Sleep." Harvard Health Publications, http://www.health.harvard.edu.

49. Morin, C. M., et al. "The Natural History of Insomnia: A Population-Based 3-Year Longitudinal Study." *Archives of Internal Medicine,* Vol. 169, No. 5, March 9, 2009, pp. 447–453.

50. Torzsa, P., et al. "Socio-Demographic Characteristics, Health Behaviour, Co-morbidity and Accidents in Snorers: A Population Survey." *Sleep and Breathing*, November 2010 (e-pub ahead of print).

51. Reishstein, J. L. "Obstructive Sleep Apnea: A Risk Factor for Cardiovascular Disease." *Journal of Cardiovascular Nursing*, November 2010 (e-pub ahead of print).

## Chapter 3

1. Casey, B. J. and R. M. Jones. "Neurobiology of the Adolescent Brain and Behavior: Implications for Substance Use Disorders." *Journal of the American Academy of Child and Adolescent Psychiatry,* Vol. 49, No. 12, December 2010, pp. 1189–1198.

2. Preidt, R. "Mental Illness Stigma Hard to Shake, Survey Finds; Awareness Campaigns Have Helped Educate Public, but Discrimination Continues, Experts Say." *HealthDay News,* Indiana University news release, September 15, 2010.

3. Hales, Robert E., et al. (eds.). *Textbook of Clinical Psychiatry*. Washington DC: American Psychiatric Press, 2008.

4. Zonzein, J., et al. "Diabetes, Depression Can Be Two-Way Street; But Experts Note Factors Such as Obesity, Inactivity Might Also Be at Play." *HealthDay News*, (e-pub November 22, 2010).

5. Reavley, N., and A. F. Jorm. "Prevention and Early Intervention to Improve Mental Health in Higher Education Students: A Review." *Early Intervention in Psychiatry,* Vol. 4, No. 2, May 2010, pp. 132–142.

6. Pryor, J. H., S. Hurtado, L. DeAngelo, L. Palucki Blake and S. Tran. *The American Freshman: National Norms for Fall 2010*. Los Angeles: University of California, Los Angeles Higher Education Research Institute, 2010.

7. American College Health Association. *National College Health Assessment Reference Group Executive Summary, Spring 2010*. Baltimore: American College Health Association, 2010.

8. American College Counseling Association, http://www.collegecounseling.org/.

9. Del Pilar, Jose. "Mental Health and Latino/a College Students: A Psychological Perspective and New Findings." *Journal of Hispanic Higher Education*, Vol. 8, 2009, p. 263.

10. American College Health Association.

11. Reavley and Jorm. "Prevention and Early Intervention to Improve Mental Health in Higher Education Students."

12. McKnight-Eily, L., et al. "9% of U.S. Adults Suffer from Depression: CDC. It's Most Prevalent in the Southeast, Perhaps Due to High Rates of Ills Like Obesity and Heart Disease, Researchers Say." *CDC's Morbidity and Mortality Weekly Report*, September 2010, *HealthDay News* (e-pub October 1, 2010).

13. Torpy, J. M., et al. "Depression." *Journal of the American Medical Association*. Vol. 303, No. 19, December 2010, p. 1994.

14. Curry, J., et al. "Nearly All Depressed Adolescents Recover with Treatment, but Half Relapse." *Archives of General Psychiatry* (e-pub November 1, 2010).

15. Parker, G., and H. Brotchie. "Gender Differences in Depression." *International Review of Psychiatry,* Vol. 22, No. 5, October 2010, pp. 429–436.

16. Schmidt, P. J., et al. "Young Women with Menopause-like Condition at Risk for Depression." *NIH News* (e-pub November 30, 2010).

17. Gelenberg, A., et al. "New Depression Guidelines Favor Tailored Treatment." *Reuters* (e-pub October 1, 2010).

18. Olfson, M. "Antidepressant Use Rising as Psychotherapy Rates Fall. Study Author Says Using Both Often the Best Treatment for Depression, Many Not Getting Optimal Care." *HealthDay News* (e-pub December 6, 2010).

19. "Mindfulness Meditation Found to Be as Effective as Antidepressant Medication in Prevention of Depression Relapse." *Biotech Week*, December 2010, p. 506; *Health Reference Center Academic* (e-pub December 21, 2010).

20. Greden, John. Personal interview.

21. Kaplan, Arline. "Task Force Proposes New Bipolar Guidelines." *Psychiatric Times*, Vol. 25, No. 4, April 2008, p. 1.

22. Fountoulakis, K., et al. "Psychotherapeutic Intervention and Suicide Risk Reduction in Bipolar Disorder: A Review of the Evidence." *Journal of Affective Disorders*, Vol. 113, No. 1, pp. 21–29.

23. Hollander, Eric, and Daphne Simeon. "Anxiety Disorders." *Textbook of Psychiatry*, 5th ed., Robert Hales, Stuart Yudolfsky, and Glen Gabbard (eds.). Washington, DC, 2008, pp. 505–608.

24. Barrera Jr., M., et al. "A Critical Analysis of Approaches to the Development of Preventative Interventions for Subcultural Groups." *American Journal of Community Psychology,* January 4, 2011 (e-pub ahead of print).

25. Visser, S., et al. "ADHD Rates Soar in U.S. Kids: Study. Better Diagnosis and Screening May Play a Role in Increase, Researchers Say." *HealthDay News* (e-pub November 10, 2010).

26. Diller, L. "ADHD in the College Student: Is Anyone Else Worried?" *Journal of Attention Disorders*, Vol. 14, No. 1, July 2010, pp. 3–6.

27. Advokat, C., et al. "College Students With and Without ADHD: Comparison of Self Report of Medication Usage, Study Habits, and Academic Achievement." *Journal of Attention Disorders* (e-pub August 2010).

28. "Transcendental Meditation Seen Promising as ADHD Therapy," January 5, 2009, www.medlineplus.gov.

29. American College Health Association.

30. Kraft, D. F. "Nonmedication Treatments for Adult ADHD: Evaluating Impact on Daily Functioning and Well-Being, by J. Russell Ramsay, Ph.D." *Journal of American College Health*, Vol. 59, No. 1, January 2011, pp. 57–59.

31. Sollman, M. J., et al. "Detection of Feigned ADHD in College Students." *Psychological Assessment*, Vol. 22, No. 2, June 2010, pp. 325–335.

32. http://cdc.gov/ncbddd/autism/topics.html

33. Landa. R., et al. "Clinical Trial of Autism Early Intervention Reveals Significant Improvements in Toddlers' Social and Communication Skills." *Journal of Child Psychology and Psychiatry*, December 2010 (e-pub ahead of print).

34. Peterson, L., et al. "Paternal Age at Birth of First Child and Risk of Schizophrenia." *American Journal of Psychiatry*, Vol. 168, No. 1, January 2011, pp. 82-88.

35. Wilcox, H. C., et al. "Prevalence and Predictors of Persistent Suicide Ideation, Plans, and Attempts during College." *Journal of Affective Disorders*, Vol. 127, No. 1–3, May 2010, pp. 287–294.

36. Toprack, S., et al. "Self-Harm, Suicidal Ideation and Suicide Attempts among College Students." *Psychiatry Research*, October 2010 (e-pub ahead of print).

37. Stewart, Victoria. "Perceived Social Support, Suicidal Ideation, Stigma, and Help-Seeking Behaviors among College Students." *Dissertation Abstracts International: Section B: The Sciences and Engineering*. Vol. 70(4-B), 2009, pp. 2589.

38. Dubovsky, Steven. "Suicide—New Data on Causes and Cures." *Journal Watch*, January 4, 2010.

39. Valenstein, M., et al. "Higher-Risk Periods for Suicide among VA Patients Receiving Depression Treatment: Prioritizing Suicide Prevention Efforts." *Journal of Affective Disorders*, Vol. 112, No. 1-3, January 2009, pp. 50–58.

40. Shafranske, E. P. "Spiritually Oriented Psychodynamic Psychotherapy." *Journal of Clinical Psychology*, Vol. 65, No. 2, pp. 147–157.

## Chapter 4

1. Lazarus, R., and R. Launier. "Stress-Related Transactions between Person and Environment." *Perspectives in Interactional Psychology*. New York: Plenum, 1978.

2. Kiecolt-Glaser, J. K. and R. Glaser. "Psychological Stress, Telomeres, and Telomerase." *Brain, Behavior, and Immunity*, Vol. 24, No. 4, May 2010, pp. 529–530.

3. Rahe, Richard. *Paths to Health and Resilience*. 2009. www.booksurge.com.

4. Kiecolt-Glaser, J. K. and R. Glaser. "Psychological Stress, Telomeres, and Telomerase." *Brain, Behavior, and Immunity*, Vol. 24, No. 4, May 2010, pp. 529–530 (e-pub 2010 February 16, 2010).

5. Kubzansky, Laura. "Aldosterone: A Forgotten Mediator of the Relationship between Psychological Stress and Heart Disease." *Neuroscience and Biobehavioral Reviews,* Vol. 34, 2010, pp. 80–86.

6. Sgoifo, A., et al. "The Inevitable Link between Heart and Behavior." *Neuroscience Biobehavior Review*, Vol. 33, No. 2, February 2009, pp. 61–62.

7. Hamer, Mark, et al. "Psychological Distress as a Risk Factor of Cardiovascular Events: Pathophysiological and Behavioral Mechanisms," *Journal of the American College of Cardiology*, Vol. 52, No. 25, December 16, 2008, pp. 2156–2162.

8. Spruill, T. M. "Chronic Psychosocial Stress and Hypertension." *Current Hypertension Reports*, Vol. 12, No. 1, February 2010, pp. 10–16.

9. Epel, E. B. "Psychological and Metabolic Stress: A Recipe for Accelerated Cellular Aging?" *Hormones*, Vol. 8, No. 1, January/March, 2009, pp. 7–22.

10. Matthews, K. A., and L.C. Gallo. "Psychological Perspectives on Pathways Linking Socioeconomic Status and Physical Health." *Annual Review of Psychology*, Vol. 62, January 2011, pp. 501–530.

11. Groër, M., et al. "An Overview of Stress and Immunity." *The Psychoneuroimmunology of Chronic Disease: Exploring the Links between Inflammation, Stress, and Illness*. Kathleen Kendall-Tackett (ed.). Washington, DC: American Psychological Association, 2010, pp. 9–22.

12. Chrousos, G.P. "Stress and Sex versus Immunity and Inflammation." www.SCIENCESIGNALING .org., Vol. 3, No. 142, October 12, 2010, pp. 36–38.

13. Heffner, K. L. "Neuroendocrine Effects of Stress on Immunity in the Elderly: Implications for Inflammatory Disease." *Immunology and Allergy Clinics of North America*, Vol. 31, No. 1, February 2011, pp. 95–108.

14. Kiecolt-Glaser, J. K. "Stress, Food, and Inflammation: Psychoneuroimmunology and Nutrition at the Cutting Edge." *Psychosomatic Medicine*. Vol. 72, No. 4, May 2010, pp. 365–369 (e-pub April 21, 2010).

15. Ulrich-Lai, Y. M., et al. "Pleasurable Behaviors Reduce Stress via Brain Reward Pathways." *Proceedings of the National Academy of Sciences Online*, Vol. 107, No. 47, September 2010, pp. 20529–20534.

16. American College Health Association. *American College Health Association-National College Health Assessment II: Reference Group Executive Summary Spring 2010*. Linthicum, MD: American College Health Association, 2010.

17. Brougham, R. R., et al. "Stress, Sex Differences, and Coping Strategies among College Students." *Current Psychology*, Vol. 28, 2009, pp. 85–97.
18. American College Health Association. *American College Health Association-National College Health Assessment II: Reference Group Data Report Fall 2009*. Baltimore: American College Health Association, 2010.
19. Barry, L. M., et al. "Differences in Self-Reported Disclosure of College Experiences by First-Generation College Student Status." *Adolescence*, Vol. 44, No. 173, Spring, 2009, pp. 55–68.
20. Brougham, "Stress, Sex Differences."
21. Magid, Viktoriya. "Negative Affect, Stress, and Smoking in College Students: Unique Associations Independent of Alcohol and Marijuana Use." *Addictive Behaviors*, Vol. 34, 2009, pp. 973–975.
22. Wichianson, J. R., et al. "Perceived Stress, Coping and Night-Eating in College Students." *Stress and Health: Journal of the International Society for the Investigation of Stress*, Vol. 25, No. 3, August 2009, pp. 235–240.
23. Nagurney, Alexander, and Brandi Bagwell. "Relations of the Gender-Related Traits and Stress to Sexual Behaviors among College Students." *North American Journal of Psychology*, Vol. 11, No. 2, 2009, pp. 85–96.
24. Bell and D'Zurilla. "The Influence of Social Problem Solving Ability."
25. mtvU/Associated Press Survey.
26. Petroff, Linda. "Stress, Adult Attachment, and Academic Success among Community College Students." Dissertation Abstracts International Section A: Humanities and Social Sciences, Vol. 69(12-A), 2009, p. 4632.
27. Bell, Alissa, and Thomas D'Zurilla. "The Influence of Social Problem-Solving Ability on the Relationship between Daily Stress and Adjustment." *Cognitive Therapy and Research*, Vol. 33, 2009, pp. 439–448.
28. Pieterse, A. L., et al. "An Exploratory Examination of the Associations among Racial and Ethnic Discrimination, Racial Climate, and Trauma-Related Symptoms in a College Student Population." *Journal of Counseling Psychology*, Vol. 57, No. 3, July 2010, pp. 255–263.
29. Walker, Rheeda, et al. "An Empirical Investigation of Acculturative Stress and Ethnic Identity as Moderators for Depression and Suicidal Ideation in College Students." *Cultural Diversity and Ethnic Minority Psychology*, Vol. 14, No. 1, 2008, pp. 75–82.
30. Goebert, Deborah. "Social Support, Mental Health, Minorities, and Acculturative Stress." In *Determinants of Minority Mental Health and Wellness*. New York: Springer, 2009.
31. Lindsey, Robert. "Sources of Stress for African American College Students." Poster Session, AAH-PERD National Convention, March 31–April 4, 2009.
32. Thomas, S. A., and Gonzalez-Pendes, A. A. "Powerlessness, Anger, and Stress in African American Women: Implications for Physical and Emotional Health." *Health Care for Women International*, Vol. 30, No. 1–2, January 2009, pp. 93–113.
33. UPI NewsTrack. "Colleges Host 'Stress-Busting' Events." *Health Reference Center Academic* (e-pub December 16, 2010).
34. "Job Losses Carry High 'Stress Tag.'" *HealthDay*, February 12, 2009, www.medlineplus.gov.
35. "Managing Your Stress in Tough Economic Times." APA Help Center, http://www.apa helpcenter.org/articles/article.php?id517.
36. "The American Freshman." *HERI Research Brief*, January 2010.
37. Bushman, Brad. Personal interview.
38. Barreira, T. V., et al. "Relationship between Objectively Measured Physical Activity and Chronic Stress Level." Poster Session, AAHPERD National Convention, March 31–April 4, 2009.
39. Furong, Xu, et al. "Relations of Physical Activity and Mental Health in University Students." Poster Session, AAH-PERD National Convention, March 31–April 4, 2009.
40. Esch, T. and G. B. Stefano. "The Neurobiology of Stress Management." *Neuroendocrinology Letters*, Vol. 31, No. 1, 2010, pp. 19–39.
41. Feldman, G., et al. "Differential Effects of Mindful Breathing, Progressive Muscle Relaxation, and Loving-Kindness Meditation on Decentering and Negative Reactions to Repetitive Thoughts." *Behaviour Research and Therapy*, Vol. 48, No. 10, October 2010, pp. 1002–1011.
42. Lutz, Antoine, et al. "Regulation of the Neural Circuitry of Emotion by Compassion Meditation: Effects of Meditative Expertise." *Public Library of Science One*, Vol. 3, No. 3: e189 7.dol:10.1371/journal.pone.0001897.
43. Chiesa, A., and A. Serretti. "A Systematic Review of Neurobiological and Clinical Features of Mindfulness Meditations." Psychological Medicine, Vol. 40, 2010, pp. 1239–1259.
44. Travis, Fred. "Effects of Transcendental Meditation Practice on Brain Functioning and Stress Reactivity in College Students." *International Journal of Psychophysiology*, Vol. 71, 2009, pp. 170–176.
45. Caldwell, K., et al. "Developing Mindfulness in College Students through Movement-Based Courses: Effects on Self-Regulatory Self-Efficacy, Mood, Stress, and Sleep Quality." *Journal of American College Health*, Vol. 58, No. 5, March/April 2010, pp. 433–442.
46. Ibid.
47. McCown, D., et al. "Mindfulness and Mindfulness-based Stress Reduction." *Integrative Psychiatry*, D. A. Monti and B.D. Beitman (eds.). 2010. New York: Oxford University Press, 2010, pp. 289–338.
48. Kiecolt-Glaser, J. K., et al. "Stress, Inflammation, and Yoga Practice." *Psychosomatic Medicine*, Vol. 72, No. 2, February 2010, pp. 113–121 (e-pub January 11, 2010).
49. "Yoga's Ability to Improve Mood and Lessen Anxiety Is Linked to Increased Levels of a Critical Brain Chemical." *Biotech Week*, December 1, 2010, p. 2009; *Health Reference Center Academic* (e-pub December, 16 2010).
50. Monk-Turner, E. and C. Turner. "Does Yoga Shape Body, Mind and Spiritual Health and Happiness? Differences between Yoga Practitioners and College Students." *International Journal of Yoga*, Vol. 3, No. 2, July 2010, pp. 48–54.
51. Kiecolt-Glaser, J. K., et al. "Stress, Inflammation, and Yoga Practice."
52. Vernon, L. L., et al. "Proactive Coping, Gratitude, and Posttraumatic Stress Disorder in College Women." *Anxiety, Stress & Coping*, Vol. 22, No. 1, January 2009, pp. 117–127.
53. Ursano, Robert, et al. "Posttraumatic Stress Disorder: Neurobiology, Psychology, and Public Health." *Psychiatric Times*, Vol. 25, No. 3, March 2008, pp. 16–20.
54. Mental Health America
55. Moore, S. A. "Cognitive Abnormalities in Post-traumatic Stress Disorder." *Current Opinion in Psychiatry*, Vol. 22, No. 1, January 2009, pp. 19–24.
56. "Posttraumatic Stress Disorder: A Growing Epidemic." *NIH Medlineplus: The Magazine*, Vol. 4, No. 1, Winter 2009, pp. 10–14.
57. Ditlevsen, D.N., and A. Elklit. "The Combined Effect of Gender and Age on Posttraumatic Stress Disorder: Do Men and Women Show Differences in the Lifespan Distribution of the Disorder?" *Annals of General Psychiatry*, Vol. 9, July 2010, p. 32.
58. Richardson, L. K., et al. "Prevalence Estimates of Combat-Related Post-Traumatic Stress Disorder: Critical Review." *Aust N Z J Psychiatry*, Vol. 44, No. 1, January 2010, pp. 4–19.
59. Levin, Aaron. "Researchers Look for Link between Brain Injury, Psychiatric Illness." *Psychiatric News*, Vol. 44, No. 1–2, January 2, 2009.
60. Heppner, P. S., et al. "The Association of Posttraumatic Stress Disorder and Metabolic Syndrome: A Study of Increased Health Risk in Veterans." *BMC Medicine*, Vol. 7, No. 1, January 9, 2009, p. 1.
61. North, C.S., et al. "Postdisaster Course of Alcohol Use Disorders in Systematically Studied Survivors of 10 Disorders." *Archives of General Psychiatry*, October 2010 (e-pub ahead of print).
62. Yoon, J., and A. S. Lau. "Maladaptive Perfectionism and Depressive Symptoms among Asian American College Students: Contributions of Interdependence and Parental Relations." *Cultural Diversity and Ethnic Minority Psychology*, Vol. 14, No. 2, April 2008, pp. 92–101.
63. Wicks, Robert. *Bounce: Living the Resilient Life*. New York: Oxford University Press, 2010.
64. Vernon, "Proactive Coping, Gratitude, and Posttraumatic Stress Disorder in College Women."
65. Rabin, L. A., et al. "Academic Procrastination in College Students: The Role of Self-Reported Executive Function." *Journal of Clinical and Experimental Neuropsychology*, November 2010, pp. 1–14 (e-pub ahead of print).
66. Ibid.

## Chapter 5

1. Christakis, N., and J. Fowler. "Connected: The Surprising Power of Our Social Networks and How They Shape Our Lives—How Your Friends' Friends' Friends Affect Everything You Feel, Think, and Do." New York: Back Bay Books, 2011.
2. Jensen-Campbell, L. A., et al. "The Psychology of Nice People." *Social and Personality Psychology Compass*, Vol. 4, No. 11, November 2010, pp. 1042–1056.
3. Ozçalişkan, S., and S. Goldin-Meadow. "Sex Differences in Language First Appear in Gesture." *Developmental Science*, Vol. 13, No. 5, September 2010, pp. 752–760.
4. Bickart, K. C., et al. "Amygdala Volume and Social Network Size in Humans." *Nature Neuroscience*, December 2010 (e-pub ahead of print).
5. Li, J., and M. Chignell. "Birds of a Feather: How Personality Influences Blog Writing and Reading." *International Journal of Human-Computer Studies*, Vol. 68, No. 9, September 2010, pp. 589–602.
6. Judd, T., and G. Kennedy. "A Five-Year Study of On-Campus Internet Use by Undergraduate Biomedical Students." *Computers and Education*, Vol. 55, No. 4, December 2010, pp. 1564–1571.
7. Junco, R., et al. "The Effect of Gender, Ethnicity, and Income on College Students' Use of Communication Technologies." *Cyberpsychology, Behavior, and Social Networking*, Vol. 13, No. 6, December 2010, pp. 619–627.
8. Patchin, J. W., and S. Hinduja. "Changes in Adolescent Online Social Networking Behaviors from 2006 to 2009." *Computers in Human Behavior*, Vol. 26, No. 6, November 2010, pp. 1818–1821.
9. Sengupta, A., and A. Chaudhuri. "Are Social Networking Sites a Source of Online Harassment for Teens? Evidence from Survey Data." *Children and Youth Services Review*, Vol. 33, No. 2, February 2011, pp. 284–290.
10. Moreno, M. A., et al. "Sexpectations: Male College Students' Views about Displayed Sexual References on Females' Social Networking Web Sites." Vol. 33, No. 2, February 2011, pp. 284–290.
11. Morgan, E. M., et al. "Image and Video Disclosure of Substance Use on Social Media Websites." *Computers in Human Behavior*, Vol. 26, No. 6, November 2010, pp. 1405–1411.
12. Kim, J., and J. R. Lee. "The Facebook Paths to Happiness." *Cyberpsychology, Behavior, and Social Networking*, November 2010 (e-pub ahead of print).
13. Lukes, C. A. "Social Media." *American Association of Occupational Health Nurses*, Vol. 58, No. 10, October 2010, pp. 415–417.
14. Kim and Lee, "The Facebook Paths to Happiness."
15. D'Amato, G., et al. "Facebook: A New Trigger for Asthma?" *Lancet*, Vol. 376, No. 9754, November 2010, pp. 1740.
16. Morgan, et al., "Image and Video Disclosure of Substance Use."
17. Moren, et al., "Sexpectations."
18. Dunbar, R. "How Many Friends Does One Person Need? Dunbar's Number and Other Evolutionary Quirks." London: Faber and Faber, 2010.

19. Ibid.
20. Kim and Lee, "The Facebook Path to Happiness."
21. Menegatos, L. M., et al. "Friends Don't Let Jane Hook Up Drunk: A Qualitative Analysis of Participation in a Simulation of College Drinking Related Decisions." *Communication Education*, Vol. 59, August 2010, pp. 374–388.
22. Nummela, O., et al. "The Effect of Loneliness and Change in Loneliness on Self-Rated Health (SRH): A Longitudinal Study among Aging People." *Archives of Gerontology and Geriatrics*, November 18, 2010 (e-pub).
23. Volbrecht, M. M., and H. H. Goldsmith. "Early Temperamental and Family Predictors of Shyness and Anxiety." *Developmental Psychology*, Vol. 46, No. 5, September 2010, pp. 1192–1205.
24. Kuo, J. R., et al. "Childhood Trauma and Current Psychological Functioning in Adults with Social Anxiety Disorder." *Journal of Anxiety Disorders*, November 26, 2010 (e-pub).
25. Hoffman, S. G., et al. "Cultural Aspects in Social Anxiety and Social Anxiety Disorder." *Depression and Anxiety*, December 3, 2010 (e-pub).
26. Gardner, A. "Web Connection Raises Chance of Romance." *Consumer Health News*, January 3, 2011 (e-pub).
27. Ross, L. L., and A. M. Bowen. "Sexual Decision Making for the 'Better Than Average' College Student." *Journal of American College Health*, Vol. 59, No. 3, November/December 2010, pp. 211–216.
28. Owen, J., and F. D. Fincham. "Young Adults' Emotional Reactions after Hooking Up Encounters." *Archives of Sexual Behavior*, August 31, 2010 (e-pub).
29. Ibid.
30. Bradshaw, C., et al. "To Hook Up or Date: Which Gender Benefits?" *Sex Roles*, Vol. 62, No. 9–10, March 2010, pp. 661–669.
31. Fielder, R. L., and M. P. Carey. "Predictors and Consequences of Sexual 'Hookups' among College Students: A Short-Term Prospective Study." *Archives of Sexual Behavior*, Vol. 39, No. 5, October 2010, pp. 1105–1119.
32. Ibid.
33. Bradshaw, et al., "To Hook Up or Date."
34. Braithwaite, S. R., et al. "Romantic Relationships and the Physical and Mental Health of College Students." *Personal Relationships*, Vol. 17, No. 1, March 2010, pp. 1–12.
35. Behen, M., et al. "Men May Be More Vulnerable to Roller Coaster Ride of Romance." *Journal of Health and Social Behavior*, Vol. 51, No. 4, December 2010, pp. 497–499.
36. Younger, J., et al. "Viewing Pictures of a Romantic Partner Reduces Experimental Pain: Involvement of Neural Rewards System." *PLoS One*, Vol. 5, No. 10, October 2010, p. e13309.
37. Fisher, Helen. Personal interview.
38. Rhoades, G. K., et al. "Physical Aggression in Unmarried Relationships: The Roles of Commitment and Constraints." *Journal of Family Psychology*, Vol. 24, No. 6, Decemeber 2010, pp. 678–687.
39. Giordano, P. C., et al. "The Characteristics of Romantic Relationships Associated with Teen Dating Violence." *Social Science Research*, Vol. 39, No. 6, November 2010, pp. 863–874.
40. American College Health Association. *American College Health Association-National College Health Assessment II: Reference Group Executive Summary Spring 2010.* Baltimore: American College Health Association, 2010.
41. Yager, Jan. Personal interview.
42. Settersten, R. A., Jr., and B. Ray. "What's Going On with Young People Today? The Long and Twisting Path to Adulthood." *Future of Children*, Vol. 20, No. 1, Spring 2010, pp. 19–41.
43. Sassler, S. "Partnering across the Life Course: Sex, Relationships, and Mate Selection." *Journal of Marriage and Family*, Vol. 72, No. 3, June 2010, pp. 557–575.
44. Furstenberg, F. F., Jr. "On a New Schedule: Transitions to Adulthood and Family Change." *Future of Children*, Vol. 20, No. 1, Spring 2010, pp. 67–87.

45. PEW Social Trends Staff. "The Decline of Marriage and Rise of New Families." 2010. Retrieved from www.pewsocialtrends.org/family.
46. Sassler, "Partnering across the Life Course."
47. PEW Social Trends Staff. "The Decline of Marriage."
48. Rhoades, G. K., et al. "The Pre-engagement Cohabitation Effect: A Replication and Extension of Previous Findings." *Journal of Family Psychology*, Vol. 23, No. 1, February 2009, pp. 107–111.
49. Munsey, C. "Does Marriage Make You Happy?" *Monitor on Psychology*, Vol. 41, No. 9, October 2010, pp. 20–23.
50. PEW Social Trends Staff. "The Decline of Marriage."
51. Wilcox, W. B. "The State of Our Unions: When Marriage Disappears." The National Marriage Project, 2010.
52. PEW Social Trends Staff. "The Decline of Marriage."
53. Henretta, J. C. "Lifetime Marital History and Mortality after Age 50." *Journal of Aging and Health*, Vol. 22, No. 8, December 2010, pp. 1198–1212.
54. Ortega, F. B., et al. "In Fitness and Health? A Prospective Study of Changes in Marital Status and Fitness in Men and Women." *American Journal of Epidemiology*, Vol. 173, No. 3, February 1, 2011, pp. 337–344.
55. Munsey, "Does Marriage Make You Happy?"
56. Crooks, Robert L., and Karla Baur. *Our Sexuality*, 10th ed. Belmont, CA: Cengage-Wadsworth, 2008.
57. Doss, D. B., et al. "Marital Therapy, Retreats and Books: The Who, What, When, and Why of Relationship Help-Seeking." *Journal of Marital and Family Therapy*, Vol. 35, No. 1, pp. 18–29.
58. Wilcox, "The State of Our Unions."
59. Motschnig-Pitrik, R., and G. Barrett-Lennard. "Coactualization: A New Construct in Understanding Well-Functioning Relationships." *Journal of Humanistic Psychology*, Vol. 50, No. 3, July 2010, pp. 374–398.
60. Parker-Pope, T. "Sustainable Love: The Happy Marriage Is the 'Me' Marriage." *New York Times.* December 31, 2010 (e-pub).
61. PEW Social Trends Staff. "The Decline of Marriage."
62. Hummer, R. A., and E. R. Hamilton. "Race and Ethnicity in Fragile Families." *Future of Children*, Vol. 20, No. 2, Fall 2010, pp. 113–131.
63. McLanahan, S., et al. "Introducing the Issue." *Future of Children*, Vol. 20, No. 2, Fall 2010, pp. 3–16.
64. Goldrick-Rab, S., and K. Sorenson. "Unmarried Parents in College." *Future of Children*, Vol. 20, No. 2, Fall 2010, pp. 179–203.
65. Ibid.

## Chapter 6

1. Park, Y., et al. "Dietary Fiber Intake and Mortality in the NIH-AARP Diet and Health Study." *Archives of Internal Medicine*, February 14, 2011 (e-pub).
2. Ruxton, C. H. S. "The Benefits of Fish Consumption." *Nutrition Bulletin*, Vol. 36, No. 1, March 2011, pp. 6–19.
3. Flegal, I. K. M., et al. "Prevalence and Trends in Obesity among U.S. Adults, 1999–2008. *Journal of the American Medical Association*, Vol. 303, No. 3, January 2010, pp. 235–241.
4. Kremer, R., et al. "Vitamin D Status and Its Relationship to Body Fat, Final Height, and Peak Bone Mass in Young Women." *Journal of Clinical Endocrinology and Metabolism*, Vol. 94, No. 1, January 2009, pp. 67–73.
5. Ross, A. C., et al. "Dietary Reference Intakes for Calcium and Vitamin D." *Institute of Medicine of the National Academies*, November 30, 2010 (e-pub).
6. Ibid.
7. Slomski, A. "IOM Endorses Vitamin D, Calcium Only for Bone Health, Dispels Deficiency Claims." *Journal of the American Medical Association*, Vol. 305, No. 5, February 2011, pp. 453–455.

8. Ross, et al., "Dietary Reference Intakes."
9. Alderman, M. H. "Reducing Dietary Sodium." *Journal of the American Medical Association*, Vol. 303, No. 5, February 3, 2010, pp. 448–449.
10. United States Department of Agriculture. *Dietary Guidelines for Americans, 2010,* January 31, 2011 (e-pub), www.cnpp.usda.gov/Publications/DietaryGuidelines/2010/PolicyDoc/PolicyDoc.pdf.
11. Ibid.
12. Ibid.
13. Ibid.
14. Schuszdziarra, V., et al. "Impact of Breakfast on Daily Energy Intake." *Nutrition Journal*, Vol. 10, No. 5, 2011, www.nutritionj.com/content/10/1/5.
15. Larson, N. I., et al. "Making Time for Meals: Meal Structure and Associations with Dietary Intake in Young Adults." *Journal of the American Dietetic Association*, Vol. 109, No. 1, January 2009, pp. 72–79.
16. Gerend, M. A. "Does Calorie Information Promote Lower Calorie Fast-Food Choices among College Students?" *Journal of Adolescent Health*, Vol. 44, No. 1, January 2009, pp. 84–86.
17. Arria, A. M., and M. C. O'Brien. "The 'High' Cost of Energy Drinks." *Journal of the American Medical Association*, Vol. 305, No. 6, February 2011, pp. 600–601.
18. Finkelstein, E. A., et al. "Mandatory Menu Labeling in One Fast-Food Chain in King County, Washington." *American Journal of Preventive Medicine*, Vol. 40, No. 2, February 2011, pp. 122–127.
19. Blumenthal, K., and K. G. Volpp. "Enhancing the Effectiveness of Food Labeling in Restaurants." *Journal of the American Medical Association*, Vol. 303, No. 6, February 2010, p. 553.
20. Voelker, R. "Experts Hope to Clear Confusion with First Guidelines to Tackle Food Allergy." *Journal of the American Medical Association*, Vol. 305, No. 5, February 2011, p. 457.
21. Boyce, J. A., et al. "Guidelines for the Diagnosis and Management of Food Allergy in the United States: Report of the NIAID-Sponsored Expert Panel." *Journal of Allergy and Clinical Immunology*, Vol. 126, No. 6, December 2010, pp. s1–58.

## Chapter 7

1. Danaei, G., et al. "National, Regional, and Global Trends in Systolic Blood Pressure since 1980: Systematic Analysis of Health Examination Surveys and Epidemiological Studies with 786 Country-Years and 5.4 Million Participants." Lancet. Vol. 377, No. 9765, February 2011, pp. 568–577.
2. Gaziano, J. M. "Fifth Phase of the Epidemiologic Transition: The Age of Obesity and Inactivity." *Journal of the American Medical Association*, Vol. 303, No. 3, January 2010, pp. 275–276.
3. "Global Strategy on Diet, Physical Activity and Health." World Health Organization, www.who.int/dietphysicalactivity/publications/facts/obesity/en/.
4. Berrington de Gonzalez, A., et al. "Body-Mass Index and Mortality among 1.46 Million White Adults." *New England Journal of Medicine*, Vol. 363, No. 23, December 2010, pp. 2211–9.
5. Gaziano, "Fifth Phase."
6. Ogden, C. L., et al. "Obesity and Socioeconomic Status in Adults: United States, 2005-2008" and "Obesity and Socioeconomic Status in Children and Adolescents: United States, 2005-2008." *National Center for Health Statistics Data Brief*. No. 50/51, December 2010, pp. 1–8.
7. Ogden, C. L., et al. "Prevalence of High Body Mass Index in U.S. Children and Adolescents, 2007-2008." *Journal of the American Medical Association*, Vol. 303, No. 3, January 2010, pp. 242–249.
8. Harris, K. M., et al. "Obesity in the Transition to Adulthood: Predictions across Race/Ethnicity, Immigrant Generation, and Sex." *Archives of Pediatrics and Adolescent Medicine*, Vol. 163, No. 11, November 2009, pp. 1022–1028.
9. Gaziano, "Fifth Phase."
10. Salamon, M. "TV: A Sneaky Part of the Food Pyramid." *HealthDay News*, January 27, 2011 (e-pub).

11. Grucza, R. A., et al. "The Emerging Link between Alcoholism Risk and Obesity in the United States." *Archives of General Psychiatry*, Vol. 67, No. 12, December 2010, pp. 1301–1308.

12. Eagle, T. F., et al. "Health Status and Behavior among Middle-School Children in a Midwest Community: What Are the Underpinnings of Childhood Obesity?" *American Heart Journal*, Vol. 160, No. 6, December 2010, pp. 1185–1189.

13. Leahey, T. M., et al. "Social Influences Are Associated with BMI and Weight Loss Intentions in Young Adults." *Obesity (Silver Spring)*, December 16, 2010 (e-pub).

14. Brown, W. J., et al. "Effects of Having a Baby on Weight Gain." *American Journal of Preventive Medicine*, Vol. 38, No. 2, February 2010, pp. 163–170.

15. United States Department of Agriculture. *Dietary Guidelines for Americans, 2010*, January 31, 2011 (e-pub). www.cnpp.usda.gov/Publications/DietaryGuidelines/2010/PolicyDoc/PolicyDoc.pdf.

16. Franco, M., et al. "Availability of Healthy Foods and Dietary Patterns: The Multi-Ethnic Study of Atherosclerosis." *American Journal of Clinical Nutrition*, Vol. 89, No. 3, March 2009, pp. 897–900.

17. Larson, N. I., et al. "Neighborhood Environments: Disparities in Access to Healthy Foods in the U.S." *American Journal of Preventive Medicine*, Vol. 36, No. 1, January 2009, pp. 74–81.

18. Sohn, S. "Sex Differences in Social Comparison and Comparison Motives in Body Image Process." *North American Journal of Psychology*. Vol. 12, No. 3, December 2010, p. 461.

19. Struble, C. B., et al. "Overweight and Obesity in Lesbian and Bisexual College Women." *Journal of American College Health*, Vol. 59, No. 1, July/August 2010, pp. 51–56.

20. Losina, E., et al. "Impact of Obesity and Knee Osteoarthritis on Morbidity and Mortality in Older Americans." *Annals of Internal Medicine*, Vol. 154, No. 4, February 2010, pp. 217–226.

21. Crimmins, E. M., et al. "Explaining Divergent Levels of Longevity in High-Income Countries." *Panel on Understanding Divergent Trends in Longevity in High-Income Countries; Division of Behavioral and Social Sciences and Education*. Washington, DC: The National Academies Press, 2011, pp. e5–26.

22. Logue, J., et al. "Obesity Is Associated with Fatal Coronary Heart Disease Independently of Traditional Risk Factors and Deprivation." *Heart*, Vol. 97, No. 7, April 2011, pp. 564–568.

23. Phipps, A., et al. "Body Size, Physical Activity, and Risk of Triple-Negative and Estrogen Receptor-Positive Breast Cancer." *Cancer Epidemiology, Biomarkers, and Prevention*, Vol. 20, No. 3, March 2011, pp. 454–463.

24. Schafer, M. H., and K. F. Ferraro. "The Stigma of Obesity: Does Perceived Weight Discrimination Affect Identity and Physical Health?" *Social Psychology Quarterly*, Vol. 74, March 2011, pp. 76–97.

25. Yancy, W. S. Jr., et al. "A Randomized Trial of a Low-Carbohydrate Diet vs Orlistat Plus a Low-Fat Diet for Weight Loss." *Archives of Internal Medicine*, Vol. 170, No. 2, January 2010, pp. 136–145.

26. Lee, M. W., and K. Fujioka. "Dietary Prescriptions for the Overweight Patient: The Potential Benefits of Low-Carbohydrate Diets in Insulin Resistance." *Diabetes, Obesity and Metabolism*, Vol. 13, No. 3, March 2011, pp. 204–206.

27. Browning, J. D., et al. "Short-Term Weight Loss and Hepatic Triglyceride Reduction: Evidence of a Metabolic Advantage with Dietary Carbohydrate Restriction." *American Journal of Clinical Nutrition*, March 2, 2011 (e-pub).

28. Busetto, L., et al. "High-Protein Low-Carbohydrate Diets: What Is the Rationale?" *Diabetes/Metabolism Research and Review*, Vol. 27, No. 3, March 2011, pp. 230–232.

29. Larsen, T. M., et al. "Diets with High or Low Protein Content and Glycemic Index for Weight-Loss Maintenance." *New England Journal of Medicine*, Vol. 363, No. 22, November 2010, pp. 2102–2113.

30. Ärnlöv, J., et al. "Impact of Body Mass Index and the Metabolic Syndrome on the Risk of Cardiovascular Disease and Death in Middle-Aged Men." *Circulation*, Vol. 121, No. 2, January 2010, pp. 230–236, e-pub December 2009.

31. Schusdziarra, V., et al. "Impact of Breakfast on Daily Energy Intake—An Analysis of Absolute Versus Relative Breakfast Calories." *Nutrition Journal*, Vol. 10, January 2011, p. 5.

32. Wasmund, S. L., et al. "Improved Heart Rate Recovery after Marked Weight Loss Induced by Gastric Bypass Surgery: Two-Year Followup in the Utah Obesity Study." *Heart Rhythm*, Vol. 8, No. 1, January 2011, pp. 84–90.

33. Chang, E. C., et al. "Complexities of Measuring Perfectionism: Three Popular Perfectionism Measures and Their Relations with Eating Disturbances and Health Behaviors in a Female College Student Sample." *Eating Behaviors*, Vol. 9, 2008, pp. 102–110.

34. Wilson, G. T., et al. "Psychological Treatments of Binge Eating Disorder." *Archives of General Psychiatry*, Vol. 67, No. 1, January 2010, pp. 94–101.

35. Rosen, D. S. "Identification and Management of Eating Disorders in Children and Adolescents." *Pediatrics*, Vol 126, No. 6, December 2010, pp. 1240–1253.

36. Greenleaf, C., et al. "Female Collegiate Athletes: Prevalence of Eating Disorders and Disordered Eating Behaviors." *Journal of American College Health*, Vol. 57, No. 5, March/April 2009, pp. 489–496.

37. Frantz, C. "'Drunkorexia' an Increasing Concern on College Campuses." *Colorado Daily*, August 10, 2009.

38. "Binges Take about One Third of Food Budgets." *HealthDay*, December 31, 2008. www.medlineplus.gov.

39. Marsh, Rachel, et al. "Deficient Activity in the Neural Systems That Mediate Self-Regulatory Control in Bulimia Nervosa." *Archives of General Psychiatry*, Vol. 66, No. 1, January 2009, pp. 51–63.

40. Mitka, M. "Report Weighs Options for Bulimia Nervosa Treatment." *Journal of the American Medical Association*, Vol. 305, No. 9, March 2011, p. 875.

## Chapter 8

1. Bungum, Tim. "Correlates of Physical Activity among Asian and African Americans." Presentation, 2009 AAHPERD National Convention, April 2009.

2. Lloyd-Jones, D., et al. "Heart Disease and Stroke Statistics 2010 Update. A Report from the American Heart Association," on behalf of the American Heart Association Statistics Committee and Stroke Statistics Subcommittee Circulation. Published online December 17, 2009.

3. www.cdc.gov

4. Stamatakis, E., et al. "Screen-Based Entertainment Time, All-Cause Mortality, and Cardiovascular Events: Population-Based Study with Ongoing Mortality and Hospital Events Follow-up." *Journal of the American College of Cardiology*, Vol. 57, No. 3, January 2011, pp. 292–297.

5. Dunstan, D. W., et al. "Television Viewing Time and Mortality: The Australian Diabetes, Obesity and Lifestyle Study (AusDiab)." *Circulation*, January 11, 2010 (e-pub ahead of print).

6. Sailors, M. H., et al. "Exposing College Students to Exercise: The Training Interventions and Genetics of Exercise Response (TIGER) Study." *Journal of American College Health*, Vol. 59, No. 1, July/August 2010, pp. 13–20.

7. Williamson, J., and M. Pahor. "Evidence Regarding the Benefits of Physical Exercise," *Archives of Internal Medicine*, Vol. 170, No. 2, January 2010, pp. 124–125.

8. Sun, Q., et al. "Physical Activity at Midlife in Relation to Successful Survival in Women at Age 70 Years or Older." *Archives of Internal Medicine*, Vol. 170, No. 2, 2010, pp. 194–201.

9. Kemmler, W., et al. "Exercise Effects on Bone Mineral Density, Falls, Coronary Risk Factors, and Health Care Costs in Older Women: The Randomized Controlled Senior Fitness and Prevention (SEFIP) Study." *Archives of Internal Medicine*, Vol. 170, No. 2, 2010, pp. 179–185.

10. Hankinson, A. L., et al. "Maintaining a High Physical Activity Level over 20 Years and Weight Gain." *Journal of the American Medical Association*, Vol. 304, No. 23, December 2010, pp. 2603–2610.

11. Nauman, J., et al. "Combined Effect of Resting Heart Rate and Physical Activity on Ischaemic Heart Disease: Mortality Follow-up in a Population Study (The HUNT Study, Norway)." *Journal of Epidemiology and Community Health*, Vol. 64, No. 2, 2010, pp. 175–181.

12. Preidt, R. "Healthier Lifestyles May Prevent 340,000 U.S. Cancers a Year: Study." *HealthDay News*, February 4, 2011 (e-pub).

13. Dotinga, R. "Brisk Walk Can Leave Common Cold Behind." *HealthDay*, October 25, 2009, www.medlineplus.gov.

14. Erickson, K. I., et al. "Exercise Training Increases Size of Hippocampus and Improves Memory." *Proceedings of the National Academy of Sciences of the United States of America,* Vol. 108, No. 7, February 2011, pp. 3017–3022.

15. Baker, L. D., et al. "Effects of Aerobic Exercise on Mild Cognitive Impairment: A Controlled Trial." *Archives of Neurology*, Vol. 67, No. 1, January 2010, pp. 71–79.

16. Liu-Ambrose, T., et al. "Resistance Training and Executive Functions: A 12-Month Randomized Controlled Trial." *Archives of Internal Medicine*, Vol. 170, No. 2, 2010, pp. 170–178.

17. Etgen, T., et al. "Physical Activity and Incident Cognitive Impairment in Elderly Persons: The INVADE Study." *Archives of Internal Medicine*, Vol. 170, No. 2, 2010, pp. 186–193.

18. Larson-Meyer, D., et al. "Caloric Restriction with or without Exercise: The Fitness versus Fatness Debate." *Medicine and Science in Sports and Exercise*, Vol. 42, No. 1, January 2010, pp. 152–159.

19. www.cdc.gov

20. "Two Deaths in One Week? It's Not Good to Play Sports with a Big Heart." Press Release, Hypertrophic Cardiomyopathy Association, January 18, 2010.

21. "Athletes' Deaths Raise Awareness of Undiagnosed Heart Conditions." Press Release, Vanderbilt University Medical Center, January 20, 2010.

22. Steinvil, A., et al. "Mandatory Electrocardiographic Screening of Athletes to Reduce Their Risk for Sudden Death: Proven Fact or Wishful Thinking?" *Journal of the American College of Cardiology*, Vol. 57, No. 11, March 2011, pp. 1291–1296.

23. Bove, A. A. "Making or Breaking Athletic Careers." *Journal of the American College of Cardiology*, Vol. 57, March 2011, pp. 1297–1298.

24. http://www.health.gov/paguidelines.

25. Van Proeyen, K., et al. "Beneficial Metabolic Adaptations Due to Endurance Exercise Training in the Fasted State." *Journal of Applied Physiology*, Vol. 110, No. 1, January 2011, pp. 236–245.

26. www.acsm.org

27. Nelson, M. E., and S. C. Folta. "Further Evidence for the Benefits of Walking." *American Journal of Clinical Nutrition*, Vol. 89, No. 1, January 2009, pp. 15–16.

28. Preidt, R. "The More You Walk, the Lower Your Diabetes Risk: Study." *HealthDay News*, January 14, 2011 (e-pub).

29. Peterson, M. D., et al. "Influence of Resistance Exercise on Lean Body Mass in Aging Adults: A Meta-analysis." *Medicine and Science in Sports and Exercise*. Vol. 43, No. 2, February 2011, pp. 249–258.

30. Osawa, Y., et al. "Effects of Whole-Body Vibration Training on Bone-Free Lean Body Mass and Muscle Strength in Young Adults." *Journal of Sports Science and Medicine*, Vol. 10, March 2011, pp. 97–104.

31. Gwebu, Amukela. "College Students' Moral Reasoning about Performance-Enhancing Drugs in Sport." Presentation, 2009 AAHPERD National Convention, April 2009.

32. American Academy of Orthopaedic Surgeons. "Stretching Before a Run Does Not Prevent Injury." *ScienceDaily*, February 20, 2011 (e-pub), www.sciencedaily.com/releases/2011/02/110218083422.htm.

33. Bergman, R. N., et al. "A Better Index of Body Adiposity." *Obesity*, March 3, 2011 (e-pub).

34. Dore, G. A., et al. "Relation between Central Adiposity and Cognitive Function in the Maine-Syracuse Study: Attenuation by Physical Activity." *Annals of Behavioral Medicine*, June 27, 2008.

35. Miller, W. C., et al. "Attitudes of Overweight and Normal Weight Adults Regarding Exercise at a Health Club." *Journal of Nutrition Education and Behavior*, Vol. 42, No. 1, January 2010, pp. 2–9.

36. Collier, R. "Low-Tech Running Shoes in High Demand." *Canadian Medical Association Journal*, Vol. 183, No. 1, January 2011, p. e20.

37. Brown, Theresa. "Perceptions of a Caring and Positive Climate in Exercise Classes." Presentation, 2009 AAHPERD National Convention, April 2009.

38. Preidt, Robert. "Winter Workouts Are Cool." *HealthyDay*, January 4, 2009, www.medlineplus.gov.

### Chapter 9

1. László, K. D., and M. S. Kopp. "Effort-Reward Imbalance and Overcommitment at Work Are Associated with Painful Menstruation: Results from the Hungarostudy Epidemiological Panel 2006." *Journal of Occupational and Environmental Medicine*, Vol. 51, No. 2, February 2009, pp. 157–163.

2. Chocano-Bedoya, P. O., et al. "Dietary B Vitamin Intake and Incident Premenstrual Syndrome." *American Journal of Clinical Nutrition*, February 23, 2011 (e-pub).

3. Khajehei, M., et al. "Effect of Treatment with Dydrogesterone or Calcium plus Vitamin D on the Severity of Premenstrual Syndromes." *International Journal of Gynecology and Obstetrics*, Vol. 105, No. 2, May 2009, pp. 158–161.

4. Busse, J. W., et al. "Psychological Intervention for Premenstrual Syndrome: A Meta-analysis of Randomized Controlled Trials." *Psychotherapeutic Psychosomatics*, Vol. 78, No. 1, 2009, pp. 6–15.

5. "Premenstrual Dysphoric Disorder (PMDD): Different from PMS?" *MedlinePlus*, www.nlm.nih.gov/medlineplus/premenstrualsyndrome.html.

6. Liebowitz, A. A., et al. "Determinants and Policy Implications of Male Circumcision in the United States." *American Journal of Public Health*, Vol. 99, No. 1, pp. 138–145.

7. Wawer, M. J., et al. "Effect of Circumcision of HIV-Negative Men on Transmission of Human Papilloma Virus to HIV-Negative Women: A Randomized Trial in Rakai, Uganda." *Lancet*, Vol. 377, No. 9761, January 2011, pp. 209–218

8. "Young Couples Often Disagree about Monogamy, Study Finds." *HealthDay*, January 21, 2011 (e-pub), www.medlineplus.gov.

9. www.cdc.gov/nchs/data/series/sr_23/sr23_030.pdf

10. Abma, J. C., et al. "Teenagers in the United States: Sexual Activity, Contraceptive Use, and Childbearing; National Survey of Family Growth 2006–2008." *National Center for Health Statistics,* June 2010 (e-pub).

11. Magnusson, B. M., et al. "Adolescent and Sexual History Factors Influencing Reproductive Control among Women Aged 18–44." *Sexual Health*, Vol. 8, No. 1, February 2011, pp. 95–101.

12. Abma, et al., "Teenagers in the United States."

13. American College Health Association. *American College Health Association-National College Health Assessment II: Reference Group Executive Summary Spring 2010,* www.acha-ncha.org/docs/ACHA-NCHA-II_ReferenceGroup_ExecutiveSummary_Spring2010.pdf.

14. Ross, L., and A. Bowen. "Sexual Decision Making for the 'Better Than Average' College Student." *Journal of American College Health*, Vol. 59, November/December 2010, pp. 211–216.

15. Caroll, Janell C. *Sexuality Now: Embracing Diversity,* 3rd ed. Belmont, CA: Cengage-Wadsworth, 2010.

16. Kaestle, C. E., and K. R. Allen. "The Role of Masturbation in Healthy Sexual Development: Perceptions of Young Adults." *Archives of Sexual Behavior*, February 4, 2011 (e-pub).

17. Henderson, A. W., et al. "Ecological Models of Sexual Satisfaction among Lesbian/Bisexual and Heterosexual Women," *Archives of Sexual Behavior*, Vol. 38, No. 1, February 2009, pp. 50–65.

18. Laumann, "A Population-Based Survey of Sexual Activity," *International Journal of Impotence Research,* 2009.

19. Lamaire, A., et al. "Why Is It That Patients with Sexual Difficulties Do Not Consult a Doctor More Frequently?" *Sexologies*, Vol. 18, No. 1, January/March 2009, pp. 14–18.

20. Bonierbale, M. "From Sexual Difficulties to Sexual Dysfunctions." *Sexologies*, Vol. 18, No. 1, January/March 2009, pp. 10–13.

21. American College Health Association, *American College Health Association-National College Health Assessment II: Reference Group Executive Summary Spring 2010.*

22. Cordell, W. H., et al. "Retinal Effects of Six Months of Daily Use of Tadalafil and Sildenafil." *Archives of Ophthalmology*, Vol. 127, No. 4, April 2009, pp. 367–373.

23. "Sexual Problems in Women." *MedLinePlus*, www.nlm.nih.gov/medlineplus/sexualproblemsinwomen.html.

### Chapter 10

1. Ness, R. B., et al. "Contraception Methods, Beyond Oral Contraceptives and Tubal Ligation, and Risk of Ovarian Cancer." *Annals of Epidemiology*, Vol. 21, No. 3, March 2011, pp. 188–196.

2. Gaydos, L. M., et al. "Racial Disparities in Contraceptive Use between Student and Nonstudent Populations." *Journal of Women's Health*, February 2010 (e-pub).

3. Buhl, E. R., et al. "The State of the Union: Sexual Health Disparities in a National Sample of U.S. College Students." *Journal of American College Health*, Vol. 58, No. 4, January/February 2010, pp. 337–346.

4. Magnusson, B. M., et al. "Adolescent and Sexual History Factors Influencing Reproductive Control among Women Aged 18–44." *Sexual Health*, Vol. 8, No. 1, February 2011, pp. 95–101.

5. Abma, J. C., et al. "Teenagers in the United States: Sexual Activity, Contraceptive Use, and Childbearing; National Survey of Family Growth 2006–2008, National Center for Health Statistics." *Vital Health Statistics*, Vol. 23, No. 30, June 2010.

6. Carroll, Janell. *Sexuality Now*, 3rd ed. Belmont, CA: Cengage-Wadsworth, 2010.

7. Carroll, *Sexuality Now*.

8. Ibid.

9. Williamson, L. M., et al. "Limits to Modern Contraceptive Use among Young Women in Developing Countries: A Systematic Review of Qualitative Research." *Reproductive Health*, Vol. 6, No. 3, February 19, 2009.

10. Ibid.

11. Nearns, J. "Health Insurance Coverage and Prescription Contraceptive Use among Young Women at Risk for Unintended Pregnancy," *Contraception*, Vol. 79, No. 2, pp. 105–110.

12. American College Health Association. *American College Health Association-National College Health Assessment II: Reference Group Executive Summary Spring 2010*, www.acha-ncha.org/.../ACHA-NCHA-II_ReferenceGroup_ ExecutiveSummary_Spring2010.pdf.

13. Ross, L., and A. Bowen. "Sexual Decision Making for the 'Better Than Average' College Student." *Journal of American College Health*, Vol. 59, November/December 2010, pp. 211–216.

14. Abma, et al., "Teenagers in the United States."

15. Tafuri, S., et al. "Determining Factors for Condom Use: A Survey of Young Italian Adults." *European Journal of Contraception and Reproductive Health Care*, Vol. 15, No. 1, February 2010, pp. 24–30.

16. Crosby, R. A., et al. "Does It Fit Okay? Problems with Condom Use as a Function of Self-Reported Poor Fit." *Sexually Transmitted Infections*, Vol. 86, No. 1, February 2010, pp. 36–38.

17. "Noncontraceptive Use of Hormonal Contraceptives." American College of Obstetricians and Gynecologists Practice Bulletin, no. 110. *Obstetrics and Gynecology*, Vol. 115, No. 1, January 2010, pp. 206–212.

18. Hannaford, P. C., et al. "Mortality among Contraceptive Pill Users: Cohort Evidence from Royal College of General Practitioners' Oral Contraception Study." *British Medical Journal*, Vol. 340, March 2010, p. c927.

19. Potter, J. E., et al. "Continuation of Prescribed Compared with Over-the-Counter Oral Contraceptives." *Obstetrics and Gynecology*. Vol. 117, March 2011, p. 551.

20. Grossman, D., et al. "Contraindications to Combined Oral Contraceptives among Over-the-Counter Compared with Prescription Users." *Obstetrics and Gynecology*. Vol. 117, March 2011, p. 558.

21. Winkler, U. H., et al. "An Open-Label, Comparative Study of the Effects of a Dose-Reduced Oral Contraceptive Containing 0.02 mg Ethinylestradiol/2 mg Chlormadinone Acetate on Hemostatic Parameters and Lipid and Carbohydrate Metabolism Variables." *Contraception*, January 2010 (e-pub).

22. Brucker, C., et al. "Long-Term Efficacy and Safety of a Monophasic Combined Oral Contraceptive Containing 0.02 mg Ethinylestradiol and 2 mg Chlormadnone Acetate Administered in a 24/4-Day Regimen." *Contraception*, February 2010 (e-pub).

23. Grimes, D. A., et al. "Progestin-Only Pills for Contraception." *Cochrane Database Systematic Reviews*, No. 1, January 20, 2010, CD007541.

24. Chakhtoura, Z., et al. "Progestogen-Only Contraceptives and the Risk of Acute Myocardial Infarction: A Meta-Analysis." *Journal of Clinical Endocrinology and Metabolism*, February 2, 2011 (e-pub).

25. Dinger, J., et al. "Effectiveness of Oral Contraceptive Pills in a Large U.S. Cohort Comparing Progestogen and Regimen." *Obstetrics and Gynecology*. Vol. 117, No. 1, January 2011, pp. 33–40.

26. Dore, D. D., et al. "Extended Case-Control Study Results on Thromboembolic Outcomes among Transdermal Contraceptive Users." *Contraception*, January 2010 (e-pub).

27. Gilliam, M. L., et al. "Adherence and Acceptability of the Contraceptive Ring Compared with the Pill among Students: A Randomized Controlled Trial." *Obstetrics and Gynecology*, Vol. 115, No. 3, March 2010, pp. 503–510.

28. Fontenot and Harris, "Latest Advances in Hormonal Contraception." *Journal of Obstetric, Gynecologic, & Neonatal Nursing*, 2008, pp. 369–374.

29. Rahman, M., et al. "Predictors of Higher Bone Mineral Density Loss and Use of Depot Medroxyprogesterone Acetate." *Obstetrics and Gynecology*, Vol. 115, No. 1, January 2010, pp. 35–40.

30. Lewis, L. N., et al. "Implanon as a Contraceptive Choice for Teenage Mothers: A Comparison of Contraceptive Choices, Acceptability and Repeat Pregnancy." *Contraception*, January 2010 (e-pub).

31. Dinger, J., et al. "Levonorgestrel-Releasing and Copper Intrauterine Devices and the Risk of Breast Cancer." *Contraception*, Vol. 83, No. 3, March 2011, pp. 211–217.

32. Black, K. "Developments and Challenges in Emergency Contraception." *Best Practice and Research Clinical Obstetrics and Gynecology*, Vol. 23, No. 2, pp. 221–231.

33. Glasier, A. F., et al. "Ulipristal Acetate versus Levonorgestrel for Emergency Contraception: A Randomized Non-inferiority Trial and Meta-Analysis." *Lancet*, Vol. 375, February 2010, pp. 555–562.

34. Fine, P., et al. "Ulipristal Acetate Taken 48–120 Hours after Intercourse for Emergency Contraception." *Obstetrics and Gynecology*, Vol. 115, No. 1, February 2010, pp. 257–263.

35. Nguyen, B. T., et al. "Pharmacy Provision of Emergency Contraception to Men: A Survey of Pharmacist Attitude." *Journal of the American Pharmacists Association*, Vol. 50, No. 1, January/February 2010, pp. 17–23.
36. Schreiber, C. A., et al. "A Randomized Controlled Trial of the Effect of Advanced Supply of Emergency Contraception in Postpartum Teens: A Feasibility Study." *Contraception*, February 2010 (e-pub).
37. Raymond, E. G., et al. "Pericoital Oral Contraception with Levonorgestrel: A Systematic Review." *Obstetrics and Gynecology*, Vol. 117, No. 3, March 2011, pp. 673–681.
38. American Society of Reproductive Medicine, www.asrm.org.

## Chapter 11

1. Tu, W., et al. "Time from First Intercourse to First Sexually Transmitted Infection Diagnosis among Adolescent Women." *Archives of Pediatrics and Adolescent Medicine*, Vol. 163, No. 1, December 2009, pp. 1106–1111.
2. Jacobs, H. S., et al. "A Closer Look at Age: Deconstructing Aggregate Gonorrhea and Chlamydia Rates, California, 1998–2007." *Sexually Transmitted Diseases*, February 23, 2010 (e-pub).
3. American College Health Association. *American College Health Association-National College Health Assessment II: Reference Group Executive Summary Spring 2010*, www.acha-ncha.org/. . ./ACHA-NCHA-II_ReferenceGroup_ExecutiveSummary_Spring2010.pdf.
4. Ibid.
5. Simons, J. S., et al. "Sexual Risk Taking among Young Adult Dual Alcohol and Marijuana Users." *Addictive Behaviors*, Vol. 35, No. 5, May 2010, pp. 533–536.
6. Wells, B. E., et al. "Patterns of Alcohol Consumption and Sexual Behavior among Young Adults in Nightclubs." *American Journal of Drug and Alcohol Abuse*, Vol. 36, No. 1, January 2010, pp. 39–45.
7. Bilardi, J. E., et al. "Experiences and Outcomes of Partner Notification among Men and Women Recently Diagnosed with Chlamydia and Their Views on Innovative Resources Aimed at Improving Notification Rates." *Sexually Transmitted Diseases*, February 23, 2010 (e-pub).
8. "STD Treatment: Time to Get on Board with Expedited Partner Therapy." *Contraceptive Technology Update*, April 1, 2011.
9. Giuliano, A. R., et al. "Incidence and Clearance of Genital Human Papillomavirus Infection in Men (HIM): A Cohort Study." *Lancet*, Vol. 377, No. 9769, March 2011, pp. 932–940.
10. Wawer, M. J., et al. "Effect of Circumcision of HIV-Negative Men on Transmission of Human Papillomavirus to HIV-Negative Women: A Randomized Trial in Rakai, Uganda." *Lancet*, Vol. 377, No. 9761, January 2011, pp. 209–218.
11. "Rise in Some Head and Neck Cancers Tied to Oral Sex." *HealthDay*, January 26, 2011, www.medlineplus.gov.
12. Committee on Infectious Diseases. "Recommended Childhood and Adolescent Immunization Schedules—United States, 2011." *Pediatrics*, Vol. 127, No. 2, February 2011, pp. 387–388.
13. Giuliano, A. R., et al. "Efficacy of Quadrivalent HPV Vaccine against HPV Infection and Disease in Males." *New England Journal of Medicine*, Vol. 364, No. 5, February 2011, pp. 401–411.
14. Lu, B., et al. "Efficacy and Safety of Prophylactic Vaccines against Cervical HPV Infection and Diseases among Women: A Systematic Review and Meta-analysis." *BMC Infectious Diseases*, Vol. 11, January 2011, p. 13.
15. Widdice, L. E., et al. "Adherence to the HPV Vaccine Dosing Intervals and Factors Associated with Completion of 3 Doses." *Pediatrics*, Vol. 127, No. 1, January 2011, pp. 77–84.
16. www.cdc.gov.
17. Tata, S., et al. "Overlapping Reactivations of Herpes Simplex Virus Type 2 in the Genital and Perianal Mucosa." *Journal of Infectious Diseases*, Vol. 201, No. 1, February 2010, pp. 499–504.

18. Hook, E. W., III. "An Evolving Understanding of Genital Herpes Pathogenesis: Is It Time for Our Approach to Therapy to Change as Well?" *Journal of Infectious Diseases*, Vol. 20, No. 1, February 2010, pp. 486–487.
19. Flagg, E. W., and H. Weinstock. "Incidence of Neonatal Herpes Simplex Virus Infections in the United States, 2006." *Pediatrics*, Vol. 127, No. 1, January 2011, pp. e1–e8.
20. Workowski, K. A., and S. Berman. "Sexually Transmitted Diseases Treatment Guidelines, 2010." *CDC Morbidity and Mortality Weekly Report; Recommendations and Reports*, Vol. 59, No. RR12, December 2010, pp. 1–110.
21. "Genital Herpes." CDC Fact Sheet, www.cdc.gov.
22. *Sexually Transmitted Disease Surveillance 2007 Supplement: Chlamydia Prevalence Monitoring Project*. Atlanta, GA: CDC Division of STD Prevention, January 2009.
23. James, et al. "Chlamydia Prevalence among College Students."
24. *Sexually Transmitted Disease Surveillance 2007 Supplement: Chlamydia Prevalence Monitoring Project.*
25. Wiehe, S. E., et al. "Chlamydia Screening among Young Women: Individual- and Provider-Level Differences in Testing." *Pediatrics*, Vol. 127, No. 2, February 2011, pp. e336–e344.
26. *Sexually Transmitted Disease Surveillance 2007 Supplement: Chlamydia Prevalence Monitoring Project.*
27. James, et al. "Chlamydia Prevalence among College Students."
28. Workowski and Berman, "Sexually Transmitted Diseases Treatment Guidelines, 2010."
29. Ibid.
30. *Sexually Transmitted Disease Surveillance 2007 Supplement: Syphilis Surveillance Report*. Atlanta, GA: CDC Division of STD Prevention, March 2009.
31. www.kff.oeg/hivaids.
32. Minichiello, V., et al. "HIV, Sexually Transmitted Infections, and Sexuality in Later Life." *Current Infectious Disease Reports*, Vol. 13, No. 2, April 2011, pp. 182–187.
33. Henry J. Kaiser Family Foundation. "The HIV/AIDS Epidemic in the United States." *HIV/AIDS Policy Fact Sheet*, March 2011, www.kff.org/hivaids/upload/3029-12.pdf.
34. Wolitski, R. J., and K. A. Fenton. "Sexual Health, HIV, and Sexually Transmitted Infections among Gay, Bisexual, and Other Men Who Have Sex with Men in the United States." *AIDS and Behavior*, February 18, 2011 (e-pub).
35. Laffoon, B., et al. "Disparities in Diagnoses of HIV Infection between Blacks/African Americans and Other Racial/Ethnic Populations—37 States, 2005–2008." *CDC Morbidity and Mortality Weekly Report*, Vol. 60, No. 4, February 4, 2011, pp. 93–98.
36. Ibid.
37. Henry J. Kaiser Family Foundation. "Women and HIV/AIDS in the United States." *HIV/AIDS Policy Fact Sheet*, March 2011, *www.kff.org/hivaids/upload/6092-09.pdf*.
38. Ketta, G. P. "New Hope in Aids Prevention." *Monitor on Psychology*, Vol. 42, No. 3, March 2011, p. 57.
39. Smith, D. K., et al. "Interim Guidance: Preexposure Prophylaxis for the Prevention of HIV Infection in Men Who Have Sex with Men." *CDC Morbidity and Mortality Weekly Report*, Vol. 60, No. 3, January 28, 2011, pp. 65–68.
40. Ovbiagele, B. and A. Nath. "Increasing Incidence of Ischemic Stroke in Patients with HIV Infection." *Neurology*, Vol. 76, No. 5, February 2011, pp. 444–450.
41. Young, B., et al. "Increased Rates of Bone Fracture among HIV-Infected Persons in the HIV Outpatient Study (HOPS) Compared with the U.S. General Population, 2000–2006." *Clinical Infectious Diseases*, March 10, 2011 (e-pub).

## Chapter 12

1. "NIDA Info Facts: High School and Youth Trends." *National Institute on Drug Abuse*, March 2011, www.drugabuse.gov.

2. Wang, D. V., and J. Z. Tsien. "Convergent Processing of Both Positive and Negative Motivational Signals by the VA Dopamine Neuronal Populations." *PLoS ONE*, Vol. 6, No. 2, February 2011, p. e17047.
3. Welte, J. W., et al. "Gambling and Problem Gambling across the Lifespan." *Journal of Gambling Studies*, Vol. 27, No. 1, March 2011, pp. 49–61.
4. Lorains, F. K., et al. "Prevalence of Comorbid Disorders in Problem and Pathological Gambling: Systematic Review and Meta-Analysis of Population Surveys." *Addiction*, Vol. 160, No. 3, March 2011, pp. 490–498.
5. Marceaux, J. C., and C. L. Melville. "Twelve-Step Facilitated versus Mapping-Enhanced Cognitive-Behavioral Therapy for Pathological Gambling: A Controlled Study." *Journal of Gambling Studies*, Vol. 27, No. 1, March 2011, pp. 171–191.
6. American College Health Association. *American College Health Association-National College Health Assessment II: Reference Group Executive Summary Spring 2010*, www.acha-ncha.org/. . ./ACHA-NCHA-II_ReferenceGroup_ExecutiveSummary_Spring2010.pdf.
7. McCauley, J. L., et al. "Non-medical Use of Prescription Drugs in a National Sample of College Women." *Addictive Behaviors*, Vol. 36, No. 7, July 2011, pp. 690–695.
8. Lord, S., et al. "Connecting to Young Adults: An Online Social Network Survey of Beliefs and Attitudes Associated with Prescription Opioid Misuse among College Students." *Substance Use and Misuse*, Vol. 46, No. 1, January 2011, pp. 66–76.
9. Rooney, M., et al. "Substance Use in College Students with ADHD." *Journal of Attention Disorders*, February 2011 (e-pub).
10. Cornelis, M.C., et al. "Genome-Wide Meta-Analysis Identifies Regions on 7P21 (AHR) and 15Q24 (CYP1A2) as Determinants of Habitual Caffeine Consumption." *PLoS Genetics*, Vol. 7, No. 4, April 2011, p. e1002033.
11. Katsky, A. "Presentation, American Heart Association Annual Conference on Cardiovascular Disease Epidemiology and Prevention." San Francisco, March 2010, pp. 3–5.
12. Lackland, D. "Presentation, American Stroke Association Stroke Conference." San Antonio, February 25, 2010.
13. Curhan, S. G., et al. "Analgesic Use and the Risk of Hearing Loss in Men." *American Journal of Medicine*, Vol. 123, No. 3, March 2010, pp. 231–237.
14. Dunn, K. M., et al. "Opioid Prescriptions for Chronic Pain and Overdose: A Cohort Study." *Annals of Internal Medicine*, Vol. 152, No. 2, January 19, 2010, pp. 85–92.
15. Lord, et al. "Connecting to Young Adults."
16. McCauley, et al. "Non-medical Use of Prescription Drugs."
17. Ibid.
18. Desantis, A. D., et al. "Aderall Is Definitely Not a Drug: Justifications for the Illegal Use of ADHD Stimulants." *Substance Use and Misuse*, Vol. 45, No. 1, January 2010, pp. 31–48.
19. Kerbs, E. E., et al. "Predictors of Long-Term Opioid Use among Patients with Painful Lumbar Spine Conditions." *Journal of Pain*, Vol. 11, No. 1, January 11, 2010, pp. 44–52.
20. "NIDA Info Facts: Drugged Driving." *National Institute on Drug Abuse*, December 2010, www.drugabuse.gov.
21. Kuepper, R., et al. "Continued Cannabis Use and Risk of Incidence and Persistence of Psychotic Symptoms: 10-Year Follow-up Cohort Study." *British Medical Journal*, Vol. 342, March 2011, p. d738.
22. Morefield, K. M., et al. "Pill Content, Dose, and Resulting Plasma Concentrations of MDMA in Recreational 'Ecstasy' Users." *Addiction*, February 14, 2011 (e-pub).
23. "ER Visits from Ecstasy Jump 75 Percent, U.S. Study Finds." *HealthDay News*, March 24, 2011, www.medlineplus.gov.
24. Shetty V., et al. "The Relationship between Methamphetamine Use and Increased Dental

Disease." *Journal of the American Dental Association*, Vol. 141, No. 3, 2010, pp. 307–318.

25. Volkow, N. "Message from the Director on 'Bath Salts'—Emerging and Dangerous Products." *National Institute on Drug Abuse*, February 2011, www.nida.gov.

26. "U.S. Children Turn to Inhaling to Get High." *HealthDay*, March 11, 2010, www.medlineplus.gov.

27. Shadley, M. "The Way It Was: Challenging the Myths of Addiction and How Treatment and Research Have Changed." *Family Therapy*, Vol. 9, No. 6, November/December 2010, pp. 16–19.

## Chapter 13

1. http://www.niaaa.nih.gov

2. "Health Behaviors of Adults: United States, 2005–2010." Atlanta: Centers for Disease Control and Prevention, *Vital and Health Statistics*, March 2010, Series 10(245).

3. "Substance Use among Black Adults." Washington, DC: U.S. SAMHSA Alcohol and Drug Information, February 18, 2010.

4. "Health Behaviors of Adults."

5. Fromme, K., et al. "Turning 21 and the Associated Changes in Drinking and Driving after Drinking among College Students." *Journal of American College Health*, Vol. 59, No. 1, July/August 2010, pp. 21–27.

6. www.collegedrinkingprevention.gov

7. "What Students' Brains Have Told Us about the Effects of Binge Drinking: Findings Are the Result of Brain and Alcohol Research Project." *Ascribe Higher Education News Service*, March 31, 2011; *Health Reference Center Academic*, April 17, 2011.

8. Tremblay, P. F., et al. "When Do First-Year College Students Drink Most during the Academic Year: An Internet-Based Study of Daily and Weekly Drinking." *Journal of American College Health*, Vol. 58, No. 5, March/April 2010, pp. 401–411.

9. Maggs, J. L., et al. "Ups and Downs of Alcohol Use among First-Year College Students: Number of Drinks, Heavy Drinking, and Stumble and Pass Out Drinking Days." *Addictive Behaviors*, Vol. 36, March 2011, pp. 197–202.

10. Glassman, T. J., et al. "Extreme Ritualistic Alcohol Consumption among College Students on Game Day." *Journal of American College Health*, Vol. 58, No. 5, March/April 2010, pp. 413–423.

11. American College Health Association. *American College Health Association-National College Health Assessment II: Reference Group Executive Summary Spring 2010*. Linthicum, MD: American College Health Association, 2010.

12. Wells, G. "The Effect of Religiosity and Campus Alcohol Culture on Collegiate Alcohol Consumption." *Journal of American College Health*, Vol. 8, No. 4, January/February 2010, pp. 295–304.

13. Logan, D. E., et al. "The Virtuous Drinker: Character Virtues as Correlates and Moderators of College Student Drinking and Consequences." *Journal of American College Health*, Vol. 58, No. 4, January/February 2010, pp. 317–324.

14. Lewis, M. A., et al. "Examining the Relationship between Typical Drinking Behavior and 21st Birthday Drinking Behavior among College Students: Implications for Event-Specific Prevention." *Addiction*, March 13, 2009.

15. Terlecki, M. A., et al. "The Role of Social Anxiety in a Brief Alcohol Intervention for Heavy-Drinking College Students." *Journal of Cognitive Psychotherapy*, Vol. 25, No. 1, February 2011, pp. 7–21.

16. Labbe, A. K., and S. A. Maisto. "Alcohol Expectancy Challenges for College Students: A Narrative Review." *Clinical Psychology Review*, Vol. 31, No. 4, June 2011, pp. 673–683 (e-pub March 1, 2011).

17. Ham, I. S., et al. "No Fear, Just Relax and Play: Social Anxiety, Alcohol Expectancies and Drinking Games among College Students." *Journal of American College Health*, Vol. 58, No. 5, March/April 2010, pp. 481–490.

18. American College Health Association, *ACHA-NCH Assessment II*.

19. Borden, L. A., et al. "The Role of College Students' Use of Protective Behavioral Strategies in the Relation between Binge Drinking and Alcohol-Related Problems." *Psychology of Addictive Behaviors*, March 28, 2011 (e-pub).

20. Naimi, T. S., et al. "The Intensity of Binge Alcohol Consumption among U.S. Adults." *American Journal of Preventative Medicine*, Vol. 38, No. 20, February 2010, pp. 201–207.

21. "Substance Use among Black Adults."

22. Ahern, N. R., et al. "Youth in Mind: Drinking Games and College Students." *Journal of Psychosocial Nursing and Mental Health Services*, January 27, 2010, pp. 1–4.

23. Cameron, J. M., et al. "Drinking Game Participation among Undergraduate Students Attending National Alcohol Screening Day." *Journal of American College Health*, Vol. 58, No. 5, March/April 2010, pp. 499–506.

24. DeJong, W., et al. "Pregaming: An Exploratory Study of Strategic Drinking by College Students in Pennsylvania." *Journal of American College Health*, Vol. 58, No. 4, January/February 2010, pp. 307–316.

25. Read, J. P., et al. "Before the Party Starts: Risk Factors and Reasons for 'Pregaming' in College Students." *Journal of American College Health*, Vol. 58, No. 5, pp. 461–472.

26. Kelly-Weeder, S. "Binge Drinking and Disordered Eating in College Students." *Journal of the American Academy of Nurse Practitioners*, Vol. 23, No. 1, January 2011, pp. 33–41.

27. "Fact Sheets: Caffeinated Alcoholic Beverages." Centers for Disease Control and Prevention, www.cdc.gov/alcohol/fact-sheets/cab.htm.

28. McGee, R., et al. "College Students' Readiness to Reduce Binge Drinking: Criterion Validity of a Brief Measure." *Addictive Behaviors*, Vol. 35, No. 3, March 2010, pp. 183–189.

29. Davis, K. C., et al. "College Women's Sexual Decision Making: Cognitive Mediation of Alcohol Expectancy Results." *Journal of American College Health*, Vol. 58, No. 5, March/April 2010, pp. 481–490.

30. Lawyer, Steven, et al. "Forcible, Drug-Facilitated, and Incapacitate Rape and Sexual Assault among Undergraduate Women." *Journal of American College Health*, Vol. 58, No. 5, March/April 2010, pp. 453–460.

31. McKinney, C. M., et al. "Does Alcohol Involvement Increase the Severity of Intimate Partner Violence?" *Alcohol: Clinical and Experimental Research*, Vol. 34, No. 4, January 2010, pp. 655–668.

32. Stappenbeck, C. A., et al. "A Longitudinal Investigation of Heavy Drinking and Physical Dating Violence in Men and Women." *Addictive Behaviors*, Vol. 35, No. 5, May 2010, pp. 479–485.

33. Fromme, et al., "Turning 21."

34. Fairlie, A. M., et al. "Sociodemographic, Behavioral and Cognitive Predictors of Alcohol-Impaired Driving in a Sample of U.S. College Students." *Journal of Health Communication*, Vol. 15, No. 2, March 2010, pp. 218–232.

35. Tsai, V. W., et al. "Alcohol Involvement among Young Female Drivers in the U.S. Fatal Crashes: Unfavourable Trends." *Injury Prevention*, Vol. 16, 2010, pp. 17–20.

36. Core Drug and Alcohol Survey, www.med.unc.edu/alcohol/prevention/coresurvey.html.

37. Mothers Against Drunk Driving, www.madd.org.

38. Terlecki, M. A., et al. "Clinical Outcomes of a Brief Motivational Intervention for Heavy Drinking Mandated College Students: A Pilot Study." *Journal of Studies on Alcohol and Drugs*, Vol. 71, No. 1, January 2010, pp. 54–60.

39. Labbe and Maisto, "Alcohol Expectancy Challenges."

40. Saylor, D. K. "Heavy Drinking on College Campuses: No Reason to Change Minimum Legal Drinking Age of 21." *Journal of American College Health*, Vol. 59, No. 4, January 2011, pp. 330–333.

41. Keathley, R. S., et al. "Knowledge of U.S. Standard Alcohol Serving Sizes among College Students." AAHPERD National Convention and Exposition Poster Session, March 19, 2010.

42. Wang, I., et al. "Alcohol Consumption, Weight Gain, and Risk of Becoming Overweight in Middle-Aged and Older Women." *Archives of Internal Medicine*, Vol. 170, March 2010, p. 453.

43. Wilson, T., et al. "Should Moderate Alcohol Consumption Be Promoted?" *Nutrition and Health: Nutrition Guide for Physicians*. Humana Press, 2010, p. 107.

44. Gruenewald, P. J., et al. "A Dose-Response Perspective on College Drinking and Related Problems." *Evidence Based Medicine*, Vol. 15, 2010, pp. 17–18.

45. Liu, B., et al. "Body Mass Index and Risk of Liver Cirrhosis in Middle-Aged UK Women: A Prospective Study." *British Medical Journal*, Vol. 11, March 2010, p. 340.

46. American Heart Association, www.americanheart.org.

47. Schütze, M., et al. "Alcohol Attributable Burden of Incidence of Cancer in Eight European Countries Based on Results from Prospective Cohort Study." *British Medical Journal*, Vol. 342, April 2011.

48. Labbe and Maisto, "Alcohol Expectancy Challenges."

49. Huebner, R. B. "Advances in Alcoholism Treatment." *Alcohol Research and Health*, Vol. 33, No. 4, 2011, pp. 295–299.

50. Kuehn, B. M. "Study Suggests Gene May Predict Success of Therapies for Alcohol Dependence." *Journal of the American Medical Association*, Vol. 305, No. 10, March 2011, pp. 984–985.

51. O'Malley, S. S., and P. G. O'Connor. "Medications for Unhealthy Alcohol Use: Across the Spectrum." *Alcohol Research and Health*, Vol. 33, No. 4, 2011, pp. 300–312.

52. Khadjessari, Z., et al. "Can Stand-Alone Computer-Based Interventions Reduce Alcohol Consumption? A Systematic Review." *Addiction*, Vol. 106, No. 2, February 2011, pp. 267–282.

53. Doumas, D. M., et al. "Reducing High-Risk Drinking in Mandated College Students: Evaluation of Two Personalized Normative Feedback Interventions." *Journal of Substance Abuse Treatment*, Vol. 40, No. 4, June 2011, pp. 376–385.

54. Pagano, M. E., et al. "Alcoholics Anonymous-Related Helping and the Helper Therapy Principle." *Alcoholism Treatment Quarterly*, Vol. 29, No. 1, January 2011, pp. 23–34.

55. Tucker, J. A., and C. A. Simpson. "The Recovery Spectrum—From Self-Change to Seeking Treatment." *Alcohol Research and Health*, Vol. 33, No. 4, 2011, pp. 371–379.

56. Casswell, S., et al. "Alcohol's Harm to Others: Reduced Well-being and Health Status for Those with Heavy Drinkers in Their Lives." *Addiction*, January 13, 2011 (e-pub).

## Chapter 14

1. Pierce, J. P., et al. "Prevalence of Heavy Smoking in California and the United States, 1965–2007." *Journal of the American Medical Association*, Vol. 305, No. 11, March 16, 2011, pp. 1106–1112.

2. Hanewinkel, R., et al. "Cigarette Advertising and Teen Smoking Initiation." *Pediatrics*, Vol. 127, February 2011, pp. e271–e278.

3. Wagner, D. D., et al. "Spontaneous Action Representation in Smokers When Watching Movie Characters Smoke." *Journal of Neuroscience*, Vol. 31, No. 3, January 2011, pp. 894–898.

4. Mutti, S., et al. "Beyond Light and Mild: Cigarette Brand Descriptors and Perceptions of Risk in the International Tobacco Control (ITC) Four Country Survey." *Addiction*, April 12, 2011 (e-pub).

5. American College Health Association. *American College Health Association-National College Health Assessment II: Reference Group Executive Summary Spring 2010*. Linthicum, MD: American College Health Association, 2010.

6. Morrell, H. E. R., et al. "Depression Vulnerability Predicts Cigarette Smoking among College Students: Gender and Negative Reinforcement Expectancies as Contributing Factors." *Addictive Behaviors*, Vol. 35, No. 6, June 2010, pp. 607–611.

7. Storr, C. L. "Smoking Estimates from Around the World: Data from the First 17 Participating Countries in the World Mental Health Survey Consortium." *Tob Control*, Vol. 19, 2010, pp. 65–74.

8. Tobacco Atlas, www.tobaccoatlas.org

9. Xue, F., et al. "Cigarette Smoking and the Incidence of Breast Cancer." *Archives of Internal Medicine*, Vol. 171, No. 2, January 24, 2011, pp. 125–133.

10. "Data on Cardiovascular Research Detailed by S. Bisanovic and Co-Authors." *Obesity, Fitness, and Wellness Week*, April 16, 2011 (e-pub).

11. "Fighting Lung Cancer: Smokers, Former Smokers, Nonsmokers." BioWorld Week, April 11, 2011; *Health Reference Center Academic*, April 21, 2011 (e-pub).

12. Weaver, K. E., et al. "Smoking Concordance in Lung and Colorectal Cancer Patient-Caregiver Dyads and Quality of Life." *Cancer Epidemiology, Biomarkers, and Prevention*, Vol. 20, No. 2, February 2011, pp. 239–248.

13. McLeish, A. C., et al. "Asthma and Cigarette Smoking in a Representative Sample of Adults." *Journal of Health Psychology*, Vol. 16, No. 4, May 2011, pp. 643–652.

14. Rodriguez, J., et al. "The Association of Pipe and Cigar Use with Cotinine Levels, Lung Function, and Airflow Obstruction: A Cross-sectional Study." *Annals of Internal Medicine*, Vol. 152, No. 4, February 16, 2010, pp. 201–210.

15. Ibid.

16. American College Health Association, *American College Health Association-National College Health Assessment II.*

17. Sutfin, E. L., et al. "Prevalence and Correlates of Waterpipe Tobacco Smoking by College Students in North Carolina." *Drug and Alcohol Dependence*, February 24, 2011 (e-pub).

18. Rodriguez et al. "The Association of Pipe and Cigar Use."

19. "Smokeless Tobacco." Smoking & Tobacco Use Fact Sheet, CDC, www.cdc.gov.

20. Post, A., et al. "Symptoms of Nicotine Dependence in a Cohort of Swedish Youths: A Comparison between Smokers, Smokeless Tobacco Users and Dual Tobacco Users." *Addiction*, Vol. 105, No. 4, February 9, 2010, pp. 740–746.

21. "New Survey Finds Menthol Smokers Feel 'Twice-Addicted.'" *Obesity, Fitness, and Wellness Week*, April 9, 2011 (e-pub).

22. Berkman, E. T., et al. "In the Trenches of Real-World Self-Control: Neural Correlates of Breaking the Link between Craving and Smoking." *Psychological Science*, Vol. 22, No. 4, April 2011, pp. 498–506.

23. Schnoll, R. A., et al. "Effectiveness of Extended-Duration Transdermal Nicotine Therapy: A Randomized Trial." *Annals of Internal Medicine*, Vol. 152, February 2, 2010, pp. 144–151.

24. Levine, M. D., et al. "Bupropion and Cognitive Behavioral Therapy for Weight-Concerned Women Smokers." *Archives of Internal Medicine*, Vol. 170, No. 6, 2010, pp. 543–550.

25. Hajek, P., et al. "Use of Varenicline for 4 Weeks Before Quitting Smoking." *Archives of Internal Medicine*, Vol. 171, No. 8, April 25, 2011, pp. 770–777.

26. Luo, J., et al. "Association of Active and Passive Smoking with Risk of Breast Cancer among Postmenopausal Women: A Prospective Cohort Study." *British Medical Journal*, Vol. 342, March 1, 2011.

27. National Cancer Institute, U.S. National Institutes of Health. NCI Fact Sheet. www.cancer .gov/cancertopics/factsheet.

28. Llewellyn, D. J., et al. "Exposure to Secondhand Smoke and Cognitive Impairment in Non-Smokers: National Cross Sectional Study with Cotinine Measurement." *British Medical Journal*, Vol. 338, February 12, 2009, p. b462.

29. Salvi, C. M., et al. "Environmental Tobacco Smoke (ETS) and Respiratory Health in Children." *Journal of Allergy and Clinical Immunology*, Vol. 123, No. 3, March 2009, pp. 575–578.

30. Rehan, V. K., et al. "Thirdhand Smoke: A New Dimension to the Effects of Cigarette Smoke on the Developing Lung." *American Journal of Physiology*, April 8, 2011 (e-pub).

31. Pierce, J., and M. León. "Effectiveness of Smoke-Free Policies." *Lancet Oncology*, Vol. 9, No. 7, pp. 614–615.

## Chapter 15

1. "1 in 5 U.S. Kids Has High Cholesterol." *Morbidity and Mortality Weekly Report*, January 22, 2010.

2. Franks, P. W., et al. "Childhood Obesity, Other Cardiovascular Risk Factors, and Premature Death." *New England Journal of Medicine*, Vol. 362, No. 6, February 2010, pp. 485–493.

3. Lloyd-Jones, D. M., et al. "Defining and Setting National Goals for Cardiovascular Health Promotion and Disease Reduction: The American Heart Association's Strategic Impact Goal Through 2020 and Beyond." American Heart Association Strategic Planning Task Force and Statistics Committee. *Circulation*, Vol. 121, No. 4, February 2010, pp. 586–613; January 20, 2010 (e-pub).

4. "Experts Push 7 Steps to Heart Health." *HealthDay*, January 20, 2010, www.medlineplus.gov.

5. Leiter, L. A., et al. "Identification and Management of Cardiometabolic Risk in Canada: A Position Paper by the Cardiometabolic Risk Working Group (Executive Summary)." *Canadian Journal of Cardiology*, Vol. 27, No. 2, March/April 2011, pp. 124–131.

6. Hayward, R. A., et al. "Optimizing Statin Treatment for Primary Prevention of Coronary Artery Disease." *Annals of Internal Medicine*, Vol. 152, No. 2, January 2010, pp. 69–77.

7. Tirosh, A., et al. "Adolescent BMI Trajectory and Risk of Diabetes versus Coronary Disease." *New England Journal of Medicine*, Vol. 364, April 2011, pp. 1315–1325.

8. Pollock, N. K., et al. "Adolescent Obesity, Bone Mass, and Cardiometabolic Risk Factors." *Journal of Pediatrics*, Vol. 158, No. 5, May 2011, pp. 727–734.

9. Logue, J., et al. "Obesity Is Associated with Fatal Coronary Heart Disease Independently of Traditional Risk Factors and Deprivation." *Heart*, Vol. 97, No. 7, February 2011, pp. 564–568.

10. Newton, R. L., et al. "Abdominal Adiposity Deposits Are Correlates of Adverse Cardiometabolic Risk Factors in Caucasian and African-American Adults." *Nutrition and Diabetes*, Vol. 1, January 31, 2011, p. e2.

11. Schneider, H. J., et al. "Measuring Abdominal Obesity: Effects of Height on Distribution of Cardiometabolic Risk Factors Risk Using Waist Circumference and Waist-to-Height Ratio." *Diabetes Care*, Vol. 34, No. 1, January 2011, p. e7.

12. "Increasing Soda Consumption Fuels Rise in Diabetes, Heart Disease." *HealthDay*, March 8, 2010, www.medlineplus.gov.

13. "TV Watching May Shorten Your Life." *HealthDay*, January 11, 2010, www.medlineplus.gov.

14. Kastorini, C. M., et al. "The Effect of Mediterranean Diet on Metabolic Syndrome and Its Components: A Meta-Analysis of 50 Studies and 534,906 Individuals." *Journal of the American College of Cardiology*, Vol. 57, March 2011, pp. 1299–1313.

15. Preidt, R. "Diabetes Soaring among American Adults." *MedlinePlus*, January 5, 2011 (e-pub).

16. "Diabetes Risk Factors." *MedlinePlus*, www.nlm .nih.gov/medlineplus/diabetes.html.

17. "More Than a Third of Adults Estimated to Have Prediabetes." *Centers for Disease Control and Prevention Press Release*, January 26, 2011 (e-pub).

18. Gakidou, E., et al. "Management of Diabetes and Associated Cardiovascular Risk Factors in Seven Countries: A Comparison of Data from National Health Examination Surveys." *Bulletin of the World Health Organization*, Vol. 89, March 2011, p. 172.

19. Barker, L. E., et al. "Geographic Distribution of Diagnosed Diabetes in the USA Diabetes Belt." *American Journal of Preventative Medicine*, Vol. 40, No, 4, April 2011, pp. 434–439.

20. Seshasai, S. R. K., et al. "Diabetes Mellitus, Fasting Glucose, and Risk of Cause-Specific Death." *New England Journal of Medicine*, Vol. 364, March 2011, pp. 829–841.

21. Wannamethee, S. G., et al. "Impact of Diabetes on Cardiovascular Disease Risk and All-Cause Mortality in Older Men." *Archives of Internal Medicine*, Vol. 171, No. 5, March 2011, pp. 404–410.

22. Kahn, S. E. "Glucose Control in Type 2 Diabetes." *Journal of the American Medical Association*, Vol. 301, No. 15, April 15, 2009, pp. 1590–1592.

23. Kuehn, B. M., et al. "Diabetes Treatment Doubles." *Journal of the American Medical Association*, Vol. 305, No. 8, February 2011, p. 770.

24. Saudek, C. D. "Can Diabetes Be Cured?" *Journal of the American Medical Association*, Vol. 301, No. 15, April 15, 2009, pp. 1588–1590.

25. Purnell, J. Q., and D. R. Flum, "Bariatric Surgery and Diabetes: Who Should Be Offered the Option of Remission?" *Journal of the American Medical Association*, Vol. 301, No. 15, April 15, 2009, pp. 1593–1595.

26. Nathan, D. N. "Progress in Diabetes Research—What's Next?" *Journal of the American Medical Association*, Vol. 301, No. 15, April 15, 2009, pp. 1599–1601.

27. Farzadfar, F., et al. "National, Regional, and Global Trends in Serum Total Cholesterol since 1980: Systematic Analysis of Health Examination Surveys and Epidemiological Studies with 321 Country-years and 3.0 Million Participants." *Lancet*, Vol. 377, No. 9765, February 2011, pp. 578–586.

28. Robertson, Rose Marie. Personal interview.

29. "Vital Signs: Prevalence, Treatment, and Control of Hypertension—United States, 1999–2002 and 2005–2008." *CDC Morbidity and Mortality Weekly Report*, February 1, 2011 (e-pub).

30. Ventura, H. and Lavie, C. "Antihypertensive Therapy for Prehypertension." *Journal of the American Medical Association*, Vol. 305, No. 9, March 2011, pp. 940–941.

31. "Top 10 Things to Know about Resistant Hypertension." American Heart Association, http://hyper.ahajournals.org/cgi/reprint/ HYPERTENSIONAHA.108.189141.

32. "Vital Signs: Prevalence, Treatment, and Control of High Levels of Low-Density Lipoprotein Cholesterol." *Journal of the American Medical Association*, Vol. 305, No. 11, March 2011, pp. 1086–1088.

33. Bambs, C., et al. "Low Prevalence of Ideal Cardiovascular Health in a Community-based Population: The Heart Strategies Concentrating on Risk Evaluation (Heart SCORE) study." *Circulation*, Vol. 123, No. 8, March 2011, pp. 850–857.

34. Heidenreich, P. A., et al. "Forecasting the Future of Cardiovascular Disease in the United States." *Circulation*, January 24, 2011 (e-pub).

35. Davidson, K. W., et al. "Don't Worry, Be Happy: Positive Affect and Reduced 10-Year Incident Coronary Heart Disease: The Canadian Nova Scotia Health Survey." *European Heart Journal*, February 17, 2010.

36. Strandhagen, E., et al. "Selection Bias in a Population Survey with Registry Linkage: Potential Effect on Socioeconomic Gradient in Cardiovascular Risk." *European Journal of Epidemiology*, February 3, 2010.

37. Mosca, L., et al. "Effectiveness-based Guidelines for the Prevention of Cardiovascular Disease in Women—2011 Updates: Guidelines from the American Heart Association." *Circulation*, Vol. 123, February 2011, pp. 1243–1262.

38. Wolff, T., et al. "Aspirin for the Primary Prevention of Cardiovascular Events: An Update of the Evidence for the U.S. Preventive Services Task Force." *Annals of Internal Medicine*, Vol. 150, No. 6, March 17, 2009, pp. 405–410.

39. Bartolucci, A. A., et al. "Meta-Analysis of Multiple Primary Prevention Trials of Cardiovascular Events Using Aspirin." *American Journal of Cardiology*, April 11, 2011 (e-pub).

40. "One Pill Might Prevent Heart Disease." *HealthDay*, March 30, 2009, www.medlineplus.gov.

41. Nawrot, T. S., et al. "Public Health Importance of Triggers of Myocardial Infarction: A Comparative Risk Assessment." *Lancet*, Vol. 377, No. 9767, February 2011, pp. 732–740.

42. "Strokes Up among the Young, Down among the Old." *HealthDay*, February 2010, www.medline.gov.

43. Alberts, M. "Preventing Death One Stroke at a Time." *Journal of the American Medical Association*, Vol. 305, No. 4, January 2011, pp. 408–409.

44. Mitka, M. "Lifestyle Changes Key to Cut Stroke Risk." *Journal of the American Medical Association*, Vol. 305, No. 6, February 2011, pp. 551–552.

45. Brown, Robert D. "'Mini Strokes' Linked to Doubled Heart Attack Risk: Study." *MedlinePlus*, March 24, 2011 (e-pub).

46. Kohler, B. A., et al. "Report to the Nation on the Status of Cancer, 1975–2007, Featuring Tumors of the Brain and Other Nervous System." *Journal of the National Cancer Institute*, March 31, 2011 (e-pub).

47. "Blacks Still Hit Hardest by Cancer." *Medline Plus*, February 1, 2011 (e-pub).

48. Preidt, R. "Healthier Lifestyles May Prevent 340,000 U.S. Cancers a Year: Study." *Medline Plus*, February 4, 2011 (e-pub).

49. "U.S. Cancer Survivors Grow to Nearly 12 Million." *Centers for Disease Control and Prevention Press Release*, March 10, 2011 (e-pub).

50. Spiegel, D. "Mind Matters in Cancer Survival." *Journal of the American Medical Association*, Vol. 305, No. 5, February 2011, pp. 502–503.

51. "Cancer Facts and Figures 2009." American Cancer Society, 2010.

52. Neugut, A. "Cancer Facts and Figures for African Americans, 2011–2012."*American Cancer Society*, http://www.cancer.org/acs/groups/content/@epidemiologysurveillance/documents/document/acspc-027765.pdf.

53. "Melanoma Update: Recent Technological Advances Are Helping Dermatologists Diagnose and Treat Early Stage Melanoma." *American Academy of Dermatology*, March 4, 2010.

54. Krieger, N., et al. "Decline in U.S. Breast Cancer Rates after the Women's Health Initiative: Socioeconomic and Racial/Ethnic Differentials." *American Journal of Public Health*. February 10, 2010 (e-pub).

55. Practice Bulletin: Breast Cancer Screening. *Obstetrics and Gynecology*, August 2011; Vol. 110; No. 12, pp. 372–382.

56. Murphy, A. M. "Mammography Screening for Breast Cancer: A View from Two Worlds." *Journal of the American Medical Association*, Vol. 303, No. 2, January 2010, pp. 166–167.

57. Berg, W. A. "Benefits of Screening Mammography." *Journal of the American Medical Association*, Vol. 303, No. 2, January 2010, pp. 168–169.

58. Rossing, M. A., et al. "Predictive Value of Symptoms for Early Detection of Ovarian Cancer." *Journal of the National Cancer Institute*, Vol. 102, No. 4, February 2010, pp. 222–229.

59. Andriole, G. L., et al. "Mortality Results from a Randomized Prostate-Cancer Screening Trial." *New England Journal of Medicine*, Vol. 360, No. 13, March 26, 2009, pp. 1310–1319.

60. Macsali, F., et al. "Oral Contraception, Body Mass Index, and Asthma: A Cross-Sectional Nordic-Baltic Population Survey." *Journal of Allergy and Clinical Immunology*, Vol. 123, No. 2, February 2009, pp. 391–397.

61. "New Treatments Improve Control for Severe Asthma." *HealthDay*, March 16, 2009, www.medlineplus.gov.

## Chapter 16

1. Adams, Troy, et al. "The Association between Mental Health and Acute Infectious Illness among a National Sample of 18- to 24-Year-Old College Students." *Journal of American College Health,* Vol. 56, No. 6, pp. 657–663.

2. Preidt, R. "Combating Myths about Seasonal Allergies." *MedlinePlus*, March 13, 2011 (e-pub).

3. "Recommended Adult Immunization Schedule—United States, 2011." *CDC Morbidity and Mortality Weekly Report*, Vol. 60, No. 4, February 4, 2011.

4. Barrett, B., et al. "Echinacea for Treating the Common Cold: A Randomized Trial." *Annals of Internal Medicine*, Vol. 153, No. 12, December 2010, pp. 769–777.

5. Singh, M., and R. R. Das. "Zinc for the Common Cold." *Cochrane Database of Systematic Reviews 2011*, June 1, 2010 (e-pub).

6. Skowronski, N. M., et al. "Effectiveness of AS03 Adjuvanted Pandemic H1N1 Vaccine: Case-Control Evaluation Based on Sentinel Surveillance System in Canada, Autumn 2009." *BMJ*, Vol. 342, February 2011, p. c7297.

7. "Meningococcal Vaccines: What You Need to Know," www.cdc.gov/meningitis/vaccine_info.html.

8. Torpy, J. M., et al. "JAMA Patient Page: Hepatitis B." *Journal of the American Medical Association*, Vol. 305, No. 14, April 2011, p. 1500.

9. Ibid.

10. Williams, I. T., et al. "Incidence and Transmission Patterns of Acute Hepatitis C in the United States, 1982–2006." *Archives of Internal Medicine*, Vol. 171, No. 3, February 2011, pp. 242–248.

11. "Epstein-Barr Virus and Infectious Mononucleosis." National Center for Infectious Diseases, http://www.cdc.gov/ncidod/diseases/ebv/htm.

12. Gerber, M. A., et al. "Prevention of Rheumatic Fever and Diagnosis and Treatment of Acute Streptococcal Pharyngitis." *Circulation*, Vol. 119, No. 11, March 24, 2009, pp. 1541–1551.

13. "Trends in Tuberculosis—United States, 2010." *CDC Morbidity and Mortality Weekly Report*, Vol. 60, No. 11, March 2011, pp. 333–337.

14. Ryan, K. A., et al. "Are Gymnasium Equipment Surfaces a Source of Staphylococcal Infections in the Community?" *American Journal of Infection Control*, Vol. 39, No. 2, March 2011, pp. 148–150.

15. "Post-Surgery Infection Can Add $60,000 to Hospital Bill." *HealthDay*, February 24, 2010, www.medline plus.gov.

16. Burton, D. C., et al. "Methicillin-Resistant *Staphylococcus aureus* Central Line-Associated Bloodstream Infections in U.S. Intensive Care Units, 1997–2007." *Journal of the American Medical Association*, Vol. 301, No. 7, February 18, 2009, pp. 727–736.

17. Datta, R., et al. "Environmental Cleaning Intervention and Risk of Acquiring Multidrug-Resistant Organisms from Prior Room Occupants." *Archives of Internal Medicine*, Vol. 171, No. 6, March 2011, pp. 491–494.

18. "Studies Highlight Challenge of Controlling Resistant Bacteria in Hospitals." *MedlinePlus*, April 13, 2011 (e-pub).

19. "Growing Number of Farm Animals Spawn New Diseases." *MedlinePlus*, February 11, 2011 (e-pub).

## Chapter 17

1. Berenson, R. A., and C. A. Cassel. "Consumer-Driven Health Care May Not Be What Patients Need—Caveat Emptor." *Journal of the American Medical Association*, Vol. 301, No. 3, January 21, 2009, pp. 321–323.

2. Food and Drug Administration, www.fda.gov/cdrh/Lasik/when.htm.

3. American Society of Plastic Surgeons, www.plasticsurgery.org.

4. Mao, J. J., et al. "Complementary and Alternative Medicine Use among Cancer Survivors: A Population-based Study." *Journal of Cancer Survivorship: Research and Practice*, Vol 5, No. 1, March 2011, pp. 8–17.

5. Niemtzow, R. C. "Acupuncture: Where Are the Data?" *Medical Acupuncture*, Vol. 23, No. 1, March 2011, p. 1.

6. Berman, B. M., et al. "Acupuncture for Chronic Low Back Pain." *New England Journal of Medicine*, Vol. 363, July 2010, pp. 454–461.

7. National Center for Complementary and Alternative Medicine, [URL].

8. "Biofeedback Now Seen as Regular Medicine." *HealthDay*, February 4, 2010, www.medlineplus.gov.

9. Holderness, J., et al. "Polysaccharides Isolated from Acai Fruit Induce Innate Immune Responses." *PLoS One*, Vol. 6, No. 2, February 2011, p. e17301.

10. Lowes, R. "Healthcare Reform's First Birthday Is No Piece of Cake." *Medscape Medical News*, March 22, 2011, www.medscape.com/viewarticle/739475.

## Chapter 18

1. National Center for Health Statistics, www.cdc.gov/nchs.

2. Ripley, Amanda. *The Unthinkable: Who Survives When Disaster Strikes—and Why.* New York: Crown, 2008.

3. "Traffic Fatalities in 2010 Drop to Lowest Level in Recorded History." National Highway Traffic Safety Administration, April 1, 2011, www.nhtsa.dot.gov.

4. AAA Foundation for Traffic Safety, www.aaafoundation.org.

5. Curry, A. E., et al. "Prevalence of Teen Driver Errors Leading to Serious Motor Vehicle Crashes." *Accident Analysis and Prevention*, Vol. 43, No. 4, July 2011, pp. 1285–1290.

6. National Highway Traffic Safety Administration, www.distraction.gov.

7. Ibid.

8. Kohnle, D. "Health Tip: Don't Drive Distracted." *HealthDay*, March 9, 2010, www.medlineplus.gov.

9. American College Health Association. *American College Health Association-National College Health Assessment II: Reference Group Executive Summary Spring 2010.* Linthicum, MD: American College Health Association; 2010.

10. Nerenberg, Arnold. Personal interview.

11. Preidt, R. "Motorcycle Deaths Drop for Second Straight Year: Report." *MedlinePlus*, April 19, 2011 (e-pub).

12. Crompton, J. G., et al. "Motorcycle Helmets Associated with Lower Risk of Cervical Spine Injury: Debunking the Myth." *Journal of the American College of Surgeons*, Vol. 212, No. 3, March 2011, pp. 295–200.

13. Ross, T. P., et al. "The Bicycle Helmet Attitudes Scale: Using the Health Belief Model to Predict Helmet Use among Undergraduates." *Journal of American College Health,* Vol. 59, No. 1, July/August 2010, pp. 29–35.

14. "Unintentional Poisoning—Keep Yourself and Others Safe." Centers for Disease Control and Prevention Features, March 21, 2011, www.cdc.gov/Features/PoisonPrevention/.

15. Franklin, C. A., and T. W. Franklin. "Predicting Fear of Crime: Considering Differences across Gender." *Feminist Criminology*, Vol. 4, No. 1, pp. 83–106.

16. "School Associated Violent Deaths." Centers for Disease Control and Prevention, www.cdc.gov/ncipc/sch-shooting-htm.

17. American College Health Association.

18. Vladutiu, C. J., et al. "College- or University-Based Sexual Assault Prevention Programs: A Review of Program Outcomes, Characteristics, and Recommendations." *Trauma, Violence, and Abuse*, Vol. 12, April 2011, pp. 67–86.

19. Potter, S. J., et al. "Using Social Self-Identification in Social Marketing Materials Aimed at Reducing Violence Against Women on Campus." *Journal of Interpersonal Violence*, Vol. 26, No. 5, March 2011, pp. 971–990.

20. Sourander, A., et al. "Psychosocial Risk Factors Associated with Cyberbullying among Adolescents: A Population-based Study." *Archives of General Psychiatry*, Vol. 67, No. 7, July 2010, 720–728.

21. Ibid.

22. Clark, S., et al. "Cyberbullying: The New Way to Bully." Sewanee The University of the South, Scholarship Sewanee 2011, April 29, 2011, http://hdl.handle.net/10090/21560.

23. Porter, J. L., and L. McQuiller-Williams. "Intimate Violence among Underrepresented Groups on a College Campus." *Journal of Interpersonal Violence*, February 28, 2011 (e-pub).

24. Buhl, E. R., et al. "Stalking Victimization among College Women and Subsequent Help-Seeking Behaviors." *Journal of American College Health*, Vol. 57, No. 4, January/February 2009, pp. 419–426.

25. Chan, K. I., et al. "Prevalence of Dating Partner Violence and Suicidal Ideation among Male and Female University Students Worldwide." *Journal of Midwifery and Women's Health*, Vol. 53, No. 6, 2008, pp. 529–537.

26. Catalozzi, M., et al. "Understanding Control in Adolescent and Young Adult Relationships." *Archives of Pediatrics and Adolescent Medicine*, Vol. 165, April 2011, pp. 313–319.

27. Hines, D. A., and E. M. Douglas. "Symptoms of Posttraumatic Stress Disorder in Men Who Sustain Intimate Partner Violence: A Study of Helpseeking and Community Samples." *Psychology of Men and Masculinity*, Vol. 12, No. 2, April 2011, pp. 112–127.

28. Fair, C. D., and J. Vanyur. "Sexual Coercion, Verbal Aggression, and Condom Use Consistency among College Students." *Journal of American College Health*, Vol. 59, No. 4, January 2011, pp. 273–280.

29. Clinton-Sherrod, M., et al. "Incapacitated Sexual Violence Involving Alcohol among College Women: The Impact of a Brief Drinking Intervention." *Violence Against Women*, Vol. 17, No. 1, January 2011, pp. 135–154.

30. Ross, L. T., et al. "Nonconsensual Sexual Experiences and Alcohol Consumption among Women Entering College." *Journal of Interpersonal Violence*, Vol. 26, No. 3, February 2011, pp. 399–413.

31. Littleton, H., and C. E. Henderson. "If She Is Not a Victim, Does That Mean She Was Not Traumatized? Evaluation of Predictors of PTSD Symptomatology among College Rape Victims." *Violence Against Women*, Vol. 15, No. 2, 2009, pp. 148–167.

32. McMahon, S. "Rape Myth Beliefs and Bystander Attitudes among Incoming College Students." *Journal of American College Health*, Vol. 59, No. 1, July/August 2010, pp. 3–11.

33. Ibid.

34. Ibid.

35. Clinton-Sherrod et al. "Incapacitated Sexual Violence Involving Alcohol."

**Chapter 19**

1. "Environmental Health." The World Health Organization, 2010, www.who.int/topics/environmental_health/en/.

2. American Association for the Advancement of Science, www.aaas.org/climate.

3. "Environmental Health." The World Health Organization, 2010, www.who.int/topics/environmental_health/en/.

4. Ziska, L., et al. "Recent Warming by Latitude Associated with Increased Length of Ragweed Pollen Season in Central North America." *Proceedings of the National Academy of Sciences of the United States of America*, Vol. 108, No. 10, March 2011, pp. 4248–4251.

5. Chen, B. Y. "Effects of Ambient Particulate Matter and Fungal Spores on Lung Function in Schoolchildren." *Pediatrics*, Vol. 127, No. 3, March 2011, pp. e690–e698.

6. Nawrot, T. S., et al. "Public Health Importance of Triggers of Myocardial Infarction: A Comparative Risk Assessment." *Lancet*, Vol. 377, No. 9767, February 2011, pp. 732–740.

7. "State of the Air 2011." American Lung Association, www.stateoftheair.org.

8. Piro, F. N., et al. "A Comparison of Self-Reported Air Pollution Problems and GIS-Modeled Levels of Air Pollution in People with and without Chronic Diseases." *Environmental Health*, Vol. 7, No. 1, February 28, 2008.

9. Pope, "Fine-Particulate Air Pollution and Life Expectancy in the United States." *New England Journal of Medicine*, pp. 376–386.

10. "FDA Regulates the Safety of Bottled Water Beverages Including Flavored Water and Nutrient-Added Water Beverages," May 3, 2010.

11. "Frequently Asked Questions about Iodine-131 Found in Surface Water." *CDC Emergency Preparedness and Response*, April 1, 2011 (e-pub).

12. "State Smoke-Free Laws for Worksites, Restaurants, and Bars—United States, 2000–2010." *CDC Morbidity and Mortality Weekly Report (MMWR)*, Vol. 60, No. 15, April 2011, pp. 472–475.

13. "Living with a Smoker May Raise Blood Pressure in Boys." *American Academy of Pediatrics, News Release*, May 1, 2011 (e-pub). http://www.aap.org/advocacy/releases/pas2011/smokersun.pdf.

14. Crane, J. M. G., et al. "Effects of Environmental Tobacco Smoke on Perinatal Outcomes: A Retrospective Cohort Study." *BJOG: An International Journal of Obstetrics and Gynaecology*, Vol. 118, No. 7, June 2011, pp. 865–871.

15. "Invisible and Odorless, Radon Poses Risks to Lungs." *MedlinePlus HealthDay*, March 11, 2011 (e-pub).

16. Knox, S. S., et al. "Implications of Early Menopause in Women Exposed to Perfluorocarbons." *Journal of Clinical Endocrinology and Metabolism*, Vol. 96, No. 6, June 2011, pp. 1747–1753.

17. Preidt, R. "Keep Safety in Mind When Cleaning House, Experts Advise." *MedlinePlus*, March 26, 2011 (e-pub).

18. Wells, E. M., et al. "Low-Level Lead Exposure and Elevations in Blood Pressure during Pregnancy." *Environmental Health Perspectives*, Vol. 119, No. 5, May 2011, pp. 664–669.

19. "Environmental Cancer Risks." *Cancer Facts and Figures 2008*. American Cancer Society, 2008.

20. Volkow, N. D., et al. "Effects of Cell Phone Radiofrequency Signal Exposure on Brain Glucose Metabolism." *Journal of the American Medical Association*, Vol. 305, No. 8, February 2011, pp. 808–813.

21. De Vocht, F., et al. "Time Trends (1998–2007) in Brain Cancer Incidence Rates in Relation to Mobile Phone Use in England." *Bioelectromagnetics*, January 28, 2011 (e-pub).

22. Djeridane, Y., et al. "Influence of Electromagnetic Fields Emitted by GSM-900 Cellular Telephones on the Circadian Patterns of Gonadal, Adrenal and Pituitary Hormones in Men." *Radiation Research*, Vol. 169, No. 3, March 2008, pp. 337–343.

23. Loeb, P. D., and W. A. Clarke. "The Cell Phone Effect on Pedestrian Fatalities." *Transportation Research Part E: Logistics and Transportation Review*, Vol. 45, No. 1, January 2009, pp. 284–290.

24. Curhan, S. G., et al. "Analgesic Use and the Risk of Hearing Loss in Men." *American Journal of Medicine*, Vol. 123, No. 3, March 2010, pp. 231–237.

25. Predit, R. "Small Study Finds Hearing Loss in 1 in 4 College Students." *MedlinePlus*, March 18, 2011 (e-pub).

26. Nash, S. D., et al. "The Prevalence of Hearing Impairment and Associated Risk Factors: The Beaver Dam Offspring Study." *Archives of Otolaryngology—Head and Neck Surgery*, Vol. 137, No. 5, May 2011, pp. 432–439.

27. Joelving, F. "Hearing Loss Common in Seniors: National Survey." *MedlinePlus*, February 28, 2011 (e-pub).

**Chapter 20**

1. Kochanek, K. D., et al. "National Vital Statistics Reports Deaths: Preliminary Data for 2009," March 16, 2011, www.cdc.gov/nchs/data/nvsr/nvsr59/nvsr59_04.pdf.

2. Ibid.

3. Danaei, G., et al. "The Promise of Prevention: The Effects of Four Preventable Risk Factors on National Life Expectancy and Life Expectancy Disparities by Race and County in the United States. *Public Library of Sciences Medicine*, Vol. 7, No. 3, March 23, 2010.

4. Viner, R. M., et al. "50-Year Mortality Trends in Children and Young People: A Study of 50 Low-Income, Middle-Income, and High-Income Countries." *Lancet*, Vol. 377, No. 9772, April 2011, pp. 1162–1174.

5. Resnick, M. D. "A Better Understanding of Mortality in Young People." *Lancet*, Vol. 377, No. 9772, April 2011, pp. 1128–1130.

6. Kochanek et al., "National Vital Statistics Reports Deaths."

7. Ibid.

8. Martin, L. G., et al. "Trends in Disability and Related Chronic Conditions among People Ages Fifty to Sixty-Four," *Health Affairs*. Vol. 29, No. 4, April 2010, pp. 725–731.

9. Rockwood, K., et al. "Changes in Relative Fitness and Frailty across the Adult Lifespan: Evidence from the Canadian National Population Health Survey." *Canadian Medical Association Journal*, Vol. 183, No. 8, May 2011, pp. e487–494.

10. Pierson, R. "Exercise Preserves, Builds Heart Muscle." *MedlinePlus*, April 2, 2011 (e-pub).

11. Clapp, W. C., et al. "Deficit in Switching between Functional Brain Networks Underlies the Impact of Multitasking on Working Memory in Older Adults." *Proceedings of the National Academy of Sciences of the United States of America*, Vol. 108, No. 17, April 2011, pp. 7212–7217.

12. Sherman, Sherry. Personal interview.

13. Speller, Marsha. Personal interview.

14. "Hot Flashes, Night Sweats Tied to Heart Risks." *MedlinePlus*, February 24, 2011 (e-pub).

15. Pinkerton, JoAnn. Personal interview.

16. "Risks of Estrogen Hormone Therapy Seen to Fade after Treatment Ends." *MedlinePlus*, April 5, 2011 (e-pub).

17. Bolaños-Díaz, R., et al. "Soy Extracts Versus Hormone Therapy for Reduction of Menopausal Hot Flushes: Indirect Comparison." *Menopause: The Journal of the North American Menopause Society*, March 3, 2011 (e-pub).

18. Pittman, G. "Mindfulness Classes Help Women with Hot Flashes." *MedlinePlus*, March 17, 2011 (e-pub).

19. Lindau, S. T., et al. "Sex, Health, and Years of Sexually Active Life Gained due to Good Health: Evidence from Two U.S. Population-Based Cross-Sectional Surveys of Ageing." *British Medical Journal*. Vol. 340, 2010, p. c810 (e-pub March 9, 2010).

20. Wilson, R. S., et al. "Cognitive Decline in Prodomal Alzheimer Disease and Mild Cognitive Impairment." *Archives of Neurology*, Vol. 68, No. 3, March 2011, pp. 351–356.

21. "Studies Find Possible New Genetic Risk Factors for Alzheimer's Disease." *NIH News Press Release*, April 4, 2011 (e-pub).

22. "2010 Alzheimer's Disease Facts and Figures." The Alzheimer's Association, www.alz.org/alzheimers_disease_fact_figures.asp?type=homepage#key.

23. Kübler-Ross, Elisabeth. *Death: The Final Stage of Growth*. Englewood Cliffs, NJ: Prentice-Hall, 1975.

24. Smith, A. K., et al. "Racial and Ethnic Differences in End-of-Life Care in Fee-for-Service Medicare Beneficiaries with Advanced Cancer." *Journal of the American Geriatrics Society*, Vol. 57, No. 1, pp. 153–158.

# Index